Nursing Interventions Classification (NIC)

THE NIC LOGO

The NIC logo of a leaf and tree appears below and on the cover of this book. The leaf is an exact replica of one from a tree in the Linnaeus Botanical Garden in Uppsala, Sweden. The leaf was picked by an artist who lived next door to the garden for an imprint on a vase she was making. The vase was a present to a team member in 1990 just when the NIC Research team was looking for a logo. Since the leaf came from Linnaeus' Garden, the team thought this would serve as a meaningful logo. Carl Linnaeus (1707–1778) was the great classifier who brought order to the plant and animal kingdoms. In the logo, the leaf is joined with the tree, the universal symbol of taxonomy.

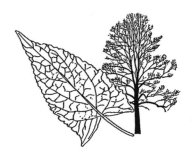

Nursing Interventions Classification (NIC)

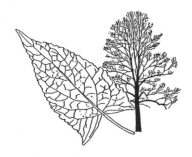

Eighth Edition

EDITORS

Cheryl M. Wagner, PhD, MBA/MSN, RN
Adjunct Assistant Professor
The University of Iowa
College of Nursing
Iowa City, Iowa
Adjunct Associate Professor, DNP Program
Chatham University
Pittsburgh, Pennsylvania

Howard K. Butcher, PhD, RN, FAAN
Professor and Director of PhD Program
Christine E. Lynn College of Nursing
Florida Atlantic University
Boca Raton, Florida
Associate Professor Emeritus
The University of Iowa
College of Nursing
Iowa City, Iowa

Mary F. Clarke, PhD, RN-BC, NE-BC
Adjunct Assistant Professor
The University of Iowa
College of Nursing
Iowa City, Iowa
Vice President of Nursing Excellence
HealthLinx
Columbus, Ohio

ELSEVIER

3251 Riverport Lane
St. Louis, Missouri 63043

NURSING INTERVENTIONS CLASSIFICATION (NIC), EIGHTH EDITION   ISBN: 978-0-323-88251-4

Notices

International Standard Book Number: 978-0-323-88251-4

Senior Content Strategist: Sandra Clark
Director, Content Development: Ellen Wurm-Cutter
Senior Content Development Specialist: Kathleen Nahm
Publishing Services Manager: Deena Burgess
Project Manager: Anne Collett
Design Direction: Margaret Reid

Printed in India

Last digit is the print number: 9   8   7   6   5   4   3   2   1

Preface

In 2022 we celebrated the 30th anniversary of the NIC and the 25th anniversary of the NOC. Since it was first conceptualized in 1987, NIC has continuously grown and evolved. This is the eighth edition of the Nursing Interventions Classification (NIC), with previous editions published in 1992, 1996, 2000, 2004, 2008, 2013, and 2018. Joanne M. Dochterman served as first editor for the first four editions and Gloria M. Bulechek for the fifth and sixth editions. Howard K. Butcher formally joined the NIC team starting with the fifth edition and served as first editor for the seventh edition. With this new edition, Cheryl M. Wagner serves as first editor, having worked on previous editions since 2004 and formally joining the NIC team for the sixth edition. We welcome Mary F. Clarke as an editor with this edition. Dr. Clarke was a member of the original NIC team in 1992 and has contributed to the CNC since its inception. Dr. Dochterman and Dr. Bulechek have formally retired from the NIC team but continue to serve when needed as consultants (see *About the Founders*).

NIC is a comprehensive classification that systematically organizes the treatments that nurses perform. Classification systems are necessary to organize knowledge so that knowledge can be managed and retrieved for knowledge building, identifying useful knowledge relationships, managing complexity, and facilitating decision-making. Classification work leads to the creation of a taxonomy, an arrangement and ordering of things, ideas, times, or places. Carl Linnaeus, widely considered the founder of scientific classifications, created a taxonomy of plants, animals, and minerals. Remarkably, in 1745, Linnaeus also created a botanical garden at Uppsala Universitet in Sweden that cultivated 1300 plant species organized according to his taxonomy of living plants. The Linnaeus Garden serves as a metaphor of the organic ever-growing nature of a classification system. The leaf that is part of the NIC logo is a replica of one from a tree in the Linnaeus Garden.

In this eighth edition of NIC, we have expanded and revised the Classification with continued research efforts and input from the professional community. The features of this edition are as follows:

- There is a total of 614 interventions in this edition. Sixty of the interventions are new, and 231 of the previously included interventions have been revised for this edition (see Appendix A for the list of new, revised, and retired interventions). Many of the new interventions were created when a need arose for unique patterns of nursing care in a pandemic. The revised interventions incorporate changes in care standards, nursing terminology, activities, and updated background readings, which we now identify as "Background Evidence". The evidence does not include, by any means, a complete reference list for any intervention. Background Evidence represents sources that were used to update the intervention's definition and activities, as well as research evidence that supports the use of the intervention in practice. We have made a focused effort to include research studies, particularly meta-analyses and systematic reviews, in the Background Evidence for the new or revised interventions. Each intervention has a unique code number to assist in computerization of NIC and facilitate reimbursement to nurses. The front matter contains a page with tips on approaches to finding an intervention.

- With this edition, we have the ability to offer use of the NIC in research projects without incurring licensure fees, in conjunction with the Center for Nursing Classification and Clinical Effectiveness, College of Nursing, Iowa City, Iowa. Approval of the use in one's research must first be obtained through the Center.

- For this edition, we reviewed and updated interventions using an approach to ensure uniqueness and similarities of activities when indicated. For example, the entire section of Medication Administration NICs (2300–2395) was revised to include the same initial activities as would occur when medications are administered by nurses.

- The class of Drug Management (H) was renamed Medication Management (H), to avoid the negative connotations associated with the word "drug", while the class Patient Education (S) was renamed Health Education, in concurrence with our belief that the education nurses provide is not limited to patients.

- An essential feature of this edition is our inspiration from the *Future of Nursing 2020-2030: Charting a Path to Achieve Health Equity* report, in directing the creation of new NICs and in revising current NICs, to reflect the need to achieve social justice. The COVID-19 pandemic exposed the breadth and depth of health inequity and its effect on the health and well-being of populations. There were strong indications that the Social Determinants of

Health (SDOH) disproportionately impacted persons of color, persons with low income, older adults, children, and those living in rural areas. The pandemic revealed not just vulnerabilities in hospital systems but the cavernous health inequalities and disparities that have always been present. In addition to the crises created by the pandemic and the trauma it caused for society at large, decades of racial injustice culminated in tragic events for persons of color. The deaths of George Floyd, Breonna Taylor, and countless others unleashed pent-up frustration and anger regarding the state of inequity in the United States and around the world. We assert that all NIC interventions must be implemented within a lens for promoting health equity. In addition, we have included a new a NIC, *Social Justice Facilitation*, as well as other socially responsible NICs, to address inequalities and social concerns (e.g., *Health Care Provider Collaboration, Human Trafficking Detection, Electronic Record Access Assistance, Readmission Prevention, Relapse Prevention, Resilience Promotion: Community, Transgender Hormone Therapy*). We also reflect this in our revisions, changing *Cultural Brokerage* to *Culture Care Negotiation*, updating *Resilience Promotion* to include activities that "strengthen coping strategies for societal stressors", and redesigning *Community Health Development* to focus on the larger needs of family and community.

- The introductory front matter section includes a short section noting what our previous editors are doing now (see *About the Founders*).
- The *Definitions of Terms* list in the front matter has been updated to include key definitions useful in the current health care environment. In our definitions and in our new and revised NICs, we have begun to replace our use of the term "patient" with the term "person", as nursing care can apply to anyone in any area of need. In addition, we have replaced our use of the term "physician" with the term "health care provider" to more accurately reflect current practice.
- The Recognition List in the front matter of the book lists individuals who assisted in updating the interventions. We were pleased to receive suggestions for new interventions from individuals in several countries. Appendix B contains the guidelines for submission of a new or revised intervention.
- In this edition, *Part One: Applying NIC to Practice, Education, and Research*, has been updated to reflect new information and publications, while *Frequently Asked Questions* remains a separate section in the front matter. Each of these sections will be of interest to both novice and experienced users of NIC.

- The NIC taxonomy, which was included for the first time in the second edition, has been updated to include all 60 new interventions. The taxonomy in this edition, as in the previous five editions, includes 7 domains and 30 classes. The taxonomy, which appears in Part Two, helps nurses to locate and choose an intervention and provides structure that can assist with curriculum design. (See the overview of the NIC taxonomy on page 32 for more detail.)
- The format for each of the interventions is the same as in previous editions. Each intervention has a label name, a definition, a list of activities that a nurse might do to carry out the intervention in the logical order that she or he might do, a publication fact line, and a short list of background evidence. The standardized language is the label name and the accompanying definition. The activities can be selected or modified as necessary to meet the specific needs of the population or individual. Thus, NIC can be used to communicate a common meaning across settings but still provide a way for nurses to individualize care.
- The specialty area core interventions section, Part Four, which helps to define the nature of the specialty, has been updated and expanded with the addition of four specialties: Disaster Nursing, Informatics Nursing, Legal Nursing, and Travel Health Nursing. There are now a total of 57 specialties with core interventions. In addition, we have renamed several specialty areas to reflect changes in the titles of specialty organizations: Ambulatory Nursing is referred to as *Ambulatory Care Nursing*, Anesthesia Nursing is now named *Postanesthesia Care Nursing and Nurse Anesthesiology*, Burn Care Nursing is now referred to as *Burn Nursing*, Correctional Facility Nursing is now renamed *Correctional Care Nursing*, Pediatric Oncology Nursing was changed to *Pediatric Hematology/Oncology Nursing*, Radiological Nursing is now *Radiology Nursing*, and Wound and Ostomy Nursing was changed to *Wound, Ostomy and Continence Nursing*. (See the introduction to the core interventions on page 470 for more information.)
- Part Five of this edition contains the estimate of time to perform an intervention and the minimum level of education that a provider needs to safely and competently administer the intervention. The levels of education were redefined to more closely reflect current education and practice patterns. The time and education level are included for all 614 interventions in this edition (See the introduction to the estimated time and education on page 502 for more information).
- This edition contains a new feature, Part Six, which includes NIC and NOC linkages to six clinical conditions. The conditions include some of the top costly, common health concerns. They are Coronary Artery

Disease, Coronavirus Disease 2019, Hyperlipidemia, Lung Cancer, Substance Use Disorder, and Ulcerative Colitis/Crohn's Disease. We are hopeful that clinical condition linkages will be a sustained section to future NIC editions, and we welcome suggestions for future linkages.

- Previous editions included a bibliography of many publications about NIC; however, the growing number of publications from multiple countries has made the task of compiling a comprehensive bibliography difficult. Publications focusing on NIC can be easily accessed using either a Cumulative Index to Nursing and Allied Health Literature (CINAHL), MedlinePlus, or PubMed database search.

In summary, NIC captures the interventions performed by all nurses. As in the past, all of the interventions included in NIC are meant to be clinically useful, although some are more general than others. Because the interventions encompass a broad range of nursing practice, no nurse could be expected to perform all interventions listed here, or even a major portion. Many of the interventions require specialized training or proper licensure, and some cannot be performed without appropriate certification. Other interventions describe basic hygiene and comfort measures that in some instances may be delegated to assistants but still need to be planned and evaluated by nurses. The use of NIC:

- helps demonstrate the impact that nurses have on the system of health care delivery,
- standardizes and defines the knowledge base for nursing curricula and practice,
- facilitates the appropriate selection of a nursing intervention,
- facilitates communication of nursing treatments to other nurses and providers,
- enables researchers to examine the effectiveness and cost of nursing care,
- assists educators to develop curricula that better align with clinical practice,
- facilitates the teaching of clinical decision making to novice nurses,
- assists administrators in planning more effectively for staff and equipment needs,
- promotes the development of a reimbursement system for nursing services,
- facilitates the development and use of nursing information systems, and
- communicates the nature of nursing to the public.

When standardized language is used to document practice, we can compare and evaluate the effectiveness of care delivered in multiple settings by different providers. The use of standardized language does not inhibit our practice; rather, it communicates the essence of nursing care to others and helps us improve our practice through research. The development and use of this classification helps to advance nursing knowledge by facilitating the clinical testing of nursing interventions. We believe the continued development and use of this classification helps in the advancement of nursing knowledge and in the efforts of nursing to gain greater voice in the health policy arena. We continue to welcome your feedback and look forward to your continued input.

Cheryl M. Wagner
Howard K. Butcher
Mary F. Clarke

About the Founders

Gloria M. Bulechek

Dr. Bulechek is enjoying her retirement years with her husband of many years, as they celebrated their 81st birthdays and 58th wedding anniversary in 2022. They like traveling, and divide their time between their lakeside home in Iowa and their winter home in Arizona. They have children and grandchildren who are frequent visitors and who help them with work around their various properties. Gloria reports that they have extended family and lifelong friends that live nearby and so are busy with social events. She notes their health is good although aging changes are catching up with her and her husband. Sometimes mobility issues are a problem, but regular exercise keeps her in shape. She continues to give input as needed to the ongoing development of the NIC.

Joanne M. Dochterman

Dr. Dochterman her husband Bruce, and cocker spaniel Wesson, live a quiet retirement life. Although both had COVID-19 in October 2021, which slowed their activities a bit, she reports a good recovery. Aging changes are also catching up with her, but she advocates water aerobics and attends three times a week to help keep moving. They sold a vacation cabin last year as the demands of taking care of two places were getting too much. At one time, Joanne was a volunteer mediator in small claims court, which she loved, but COVID-19 and the difficulty walking ended that experience. They help with delivery of Meals on Wheels once a week and enjoy sports on TV as well as Netflix. Joanne enjoys square dancing, knitting, counted cross-stitching, and doing jigsaw puzzles. They have visits with four children and grandchildren as often as possible. They took a small ship cruise in 2021 with friends and go north for a week's fishing every year. She reports that they are thankful to be able to enjoy each day. She continues to give input as needed to the ongoing development of the NIC.

Strengths of the Nursing Interventions Classification

- *Comprehensive*—NIC includes the full range of nursing interventions for general practice as well as specialty areas. Interventions include the following areas: physiological and psychosocial; illness treatment and prevention; health promotion; those for individuals, families, and communities; and indirect care. Both independent and collaborative interventions are included; they can be used in any practice setting regardless of philosophical orientation, including areas of social concern.

- *Research based*—The research to develop NIC used a multimethod approach; methods included content analysis, questionnaire survey to experts, focus group review, similarity analysis, hierarchical clustering, multidimensional scaling, and clinical field testing. The early research was partially funded by the National Institutes of Health and the National Institute of Nursing Research. Ongoing work to update the classification builds on contemporary evidence-based developments in the nursing field, expert opinion, and research-based publications.

- *Developed inductively based on existing practice*—Original sources include current textbooks, care planning guides, and nursing information systems from clinical practice, augmented by the clinical practice expertise of team members and experts in specialty areas of practice. The new additions and refinements are the result of current nursing and healthcare literature, suggestions from users, and peer reviewers.

- *Reflects current practice and research*—All interventions are accompanied by a list of background evidence that supports the development and research substantiation of the intervention. All interventions have been reviewed by experts in clinical practice and many by relevant clinical practice specialty organizations. A feedback process is used to incorporate suggestions from users in practice.

- *Has easy-to-use organizing structure* (domains, classes, interventions, activities)—All domains, classes, and interventions have definitions. Principles have been developed to maintain consistency and cohesion within the Classification; interventions are numerically coded.

- *Uses language that is clear and clinically meaningful*—Throughout the work, the language most useful in clinical practice has been selected. The language is intuitive and reflects clarity in conceptual issues, such as including only interventions, not diagnoses or outcomes.

- *Has established process and structure for continued refinement*—Suggestions for refinement are accepted from users around the world. The continued refinement of NIC is facilitated by the Center for Nursing Classification and Clinical Effectiveness, established in the College of Nursing at the University of Iowa in 1995 by the Iowa Board of Regents.

- *Has been field tested*—The process of implementation was initially studied in five field sites representing the various settings where nursing care takes place; hundreds of other clinical and educational agencies are also implementing the Classification. Steps for implementation have been developed to assist in the change process.

- *Accessible through numerous publications and media*—In addition to the classification itself, numerous articles and chapters have been published since 1990. Book and article reviews and publications about the use and value of NIC attest to the significance of the work.

- *Linked to other nursing classifications*—NIC has been linked to NANDA International (NANDA-I) diagnoses in the previous sixth edition of this book to assist with clinical decision making. A third edition of a book linking Nursing Outcomes Classification (NOC) outcomes and NIC interventions to NANDA-I diagnoses, and other clinical conditions is available from Elsevier. Earlier editions of NIC were linked to Omaha system problems, NOC outcomes, Resident Assessment Protocols (RAP) in long-term care, and Outcome and Assessment Information Set (OASIS) for home health.

- *Recipient of national recognition*—NIC is recognized by the American Nurses Association, is included in the National Library of Medicine's *Meta-thesaurus for a Unified Medical Language*, is included in indexes of CINAHL, is mapped into SNOMED CT (Systemized Nomenclature of Medicine Clinical Terms) and is registered in HL7 (Health Level Seven International).

- *Developed at same site as outcomes classification*—The NOC of patient outcomes sensitive to nursing practice has also been developed at the University of Iowa College of Nursing; both NIC and NOC are housed in the Center for Nursing Classification and Clinical Effectiveness (https://nursing.uiowa.edu/center-for-nursing-classification-and-clinical-effectiveness).

- *Included in a growing number of vendor software clinical information systems*—The SNOMED CT has included NIC in its multidisciplinary record system. There are vendors who have licensed NIC for inclusion in their software, targeted at hospital and community settings, as well as practitioners in either general or specialty practice. NIC is used in many nursing textbooks, electronic dictionaries, and clinical search engines that are used to define and plan treatment for a variety of conditions.

- *Global use*—NIC is an established classification of nursing interventions with 20 years of use in multiple countries. Translations are complete or in process for the following languages: Chinese, Dutch, French, German, Indonesian, Italian, Japanese, Korean, Norwegian, Portuguese, Spanish, and Turkish.

Acknowledgments

The Classification is continuously improved to better reflect clinical practice and best practices through the participation of many. As in past editions, individuals and groups from around the globe have submitted suggestions for new interventions. In addition, there are individuals who have reviewed and revised interventions for this edition. The names of individuals who have contributed to this edition appear in the recognition list in the preliminary pages.

We thank the University of Iowa College of Nursing for support of the Center for Nursing Classification and Clinical Effectiveness, founded in 1995, to facilitate ongoing development of the Nursing Interventions Classification (NIC) and the Nursing Outcomes Classification (NOC). We are grateful to individual donors to the endowment at the University of Iowa Foundation, which provides permanent support for the continued advancement and upkeep of the Classification.

Our editor, Sandra Clark at Elsevier, has guided this classification through this edition, as well as the three previous editions. We thank Kathleen Nahm at Elsevier, our senior content development specialist, and Anne Collett, our senior project manager, who assisted in getting the classification in its final format. We thank Bonita Allen, our licensing specialist, for all her work with vendors and agencies who are implementing NIC into the electronic world. We also appreciate all the efforts made by many individuals at Elsevier for their wide-ranging marketing strategies designed to inform the professional community about the content and value of this work in advancing nursing knowledge and the quality of nursing care.

The assistance of Noriko Abe, MSN, CNC Coordinator, Center for Nursing Classification and Clinical Effectiveness at the University of Iowa College of Nursing, has been invaluable in assisting with our NIC team meetings, keeping detailed minutes, tracking all revisions, maintaining electronic documents, and preparing the manuscript for submission. This is a time-consuming and complicated job, and she has managed this work well.

Individuals at NANDA International and the researchers for the Nursing Outcomes Classification continue to be invaluable to us through their ongoing support as we work together to facilitate linkages among NANDA-I diagnoses, NOC outcomes, and NIC interventions for the purpose of implementing standardized nursing languages into nursing education and practice. We also appreciate other authors who have incorporated NIC in multiple health care textbooks.

Most of all, we thank the nurses around the world who have enthusiastically embraced the Classification in a variety of ways: by documenting their care in practice; by helping students learn how to plan and implement nursing care; by engaging in research designed to validate interventions and demonstrate the effectiveness of nursing interventions; and by striving to integrate NIC into electronic health care information systems for planning, implementing, documenting, and evaluating the care that nurses provide to all.

Recognition List, Eighth Edition

The following individuals contributed to this edition of NIC in multiple ways. Some submitted new interventions for consideration or suggested revisions to existing interventions. Some assisted in reviewing additions or revisions to the Classification. Others submitted examples of how they have implemented NIC in practice or education. All have made a valuable contribution to the users of NIC.

Miriam de Abreu Almeida, PhD, RN, Professor, School of Nursing, Graduate Program in Nursing, Universidade Federal do Rio Grande do Sul (UFRGS), Porto Alegre, Brazil

Fernanda de Souza Freitas Abbud, RN, Obstetrics and Gynecology Nurse Practitioner, Member of Research Group on Women's and Newborn Health, School of Nursing, University of Campinas (UNICAMP), São Paulo, Brazil

Nahid Aghebati, PhD, MSc, BSc, Assistant Professor, Department of Medical Surgical Nursing, School of Nursing and Midwifery, Mashhad University of Medical Sciences, Mashhad, Iran

Priscilla Alfradique de Souza, PhD, RN, Assistant Professor, Universidade Federal do Rio de Janeiro (UFRJ), Rio de Janeiro, Brazil

Regina Allande-Cusso, PhD, RN, Associate Professor, Nursing Department, Universidad de Sevilla, Research Group PAIDI-CTS, Seville, Spain

Maria Milagros Amundarain-Lejarza, RN, Mental Health Nurse, Osakidetza Basque Health Service, Bizkaia Mental Health Network, Durango Mental health Center, Basque Country, Spain

Leslie Arends, DNP, ARNP, CPNP, Assistant Professor (Clinical), College of Nursing, University of Iowa, Iowa City, Iowa

Amaia Arzubia-Aroma, RN, Nursing Supervisor of Barrualde, Osakidetza Basque Health Service, Bizkaia Mental Health Network, Basque Country, Spain

Graziele R. Bitencourt, PhD, RN, Adjunct Professor, Universidade Federal do Rio de Janeiro (UFRJ), Rio de Janeiro, Brazil

Maria Teresa Del Campo-Gonzalo, RN, Mental Health Nurse, Osakidetza Basque Health Service, Bizkaia Mental Health Network, Santurtzi Mental health Center, Basque Country, Spain

Gregory M. Clancy, DNP, MSN, BSN, RN, Iowa City, Iowa

Erin Cullen, DNP, FNP-C, University of Iowa Hospital and Clinics, Department of Family Medicine, Muscatine Family Care center, Muscatine, Iowa

Alyssa Davis, BSN, RN, Staff Nurse, University of Iowa Health Care, Iowa City, Iowa

Maria Teresa Del Campo-Gonzalo, RN, Mental Health Nurse, Osakidetza Basque Health Service, Bizkaia Mental Health Network, Santurtzi Mental health Center, Basque Country, Spain

Patrizia Di Giacomo, PhD, MSN, RN, Nursing Tutor, University of Bologna, Bologna, Italy

Suellen Cristina Dias Emidio, PhD, Assistant Professor at Federal University of Tocantins, Nursing Department, Master in Science, Nurse Specialist in Pediatrics and Neonatology, Tocantins, Brazil

Karen Dunn Lopez, PhD, MPH, RN, FAAN, Associate Professor, Director for the Center for Nursing Classification & Clinical Effectiveness, College of Nursing, University of Iowa, Iowa City, Iowa

Maria Izaskun Eraña-Aranaga, RN, Deputy Head of Nursing of Community, Osakidetza Basque Health Service, Bizkaia Mental Health Network, Basque Country, Spain

Özüm Erkin Geyiktepe, PhD, RN, Associate Professor, İzmir Demokrasi University, Faculty of Health Sciences, Department of Nursing, Turkey

Zahra Fekri, MSc of Elderly Nursing, Department of Medical Surgical Nursing, School of Nursing and Midwifery, Mashhad University of Medical Sciences, Mashhad, Iran

Leire Fentanes-Hernandez, RN, Nursing Supervisor of Acute Psychiatric Unit, Osakidetza Basque Health Service Ezkerraldea-Enkarterri-Cruces Integrated Health Organization, Basque Country, Spain

Fritz Frauenfelder, PhD, RN Deputy Director of Nursing, Therapy, and Social Work Psychiatric University Hospital Zürich, Switzerland

Clara Fróes de Oliveira Sanfelice, PhD, RN, Obstetrics and Gynecology Nurse Practitioner, Assistant Professor and Vice Leader of Research Group on Women's and Newborn Health, School of Nursing, University of Campinas (UNICAMP), São Paulo, Brazil

Amalia Gedney-Lose, DNP, ARNP, FNP-C, Assistant Professor (Clinical), Assistant Director, DNP-FNP Program, College of Nursing, University of Iowa, Iowa City, Iowa

Farneti Giulia, RN, Clinical Nurse, Hospital of Rimini, Rimini, Italy

Ana Manzanas, Gutiérrez, Asociación Española de Enfermería en Cuidados Paliativos (AECPAL), Madrid, Spain

Sonia Herrera-Anaya, Nursing Supervisor of Bilbao, Osakidetza Basque Health Service, Bizkaia Mental Health Network, Basque Country, Spain

Brenda Krogh Duree, PhD, RN, Associate Professor (Instructional), University of Iowa, College of Nursing, Iowa City, Iowa

Mary Jahrsdoerfer, PhD, RN, Chief Nursing Information Officer, Bernoulli Health, Milford, Connecticut, and Director of Graduate Studies Healthcare Informatics, Assist. Clinical Professor of Healthcare Informatics, College of Nursing and Public Health, Adelphi University, Garden City, New York

M. Lindell Joseph, PhD, RN, FAAN, FAONL, Professor (Clinical), Director, Health Systems/Administration Program, College of Nursing, University of Iowa, Iowa City, Iowa

Elem Kocacal, PhD, RN, Associate Professor, İzmir Demokrasi University, Faculty of Health Sciences, Department of Nursing, Turkey

Maria del Puy Lopez-Zabarte, RN, Mental Health Nurse of Osasun Eskola, Osakidetza Basque Health Service, Subdirectorate of Coordination of Primary Care, Directorate General, Basque Country, Spain

Pilar Lozano, PhD, RN, Therapeutic Community of Mental Health, Cádiz, School of Nursing and Physiotherapy, University Hospital of Puerto Real University of Cádiz, Cádiz, Spain

Juana Macias-Seda, PhD, RN, Associate Professor, Nursing Department, Universidad de Sevilla/University of Seville, Research Group PAIDI-CTS, Seville, Spain

María del Pilar Vallés Martínez, Asociación Española de Enfermería en Cuidados Paliativos (AECPAL), Madrid, Spain

Özlem Metreş PhD, RN, The Turkısh Republıc of Demiroglu Bilim University, Faculty of Health Sciences, İstanbul, Turkey

Janice Miller, MSN, RN, Lecturer (Instructional), University of Iowa, College of Nursing, Iowa City, Iowa

Vanessa Monteiro Mantovani, PhD, MSc. RN, Social Projects Nurse, Hospital Moinhos de Vento, Port Alegre, Rio Grande do Sul, Brazil

Vítor Monteiro Moraes, RN, Critical Care Nursing Specialist, Master's degree student in Nursing, School of Nursing, Universidade Federal do Rio Grande do Sul (UFRGS), Brazil

Elizabeth Moore, BSN, RN, MBA, Associate Director, Heart and Vascular Center, University of Iowa Health Care, Iowa City, Iowa

Sue Moorhead, PhD, FAAN, RN, Associate Professor Emerita, University of Iowa, College of Nursing, Iowa City, Iowa

Begoña Morales-Domaica, Deputy Head of Nursing of Zamudio Hospital, Osakidetza Basque Health Service, Bizkaia Mental Health Network, Basque Country, Spain

Maria Concepcion Moreno-Calvete, RN, Deputy Director of Research and Innovation, Biocruces Bizkaia Health Research Institute, Osakidetza Basque Health Service, Bizkaia Mental Health Network, Basque Country, Spain

Megyn L. Moser, RN, BSN, Labor and Delivery Nurse, Davenport, IA

Maritza Barroso Niño, Docente, Escuela de Enfermería, Fundación Universitaria Juan N Copras, Bogota, Columbia

Maria Antonina Roman Ochoa, Dean, Escuela de Enfermería, Fundacion Unviersitaria Juan N Corpas, Bogota, Columbia

Aurora Oña-Garcia, RN, Nursing Supervisor of Uribe, Osakidetza Basque Health Service, Bizkaia Mental Health Network, Basque Country, Spain

Nilüfer Özgürbüz, PhD, RN, Assistant Professor, İzmir Tınaztepe University, Faculty of Health Sciences, Department of Nursing, Turkey

Ana María Porcel- Gálvez, PhD, RN Associate Professor, Nursing Department, Universidad de Sevilla/ University of Seville, Research Group PAIDI-CTS, Seville, Spain

Luisa Anna Rigon, MSN, RN, President and CEO of Formazione in Agorà – Scuola di Formazione alla Salute-Padua, Padua, Italy

Luciane Cristina Rodrigues Fernandes, Obstetrics and Gynecology Nurse Practitioner, Doctoral Student and Member of Research Group on Women's and Newborn Health, School of Nursing, University of Campinas-UNICAMP, São Paulo, Brazil

Ana Isabel Rodriguez-Iturrizar, RN, Director of Nursing, Osakidetza Basque Health Service, Bizkaia Mental Health Network, Basque Country, Spain

Isidro Garcia Salvador, Asociación Española de Enfermería en Cuidados Paliativos (AECPAL), Madrid, Spain

Cristina Santin, Doctoral student, MSN, RN, Nursing Tutor, University of Padua, Padua, Italy

Clarissa Shaw, PhD, RN, Assistant Professor, University of Iowa College of Nursing, Iowa City, Iowa

Definitions of Terms

CLASSIFICATION TERMS
Nursing Intervention

Any treatment, based upon clinical judgment and knowledge that a nurse performs to enhance health outcomes. Nursing interventions include both direct and indirect care; those aimed at individuals, families, and the community; and those for nurse-initiated, physician-initiated, and other provider-initiated treatments.

A *direct care intervention* is a treatment performed through interaction with the person or group of persons. Direct care interventions include both physiological and psychosocial nursing actions; both actions involving the "laying-on of hands" and those that are more supportive in nature, including counseling.

An *indirect care intervention* is a treatment performed away from the person but on behalf of a person or group of persons. Indirect care interventions include nursing actions aimed at management of the care environment and interdisciplinary collaboration. These actions support the effectiveness of the direct care interventions.

A *community (or public health) intervention* is targeted to promote and preserve the health of populations. Community interventions emphasize health promotion, health maintenance, and disease prevention of populations and include strategies to address the social and political climate in which the population resides.

A *nurse-initiated treatment* is an intervention initiated by the nurse in response to a nursing diagnosis. It is an autonomous action based on scientific rationale that is executed to benefit the person in a predicted way related to the nursing diagnosis and projected outcomes. These actions would include those treatments initiated by advanced nurse practitioners.

A *health care provider-initiated treatment* is an intervention initiated by a health care provider in response to a medical diagnosis but carried out by a nurse in response to a "provider's prescription." Nurses may also implement treatments initiated by other providers, such as advanced practice nurses, pharmacists, respiratory therapists, or physician assistants.

Nursing Activities

The specific behaviors or actions that nurses do to implement an intervention and which assist persons to move toward a desired outcome. Nursing activities are at the concrete level of action. A series of activities is necessary to implement an intervention.

Classification of Nursing Interventions

The ordering or arranging of nursing activities into groups or sets on the basis of their relationships and the assigning of intervention labels to these groups of activities.

Taxonomy of Nursing Interventions

A systematic organization of the interventions based upon similarities into a conceptual framework. The NIC taxonomy structure has three levels: domains, classes, and interventions.

OTHER TERMS
Caregiver

A family member, significant other, friend, or other person who cares for or acts on behalf of someone else.

Community

An interactive population with relationships that emerge and the relationships that develop among them as they share in common a physical environment; some agencies and institutions (e.g., school, fire department, voting place).

Family

Two or more individuals related biologically, legally or by choice who have a societal expectation to socialize, enculturate and care for its members.

Health Care Providers

Professional and assistive personnel who are reimbursed for providing health care services.

Parent

Mother, father, or other individual assuming the child-rearing role.

Person or Patient

A person is any individual, group, family, or community who is the focus of the nursing intervention. The terms *patient, individual, health care consumer, care recipient,* and *person* are used in this book, but in some settings, *client* or another word may be the preferred term. Our preferred term is *person*. Users should feel free to use the term that is most relevant to their care setting.

How to Find an Intervention

This edition of the Classification contains 614 interventions. There are several methods available for finding the desired intervention:

Choose **alphabetically** if one knows the name of the intervention and desires to see the entire listing of activities and background readings (see Part Three).

Use the **NIC Taxonomy** if one wishes to identify related interventions in particular topic areas (see Part Two).

Review the **NIC Core Interventions by Specialty** if one is designing a course or information system for a particular specialty group (see Part Four).

Select the **Clinical Condition Linkages** if one is interested in a condition that is listed (see Part Six).

An individual should not be overwhelmed by the size of the Classification, as it is intended to be comprehensive for all specialties and all disciplines. It does not take long to become familiar with the Classification and to locate the interventions most relevant to one's own practice. The selection of a nursing intervention for a particular patient is part of the clinical decision making of the nurse.

Six factors should be considered when choosing an intervention: (1) desired outcomes, (2) characteristics of the nursing diagnosis, (3) research base for the intervention, (4) feasibility for doing the intervention, (5) acceptability to the person, and (6) capability of the nurse. These are explained in Part One.

Frequently Asked Questions

Understanding the reasons things were done in a certain way will assist in better use of the Classification. Here we have grouped the questions individuals may have under five related topics: (1) types of interventions, (2) choosing an intervention, (3) activities, (4) implementing or computerizing NIC, and (5) other.

Types of Interventions

1. Does NIC cover treatments used by nurses practicing in specialty areas and advanced practice? Most definitely yes. Part Four lists 57 nursing specialty areas, and in each area, the core (or most common) NIC interventions that would be used by practicing nurses in the specialty are listed. Furthermore, many of the specialty areas such as Nurse Anesthesiology/Post Anesthesia Care Nursing, Midwifery Nursing, and Oncology Nursing require an advanced practice licensure, certification, or advanced experience in the clinical specialty area with a master's degree or doctorate in nursing practice (DNP). For example, the following interventions may reflect the practice of a certified nurse working in obstetrics: *Amnioinfusion, Birthing, Electronic Fetal Monitoring: Antepartum, High-Risk Pregnancy Care, Labor Induction, Labor Pain Management, Labor Suppression, Reproductive Technology Management,* and *Ultrasonography: Obstetric and Gynecologic.* A similar list can be identified for most specialties. There are also interventions that require an advanced practice license such as *Prescribing: Diagnostic Testing, Medication Prescribing, Medication Deprescribing,* and *Anesthesia Administration.*

2. Does NIC include the important monitoring functions of the nurse? Very definitely yes. NIC includes many monitoring interventions (e.g., *Acid-Base Monitoring, Electronic Fetal Monitoring: Antepartum, Health Policy Monitoring, Intracranial Pressure [ICP] Monitoring, Invasive Hemodynamic Monitoring, Neurologic Monitoring, Surveillance, Surveillance: Late Pregnancy, Surveillance: Remote Monitoring,* and *Vital Signs Monitoring*). These interventions consist mostly of monitoring activities but also include some activities to reflect the clinical judgment process, or what nurses are thinking and anticipating when they monitor. These interventions define what to look for and what to do when an anticipated event occurs. In addition, all interventions in NIC include monitoring activities

when these are done as part of the intervention. We use the words *monitor* and *identify* to mean assessment activities that are part of an intervention. We have tried to use these words rather than the word *assess* in this intervention classification because *assessment* is the term used in the nursing process to refer to those activities that take place before diagnosis and therefore before the intervention.

3. Does NIC include interventions that would be used by a primary care practitioner, especially interventions designed to promote health? Yes indeed. There is an entire class of *Health Education* interventions focused on promoting health, which includes interventions such as *Health Education, Teaching: Individual,* and *Teaching: Disease Process.* Many other health-promotion interventions are included across classes. Examples include *Adolescent Care, Anticipatory Guidance, Child Care, Decision-Making Support, Exercise Promotion, Health Coaching, Health Screening, Learning Facilitation, Nutrition Management, Oral Health Promotion, Parent Education: Adolescent, Parent Education: Childrearing Family, Parent Education: Infant, Risk Identification, Smoking Cessation Assistance, Substance Use Prevention, Self-Responsibility Facilitation, Vaccination Management,* and *Weight Management. Medication Prescribing, Medication Deprescribing,* and *Prescribing: Diagnostic Testing* are interventions used by many advanced practice nurses working in primary care.

4. Does NIC include alternative therapies? We assume this question refers to treatments that are not part of mainstream health care in the United States but may be more common in other countries. Interventions in NIC that might be listed as alternative therapies include *Acupressure, Aromatherapy, Autogenic Training, Biofeedback, Dance Therapy, Garden Therapy, Guided Imagery, Healing Touch, Hypnosis, Laughter Yoga, Massage, Meditation Facilitation, Phytotherapy, Reiki, Relaxation Therapy, Therapeutic Touch,* and *Yoga.* Many of these interventions are located in the class *Psychological Comfort Promotion.* Other alternative therapies will be added to NIC as they become part of accepted nursing practice.

5. Does the Classification include administrative interventions? The Classification includes indirect care interventions done by first-line staff or advance practice nurses but does not include, for the most part, those behaviors that are administrative in nature. An indirect care intervention is a treatment performed by a direct care provider away from the person but on behalf of a person or group of persons, while an administrative intervention is an action performed by a nurse administrator (nurse manager or other nurse administrator) to enhance the performance of staff members to promote better outcomes. Some of the interventions in NIC, when used by an administrator to enhance staff performance, would then be administrative interventions. Most of these are located in the taxonomy in the Health System domain, for example, *Competency Management, Delegation, Peer Review, Quality Monitoring, Safety Huddle, Staff Supervision*, and *Supply Chain Management*. It should be noted that the borders between direct, indirect, and administrative interventions are not firm and some NIC interventions may be used in various contexts. For example, the nurse in the hospital may provide *Caregiver Support* as an indirect intervention administered to a relative of the person being cared for, but the nurse in the home, treating the whole family, may provide this intervention as direct care. We have also included interventions for communities, such as *Community Health Development, Program Development*, and *Social Marketing*. However, these interventions are often delivered by the primary care nurse in the community setting or by the case manager.

Choosing an Intervention

6. How do I find the interventions I use when there are so many interventions in NIC? At first glance, NIC, with 614 interventions, may seem overwhelming. Remember, however, that NIC covers the practice domain of all nurses. An individual nurse will use only a portion of the interventions in NIC on a regular basis. These can be identified by reviewing the classes in the taxonomy that are most relevant to an individual's practice area or by reviewing the list of core interventions for one's specialty (see Part Four). In those agencies with nursing information systems, the interventions can be grouped or bundled together by taxonomy class, nursing diagnosis, various types of populations (e.g., burn, cardiac, maternity), nursing specialty area, or unit. Many computer systems will also allow individual nurses to create and maintain a personal library of most-used interventions. We have been told by nurses using the Classification that they quickly identify a relatively small number of interventions that reflect the core of their practice.

7. How do I decide which intervention to use when one intervention includes an activity that refers to another intervention? In some NIC interventions, there is reference in the activity list to another intervention. For example, the intervention of *Airway Management* contains an activity that says, "Remove secretions through appropriate means (e.g., coughing, suctioning: oropharynx, nasopharynx, tracheal, endotracheal)." There is another intervention in NIC, *Airway Suctioning*, which is defined as "Removal of secretions by inserting a suction catheter into the person's oral, nasopharyngeal, or tracheal airway" and has more than 20 activities listed under it. Another example is the intervention of *Pain Management: Chronic*, which contains an activity that says: "Encourage appropriate use of nonpharmacological techniques (e.g., biofeedback, TENS, hypnosis, relaxation, guided imagery, music therapy, distraction, play therapy, activity therapy, acupressure, heat and cold application, massage) and pharmacological options as pain control measures." Nearly all of the techniques listed in the parentheses of this activity are listed in NIC as interventions, each with a definition and a set of defining activities. The two examples demonstrate that the more abstract, more global interventions sometimes refer to other interventions. Sometimes one needs the more global intervention, sometimes the more specific one, and sometimes both. The selection of nursing interventions for use with an individual is part of the clinical decision-making process of the nurse. NIC reflects all possibilities. The nurse should choose the intervention(s) to use for a particular person using the six factors discussed in *Use of NIC in Practice: Selecting an Intervention* in Part One.

8. When is a new intervention developed? We believe that each of our interventions is different from others in the Classification. We developed the guiding principle that a new intervention is added if 50% or more of the activities are different from another related intervention. Thus, each time a new intervention is proposed, it is compared with other existing interventions. If 50% or more of the activities are different, it is viewed as significantly different and therefore is added to the Classification.

With interventions that are types of a more general intervention (e.g., *Sexual Counseling* is a type of *Counseling*; *Tube Care: Gastrointestinal* is a type of *Tube Care*), the most pertinent activities are included in the more concrete intervention so that this intervention can stand alone. The more concrete intervention should not list all the activities from the more general intervention, rather just those that are essential to carrying out the intervention. In addition, the new intervention must have at least 50% new activities.

With this edition, we have implemented a process of reviewing classes of closely related interventions as new interventions are submitted, to further ensure uniqueness. For example, when considering the new NIC *Surveillance: Video Monitoring*, we reviewed all of the existing surveillance NICs, to confirm that the new content was not contained in any existing NIC. This process generated an update to all of the surveillance NICs.

9. *In initiating a plan of care, what's the structure for NIC and NOC? What do you choose and think about first?* The answer to this reflects the clinical decision making of the provider who is planning and delivering the care. Individuals have different approaches to planning care, reflecting what they learned in school and refined by what they find works best for them and their typical population. As a general approach, we suggest first making the diagnosis (or diagnoses), then selecting outcomes and indicators, rating the person on these, then selecting the interventions and appropriate activities, implementing these, and then rating the outcomes again. If one wants to set goals, these can be derived from the NOC outcomes (e.g., the person is at 2 on X outcome and by discharge he should be at a level of 4). In some situations, this process is not possible or even desirable and one would want to use a different order. For example, in a crisis, one would move immediately to the implementation of the intervention, with the diagnosis and outcome left for later. The advantage of the standardized classifications is that they provide the language for the knowledge base of nursing. Educators and others can now focus on teaching and practice of skills in clinical decision making; researchers can focus on examining the effects of interventions on outcomes in real practice situations. See the model in Part One that shows how standardized language can be used at the individual level, the unit/organizational level, and the network/state/country level.

Activities

10. *Why are certain basic activities included in the activity list for some interventions but not others?* For example, why should an activity related to documentation be included in *Discharge Planning* and *Referral* and not in every intervention? Or, why should an activity related to evaluation of outcomes be included in *Discharge Planning* and not in all interventions? Or, why should an activity on establishing trust be included in *Reminiscence Therapy* or *Support Group* but not in other interventions?

Basic activities are included when they are critical for the implementation of that intervention (i.e., absolutely essential to communicate the essence of the intervention). They are not included when they are part of the routine actions of the nurse but not a critical piece of the intervention. For example, hand washing is a routine part of many physical interventions but is not critical to interventions such as *Bathing or Skin Care: Topical Treatment*. (We are not saying that washing one's hands should not be done for these interventions, just that this is not a critical activity.) Hand washing is a critical part, however, of such interventions as *Infection Control and Contact Lens Care*. Some activities are of such importance that they may also be NIC interventions. For example, *Patient Identification* is a critical activity for most interventions; however, the importance of person identification

for current safety initiatives and the use of many new techniques and electronic devices elevates this activity to intervention status.

11. *Can I change the activities in an intervention when I use it in practice?* Yes. The standardized language is the label name and the definition, and these should remain the same for all persons and all situations. Individualization of care is a core value of nursing. NIC activities help nurses to individualize care by selecting activities to reflect the needs of the particular situation. These are advantages of NIC: it provides both a standardized language that will help nurses communicate across settings about our interventions and it allows for individualized care. The NIC activities use the modifiers *as appropriate, as needed*, and *as indicated* to reflect the fact that individuals are unique and may require different approaches. The NIC activities include all ages of persons; however, when used with adults, some of the activities directed at children may not be appropriate (and vice versa). In this case, these can be omitted from an agency's list of activities. Also, the NIC interventions are not at the procedure level of specificity, and some agencies may wish to be more specific to reflect particular protocols developed for their populations. The activities can easily be modified to reflect this. At the same time, we believe activities can and should be modified to meet individual needs, but we caution that activities should not be changed so much that the original NIC list is unrecognized. If this is done, then the intervention may in fact not be the same. Any modified or new activities should fit the definition of the intervention. In addition, when an activity is being added consistently for most persons and populations, then it may be needed in NIC's general listing of activities. In this case, we would urge the clinician to submit the proposed activity as an addition or change. In this way, the activity list continues to reflect the best of current practice and is most useful in teaching the interventions to new practitioners.

12. *Why are the activities not standardized?* Increasingly, as NIC is entered into computer systems, we are asked this question. Those who design computer systems would like similar activities listed under different interventions to be worded the same so that it would be easier for them to create and use databases. We launched a project to systematically evaluate the feasibility of standardizing the activities using the fourth edition (2004). Two approaches were used. First, all of the nearly 13,000 activities in NIC were printed alphabetically using the first word (a verb) in the activities. One of the team members reviewed these and brought a sample to the NIC team for review. This approach revealed a small number of editorial concerns (e.g., missing commas before "as appropriate" or "as needed") and a very limited number of activities whose wording could be made identical to similar activities without changing the meaning.

The second approach was to identify frequently addressed topics (nouns) such as referral, medication side effects, environment, procedure or treatment, intake and output, privacy, approach, trust, listener, relationship, support, and vital signs. Using a computer search program, activities that included the identified topic (e.g., referral) were printed. These topic searches resulted in lists of anywhere from 100 to several hundred activities. One of the team members reviewed the topic listings, and two of these were taken to the NIC team for discussion. Various approaches to standardization were proposed, but team members agreed that rewording activities would result in loss of meaning and content. After this systematic review and deliberation, it was decided not to pursue standardization of activities any further.

The reasons that NIC activities are not standardized are listed subsequently:

a. As we have emphasized in the past, the focus and standardization of NIC is at the intervention label level. Activities can be added, deleted, or modified for each intervention as the situation requires. Further standardization of activities would defeat the nursing value of individualized care.

b. Each activity was written for a specific intervention and has meaning for the context of the specific intervention.

c. The activities already have a standard format and follow rules for development (i.e., begin with a verb, list in order of doing, meet the definition of the intervention, use an already worded activity from a related intervention if the activity is one that also fits the new intervention). Indeed, many activities already are worded the same across similar interventions.

Implementing or Computerizing NIC

13. *Does my health care agency need to be computerized to use NIC?* No, NIC can be used in a manual care planning and documentation system. If the system is manual, nurses unfamiliar with NIC will need ready access to the NIC book. The book should also be available for nurses working in agencies that have computerized NIC (we think every unit should have a book and encourage individual nurses to have their own copies); with a computer, however, NIC can be stored and accessed electronically. Portable devices such as smart phones and tablets can also be used for accessing an electric version of NIC for planning and documentation. Ideally, these portable and computer versions of NIC should be integrated into the facility's electronic health care system. Computers make it easy to access NIC interventions in a variety of ways (for now, by taxonomic classes and nursing diagnoses, but it is also possible by population type, unit type, outcome, clinical path, etc.). Computers can easily accommodate a variety of clinical decision support screens for nurses. Documenting what we do for persons using a standardized language on computers makes it possible for nursing to build agency, state, regional, and national databases to do effectiveness research. If one's agency is not computerized, help it to become computerized, but do not wait for a computer before using NIC. NIC is helpful to communicate nursing care with or without a computer.

14. *How should NIC be included in my computer system?* We urge that computer systems be built that use the standardized intervention label, with the list of nursing activities for each specific intervention under the intervention label. The activities are most often accessed as a pull-down menu linked to the intervention label. Nurses should plan, document, and communicate care at intervention level. If one also wishes to document the activities, this, of course, can be done either by indicating those activities that were implemented or by charting by exception for those activities not implemented. Some agencies only wish to document a short list of those activities that are essential for legal purposes or those that need further follow-up as "orders" for nursing assistants. Overall, however, we must begin to acknowledge that the standard of care for the delivery of a particular intervention involves the nurse doing the listed activities as they are appropriate for the particular person and situation.

15. *What is the best way to go about implementation of NIC in my agency?* Other related questions include the following: Should I implement NIC and NOC together? Should I implement NIC at the same time I orient nurses to a new computer system? Should we do this on just a pilot unit first or put this up "live" for everyone at the same time? Part One lists helpful steps for implementation for practice agencies (see Box 2) as well as steps for implementation for educational facilities (see Box 6).

As for the questions related to how much to do at one time, there is no one right way; it truly does depend on the situation and the amount and nature of the changes, the resources and support available, and the time constraints. The companion NOC book has many helpful suggestions about implementation of NOC. We would caution not to make too many changes at once for this is often more than most can handle. On the other hand, it may not be wise to delay change by doing only small pieces over an extended time. Duplicate charting (recording the same thing in more than one place) is discouraged. Piloting is a chance to work the bugs out (say, starting on one unit where the nurse manager and staff are supportive) and is always a good idea. Providing time for training and having support available when the change is first made is important. It is also important in the beginning to think about the uses of the data in the future, beyond the initial care planning or documentation purposes. Part One covers the idea of setting up a comprehensive database for effectiveness research in the future.

16. *When do I need to obtain a license?* Other related questions include the following: Why do I need a license? Why isn't NIC in the public domain? Why is the copyright for NIC held by a publisher? A license is needed if one puts NIC on a nursing information system or if one will use a substantial part of the Classification for commercial gain or advantage. NIC is published and copyrighted by Elsevier, and this organization processes requests for permissions to use the Classification. See the inside front cover of this text for directions on whom to contact for permission to use or licensing.

When we first began working on the NIC classification, we had little idea of the magnitude of the work or its current widespread use or that it would be followed by NOC. We were looking for a way to get the work in print and disseminated quickly. As academics, we were familiar with the book publishing world, and after some very serious review of alternative mechanisms and talks with other publishers, we selected Mosby (now Elsevier) as the publisher. Publication with Elsevier has several advantages. First, they have the resources and the contacts to produce a book, to market it, and to sell it. In addition, they have the legal staff and resources to process requests for permission and protect the copyright. This is especially important with standardized language, where alteration of terms will impede the goal of communication among nurses across specialties and between delivery sites. We view our relationship with Elsevier as a partnership.

Copyright does not restrict fair use. According to guidelines by the American Library Association, fair use allows materials to be copied if: (1) the portion copied is selective and sparing in comparison to the whole work; (2) the materials are not used repeatedly; (3) no more than one copy is made for each person; (4) the source and copyright notice is included on each copy; and (5) persons are not assessed a fee for the copy beyond the actual cost of reproduction. The determination of the amount that can be copied under fair use policies has to do with the effect of the copying on sales of the original material. The American Library Association states that no more than 10% of a work should be copied.

When someone puts NIC in an information system that will be used by multiple users, copyright is violated (a book is now being "copied" for use by hundreds of nurses), so a licensing agreement is needed. Also, when someone uses large amounts of NIC in a book or software product that is then sold and makes money for that individual, then a permissions fee is necessary. Schools of nursing and health care agencies that want to use NIC in their own organizations and have no intention of selling a resulting product are free to do so. Fair use policies exist, however. For example, NIC and NOC should not be photocopied and used in syllabi semester after semester; instead, the classification books should be adopted for use. Similarly, health care agencies should purchase a reasonable number of books (say, one per unit) rather than copy the interventions and place them in some procedure manual.

With this edition, we have the ability to offer use of the NIC in research projects without incurring licensure fees, in conjunction with the Center for Nursing Classification and Clinical Effectiveness, College of Nursing, Iowa City, Iowa. Approval of the use in one's research must first be obtained through the Center.

Requests for use of NIC and NOC should be sent to the permissions department of Elsevier. Many requests for permission to use do not violate copyright, and permission is given with no fee. Fees for use in a book depend on the amount of material used. Fees for use in information systems depend on the number of users. There is a flat fee for incorporating NIC into a vendor's database and then a sublicense fee for each sublicense undertaken based on the number of users. The fees are reasonable, and a substantial portion of the fees are being forwarded to the Center for Nursing Classification and Clinical Effectiveness to help support the ongoing development and use of NIC. The Classification is only useful if it reflects current practice; upkeep is time consuming and expensive, and the fees generated from usage support this work.

17. *How do I explain to the administrator at my institution that a license is needed?* First, one wants to repeat that only use in an information system requires a license and a fee; if you want to use NIC manually or for a particular project that does not violate copyright, please go ahead. In our experience, it is nurses and not health care administrators who are unfamiliar with licenses and fees. Most other health care classifications are copyrighted, and fees are required for use. For example, the *Current Procedural Terminology (CPT)* is copyrighted by the American Medical Association, and the *Diagnostic and Statistical Manual of Mental Disorders 5th edition (DSM 5)* is copyrighted by the American Psychiatric Association. Health care institutions regularly pay license fees for these classifications now, but most nurses are not aware of these usage fees.

License fees are often included as part of the software costs. NIC can be licensed from Elsevier (use of the language) for incorporation in an existing information system or purchased from a vendor with software (the vendor has purchased the license from Elsevier, and the software price includes the cost of the license). As more nurses understand the advantages of using standardized language and desire this in purchases of new information systems, more vendors will include NIC in their products.

In nursing, none of the professional organizations have the resources to maintain NIC, so another avenue was needed. We have been told by those in the health care field that having the Classification housed in a university setting has advantages over the professional organizational model, in which politics (what is in and what is out) may play a part. Ongoing development and maintenance, however, require resources. Classifications and other works in the public domain are often those for which there will be no upkeep, so one can use what is there but does not expect it to be kept current. We have attempted to make NIC as accessible as possible but to also collect fees so that we can have a revenue stream to finance the maintenance work that must continue.

18. What is a reference terminology model? Why are these being developed? Will they make classifications such as NIC obsolete? A reference terminology (RT) model identifies the parts of a concept (e.g., the parts of any diagnosis or any intervention) that can be used behind the screens in computer systems to assist these systems to talk with each other. For example, an intervention might consist of an action, a recipient, and a route. Theoretically, an RT model enables differing vocabularies (e.g., NIC and Omaha) to be mapped to one RT model and, thus, compared with each other. We say theoretically because this approach has not yet been tested in practice. In the late 1990s and early 2000s, there was a mushrooming of terminology models. Examples include HL7 (in the United States for all of health care), CEN (in Europe for all of health care), SNOMED CT (for use in the United States and Europe), and ISO-Nursing (for nursing internationally). We consider the International Classification of Nursing Practice (ICNP), with its axes, an RT model that is more helpful behind the screens than useful to practicing nurses as a front-end terminology.

A second part of this question is whether the creation of an RT model will make classifications such as NIC obsolete. No, NIC is a front-end language designed for communication among nurses and between nurses and other providers. We want nurses to be able to write and talk NIC. On the other hand, RT models are for use behind the screens: if they do succeed, they will help vendors to build computer systems that can use and compare different front-end languages. RT models are often difficult to understand and not clinically useful. Even if they allow users to document care in their own words (versus standardized language), this is not desirable for the profession (except in a free-text notes section that supplements and elaborates on the standardized language) because we would still have the problem of lack of communication among ourselves and between ourselves and others as to what we do. We will always need a standardized language to communicate the work of nursing. NIC is intended to be just that.

19. Is there commercial software available with NIC in it? Are there vendors that have clinical nursing software with NIC? Yes. This is a growing area. When a licensing agreement for NIC is made with Elsevier, the user is sent a CD to make it easier to transfer the language to a computer system. A growing number of vendors are including NIC in their information systems, and website information for them is listed in Part One, Box 1.

When individuals are considering selecting a particular vendor for implementing in a facility, we suggest choosing a vendor that already has nursing languages built into the system. If vendors do not have NIC included in their electronic health system, ask them to build the system so that nurses can use NIC nursing terminology in the planning and documenting of care. Vendors will build their products according to user demand. Nurses need to speak up and ask for standardized language to be included in clinical information systems.

Other

20. How does NIC compare to other classifications? The American Nurses Association recognizes 12 terminologies for nursing practice information infrastructure. Some are data element sets, some are interface terminologies, and some are multidisciplinary terminologies. Compared with the other classifications, NIC is the most comprehensive for interventions. Of all the classifications, only NANDA-I, NIC, and NOC are comprehensive and have ongoing efforts to keep them current. Numerous publications exist documenting the use and relationship among the three classification systems.

21. Should we use a nursing classification when most of health care is being delivered by interprofessional teams? Occasionally, we hear something like "we can't use anything that is labeled *nursing* and comes from nursing when everything is now going to be *interprofessional*." We hear this, by the way, from nurses rather than from physicians or other power holders in the interprofessional arena. At the same time, it is assumed that using medical language does not violate this artificial interprofessional principle. We believe that nurses who are members of an interprofessional team addressing the development and implementation of a computerized integrated care record should be, in fact must be, the spokespersons for use of NIC and NOC. Yes, these have the nursing word in their titles because they were developed inductively through research based on the work of nurses by nurses. Taken as a whole, they reflect the discipline of nursing, but any one individual intervention may be done by other types of providers, and any one outcome may be influenced by the treatments of other providers or by many other factors. This is a situation in which nursing has something of value that the other providers, for the most part, do not. NIC and NOC document the contributions of nurses and can be used, or adapted and used, by others if they wish. Nurses should not avoid talking about these nursing initiatives; rather they should assertively offer them as the nursing contribution to the interprofessional goal of a computerized health care record that can cross settings and specialties.

We have heard a few individuals say that there should be only one language that is shared by all health disciplines. If this is possible, we believe that the one language should develop inductively through sharing and adding to the current languages that exist. Perhaps, over time, we will build one large common language whereby some intervention and outcome terms are shared by many providers. But even if we can build one large common language, it will always be used in parts because the whole is too great to learn, communicate, and study, and all interventions and outcomes are not the business of every discipline. The one very large language will be broken down and used in parts for the same reasons that there are disciplines; the whole is too large and complex to be mastered by any one individual. Hence, different disciplines represent different specialized perspectives.

22. How does NIC contribute to theory development in nursing? The intervention labels are the concepts, or the names of the treatments provided by nurses. The definitions and activities that accompany the labels provide for definition and description of the interventions. Clarification of intervention concepts contributes to the development of nursing knowledge and facilitates communication within the discipline. As nursing's ability to link diagnoses, interventions, and outcomes grows, prescriptive theory for nursing practice will evolve. The NIC is a crucial development because it provides the lexical elements for middle-range theories in nursing that will link diagnoses, interventions, and outcomes. Interventions are the key element in nursing. All other aspects of nursing practice are contingent upon, and secondary to, the treatments that identify and delineate our discipline. This intervention-centric approach does not diminish the importance of the person; but from a disciplinary perspective, the person is important because he or she can be affected by nursing action. We believe that use of standardized languages for nursing diagnoses, interventions, and outcomes heralds a new era in the development of nursing theory. NIC can be included in most all practice models derived from nursing conceptual models and theories. Furthermore, NIC can be used by any institution, nursing specialty, or care delivery model regardless of philosophical orientation.

Contents

Detailed Contents

PART FOUR Core Interventions for Nursing Specialty Areas, 469

Core Interventions for Nursing Specialty Areas, 470

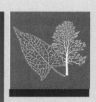

## PART ONE

Overview and Application of the NIC in Practice, Education, and Research

DESCRIPTION OF NIC

Interventions are the quintessence of nursing and the profession's *raison d'être* (reason for being). The professional responsibility of nursing focuses on providing safe, high quality, evidence-based interventions to address important nursing situations for the purpose of promoting health, well-being, and positive health outcomes. Health professionals engage with persons in making health decisions related to their care by selecting treatments of interventions and monitoring responses to interventions. Interventions are the "central elements of healthcare, and their careful selection and their appropriate delivery form the basis of high-quality care"[104] (p. 3). Accurate, safe, and effective decision-making requires that health care providers are aware of and have knowledge of the evidence-based interventions and actions designed to treat health concerns. The Nursing Interventions Classification (NIC) is a comprehensive standardized classification of interventions that nurses perform. It is useful for care planning, clinical documentation, communication of care across settings, integration of data across systems and settings, effectiveness research, productivity measurement, competency evaluation, reimbursement, teaching, and curricular design.

The development and use of nursing classification systems is a hallmark of success in the evolution of nursing science and practice.[35] All sciences order accumulated knowledge through systems of classification.[88] These classifications and taxonomies identify the phenomena central to the discipline's concern, provide a name for the phenomena to create a common language, and use definitions or descriptions of terms in the classification to give names meaning. A classification is a broad term referring to a systematic arrangement of groups or categories according to established criteria. A taxonomy is the orderly classification, arrangement, and naming of concepts of knowledge into a hierarchical structure of categories. Lambe[69] points out that a classification system makes knowledge visible and serves to organize knowledge so we can manage and retrieve information. A taxonomy is identified by its nomenclature or arrangement into classes and its terminology. As society becomes more information intensive and more technological, the need to organize knowledge is increasingly essential.[14,44,54,69] "Knowledge organization is a fundamental precondition for managing knowledge effectively"[69] (p. 3).

Along with classification systems for nursing diagnoses and nursing outcomes, the NIC form the knowledge base that supports professional nursing practice. While nursing classification systems form the substance of nursing, discipline-specific conceptual frameworks and theories provide the conceptual and scientific foundation for linking diagnoses, interventions, and outcomes.

NIC is a means to identify the treatments nurses perform, organize this information into a coherent structure, and provide the language to communicate with individuals, families, communities, members of other disciplines, and the public. When NIC is used to document the work of nurses in practice, then we have the ability to determine the impact of nursing care on health outcomes. Building on Clark and Lang's statement[25] on the importance of nursing languages and classifications, we assert if we cannot name it, we cannot plan and manage it, finance it, teach it, research it, synthesize it, or put it into public policy.

NIC, like all classifications, accomplishes its goals first by reflecting the work that nurses perform and second by carefully organizing and categorizing that work. In other words, NIC is useful when the interventions reflect and are connected to the real world of nursing practice. The Classification includes the interventions that nurses perform on behalf of persons, both independent and collaborative interventions, and both direct and indirect care. An *intervention* is defined as *any treatment based upon clinical judgment and knowledge that a nurse performs to enhance health outcomes.* Although individual nurses will have expertise in only a limited number of interventions reflecting their specialty, the entire Classification captures the expertise of *all* nurses. NIC can be used in *all settings* (from acute care to intensive care units to primary to home care to hospice care) and *all specialties* (from emergency care to critical care nursing to pediatric nursing to gerontological nursing). The entire Classification describes the domain of nursing; however, some of the interventions in the Classification may also be useful to other providers and members of the interprofessional team. All health care providers are welcome to use NIC to describe their treatments.

NIC interventions include both the physiological (e.g., Airway Management) and the psychosocial (e.g., Anxiety Reduction). Interventions are included for illness treatment (e.g., Hyperglycemia Management), prevention (e.g., Fall

Prevention), and health promotion (e.g., Exercise Promotion). Most of the interventions are for use with individuals, but many are for use with families (e.g., Family Support), and some are for entire communities (e.g., Communicable Disease Management). Indirect care interventions (e.g., Competency Management) are also included.

Each intervention as it appears in the Classification is listed with a label name, a definition, a set of activities to carry out the intervention, and references of background evidence supporting the intervention. A notation that appears with each intervention (just before the listing of background evidence) lists the edition where the intervention was originally developed and when it was revised.

Central to any scientific system of knowledge is having a means to classify and structure categories of information. The creation of this classification of nursing interventions begins with naming or providing a standardized and distinct linguistic label designating a treatment or an intervention that the nurse performs. The identification of nursing interventions is inductively derived by examining, describing, and naming in a systematic way, what is embedded in nursing practice. Lunney points out "naming is classifying so every time a name is given to a phenomenon, classification is occurring"[73] (p. 37). Ohl, in his book *The Art of Naming*,[86] explains that scientific naming becomes part of our perception, and names are verbal tags that give meaning and understanding to the world around us. Scientific names, like the label for each nursing intervention, in Ohl's words[86] are "linguistic beauties" and behind all scientific NIC labels are the stories and knowledge reflecting nursing practice. Although a "label" or name of an intervention does not by itself include a depth of understanding and meaning, all intervention labels call forth and connect the person to all the beliefs, narratives, and practices associated with the label name. In other words, every nursing intervention is associated with a whole universe of meanings, perceptions, skills, emotions, and action embedded in the nurse-person caring experience. NIC makes the hidden work of nursing visible by identifying the knowledge embedded in nursing practice.

In this edition, there are 614 interventions and approximately 15,000 activities. The intervention labels and the definitions are standardized; therefore, the label name and definition **should not** be changed when they are used. This allows for communication across settings and comparison of outcomes.[114] However, care is individualized by selecting the activities relevant for each nursing situation. From a list of approximately 20 to 30 activities per intervention, the provider selects the activities that are appropriate for the specific individual, family, or community, and then can add new activities if desired. However, all modifications or additions to activities should be congruent with the definition of the intervention.

For each intervention, the activities are listed in logical order, from what a nurse would do first to what the nurse would do last. For many activities, the placement is not crucial, but for others, the time sequence is important. The lists of activities are comprehensive because the Classification is designed to meet the needs of multiple users including students and novices who often require more specific knowledge and directions about nurse activities than experienced nurses. The activities are not standardized. Each activity has particular meaning within the context of each intervention. In addition, standardizing activities would defeat the purpose of using them to individualize care. At the end of the list of activities is a short list of selected background evidence references found helpful in developing the intervention, including research evidence supporting the use of the intervention in achieving desired health outcomes. The references can serve as background if one is unfamiliar with the intervention, but they are not intended to be a complete reference list, nor are they inclusive of all the research on the intervention.

Although the lists of activities are very helpful for the teaching of an intervention and for implementation of the delivery of the intervention, they are not the essence of the Classification. The intervention label names and definitions are the key to the Classification; the names provide a summary label for the discrete activities and allow nurses to identify and communicate the nature of their work. Before NIC, nurses only had long lists of discrete activities and no organizing structure; with NIC, nurses can easily communicate their interventions with the label name that is defined with both a formal definition and a list of implementation activities.

The interventions are grouped into 7 domains and 30 classes for ease of use. The 7 domains are: (1) Physiological: Basic, (2) Physiological: Complex, (3) Behavioral, (4) Safety, (5) Family, (6) Health System, and (7) Community (see the Taxonomy beginning on p. 34). A few interventions are in more than one class, but each has a unique number (code) that identifies the primary class and is not used for any other intervention. The NIC taxonomy is coded for several reasons: (1) to facilitate computer use, (2) to facilitate ease of data management, (3) to enhance linking NIC intervention with other coded systems (e.g., Systematized Nomenclature of Medicine Clinical Terms [SNOMED CT]), and (4) to allow for use in reimbursement of nursing care.[113] The codes for the 7 domains are 1 to 7; the codes for the 30 classes are A to Z, a, b, c, d. Each intervention is assigned a unique four-digit code.

Although the activities in this edition are not coded, **activities can be coded** sequentially using two digits after the four-digit code (numbers are not included in the text so as not to distract the reader). An example of a complete code for the second activity of Fall Prevention would be 4V649002, which is 4 for the Safety domain, V for the Risk Management class, 6490 for the Fall Prevention intervention, and 02 for second activity: "Identify behaviors and factors that affect risk of falls."

The language used in the Classification is designed to be clear, concise, consistent, and carefully phrased, reflecting language used in practice. Surveys to clinicians and 30 years of use of the Classification have demonstrated that all the interventions are used in practice. Although the overall listing of 614 interventions may seem overwhelming at first, we have seen that nurses soon discover those interventions that are used most often in their specialty or with their population. Often, specialty practice areas will create easily retrievable lists or "bundles" of the most frequently used interventions linked to specific diagnoses and outcomes used for providing care in their setting. Other ways to locate the desired interventions include the taxonomy, computer programs, and tools that include linkages to nursing diagnoses and outcomes or to clinical conditions (see Part Six); and the core interventions for specialties (see Part Four).

The Classification is continually updated and has an ongoing process for feedback and review. Appendix B includes instructions for users to submit suggestions for modifications to existing interventions or to propose a new intervention. Many of the changes in the 8th edition have come about due to clinicians and researchers taking time to submit suggestions for modifications based upon their use in practice and research. The submissions undergo a rigorous review process by the editors of NIC, including clinical experts when required, for additional revisions and final approval. All reviewers whose changes are included in the edition are acknowledged in the Recognitions List. New editions of the Classification are planned for approximately every 5 years. In addition, there are multiple publications, many in the *International Journal of Nursing Knowledge* and the *International Journal of Nursing Terminologies and Classifications*, describing various applications of using NIC in practice, research, and education.

NIC interventions have been linked with NANDA International (NANDA-I) nursing diagnoses (included in NIC 6th edition, Part Six), Omaha System problems,[52] resident assessment protocols (RAP) used in nursing homes,[21] and Outcome and Assessment Information Set (OASIS),[22] currently mandated for collection for Medicare/Medicaid-covered persons receiving nursing home care. The new 7th edition of the Nursing Outcomes Classification (NOC) is also published by Elsevier at the same time as the current 8th edition of NIC and can be used in conjunction with the NIC for planning nursing care.

Several tools are available that assist in the implementation of the Classification. Included in this book are the taxonomic structure (Part Two) to assist a user to find the intervention of choice, the core intervention lists for areas of specialty practice (Part Four), the amount of time and level of education needed to perform each intervention (Part Five), and linkages to six common clinical conditions (Part Six). Permission to use NIC in publications, information systems, and web courses can be acquired from Elsevier (see the inside front cover). Part of the money to purchase a license returns to the Center for Nursing Classification and Clinical Effectiveness (CNC) to help with ongoing development and upkeep of the Classification.

CENTER FOR NURSING CLASSIFICATION AND CLINICAL EFFECTIVENESS

NIC is housed in the CNC at the University of Iowa, College of Nursing. The CNC was approved by the Iowa Board of Regents (the governing body that oversees the state's three public universities) in 1995. The CNC has had three directors since its inception: Joanne Dochterman (1995–2004), Sue Moorhead (2004–2020), and Karen Dunn Lopez (2020–present). The CNC provides a structure for the continued upkeep of the Classifications and for communication with the many nurses and others in education and healthcare facilities who are using the languages in their curricula and documentation systems. The overarching goal of the CNC is: *To expand adoption of the Nursing Interventions Classification and Nursing Outcomes Classifications to advance nursing science, practice, and person-centered care.* The CNC seeks to develop and enhance relevant, easy to use products; create opportunities for synergy with research, education, and practice; expand the context for use of the classifications; and influence policy makers and regulatory bodies to promote the use of terminologies. The CNC also conducts research, disseminates materials related to the Classifications, provides educational opportunities for national and international students, faculty, fellows, and visiting professors, provides consultation for implementation and use of the Classifications in clinical practice and educational settings, and assists faculty and students with projects and research using the Classifications.

Financial support for the CNC comes from a variety of sources, including university and college funds, licensing, permission, and product revenue from NIC, NOC, and related publications, grants, and income from Center initiatives. A substantial endowment for the support of the CNC has been raised through donations. The endowment provides some permanent long-range security for the work of the CNC. Information about the CNC happenings can be found on the website https://nursing.uiowa.edu/center-for-nursing-classification-and-clinical-effectiveness.

DEVELOPMENT OF THE NIC CLASSIFICATION

The research to develop NIC began in 1987 and has progressed through four phases, each with some overlap in time:

Phase I: Construction of the Classification (1987–1992)
Phase II: Construction of the Taxonomy (1990–1995)
Phase III: Clinical Testing and Refinement (1993–1997)
Phase IV: Use and Maintenance (1996–ongoing)

Work conducted in each of these phases is described in previous editions of this book and in many other publications.[16,26,50,51,79] The research was initiated with 7 years of funding from the National Institute of Nursing at the National Institutes of Health. NIC was developed by a large research team whose members represented multiple areas of clinical and methodological expertise.

Multiple research methods were used in the original development of NIC. An inductive approach was used in Phase I to build the Classification based on existing practice. Original sources included textbooks, care planning guides, and nursing information systems to identify interventions and associated nursing activities. Experts in specialty areas of practice were used to augment the clinical practice expertise of team members who engaged in content analysis, focus group review, and questionnaires to identify and validate the identification of interventions. Phase II was characterized by deductive methods. Methods to construct the taxonomy included similarity analysis, hierarchical clustering, and multidimensional scaling. Through clinical field-testing, steps for implementation were developed and tested and the need for linkages between NANDA-I diagnoses, NIC, and NOC were identified. More than 1000 nurses completed questionnaires and approximately 50 professional associations have provided input about the creation of the classification. More details are found in chapters in the earlier editions of NIC, especially in the first four editions and in numerous articles, book chapters, and publications describing NIC.

INDICATIONS OF NIC's USEFULNESS

Indications of NIC's usefulness include its national and increasing international recognition. In 2006 the American Nurses Association (ANA)'s Committee for Nursing Practice Information Infrastructure recognized NIC as a standardized nursing language or terminology that met the uniform guidelines for information system vendors in the ANA's Nursing Information and Data Set Evaluation Center (NIDSEC). The ANA criteria that the NIC met included that the classification was being periodically updated; there was a rationale for its development; and that the classification supports the nursing process by providing clinically useful terminology. As noted by Keenan, a standardized nursing language is a "common language, readily understood by all nurses, to describe care"[59] (p. 12). In addition, the classification concepts must be clear and unambiguous, and there must be documentation of utility in practice as well as validity and reliability. Finally, there must be a named group who will be responsible for maintaining and revising the system.[99]

NIC is licensed for inclusion in Systematized Nomenclature of Medicine Clinical Terms (SNOMED CT). NIC interventions are included in the National Library of Medicine's Meta-Thesaurus for a Unified Medical Language System (UMLS) and is included in the Cumulative Index to Nursing and Allied Health Literature (CINAHL) Database, available via Elton B. Stephens Company (EBSCO) host in its indexes. NIC is registered in Health Level 7 (HL7), the U.S. standards organization for healthcare. Growing international use of NIC is occurring, and it is currently translated into Chinese, Dutch, French, Italian, German, Indonesian, Japanese, Korean, Norwegian, Spanish, Portuguese, and Turkish (see Appendix E).

The best indication of usefulness, however, is the impressive list of individuals and healthcare agencies that use NIC. Many healthcare agencies have adopted NIC for use in policy standards, care planning, competency evaluation, and nursing information systems. NIC is used globally in nursing education programs to structure curricula and identify competencies for nursing students, teach clinical reasoning using the nursing process, and to teach nursing care for the treatment of clinical conditions. Authors of major texts are using NIC to describe nursing treatments, and researchers are using NIC to study the effectiveness of nursing care. Vendors of information systems are incorporating NIC in their software for the planning and documentation of nursing care. A CINAHL search of the term *"nursing interventions classification"* revealed more than 1000 journal publications, and nearly 700 journal publications in PubMed, with the majority occurring since 2016. Since 2012, NIC textbooks in English, Spanish, and Portuguese alone have been referenced more than 5000 times according to Google Scholar.

USE OF NIC IN PRACTICE
Selecting an Intervention

Nursing is a learned profession that reflects multiple ways of knowing and

> "integrates the art and science of caring and focusing on the protection, promotion, and optimization of health and human functioning; prevention of illness and injury; facilitation of healing; and alleviation of suffering through compassionate presence. Nursing is the diagnosis and treatment of human response and advocacy in the care of individuals, families, groups, communities, and populations in recognition of the connection of all humanity"[4] (p. 1).

Registered nurses integrate objective data with knowledge from assessments, which include subjective experiences to make health decisions rooted in evidenced based knowledge. These decisions are designed to promote positive health outcomes delivered in the context of caring, culture, and a supportive environment. Nurses develop individualized, holistic, evidence-based plans of care in partnership with persons, families, significant others, and the interprofessional team. They do this by selecting innovative nursing interventions and practices that are designed to promote health; prevent illness, injury, disease, and complications; enhance quality of life; alleviate suffering; promote wholeness, comfort, and growth; mitigate environment and occupational risks; and advocate for transformative, action-orientated policies and initiatives that alleviate inequality and promote social justice. Selecting evidence-based nursing interventions is part of the clinical reasoning and decision-making of the nurse. Six factors should be considered when choosing an intervention: (1) desired outcomes, (2) characteristics of the nursing diagnosis, (3) research base for the intervention, (4) feasibility for performing the intervention, (5) acceptability to the person, and (6) capability of the nurse.[15]

Desired Outcomes. Person outcomes should be specified before an intervention is chosen. They serve as the criteria against which to judge the success of a nursing intervention. Outcomes describe behaviors, responses, and feelings of the person in response to the care provided. Many variables influence outcomes, including the clinical problem; interventions prescribed by the health care providers; the health care providers themselves; the environment in which care is received; health care consumer's own motivation, genetic structure, and pathophysiology; and their significant others. There are many intervening or mediating variables in each situation, making it difficult to establish a causal relationship between nursing interventions and outcomes in some instances. The nurse must identify outcomes that can be reasonably expected and can be attained as the result of the nursing care.

The most effective way to specify outcomes is by use of NOC. NOC contains outcomes for individuals, families, and communities that are representative for all settings and clinical specialties.[83] Each NOC outcome describes person states at a conceptual level, with indicators expected to be responsive to nursing intervention. The indicators for each outcome allow measurement of the outcomes at any point on a 5-point Likert scale, from most negative to most positive. Repeated ratings over time provide identification of changes in the person's condition. Thus, NOC outcomes are used to monitor the extent of progress or lack of progress throughout an episode of care. NOC outcomes have been developed to be used in all settings, all specialties, and across the continuum of care.

Characteristics of the Nursing Diagnosis. Outcomes and interventions are selected in relationship to particular nursing diagnoses. The use of standardized nursing language began in the early 1970s with the development of the NANDA-I nursing diagnosis classification. A nursing diagnosis according to NANDA-I is "a clinical judgment concerning a human response to health conditions/life processes, or vulnerability for that response by an individual, caregiver, family, group, or community"[46] (p. 85). A nursing diagnosis provides the basis for selection of nursing interventions to achieve outcomes for which the nurse has accountability. The elements of the NANDA-I diagnosis statement are the label, the related factors (causes or associated factors), and the defining characteristics (signs and symptoms). Interventions are directed toward altering the etiological factors (related factors) or causes of the diagnosis. If the intervention is successful in altering the etiology, the care recipient's status can be expected to improve. It may not always be possible to change the etiological factors and when this is the case, it is necessary to treat the defining characteristics (signs and symptoms).

Creating linkages between specific nursing diagnoses or clinical conditions, outcomes, and interventions is a strategy that assists in selecting appropriate nursing interventions. The *NOC and NIC Linkages to NANDA-I and Clinical Conditions: Supporting Clinical Reasoning and Quality Care*[55] text remains a valuable resource and can serve as a template for identifying outcomes and interventions for NANDA-I nursing diagnoses as well as for the 10 common clinical conditions of asthma, chronic obstructive pulmonary disease, colon and rectal cancer, depression, diabetes mellitus, heart failure, hypertension, pneumonia, stroke, and total joint replacement: hip/knee. In this text (see Part Six), we have added linkages for six additional clinical conditions: coronary artery disease, coronavirus disease 2019 (COVID-19), hyperlipidemia, lung cancer, substance use disorder, and ulcerative colitis/Crohn disease as examples of how NIC can be linked to NOC outcomes for specific conditions.

Ros et al.'s Spanish text *NIC para el Aprendizaje Teorico-Practico en Enfermeria* (NIC for Theoretical-Practical Learning in Nursing)[98] is a valuable resource that links NIC interventions to nursing situations, including such fundamentals as promoting comfort, safety, and mobility; health conditions such as wound care; and acute and critical care such as persons on mechanical ventilation and cardiac monitoring. There are many publications that have identified the most common NIC interventions for a variety of nursing situations. For example, a team of nurses at the Center for Nursing Classification and Effectiveness published a series of articles identifying common NANDA-I diagnoses, NIC, and NOC linkages in relation to the COVID-19 pandemic at the community level;[82] the level of individuals;[109] and for families.[117] In addition, the Brazilian Nursing Process

Research Network, a team of 26 researchers from across Brazil, identified NANDA-I diagnoses, NOC, and NIC activities for treating persons with COVID-19 in communities; for persons with suspected or mild, moderate, and critical COVID-19 infections, and residents in nursing homes.[10] The findings are also available as a download from the Brazilian Nursing Process Research Network website in English, Spanish, and Portuguese (https://repperede.org/). There are also several electronic tools that are available to assist nurses in making linkages between NANDA-I diagnoses, NIC, and NOC. For example, NNN Consult (https://www.nnnconsult.com) is a Spanish Elsevier electronic product for teaching and consulting in clinical practice linking NANDA-I diagnoses, NIC, and NOC.

Research Base for the Intervention. Butcher asserted, "Nurses are living in the age of evidence-based practice (EBP)"[17] (p. 25). EBP is a problem-solving approach to delivering care that integrates: (1) the best evidence from well-designed research studies and evidence-based theories; (2) the clinician's expertise and evidence from assessment of the person's history and condition as well as healthcare resources; and (3) the person, family, group, and population preferences and resources.[4,81] The Nursing: Scope and Standards of Practice[4] lists the use of evidence-based interventions and strategies to achieve mutually identified goals and outcomes as a competency for implementation for all registered nurses. The new Essentials: Core Competencies for Professional Nursing Education includes "evidence-based interventions to improve outcomes and safety" as a core competency in Domain 2: Person Centered Care[3] (p. 31). In the American Association of Colleges of Nursing (AACN)'s description of person-centered care,[3] there is an emphasis on diversity, equity, and inclusion based on best evidence and clinical judgment in the planning and delivery of care across time, spheres of care, and developmental levels.

The Agency for Healthcare Research and Quality (AHRQ), the National Academy of Medicine (NAM; previously called *the Institute of Medicine [IOM]*), American Nurses Association (ANA), and American Association of College of Nursing (AACN) are just some of the agencies and professional associations who have long endorsed the use of EBP as the basis for all healthcare delivery. They have emphasized that interventions supported by research evidence improve person outcomes and clinical practice. It is essential now that nurses develop clinical inquiry skills, which requires nurses to continually question whether the care being given is the best possible practice.

To determine the best practice, evidence that is based on research needs to be assimilated and used in choosing interventions. Thus, the nurse who uses an intervention needs to be familiar with its research base. The research will indicate the effectiveness of using the intervention with certain types of conditions. Some interventions and their corresponding nursing activities have been widely tested for specific populations, whereas others need to be tested and are based on expert clinical knowledge.

To successfully implement EBP, nurse leaders need to place mentors at the bedside who can work side by side with clinicians to help them learn these skills and implement EBP consistently.[17] One way to facilitate EBP is the use of evidence-based guidelines, clinical pathways, evidence-based protocols, and best practices statements. Evidence-based guidelines use systematic reviews to inform specific clinical circumstances. Guidelines are developed to promote accurate assessment, diagnosis, and effective management of the condition. The Cochrane Library and the Joanna Briggs Institute (JBI) each have established clear criteria for developing evidence-based guidelines and have websites where one can access the guidelines. However, typically evidence-based guidelines do not incorporate standardized nursing language such as NANDA-I diagnoses, NIC, and NOC. The integration of NIC would serve to strengthen the evidence base guiding nursing practice.

There are a wide range of models designed to promote evidence-based nursing care in practice settings. For example, *Evidence-based Practice in Action: Comprehensive Strategies, Tools, and Tips from the University of Iowa Hospital and Clinics*[30] offers a detailed plan to nurses and health care leaders in promoting EBP adoption and implementation, including the process of assembling evidence for treating a particular clinical problem and deciding on a practice protocol.

Nursing diagnosis handbooks such as Makic and Martinez-Karatz[77] provide research references from case studies to systematic reviews that provide additional evidence related to NIC interventions and activities. Nurses learn about the research related to particular interventions through their education programs and learn how to keep their knowledge current by finding and evaluating research studies. If there is no research base for an intervention to assist a nurse in choosing an intervention, then the nurse would use scientific principles (e.g., infection transmission) or would consult an expert about the specific populations for which the intervention might work.

Feasibility for Performing the Intervention. Feasibility concerns include the ways in which the intervention interacts with other interventions, both those of the nurse and those of other health care providers. It is important that the nurse is involved in the total plan of care for the person. Other feasibility concerns, critical in today's healthcare environment, are the cost of the intervention and the amount of time required for implementation. The nurse needs to consider the interventions of other providers, the cost of the intervention, the environment, and the time needed to adequately implement an intervention when choosing a course of action.

Acceptability to the Care Recipient. An intervention must be acceptable to the health care consumer and family. The nurse is frequently able to recommend a choice of interventions to assist in reaching a particular outcome. To facilitate an informed choice, the care recipient should be given information about each intervention and how they are expected to participate. Most importantly, the person's values, beliefs, and culture must all be considered when choosing an intervention.

Capability of the Nurse. The nurse must be competent to implement the intervention and must: (1) have knowledge of the scientific rationale for the intervention, (2) possess the necessary psychomotor and interpersonal skills, and (3) be able to function within the particular setting to effectively use healthcare resources.[15] It is clear from just glancing at the total list of 614 interventions that no one nurse has the capability of implementing all the interventions. Nursing, like other health disciplines, is specialized, and individual nurses perform within their specialty and refer or collaborate when other skills are needed.

After considering each of these factors for a particular care recipient, the nurse would select the intervention(s). This is not as time consuming as it sounds when elaborated in writing. With experience, the nurse synthesizes this information and can recognize patterns rapidly. One advantage of the classification is that it facilitates the teaching and learning of decision-making for the novice nurse. Using standardized language to communicate the nature of our interventions does not mean that we stop delivering individualized care. Interventions are tailored to individuals by selective choice of the activities and by modification of the activities as appropriate for the health care consumer's age and their family's physical, social, emotional, and spiritual status. These modifications are made by the nurse, using sound clinical judgment.

Implementing NIC in a Health Care Agency

A number of vendors who develop computerized clinical information systems (CIS) and electronic health records (EHR) are including standardized nursing terminologies in hospital and healthcare settings. It is not surprising that NIC is being implemented into a wide range of computer information systems in the United States as well as countries around the world, including Belgium, Brazil, Canada, China, Denmark, England, France, Germany, Iceland, Indonesia, Italy, Japan, Korea, Norway, Portugal, Spain, Switzerland, The Netherlands, and Turkey. Box 1 lists some of the healthcare

Box 1

Vendors Who Have Licenses for NIC

Vendor	Description
Clinical Architecture Carmel, IN https://clinicalarchitecture.com/symedical-healthcare-terminology-management-software	NIC and NOC integrated within their Symedical, a health care content management software.
Computer Program and System Inc. (CPSI) Mobile, AL www.cpsi.com	NIC and NOC integrated within their Electronic Patient Record system for care planning. The system is used by small to midsize hospitals.
DIPS ASA Bodø, Norway www.dips.com	NIC integrated within their Electronic Patient Record System for care planning. Company located in Bodo, Norway.
Robin Technologies, Inc Worthington, OH www.careplans.com	NIC and NOC are used within plans of care for use by students and nurses in long-term care facilities.

The list of vendors provided in March 2022 by Bonita Allen, Elsevier, 3251 Riverport Lane Maryland Heights, MO 63043 USA
NOTE: Translated electronic versions of NIC for licensure are also available from Elsevier Japan, Elsevier Spain, Elsevier Netherlands, and Hogefe Verlagsgruppe in Bern, Switzerland. Other vender platforms (EPIC, Cerner) have incorporated NIC at the request of the local facility. Vendors will respond to customer requests to incorporate NIC into their products.

system computer vendors who have licensed NIC for incorporation into their software products. Computer documentation systems, including NIC and NOC, are currently being used in many diverse healthcare settings. Such systems can assist health care professionals to plan and document nursing care as well as provide a way to enhance clinical decision-making, share information, and track the achievement of outcomes.[37] Vendors have employed NIC in a variety of ways to customize the EHR for various clinical agencies. It is important to note that clinical decision-making and the individualization of care are enhanced when both the NIC label name and related activities appear as choices in the electronic information system.

The omission of rigorously developed standardized nursing languages from EHR systems is a concerning trend that creates a barrier to identifying nursing's intellectual contribution to healthcare. When standardized nursing classifications are not included in the EHR, nursing care may be inaccurately and inconsistently depicted in the documentation system. Importantly, this absence limits the ability of the nurse to accurately indicate the care provided, readily access nursing care provided in other settings, and to provide nursing care continuity across settings. Terms and phrases developed by vendors have the potential to be interoperable within the vendor clients but have not been developed through decades of research and may not be validated by nursing's scholars and practicing nurses.[110]

Electronic checklists, flow charts, ratings, or checklists for delivering health care provider prescriptions included in EHR for documenting nursing care are not adequate replacements for nurses' intellectual contributions to person centered care. Nursing care is rendered invisible when NIC and other nursing languages are not included in the EHR. Not only does the absence of nursing content inaccurately depict what transpired during the care episode, but it removes the ability of nurses to properly research their actions and strengthen their EBP when there is no meaningful nursing data in the health record to be gathered and analyzed. Since technology drives the data essential for determining practice, nurses need to proactively advocate for the inclusion of meaningful nursing languages in the EHR system.

According to the IOM report *The Future of Nursing: Leading Change, Advancing Health*, there is "no greater opportunity to transform practice than through technology"[49] (p. 136). As Gleick[39] points out, placing information in mathematical and electronic form allows computers to rapidly process, store, and retrieve information. Automated CIS contribute to reduced errors, increased access to diagnostic tests and treatment results, and improved communication and coordination of care.[48] Information systems also aid in clinical decision-making, documentation of care, and determination of the cost of care. Nursing elements of electronic records refer to any information related to the nursing diagnosis, treatment, and outcomes relevant to nursing. EHRs will not benefit nursing until nurses are better able to describe their work, which will guide the design of information systems.[19] Furthermore, nursing content in the EHR must be standardized and based on EBP. The ANA Standards of Practice[4] include the use of information systems, along with EBP, as a core practice in describing the "how" of nursing practice (p. 32). The *Essentials: Core Competencies for Professional Nursing Education*[3] has core competencies concerning the use of electronic information and communication tools in the planning, delivery, and documentation of care, and lists the ability to "describe the importance of standardized nursing data to reflect the unique contribution of nursing practice" as an entry level competency for professional nurses (p. 47).

NIC is standardized and available in electronic form and ready to be integrated into health information systems. Many agencies have integrated NIC into their hospital based EHR[62,89] while other programs, such as Hands-on Automated Nursing Data System (HANDS), operate on standalone devices.[60] The use of NIC provides terms for clinical decision-making support and enables the documentation, storage, and retrieval of clinical information about nursing treatments. Electronic implementation of standardized nursing languages facilitates the communication of nursing care to other nurses and health care providers; makes feasible a means for billing and the reimbursement for the provision of nursing care; and allows for the evaluation of the achievement of nursing outcomes and quality of nursing care.

The time and cost for implementation of NIC into a nursing information system in a clinical practice agency depends on the agency's selection and use of an EHR, a nursing information system, the computer competency of nurses, and the nurses' previous use and understanding of standardized nursing language. The change to entering standardized nursing language into a computer represents, for many, a major change in the way in which nurses have traditionally documented care, and effective change strategies need to be followed, for example, the use of the Systems Development Life Cycle (SDLC).[80] Complete implementation of NIC throughout an agency may take months to several years; the agency should devote resources for computer programming, education, and training. As major vendors design and update clinical nursing information systems that include NIC, implementation will be easier.

We have included several guides to assist in implementation of NIC into practice settings. Box 2 provides steps for implementation of NIC in a clinical practice agency. Although not all the steps must be followed in every institution, the list is helpful in planning for implementation. We have found that successful implementation of the steps requires knowledge about change and nursing information systems. In addition, it is a good idea to have an evaluation process established. There are numerous publications that describe the processes of implementing NIC into a wide variety of practice settings; these can be located by a computer search of nursing literature. Those leaders who are directing the implementation effort as well as administrators, computer information system designers, and practicing nurses will benefit from reading the literature describing the implementation process. Box 3 includes "rules of thumb" for using NIC in an information system. Following these will help ensure that data are captured in a consistent manner. In some computer systems, due to space restrictions, there is a need to shorten some of the NIC activities. Although this is becoming less of a necessity as computer space for nursing expands, Box 4 provides guidelines for shortening NIC activities to fit in a computer system.

Box 2

Steps for Implementation of NIC in a Clinical Practice Agency

A. Establish organizational commitment to NIC
- Identify the key person responsible for implementation (e.g., person in charge of nursing informatics).
- Create an implementation task force with representatives from key areas.
- Provide NIC materials to all members of the task force.
- Purchase copies of the NIC book and circulate readings about NIC to units.
- Have members of the task force begin to use the NIC language in everyday discussion.
- Access the Center of Nursing Classification website at the University of Iowa.

B. Prepare an implementation plan
- Write the specific goals to be accomplished.
- Do a force field analysis to determine driving and restraining forces.
- Determine whether an in-house evaluation will be done and the nature of the evaluation effort.
- Identify which of NIC interventions are most appropriate for the agency/unit.
- Determine the extent to which NIC is to be implemented (e.g., in standards, care planning, documentation, discharge summary, performance evaluation).
- Prioritize the implementation efforts.
- Choose 1–3 pilot units. Get members from these units involved in the planning.
- Develop a written timeline for implementation.
- Review current system and determine the logical sequence of actions to integrate NIC.
- Create work groups of expert clinical users to review NIC interventions and activities, determine how these will be used in agency, and develop needed forms.
- Distribute the work of the expert clinicians to other users for evaluation and feedback before implementation.

- Encourage the development of an *NIC champion* on each of the units.
- Keep other key decision makers in agency informed.
- Determine the nature of the total nursing data set. Work to ensure that all units are collecting data on all variables in a uniform manner so that future research can be done.
- Make plans to ensure that all nursing data are retrievable.
- Identify learning needs of staff and plan ways to address these.

C. Carry out the implementation plan
- Develop the screens/forms for implementation. Review each NIC intervention and decide whether all parts (e.g., label, definition, activities, references) are to be used. Determine whether there are critical activities to document and whether further details are desired.
- Provide training time for staff.
- Implement NIC in the pilot unit(s) and obtain regular feedback.
- Update content or create new computer functions as needed.
- Use focus groups to clarify issues and address concerns/questions.
- Use data on positive aspects of implementation in house-wide presentations.
- Implement NIC house-wide.
- Collect postimplementation evaluation data and make changes as needed.
- Identify key markers to use for ongoing evaluation and continue to monitor and maintain the system.
- Provide feedback to the Iowa intervention project.

Box 3

Implementation Rules of Thumb for Using NIC in a Nursing Information System

1. The information system should clearly indicate that NIC is being used.
2. NIC intervention labels and definitions should appear in whole and should be clearly labeled as interventions and definitions.
3. Activities are not interventions and should not be labeled as such on the screens.
4. Documentation that the intervention was planned or delivered should be captured at the intervention label level. In addition, an agency may choose to have nurses identify specific activities within the intervention for patient care planning and documentation.
5. The number of activities required in an information system should be kept as few as possible for each intervention so as not to overburden the provider.

6. If activities are included in the information system, they should be written to the extent possible (given the constraints of the data structure) as they appear in NIC. Activities that must be rewritten to fit short field constraints should reflect the intended meaning.
7. All additional or modified activities should be consistent with the definition of the intervention.
8. Modification of NIC activities should be done sparingly and only as needed in the practice situation.
9. NIC interventions should be a permanent part of the patient's record with capability to retrieve this information.

Box 4

Guidelines for Shortening NIC Activities to Fit in a Computer System

<u>Introduction:</u> While electronic database systems are changing, some computer systems still restrict space, thereby not allowing for the number of characters necessary for including the entire length of the NIC activities. If this is the case, we would advise requesting more space. However, for whatever reason this is not possible, the following guidelines should be used to decrease the length of the activities. If these guidelines are followed, all activities could be less than 125 characters.

Guidelines

1. Eliminate all "as appropriates" and "as needed" found after a comma at the end of some activities.
2. Remove all e.g. found inside of parentheses.
3. Delete words or dependent clauses that describe other parts of an activity.

4. Use the abbreviation "pt" for patient and "nse" for nurse.
5. Do NOT create new language and do not replace words.

(Note: We have decided not to suggest additional word abbreviations more than what is already in NIC as most agencies have an agreed-upon list of abbreviations that they are required to use; these lists are not uniform across agencies and creating yet another list may lead to further confusion.)

Examples

Monitor core body temperature.
Perform and document the patient's health history and physical assessment.
Deliver anesthetic consistent with patient's needs, clinical judgment, and Standards.
Obtain ordered specimen for laboratory analysis of acid-base.
Screen for symptoms of a history of domestic abuse.

Many healthcare organizations have implemented EHRs; however, manual nursing care plans are still used in many settings. It is very feasible to use standardized language in a manual/paper or noncomputer system. In fact, implementation is easier if the nursing staff can learn to use standardized language before introduction of an electronic system.

Use of a Standardized Language Model

The model depicted in Figure 1 illustrates the use of standardized language to document actual care delivered by the nurse, which in turn generates data for decision making about cost and quality issues in the healthcare agency. The data are also useful for making health policy decisions. The three-level model indicates that use of standardized language for documentation of care not only assists the practicing nurse to communicate to others but also leads to several other important uses.

At the individual level, each nurse uses standardized language in the areas of diagnoses, interventions, and outcomes to communicate care plans and to document care delivered. Individual nurses working with an individual or group of persons ask themselves several questions according to the steps of the nursing process: (1) What are the nursing diagnoses? (2) What are the outcomes that I am trying to achieve? (3) What interventions do I use to obtain these outcomes? The identified diagnoses, outcomes, and interventions are then documented using the standardized language in these areas. A nurse working with an information system that includes NIC will document the care provided by choosing the intervention. Not all of the activities will be done for every person. To indicate which activities were done, the nurse could either highlight those done or simply

document the exceptions, depending on the existing documentation system. A nurse working with a manual information system will write in the chosen NIC intervention labels as care planning and documentation are done. The activities can also be specified depending on the agency's documentation system. Although the activities may be important in communicating the care, the intervention label is the place to begin when planning care.

The individual level part of the model can be thought of as documentation of the key decision points of the nursing process using standardized language. It makes apparent the importance of nurses' skills in clinical decision-making. We have found that, even though NIC requires nurses to learn a new language and a different way to conceptualize what they do (naming the intervention concept rather than listing a series of discrete behaviors), they quickly adapt and in fact become the driving force to implement the language. With or without computerization, the adoption of NIC makes it easier for nurses to communicate what they do, with each other and with other providers. Plans of care are much shorter, and interventions can be linked to diagnoses and outcomes. Because an individual nurse's decisions about diagnoses, interventions, and outcomes are collected in a uniform way, the information can be aggregated to the level of the unit or organization.

At the unit or organizational level, the information about the individual is aggregated for all the persons in the unit (or other group) and, in turn, in the entire facility. This aggregated nursing practice data can then be linked to information contained in the nursing management database. The management database includes data about the nurses and others who provide care and the means of care delivery.

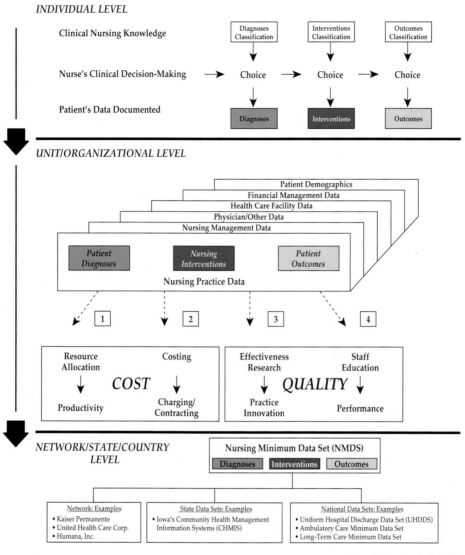

Fig. 1 Nursing Practice Data: Three Levels.

In turn, the nursing practice and management data can be linked with data about the treatments by health care providers, facility information, person information, and financial data. Most of these data, except for some of the data about treatments by providers other than physicians, are already collected in a uniform way and are available for use.

The model illustrates how the clinical practice data linked with other data in the agency's information system can be used to determine both cost and quality of nursing care. The cost side of the model addresses resource allocation and costing out of nursing services; the quality side of the model addresses effectiveness research and nursing personnel education. The use of standardized language to plan and document care does not automatically result in knowledge about cost and quality but provides the potential for data for decision making in these areas. The steps to determining cost through resource allocation and costing out of nursing services, and the steps to assure quality through effectiveness research and nursing personnel education are outlined in the following list. An excellent source for ensuring employee competence was published by Nolan[85] and outlines a step-by-step process incorporating NICs into personnel competencies and performance evaluations. Explanation of some managerial and financial terms is provided in parentheses for those not familiar with these areas.

Cost

Resource allocation—distributing nursing personnel and supplies

- Determine the interventions and related outcomes/type of population.
- Determine and apply the rules for personnel mix (ratio of professional to nonprofessional nursing care providers) per type of population.
- Allocate other resources (supplies and equipment) accordingly.
- Determine productivity (ratio of output to input or the ratio of work produced to people and supplies needed to produce the work) of the nursing personnel.

Costing—determining the cost of nursing services rendered

- Identify the interventions delivered.
- Affix a price per intervention, taking into account the level of provider and time spent.
- Determine an overhead charge (amount billed for business expenses that are not chargeable to a particular service but are essential to the production of services, such as heat, light, building, and repairs); allocate evenly to all and be able to provide justification.
- Determine the cost of care delivery (direct care interventions plus overhead).
- Determine the charge for each person or use the information to contract for nursing services (establishing a business arrangement for the delivery of nursing services at a fixed price).

Quality

Effectiveness research—determining effects or outcomes of nursing interventions

- Identify the research questions (e.g., what combination of interventions gives the best outcomes for a particular type of condition?).
- Select the outcomes to be measured.
- Identify and collect the intervening variables (e.g., care recipient's characteristics, physician treatments, staff mix, workload).
- Analyze the data.
- Make recommendations for practice innovations.

Employee education—ensuring competency to deliver the needed interventions

- Determine the level of competence of the nurses related to particular interventions.
- Provide education as needed and repeat measure of competence.
- Determine the nurse's level of accountability for the interventions and whether the intervention or part of the intervention is delegated.
- Provide education as needed related to decision making, delegation, and team building.
- Evaluate performance in terms of achievement of outcomes.
- Use information in nurse's performance evaluation, taking into consideration the nurse's ability to competently perform the intervention and overall level of professional accountability.

The two sides of the model are interactive. Cost and quality should always be considered hand in hand. In addition, the four paths do not mean to imply that these are mutually exclusive. Research can be conducted on the cost side, and costs can be determined for research and education. The four distinct paths, however, are helpful to indicate the main areas of use of these data at an organizational level.

The *network/state/country level* of the model involves the "sending forward" of nursing data to be included in large databases that are used to set benchmarks for determination of quality and for health policy making. In a classic and highly influential article, Werley and Lang[118] described the Nursing Minimum Data Set (NMDS) and identified 16 variables that should be included in large policy-making databases. These include the three clinical variables of diagnoses, interventions, and outcomes; nursing intensity (defined as staff mix and hours of care), which will be collected in the nursing management database; and 12 other variables, such as the age, sex, and race, and the expected payer of the bill, which are available from other parts of the clinical record. The model indicates that the nursing data on diagnoses, interventions, and outcomes are aggregated by facility and then included in the larger regional and national databases. A growing number of networks of care providers also are constructing databases. According to Jacox,[53] nursing has remained essentially invisible in these clinical and administrative databases. She listed the following ramifications of the invisibility of nursing and nursing care in the databases nearly three decades ago, and yet they remain even more relevant today:

- We cannot describe the nursing care received by persons in most healthcare settings.
- Much of nursing practice is described as the practice of others, especially physicians.

- We cannot describe the effects of nursing practice on outcomes.
- We often cannot describe nursing care within a single setting, let alone across settings.
- We cannot identify what nurses do so that they may be reimbursed for it.
- We cannot tell the difference in care and costs when care is delivered by physicians as contrasted with nurses.
- This invisibility perpetuates the view of nursing as a part of medicine that does not need to be separately identified.

Estimating nursing care requirements and projecting these requirements to determine staffing levels are challenges for nurse managers. Although many agencies continue to develop tools to determine staffing and acuity levels, typically these are not usable across different settings. To fill this void, the acuity scale shown in Box 5 was developed with help from individuals in different settings as an easy-to-use acuity scale that can be used across settings. Although testing of the scale has been limited, its usefulness in all settings has been demonstrated. Nurse-to-person ratios could also be determined by identifying the major interventions for persons at the unit level and identifying and calculating the estimated time and level of education required to safely implement the interventions as identified in Part Five of this book.

There is strong evidence of a relationship between nurse staffing, person safety, and quality of care. Low RN staffing levels are associated with increased mortality rates.[43] Rae et al.[94] found significant associations between lower levels of critical care nurse staffing and increased odds of both mortality and nosocomial infection, increased hospital costs, lower nurse-perceived quality of care and lower family satisfaction. Griffiths et al.[41] reported low RN staffing is associated with reports of missed nursing care in hospitals. The Aiken et al. study[1] across 300 hospitals in nine countries determined that an increase in a nurses' workload by one person increased by 7% the likelihood of an inpatient dying within 30 days of admission, and every 10% increase in nurses with bachelor's degrees was associated with a decrease in the likelihood of mortality. Kane et al.[56] found adding RNs to unit staffing eliminated one-fifth of all hospital deaths and reduced relative risk of adverse events such as bleeding and infection.

Box 5

NIC Patient Acuity Scale

Instructions: Rate each patient on this scale once a day (or as appropriate in your practice).

Acuity level of patient (circle one)

1. The self-care patient is primarily in contact with the health-care system for assistance with health promotion activities. The patient may require some assistance to cope with the effects of disease or injury, but the amount of treatment provided is not more than that which could be provided on a brief outpatient visit. *The patient in this category is often seeking routine health screening tests, such as mammograms, pap smears, parenting instructions, weight loss and blood pressure checks, sports physicals, and well-baby check-ups. The teaching aspects of care are usually brief and often limited to take-home written instructions.*

2. The patient is relatively independent as a self-care agent but may have some limitations in total self-care. The patient requires periodic nursing assessment and interventions for needs that may be simple or complex. Teaching activities form a good part of the care delivered, and health care requirements include the need for education about prevention. *Examples of patients that may fit in this category include women at high risk for a complicated pregnancy, individuals with hard-to-control diabetes or newly diagnosed diabetics, individuals who have a stable psychiatric illness, a family with a child with attention deficit disorder, and cardiac patients in the rehabilitation stage.*

3. The patient is unable to find enough resources or energies to meet his or her own needs and is dependent on others for self-care requirements. This person requires continuing nursing intervention, but the care is predictable and not in the nature of an emergency. *Examples of patients who fit this category are someone with an unstable or energy-draining chronic illness, a woman in active labor, a long-term care patient, a hospice patient, a depressed psychiatric patient, and a stabilized postoperative patient.*

4. The patient is acutely ill and dependent on others for self-care requirements with needs that may change quickly. The patient requires continuing nursing assessment and intervention, and care requirements are not predictable. *Examples of patients in this category are a postoperative patient recovering from major surgery during the first 24–36 hours, someone suffering from an acute psychiatric episode, and a woman in the high-risk pregnancy category in active labor.*

5. The patient is critically ill and requires life-saving measures to maintain life. The patient has no ability to act as his or her own self-care agent and requires constant assessment and nursing intervention to maintain an existence. *Examples of patients in this category are patients in intensive care receiving full life support, psychiatric patients in intensive care, low birthweight preemies, head-injury accident victims, and, in general, those individuals with multisystem failures.*

Increasing the number of RNs can yield cost savings of nearly 3 billion dollars from more than 4 million avoided extra hospital stays for adverse events in the United States alone.[84] Several states have enacted safe staffing legislation using the approach set forth in the American Nurses' Association.[4] Although California and Massachusetts are the only states to pass laws governing safe staffing policies, 12 other states have introduced statewide regulations that address nurse staffing in hospitals. These states are Connecticut, Illinois, Minnesota, Nevada, New Jersey, New York, Ohio, Oregon, Rhode Island, Texas, Vermont, and Washington. Of those states, Connecticut, Illinois, New York, Nevada, Ohio, Oregon, Texas, and Washington require hospitals to form staffing committees to develop plans and policies to direct the implementation of optimal staffing practices. Beyond these states, New Mexico and North Carolina have also started the assessment process by requesting studies that will gather and report information that can be used to develop future staffing mandates and policies. Although this research is noteworthy, integration of a standardized method to document the treatments that nurses provide (such as NIC) in CIS will provide the databases with information that can be used to determine the specific contributions of RNs to safety and quality of care. The use of standardized languages to correlate staffing and outcome data has been mentioned in several recent studies as a method of strengthening design and allowing for better interpretation of data.[87,116]

EBP is the integration of best research evidence with clinical expertise and person values to facilitate clinical decision making.[100] While EBP has been embraced and achieved widespread acceptance by being integrated into bachelor's, master's and doctoral curricula,[3] the call to fully implement EBP into practice has been more challenging.[17] The use of EBP guidelines is enhanced when NIC interventions are included as recommendations for effective nursing treatments. Guidelines are created in the form of protocols or evidence-based parameters that convert scientific knowledge into clinical actions in a form that is available to clinicians. Guidelines describe a process of care management that has the potential to improve the quality of clinical and consumer decision making. Advocates of EBP believe interventions found to be effective and safe that are based on the best available evidence need to be delivered in a consistent manner to produce the same desired outcomes for the same problem. After the Agency for Health Care Policy and Research (AHCPR),[111] now known as Agency for Healthcare Research and Quality (AHRQ), published its national initiative, starting in the 1990s the nursing profession has focused on development and use of guidelines. Because the focus of a guideline is management of a clinical condition, incorporating NIC into protocols is very useful in describing the nurs-ing interventions contained in the guideline and needed to standardize languages for use in effectiveness research.

USE OF NIC IN EDUCATION

The AACN called for the use of standardized terminologies as foundational to the development of effective CIS.[3] Integration of standardized terminologies into the CIS not only supports day-to-day nursing practice but also the capacity to enhance interprofessional communication and automatically generate standardized data to continuously evaluate and improve practice.[4]

Nursing diagnoses have been included in most of the major care planning textbooks since the 1980s, and NIC has been incorporated in a wide variety of nursing specialty textbooks as well as books that help students with the planning of care. Inclusion of standardized nursing language in a curriculum focuses the teaching on clinical decision making (the selection of the appropriate nursing diagnoses, outcomes, and interventions for a particular nursing situation). These resources are rapidly expanding as more educational programs teach standardized nursing language as the knowledge base of nursing. Every major nursing publishing company is incorporating standardized nursing language in both printed and electronic resources.

NANDA-I diagnoses, NIC, and NOC are the most frequently used classifications internationally with the most comprehensive, researched, and evidence-based nursing languages.[5,45] In a study comparing the usefulness of NIC to other terminologies such as the International Classification for Nursing Practice (ICNP), Omaha System, Clinical Care Classification/Home Health Care Classification, Perioperative Nursing Data Set, and other nursing standardized languages, Tastan et. al.[110] found the majority of the research was focused on NANDA-I diagnoses, NIC, and NOC (NNN) languages, and indicated that NNN was one of two standardized nursing languages that had successful integration and use in EHRs for person care. Thus, NIC can assist faculty in organizing the curricular content in all clinical courses. Specialty course content can be structured around the core interventions for specific clinical conditions and their associated nursing diagnoses.

Nonetheless, change can be a challenge in academic settings. But implementing NIC in an educational setting can be easier than in a practice setting because fewer individuals are involved and there are usually no issues related to use in an information system. We have included some guidelines to help in making the change. Box 6 is a guide that lists steps for implementing NIC in an educational setting. These are like Steps for Implementation of NIC in a Clinical Practice Agency (see Box 2), but the specific actions relate to the academic setting and course development. The central decision that must be made is for faculty members to adopt a nursing

Steps for Implementation of NIC in an Educational Setting

A. Establish organizational commitment to NIC

- Identify the key person responsible for implementation (e.g., head of curriculum committee).
- Create an implementation task force with representatives from key areas.
- Access the Center for Nursing Classification website.
- Provide NIC materials to all members of the task force.
- Purchase and distribute copies of the latest edition of NIC.
- Circulate readings about NIC to faculty.
- Examine the philosophical issues regarding the centrality of nursing interventions in nursing.
- Have members of the task force and other key individuals begin to use the NIC language in everyday discussion.

B. Prepare an implementation plan

- Write specific goals to be accomplished.
- Do a force field analysis to determine driving and restraining forces.
- Determine whether an in-house evaluation will be done and the nature of the evaluation.
- Determine the extent to which NIC is to be implemented (e.g., in graduate as well as undergraduate programs, in philosophy statements, in process recordings, care plans, case studies, in orientation for new faculty).
- Prioritize the implementation efforts.
- Develop a written timeline for implementation.
- Create work groups of faculty and perhaps students to review NIC interventions and activities, determine where these will be taught in the curriculum and how

they relate to current materials, and develop or redesign any needed forms.
- Identify which NIC interventions should be taught at the graduate level and at the undergraduate level.
- Identify which interventions should be taught in which courses.
- Distribute the drafts of decisions to other faculty for evaluation and feedback.
- Encourage the development of an *NIC champion* in each department or course group.
- Keep other key decision makers informed of your plans.
- Identify learning needs of faculty and plan ways to address these.

C. Carry out the implementation plan

- Revise the syllabi, order the NIC textbook for students, and ask the library to order books.
- Provide time for discussion and feedback in course groups.
- Implement NIC one course at a time and obtain feedback from both faculty and students.
- Update course content as needed.
- Determine impact on and implications for supporting courses and prerequisites and restructure these as needed.
- Report progress on implementation regularly at faculty meetings.
- Collect postimplementation evaluation data and make changes in curriculum as needed.
- Identify key markers to use for ongoing evaluation and continue to monitor and maintain the system.
- Provide feedback to the Iowa intervention project team.

---

philosophical orientation and focus, rather than the more traditional medical orientation with nursing implications added.

Teaching clinical reasoning and decision making is enhanced when nurses are taught to use standardized nursing languages including NIC. In addition, texts that use case studies that incorporate NIC, such as Lunney's *Critical Thinking to Achieve Positive Health Outcomes: Nursing Case Studies and Analyses,*[75] as well as research on the use of case studies with NANDA-I diagnoses, NIC, and NOC to teach clinical reasoning,[105] are useful sources. Faculty and students can develop their own case studies incorporating standardized nursing languages, and faculty can teach students to integrate NIC interventions into the plans of care developed for their assigned persons. NNN can be integrated into well-designed simulation scenarios teaching clinical reasoning, either when using manikin-based simulations, video depictions, or actors simulating nursing situations.[96] There are multiple

published resources for teaching clinical reasoning using NIC and integrating standardized nursing languages into the curriculum.[32,65,74,77] Perry and Potter's widely used *Fundamentals in Nursing* textbook[90] integrates NIC and NOC into care planning throughout the text. In addition, colleges and schools of nursing are increasingly developing and using software programs that include NIC along with NANDA-I diagnoses and NOC to teach students clinical reasoning for the planning and documenting nursing care, such as Elsevier's NNN Consult or Clinical Key (https://www.elsevier.com/solutions/clinicalkey/nurses).

Not all interventions can or should be addressed at the undergraduate level; faculty must decide which interventions should be learned by all undergraduate students and which require advanced education and should be learned in a master's program. Some interventions are unique to specialty areas and perhaps are best taught only in specialty elective courses. Connie Delaney, while a professor at The University of Iowa, elaborated the steps to identify which interventions are taught in what courses. Delaney recommended the following steps, which we have expanded:

1. Identify the NIC interventions that are never taught in the curriculum (e.g., associate, baccalaureate, master's) and eliminate these from further action.
2. Using the remaining interventions, have each course group identify the interventions that are taught in their course or area of teaching responsibility. That is, match what is currently taught with the NIC intervention terms.
3. Compile this information into a master grid (interventions on one axis and each course on the other axis) and distribute it to all faculty members.
4. Have a faculty discussion, noting the interventions that are unique to certain courses and those that are taught in more than one course. Clearly articulate the unique perspective offered by each course for each intervention that is taught in more than one place (e.g., is the intervention being delivered to a different population?). Should both courses continue to teach the intervention, or should content be deleted from one course? Review interventions that are not located in any courses, but that faculty believe should be taught at this level. Should content be added?
5. Affirm consensus of the faculty on what interventions are taught in which courses.
6. The same process can, of course, be completed with nursing diagnoses (using NANDA-I diagnoses) and with outcomes (using NOC). Many educational programs already use NANDA-I diagnoses and can implement NIC by reviewing the NANDA-I–to–NIC linkages and determining the interventions that might be taught in relationship with NANDA-I diagnoses.

Using NIC in Clinical Reasoning Models

Decision-making models provide the structure and process that facilitate clinical reasoning. Clinical reasoning is the effective use of knowledge using reflective, creative, concurrent, and critical-thinking processes to achieve desired outcomes. Since the 1950s, the nursing process has provided the structure for facilitating clinical reasoning in the education of student nurses. The nursing process 5-step model (assessment, diagnosis, planning, intervention, and evaluation [ADPIE]) is a standard of nursing practice. Standardized language facilitates the teaching of the nursing process when fully integrated into each of the five steps. Assessment leads to the identification of NANDA-I diagnoses[46] in the Diagnostic phase; Planning care for each diagnosis involves choosing relevant NIC interventions and selected activities and selecting nursing-sensitive NOC outcomes and indicators; the Intervention

phase is the process of implementing NIC interventions and activities; and Evaluation is the process of determining the changes in the NOC outcomes. The ANA Scope and Standards of Practice's "Professional Nursing Model"[4] includes cyclic, iterative, and interactive nursing processes consisting of six components: assessment, diagnosis, outcomes-identification, planning, implementation, and evaluation that are undergirded by the nurse's caring, values, wisdom, energy, and ethics. In this nursing process model, NIC interventions would be identified in the planning phase and be applied in the next phase, implementation. The model supports EBP and includes bidirectional feedback loops between each of the six components.

Although the nursing process has demonstrated its usefulness as a clinical decision-making method, the traditional nursing process presents several limitations for contemporary nursing practice. Today, nursing practice calls for an emphasis on knowing the person's "story," thereby placing their situation in a meaningful context. Pesut and Herman[92] point out that the traditional nursing process does not explicitly focus on outcomes; it deemphasizes reflective and concurrent creative thinking; it is more procedure-oriented rather than focusing on the structures and processes of thinking; it uses stepwise and linear thinking that limits the relational thinking needed to understand the complex interconnections among their presenting problems; and it limits the development of practice-relevant theory. In response to the need for a more contemporary model for clinical reasoning, Pesut and Herman[92] developed the Outcome Present State Test (OPT) model of reflective clinical reasoning. Kuiper et al.[65] updated the OPT model and applied the model using NIC in neonatal, adolescent, young adult, women's health, men's health, older adult, and hospice and palliative care nursing situations.

The OPT model (Figure 2) is a major advancement in the teaching and practice of clinical decision-making by using a clinical reasoning structure. There is evidence that the OPT model and its associated teaching-learning strategies positively enhance the development of clinical reasoning in nursing students.[11,42,64,66,68] Contrary to the traditional nursing process, the OPT model of reflective clinical reasoning provides a structure for clinical thinking with a focus on outcomes, not as a sequential process. Clinical reasoning that focuses on outcomes improves quality by evaluating effectiveness rather than focusing primarily on problems. In the OPT model of clinical reasoning, the nurse *simultaneously* focuses on problems and outcomes in juxtaposition. The OPT model requires that nurses simultaneously consider relationships among diagnoses, interventions, and outcomes with attention to the evidence. Rather than considering one problem at a time, the OPT requires the nurse to consider several identified problems simultaneously and to discern which problem or issue is central and most

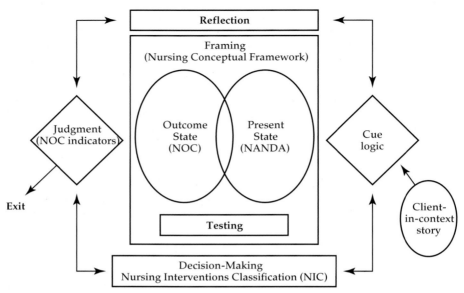

Fig. 2 Integrating Outcome Present State Test (OPT) Model with NANDA-I, NIC, and NOC. (*Modified from* Kuiper, R., Donnell, S., Pesut, D., & Turrise, S. [2017]. *The essentials of clinical reasoning for nurses: Using the Outcome-Present State-Test Model for reflective practice. Reprinted with permission of* Sigma Theta Tau International.)

important in relationship with all the other problems. Our modified version of the OPT model emphasizes listening to the person's story; using NANDA-I diagnoses to describe the present state; framing the story in a discipline-specific *nursing* conceptual framework; using NOC to describe the outcome state; mapping the web of relationships among the NANDA-I diagnoses for identifying the keystone issue; and using NIC in decision-making to move the person from the present state to the outcome state. As an emerging clinical decision-making model, the OPT model provides a new and more effective process for teaching, learning, and practicing nursing.[13,42,57]

Kuiper et al.'s *Clinical Reasoning and Care Coordination in Advanced Practice Nursing*[67] consists of an update of the OPT model with applications of the model to specific case studies in acute care, long-term care, rehabilitation, mental health, pediatrics, neonate, and in primary community health. Pesut asserts that "clinical thinking and reasoning presupposes the use of a standardized nursing language.... nursing knowledge classification systems provide the vocabulary for clinical thinking"[91] (p. 3). Within the OPT model, NIC can be used in conjunction with NANDA-I diagnoses and NOC to assist students in developing the skills necessary for clinical decision making. Kautz et al. conducted extensive research into the teaching of clinical reasoning using standardized nursing languages with the OPT model, noting that "students who consistently used NNN language with OPT models were the students

who performed well in the clinical area and did better in completing their clinical reasoning webs and OPT model worksheets"[58] (p. 137).

USE OF NIC IN RESEARCH

Nursing is a scientific discipline; to preserve the recognition of nursing as a science, nurses must generate, expand, and refine the knowledge base that demonstrates the discipline's unique contribution toward providing safe, high-quality care that enhances health and produces beneficial health outcomes. Nursing interventions need to be carefully designed, systematically evaluated, and successfully translated into practice to ensure that the interventions are effective in producing intended outcomes.

Healthcare finance is being driven by outcome-oriented healthcare delivery systems, quality of care, and cost-effective health care dependent on the use of the interventions that are most effective in achieving desired outcomes. Providing and maintaining cost-effective optimal quality care requires designing and evaluating interventions to establish a sound knowledge base to guide clinical decision making regarding the selection and implementation of interventions that are most effective in improving the health-illness conditions people experience.

We believe that NIC provides the *concepts* and *language* for identifying and defining interventions for all forms of nursing intervention research. Using a standardized language in nursing intervention research assures that research findings by multiple research teams can be systematically compared. Furthermore, using NIC intervention concept labels as the basis of nursing intervention research enables researchers to work together, grounds the focus of the research in a primary source of knowledge on nursing interventions, and contributes to the development of discipline-specific knowledge. Chae et al.[23] conducted an integrative review on the effectiveness of NIC interventions, finding 18 studies, which measured the effect of NIC interventions on specific outcomes. Examples of testing specific NIC interventions include: (1) Aríztegui Echenique et al.[6] tested the effect of NIC interventions in persons with type 2 diabetes; (2) de Araujo et al.[31] tested effectiveness of the NIC intervention Eye Care in preventing dry eye in intensive care units; and (3) Azzolin et al.[8] tested the effectiveness of NIC interventions for treating heart failure.

Research on the use of NIC is expanding. Fennelly et al.[37] conducted a scoping review on the use of NIC and other standardized nursing languages in practice and identified 33 studies focusing on NIC in relation to NANDA-I diagnoses and NOC, and an additional 5 studies on NIC alone. The review is useful for identifying the type of research being conducted with NIC. Research studies on nursing languages typically focus on evaluating the validity, reliability, responsiveness, useability, time efficiency, user perception, applicability, interoperability, documentation quality, impact on care, knowledge generation, and impact on student learning. Intervention research using large databases is increasingly becoming essential in determining which interventions are most useful in treating specific conditions. Research focusing on NIC interventions generally involves descriptive research, intervention testing, or effectiveness research. Each approach is discussed with examples of studies that serve as models for conducting research on NIC interventions.

Descriptive Research. Descriptive nursing intervention research has focused primarily on: (1) validating nursing interventions in specific populations, (2) identifying the most common or core interventions in specific populations, and (3) using NIC interventions in determining nursing workload. A wide range of studies validate the content of nursing intervention labels and activities in specific populations.[28,71,72] Fehring's model,[36] originally designed to validate nursing diagnoses, is a common and appropriate method for research designed to validate NIC interventions. However, other validation methods such as Carlson's consensus-validation method[18] have also been used to validate NIC interventions.[76] Validating research involves asking clinical experts to rate the usefulness of specific interventions and nursing activities in a specific population. For example, Silva and Ferreira[106] used Fehring's model[36] to validate NIC interventions for preventing cardiovascular

events in outpatients with diabetes by asking 14 clinical experts. In an example of research validating nursing activities, Lopes et al.[70] examined the 83 nursing activities for Fluid Management, Fluid Monitoring, and Hypervolemia Management in cardiac patients.

Another area of much needed research involves identifying core interventions that provide evidence of the effects and contributions that nursing care provides. Identifying the most frequently used interventions, along with nursing diagnoses and nursing outcomes, provides a knowledge base for identifying optimal nursing interventions for clinical decision making when planning; it also contributes to building EBP and costing out nursing care. Escalada-Hernández et al.[34] examined 690 records in psychiatric clinics and found 13,396 NIC interventions were recorded. They identified the most common NIC interventions in persons diagnosed with schizophrenia, organic mental disorders, intellectual disability, affective disorders, disorders of adult personality and behavior, mental and behavioral disorders due to psychoactive substance use, and neurotic, stress-related, and somatoform disorders. Shin et al.[103] identified NANDA-I diagnoses, NOC, NIC, and NNN linkages for 57 residents in 25 nursing homes in Korea. Initially, the researchers identified 82 core nursing intervention that were sent to nurses working in the facilities. There were NICs selected in greater that 90% of the residents, which included Medication Management, Vital Signs Monitoring, Environment Management: Comfort, Fall Prevention, Surveillance: Safety, Cognitive Stimulation, and Environment Management: Safety.

An additional thread of needed research involves identifying workforce planning by identifying nursing workload. Workload is usually defined as the nursing service volume in a particular setting and can be obtained by determining the time spent implementing nursing activities and multiplying it by the number of persons receiving care. Using NIC as a standardized nursing language in the provision of care creates the opportunity to collect data measuring the amount of time implementing nursing interventions and activities in specific settings and populations. In an integrative review of studies based on NIC to determine workload, Cruz and colleagues[29] identified 10 studies published between 2006 and 2013, and concluded more studies are needed. Studies that subsequently investigated workload using the NIC terms and activities in a wide variety of settings,[24,93,108,115] found such things as average time of admissions, excessive nursing workload and underpayment, workload distribution among nurses, and productivity.

Intervention Testing. If nursing interventions are the profession's *raison d'être*, then it follows that intervention testing research is our *appel à l'action* (call-to-action).

Nursing research is a systematic process of inquiry used to generate a significant new body of knowledge, seek understanding, validate existing knowledge, develop the evidence for guiding nursing practice, shape health policy, and promote the health and well-being of persons, families, and communities. We hold the stance that nursing research be guided by discipline specific knowledge in the form of nursing theoretical perspectives and standardized nursing languages. Although descriptive research has value in developing and refining interventions, nursing practice must be based on interventions with the best research evidence supporting their use and evaluating their effectiveness for achieving positive health outcomes.

Testing nursing interventions began with Rita Dumas' classic work in the 1960s. Although there has been a multitude of intervention studies since then, nursing intervention testing is the greatest research priority in establishing the effect of interventions on desired outcomes. Intervention testing research using experimental designs leads to establishing the strongest level of evidence for delivering high-quality, safe, and cost-effective care.

There are several excellent comprehensive resources for developing rigorous and relevant intervention testing research. Melnyk and Morrison-Beedy's *Intervention Research and Evidence-based Quality Improvement: Designing, Conducting, Analyzing, and Funding*[81] text has chapters on how to design intervention studies, implement the studies, and analyze the data from intervention testing studies. There are also chapters on writing successful grant proposals. Sidani and Braden's *Nursing and Health Interventions: Design, Evaluation, and Implementation*[104] is an intervention theory-based text with chapters on designing studies that evaluate the impact of interventions on health outcomes. Gray and Grove's *Burns and Grove: The Practice of Nursing Research: Appraisal, Synthesis, and Generation of Evidence*[40] includes a chapter that offers a step-by-step process of conducting intervention testing studies. It is notable that this chapter names NIC as a source for identifying interventions for research. An additional resource that can be used in designing intervention testing studies is the Consolidated Standards of Reporting Trials (CONSORT).[27] CONSORT was developed to enable transparent reporting of clinical trial findings that can be accurately assessed and compared to other studies.[27] The CONSORT guideline can also be used as a guide when designed randomized controlled trials. Transparent Reporting of Evaluation with Nonrandomized Designs (TREND)[20] is another useful checklist of criteria that can be used by nurse researchers in designing intervention test studies.

Enderlin and Richards[33] point out that when considering implementing an intervention, the intervention's efficacy is of paramount importance. Efficacy refers to the degree to which an intervention causes the intended effects under ideal conditions. Ideal conditions are those that minimize the potential influence of any factors other than the intervention that may contribute to the outcomes.[106] Recent advances in nursing intervention research suggest the need to test interventions that are either targeted or tailored. Targeted interventions are those designed to address a single characteristic of a group, such as gender, age, ethnicity, diagnosis, culture, or health literacy.[12] Tailored interventions are those designed to address individual characteristics of persons within a sample, such as personality factors, goals, needs, preferences, and resources, which can promote the adaptability and feasibility of the intervention and enhance the participant's motivation and engagement with the intervention.[104] NIC interventions in both a research and practice context can be tailored by selecting and focusing on the effect of specific activities on health outcomes. The NIC taxonomy offers researchers a source for identifying standardized nursing interventions that can be individualized for designing targeted and tailored intervention-testing research. Even if standardized interventions are found to be effective, a tailored or targeted intervention may promote better adherence, achieve better outcomes, and be more cost efficient. A wide range of studies need to be conducted based on the use of NIC interventions to assist with targeting and tailoring of nursing interventions.

Maintaining the integrity of the intervention across participants and settings is also important because inconsistent intervention delivery may result in variability in the outcomes achieved.[33] Using NIC, this means that a substantial number of the activities listed for a particular intervention should be done and that all activities that are done should be consistent with the definition of the intervention. It is important that the activities be tailored for individual care, but they must not vary so much that the intervention is no longer the same.

Determining the dose of an intervention is also important in determining the effect of an intervention in practice. In other words, it is essential that nurse researchers make well-grounded decisions about which nursing interventions to test, as well as how much of each intervention should be provided to achieve a desired outcome. Reed et al.[97] discuss dose in terms of the amount, frequency, and duration of the intervention. They suggest that counting the number of activities in a NIC intervention is a way of determining the amount. Duration can be determined by noting the total time spent on all activities. Further granularity can be achieved by weighting each activity as to its strength, so different activities can have their own assigned value; the values would then be summed to determine the dose of the intervention. The authors conclude that measuring and reporting the dose of an intervention in research is essential to the development of an evidence base to support practice.

For example, Shever[101] examined the NIC intervention Surveillance and found when surveillance nurse activities were delivered in a high dose (more than 12 times a day), there was a significant decrease in the odds of experiencing a failure to rescue episode, compared to administering Surveillance less than 12 times a day.

At present, there is no solution to the issue of dose of the intervention. A proxy measure, such as the amount of time a practitioner uses when doing the intervention, is helpful and may suffice as a measure of dose in some studies. Another solution is to know the number and extent of the specific activities that are done. Although the documentation of the intervention label is most important for comparison of data across sites, it is also important to have a way to ascertain the consistent implementation of the intervention. This can be done by an agency's adoption of a standard protocol for the delivery of the intervention, collection of the time spent for intervention delivery, or documentation of the activities related to the intervention.

Effectiveness Intervention Research. In effectiveness research, nurse researchers use actual clinical data contained in the agency databases as the variables (e.g., interventions, outcomes, specific person characteristics, specific provider characteristics, specific treatment setting characteristics) and their measures to evaluate the effectiveness of the intervention. Effectiveness research is often designed to study the effect of provider interventions on person outcomes for the purpose of facilitating better clinical decision making and to make better use of resources. To analyze data about the use and effectiveness of nursing interventions, it is necessary to collect, in a systematic way, other information that can be used in conjunction with the NIC data about interventions to address a variety of questions. Early in the process of implementation, an institution should identify key research questions to be addressed with clinical data contained in an electronic documentation system. After the research questions are identified, researchers can determine the variables needed to address the questions and whether the data are currently collected or should be collected in the new system. The data that will be obtained from the identified variables must be linked at the individual person level. One should address these concerns when setting up a nursing information system to prevent problems later.

The following three questions are examples of types of questions that can be studied using actual clinical data:

1. *What interventions typically occur together?* When information is systematically collected about the treatments nurses perform, clusters of interventions that typically occur together for certain types of persons can be identified. We need to identify interventions that are frequently used together for certain types of persons so we can study their interactive effects. This information will also be useful in constructing standardized protocols, determining costs of services, and planning for resource allocation.

2. *Which nurses use which interventions?* Systematic documentation of intervention use will allow nurses to study and compare the use rate of particular interventions by type of unit and facility. Implementation of NIC will allow nurses to learn which interventions are used by which nursing specialties. Determining the interventions used most frequently on a specific type of unit or in a certain type of agency will help determine which interventions should be on that unit or agency's nursing information system. It will also help in the selection of personnel to staff that unit and in the structuring of continuing education provided to the personnel on these units.

3. *What are the related diagnoses and outcomes for particular interventions?* Knowing which interventions work best for specific diagnoses and lead to certain outcomes can be used to assist nurses to make better clinical decisions. In addition, this information can help nurses to design treatment plans that will have the best chances of success.

The recommended data elements to address these questions are listed in Box 7 and include both a definition and the proposed measurement. Consistent definition and measurement are necessary to aggregate and compare data from different units in different settings. These variables and their measures have been discussed with representatives from several types of agencies and care settings to make them meaningful in all settings. As can be seen from the list, more than clinical nursing data are needed. The identity number is needed to link information; age, gender, and race/ethnicity are included to provide some demographic information on the population; and the health care provider's diagnoses and medical interventions, medications, and the work unit's type, staff mix, average acuity, and workload are included for controls. This is because for some analyses we may need to control one or more of these to determine whether the nursing intervention was the cause of the effect on the outcome.

Work with these variables demonstrates that the profession still must grapple with several issues related to the collection of standardized data. One issue is that the collection and coding of medications (Number 8) in easily retrievable form is still not yet available in many facilities. Although nursing research can be done without the knowledge of medications, many of the outcomes that are achieved by nurses are also influenced by certain medications, so the control for medication effect is desirable. If there is no unique number that identifies the primary nurse (Number 13), it is not possible to attribute clinical interventions or outcomes to particular nurses based on documentation data. Another issue arises when healthcare facilities do not collect the unit data (Numbers 20 through 24) in a standardized way. If one wished to compare these data across facilities, the data

Data Elements for Effectiveness Research in Nursing

Definitions and Measurement

Facility Data

1. **Facility Identification Number**
   Definition: a number that identifies the organization where the patient or client was provided nursing care
   Measurement: Use Medicare identification number.

Admission Data

2. **Patient Identification Number**
   Definition: the unique number assigned to each patient or client within a healthcare facility that distinguishes and separates one patient record from another in that facility
   Measurement: Use the facility's record number.

3. **Date of Birth**
   Definition: the day of the patient's birth
   Measurement: month, day, and year of birth

4. **Gender**
   Definition: the patient's sex
   Measurement: male, female, unknown

5. **Race**
   Definition: a class or kind of people unified by community of interests, habits, or characteristics
   Measurement: use Uniform Hospital Discharge Data Set (UHDDS) codes: 1. American Indian or Alaska Native; 2. Asian/Pacific Islander; 3. black, not Hispanic; 4. Hispanic; 5. white, not Hispanic; 6. other (please specify); 7. unknown

6. **Marital Status**
   Definition: legally recognized union of two people
   Measurement: 1. married; 2. widowed; 3. divorced; 4. separated; 5. never married; 6. unknown

7. **Admission Date**
   Definition: date of initiation of care
   Measurement: month, day, year

Medications

8. **Medications**
   Definition: a medicinal substance used to cure disease or relieve symptoms
   Measurement: 1. name of drug; 2. route of administration: a. PO; b. IM/SC; c. IV; d. aerosol; e. rectal; f. eye drops; g. other; 3. dose: amount of drug prescribed; 4. frequency: number of times per day given; 5. start date: date drug began this episode of care: month, day, year; 6. stop date: date drug was discontinued this episode of care: month, day, year

Physician Data

9. **Physician Identification Number**
   Definition: a number across settings that identifies the physician who is primarily responsible for the medical care of the patient or client during the care episode
   Measurement: unique number used by provider to bill for services (UHDDS uses attending and operating)

10. **Medical Diagnosis**
    Definition: the medical conditions that coexist at the time of admission, that develop subsequently, or that affect the treatment received and/or the length of stay; all diagnoses that affect the current episode of care
    Measurement: names of medical diagnoses as listed on the patient's bill using ICD-9-CM codes

11. **Diagnosis Related Group (DRG)**
    Definition: the U.S. prospective payment system used for reimbursement of Medicare patients; categorizes discharged patients into approximately 500 groups based upon medical diagnosis, age, treatment procedure, discharge status, and sex
    Measurement: the three-digit number and name of the DRG to which this patient was assigned

12. **Medical Intervention**
    Definition: a treatment prescribed by a physician; all significant procedures for the current episode of care
    Measurement: 1. names of physician procedures listed on the patient bill using CPT codes; 2. start date: date procedure began this episode of care: month, day, year; 3. stop date: date procedure was discontinued this episode of care: month, day, year

Nursing Data

13. **Nurse Identification Number**
    Definition: a number across settings that identifies the nurse who is primarily responsible for the nursing care of the patient or client during the care episode
    Measurement: does not exist at this time; make own codes

14. **Nursing Diagnosis**
    Definition: a clinical judgment made by a nurse about the patient's response to an actual or potential health problem or life process during this episode of care that affects the treatments received and/or the length of stay
    Measurement: names of nursing diagnoses using NANDA-I terms and codes

15. **Nursing Intervention**
    Definition: a treatment performed by a nurse
    Measurement: 1. names of treatments delivered to patient during episode of care using NIC terms and codes; 2. start date: date intervention began this episode of care: month, day, year; 3. stop date: date intervention was discontinued this episode of care: month, day, year

Outcomes

16. **Patient Outcomes**
    Definition: an aspect of patient or client health status that is influenced by nursing intervention during this episode of care
    Measurement: 1. names of outcomes using NOC terms, 2. date identified, 3. date outcome is stopped, 4. status of outcome at beginning and end of episode of care (use NOC scale)

17. **Discharge Date**
    Definition: date of termination of an episode of care
    Measurement: month, day, and year

Box 7

Data Elements for Effectiveness Research in Nursing—cont'd

18. **Disposition**

Definition: plan for continuing health care made upon discharge

Measurement: use NMDS with modification: 1. discharged to home or self-care (routine discharge); 2. discharged to home with referral to organized community nursing service; 3. discharged to home with arrangements to see nurse in ambulatory setting; 4. transfer to a short-term hospital; 5. transfer to a long-term institution; 6. died; 7. left against medical advice; 8. still a patient; 9. other

19. **Cost of Care**

Definition: provider's charges for the services rendered to the client incurred during the episode of care

Measurement: total charges billed for episode of care (from patient's bill)

Unit Data

20. **Unit Type**

Definition: name of type of unit or specialty area, which best characterizes where majority of patient care is delivered

Measurement: All units answer both parts A and B.

A. Where is the location of nursing care? (Check only one site.)

_____ Ambulatory care/Outpatient
_____ Community
_____ Home
_____ Hospital
_____ Long-term care setting/Nursing home
_____ Occupational health
_____ Rehabilitation agency
_____ School
_____ Other: Please describe_____

B. What is the specialty that best characterizes the type of care being delivered? (Choose only one.)

_____ General medical
_____ General surgical
_____ General medical surgical
_____ Geriatric
_____ Intensive or emergency care (e.g., CCU, MICU, PICU, SICU, ER, OR)
_____ Maternal-child
_____ Psychiatric (adult or child, including substance abuse)
_____ Specialty medicine (e.g., bone marrow, cardiology, dermatology, hematology, hemodialysis, neurology, oncology, pulmonary, radiology)
_____ Specialty surgery (e.g., EENT, neurosurgery, orthopedics, urology)
_____ Other (Please describe):_____

21. **Staff Mix**

Definition: ratio of professional to nonprofessional nursing care providers in the unit/clinic/group where care is being provided

Measurement: number of RNs to nonprofessional staff *worked* on unit/clinic/group each day of patient's stay (Collect daily for patient's length/episode of care; if cannot get daily, take weekly average.) Allocate 12-hour shifts or other irregular shifts to times actually worked (i.e., a person who works 12 hours 7:30 a.m. to 7:30 p.m. is allocated 8 hours (1 FTE) on days and 4 hours (.5 FTE) on evenings. Count only actual direct-care hours (i.e., remove the head nurse and charge nurse unless they are providing direct care, remove the unit secretary, and do not include nonproductive hours such as orientation and continuing education).

# of FTE RNs days _____
# of FTE RNs evenings _____
# of FTE RNs nights _____
# of FTE LPN/LVNs days _____
# of FTE LPN/LVNs evenings _____
# of FTE LPN/LVNs nights _____
# of FTE aides days _____
# of FTE aides evenings _____
# of FTE aides nights _____
others days (please identify) _____
others evenings (please identify) _____
others nights (please identify) _____

22. **Hours of Nursing Care**

Definition: hours of nursing care administered per patient day in unit/clinic/group where care is delivered

Measurement: hours of care (actual staffing) by RNs, LPNs, and aides

Days: RN hours _____ LPN hours _____ aide hours _____ others hours _____
Evenings: RN hours _____ LPN hours _____ aide hours _____ others hours _____
Nights: RN hours _____ LPN hours _____ aide hours _____ others hours _____
NOTE: These are the same people as in number 21.

23. **Patient Acuity**

Definition: average illness level of patients cared for on the unit

Measurement: Patient is rated on agreed-upon patient acuity scale.

24. **Workload**

Definition: the amount of nursing service provided on a unit

Measurement: the average patient acuity (number 23) times the number of occupied beds per day (or number of patients seen in ambulatory) divided by the number of RNs working or number of total nursing personnel working (number 21)

Midnight census or number of patients encountered per day

would need to be translated facility by facility to common measures such as those proposed in Box 7. Integrating NIC in the EHR is what makes effectiveness research possible.

The method to conduct effectiveness research with actual clinical data is outlined in a monograph based on research conducted by a team at Iowa.[114] This publication outlines methods for retrieving clinical nursing data from electronic systems, storing it according to privacy requirements, applying risk adjustment techniques, and analyzing the impact of nursing treatments. This research resulted in several publications that demonstrate the effect of NIC interventions on outcomes. For example, in a publication examining patterns of nursing interventions in persons hospitalized with heart failure and hip procedures and who were at risk for falling, Shever et al.[102] concluded that not only did the use of NIC allow for the extraction of data from the EHR, but found that Surveillance, Intravenous Therapy, Fluid Management, and Diet Staging were the four most frequent interventions implemented in all four groups of older adults in an acute care setting. They also identified which interventions were unique and specific to each adult group and concluded that nursing intervention data using NIC provides administrators with information about the care provided that is useful for evaluating staffing, allocating resources, educating nursing staff, and evaluating nursing competency.

Chae et al.[23] conducted a comprehensive integrative review of the effectiveness research using NIC interventions on specific outcomes. The review focused on studies using NNN, since it is one of the most commonly used terminologies globally.[112] Although 22 studies met the selection criteria, they were only able to identify the cost-effectiveness of nursing interventions in the hospital that used NNN. This affirmed Hong and Lee's assertion[47] that when nursing care data in standardized databases are retrievable, knowledge that has potential to improve the quality of care can be discovered using statistical or data mining tools.

Akkuş and Akdemir,[2] in a study of 45 persons living at home with multiple sclerosis (MS) who were receiving a health education program consisting of eight home visits over 4 months, used a wide range of NIC interventions information about treatment, care, exercise, nutrition, excretion, activity, sleep and rest, cognitive functions, communication, and sexuality in their health education program. While not explicitly identified, Nutritional Counseling, Self-Care Assistance, Exercise Promotion, Coping Enhancement, Socialization Enhancement, and Environmental Management: Safety are some of the interventions implemented by those visiting nurses. In a study with visiting nurses and persons diagnosed with heart failure, Azzolin et al.[7] tested the effect of *Self-Modification Assistance, Behavior Modification, Health Education, Teaching: Prescribed Medication*, and *Teaching: Disease Process* on specific NOCs. Findings revealed an improved

knowledge of heart failure and a strong correlation between NOC indicator scores and Knowledge Questionnaire scores. Ferreira Santana et al.[38] tested NIC interventions in the Cognitive Therapy class with 67 older adults and found cognitive stimulation activities were effective in maintaining the functional capacity of participants, and were configured as an effective strategy for socialization and health promotion.

Comparative Effectiveness Research. Funding agencies are increasingly interested in comparative effectiveness research (CER), which is the comparison of effective interventions among persons in care settings. CER addresses whether an intervention works better than other interventions in a practice where persons are more heterogeneous than those recruited and accepted in clinical trials. Nurse researchers need to engage in the methods of CER because it provides the means to identify which interventions work for what persons under specific circumstances. Key elements in CER are direct comparison of effective interventions, the study of persons in typical clinical care situations, and tailoring the intervention to the needs of individuals. However, it is important to note, using standardized interventions such as those provided in NIC makes comparisons of interventions among populations and across settings possible when designing CER studies.

Designing and Testing Complex Interventions. Persons reside in complex environments where multiple factors contribute to their health. In addition, people may experience more than one health issue concurrently, or it is apparent that successful treatment of a single condition requires a combination of interventions. Complex health conditions require complex solutions or complex interventions. The Medical Research Council (MRC)[107] describes complex interventions as interventions that consist of multiple components. A method of developing a complex intervention consists of developing a multi-component intervention containing several NIC interventions. Sidani and Braden[104] note complex interventions can be delivered in a standardized method where all persons are given all components, or the complex intervention can be tailored to the person's unique experience of the health situation. Persons in this case could be provided one NIC or a combination of NICs that are most appropriate in the treatment of the health conditions. Each component of the intervention targets a particular aspect of the health issue. Outcomes measures are selected that are sensitive to the specific interventions. In a research context, components often work independently, producing complex, multiple causal pathways that have effects on outcomes. It is essential to have a "theory of change" that provides an explanation of the "web of causation," as understanding these inter-relations is essential for designing the complex intervention and determining which outcomes are most sensitive to the intervention. The MRC has developed a comprehensive 12-phase tool for developing, designing, and implementing complex interventions in a systematic, rigorous, yet flexible and iterative way.[107] In the MRC framework[107], context is central to the design and evaluation of the intervention, and the social determinants of health (characteristics of populations such as race, ethnicity, socioeconomic background, access and quality of health service systems) must be incorporated.

Big Data Analytics. The healthcare data revolution fueled by "big data analytics" will transform nursing. In The Inevitable: Understanding the 12 Technological Forces That Will Shape Our Future, Kelly identified 12 influential technological trends, including one he refers to as "cognifying."[61] Cognifying is the process of using supercomputers to add "additional intelligence"[61] (p. 26) to maximize multiple benefits from the new technology. He describes possible cognifying applications that will "change everything" including healthcare. Remarkably, Kelly, a founder and the executive editor of Wired magazine for its first 7 years, specifically identified nursing as a "realm waiting to be cognitively enhanced"[61] (p. 36). As an example, Kelly describes how persons can be outfitted with sensors that track their biomarkers 24 hours a day so treatments can be highly personalized, adjusted, and refined daily. Over the next 30 years, digital sensors will be enhanced by smaller chips, stronger batteries, and cloud connectivity while coupled with massive databases allowing for "big data analytics" and "deeper algorithms," which can track and monitor hundreds of health parameters relevant to nursing care[61] (p. 40).

In their book *Big Data: A Revolution That Will Transform How We Live, Work, and Think*, Mayer-Schonberger and Cukier stated that "big data refers to things one can do at a large scale that cannot be done at a smaller one, to extract new insights or create new forms of value"[78] (p. 8). The current trend toward rapid digitization of large amounts of person and healthcare data in EHRs creates the possibility for the data to be synthesized and analyzed for the purpose of identifying patterns and trends. Raghupathi and Raghupathi[95] demonstrate how big data analytics can be used to support a wide range of health care activities including clinical decision support, population health management, and health surveillance. Big data analytics can assist health care providers to develop more insightful diagnoses and treatments, which one would expect to lead to enhanced desired outcomes and a higher quality of care at lower cost. NIC, as a standardized nursing language, makes cognifying nursing and big data analytics possible because NIC intervention labels and activities can be used in EHRs to plan and document the work of nurses in practice. Coded NIC labels and activities in the EHRs can be stored, retrieved, analyzed, and shared in ways designed to enhance clinical decision making, evaluate the quality and effectiveness of nursing treatments, promote the achievement of optimal outcomes, and manage healthcare costs.

Natural Language Processing. The use of novel technology in healthcare, such as natural language processing (NLP), is in early developmental phases. NLP technology enables computers to derive computable and actionable data from text, especially when text is recorded in the form of natural human language (i.e., phrases, sentences, paragraphs). An example of using NLP includes extracting information from narrative documentation in health records about symptoms that can be used for illness prediction.[63] Bako et al.[9] used NLP to extract, identify, and categorize interventions that social workers used to address the social needs of persons. While NLP is not a substitute for using standardized nursing languages, NLP can be used to create algorithms to link unstructured narrative health documentation to NIC interventions. Our hope is NLP can be leveraged to gain better insight into selecting evidence-based nursing interventions needed to provide optimal quality care for person populations.

CONCLUSION

Nursing is a branch of knowledge comprised of information about the nature of health and illness, as well as the strategies and treatments to promote health and well-being. As a classification system, NIC identifies the treatments nurses perform, organizes this information into a coherent structure, and provides the language to communicate with individuals, families, communities, members of other disciplines, and the public.

Nurses are information and knowledge users, and NIC facilitates the use of knowledge about nursing interventions in practice, education, and research. NIC is a primary source for intervention knowledge development in nursing and provides the knowledge content for guiding nursing treatments. As the largest group of health care knowledge workers, nurses rely on extensive clinical information to implement and evaluate the processes and outcomes of their clinical decision-making care. Standardized NIC interventions facilitate the knowledge-user role by structuring nursing treatments designed to achieve desired outcomes. Furthermore, computerized mechanisms greatly assist nurse knowledge users by bringing knowledge resources to the point of care so they can be quickly accessible during the actual clinical decision-making process. NIC interventions are already in a wide variety of healthcare information systems that are used at the point of care for planning and documenting nursing care. When nursing care is documented and stored in data warehouses, the data can be retrieved for evaluations of effectiveness and for comparative effectiveness research.

Nurses are committed to delivering high-quality nursing interventions. The benefits of using NIC are clear and well established. Since NIC was first developed in 1992, there has been rapid movement incorporating NIC in nursing practice, education, and research. Each edition of NIC offers new advances, including new and revised interventions, new uses of NIC in nursing education, new applications of NIC in practice settings that enhance clinical decision making and documentation of nursing care, and new knowledge generated through the use of NIC in effectiveness research. We continually work to advance and improve NIC and look forward to any feedback, recommendations, and suggestions that readers and users have for improvement.

References

1. Aiken, L. H., Sloane, D. M., Bruyneel, L., Van den Heede, K., Griffiths, P., Busse, R., Diomidous, M., Kinnunen, J., Kózka, M., Lesaffre, E., McHugh, M. D., Moreno-Casbas, M. T., Rafferty, A. M., Schwendimann, R., Scott, P. A., Tishelman, C., van Achterberg, T., Sermeus, W., & RN4CAST consortium, (2014). Nurse staffing and education and hospital mortality in nine European countries: a retrospective observational study. Lancet, 383(9931), 1824–1830. https://doi.org/10.1016/S0140-6736(13)62631-8

2. Akkuş, Y., & Akdemir, N. (2012). Improving the quality of life for multiple sclerosis patients using the nurse-based home visiting model. Scandinavian Journal of Caring Sciences, 26(2), 295–303. https://doi.org/10.1111/j.1471-6712.2011.00933.x

3. American Association of Colleges of Nursing. (2021). The essentials: Core competencies for professional nursing education.

4. American Nurses Association (2021). Nursing: Scope and standards of practice. (4th ed.).

5. Anderson, C. A., Keenan, G., & Jones, J. (2009). Using bibliometrics to support your selection of a nursing terminology set. CIN: Computers, Informatics, Nursing, 27(2), 82–90.

6. Ancízar Echenique, A. M., San Martín Rodríguez, L., & Marín Fernández, B. (2020). Effectiveness of nursing interventions in the control of type 2 diabetes mellitus. Anales del sistema sanitario de Navarra, 43(2), 159–167. https://doi.org/10.23938/ASSN.0860

7. Azzolin, K., Lemos, D. M., Lucena, A., & Rabelo-Silva, E. R. (2015). Home-based nursing interventions improve knowledge of disease and management in patients with heart failure. Revista latino-americana de enfermagem, 23(1), 44–50. https://doi.org/10.1590/0104-1169.0144.2523

8. Azzolin, K., Mussi, C. M., Ruschel, K. B., de Souza, E. N., de Fátima Lucena, A., & Rabelo-Silva, E. R. (2013). Effectiveness of nursing interventions in heart failure patients in home care using NANDA-I, NIC, and NOC. Applied Nursing Research, 26(4), 239–244. https://doi.org/10.1016/j.apnr.2013.08.003

9. Bako, A. T., Taylor, H. L., Wiley, K., Jr., Zheng, J., Walter-McCabe, H., Kasthurirathne, S. N., & Vest, J. R. (2021). Using natural language processing to classify social work interventions. The American Journal of Managed Care, 27(1), e24–e31. https://doi.org/10.37765/ajmc.2021.88580

10. Barros, A. L. B. L., Silva, V. M., Santana, R. F., Cavalcante, A. M. R. Z., Vitor, A. F., Lucena, A. F., Napoleão, A. A., Lopes, C. T., Primo, C. C., Carmona, E. V., Duran, E. C. M., Butcher, H. K., Lopes, J. L., Díaz, L. J. R., Cubas, M. R., Brandão, M. A. G., Lopes, M. V. O., Nóbrega, M. M. L., Almeida, M. A., Souza, P. A., Butcher, R. C. G. S., Jensen, R., Silva, R. S., Morais, S.

C. R. V., & Santos, V. B. (2020). Brazilian Nursing Process Research Network contributions for assistance in the COVID pandemic. Revista Brasileira de Enfermagem, 73(Suppl 2), e20200798. https://doi.org/10.1590/0034-7167-2020-0798

11. Bartlett, R., Bland, A., Rossen, E., Kautz, D., Benfield, S., & Carnevale, T. (2008). Evaluation of the Outcome-Present State Test Model as a way to teach clinical reasoning. Journal of Nursing Education, 47(8), 337–344. https://doi.org/10.3928/01484834-20080801-01

12. Beck, C., McSweeney, J., Richards, K., Robinson, P., Tsai, P. -F., & Souder, E. (2010). Challenges in tailored intervention research. Nursing Outlook, 58(2), 104–110.

13. Bland, A., Rossen, E., Bartlett, R., Kautz, D., Carnevale, T., & Benfield, S. (2009). Implementation and testing of the OPT Model as a teaching strategy in an undergraduate psychiatric nursing course. Nursing Education Perspectives, 30(1), 14–21.

14. Bowker, G. C., & Starr, S. L. (1999). Sorting things out: Classification and its consequences. The MIT Press.

15. Bulechek, G., & McCloskey, J. (Eds.). (2000). Nursing interventions: Effective nursing treatments (3rd ed.). W. B. Saunders.

16. Bulechek, G., & McCloskey, J. (Guest Eds.). (1992). Symposium on nursing interventions. Nursing Clinics of North America, 27(2). W.B. Saunders.

17. Butcher, H. (2016). Development and use of gerontological evidence-based practice guidelines. Journal of Gerontological Nursing, 42(7), 25–32.

18. Carlson, J. (2006, March). Total consensus validation process: A standardized research method to identify and link relevant NNN terms for professional practice. Philadelphia, PA: Paper presented at the NANDA, NIC, and NOC 2006: Electronic Use of Clinical Nursing Data Conference.

19. Casey, A. (2011). Global challenges of electronic records for nursing. In P. S. Cowen & S. Moorhead (Eds.), Current Issues in Nursing (8th ed., pp. 340–347). Mosby Elsevier.

20. Center for Disease Control and Prevention. Transparent Reporting of Evaluation with Nonrandomized Designs (TREND) (2018). https://www.cdc.gov/trendstatement/index.html#:~:text=Transparent%20Reporting%20of%20Evaluations%20with%20Nonrandomized%20Designs%20

21. Center for Nursing Classification. (2000a). NIC interventions and NOC outcomes linked to the OASIS Information Set. Iowa City, IA.

22. Center for Nursing Classification. (2000b). Standardized nursing language in long-term care [R. Cox, preparer]. Iowa City, IA.

23. Chae, S., Oh, H., & Moorhead, S. (2020). Effectiveness of nursing interventions using standardized nursing terminologies: An integrative review. Western Journal of Nursing Research, 42, 963–973.

24. Chang, L. Y., Yu, H. H., & Chao, Y. C. (2019). The relationship between nursing workload, quality of care, and nursing payment in intensive care units. The Journal of Nursing Research: JNR, 27(1), 1–9.

25. Clark, J., & Lang, N. (1992). Nursing's next advance: An international classification for nursing practice. International Nursing Review, 39(4), 109–112.

26. Cohen, M., Kruckeberg, T., McCloskey, J., Bulechek, G., Craft, M., Crossley, J., Denehy, J. A., Glick, O. J., Maas, M., & Prophet, C. M. (1991). Inductive methodology and a research team. Nursing Outlook, 39(4), 162–165.

27. CONSORT: Transparent Reporting of Trials (n.d.). http://www.consort-statement.org

28. Costa, R., dos Santos, E., Lopes, C., & Bergamasco, E. (2015). Adequacy of the activities in the nursing intervention exercise therapy: Ambulation for medical-surgical patients with

impaired physical mobility. *International Journal of Nursing Knowledge, 27*(4), 201–204.

29. Cruz, C., Bonfim, D., Galdzinski, R., Fuqulin, F., & Laus, A. (2014). The use of nursing interventions classification (NIC) in identifying the workload of nursing: An integrative review. *International Journal of Nursing Knowledge, 25*(3), 154–160.

30. Cullen, L., Hanrahan, K., Farrington, M., DeBerg, J., Tucker, S., & Kleiber, C. (2018). *Evidence-based practice in action. Comprehensive strategies, tools, and tips from the University of Iowa Hospitals and Clinics.* Sigma Theta Tau International.

31. de Araujo, D. D., Silva, D., Rodrigues, C., Silva, P. O., Macieira, T., & Chianca, T. (2019). Effectiveness of nursing interventions to prevent dry eye in critically ill patients. *American Journal of Critical Care: An Official Publication, American Association of Critical-Care Nurses, 28*(4), 299–306. https://doi.org/10.4037/ajcc2019360

32. Doenges, M. E., Moorhouse, F., & Murr, A. C. (2019). *Nursing care plans: Guidelines for individualizing client care across the life span* (10th ed.). F.A. Davis.

33. Enderlin, C., & Richards, K. (2006). Research testing of tailored interventions. *Research and Theory for Nursing Practice, 20*(4), 317–324.

34. Escalada-Hernández, P., Muñoz-Hermoso, P., González-Fraile, E., Santos, B., González-Vargas, J. A., Feria-Raposo, I., Girón-García, J. L., & García-Manso, M. (2015). A retrospective study of nursing diagnoses, outcomes, and interventions for patients with mental disorders. *Applied Nursing Research, 28*(2), 92–98.

35. Fawcett, J., & Carino, C. (1989). Hallmarks of success in nursing practice. *Advances in Nursing Science, 11*(4), 1–8.

36. Fehring, R. (1987). Methods to validate nursing diagnoses. *Heart and Lung, 16*, 625–629.

37. Fennelly, O., Grogan, L., Reed, A., & Hardiker, N. R. (2021). Use of standardized terminologies in clinical practice: A scoping review. *International Journal of Medical Informatics, 149*, 104431. https://doi.org/10.1016/j.ijmedinf.2021.104431

38. Ferreira Santana, R., Batista Rosa, T., Gonçalves Aquino, R., Araújo de Alexandrino, S., Alves Santos, G. L., & Araújo Lobato, H. (2016). Maintenance of functional capacity in cognitive stimulation subgroups. *Investigacion y Educacion en Enfermeria, 34*(3), 493–501.

39. Gleick, J. (2011). *The information: A history, a theory, a flood.* Pantheon.

40. Gray, J. R., & Grove, S. K. (2021). *Burns and Grove's The practice of nursing research: Appraisal, synthesis, and generation of evidence* (9th ed.). Elsevier.

41. Griffiths, P., Recio-Saucedo, A., Dall'Ora, C., Briggs, J., Maruotti, A., Meredith, P., Smith, G. B., & Ball, J. (2018). The association between nurse staffing and omissions in nursing care: A systematic review. *Journal of Advanced Nursing (John Wiley & Sons, Inc.), 74*(7), 1474–1487. https://doi.org/10.1111/jan.13564

42. Griggs, K., Arms, T., & Turrise, S. (2019). Outcome-Present State Test Model for expanding students' clinical reasoning. *Nurse Educator, 44*(3), 174. https://doi.org/10.1097/NNE.0000000000000578

43. Haegdorens, F., Van Bogaert, P., De Meester, K., & Monsieurs, K. G. (2019). The impact of nurse staffing levels and nurse's education on patient mortality in medical and surgical wards: An observational multicentre study. *BMC Health Services Research, 19*(1), 864. https://doi.org/10.1186/s12913-019-4688-7

44. Hedden, H. (2010). *The accidental taxonomist.* Information Today.

45. Herdman, T. H., & Kamitsuru, S. (2014). Frequently asked questions. In T. H. Herdman & S. Kamitsuru (Eds.), *NANDA International nursing diagnoses: Definitions & classification, 2015–2017* (10th ed., pp. 105–130). Wiley Blackwell.

46. Herdman, T. H., Kamitsuru, S., & Lopes, C. T. (2021). *Nursing diagnoses: Definitions and classification 2021–2023* (12th ed.). Thieme.

47. Hong, S. -J., & Lee, E. (2012). Korean and United States: Comparison of costs of nursing interventions. *Korean Journal of Adult Nursing, 24*(4), 358–369. https://doi.org/10.7475/kjan.2012.24.4.358

48. Institute of Medicine, (2001). *Crossing the quality chasm: A new health system for the 21st century.* The National Academies Press.

49. Institute of Medicine. (2011). *The future of nursing: Leading change, advancing health.* The National Academies Press.

50. Iowa Intervention Project. (1993). The NIC taxonomy structure. *Image: Journal of Nursing Scholarship, 25*(3), 187–192.

51. Iowa Intervention Project. (1995). Validation and coding of the NIC taxonomy structure. *Image: Journal of Nursing Scholarship, 27*(1), 43–49.

52. Iowa Intervention Project. (1996). *NIC interventions linked to Omaha system problems.* Iowa City, IA: Center for Nursing Classification.

53. Jacox, A. (1995). Practice and policy implications of clinical and administrative databases. In N. M. Lang (Ed.), *Nursing data systems: The emerging framework.* American Nurses Association.

54. Jagerman, E.J. (2006). *Creating, maintaining and applying quality taxonomies.*

55. Johnson, M., Moorhead, S., Bulechek, G., Butcher, H., Maas, M., & Swanson, E. (Eds.), (2012). *NOC and NIC linkages to NANDA-I and clinical conditions: Supporting critical reasoning and quality care.* Elsevier Mosby.

56. Kane, R., Shamliyan, T., Mueller, C., Duval, S., & Wilt, T. (2007). The association of registered nurse staffing levels and patient outcomes: A systematic review and meta-analysis. *Medical Care, 45*(12), 1195–1204.

57. Kautz, D. D., Kuiper, R., Pesut, D. J., Knight-Brown, P., & Daneker, D. (2005). Promoting clinical reasoning in undergraduate nursing students: Application and evaluation of Outcome Present State Test (OPT) model of clinical reasoning. *International Journal of Nursing Education Scholarship, 2*(1). https://doi.org/10.2202/1548-923X.1052

58. Kautz, D. D., Kuiper, R., Pesut, D. J., & Williams, R. L. (2006). Using NANDA, NIC, and NOC (NNN) language for clinical reasoning with the Outcome-Present State-Test (OPT) model. *International Journal of Nursing Terminologies and Classifications: The Official Journal of NANDA International, 17*(3), 129–138. https://doi.org/10.1111/j.1744-618X.2006.00033.x

59. Keenan, G. (1999). Use of standardized nursing language will make nursing visible. *Michigan Nurse, 72*(2), 12–13.

60. Keenan, G. M., Yakel, E., Yao, Y., Xu, D., Szalacha, L., Tschannen, D., Ford, Y., Chen, Y. -C., Johonson, A., Dunn Lopez, K., & Wilkie, D. J. (2012). Maintaining a consistent big picture: Meaningful use of a web-based POC EHR system. *International Journal of Nursing Knowledge, 23*(3), 119–133. https://doi.org/10.1111/j.2047-3095.2012.01215.x

61. Kelly, K. (2016). *The inevitable: Understanding the 12 technological forces that will shape our future.* Viking.

62. Klehr, J., Hafner, J., Spelz, L. M., Steen, S., & Weaver, K. (2009). Implementation of standardized nomenclature in the electronic medical record. *International Journal of Nursing Terminologies and Classifications, 20*, 169–180. https://doi.org/10.1111/j.1744-618X.2009.01132.x

63. Koleck, T. A., Tatonetti, N. P., Bakken, S., Mitha, S., Henderson, M. M., George, M., Miaskowski, C., Smaldone, A., & Topaz, M. (2021). Identifying symptom information in clinical notes using Natural Language Processing. *Nursing Research*, *70*(3), 173–183.

64. Kuiper, R. (2008). Use of personal digital assistants to support clinical reasoning in undergraduate baccalaureate nursing students. *Computers Informatics*, *26*(2), 90–98.

65. Kuiper, R., Donnell, S., Pesut, D., & Turrise, S. (2017). *The essentials of clinical reasoning for nurses: Using the Outcome-Present State-Test Model for reflective practice*. Sigma Theta Tau International.

66. Kuiper, R., Heinrich, C., Matthias, A., Graham, M., & Bell-Kotwall, L. (2008). Evaluating situated cognition during simulation: Debriefing with the OPT model of clinical reasoning. *International Journal of Nursing Education Scholarship*, *5*(1). https://doi.org/10.2202/1548-923X.1466

67. Kuiper, R., Pesut, D., & Arms, T. (2016). *Clinical reasoning and care coordination in advanced practice nursing*. Springer.

68. Kuiper, R., Pesut, D., & Kautz, D. (2009). Promoting self-regulation of clinical reasoning skills in nursing students. *Open Nursing Journal*, *3*, 76–85. https://doi.org/10.2174/1874434600903010076

69. Lambe, P. K. (2007). *Organising knowledge: Taxonomies, knowledge, and organizational effectiveness*. Chandos.

70. Lopes, J., de Barros, A., & Michel, J. (2009). A pilot study to validate the priority nursing interventions classification and nursing outcomes classification outcomes for the nursing diagnosis "excess fluid volume" in cardiac patients. *International Journal of Nursing Terminologies and Classifications*, *20*(2), 76–88.

71. Lozano, P., Butcher, H. K., Serrano, C., Carrasco, A., Lagares, C., Lusilla, P., & O'Ferrall, C. (2021). Motivational interviewing: Validation of a proposed NIC nursing intervention in persons with a severe mental illness. *International Journal of Nursing Knowledge*, *32*(4), 240–252.

72. Lucena, A., de, F., Magro, C. Z., da Costa Proença, M. C., Bertoldo Pires, A. U., Monteiro Moraes, V., & Badin Aliti, G. (2017). Validation of the nursing interventions and activities for patients on hemodialytic therapy. *Revista Gaucha de Enfermagem*, *38*(3), 1–9.

73. Lunney, M. (2003). Theoretical explanations for combining NANDA, NIC, and NOC. In J. M. Dochterman & D. A. Jones (Eds.), *Unifying nursing languages: The harmonization of NANDA, NIC, and NOC* (pp. 35–45). American Nurses Association.

74. Lunney, M. (2006). Helping nurses use NANDA, NOC, and NIC: Novice to expert. *Nurse Educator*, *31*(1), 40–46.

75. Lunney, M. (Ed.), (2009). *Critical thinking to achieve positive health outcomes: Nursing case studies and analyses*. Wiley-Blackwell.

76. Lunney, M., McGuire, M., Endozo, N., & McIntosh-Waddy, D. (2010). Consensus-validation study identifies relevant nursing diagnoses, nursing interventions, and health outcomes for people with traumatic brain injuries. *Rehabilitation Nursing*, *35*(4), 161–166.

77. Makic, B. F. M., & Martinez-Karatz, M. R. (2022). *Ackley and Ladwig's nursing diagnosis handbook: An evidence-based guide to planning care* (13th ed.). Elsevier.

78. Mayer-Schonberger, V., & Cukier, K. (2013). *Big data: A revolution that will transform how we live, work, and think*. Eamon Dolan.

79. McCloskey, J. C., Bulechek, G. M., & Donahue, W. (1998). Nursing interventions core to specialty practice. *Nursing Outlook*, *46*(2), 67–76.

80. McGonigle, D., & Mastrian, K. D. (2022). Systems Development Life Cycle: Nursing informatics and organizational decision making: *Nursing informatics and the foundation of knowledge* (pp. 191–204) (5th ed.). Jones & Bartlett Learning.

81. Melnyk, B. M., & Morrison-Beedy, D. (2019). *Intervention research and evidence-based quality improvement: Designing, conducting, analyzing, and funding* (2nd ed.). Springer.

82. Moorhead, S., Macieira, T. G. R., Lopez, K. D., Mantovani, V. M., Swanson, E., Wagner, C., & Abe, N. (2021). NANDA-I, NOC, and NIC Linkages to SARS-Cov-2 (COVID-19): Part 1. Community response. *International Journal of Nursing Knowledge*, *32*(1), 59–67. https://doi.org/10.1111/2047-3095.12291

83. Moorhead, S., Swanson, E., & Johnson, M. (2024). *Nursing outcomes classification: Measurement of health outcomes* (7th ed.). Elsevier.

84. Needleman, J., Buerhaus, P., Pankratz, V., Leibson, C., Stevens, S., & Harris, M. (2011). Nurse staffing and inpatient hospital mortality. *The New England Journal of Medicine*, *364*(11), 1037–1045.

85. Nolan, P. (1998). Competencies drive decision making. *Nursing Management*, *29*(3), 27–29.

86. Ohl, M. (2018). *The art of naming*. The MIT Press.

87. Olley, R., Edwards, I., Avery, M., & Cooper, H. (2019). Systematic review of the evidence related to mandated nurse staffing ratios in acute hospitals. *Australian Health Review*, *43*(3), 288–293. https://doi.org/10.1071/AH16252

88. Peplau, H. E. (1987). Nursing science: A historical perspective. In R. R. Parse (Ed.), *Nursing science: Major paradigms, theories, and critiques* (pp. 13–29). Saunders.

89. Peres, H. H., de Almeida Lopes M da Cruz, D., Tellez, M., de Cassia Gengo e Silva, R., dos S Diogo, R. C., Ortiz, D. C., & Ortiz, D. R. (2015). Nursing clinical documentation system structured on NANDA-I, NOC, and NIC classification systems. *Studies in Health Technology and Informatics*, *216*, 943.

90. Perry, P. A., Potter, A. G., Stockert, P. A., & Hall, A. M. (2021). *Fundamentals of nursing* (10th ed.). Elsevier.

91. Pesut, D. (2002). Nursing nomenclatures and eye-roll anxiety control. *Journal of Professional Nursing*, *18*(1), 3–4.

92. Pesut, D., & Herman, J. (1999). *Clinical reasoning: The art and science of critical and creative thinking*. Delmar.

93. Possari, J. F., Gaidzinski, R. R., Lima, A. F., Fugulin, F. M., & Herdman, T. H. (2015). Use of the nursing intervention classification for identifying the workload of a nursing team in a surgical center. *Revista Latino-Americana de Enfermagem*, *23*(5), 781–788. https://doi.org/10.1590/0104-1169.0419.2615

94. Rae, P. J. L., Pearce, S., Greaves, P. J., Dall'Ora, C., Griffiths, P., & Endacott, R. (2021). Outcomes sensitive to critical care nurse staffing levels: A systematic review. *Intensive & Critical Care Nursing*, *67*, 103110. https://doi.org/10.1016/j.iccn.2021.103110

95. Raghupathi, W., & Raghupathi, V. (2014). Big data analytics in healthcare: Promise and potential. *Health Information Science and Systems*, *2*(3), 1–29. https://doi.org/10.1186/2047-2501-2-3

96. Raurell-Torredà, M., Llauradó-Serra, M., Lamoglia-Puig, M., Rifà-Ros, R., Díaz-Agea, J. L., García-Mayor, S., & Romero-Collado, A. (2020). Standardized language systems for the design of high-fidelity simulation scenarios: A Delphi study. *Nurse Education Today*, *86*, 104319. https://doi.org/10.1016/j.nedt.2019.104319

97. Reed, D., Titler, M., Dochterman, J., Shever, L., Kanak, M., & Picone, D. (2007). Measuring the dose of nursing intervention. *International Journal of Nursing Terminologies and Classifications*, *18*(4), 121–130.

98. Ros, R. R., Adrados, C. O., & Lenguaje Puig, M. (2020). *NIC para el aprendizaje teorico-practico en enfermeria* (2nd ed.). Elsevier.

99. Rutherford, M. A. (2008). Standardized Nursing Language: What does it mean for nursing practice. *OJIN: The Online Journal of Issues in Nursing, 13*(1). https://doi.org/10.3912/OJIN.Vol13No01PPT05

100. Sackett, D., Straus, S., Richardson, W., Rosenberg, W., & Haynes, R. (2000). *Evidence-based medicine: How to practice and teach EBM* (2nd ed.). Churchill Livingstone.

101. Shever, L. L. (2011). The impact of nursing surveillance on failure to rescue. *Research and Theory for Nursing Practice, 25*(2), 107–126. https://doi.org/10.1891/1541-6577.25.2.10

102. Shever, L. L., Titler, M., Dochterman, J., Fei, Q., & Picone, D. (2007). Patterns of nursing intervention use across 6 days of acute care hospitalization for three older patient populations. *International Journal of Nursing Terminologies and Classifications, 18*(1), 18–29. https://doi.org/10.1111/j.1744-618X.2007.00044.x

103. Shin, J. H., Choi, G. Y., & Lee, J. (2021). Identifying frequently used NANDA-I nursing diagnoses, NOC outcomes, NIC interventions, and NNN linkages for nursing home residents in Korea. *International Journal of Environmental Research and Public Health, 18*(21), 11505. https://doi.org/10.3390/ijerph182111505

104. Sidani, S., & Braden, C. J. (2021). *Nursing and health interventions: Design, evaluation, and implementation* (2nd ed.). Wiley Blackwell.

105. Silva de Melo, L., da Silva Figueiredo, L., de Melo Vellozo Pereira, J., Peclat Flores, P. V., Barbosa Siqueira, M. E., & Dantas Cavalcanti, A. C. (2017). Educational strategies used in standardized language systems by nurses: An integrative review. *Online Brazilian Journal of Nursing, 16*(3), 4. https://doi.org/10.17665/1676-4285.20175549

106. Silva, R., & Ferreira, N. (2016). Content validation study of nursing interventions intended to prevent cardiovascular events in diabetic patients. *Journal of Clinical Nursing, 26*(3–4), 366–368. https://doi.org/10.1111/jocn13181

107. Skivington, K., Matthews, L., Simpson, S. A., Craig, P., Baird, J., Blazeby, J. M., Boyd, K. A., Craig, N., French, D. P., McIntosh, E., Petticrew, M., Rycroff-Malone, J., White, M., & Moore, L. (2021). A new framework for developing and evaluating complex interventions: Update of Medical Research Council guidance. *BMI, 374*(2061). https://doi.org/10.1136/bmj.n2061

108. Sun, J., Li, Y., & Shen, N. (2021). The use of the Nursing Interventions Classification in identifying the workload of a nursing team in a pediatric oncology center. *Studies in Health Technology and Informatics, 284*, 83–84. https://doi.org/10.3233/SHTI210673

109. Swanson, E., Mantovani, V. M., Wagner, C., Moorhead, S., Lopez, K. D., Macieira, T. G. R., & Abe, N. (2021). NANDA-I, NOC, and NIC linkages to SARS-CoV-2 (COVID-19): Part 2. Individual response. *International Journal of Nursing Knowledge, 32*(1), 68–83. https://doi.org/10.1111/2047-3095.12307

110. Tastan, S., Linch, G. C., Keenan, G. M., Stifter, J., McKinney, D., Fahey, L., Lopez, K. D., Yao, Y., & Wilkie, D. J. (2014). Evidence for the existing American Nurses Association-recognized standardized nursing terminologies: A systematic review. *International Journal of Nursing Studies, 51*(8), 1160–1170. https://doi.org/10.1016/j.ijnurstu.2013.12.004

111. The Agency for Health Care Policy and Research Reauthorization Act of 1992 (P.L. 102-410).

112. Thede, L. Q., & Schwirian, P. M. (2016). Informatics: The standardized nursing terminologies: A national survey of nurses' experience and attitudes—SURVEY II: Evaluation of standardized nursing terminologies. *Online Journal of Issues in Nursing, 21*(1), 6. https://doi.org/10.3912/OJIN.Vol21No01InfoCol01

113. Titler, M., Dochterman, J., Kim, T., Kanak, M., Shever, L., Picone, D., Everett, L., & Budreau, G. (2007). Costs of care for seniors hospitalized for hip fractures and related procedures. *Nursing Outlook, 55*(1), 5–14. https://doi.org/10.1016/j.outlook.2006.06.006

114. Titler, M., Dochterman, J., & Reed, D. (2004). *Guideline for conducting effectiveness research in nursing and other health-care services.* The University of Iowa, College of Nursing, Center for Nursing Classification and Clinical Effectiveness.

115. Trovó, S. A., Cucolo, D. F., & Perroca, M. G. (2020). Time and quality of admissions: Nursing workload. *Revista brasileira de enfermagem, 73*(5), e20190267. https://doi.org/10.1590/0034-7167-2019-0267

116. Twigg, D. E., Whitehead, L., Doleman, G., & El, Z. S. (2021). The impact of nurse staffing methodologies on nurse and patient outcomes: A systematic review. *Journal of Advanced Nursing, 77*(12), 4599–4611. https://doi.org/10.1111/jan.14909

117. Wagner, C. M., Swanson, E. A., Moorhead, S., Mantovani, V. M., Dunn, L. K., Macieira, T. G. R., Abe, N., & Breitenstein, S. (2022). NANDA-I, NOC, and NIC linkages to SARS-CoV-2 (COVID-19): Part 3. Family response. *International Journal of Nursing Knowledge, 33*(1), 5–17. https://doi.org/10.1111/2047-3095.12323

118. Werley, H. H., & Lang, N. M. (Eds.). (1988). *Identification of the nursing minimum data set.* Springer.

## PART TWO

Taxonomy of Nursing Interventions

Overview of the NIC Taxonomy

This 8th edition of the *Nursing Interventions Classification* has 614 interventions organized, as in the last five editions, into 7 domains and 30 classes. This three-level taxonomic structure is included on the following pages. At the topmost abstract level are 7 *domains* (numbered 1 to 7). Each domain includes *classes* (assigned alphabetical letters) that are at the second level of abstraction of the taxonomy and are groupings of similar interventions. The third level contains the *intervention* labels, each with a unique code of four numbers. Only intervention label names are used in the taxonomy. Refer to the alphabetical listing in the book for the definition and defining activities for each intervention. The taxonomy was originally constructed using the methods of similarity analysis, hierarchical clustering, clinical judgment, and expert review. Refer to previous editions for more details on the construction, validation, and coding of the taxonomy.

The taxonomy clusters related interventions for ease of use. The groupings represent all areas of nursing practice. Nurses in any specialty should remember that they should use the whole taxonomy with a particular person, not just interventions from one class or domain. The taxonomy is theory neutral; the interventions can be used with any nursing theory and in any of the various nursing settings and healthcare delivery systems. The interventions can also be used with various diagnostic classifications, including NANDA International, International Classification of Diseases (ICD), Diagnostic and Statistical Manual of Mental Disorders (DSM), and the Omaha System Problem List.

Each of the interventions has been assigned a unique number to facilitate computerization. Identify the class and domain of the intervention using six digits (i.e., 1A-1040 is Body Mechanics Promotion and is located in the Activity and Exercise Management class in the Physiological: Basic domain). Activity codes are not included in this book. To assign codes to the activities, each intervention's activities can be numbered using two spaces after a decimal (i.e., 1A-0140.01 designates the first activity in Body Mechanics Promotion). If activities are coded in a particular facility, they need to be used together with the related intervention code.

Some interventions have been included in two classes but are coded according to the primary class. We have attempted to keep cross-referencing to a minimum because the taxonomy could easily become long and unwieldy. Interventions are listed in another class only if they were

judged to be sufficiently related to the interventions in that class. No intervention is listed in more than two classes. Occasionally, an intervention is located in only one class but has a code that is assigned to another class (i.e., Nutritional Counseling is located in class D, Nutrition Support, but is coded 5246 to indicate that it is a counseling intervention). The interventions in each class are listed alphabetically, but the numbers may not be sequential because of additions, deletions, and cross-referencing. The last two classes in the domain Health System (Health System Management, coded a, and Information Management, coded b) contain many of the indirect care interventions (i.e., those that would be included in overhead costs).

The taxonomy first appeared in the second edition of NIC in 1996 with 6 domains and 27 classes. The third edition, published in 2000, included one new domain (Community) and three new classes: Childrearing Care (coded Z) in the Family domain and Community Health Promotion and Community Risk Management in the Community domain (c and d). No new domains or classes were added in this edition; the 60 new interventions were easily placed in the existing classes. The class Drug Management (H) was renamed Medication Management in this issue, to avoid the negative connotation of the term "*drug*", while the class Patient Education (S) was renamed Health Education, in concurrence with our belief that the education nurses provide is not limited to patients.

The coding guidelines used for this and previous editions are summarized as follows:

- Each intervention is assigned a unique four-digit code, which belongs to the intervention as long as the intervention exists, regardless of whether it should change class in some future edition.
- Codes are retired when interventions are retired; no code is used more than once.
- Interventions that have a modification in label name only that *does not* change the nature of the intervention will keep the same code number. In this case, the label name change does not affect the intervention, but the change was needed for a compelling reason (e.g., Abuse Protection was changed to Abuse Protection Support in the third edition to distinguish the intervention from an outcome in NOC that had the same name; Conscious Sedation was changed in the fourth edition to Sedation Management to better reflect current practice; Shift

Report was changed to Handoff Report in the seventh edition to reflect that this intervention is used in other settings besides hospitals, and Rape-Trauma Treatment was changed to Sexual Assault Trauma Care in this edition to better reflect current terminologies).

- Interventions that have a modification in label name only that *does* change the nature of the intervention are assigned a new code, and the previous code is retired (i.e., in the third edition, Triage was retired and a new intervention Triage: Disaster was added, indicating the more discrete nature of this intervention and distinguishing it from the interventions of Triage: Emergency Center and Triage: Telecommunication; in the seventh edition Pain Management was retired and two new more discrete interventions, Pain Management: Acute and Pain Management: Chronic, were added; and in this edition Physician Support was retired and a new intervention Health Care Provider Collaboration was added, more accurately reflecting the current collaborative nature of nursing practice).
- Cross-referencing is avoided if possible, and no intervention is cross-referenced in more than two classes; the number assigned is selected from the primary class.
- Interventions are listed alphabetically within each class; the code numbers may not be sequential because of changes, additions, and deletions.
- Although the codes originally begun in the second edition were assigned logically and this logical order is being continued, when possible, *codes are context free* and should not be interpreted to have any meaning except as a four-digit number.
- Activities are not coded, but if one desires to do this, use two (or more if indicated in your computer system) spaces to the right of a decimal and number the activities as they appear in each intervention (e.g., 0140.01, 0140.02).

NIC Taxonomy

	Domain 1	Domain 2	Domain 3
Level 1 Domains	**1. Physiological: Basic** Care that supports physical functioning	**2. Physiological: Complex** Care that supports homeostatic regulation	**3. Behavioral** Care that supports psychosocial functioning and facilitates lifestyle changes
Level 2 Classes	**A. Activity and Exercise Management** Interventions to organize or assist with physical activity and energy conservation and expenditure	**G. Electrolyte and Acid-Base Management** Interventions to regulate electrolyte/acid base balance and prevent complications	**O. Behavior Therapy** Interventions to reinforce or promote desirable behaviors or alter undesirable behaviors
	B. Elimination Management Interventions to establish and maintain regular bowel and urinary elimination patterns and manage complications due to altered patterns	**H. Medication Management** Interventions to facilitate desired effects of pharmacological agents	**P. Cognitive Therapy** Interventions to reinforce or promote desirable cognitive functioning or alter undesirable cognitive functioning
	C. Immobility Management Interventions to manage restricted body movement and the sequelae	**I. Neurologic Management** Interventions to optimize neurologic function	**Q. Communication Enhancement** Interventions to facilitate delivering and receiving verbal and nonverbal messages
	D. Nutrition Support Interventions to modify or maintain nutritional status	**J. Perioperative Care** Interventions to provide care before, during, and immediately after surgery	**R. Coping Assistance** Interventions to assist another to build on own strengths, to adapt to a change in function, or achieve a higher level of function
	E. Physical Comfort Promotion Interventions to promote comfort using physical techniques	**K. Respiratory Management** Interventions to promote airway patency and gas exchange	**S. Health Education** Interventions to facilitate learning
	F. Self-Care Facilitation Interventions to provide or assist with routine activities of daily living	**L. Skin/Wound Management** Interventions to maintain or restore tissue integrity	**T. Psychological Comfort Promotion** Interventions to promote comfort using psychological techniques
		M. Thermoregulation Interventions to maintain body temperature within a normal range	
		N. Tissue Perfusion Management Interventions to optimize circulation of blood and fluids to the tissue	

Domain 4	Domain 5	Domain 6	Domain 7
4. Safety Care that supports protection against harm	**5. Family** Care that supports the family	**6. Health System** Care that supports effective use of the healthcare delivery system	**7. Community** Care that supports the health of the community
U. Crisis Management Interventions to provide immediate short-term help in both psychological and physiological crises **V. Risk Management** Interventions to initiate risk reduction activities and continue monitoring risks over time	**W. Childbearing Care** Interventions to assist in the preparation for childbirth and management of the psychological and physiological changes before, during, and immediately following childbirth **Z. Childrearing Care** Interventions to assist in raising children **X. Lifespan Care** Interventions to facilitate family unit functioning and promote the health and welfare of family members throughout the lifespan	**Y. Health System Mediation** Interventions to facilitate the interface between person/family and the healthcare system **a. Health System Management** Interventions to provide and enhance support services for the delivery of care **b. Information Management** Interventions to facilitate communication about health care	**c. Community Health Promotion** Interventions that promote the health of the whole community **d. Community Risk Management** Interventions that assist in detecting or preventing health risks to the whole community

Level 1 Domains	1. **Physiological: Basic** **Care that supports physical functioning**	

Level 2 Classes

A. **Activity and Exercise Management** Interventions to organize or assist with physical activity and energy conservation and expenditure	B. **Elimination Management** Interventions to establish and maintain regular bowel and urinary elimination patterns and manage complications due to altered patterns	C. **Immobility Management** Interventions to manage restricted body movement and the sequelae

Level 3 Interventions

A	B	C
0140 Body Mechanics Promotion 0180 Energy Management 0200 Exercise Promotion 0201 Exercise Promotion: Strength Training 0202 Exercise Promotion: Stretching 0221 Exercise Therapy: Ambulation 0222 Exercise Therapy: Balance 0224 Exercise Therapy: Joint Mobility 0226 Exercise Therapy: Muscle Control 5612 Teaching: Prescribed Exercise **S***	0550 Bladder Irrigation 0410 Bowel Incontinence Care 0412 Bowel Incontinence Care: Encopresis **Z** 0430 Bowel Management 0450 Constipation Management 0460 Diarrhea Management 0466 Enema Administration 0470 Flatulence Reduction 0480 Ostomy Care **L** 0560 Pelvic Muscle Exercise 0630 Pessary Management 0640 Prompted Voiding 0490 Rectal Prolapse Management 1804 Self-Care Assistance: Toileting **F** 1876 Tube Care: Urinary 0565 Ultrasonography: Bladder 0570 Urinary Bladder Training 0580 Urinary Catheterization 0581 Urinary Catheterization: External 0582 Urinary Catheterization: Intermittent 0590 Urinary Elimination Management 0600 Urinary Habit Training 0610 Urinary Incontinence Care 0612 Urinary Incontinence Care: Enuresis **Z** 0620 Urinary Retention Care	0740 Bed Rest Care 0762 Cast Care: Maintenance 0764 Cast Care: Wet 6580 Physical Restraint **V** 0840 Positioning 0846 Positioning: Wheelchair 1806 Self-Care Assistance: Transfer **F** 0910 Splinting 0940 Traction/Immobilization Care 0970 Transfer
0100 to 0399	0400 to 0699	0700 to 0999

*Letter indicates another class where the intervention is also included.

D. Nutrition Support

Interventions to modify or maintain nutritional status

1020 Diet Staging
1024 Diet Staging: Weight Loss Surgery
1030 Eating Disorders Management
1056 Enteral Tube Feeding
1050 Feeding **F**
1080 Nasogastric Intubation
1100 Nutrition Management
1120 Nutrition Therapy
5246 Nutritional Counseling
1160 Nutritional Monitoring
1860 Swallowing Therapy **F**
5614 Teaching: Prescribed Diet **S**
1200 Total Parenteral Nutrition (TPN)
   Administration **G**
1874 Tube Care: Gastrointestinal
1240 Weight Gain Assistance
1260 Weight Management
1280 Weight Reduction Assistance

E. Physical Comfort Promotion

Interventions to promote comfort using physical techniques

1310 Abdominal Massage
1320 Acupressure
1330 Aromatherapy
6482 Comfort Management
1340 Cutaneous Stimulation
1350 Dry Eye Prevention
1360 Endotracheal Extubation: Palliative
1380 Heat/Cold Application
1390 Healing Touch
6855 Labor Pain Management **W**
1480 Massage
1450 Nausea Management
1410 Pain Management: Acute
1415 Pain Management: Chronic
1440 Premenstrual Syndrome (PMS)
   Management
1460 Progressive Muscle Relaxation
3550 Pruritus Management **L**
1520 Reiki
5465 Therapeutic Touch
1540 Transcutaneous Electrical Nerve
   Stimulation (TENS)
1570 Vomiting Management

F. Self-Care Facilitation

Interventions to provide or assist with routine activities of daily living

1610 Bathing
1620 Contact Lens Care
6462 Dementia Management: Bathing **V**
1630 Dressing
1640 Ear Care
1645 Ear Irrigation
1650 Eye Care
1655 Eye Irrigation
1050 Feeding **D**
1660 Foot Care
1665 Functional Ability Enhancement
1670 Hair and Scalp Care
1680 Nail Care
1710 Oral Health Maintenance
1720 Oral Health Promotion
1730 Oral Health Restoration
1750 Perineal Care
1770 Postmortem Care
1800 Self-Care Assistance
1804 Self-Care Assistance: Toileting **B**
1806 Self-Care Assistance: Transfer **C**
1850 Sleep Enhancement
1860 Swallowing Therapy **D**
1870 Tube Care

Level 1 Domains

2. PHYSIOLOGICAL: COMPLEX
Care that supports homeostatic regulation

Level 2 Classes

G. Electrolyte and Acid-Base Management
Interventions to regulate electrolyte/acid base balance and prevent complications

H. Medication Management
Interventions to facilitate desired effects of pharmacological agents

Level 3 Interventions

1910 Acid-Base Management
1911 Acid-Base Management: Metabolic Acidosis
1912 Acid-Base Management: Metabolic Alkalosis
1913 Acid-Base Management: Respiratory Acidosis **K***
1914 Acid-Base Management: Respiratory Alkalosis **K**
1920 Acid-Base Monitoring
2000 Electrolyte Management
2001 Electrolyte Management: Hypercalcemia
2002 Electrolyte Management: Hyperkalemia
2003 Electrolyte Management: Hypermagnesemia
2004 Electrolyte Management: Hypernatremia
2005 Electrolyte Management: Hyperphosphatemia
2006 Electrolyte Management: Hypocalcemia
2007 Electrolyte Management: Hypokalemia
2008 Electrolyte Management: Hypomagnesemia
2009 Electrolyte Management: Hyponatremia
2010 Electrolyte Management: Hypophosphatemia
2020 Electrolyte Monitoring
2080 Fluid/Electrolyte Management N
2100 Hemodialysis Therapy
2110 Hemofiltration Therapy
2120 Hyperglycemia Management
2125 Hyperlipidemia Management
2130 Hypoglycemia Management
2150 Peritoneal Dialysis Therapy
4232 Phlebotomy: Arterial Blood Sample **N**
1200 Total Parenteral Nutrition (TPN) Administration **D**

2210 Analgesic Administration
2214 Analgesic Administration: Intraspinal
2840 Anesthesia Administration **J**
4054 Central Venous Access Management: Central Insertion **N**
4220 Central Venous Access Management: Peripheral Insertion **N**
6430 Chemical Restraint **V**
2240 Chemotherapy Management **S**
2280 Hormone Replacement Therapy
2300 Medication Administration
2321 Medication Administration: Continuous Subcutaneous Infusion
2308 Medication Administration: Ear
2301 Medication Administration: Enteral
2310 Medication Administration: Eye
2311 Medication Administration: Inhalation
2302 Medication Administration: Interpleural
2312 Medication Administration: Intradermal
2313 Medication Administration: Intramuscular (IM)
2322 Medication Administration: Intraocular Disk
2303 Medication Administration: Intraosseous
2319 Medication Administration: Intraspinal
2314 Medication Administration: Intravenous (IV)

2320 Medication Administration: Nasal
2304 Medication Administration: Oral
2315 Medication Administration: Rectal
2316 Medication Administration: Skin
2317 Medication Administration: Subcutaneous
2318 Medication Administration: Vaginal
2307 Medication Administration: Ventricular Reservoir
2370 Medication Deprescribing
2380 Medication Management
2385 Medication Management: Medical Cannabis
2390 Medication Prescribing
2395 Medication Reconciliation **V**
2398 Medication Management: Wearable Infusion Device
2400 Patient-Controlled Analgesia (PCA) Assistance
2420 Phytotherapy
2260 Sedation Management
5616 Teaching: Prescribed Medication **S**
4270 Thrombolytic Therapy Management **N**
2430 Transgender Hormone Therapy

1900 to 2199

2200 to 2499

*Letter indicates another class where the intervention is also included.

I. Neurologic Management

Interventions to optimize neurologic function

2540 Cerebral Edema Management
2550 Cerebral Perfusion Promotion
2560 Dysreflexia Management
2570 Electroconvulsive Therapy (ECT) Management
2590 Intracranial Pressure (ICP) Monitoring
2620 Neurologic Monitoring
2660 Peripheral Sensation Management
0844 Positioning: Neurologic
2680 Seizure Management **V**
2690 Seizure Precautions
2720 Subarachnoid Hemorrhage Precautions
1878 Tube Care: Ventriculostomy/Lumbar Drain
2760 Unilateral Neglect Management

J. Perioperative Care

Interventions to provide care before, during, and immediately after surgery

2840 Anesthesia Administration **H**
2860 Autotransfusion **N**
3000 Circumcision Care **W**
6545 Infection Control: Intraoperative
6560 Laser Precautions **V**
2865 Pneumatic Tourniquet Management
0842 Positioning: Intraoperative
2870 Postanesthesia Care
2880 Preoperative Coordination **Y**
3582 Skin Care: Donor Site **L**
3583 Skin Care: Graft Site **L**
2900 Surgical Assistance
2910 Surgical Instrumentation Management
2920 Surgical Precautions **V**
2930 Surgical Preparation
5610 Teaching: Preoperative **S**
3902 Temperature Regulation: Perioperative **M**

Level 1 *Domains*	**2. PHYSIOLOGICAL: COMPLEX—cont'd** **Care that supports homeostatic regulation**	
Level 2 *Classes*	**K. Respiratory Management** Interventions to promote airway patency and gas exchange	**L. Skin/Wound Management** Interventions to maintain or restore tissue integrity
Level 3 *Interventions*	1913 Acid-Base Management: Respiratory Acidosis **G*** 1914 Acid-Base Management: Respiratory Alkalosis **G** 3120 Airway Insertion and Stabilization 3140 Airway Management 3160 Airway Suctioning 6412 Anaphylaxis Management **V** 3180 Artificial Airway Management 3200 Aspiration Precautions **V** 3210 Asthma Management 3230 Chest Physiotherapy 3250 Cough Enhancement 4106 Embolus Care: Pulmonary **N** 3270 Endotracheal Extubation 3300 Mechanical Ventilation Management: Invasive 3302 Mechanical Ventilation Management: Noninvasive 3304 Mechanical Ventilation Management: Pneumonia Prevention **V** 3310 Mechanical Ventilatory Weaning 3316 Nasal Irrigation 3320 Oxygen Therapy 3330 Positioning: Prone 3340 Rapid Sequence Induction and Intubation 3350 Respiratory Monitoring 1872 Tube Care: Chest 3390 Ventilation Assistance	3420 Amputation Care 3440 Incision Site Care 3460 Leech Therapy 3480 Lower Extremity Monitoring 0480 Ostomy Care **B** 3510 Phototherapy: Skin 3520 Pressure Injury Care 3540 Pressure Injury Prevention **V** 3550 Pruritus Management **E** 3570 Skin Care: Absorbent Products 3582 Skin Care: Donor Site **J** 3583 Skin Care: Graft Site **J** 3584 Skin Care: Topical Treatment 3590 Skin Surveillance 3620 Suturing 3660 Wound Care 3661 Wound Care: Burns 3662 Wound Care: Closed Drainage 3664 Wound Care: Nonhealing 3670 Wound Care: Protection 3680 Wound Irrigation
	3100 to 3399	3400 to 3699

*Letter indicates another class where the intervention is also included.

M. Thermoregulation

Interventions to maintain body temperature within a normal range

3786 Hyperthermia Management
3790 Hypothermia Induction Therapy
3800 Hypothermia Treatment
3840 Malignant Hyperthermia Precautions **U**
3900 Temperature Regulation
3910 Temperature Regulation: Newborn
3902 Temperature Regulation: Perioperative **J**
3920 Thermoregulation Management

N. Tissue Perfusion Management

Interventions to optimize circulation of blood and fluids to the tissue

2860 Autotransfusion **J**
4010 Bleeding Precautions
4020 Bleeding Reduction
4021 Bleeding Reduction: Antepartum Uterus **W**
4022 Bleeding Reduction: Gastrointestinal
4024 Bleeding Reduction: Nasal
4026 Bleeding Reduction: Postpartum Uterus **W**
4028 Bleeding Reduction: Wound
4030 Blood Products Administration
4035 Capillary Blood Sample
4040 Cardiac Care
4044 Cardiac Care: Acute
4046 Cardiac Care: Rehabilitative
4050 Cardiac Risk Management
4054 Central Venous Access Management: Central Insertion **H**
4220 Central Venous Access Management: Peripheral Insertion **H**
4062 Circulatory Care: Arterial Insufficiency
4064 Circulatory Care: Mechanical Assist Device
4066 Circulatory Care: Venous Insufficiency
4070 Circulatory Precautions
4095 Defibrillator Management: External **U**
4096 Defibrillator Management: Internal
4240 Dialysis Access Maintenance
4090 Dysrhythmia Management
4104 Embolus Care: Peripheral
4106 Embolus Care: Pulmonary **K**
4110 Embolus Precautions

4115 Extracorporeal Membrane Oxygenation (ECMO) Therapy
2080 Fluid/Electrolyte Management **G**
4120 Fluid Management
4130 Fluid Monitoring
4140 Fluid Resuscitation
4150 Hemodynamic Regulation
4162 Hypertension Management
4170 Hypervolemia Management
4175 Hypotension Management
4180 Hypovolemia Management
4190 Intravenous (IV) Insertion
4200 Intravenous (IV) Therapy
4210 Invasive Hemodynamic Monitoring
4091 Pacemaker Management: Permanent
4092 Pacemaker Management: Temporary
4232 Phlebotomy: Arterial Blood Sample **G**
4234 Phlebotomy: Blood Acquisition
4238 Phlebotomy: Venous Blood Sample
4250 Shock Management
4254 Shock Management: Cardiac
4255 Shock Management: Sepsis
4256 Shock Management: Vasogenic
4258 Shock Management: Volume
4260 Shock Prevention
4266 Stem Cell Infusion
4270 Thrombolytic Therapy Management **H**

Level 1 Domains	3. BEHAVIORAL	
	Care that supports psychosocial functioning and facilitates lifestyle changes	

Level 2 Classes	O. **Behavior Therapy**	P. **Cognitive Therapy**
	Interventions to reinforce or promote desirable behaviors or alter undesirable behaviors	Interventions to reinforce or promote desirable cognitive functioning or alter undesirable cognitive functioning

Level 3 Interventions

O. Behavior Therapy:

4310 Activity Therapy
4320 Animal-Assisted Therapy **Q***
4330 Art Therapy **Q**
4340 Assertiveness Training
4420 Behavior Contracting
4350 Behavior Management
4352 Behavior Management: Inattention and Hyperactivity
4354 Behavior Management: Self-Harm
4356 Behavior Management: Sexual
4360 Behavior Modification
4362 Behavior Modification: Social Skills
4364 Commendation
4367 Dance Therapy
4368 Gardening Therapy
4370 Impulse Control Training
4380 Limit Setting
4390 Milieu Therapy
4395 Motivational Interviewing
4400 Music Therapy **Q**
4410 Mutual Goal Setting
6926 Phototherapy: Mood Regulation
4470 Self-Modification Assistance
4480 Self-Responsibility Facilitation
4490 Smoking Cessation Assistance
4500 Substance Use Prevention
4510 Substance Use Treatment
4512 Substance Use Treatment: Alcohol Withdrawal
4514 Substance Use Treatment: Drug Withdrawal
4516 Substance Use Treatment: Overdose
4430 Therapeutic Play **Q**

P. Cognitive Therapy:

4640 Anger Control Assistance
4680 Bibliotherapy
4700 Cognitive Restructuring
4720 Cognitive Stimulation
4730 Guided Reflection
4740 Journaling
5520 Learning Facilitation **S**
4760 Memory Training
4820 Reality Orientation
4860 Reminiscence Therapy

4300 to 4599   4600 to 4899

*Letter indicates another class where the intervention is also included.

Q. Communication Enhancement

Interventions to facilitate delivering and receiving
verbal and nonverbal messages

4920 Active Listening
4320 Animal-Assisted Therapy **O**
4330 Art Therapy **O**
5000 Caring Interaction Development
4974 Communication Enhancement: Hearing Deficit
4976 Communication Enhancement: Speech Deficit
4978 Communication Enhancement: Visual Deficit
5020 Conflict Mediation
5328 Listening Visits **R**
4400 Music Therapy **O**
5100 Socialization Enhancement
4430 Therapeutic Play **O**
6675 Vision Screening **V**

Level 1 Domains	**3. BEHAVIORAL—cont'd**
	Care that supports psychosocial functioning and facilitates life style changes

Level 2 Classes	**R. Coping Assistance**	**S. Health Education**
	Interventions to assist another to build on own strengths, to adapt to a change in function, or achieve a higher level of function	Interventions to facilitate learning

Level 3 Interventions		
	5210 Anticipatory Guidance **Z***	2240 Chemotherapy Management **H**
	5215 Bereavement Care	6784 Family Planning: Contraception **W**
	5220 Body Image Enhancement	5510 Health Education **c**
	5230 Coping Enhancement	5515 Health Literacy Enhancement
	5240 Counseling	5520 Learning Facilitation **P**
	6160 Crisis Intervention **U**	5562 Parent Education: Adolescent **Z**
	5250 Decision-Making Support **Y**	5566 Parent Education: Childrearing Family **Z**
	5260 Dying Care	5568 Parent Education: Infant **Z**
	5270 Emotional Support	5580 Preparatory Sensory Information
	5280 Forgiveness Facilitation	5670 Teaching: Adolescent Development 12–21 Years **Z**
	5242 Genetic Counseling **W**	5672 Teaching: Adolescent Nutrition 12–21 Years **Z**
	5290 Grief Work Facilitation	5674 Teaching: Adolescent Safety 12–21 Years **Z**
	5294 Grief Work Facilitation: Perinatal Death **W**	5602 Teaching: Disease Process
	5300 Guilt Work Facilitation	5680 Teaching: Early Childhood Development 1–5 Years
	5305 Health Coaching	5682 Teaching: Early Childhood Nutrition 1–5 Years
	5310 Hope Inspiration	5684 Teaching: Early Childhood Safety1–5 Years
	5320 Humor	5604 Teaching: Group
	5326 Life Skills Enhancement	5606 Teaching: Individual
	5328 Listening Visits **Q**	5655 Teaching: Infant Development 0–3 Months **Z**
	5330 Mood Management	5658 Teaching: Infant Development 4–6 Months **Z**
	5340 Presence	5656 Teaching: Infant Development 7-9 Months **Z**
	5360 Recreation Therapy	5657 Teaching: Infant Development 10–12 Months **Z**
	5235 Relapse Prevention	5640 Teaching: Infant Nutrition 0–3 Months **Z**
	5422 Religious Addiction Therapy	5641 Teaching: Infant Nutrition 4–6 Months **Z**
	5424 Religious Ritual Enhancement	5642 Teaching: Infant Nutrition 7–9 Months **Z**
	5350 Relocation Stress Reduction	5643 Teaching: Infant Nutrition 10–12 Months **Z**
	5370 Role Enhancement **X**	5645 Teaching: Infant Safety 0–3 Months **Z**
	5390 Self-Awareness Enhancement	5646 Teaching: Infant Safety 4–6 Months **Z**
	5395 Self-Efficacy Enhancement	5647 Teaching: Infant Safety 7–9 Months **Z**
	5400 Self-Esteem Enhancement	5648 Teaching: Infant Safety 10–12 Months **Z**
	5248 Sexual Counseling	5649 Teaching: Infection Control **V**
	5426 Spiritual Growth Facilitation	5650 Teaching: Middle Childhood Development 6–12 Years **Z**
	5420 Spiritual Support	5652 Teaching: Middle Childhood Nutrition 6–12 Years **Z**
	5430 Support Group	5654 Teaching: Middle Childhood Safety 6–12 Years **Z**
	5440 Support System Enhancement	5610 Teaching: Preoperative **J**
	5450 Therapy Group	5614 Teaching: Prescribed Diet **D**
	5460 Touch	5612 Teaching: Prescribed Exercise **A**
	5410 Trauma Therapy: Child	5616 Teaching: Prescribed Medication **H**
	5470 Truth Telling	5618 Teaching: Procedure or Treatment
	5480 Values Clarification	5620 Teaching: Psychomotor Skill
		5622 Teaching: Safe Sex
		5624 Teaching: Sexuality
		5660 Teaching: Toddler Nutrition 13–18 Months **Z**
		5661 Teaching: Toddler Nutrition 19–24 Months **Z**
		5662 Teaching: Toddler Nutrition 25–36 Months **Z**
		5665 Teaching: Toddler Safety 13–18 Months **Z**
		5666 Teaching: Toddler Safety 19–24 Months **Z**
		5667 Teaching: Toddler Safety 25–36 Months **Z**
		5634 Teaching: Toilet Training **Z**
	5200 to 5499	**5500 to 5799**

*Letter indicates another class where the intervention is also included.

T. Psychological Comfort Promotion
Interventions to promote comfort using psychological techniques

5820 Anxiety Reduction
5840 Autogenic Training
5860 Biofeedback
5880 Calming Technique
5900 Distraction
6000 Guided Imagery
5920 Hypnosis
5930 Laughter Yoga
5960 Meditation Facilitation
6040 Relaxation Therapy
5922 Self-Hypnosis Facilitation
6050 Yoga

Level 1
Domains

4. SAFETY
Care that supports protection against harm

Level 2
Classes

U. **Crisis Management**

Interventions to provide immediate short-term help in both psychological and physiological crises

Level 3
Interventions

6140 Code Management
6160 Crisis Intervention **R***
6170 De-Escalation Management
4095 Defibrillator Management: External **N**
6200 Emergency Care
7170 Family Presence Facilitation **X**
6240 First Aid
3840 Malignant Hyperthermia Precautions **M**
6260 Organ Procurement
6320 Resuscitation
6300 Sexual Assault Trauma Care
6340 Suicide Prevention **V**
6362 Triage: Disaster
6364 Triage: Emergency Center
6366 Triage: Telecommunication

6100 to 6399

*Letter indicates another class where the intervention is also included.

V. Risk Management

Interventions to initiate risk reduction activities and continue monitoring risks over time

6400 Abuse Protection Support
6402 Abuse Protection Support: Child **Z**
6403 Abuse Protection Support: Domestic Partner
6404 Abuse Protection Support: Elder
6408 Abuse Protection Support: Religious
6410 Allergy Management
6412 Anaphylaxis Management **K**
6420 Area Restriction
3200 Aspiration Precautions **K**
6425 Body Search
6522 Breast Examination
6430 Chemical Restraint **H**
6440 Delirium Management
6450 Delusion Management
6460 Dementia Management
6462 Dementia Management: Bathing **F**
6466 Dementia Management: Wandering
6470 Elopement Precautions
6480 Environmental Management
6486 Environmental Management: Safety
6487 Environmental Management: Violence Prevention
6490 Fall Prevention
6500 Fire-Setting Precautions
6510 Hallucination Management
6520 Health Screening **d**
6525 Human Trafficking Detection
6540 Infection Control
6550 Infection Protection

6560 Laser Precautions **J**
6570 Latex Precautions
3304 Mechanical Ventilation Management: Pneumonia Prevention **K**
2395 Medication Reconciliation **H**
6580 Neutropenic Precautions
6592 Pandemic Precautions
6574 Patient Identification
6576 Physical Accompaniment
6594 Physical Distancing Facilitation
6580 Physical Restraint **C**
3540 Pressure Injury Prevention **L**
6596 Quarantine Facilitation
6600 Radiation Therapy Management
6610 Risk Identification **d**
6620 Risk Identification: Infectious Disease
6630 Seclusion
2680 Seizure Management **I**
6340 Suicide Prevention **U**
2920 Surgical Precautions **J**
6650 Surveillance
6660 Surveillance: Video Monitoring
5649 Teaching: Infection Control **S**
6648 Teaching: Sports Injury Prevention **Z**
6530 Vaccination Management **c**
6670 Validation Therapy
9050 Vehicle Safety Promotion **d**
6675 Vision Screening **Q**
6680 Vital Signs Monitoring

Level 1
Domains

Level 2
Classes

Level 3
Interventions

5. FAMILY
Care that supports the family

W. Childbearing Care

Interventions to assist in the preparation for childbirth and management of the psychological and physiological changes before, during, and immediately following childbirth

6700 Amnioinfusion
6720 Birthing
4021 Bleeding Reduction: Antepartum Uterus **N***
4026 Bleeding Reduction: Postpartum Uterus **N**
6750 Cesarean Birth Care
6760 Childbirth Preparation
3000 Circumcision Care **J**
6771 Electronic Fetal Monitoring: Antepartum
6772 Electronic Fetal Monitoring: Intrapartum
7104 Family Integrity Promotion: Childbearing Family
6784 Family Planning: Contraception **S**
6786 Family Planning: Infertility
6788 Family Planning: Unplanned Pregnancy
7160 Fertility Preservation
5242 Genetic Counseling **R**
5294 Grief Work Facilitation: Perinatal Death **R**
6800 High-Risk Pregnancy Care
6824 Infant Care: Newborn
6826 Infant Care: Preterm
6830 Intrapartal Care
6834 Intrapartal Care: High-Risk Delivery
6840 Kangaroo Care
6850 Labor Induction
6855 Labor Pain Management **E**
6860 Labor Suppression
6870 Lactation Suppression
6900 Nonnutritive Sucking
6924 Phototherapy: Neonate
6930 Postpartal Care
5247 Preconception Counseling
6950 Pregnancy Termination Care
6960 Prenatal Care
6965 Procedural Support: Infant
7886 Reproductive Technology Management
6972 Resuscitation: Fetus
6974 Resuscitation: Neonate
6612 Risk Identification: Childbearing Family
6656 Surveillance: Late Pregnancy
1875 Tube Care: Umbilical Line
6982 Ultrasonography: Obstetric and Gynecologic

*Letter indicates another class where the intervention is also included.

Z. Childrearing Care

Interventions to assist in raising children

6402 Abuse Protection Support: Child V
8272 Adolescent Care
5210 Anticipatory Guidance **R**
6710 Attachment Promotion
1052 Bottle Feeding
0412 Bowel Incontinence Care: Encopresis **B**
8274 Child Care
8240 Cup Feeding: Newborn
8278 Developmental Enhancement: Infant
6820 Infant Care
6810 Infant Care: Eye Examination Support
5244 Lactation Counseling
7200 Normalization Promotion
5562 Parent Education: Adolescent **S**
5566 Parent Education: Childrearing Family **S**
5568 Parent Education: Infant **S**
8300 Parenting Promotion
8340 Resilience Promotion
7280 Sibling Support
5670 Teaching: Adolescent Development 12–21 Years **S**
5672 Teaching: Adolescent Nutrition 12–21 Years **S**
5674 Teaching: Adolescent Safety 12–21 Years **S**
5680 Teaching: Early Childhood Development 1–5 Years **S**
5682 Teaching: Early Childhood Nutrition 1–5 Years **S**
5684 Teaching: Early Childhood Safety 1––5 Years **S**
5655 Teaching: Infant Development 0–3 Months **S**
5658 Teaching: Infant Development 4–6 Months **S**
5656 Teaching: Infant Development 7–9 Months **S**
5657 Teaching: Infant Development 10–12 Months **S**
5640 Teaching: Infant Nutrition 0–3 Months **S**
5641 Teaching: Infant Nutrition 4–6 Months **S**
5642 Teaching: Infant Nutrition 7–9 Months **S**
5643 Teaching: Infant Nutrition 10–12 Months **S**
5645 Teaching: Infant Safety 0–3 Months **S**
5646 Teaching: Infant Safety 4–6 Months **S**
5647 Teaching: Infant Safety 7–9 Months **S**
5648 Teaching: Infant Safety 10–12 Months **S**
5650 Teaching: Middle Childhood Development 6–12 Years **S**
5652 Teaching: Middle Childhood Nutrition 6–12 Years **S**
5654 Teaching: Middle Childhood Safety 6–12 Years **S**
6648 Teaching: Sports Injury Prevention **V**
5660 Teaching: Toddler Nutrition 13–18 Months **S**
5661 Teaching: Toddler Nutrition 19–24 Months **S**
5662 Teaching: Toddler Nutrition 25–36 Months **S**
5665 Teaching: Toddler Safety 13–18 Months **S**
5666 Teaching: Toddler Safety 19–24 Months **S**
5667 Teaching: Toddler Safety 25–36 Months **S**
5634 Teaching: Toilet Training **S**
0612 Urinary Incontinence Care: Enuresis **B**

X. Lifespan Care

Interventions to facilitate family unit functioning and promote the health and welfare of family members throughout the lifespan

7040 Caregiver Support
7100 Family Integrity Promotion
7110 Family Involvement Promotion
7120 Family Mobilization
7170 Family Presence Facilitation **U**
7130 Family Process Maintenance
7140 Family Support
7150 Family Therapy
7180 Home Maintenance Assistance
7260 Respite Care
6614 Risk Identification: Genetic
5370 Role Enhancement **R**

Level 1 *Domains*	**6. HEALTH SYSTEM** **Care that supports effective use of the healthcare delivery system**
Level 2 *Classes*	**Y. Health System Mediation** Interventions to facilitate the interface between person/family and the healthcare system
Level 3 *Interventions*	7300 Advanced Care Planning 7310 Admission Care 7320 Case Management **c*** 7330 Cultural Care Negotiation 5250 Decision-Making Support **R** 7370 Discharge Planning 6485 Discharge Planning: Home Preparation 7380 Financial Resource Assistance 7400 Health System Guidance 7410 Insurance Authorization 7440 Pass Facilitation 7460 Patient Rights Protection 2880 Preoperative Coordination **J** 7470 Readmission Prevention 7500 Sustenance Support 7560 Visitation Facilitation

7300 to 7599

*Letter indicates another class where the intervention is also included.

a. Health System Management

Interventions to provide and enhance support services for the delivery of care

7615 Collaboration Enhancement
7850 Competency Management
7620 Controlled Substance Checking
7630 Cost Containment
7640 Critical Path Development
7650 Delegation
7660 Emergency Cart Checking
7680 Examination Assistance
8550 Fiscal Resource Management **c**
7685 Healthcare Provider Collaboration
7690 Laboratory Data Interpretation
7700 Peer Review
7610 Point of Care Testing
7722 Preceptor: Employee
7726 Preceptor: Student
7760 Product Evaluation
7770 Professional Development Facilitation
7800 Quality Monitoring
7810 Safety Huddle
7820 Specimen Management
7830 Staff Supervision
7840 Supply Chain Management
7880 Technology Management
7890 Transport: Interfacility
7892 Transport: Intrafacility

b. Information Management

Interventions to facilitate communication about health care

7910 Consultation
7930 Deposition
8190 Discharge Follow-Up
7920 Documentation
7926 Documentation: Meetings
8070 Electronic Health Record Access Assistance
7940 Forensic Data Collection
8140 Handoff Report
7960 Healthcare Information Exchange
7970 Health Policy Monitoring **c**
7980 Incident Reporting
8020 Multidisciplinary Care Conference
8060 Order Transcription
8080 Prescribing: Diagnostic Testing
8086 Prescribing: Nonpharmalogic Treatment
8100 Referral
8130 Research Protocol Management
6658 Surveillance: Remote Monitoring
8180 Telecommunication Consultation

Level 1
Domains

Level 2
Classes

Level 3
Interventions

7. **COMMUNITY**
Care that supports the health of the community

c. **Community Health Promotion**
   Interventions that promote the health of the whole community

7320 Case Management **Y***
8510 Community Health Advocacy
8500 Community Health Development
8550 Fiscal Resource Management **a**
5510 Health Education **S**
7970 Health Policy Monitoring **b**
8700 Program Development
8720 Resilience Promotion: Community
8740 Social Justice Facilitation
8750 Social Marketing
6530 Vaccination Management **V**

8500-8799

*Letter indicates another class where the intervention is also included.

d. Community Risk Management

Interventions that assist in detecting or preventing health risks to the whole community

8810 Bioterrorism Preparedness
8820 Communicable Disease Management
8840 Community Disaster Preparedness
6484 Environmental Management: Community
6489 Environmental Management: Worker Safety
8880 Environmental Risk Protection
6520 Health Screening **V**
6610 Risk Identification **V**
6652 Surveillance: Community
9050 Vehicle Safety Promotion **V**

PART THREE

The Classification

A

Abdominal Massage 1310

Definition: The process of circular hand movements to the abdomen to reduce pain, decrease bloating, and improve constipation

Activities:

- Screen for contraindications (e.g., decreased platelets, decreased skin integrity, deep vein thrombosis, areas with open lesions, redness or inflammation, tumors, hypersensitivity to touch)
- Place in supine position in relaxed manner
- Explain procedure and benefits of abdominal massage
- Instruct on diaphragmatic breathing technique
- Maintain privacy before exposing abdomen
- Warm hands
- Move hands in clockwise or counterclockwise motions, or form the letters I, L, U, and O with hand motions
- Perform abdominal massage at least 2 hours after having meal
- Instruct on appropriate volume of daily fluid intake if there is no fluid limitation
- Instruct on appropriate amount of fiber
- Use essential oils during massage to enhance reduced symptoms (e.g., peppermint, fennel, ginger, anise, cinnamon)
- Instruct to defecate by sitting in position with hip bent in 90-degree angle while body upright, if possible
- Instruct person on complete bed rest to defecate in lateral position with hip and knee flexed
- Monitor bowel habits and any distention after abdominal massage daily
- Document massage and response

Background Evidence:

Birimoglu Okuyan, C., & Bilgili, N. (2019). Effect of abdominal massage on constipation and quality of life in older adults: A randomized controlled trial. *Complementary Therapies in Medicine, 47*, 102219. https://doi.org/10.1016/j.ctim.2019.102219

Çevik, K., Çetinkaya, A., Yiğit Gökbel, K., Menekşe, B., Saza, S., & Tıkız, C. (2018). The effect of abdominal massage on constipation in the elderly residing in rest homes. *Gastroenterology Nursing, 41*(5), 396–402. https://doi.org/10.1097/sga.0000000000000343

Dehghan, M., Mehdipoor, R., & Ahmadinejad, M. (2018). Does abdominal massage improve gastrointestinal functions of intensive care patients with an endotracheal tube? A randomized clinical trial. *Complementary Therapies in Clinical Practice, 30*, 122–128. https://doi.org/10.1016/j.ctcp.2017.12.018

Fekri, Z., Aghebati, N., Sadeghi, T., & Farzadfard, M. T. (2021). The effects of abdominal "I LOV U" massage along with lifestyle training on constipation and distension in the elderly with stroke. *Complementary Therapies in Medicine, 57*, 102665. https://doi.org/10.1016/j.ctim.2021.102665

Forootan, M., Bagheri, N., & Darvishi, M. (2018). Chronic constipation: A review of literature. *Medicine, 97*(20), e10631–e10631. https://doi.org/10.1097/MD.0000000000010631

Li, J., Yuan, M., Liu, Y., Zhao, Y., Wang, J., & Guo, W. (2017). Incidence of constipation in stroke patients: A systematic review and meta-analysis. *Medicine, 96*(25). https://doi.org/10.1097/MD.0000000000007225

8th edition 2024

Abuse Protection Support 6400

Definition: Identification of high-risk dependent relationships and actions to prevent further infliction of physical or emotional harm

Activities:

- Identify individuals who are at risk for possible abuse (e.g., pregnancy complications, low birth weight, disability, history associated with abuse or neglect, rejection, excessive criticism, feelings of being worthless and unloved, dependency upon another for cares)
- Consider parental risk factors for possible abuse (e.g., substance abuse, criminal behavior, family conflict or violence, mental health issues, child being perceived as problem by parents, unplanned pregnancy, youth pregnancy, single or unmarried parents, parental temperament, use of physical punishment)
- Identify social and environmental factors that may be indicators for possible abuse (e.g., social isolation, low self-esteem, physical health conditions, housing stress, socioeconomic stressors, parental unemployment, lack of prenatal care, low social support, neighborhood violence, community disadvantage)
- Identify persons who have difficulty trusting others or feel disliked by others
- Identify if person feels asking for help is indicator of personal incompetence
- Determine whether family needs periodic relief from care responsibilities
- Identify whether adult at risk has close friends or family available to help with dependents
- Determine relationship between caregivers and individuals
- Determine whether adults can take over for each other when needed to deal with dependent family member
- Determine whether child or dependent adult is viewed differently by adult based on sex, appearance, or behavior
- Identify crisis situations that may trigger abuse (e.g., poverty, unemployment, divorce, loss)
- Monitor for signs of neglect in high-risk families
- Observe ill or injured child or dependent adult for signs of abuse
- Listen to explanation of how illness or injury happened
- Identify when explanation of cause of injury is inconsistent among those involved
- Encourage admission of child or dependent adult for further observation and investigation, as appropriate
- Record times and duration of visits during hospitalization
- Monitor parent-child interactions and record observations, as appropriate
- Monitor for underreactions or overreactions on part of adult
- Monitor child or dependent adult for extreme compliance, such as passive submission to hospital procedures

- Monitor child for role reversal such as comforting parent, or overactive or aggressive behavior
- Listen attentively to adult who begins to talk about own problems
- Listen to pregnant woman's feelings about pregnancy and expectations about unborn child
- Monitor new parent's reactions to infant, observing for feelings of disgust, fear, or unrealistic expectations
- Monitor parent who holds newborn at arm's length, handles newborn awkwardly, or asks for excessive assistance
- Monitor for repeated visits to clinic, emergency room, or health care provider office for minor problems
- Monitor for progressive deterioration in physical and emotional care provided to child or dependent adult in family
- Monitor child for signs of failure to thrive, depression, apathy, developmental delay, or malnutrition
- Determine expectations adult has for child to determine whether expected behaviors are realistic
- Instruct parents on realistic expectations of child based on developmental level
- Establish rapport with families with history of abuse for long-term evaluation and support
- Help families identify coping strategies for stressful situations
- Instruct adult family members on signs of abuse
- Refer person at risk to appropriate specialists
- Inform appropriate health care provider of observations indicative of abuse
- Report any situations in which abuse suspected to proper authorities
- Refer person to shelters for abused spouses, as appropriate
- Refer parents to support group support, as appropriate
- Encourage person to contact police when physical safety threatened
- Inform person of laws and services relevant to abuse

1st edition 1992; revised 2000, 2004, 2024

Background Evidence:

Berkowitz, C. D. (2017). Physical abuse of children. *The New England Journal of Medicine, 376*(17), 1659–1666. https://doi.org/10.1056/NEJMcp1701446

Centers for Disease Control and Prevention. (2021, March 15). *Child abuse and neglect prevention.* https://www.cdc.gov/violenceprevention/childabuseandneglect/index.html

Centers for Disease Control and Prevention. (2021, June 2). *Elder abuse.* https://www.cdc.gov/violenceprevention/elderabuse/index.html

Hoehn, E. F., Wilson, P. M., Riney, L. C., Ngo, V., Bennett, B., & Duma, E. (2018). Identification and evaluation of physical abuse in children. *Pediatric Annals, 47*(3), e97–e101. https://doi.org/10.3928/19382359-20180227-01

Hoft, M., & Haddad, L. (2017). Screening children for abuse and neglect: A review of the literature. *Journal of Forensic Nursing, 13*(1), 26–34. https://doi.org/10.1097/JFN.0000000000000136

Pickering, C. E., Ridenour, K., Salaysay, Z., Reyes-Gastelum, D., & Pierce, S. J. (2017). Identifying elder abuse & neglect among family caregiving dyads: A cross sectional study of psychometric properties of the QualCare scale. *International Journal of Nursing Studies, 69*, 41–46. https://doi.org/10.1016/j.ijnurstu.2017.01.012

Raz, M., Dettlaff, A., & Edwards, F. (2021). The perils of child "protection" for children of color: Lessons from history. *Pediatrics, 148*(1), 1–4. https://doi.org/10.1542/peds.2021-050237

Read, J., Harper, D., Tucker, I., & Kennedy, A. (2018). Do adult mental health services identify child abuse and neglect? A systematic review. *International journal of Mental Health Nursing, 27*(1), 7–19. https://doi.org/10.1111/inm.12369

Teeuw, A. H., Kraan, R., van Rijn, R. R., Bossuyt, P., & Heymans, H. (2019). Screening for child abuse using a checklist and physical examinations in the emergency department led to the detection of more cases. *Acta Paediatrica, 108*(2), 300–313. https://doi.org/10.1111/apa.14495

Williams, P. (2020). *Basic geriatric nursing* (7th ed.). Elsevier.

Abuse Protection Support: Child   6402

Definition: Identification of high-risk, dependent child relationships and actions to prevent possible or further infliction of physical, sexual, or emotional harm or neglect of basic necessities of life

Activities:

- Identify mothers who have a history of no or late (4 months or later) prenatal care
- Identify parents who have had another child removed from the home or have placed previous children with relatives for extended periods
- Identify parents who have a history of substance abuse, depression, or major psychiatric illness
- Identify parents who demonstrate an increased need for parent education (e.g., parents with learning problems, parents who verbalize feelings of inadequacy, parents of a first child, teen parents)
- Identify parents with a history of domestic violence or a mother who has a history of numerous "accidental" injuries
- Identify parents with a history of unhappy childhoods associated with abuse, rejection, excessive criticism, or feelings of being worthless and unloved
- Identify crisis situations that may trigger abuse (e.g., poverty, unemployment, divorce, homelessness, domestic violence)
- Determine whether the family has an intact social support network to assist with family problems, respite child care, and crisis child care

- Identify infants and children with high-care needs (e.g., prematurity, low birth weight, colic, feeding intolerances, major health problems in the first year of life, developmental disabilities, hyperactivity, attention deficit disorders)
- Identify caretaker explanations of child's injuries that are improbable or inconsistent, allege self-injury, blame other children, or demonstrate a delay in seeking treatment
- Determine whether a child demonstrates signs of physical abuse (e.g., numerous injuries, unexplained bruises and welts, burns, fractures, unexplained facial lacerations and abrasions, human bite marks, whiplash, shaken infant syndrome)
- Determine whether the child demonstrates signs of neglect (e.g., failure to thrive, wasting of subcutaneous tissue, consistent hunger, poor hygiene, constant fatigue and listlessness, skin afflictions, apathy, unyielding body posture, inappropriate dress for weather conditions)
- Determine whether the child demonstrates signs of sexual abuse (e.g., difficulty walking or sitting, torn or bloody underclothing, reddened or traumatized genitals, vaginal or anal lacerations, recurrent urinary tract infections, poor sphincter tone, acquired sexually transmitted diseases, pregnancy, promiscuous behavior, history of running away)

A

- Determine whether the child demonstrates signs of emotional abuse (e.g., lags in physical development, habit disorders, conduct learning disorders, neurotic traits or psychoneurotic reactions, behavioral extremes, cognitive developmental lags, attempted suicide)
- Encourage admission of child for further observation and investigation, as appropriate
- Record times and durations of visits during hospitalizations
- Monitor parent-child interactions and record observations
- Determine whether acute symptoms in child abate when child is separated from family
- Determine whether parents have unrealistic expectations or negative attributions for their child's behavior
- Monitor child for extreme compliance, such as passive submission to invasive procedures
- Monitor child for role reversal, such as comforting the parent, or overactive or aggressive behavior
- Listen to pregnant woman's feelings about pregnancy and expectations about the unborn child
- Monitor new parents' reactions to their infant, observing for feelings of disgust, fear, or disappointment in gender
- Monitor for a parent who holds newborn at arm's length, handles newborn awkwardly, asks for excessive assistance, and verbalizes or demonstrates discomfort in caring for the child
- Monitor for repeated visits to clinics, emergency rooms, or physicians' offices for minor problems
- Establish a system to flag the records of children who are suspected victims of child abuse or neglect
- Monitor for a progressive deterioration in the physical and emotional state of the infant or child
- Determine parent's knowledge of basic care needs and provide appropriate childcare information, as indicated
- Instruct parents on problem solving, decision making, and childrearing and parenting skills, or refer parents to programs in which these skills can be learned
- Help families identify coping strategies for stressful situations
- Provide parents with information on how to cope with protracted infant crying, emphasizing that they should not shake the baby
- Provide the parents with noncorporal punishment methods for disciplining children
- Provide pregnant women and their families with information on the effects of smoking, poor nutrition, and substance abuse on both the baby's and their health
- Engage parents and child in attachment-building exercises
- Provide parents and their adolescents with information on decision-making and communication skills, and refer to youth services counseling, as appropriate

- Provide older children with concrete information on how to provide for the basic care needs of their younger siblings
- Provide children with positive affirmations of their worth, nurturing care, therapeutic communication, and developmental stimulation
- Provide children who have been sexually abused with reassurance that the abuse was not their fault and allow them to express their concerns through play therapy appropriate for age
- Refer at-risk pregnant women and parents of newborns to nurse home visitation services
- Provide at-risk families with a Public Health Nurse referral to ensure that the home environment is monitored, that siblings are assessed, and that families receive continued assistance
- Refer families to human services and counseling professionals, as needed
- Provide parents with community resource information (e.g., addresses and phone numbers of agencies that provide respite care, emergency child care, housing assistance, substance abuse treatment, sliding-fee counseling services, food pantries, clothing distribution centers, domestic abuse shelters)
- Inform physician of observations indicative of abuse or neglect
- Report suspected abuse or neglect to proper authorities
- Refer a parent who is being battered and at-risk children to a domestic violence shelter
- Refer parents to Parents Anonymous for group support, as appropriate

2nd edition 1996; revised 2000, 2013

Background Evidence:

Asgeirsdottir, B. B., Sigfusdottir, I. D., Gudjonsson, G. H., & Sigurdsson, J. F. (2011). Associations between sexual abuse and family conflict/violence, self-injurious behavior, and substance use: The mediating role of depressed mood and anger. *Child Abuse and Neglect, 35*(3), 210–219.

Bylander, M., & Kydd, J. (2008). Violence to children, definition and prevention of. In L. Kurtz (Ed.), *Encyclopedia of violence, peace, and conflict* (2nd. ed., pp. 2318–2330). Academic Press.

Cowen, P. S. (2006). Child maltreatment: Developmental and health effects. In P. S. Cowen & S. Moorhead (Eds.), *Current issues in nursing* (7th ed., pp. 684–701). Mosby Elsevier.

Cowen, P. S. (2006). Child neglect prevention: The pivotal role of nursing. In P. S. Cowen & S. Moorhead (Eds.), *Current issues in nursing* (7th ed., pp. 702–726). Mosby Elsevier.

Dubowitz, H., Kim, J., Black, M., Weisbart, C., Semiatin, J., & Magder, L. (2011). Identifying children at high risk for a child maltreatment report. *Child Abuse and Neglect, 35*(2), 96–104.

Scannapieco, M., & Connell-Carrick, K. (2005). *Understanding child maltreatment: An ecological and developmental perspective.* Oxford University Press.

Abuse Protection Support: Domestic Partner   6403

Definition: Identification of high-risk, dependent domestic relationships and actions to prevent possible or further infliction of physical, sexual, or emotional harm or exploitation of a domestic partner

Activities:
- Screen for risk factors associated with domestic abuse (e.g., history of domestic violence, abuse, rejection, excessive criticism, or feelings of being worthless and unloved; difficulty trusting others or feeling disliked by others; feeling that asking for help is an indication of personal incompetence; high physical care needs; intense family care responsibilities; substance abuse; depression; major psychiatric illness; social isolation; poor relationships between domestic partners; multiple marriages; pregnancy; poverty; unemployment; financial dependence; homelessness; infidelity; divorce; or death of a loved one)
- Screen for symptoms of a history of domestic abuse (e.g., numerous accidental injuries, multiple somatic symptoms, chronic abdominal pain, chronic headaches, pelvic pain, anxiety, depression, posttraumatic stress syndrome, and other psychiatric disorders)

- Monitor for signs and symptoms of physical abuse (e.g., numerous injuries in various stages of healing; unexplained lacerations, bruises or welts, patches of missing hair, restraining marks on wrists or ankles, "defensive" bruises on forearms, human bite marks)
- Monitor for signs and symptoms of sexual abuse (e.g., presence of semen or dried blood, injury to external genital, acquired sexually transmitted diseases,or dramatic behavioral or health changes of an undetermined etiology)
- Monitor for signs and symptoms of emotional abuse (e.g., low self-esteem, depression, humiliation, and defeat; overly cautious behavior around partner; aggression against self or suicide gestures)
- Monitor for signs and symptoms of exploitation (e.g., inadequate provision for basic needs when adequate resources are available; deprivation of personal possessions; unexplained loss of social support checks; lack of knowledge of personal finances or legal matters)
- Document evidence of physical or sexual abuse using standardized assessment tools and photographs
- Listen attentively to individual who begins to talk about own problems
- Identify inconsistencies in explanation of cause of injury(ies)
- Determine congruence between the type of injury and the description of cause
- Interview patient or knowledgeable other about suspected abuse in the absence of partner
- Encourage admission to a hospital for further observation and investigation, as appropriate
- Monitor partner interactions and record observations, as appropriate (e.g., record times and duration of partner visits during hospitalization, underreactions or overreactions by partner)
- Monitor the individual for extreme compliance, such as passive submission to hospital procedures
- Monitor for progressive deterioration in the physical and emotional state of individuals
- Monitor for repeated visits to a clinic, emergency room, or physician's office for minor problems
- Establish a system to flag individual records in which there is suspicion of abuse
- Provide positive affirmation of worth
- Encourage expression of concerns and feelings, which may include fear, guilt, embarrassment, and self-blame

- Provide support to empower victims to take action and make changes to prevent further victimization
- Assist individuals and families in developing coping strategies for stressful situations
- Assist individuals and families to objectively evaluate strengths and weaknesses of relationships
- Refer individuals at risk for abuse or who have suffered abuse to appropriate specialists and services (e.g., public health nurse, human services, counseling, legal assistance)
- Refer abusive partner to appropriate specialists and services
- Provide confidential information regarding domestic violence shelters, as appropriate
- Initiate development of a safety plan for use in the event that violence escalates
- Report any situations in which abuse is suspected in compliance with mandatory reporting laws
- Initiate community education programs designed to decrease violence
- Monitor use of community resources

3rd edition 2000; revised 2004, 2013

Background Evidence:

Boursnell, M., & Prosser, S. (2010). Increasing identification of domestic violence in emergency departments: A collaborative contribution to increasing the quality of practice of emergency nurses. *Contemporary Nurse, 35*(1), 35–46.

Garcia-Moreno, C., Heise, L., Jansen, H., Ellsberg, M., & Watts, C. (2005). Violence against women. *Science, 310*(5752), 1282–1283.

Klein, A. R. (2009). *Practical implications of current domestic violence research: For law enforcement, prosecutors and judges.* National Institute of Justice.

Pillitteri, A. (2007). *Maternal and child health nursing: Care of the childbearing and childrearing family* (5th ed.). Lippincott Williams & Wilkins.

Smith, J. S., Rainey, S. L., Smith, K. R., Alamares, C., & Grogg, D. (2008). Barriers to the mandatory reporting of domestic violence encountered by nursing professionals. *Journal of Trauma Nursing, 15*(1), 9–11.

Taylor, J. Y. (2006). Care of African American women survivors of intimate partner violence. In P. S. Cowen & S. Moorhead (Eds.), *Current issues in nursing* (7th ed., pp. 727–731). Mosby Elsevier.

Abuse Protection Support: Elder   6404

Definition: Identification of high-risk, dependent elder relationships and actions to prevent possible or further infliction of physical, sexual, or emotional harm; neglect of basic necessities of life; or exploitation

Activities:
- Identify elder patients who perceive themselves to be dependent on caretakers due to impaired health status, limited economic resources, depression, substance abuse, or lack of knowledge of available resources and alternatives for care
- Identify care arrangements that were made or continue under duress with only minimal consideration of the elder's care needs (e.g., the caregivers' abilities, characteristics, and competing responsibilities; need for environmental accommodations; and the history and quality of the relationships between the elder and the caregivers)
- Identify family crisis situations that may trigger abuse (e.g., poverty, unemployment, divorce, homelessness, death of a loved one)

- Determine whether the elder patient and their caretakers have a functional social support network to assist the patient in performing activities of daily living and in obtaining health care, transportation, therapy, medications, community resource information, financial advice, and assistance with personal problems
- Identify elder patients who rely on a single caretaker or family unit to provide extensive physical care assistance and monitoring
- Identify caretakers who demonstrate impaired physical or mental health (e.g., substance abuse, depression, fatigue, back injuries due to unassisted lifting, injuries that were inflicted by patient); financial problems or dependency; failure to understand patient's condition or needs; intolerant or hypercritical attitudes toward patient; burnout; or those who threaten patient with abandonment, hospitalization, institutionalization, or painful procedures

A

- Identify family caretakers who have a history of being abused or neglected in childhood
- Identify caretaker explanations of patient's injuries that are improbable, inconsistent, allege self-injury, blame others, include activities beyond elder's physical abilities, or demonstrate a delay in seeking treatment
- Determine whether elder patient demonstrates signs of physical abuse (e.g., numerous injuries in various stages of healing; unexplained lacerations, abrasions, bruises, burns or fractures; patches of missing hair; human bite marks)
- Determine whether the elder patient demonstrates signs of neglect (e.g., poor hygiene, inadequate or inappropriate clothing, untreated skin lesions, contractures, malnutrition, inadequate aids to mobility and perception [canes, glasses, hearing aids], no dentures or decayed fractured teeth, vermin infestation, medication deprivation or oversedation, deprivation of social contacts)
- Determine whether the elder patient demonstrates signs of sexual abuse (e.g., presence of semen or dried blood, injury to external genitals, acquired sexually transmitted diseases, dramatic behavioral or health changes of undetermined etiology)
- Determine whether the elder patient demonstrates signs of emotional abuse (e.g., low self-esteem, depression, humiliation and defeat, overly cautious behavior around caretaker, aggression against self or suicide gestures)
- Determine whether the elder patient demonstrates signs of exploitation (e.g., inadequate provision for basic needs when adequate resources are available, deprivation of personal possessions, unexplained loss of Social Security or pension checks, lack of knowledge of personal finances or legal matters)
- Encourage admission of patient for further observation and investigation, as appropriate
- Monitor patient-caretaker interactions and record observations
- Determine whether acute symptoms in patient abate when they are separated from caretakers
- Determine whether caretakers have unrealistic expectations for patient's behavior or if they have negative attributions for the behavior
- Monitor for extreme compliance to caretakers' demands or passive submission to invasive procedures
- Monitor for repeated visits to clinics, emergency rooms, or physicians' offices for injuries, inadequate health care monitoring, inadequate surveillance, or inadequate environmental adaptations
- Provide patients with positive affirmation of their worth and allow them to express their concerns and feelings, which may include fear, guilt, embarrassment, and self-blame
- Assist caretakers to explore their feelings about relatives or patients in their care and to identify factors that are disturbing and appear to contribute to abusive and neglectful behaviors
- Assist patients in identifying inadequate and harmful care arrangements, and help them and their family members identify mechanisms for addressing these problems
- Discuss concerns about observations of at-risk indicators separately with the elder patient and the caretaker
- Determine the patient's and caretaker's knowledge and ability to meet the patient's care and safety needs, and provide appropriate teaching
- Help patients and their families identify coping strategies for stressful situations, including the difficult decision to discontinue home care

- Determine deviations from normal aging and note early signs and symptoms of ill health through routine health screenings
- Promote maximum independence and self-care through innovative teaching strategies and the use of repetition, practice, reinforcement, and individualized pacing
- Provide environmental assessment and recommendations for adapting the home to promote physical self-reliance or refer to appropriate agencies for assistance
- Assist with restoration of full range of activities of daily living, as possible
- Instruct on the benefits of a routine regimen of physical activity, provide tailored exercise regimens, and refer to physical therapy or exercise programs as appropriate in order to prevent dependency
- Implement strategies to enhance critical thinking, decision-making, and remembering
- Provide a public health nurse referral to ensure that the home environment is monitored and that patient receives continued assistance
- Provide referrals for patients and their families to human services and counseling professionals
- Provide elder patients and their caretakers with community resource information (e.g., addresses and phone numbers of agencies that provide senior service assistance, home health care, residential care, respite care, emergency care, housing assistance, transportation, substance abuse treatment, sliding-fee counseling services, food pantries and Meals on Wheels, clothing distribution centers)
- Caution patients to have their Social Security or pension checks directly deposited, not to accept personal care in return for transfer of assets, and not to sign documents or make financial arrangements before seeking legal advice
- Encourage patients and their families to plan in advance for care needs, including who will assume responsibility if the patient becomes incapacitated and how to explore abilities, preferences, and options for care
- Consult with community resources for information
- Inform physician of observations indicative of abuse or neglect
- Report suspected abuse or neglect to proper authorities

2nd edition 1996; revised 2000, 2004, 2013

Background Evidence:

Brandl, B., Dyer, C., Heisler, C., Otto, J., Stiegel, L., & Thomas, R. (2007). *Elder abuse detection and intervention: A collaborative approach.* Springer.

Cohen, M., Halevy-Levin, S., Gagin, R., Priltuzky, D., & Friedman, G. (2010). Elder abuse in long-term care residences and the risk indicators. *Ageing and Society, 30*(6), 1027–1040.

Fraser, A. (2010). Preventing abuse of older people. *Nursing Management, 17*(6), 26–29.

Gorbien, M. J., & Eisenstein, A. R. (2005). Elder abuse and neglect: An overview. *Clinics in Geriatric Medicine, 21*(2), 279–292.

Lemko, K., & Fulmer, T. (2006). Nursing care: Victims of violence—elder mistreatment. In P. S. Cowen & S. Moorhead (Eds.), *Current issues in nursing* (7th ed., pp. 732–737). Mosby Elsevier.

Post, L., Page, C., Conner, T., Prokhorov, A., Fang, Y., & Biroscak, B. J. (2010). Elder abuse in long-term care: Types, patterns, and risk factors. *Research on Aging, 32*(3), 323–348.

Abuse Protection Support: Religious   6408

Definition: Identification of high-risk, controlling religious relationships and actions to prevent infliction of physical, sexual, or emotional harm, or exploitation

Activities:
- Identify individuals who are dependent on religious "leader" due to impaired or altered religious development, mental or emotional impairment, depression, substance abuse, lack of social resources, or financial issues
- Identify patterns of behavior, thinking, and feeling in which person experiences "control over" their religious journey by another
- Determine whether individual demonstrates signs of physical abuse, emotional abuse, exploitation, or religious addiction
- Report suspected abuse to proper church and legal authorities
- Determine whether individual has religious functional network to assist in meeting needs for belonging, care, and transcendence in healthy manner
- Offer prayer and healing services for person and healing of family or congregation, if comfortable doing so and if individual chooses
- Help identify resources to meet religious "safety" and support of individual and group
- Provide interpersonal support on regular basis, as needed
- Refer for appropriate religious counseling focusing on needs of individual
- Provide resources to victimized individual on benefits of forgiveness, when and if appropriate
- Refer to professional specialist if occult or satanic ritual abuse suspected
- Document interactions per organizational policy

3rd edition 2000; revised 2024

Background Evidence:

Davis, M., & Johnson, M. (2021). Exploring black clergy perspectives on religious/spiritual related domestic violence: First steps in facing those who wield the sword abusively. *Journal of Aggression, Maltreatment & Trauma, 30*(7), 950–971. https://doi.org/10.1080/10926771.2020.1738615

Dayan, H. (2018). Sexual abuse and charismatic cults. *Aggression & Violent Behavior, 41*, 25–31. https://doi.org/10.1016/j.avb.2018.04.004

Oakley, L., Kinmond, K., & Humphreys, J. (2018). Spiritual abuse in Christian faith settings: Definition, policy and practice guidance. *Journal of Adult Protection, 20*(3), 144–154. https://doi.org/10.1080/10926771.2011.627914

Proctor, M-T., Cleary, M., Kornhaber, R., & McLean, L. (2019). Christians with chronic complex trauma and relationally focused spiritual difficulties: A conversational model perspective. *Journal of Spirituality in Mental Health, 21*(2), 77–110. https://doi.org/10.1080/19349637.2018.1460228

Videbeck, S. H. (Ed.). (2020). *Psychiatric-mental health nursing* (8th ed.). Lippincott Williams & Wilkins.

Acid-Base Management   1910

Definition: Promotion of acid-base balance and prevention of complications resulting from acid-base imbalance

Activities:
- Maintain a patent airway
- Position to facilitate adequate ventilation (e.g., open airway and elevate head of bed)
- Maintain patent IV access
- Monitor trends in arterial pH, $PaCO_2$, and HCO_3 to determine particular type of imbalance (e.g., respiratory or metabolic) and compensatory physiological mechanisms present (e.g., pulmonary or renal compensation, physiological buffers)
- Maintain concurrent examination of arterial pH and plasma electrolytes for accurate treatment planning
- Monitor arterial blood gases (ABGs) and serum and urine electrolyte levels, as appropriate
- Obtain ordered specimen for laboratory analysis of acid-base balance (e.g., ABGs, urine, and serum), as appropriate
- Monitor for potential etiologies before attempting to treat acid-base imbalances as it is more effective to treat etiology than imbalance
- Determine pathologies needing direct intervention versus those requiring supportive care
- Monitor for complications of corrections of acid-base imbalances (e.g., rapid reduction in chronic respiratory alkalosis resulting in metabolic acidosis)
- Monitor for mixed acid-base derangements (e.g., primary respiratory alkalosis and primary metabolic acidosis)
- Monitor respiratory pattern
- Monitor determinants of tissue oxygen delivery (e.g., PaO_2, SaO_2, and hemoglobin levels and cardiac output), if available
- Monitor for symptoms of respiratory failure (e.g., low PaO_2 and elevated $PaCO_2$ levels, and respiratory muscle fatigue)
- Monitor determination of oxygen consumption (e.g., SvO_2 and $avDO_2$ levels), if available
- Monitor intake and output
- Monitor hemodynamic status, including CVP, MAP, PAP, and PCWP levels, if available
- Monitor for loss of acid (e.g., vomiting, nasogastric output, diarrhea, and diuresis), as appropriate
- Monitor for loss of bicarbonate (e.g., fistula drainage and diarrhea), as appropriate
- Monitor neurological status (e.g., level of consciousness and confusion)
- Provide mechanical ventilatory support, if necessary
- Provide for adequate hydration and restoration of normal fluid volumes, if necessary
- Provide for restoration of normal electrolyte levels (e.g., potassium and chloride), if necessary
- Administer prescribed medications as based on trends in arterial pH, $PaCO_2$, HCO_3, and serum electrolytes, as appropriate
- Instruct patient to avoid excessive use of medications containing HCO_3, as appropriate
- Sedate patient to reduce hyperventilation, if appropriate
- Treat fever, as appropriate
- Administer pain medication, as appropriate
- Administer oxygen therapy, as appropriate
- Administer microbial agents and bronchodilators, as appropriate

A

- Administer low flow oxygen and monitor for CO_2 narcosis in case of chronic hypercapnia
- Instruct the patient and/or family on actions instituted to treat the acid-base imbalance

1st edition 1992; revised 2013

Background Evidence:
American Association of Critical-Care Nurses, & Alspach, J. G. (2006). *Core curriculum for critical care nursing* (6th ed.). Elsevier.

Appel, S. J., & Downs, C. A. (2007). Steady a disturbed equilibrium: Accurately interpret the acid-base balance of acutely ill patients. *Nursing Critical Care, 2*(4), 45–53.

Clancy, J., & McVicar, A. (2007). Intermediate and long-term regulation of acid-base homeostasis. *British Journal of Nursing, 16*(17), 1076–1079.

Isenhour, J. L., & Slovis, C. M. (2008). Arterial blood gas analysis: A 3-step approach to acid-base disorders. *The Journal of Respiratory Diseases, 29*(2), 74–82.

Kraut, J. A., & Madeas, N. E. (2001). Approach to patients with acid-base disorders. *Respiratory Care, 46*(4), 392–402.

Lian, J. X. (2010). Interpreting and using the arterial blood gas analysis. *Nursing Critical Care, 5*(3), 26–36.

Porth, C. M. (2007). *Essentials of pathophysiology: Concepts of altered health states* (2nd ed.). Lippincott Williams & Wilkins.

Powers, F. (1999). The role of chloride in acid-base balance. *Journal of Intravenous Nursing, 22*(5), 286–290.

Smeltzer, S. C., & Bare, B. G. (2004). *Brunner & Suddarth's textbook of medical surgical nursing* (Vol. 1) (10th ed.). Lippincott Williams & Wilkis.

Acid-Base Management: Metabolic Acidosis   1911

Definition: Promotion of acid-base balance and prevention of complications resulting from serum HCO_3 levels lower than desired or serum hydrogen ion levels higher than desired

Activities:
- Maintain a patent airway
- Monitor respiratory pattern
- Maintain patent IV access
- Monitor for potential etiologies before attempting to treat acid-base imbalances (i.e., it is more effective to treat etiology than imbalance)
- Determine pathologies needing direct intervention versus those requiring supportive care
- Monitor for causes of HCO_3 deficit or hydrogen ion excess (e.g., methanol or ethanol ingestion, uremia, diabetic ketoacidosis, alcoholic ketoacidosis, lactic acidosis, sepsis, hypotension, hypoxia, ischemia, isoniazid or iron ingestion, salicylate toxicity, diarrhea, hyperalimentation, hyperparathyroidism)
- Calculate anion gap to assist in determining causes of metabolic acidosis (e.g., nonanion gap indicates electrolyte influenced causes; anion gap indicates loss of bicarbonate causes)
- Use mnemonics to assist in determining causes of metabolic acidosis (e.g., MUDPILES: Methanol ingestion, Uremia, Diabetic, alcoholic, or starvation ketoacidosis, Paraldehyde ingestion, Isoniazid or iron poisoning, Lactic acidosis, Ethylene glycol ingestion, Salicylate ingestion; HARDUP: Hyperalimentation, Acetazolamide, Renal tubular acidosis, renal insufficiency, Diarrhea and diuretics, Ureteroenterostomy, Pancreatic fistula)
- Monitor for electrolyte imbalances associated with metabolic acidosis (e.g., hyponatremia, hyperkalemia or hypokalemia, hypocalcemia, hypophosphatemia, and hypomagnesemia), as appropriate
- Monitor for signs and symptoms of worsening HCO_3 deficit or hydrogen ion excess (e.g., Kussmaul-Kien respirations, weakness, disorientation, headache, anorexia, coma, urinary pH level less than 6, plasma HCO_3 level less than 22 mEq/L, plasma pH level less than 7.35, base excess less than −2 mEq/L, associated hyperkalemia, and possible CO_2 deficit)
- Administer fluids as indicated for excessive losses from underlying condition (e.g., diarrhea, diuretics, hyperalimentation)
- Administer oral or parenteral HCO_3 agents, if appropriate
- Use parenteral HCO_3 agents cautiously in premature infants, neonates, and small children
- Avoid administration of medications resulting in lowered HCO_3 level (e.g., chloride-containing solutions and anion exchange resins), as appropriate
- Prevent complications from excessive HCO_3 administration (e.g., metabolic alkalosis, hypernatremia, volume overload, decreased oxygen delivery, decreased cardiac contractility, and enhanced lactic acid production)
- Administer prescribed insulin, fluid hydration (isotonic and hypotonic) and potassium for treatment of diabetic ketoacidosis, as appropriate
- Administer prescribed medications for treatment of inappropriate substance ingestion (e.g., alcohol, salicylate, ethylene glycol) or renal insufficiency
- Monitor intake and output
- Monitor determinants of tissue oxygen delivery (e.g., PaO_2, SaO_2, hemoglobin levels, and cardiac output), as appropriate
- Reduce oxygen consumption (e.g., promote comfort, control fever, and reduce anxiety), as appropriate
- Monitor loss of bicarbonate through the GI tract (e.g., diarrhea, pancreatic fistula, small bowel fistula, and ileal conduit), as appropriate
- Monitor for decreasing bicarbonate and acid buildup from excessive nonvolatile acids (e.g., renal failure, diabetic ketoacidosis, tissue hypoxia, and starvation), as appropriate
- Prepare renal failure patient for dialysis (i.e., assist with catheter placement for dialysis), as appropriate
- Assist with dialysis (e.g., hemodialysis or peritoneal dialysis), as appropriate
- Institute seizure precautions
- Provide frequent oral hygiene
- Maintain bed rest, as indicated
- Monitor for CNS manifestations of worsening metabolic acidosis (e.g., headache, drowsiness, decreased mentation, seizures, and coma), as appropriate
- Monitor for cardiopulmonary manifestations of worsening metabolic acidosis (e.g., hypotension, hypoxia, arrhythmias, and Kussmaul-Kien respiration), as appropriate
- Monitor for GI manifestations of worsening metabolic acidosis (e.g., anorexia, nausea, and vomiting), as appropriate

- Provide adequate nutrition for patients experiencing chronic metabolic acidosis
- Provide comfort measures to deal with the GI effects of metabolic acidosis
- Encourage diet low in carbohydrate to decrease CO_2 production (e.g., administration of hyperalimentation and total parenteral nutrition), as appropriate
- Monitor calcium and phosphate levels for patients experiencing chronic metabolic acidosis to prevent bone loss
- Instruct the patient and/or family on actions instituted to treat the metabolic acidosis

1st edition 1992; revised 2013

Background Evidence:

Appel, S. J., & Downs, C. A. (2007). Steady a disturbed equilibrium: Accurately interpret the acid-base balance of acutely ill patients. *Nursing Critical Care, 2*(4), 45–53.

Aschner, J. L., & Poland, R. L. (2008). Sodium bicarbonate: Basically useless therapy. *Pediatrics, 122*(4), 831–835.

Clancy, J., & McVicar, A. (2007). Intermediate and long-term regulation of acid-base homeostasis. *British Journal of Nursing, 16*(17), 1076–1079.

Isenhour, J. L., & Slovis, C. M. (2008). Arterial blood gas analysis: A 3-step approach to acid-base disorders. *The Journal of Respiratory Diseases, 29*(2), 74–82.

Jones, M. B. (2010). Pediatric care: Basic interpretation of metabolic acidosis. *Critical Care Nurse, 30*(5), 63–70.

Kovacic, V., Roguljic, L., & Kovacic, V. (2003). Metabolic acidosis of chronically hemodialyzed patients. *American Journal of Nephrology, 23*(3), 158–164.

Lian, J. X. (2010). Interpreting and using the arterial blood gas analysis. *Nursing Critical Care, 5*(3), 26–36.

Porth, C. M. (2007). *Essentials of pathophysiology: Concepts of altered health states* (2nd ed.). Lippincott Williams & Wilkins.

Powers, F. (1999). The role of chloride in acid-base balance. *Journal of Intravenous Nursing, 22*(5), 286–290.

Acid-Base Management: Metabolic Alkalosis   1912

Definition: Promotion of acid-base balance and prevention of complications resulting from serum HCO_3 levels higher than desired

Activities:

- Maintain a patent airway
- Monitor respiratory pattern
- Maintain patent IV access
- Monitor for potential etiologies before attempting to treat acid-base imbalances (i.e., it is more effective to treat etiology than imbalance)
- Determine pathologies needing direct intervention versus those requiring supportive care
- Monitor for causes of HCO_3 buildup or hydrogen ion loss (e.g., gastric fluid loss, vomiting, NG drainage, persistent diarrhea, loop or thiazide diuretics, cystic fibrosis, posthypercapnia syndrome in mechanically ventilated patients, primary aldosteronism, excessive ingestion of licorice)
- Calculate urine chloride concentration to assist in determining causes of metabolic alkalosis (e.g., saline responsive is indicated when urine chloride concentration is less than 15 mmol/L; nonsaline responsive is indicated when urine chloride concentration is greater than 25 mmol/L)
- Use mnemonics to assist in determining causes of metabolic alkalosis (e.g., DAMPEN: Diuretics, Adenoma secretor, Miscellaneous including Bartter's syndrome, penicillin, potassium deficiency, bulimia, Posthypercapnia, Emesis, Nasogastric tube; A BELCH: Alkali ingestion with decreased glomerular filtration rate, 11-B-hydroxylase deficiency, Exogenous steroids, Licorice ingestion, Cushing's syndrome and disease, Hyperaldosteronism)
- Obtain ordered specimen for laboratory analysis of acid-base balance, as appropriate
- Monitor arterial blood gases and serum and urine electrolyte levels, as appropriate
- Administer dilute acid (e.g., isotonic hydrochloride, arginine monohydrochloride), as appropriate
- Administer H_2 receptor antagonist (e.g., ranitidine and cimetidine) to block hydrochloride secretion from the stomach, as appropriate
- Administer carbonic anhydrase-inhibiting diuretics (e.g., acetazolamide and methazolamide) to increase excretion of bicarbonate, as appropriate
- Administer chloride to replace deficient anion (e.g., ammonium chloride, arginine hydrochloride, normal saline), as appropriate
- Administer prescribed IV potassium chloride until underlying hypokalemia is corrected
- Administer potassium-sparing diuretics (e.g., spironolactone and triamterene), as appropriate
- Administer antiemetics to reduce loss of HCl in emesis, as appropriate
- Replace extracellular fluid deficit with IV saline, as appropriate
- Irrigate NG tube with isotonic saline to avoid electrolyte washout, as appropriate
- Monitor intake and output
- Monitor for complications of corrections of acid-base imbalances (i.e., rapid reduction in metabolic alkalosis results in metabolic acidosis)
- Monitor for mixed acid-base derangements (e.g., primary metabolic alkalosis and primary respiratory acidosis) presenting as inappropriate metabolic compensations shrouding a primary respiratory disorder
- Calculate differences in observed HCO_3 and expected change in HCO_3 to determine presence of mixed acid-base derangement
- Monitor determinants of tissue oxygen delivery (e.g., PaO_2, SaO_2, hemoglobin levels, cardiac output), if available
- Avoid administration of alkaline substances (e.g., IV sodium bicarbonate, PO, or NG antacids), as appropriate
- Monitor for electrolyte imbalances associated with metabolic alkalosis (e.g., hypokalemia, hypercalcemia, hypochloremia), as appropriate
- Monitor for associated excesses of bicarbonate (e.g., hyperaldosteronism, glucocorticoid excess, licorice abuse), as appropriate
- Monitor for renal loss of acid (e.g., diuretic therapy), as appropriate

A

- Monitor for GI loss of acid (e.g., vomiting, NG suctioning, high chloride content diarrhea), as appropriate
- Monitor patient receiving digitalis for toxicity resulting from hypokalemia associated with metabolic alkalosis, as appropriate
- Monitor for neurological and/or neuromuscular manifestations of metabolic alkalosis (e.g., seizures, confusion, stupor, coma, tetany, hyperactive reflexes)
- Monitor for pulmonary manifestations of metabolic alkalosis (e.g., bronchospasm, hypoventilation)
- Monitor for cardiac manifestations of metabolic alkalosis (e.g., arrhythmias, reduced contractility, decreased cardiac output)
- Monitor for GI manifestations of metabolic alkalosis (e.g., nausea, vomiting, diarrhea)
- Instruct the patient and/or family on actions instituted to treat the metabolic alkalosis

1st edition 1992; revised 2004, 2013

Background Evidence:

Appel, S. J., & Downs, C. A. (2007). Steady a disturbed equilibrium: Accurately interpret the acid-base balance of acutely ill patients. *Nursing Critical Care, 2*(4), 45–53.

Clancy, J., & McVicar, A. (2007). Intermediate and long-term regulation of acid-base homeostasis. *British Journal of Nursing, 16*(17), 1076–1079.

Huang, L.H., & Priestley, M.A. (2008). *Pediatric metabolic alkalosis.* http://emedicine.medscape.com/article/906819-overview

Isenhour, J. L., & Slovis, C. M. (2008). Arterial blood gas analysis: A 3-step approach to acid-base disorders. *The Journal of Respiratory Diseases, 29*(2), 74–82.

Khanna, A., & Kurtzman, N. A. (2001). Metabolic alkalosis. *Respiratory Care, 46*(4), 354–365.

Kraut, J. A., & Madias, N. E. (2001). Approach to patients with acid-base disorders. *Respiratory Care, 46*(4), 392–403.

Lian, J. X. (2010). Interpreting and using the arterial blood gas analysis. *Nursing Critical Care, 5*(3), 26–36.

Lynch, F. (2009). Arterial blood gas analysis: Implications for nursing. *Paediatric Nursing, 21*(1), 41–44.

Porth, C. M. (2007). *Essentials of pathophysiology: Concepts of altered health states* (2nd ed.). Lippincott Williams & Wilkins.

Ruholl, L. (2006). Arterial blood gases: Analysis and nursing responses. *MEDSURG Nursing, 15*(6), 343–351.

Acid-Base Management: Respiratory Acidosis   1913

Definition: Promotion of acid-base balance and prevention of complications resulting from serum $PaCO_2$ levels higher than desired or serum hydrogen ion levels higher than desired

Activities:

- Maintain a patent airway
- Maintain airway clearance (e.g., suction, insert or maintain artificial airway, chest physiotherapy, and cough-deep breath), as appropriate
- Monitor respiratory pattern
- Maintain patent IV access
- Obtain ordered specimen for laboratory analysis of acid-base balance (e.g., ABG, urine, and serum levels), as appropriate
- Monitor for potential etiologies before attempting to treat acid-base imbalances (i.e., it is more effective to treat etiology than imbalance)
- Monitor for possible causes of carbonic acid excess and respiratory acidosis (e.g., airway obstruction, depressed ventilation, CNS depression, neurological disease, chronic lung disease, musculoskeletal disease, chest trauma, pneumothorax, respiratory infection, ARDS, cardiac failure, acute opioid ingestion, use of respiratory depressant drugs, obesity hypoventilation syndrome)
- Determine pathologies needing direct intervention versus those requiring supportive care
- Monitor for signs and symptoms of carbonic acid excess and respiratory acidosis (e.g., hand tremor with extensions of arms, confusion, drowsiness progressing to coma, headache, slowed verbal response, nausea, vomiting, tachycardia, warm sweaty extremities, pH level less than 7.35, $PaCO_2$ level greater than 45 mm Hg, associated hypochloremia, and possible HCO_3 excess)
- Support ventilation and airway patency in the presence of respiratory acidosis and rising $PaCO_2$ level, as appropriate
- Administer oxygen therapy, as appropriate
- Administer microbial agents and bronchodilators, as appropriate
- Administer medication therapy aimed at reversing the effects of inappropriate sedative drugs (e.g., naloxone to reverse narcotics, flumazenil to reverse benzodiazepines), as appropriate
- Maintain caution when reversing the effects of benzodiazepines to avoid seizures if reversal is accomplished too vigorously
- Administer low flow oxygen and monitor for CO_2 narcosis in cases of chronic hypercapnia (e.g., COPD)
- Administer noninvasive, positive-pressure ventilation techniques (e.g., nasal continuous positive-pressure ventilation, nasal bilevel ventilation) for hypercapnia related to obesity hypoventilation syndrome or musculoskeletal disease
- Monitor for hypoventilation and treat causes (e.g., inappropriate low-minute mechanical ventilation, chronic reduction in alveolar ventilation, COPD, acute opioid ingestion, obstructive or restrictive airway diseases)
- Monitor ABG levels for decreasing pH level, as appropriate
- Monitor for indications of chronic respiratory acidosis (e.g., barrel chest, clubbing of nails, pursed-lips breathing, and use of accessory muscles), as appropriate
- Monitor determinants of tissue oxygen delivery (e.g., PaO_2, SaO_2, hemoglobin levels, cardiac output) to determine the adequacy of arterial oxygenation
- Monitor for symptoms of respiratory failure (e.g., low PaO_2, elevated $PaCO_2$ levels, respiratory muscle fatigue)
- Position patient for optimum ventilation-perfusion matching (e.g., good lung down, prone, semi-Fowler's), as appropriate
- Monitor work of breathing (e.g., respiratory rate, heart rate, use of accessory muscles, diaphoresis)
- Provide mechanical ventilatory support, if necessary
- Provide low-carbohydrate, high-fat diet to reduce CO_2 production, if indicated
- Provide frequent oral hygiene
- Monitor GI functioning and distention to prevent reduced diaphragmatic movement, as appropriate
- Promote adequate rest periods (e.g., 90 minutes of undisturbed sleep, organize nursing cares, limit visitors, coordinate consults), as appropriate

- Monitor neurological status (e.g., level of consciousness and confusion)
- Instruct the patient and/or family on actions instituted to treat the respiratory acidosis
- Contract with patient's visitors for limited visitation schedule to allow for adequate rest periods to reduce respiratory compromise, if indicated

1st edition 1992; revised 2004, 2013

Background Evidence:

Appel, S. J., & Downs, C. A. (2007). Steady a disturbed equilibrium: Accurately interpret the acid-base balance of acutely ill patients. *Nursing Critical Care, 2*(4), 45–53.

Clancy, J., & McVicar, A. (2007). Intermediate and long-term regulation of acid-base homeostasis. *British Journal of Nursing, 16*(17), 1076–1079.

Isenhour, J. L., & Slovis, C. M. (2008). Arterial blood gas analysis: A 3-step approach to acid-base disorders. *The Journal of Respiratory Diseases, 29*(2), 74–82.

Kraut, J. A., & Madias, N. E. (2001). Approach to patients with acid-base disorders. *Respiratory Care, 46*(4), 392–403.

Lian, J. X. (2010). Interpreting and using the arterial blood gas analysis. *Nursing Critical Care, 5*(3), 26–36.

Lynch, F. (2009). Arterial blood gas analysis: Implications for nursing. *Paediatric Nursing, 21*(1), 41–44.

Porth, C. M. (2007). *Essentials of pathophysiology: Concepts of altered health states* (2nd ed.). Lippincott Williams & Wilkins.

Ruholl, L. (2006). Arterial blood gases: Analysis and nursing responses. *MEDSURG Nursing, 15*(6), 343–351.

Acid-Base Management: Respiratory Alkalosis   1914

Definition: Promotion of acid-base balance and prevention of complications resulting from serum $PaCO_2$ levels lower than desired

Activities:

- Maintain a patent airway
- Monitor respiratory pattern
- Maintain patent IV access
- Monitor for potential etiologies before attempting to treat acid-base imbalances (i.e., it is more effective to treat etiology than imbalance)
- Determine pathologies needing direct intervention versus those requiring supportive care
- Monitor for hyperventilation and treat causes (e.g., inappropriate high-minute mechanical ventilation, anxiety, hypoxemia, lung lesions, severe anemia, salicylate toxicity, CNS injury, hypermetabolic states, GI distention, pain, high altitude, septicemia, stress)
- Reduce oxygen consumption by promoting comfort, controlling fever, and reducing anxiety to minimize hyperventilation, as appropriate
- Provide rebreather mask for hyperventilating patient, as appropriate
- Sedate patient to reduce hyperventilation, if appropriate
- Reduce high-minute ventilation (e.g., rate, mode, tidal volume) in mechanically overventilated patients, as appropriate
- Monitor end-tidal CO_2 level, as appropriate
- Promote adequate rest periods of at least 90 minutes of undisturbed sleep (e.g., organized nursing cares, limited visitors, coordinated consults), as appropriate
- Administer parenteral chloride solutions to reduce HCO_3 when correcting the cause of respiratory alkalosis, as appropriate
- Monitor trends in arterial pH, $PaCO_2$, and HCO_3 to determine effectiveness of interventions
- Monitor for symptoms of worsening respiratory alkalosis (e.g., alternating periods of apnea and hyperventilation, increasing anxiety, increased heart rate without increased blood pressure, dyspnea, dizziness, tingling in extremities, hyperreflexia, frequent sighing and yawning, blurred vision, diaphoresis, dry mouth, pH level of greater than 7.45, $PaCO_2$ less than 35 mm Hg, associated hyperchloremia, HCO_3 deficit)
- Obtain ordered specimen for laboratory analysis of acid-base balance (e.g., ABGs, urine, serum), as appropriate
- Maintain concurrent examination of arterial pH and plasma electrolytes for accurate treatment planning
- Monitor arterial blood gases and serum and urine electrolyte levels, as appropriate
- Monitor for hypophosphatemia and hypokalemia associated with respiratory alkalosis, as appropriate
- Monitor for complications of corrections of acid-base imbalances (e.g., rapid reduction in chronic respiratory alkalosis resulting in metabolic acidosis)
- Monitor for mixed acid-base derangements (e.g., primary respiratory alkalosis and primary metabolic acidosis) presenting as inappropriate respiratory compensations shrouding a primary metabolic disorder
- Calculate differences in observed $PaCO_2$ and expected change in $PaCO_2$ to determine presence of mixed acid-base derangement
- Monitor for indications of impending respiratory failure (e.g., low PaO_2 level, respiratory muscle fatigue, low SaO_2/SvO_2 level)
- Provide oxygen therapy, if necessary
- Provide mechanical ventilatory support, if necessary
- Position to facilitate adequate ventilation (e.g., open airway, elevate head of bed)
- Monitor intake and output
- Monitor for neurological and/or neuromuscular manifestations of respiratory alkalosis (e.g., paresthesias, tetany, seizures), as appropriate
- Monitor for cardiopulmonary manifestations of respiratory alkalosis (e.g., arrhythmias, decreased cardiac output, hyperventilation)
- Administer sedatives, pain relief, and antipyretics, as appropriate
- Administer neuromuscular-blocking agents only if patient is mechanically ventilated, if indicated
- Promote stress reduction
- Provide frequent oral hygiene
- Promote orientation
- Instruct the patient and/or family on actions instituted to treat the respiratory alkalosis
- Contract with patient's visitors for limited visitation schedule to allow for adequate rest periods to reduce respiratory compromise, if indicated

1st edition 1992; revised 2013

A

Background Evidence:

Appel, S. J., & Downs, C. A. (2007). Steady a disturbed equilibrium: Accurately interpret the acid-base balance of acutely ill patients. *Nursing Critical Care, 2*(4), 45–53.

Clancy, J., & McVicar, A. (2007). Intermediate and long-term regulation of acid-base homeostasis. *British Journal of Nursing, 16*(17), 1076–1079.

Foster, G. T., Vaziri, N. D., & Sassoon, C. S. (2001). Respiratory alkalosis. *Respiratory Care, 46*(4), 384–391.

Isenhour, J. L., & Slovis, C. M. (2008). Arterial blood gas analysis: A 3-step approach to acid-base disorders. *The Journal of Respiratory Diseases, 29*(2), 74–82.

Kraut, J. A., & Madias, N. E. (2001). Approach to patients with acid-base disorders. *Respiratory Care, 46*(4), 392–403.

Lian, J. X. (2010). Interpreting and using the arterial blood gas analysis. *Nursing Critical Care, 5*(3), 26–36.

Lynch, F. (2009). Arterial blood gas analysis: Implications for nursing. *Paediatric Nursing, 21*(1), 41–44.

Ruholl, L. (2006). Arterial blood gases: Analysis and nursing responses. *MEDSURG Nursing, 15*(6), 343–351.

Acid-Base Monitoring   1920

Definition: Collection and analysis of patient data to regulate acid-base balance

Activities:

- Obtain ordered specimen for laboratory analysis of acid-base balance (e.g., ABGs, urine, and serum) in at-risk populations, as appropriate
- Obtain sequential specimens to determine trends
- Analyze trends in serum pH in the patient experiencing conditions with escalating effects on pH levels (e.g., hyperventilating patients, diabetic or alcoholic ketoacidosis patients, septic patients)
- Analyze trends in serum pH in at-risk populations (e.g., patients with compromised respiratory status, renal impairment, diabetes mellitus, prolonged diarrhea or vomiting, Cushing's syndrome)
- Note if arterial pH level is on the alkaline or acidotic side of the mean (7.35–7.45)
- Note if $PaCO_2$ level shows respiratory acidosis, respiratory alkalosis, or normalcy
- Note if the HCO_3 level shows metabolic acidosis, metabolic alkalosis, or normalcy
- Examine trends in serum pH in conjunction with $PaCO_2$ and HCO_3 trends to determine whether the acidosis or alkalosis is compensated or uncompensated
- Note if the compensation is pulmonary, metabolic, or is physiologically buffered
- Identify potential etiologies before attempting to treat acid-base imbalances as it is more effective to treat etiology than imbalance
- Identify the presence or absence of an anion gap (greater than 14 mEq/L) signaling an increased production or decreased excretion of acid products
- Monitor for signs and symptoms of HCO_3 deficit and metabolic acidosis (e.g., Kussmaul-Kien respirations, weakness, disorientation, headache, anorexia, coma, urinary pH level less than 6, plasma HCO_3 level less than 22 mEq/L, plasma pH level less than 7.35, base excess less than −2 mEq/L, associated hyperkalemia, and possible CO_2 deficit)
- Monitor for causes of metabolic acidosis (e.g., methanol or ethanol ingestion, uremia, diabetic ketoacidosis, alcoholic ketoacidosis, paraldehyde ingestion, lactic acidosis, sepsis, hypotension, hypoxia, ischemia, malnutrition, diarrhea, renal failure, hyperalimentation, hyperparathyroidism, salicylate toxicity, ethylene glycol ingestion)
- Monitor for signs and symptoms of HCO_3 excess and metabolic alkalosis (e.g., numbness and tingling of the extremities, muscular hypertonicity, shallow respirations with pause, bradycardia, tetany, urinary pH level greater than 7, plasma HCO_3 level greater than 26 mEq/L, plasma pH level greater than 7.45, BE greater than 2 mEq/L, associated hypokalemia, and possible CO_2 retention)
- Monitor for causes of metabolic alkalosis (e.g., diuretics, emesis, nasogastric tube, posthypercapnia, potassium deficiency, alkali ingestion, Cushing's syndrome, hyperaldosteronism, hypochloremia, excessive ingestion of medications containing HCO_3)
- Monitor for signs and symptoms of $PaCO_2$ level deficit and respiratory alkalosis (e.g., frequent sighing and yawning, tetany, paresthesia, muscular twitching, palpitations, tingling and numbness, dizziness, blurred vision, diaphoresis, dry mouth, convulsions, pH level greater than 7.45, $PaCO_2$ less than 35 mm Hg, associated hyperchloremia, and possible HCO_3 deficit)
- Monitor for causes of respiratory alkalosis (e.g., hyperventilation, mechanical overventilation, hepatic disease, pregnancy, septicemia, pain, CNS lesions, and fever)
- Monitor for signs and symptoms of $PaCO_2$ level excess and respiratory acidosis (e.g., hand tremor with extensions of arms, confusion, drowsiness progressing to coma, headache, slowed verbal response, nausea, vomiting, tachycardia, warm sweaty extremities, pH level less than 7.35, $PaCO_2$ level greater than 45 mm Hg, associated hypochloremia, and possible HCO_3 excess)
- Monitor for possible causes of respiratory acidosis (e.g., airway obstruction, depressed ventilation, CNS depression, neurological disease, chronic lung disease, musculoskeletal disease, chest trauma, infection, ARDS, cardiac failure, acute opioid ingestion, and use of respiratory depressant drugs)
- Compare current status with previous status to detect improvements and deterioration in patient's condition
- Initiate and/or change medical treatment to maintain patient parameters within limits ordered by the physician, using established protocols

1st edition 1992; revised 2013

Background Evidence:

Appel, S. J., & Downs, C. A. (2007). Steady a disturbed equilibrium: Accurately interpret the acid-base balance of acutely ill patients. *Nursing Critical Care, 2*(4), 45–53.

Clancy, J., & McVicar, A. (2007). Intermediate and long-term regulation of acid-base homeostasis. *British Journal of Nursing, 16*(17), 1076–1079.

Coombs, M. (2001). Making sense of arterial blood gases. *Nursing Times, 97*(27), 36–38.

Isenhour, J. L., & Slovis, C. M. (2008). Arterial blood gas analysis: A 3-step approach to acid-base disorders. *The Journal of Respiratory Diseases, 29*(2), 74–82.

Lian, J. X. (2010). Interpreting and using the arterial blood gas analysis. *Nursing Critical Care, 5*(3), 26–36.

Powers, F. (1999). The role of chloride in acid-base balance. *Journal of Intravenous Nursing, 22*(5), 286–290.

Smeltzer, S. C., & Bare, B. G. (2004). *Brunner & Suddarth's textbook of medical surgical nursing* (Vol. 1) (10th ed.). Lippincott Williams & Wilkis.

A

Active Listening 4920

Definition: Attending closely to and attaching significance to verbal and nonverbal messages

Activities:
- Establish purpose for interaction
- Display interest in person
- Use open-ended questions or statements to encourage expression of thoughts, feelings, and concerns
- Refrain from making any judgments about person and their experience (e.g., prejudice, bias, assumptions)
- Focus on interaction by suppressing personal concerns and other distractions
- Avoid barriers to active listening (e.g., minimizing feelings, offering easy solutions, interrupting, talking about self, premature closure)
- Display awareness of and sensitivity to emotions
- Use nonverbal behavior to facilitate communication (i.e., be aware of physical stance conveying nonverbal messages)
- Use silence to encourage expression of feelings, thoughts, and concerns
- Listen for unexpressed message and feeling, as well as content, of conversation
- Be aware of which words are avoided, as well as nonverbal message that accompanies expressed words
- Be aware of tone, tempo, volume, pitch, and inflection of voice
- Mirror and reflect on information and emotions by periodically paraphrasing key points
- Identify predominant themes
- Determine meaning of message by reflecting on attitudes, past experiences, and current situation
- Time response so that it reflects understanding of received message
- Clarify message through use of probing questions and feedback
- Verify understanding of messages through use of questions or feedback
- Use series of interactions to discover meaning of behavior
- Summarize by restating key themes
- Arrange for any mutual responsibilities and follow-up, if needed

1st edition 1992; revised 1996, 2004, 2024

Background Evidence:

Ellis, P., & Abbott, J. (2018). Active listening, Part one: How and where. *Journal of Kidney Care, 3*(2), 126–128. https://doi.org/10.12968/jokc.2018.3.2.126

Ellis, P., & Abbott, J. (2018). Active listening, Part two: Showing empathy. *Journal of Kidney Care, 3*(3), 193–195. https://doi.org/10.12968/jokc.2018.3.3.193

Fitzgerald, D. T. (2020). Using online active listening to facilitate student communication skills. *The Journal of Nursing Education, 59*(2), 117. https://doi.org/10.3928/01484834-20200122-13

Jonsdottir, I. J., & Kristinsson, K. (2020). Supervisors' active-empathetic listening as an important antecedent of work engagement. *International Journal of Environmental Research and Public Health, 17*(21), 7976. https://doi.org/10.3390/ijerph17217976

Kilgore, C. (2017). Active listening key to quality palliative care. *Caring for the Ages, 18*(10), 15.

Payton, J. (2018). Improving communication skills within the nephrology unit. *Nephrology Nursing Journal: Journal of the American Nephrology Nurses' Association, 45*(3), 269–280.

Pangh, B., Jouybari, L., Vakili, M. A., Sanagoo, A., & Torik, A. (2019). The effect of reflection on nurse-patient communication skills in emergency medical centers. *Journal of Caring Sciences, 8*(2), 75–81. https://doi.org/10.15171/jcs.2019.011

Activity Therapy 4310

Definition: Prescription of and assistance with specific physical, cognitive, social, and spiritual activities to increase the range, frequency, or duration of an individual's or group's activity

Activities:
- Determine patient ability to participate in specific activities
- Collaborate with occupational, physical, or recreational therapists in planning and monitoring an activity program, as appropriate
- Determine patient's commitment to increasing frequency and range of activity
- Assist patient to explore the personal meaning of usual activity (e.g., work) and favorite leisure activities
- Assist patient to choose activities and achievement goals for activities consistent with physical, psychological, and social capabilities
- Assist patient to focus on abilities rather than on deficits
- Assist patient to identify and obtain resources required for the desired activity
- Encourage creative activities, as appropriate
- Assist patient to obtain transportation to activities, as appropriate
- Assist patient to identify preferences for activities
- Assist patient to identify meaningful activities
- Assist patient to schedule specific periods for activities into daily routine
- Assist patient and family to identify deficits in activity level
- Identify strategies to promote patient participation in desired activities

A

- Instruct patient and family regarding the role of physical, social, spiritual, and cognitive activity in maintaining function and health
- Instruct patient and family how to perform desired or prescribed activity
- Coordinate patient selection of age-appropriate activities
- Assist patient and family to adapt environment to accommodate desired activity
- Provide activities to increase attention span in consultation with occupational therapist
- Facilitate activity substitution when patient has limitations in time, energy, or movement, in consultation with occupational, physical, or recreational therapists
- Encourage involvement in group activities or therapies, as appropriate
- Refer to community centers or activity programs, as appropriate
- Assist with regular physical activities (e.g., ambulation, transfers, turning, and personal care), as needed
- Provide gross motor activities for hyperactive patient
- Promote a physically active lifestyle to avoid unneeded weight gain, as appropriate
- Suggest methods of increasing daily physical activity, as appropriate
- Make environment safe for continuous large muscle movement, as indicated
- Provide motor activity to relieve muscle tension
- Provide activities with implicit and emotional memory components (e.g., specially selected religious activities) for dementia patients, as appropriate
- Provide noncompetitive, structured, and active group games
- Promote engagement in recreational and diversional activities aimed at reducing anxiety (e.g., group singing; volleyball; table tennis; walking; swimming; simple, concrete tasks; simple games; routine tasks; housekeeping chores; grooming; and puzzles and cards)
- Employ animal-assisted activity programs, as appropriate
- Provide positive reinforcement for participation in activities

- Instruct family to provide positive reinforcement for participation in activities
- Allow for family participation in activities, as appropriate
- Assist patient to develop self-motivation and reinforcement
- Monitor emotional, physical, social, and spiritual response to activity
- Assist patient and family to monitor own progress toward goal achievement

1st edition 1992; revised 2013

Background Evidence:

Chilvers, R., Corr, S., & Singlehurst, H. (2010). Investigation into the occupational lives of healthy older people through their use of time. *Australian Occupational Therapy Journal, 57*(1), 24–33.

Chu, C., Liu, C., Sun, C., & Lin, J. (2009). The effect of animal-assisted activity on inpatients with schizophrenia. *Journal of Psychosocial Nursing & Mental Health Services, 47*(12), 42–48.

Dorrestein, M. (2006). Leisure activity assessment in residential care: Improving occupational outcomes for residents. *New Zealand Journal of Occupational Therapy, 53*(2), 20–26.

Griffiths, S. (2008). The experience of creative activity as a treatment medium. *Journal of Mental Health, 17*(1), 49–63.

Ketteridge, A., & Boshoff, K. (2008). Exploring the reasons why adolescents participate in physical activity and identifying strategies that facilitate their involvement in such activity. *Australian Occupational Therapy Journal, 55*(4), 273–282.

Lloyd, C., Williams, P. L., Simpson, A., Wright, D., Fortune, T., & Lal, S. (2010). Occupational therapy in the modern adult acute mental health setting: A review of current practice. *International Journal of Therapy & Rehabilitation, 17*(9), 483–493.

Shirley, D., van der Ploeg, H. P., & Bauman, A. E. (2010). Physical activity promotion in the physical therapy setting: Perspectives from practitioners and students. *Physical Therapy, 90*(9), 1311–1322.

Vance, D. E., Eaves, Y. D., Keltner, N. L., & Struzick, T. S. (2010). Practical implications of procedural and emotional religious activity therapy for nursing. *Journal of Gerontological Nursing, 36*(8), 22–29.

Acupressure   1320

Definition: Application of firm, sustained pressure to special points on the body for therapeutic effect

Activities:

- Screen for contraindications (e.g., serious medical conditions such as arteriosclerosis, cardiac conditions, contusions, scar tissue, infection, young children)
- Decide on purpose of acupressure for prevention or treatment of a particular individual (e.g., pain, headaches, nausea, asthma, colds and flu, arthritis, allergies, nervous tension, menstrual cramps, sinus problems, sprains, tennis elbow)
- Describe the rationale, benefits, limits, and types of acupressure available (e.g., Shiatsu, Tui Na, Sujok, Jin Shin, Atmena)
- Provide detailed description of chosen acupressure technique
- Determine individual's degree of psychological comfort with touch
- Determine desired outcomes
- Determine which acupoints to stimulate, depending on desired outcome
- Create a quiet, nondisrupting environment, when possible
- Suggest that the individual assume a comfortable position with unrestricted clothing
- Explain to individual that you will be searching for a tender area

- Encourage individual to relax during the stimulation
- Apply firm finger pressure in a slow, rhythmic manner to enable the layers of tissue to respond
- Use thumbs, fingers, palms, the side of the hand, or knuckles to apply steady, stationary pressure at the pressure sensitive spot in the general location of the acupoint by using one's body weight to lean into the point to which pressure is applied
- Apply pressure gradually and hold without any movement for several minutes at a time to relax an area or relieve pain
- Apply steady pressure over hypertonic muscle tissue for pain until relaxation is felt or pain is reported to have decreased, usually 15 to 20 seconds
- Repeat procedure over same point on opposite side of body
- Apply steady pressure until the nausea subsides or maintain wristbands indefinitely during actual or anticipated nausea
- Observe verbal or postural cues (e.g., wincing, "ouch") to identify desired point or location
- Treat the contralateral points first when there is extreme tenderness at any one point

A

- Use daily acupressure applications during the first week of treatment for pain
- Recommend use of progressive relaxation techniques and stretching exercises between treatments
- Instruct family/significant other(s) to provide acupressure treatments
- Document action and individual response to acupressure

2nd edition 1996; revised 2018

Background Evidence:

Chen, Y. W., & Wang, H. H. (2014). The effectiveness of acupressure on relieving pain: A systematic review. *Pain Management Nursing, 15*(2), 539–550.

Gach, M. (2014). *Acupressure.com.* http://acupressure.com/index.htm

Matsubara, T., Arai, Y-C. P., Shiro, Y., Shimo, K., Nishihara, M., Santo, J., & Ushida, T. (2011). Comparative effects of acupressure at local and distal acupuncture points on pain conditions and autonomic function in females with chronic neck pain. *Evidenced Based Complementary and Alternative Medicine, 2011.* https://doi.org/10.1155/2011/543291

Robinson, N., Lorenc, A., & Liao, X. (2011). The evidence for Shiatsu: A systematic review of Shiatsu and acupressure. *BMC: Complementary & Alternative Medicine, 11,* 1–15.

Yeung, W., Chung, K., Poon, M., Ho, F., Zhang, S., Zhang, Z., Ziea, E. T-C., & Won+g, V. (2012). Acupressure, reflexology, and auricular acupressure for insomnia: A systematic review of randomized controlled trials. *Sleep Medicine, 13*(8), 971–984.

Admission Care 7310

Definition: Facilitating entry of a person into a healthcare facility

Activities:

- Introduce self and role in providing care
- Identify using at least two identifiers (e.g., name, date of birth)
- Place in appropriate receiving area
- Provide appropriate privacy
- Determine if has sensory or communication need (e.g., glasses, hearing aid, need for an interpreter) or preferred communication method
- Provide professional translator or telephone interpreter services if does not speak, read, or understand English
- Determine educational background, health literacy level, and ability to understand instructions
- Provide with patient bill of rights
- Provide with advance care directive information (e.g., living will, durable power of attorney for health care)
- Obtain copies of advance care directives, if available
- Orient to expectations of care, including relevant healthcare agency policies and procedures
- Orient to immediate environment, including call lights, bathroom facilities, and equipment
- Orient to agency facilities
- Review health history including past medical illnesses, medications, and allergies
- Review physical, financial, psychosocial, and religious assessments, as appropriate
- Determine cultural variables that require accommodation or adaptation (e.g., dietary preferences, clothing requirements, beliefs about healing and wellness)
- Review medications including herbal or OTC medications
- Review risk status (e.g., risk for falls, tuberculosis screening, skin assessment)
- Determine if uses any assistive devices and provide, after assuring devices safe to use
- Perform preliminary testing and screening per agency policies and person condition
- Note verbal and nonverbal behaviors and responses
- Determine perception of illness, health care needs, knowledge of health problems and expectations of care
- Identify persons at high risk for readmission based on condition, previous hospitalizations, emergency department visits, and social determinants of health (e.g., **LACE** criteria [**L**ength of stay during index admission, **A**cute [emergent admissions], **C**harlson comorbidity index, **E**D visits])
- Initiate ongoing flexible plan for discharge at admission (e.g., regular evaluation of discharge readiness, periodic discussions related to discharge plans)
- Determine home resources including family or caregiver availability, as early as possible
- Encourage early involvement in all interactions related to home care and discharge needs
- Implement safety precautions, as appropriate (e.g., fall protocol, isolation precautions)
- Label clinical record, room door, and head of bed with safety alerts, including wrist band identification, as indicated
- Notify health care provider of admission and status
- Obtain health care provider orders for care
- Document pertinent information
- Maintain confidentiality of information

1st edition 1992; revised 2004, 2024

Background Evidence:

Berman, A., Snyder, S. J., & Frandsen, G. (2021). *Kozier and Erb's Fundamentals of nursing: Concepts, process and practice* (11th ed.). Pearson.

Jensen, S. (2021). Health assessment. In R. F. Craven, C. J. Hirnle, & C. J. Henshaw (Eds.), *Fundamentals of nursing: Human health and function* (9th ed., pp. 319–370). Wolters-Kluwer.

Potter, P. A., Ostendorf, W. R., & LaPlante, N. (2018). *Admitting patients. Clinical nursing skills and techniques* (pp. 13–19) (9th ed.). Mosby.

Smith, S. F., Duell, D. J., Martin, B. C., Aebersold, M. L., & Gonzalez, L. (2017). *Admission, transfer and discharge. In Clinical nursing skills: Basic to advanced skills* (pp. 84–100) (9th ed.). Pearson.

Williams, P. (2020). *Basic geriatric nursing* (7th ed.). Elsevier.

A

Adolescent Care 8272

Definition: Facilitating developmentally appropriate care to support the physical, cognitive, social, and emotional growth during the transition from childhood to adulthood

Activities:
- Build trusting relationship with adolescent
- Encourage adolescent to be actively involved in decisions regarding own health care
- Discuss developmental milestones and associated behaviors with adolescent and parent
- Screen for health problems relevant to adolescent and suggested by history (e.g., anemia; hypertension; hearing and vision disorders; hyperlipidemia; oral health problems; abnormal sexual maturation; abnormal physical growth; body image disturbances; eating disorders; poor nutrition; alcohol, tobacco, or drug use; unhealthy sexual behavior; infectious disease; poor self-concept; low self-esteem; depression; difficult relationships; abuse; learning problems; work problems)
- Encourage yearly physical and vision screening
- Instruct on self-breast or self-testicle exam, as indicated
- Encourage dental exam twice per year
- Encourage to practice good dental hygiene
- Provide education and encourage age-appropriate immunizations
- Provide health counseling and guidance to adolescent and parent, as needed
- Acknowledge pubertal development stage and provide education on developmental process
- Promote personal hygiene and grooming
- Provide privacy
- Promote independence with ADLs, as appropriate
- Encourage participation in safe exercise on regular basis
- Promote healthy diet
- Facilitate development of sexual identity
- Encourage responsible sexual behavior and screen for STDs
- Provide contraceptives with instruction for use, if needed
- Promote avoidance of alcohol, tobacco, and drugs
- Promote vehicle safety

- Facilitate decision-making ability
- Enhance communication and assertiveness skills
- Facilitate sense of responsibility for self and others
- Encourage nonviolent responses to conflict resolution
- Encourage goal setting
- Encourage development and maintenance of social relationships
- Encourage participation in school, extracurricular, and community activities
- Enhance parental effectiveness of adolescents
- Evaluate teen for stressors and stress management techniques
- Evaluate mood and provide resources for concerns (e.g., depression, suicidal ideation) as needed
- Discuss body modification, such as tattoos and piercings
- Refer for counseling, as needed
- Use teach-back to ensure understanding

3rd edition 2000; revised 2024

Background Evidence:

Garzon Maaks, D. L., Barber Starr, N., Brady, M. A., Gaylord, N. M., Driessnack, M., & Duderstadt, K. (2021). *Burns' pediatric primary care* (7th ed.). Elsevier.

Hagan, J. F., Shaw, J. S., & Duncan, P. M. (2017). *Bright futures: Guidelines for health supervision of infants, children, and Adolescents* (4th ed.). American Academy of Pediatrics.

Hockenberry, M. J., Wilson, D., & Rodgers, C. (2019). *Wong's nursing care of infants and children* (11th ed.). Elsevier.

Perry, S. E., Hockenberry, M. J., Lowdermilk, D. L., & Wilson, D. (2018). *Maternal child nursing care* (6th ed.). Elsevier.

Richardson, B. (2020). *Pediatric primary care: Practice guidelines for nurses* (4th ed.). Jones & Bartlett Learning.

Advance Care Planning 7300

Definition: Providing support to develop a plan for end of life decisions that incorporates personal values, life goals, and preferences

Activities:
- Determine readiness to receive information
- Facilitate discussions about preferences regarding future health care
- Facilitate decision-making and informed choices based on preferences
- Encourage expression of feelings and emotions during discussions
- Identify hopes, fears, and personal life goals and values related to future health care
- Discuss treatment, risks and benefits, and symptom management
- Respect right to receive or not receive information about health and prognosis
- Assist to identify surrogate decision maker when unable to make own decisions

- Facilitate decision-making hierarchy with durable power of attorney for health care
- Include other health care professionals in discussions including spiritual and religious support
- Assist in filing legally recognized advanced directives if appropriate
- Refer to legal aid if indicated
- Refer to hospice services as indicated
- Revisit discussion and update over time as health condition changes
- Document discussions, preferences, and decisions

8th edition 2024

Background Evidence:

Arruda, L. M., Abreu, K., Santana, L., & Sales, M. (2019). Variables that influence the medical decision regarding Advance Directives and their impact on end-of-life care. *Einstein (Sao Paulo, Brazil)*, 18, eRW4852. https://doi.org/10.31744/einstein_journal/2020RW4852

Dingfield, L. E., & Kayser, J. B. (2017). Integrating advance care planning into practice. *Chest*, 151(6), 1387–1393. https://doi.org/10.1016/j.chest.2017.02.024

Nierop-van Baalen, C., Grypdonck, M., Hecke, A., & Verhaeghe, S. (2020). Associated factors of hope in cancer patients during treatment: A systematic literature review. *Journal of Advanced Nursing*, 76(7), 1520–1537. https://doi.org/10.1111/jan.14344

Sudore, R. L., Lum, H. D., You, J. J., Hanson, L. C., Meier, D. E., Pantilat, S. Z., Matlock, D. D., Rietjens, J. A. C., Korgfage, I., Ritchie, C., Kutner, J. S., Teno, J. M., Thomas, J., McMahan, R. D., & Heyland, D. K. (2017). Defining advance care planning for adults: A consensus definition from a multidisciplinary Delphi panel. *Journal of Pain and Symptom Management*, 53(5), 821–832.e821. https://doi.org/10.1016/j.jpainsymman.2016.12.331

Weaver, M. S., Anderson, B., Cole, A., & Lyon, M. E. (2019). Documentation of advance directives and code status in electronic medical records to honor goals of care. *Journal of Palliative Care*, 2019. https://doi.org/10.1177/0825859719860129. 825859719860129

Airway Insertion and Stabilization   3120

Definition: Insertion or assistance with insertion and stabilization of an artificial airway

Activities:

- Perform hand hygiene
- Use personal protective equipment (PPE) (gloves, goggles, and mask), as appropriate
- Select the correct size and type of oropharyngeal or nasopharyngeal airway
- Position patient and head, as appropriate
- Suction mouth and oropharynx
- Insert oro/nasopharyngeal airway, ensuring that it reaches to the base of the tongue, supporting the tongue in a forward position
- Tape the oro/nasopharyngeal airway in place
- Monitor for dyspnea, snoring, or inspiratory crowing when oro/nasopharyngeal airway is in place
- Change the oro/nasopharyngeal airway daily and inspect mucosa
- Insert a laryngeal mask airway (LMA), as appropriate
- Insert an esophageal obturator airway (EOA), as appropriate
- Auscultate for breath sounds bilaterally before inflating the esophageal cuff of the EOA
- Collaborate with the physician to select the correct size and type of endotracheal (ET) or tracheostomy tube
- Select artificial airways with high-volume, low-pressure cuffs
- Limit insertion of ETs and tracheostomies to qualified and credentialed personnel
- Encourage physicians to place ETs via the oropharyngeal route, as appropriate
- Assist with insertion of an ET by gathering necessary intubation and emergency equipment, positioning patient, administering medications as ordered, and monitoring the patient for complications during insertion
- Assist with emergent tracheostomy by setting up appropriate support equipment, administering medications, providing a sterile environment, and monitoring for changes in the patient's condition
- Instruct patient and family about the intubation procedure
- Hyperoxygenate with 100% oxygen for 3 to 5 minutes, as appropriate
- Auscultate the chest after intubation
- Observe for systematic chest wall movement
- Monitor oxygen saturation (SpO_2) by noninvasive pulse oximetry and CO_2 detection
- Monitor respiratory status, as appropriate
- Inflate endotracheal/tracheostomy cuff, using minimal occlusive volume technique or minimal leak technique
- Stabilize endotracheal/tracheostomy tube with adhesive tape, twill tape, or commercially available stabilizing device
- Mark ET at the position of the lips or nares, using the centimeter markings on the ET, and document
- Verify tube placement with a chest radiograph, ensuring cannulation of the trachea 2 to 4 cm higher than the carina
- Minimize leverage and traction of the artificial airway by suspending ventilator tubing from overhead supports, using flexible catheter mounts and swivels, and supporting tubes during turning, suctioning, and ventilator disconnection/reconnection

1st edition 1992; revised 2013

Background Evidence:

Day, M. W. (2005). Laryngeal mask airway. In D. Wiegand & K. Carlson (Eds.), *AACN procedure manual for critical care* (5th ed., pp. 4252). Elsevier Saunders.

Evans-Smith, P. (2005). *Taylor's clinical nursing skills: A nursing process approach*. Lippincott Williams & Wilkins.

Goodrich, C., & Carlson, K. K. (2005). Endotracheal intubation (perform). In D. Wiegand & K. Carlson (Eds.), *AACN procedure manual for critical care* (5th ed., pp. 9–20). Saunders.

Scott, J. M. (2005). Endotracheal intubation (assist). In D. Wiegand & K. Carlson (Eds.), *AACN procedure manual for critical care* (5th ed., pp. 20–27). Elsevier Saunders.

Skillings, K. N., & Curtis, B. L. (2005). Nasopharyngeal airway insertion. In D. Wiegand & K. Carlson (Eds.), *AACN procedure manual for critical care* (5th ed., pp. 53–56). Elsevier Saunders.

Skillings, K. N., & Curtis, B. L. (2005). Oropharyngeal airway insertion. In D. Wiegand & K. Carlson (Eds.), *AACN procedure manual for critical care* (5th ed., pp. 57–61). Elsevier Saunders.

Airway Management 3140

Definition: Facilitation of patency of air passages

Activities:

- Determine if breathing absent or inadequate
- Determine if airway insertion required
- Use hand hygiene and personal protective equipment (PPE) (e.g., gloves, goggles, mask, face shield), as appropriate
- Provide rescue breaths using available equipment (e.g., one-way valve CPR mask, bag mask) if breathing absent
- Determine cause of airway patency issue (e.g., cardiac arrest, drug overdose, upper airway obstruction, trauma, lung disease, congestive heart failure)
- Open airway, using chin lift or jaw thrust technique, as appropriate
- Remove foreign bodies from airway if visible
- Make sure mask has proper seal
- Ensure rescue breath volume associated with chest rise
- Administer intramuscular or intranasal naloxone for person with known or suspected opioid overdose-induced respiratory arrest, as appropriate
- Insert artificial airway device (e.g., oral, nasopharyngeal, tracheal), as appropriate
- Position to maximize ventilation potential (i.e., position to alleviate dyspnea)
- Auscultate breath sounds, noting areas of decreased or absent ventilation and presence of adventitious sounds
- Remove secretions through appropriate means (e.g., coughing; suctioning of oropharynx, nasopharynx, trachea, endotracheal areas)
- Perform chest physical therapy, as appropriate
- Monitor respiratory and oxygenation status, as appropriate
- Encourage slow, deep breathing, turning, and coughing
- Use age appropriate and interactive techniques to encourage deep breathing for children (e.g., blow bubbles with bubble blower; blow on pinwheel, balloons, party blowers; feathers)
- Instruct how to cough effectively
- Assist with incentive spirometer, as appropriate
- Administer bronchodilators or other treatments via aerosol treatments or ultrasonic nebulizer treatments, as prescribed
- Instruct how to use prescribed respiratory treatments, as appropriate
- Administer humidified air or oxygen, as appropriate
- Regulate fluid intake to optimize fluid balance
- Use teach-back to ensure understanding

1st edition 1992; revised 2000, 2004, 2024

Background Evidence:

Burns, S. M., & Delgado, S. A. (2019). *AACN essentials of critical care nursing.* McGraw Hill Education.

Hartjes, T. M. (2017). *Core curriculum for high acuity, progressive and critical care nursing.* American Association of Critical Care Nursing. Elsevier.

Perry, A. G., Potter, P. A., Ostendorf, W., & Laplante, N. (2021). *Clinical nursing skills and techniques* (10th ed.). Elsevier.

Sole, M. L., Klein, D. G., & Moseley, M. J. (2021). *Introduction to critical care nursing* (8th ed.). Elsevier.

Airway Suctioning 3160

Definition: Removal of secretions by inserting a suction catheter into the patient's oral, nasopharyngeal, or tracheal airway

Activities:

- Perform hand hygiene
- Use universal precautions
- Use personal protective equipment (e.g., gloves, goggles, and mask), as appropriate
- Determine the need for oral and/or tracheal suctioning
- Auscultate breath sounds before and after suctioning
- Inform the patient and family about suctioning
- Aspirate the nasopharynx with a bulb syringe or suction device, as appropriate
- Provide sedation, as appropriate
- Insert a nasal airway to facilitate nasotracheal suctioning, as appropriate
- Instruct the patient to take several deep breaths before nasotracheal suctioning and use supplemental oxygen, as appropriate
- Hyperoxygenate with 100% oxygen for at least 30 seconds, using the ventilator or manual resuscitation bag before and after each pass
- Hyperinflate using tidal volumes that are indexed to the size of the patient, as appropriate
- Use closed-system suctioning, as indicated
- Use sterile disposable equipment for each tracheal suction procedure
- Select a suction catheter that is one half the internal diameter of the endotracheal tube, tracheostomy tube, or patient's airway
- Instruct the patient to take slow, deep breaths during insertion of the suction catheter via the nasotracheal route
- Leave the patient connected to the ventilator during suctioning, if a closed tracheal suction system or an oxygen insufflation device adaptor is being used
- Use the lowest amount of wall suction necessary to remove secretions (e.g., 80–120 mm Hg for adults)
- Monitor for presence of pain
- Monitor patient's oxygen status (SaO_2 and SvO_2 levels), neurological status (e.g., mental status, ICP, cerebral perfusion pressure [CPP]) and hemodynamic status (e.g., MAP level and cardiac rhythms) immediately before, during, and after suctioning
- Base the duration of each tracheal suction pass on the necessity to remove secretions and the patient's response to suctioning
- Suction the oropharynx after completion of tracheal suctioning
- Clean area around tracheal stoma after completion of tracheal suctioning, as appropriate
- Stop tracheal suctioning and provide supplemental oxygen if patient experiences bradycardia, an increase in ventricular ectopy, and/or desaturation
- Vary suctioning techniques based on the clinical response of the patient

- Monitor and note secretion color, amount, and consistency
- Send secretions for culture and sensitivity tests, as appropriate
- Instruct the patient and/or family how to suction the airway, as appropriate

1st edition 1992; revised 2013

Background Evidence:

Chulay, M. (2005). Suctioning: Endotracheal or tracheostomy tube. In D. Wiegand & K. Carlson (Eds.), *AACN procedure manual for critical care* (5th ed., pp. 63–70). Elsevier Saunders.

Evans-Smith, P. (2005). *Taylor's clinical nursing skills: A nursing process approach.* Lippincott Williams & Wilkins.

Sole, M. L., Byers, J. F., Ludy, J. E., Zhang, Y., Banta, C. M., & Brummel, K. (2003). A multisite survey of suctioning techniques and airway management practices. *American Journal of Critical Care, 12*(3), 220–230.

Stone, K., Preusser, B., Groch, K., Karl, J., & Gonyon, D. (1991). The effect of lung hyperinflation and endotracheal suctioning on cardiopulmonary hemodynamics. *Nursing Research, 40*(2), 76–80.

Thompson, L. (2000). *Suctioning of adults with an artificial airway: A systematic review. Review No. 9.* The Joanna Briggs Institute.

Allergy Management   6410

Definition: Identification, treatment, and prevention of allergic responses to food, medications, insect bites, and other substances

Activities:

- Identify known allergies (e.g., medication, food, insect, environmental) and usual reaction
- Notify caregivers and health care providers of known allergies
- Document all allergies in clinical record, according to policy
- Place allergy band on person, as appropriate
- Monitor for allergic reactions to new medications, formulas, foods, latex, and test dyes
- Monitor after exposures to agents known to cause allergic responses, for signs of generalized flush, angioedema, urticaria, paroxysmal coughing, severe anxiety, dyspnea, wheezing, orthopnea, vomiting, cyanosis, or shock
- Observe for 30 minutes after administration of agent known to be capable of inducing allergic response
- Determine level of threat allergic reaction presents to health status
- Monitor for reoccurrence of anaphylaxis within 24 hours
- Provide life-saving measures during anaphylactic shock or severe reactions
- Provide medication to reduce or minimize allergic response
- Assist with allergy testing, as appropriate
- Instruct on all new allergies
- Encourage to wear medical alert tab, as appropriate
- Administer allergy injections, as needed
- Watch for allergic responses during immunizations
- Instruct person with new medication prescriptions to monitor for potential allergic reactions
- Instruct how to read food labels for hidden ingredients
- Instruct how to treat rashes, vomiting, diarrhea, or respiratory problems
- Discuss methods to control environmental allergens (e.g., dust, mold, pollen)
- Instruct how to avoid allergens, situations, or substances that cause risk
- Instruct how to respond if anaphylactic reaction occurs
- Instruct on use of epinephrine pen
- Encourage use of healthy coping strategies (e.g., problem-solving, seeking information, sharing feelings)
- Use teach-back to ensure understanding

1st edition 1992; revised 1996, 2000, 2024

Background Evidence:

DunnGalvin, A., Roberts, G., Regent, L., Austin, M., Kenna, F., Schnadt, S., Sanchez, S. A., Hernandez, P., Hjorth, B., Fernandez, R. M., Taylor, S., Baumert, J., Sheikh, A., Astley, S., Crevel, R., & Mills, C. (2019). Understanding how consumers with food allergies make decisions based on precautionary labelling. *Clinical & Experimental Allergy, 49*(11), 1446–1454. https://doi.org/10.1111/cea.13479

Muzalyova, A., & Brunner, J. O. (2020). Determinants of the utilization of allergy management measures among hay fever sufferers: A theory-based cross-sectional study. *BMC Public Health, 20*(1), 1876. https://doi.org/10.1186/s12889-020-09959-w

Saha, S., Vaidyanathan, A., Lo, F., Brown, C., & Hess, J. J. (2021). Short term physician visits and medication prescriptions for allergic disease associated with seasonal tree, grass, and weed pollen exposure across the United States. *Environmental Health: A Global Access Science Source, 20*(1), 1–12. https://doi.org/10.1186/s12940-021-00766-3

Vyles, D., Mistry, R. D., Heffner, V., Drayna, P., Chiu, A., Visotcky, A., Fraser, R., & Brousseau, D. C. (2019). Reported knowledge and management of potential penicillin allergy in children. *Academic Pediatrics, 19*(6), 684–690. https://doi.org/10.1016/j.acap.2019.01.002

Amnioinfusion   6700

Definition: Infusion of fluid into the uterus during labor to relieve umbilical cord compression or to dilute meconium-stained fluid

Activities:

- Observe for signs of inadequate amniotic fluid volume (e.g., oligohydramnios, asymmetrical intrauterine growth retardation, postdatism, known fetal urinary tract abnormalities, prolonged rupture of membranes)
- Recognize potential contraindications for amnioinfusion (e.g., amnionitis, polyhydramnios, multiple gestation, severe fetal distress, fetal scalp pH less than 7.20, known fetal anomaly, known uterine anomaly)

- Observe for variable or prolonged fetal heart decelerations during intrapartal electronic monitoring
- Document presence of thick meconium fluid with rupture of membranes
- Ensure informed consent
- Prepare equipment needed for amnioinfusion
- Flush intrauterine catheter with infusate
- Place intrauterine catheter using sterile technique
- Calibrate and flush catheter after placement
- Infuse isotonic IV solution rapidly into uterine cavity, as prescribed
- Lower head of bed 15 to 30 degrees or place supine with feet elevated higher than heart level
- Maintain continuous infusion at prescribed rates
- Monitor intrauterine pressure readings
- Observe characteristics of return fluid
- Change perineal pads, as appropriate
- Document changes in intrapartal electronic monitor tracings
- Observe for signs of adverse reaction (e.g., uterine overdistension, umbilical cord prolapse, amniotic fluid embolism)

- Obtain cord blood gas levels at time of delivery to evaluate effectiveness of intervention

2nd edition 1996; revised 2004, 2024

Background Evidence:

Ahmed, B. (2021). Amnioinfusion in severe oligohydramnios with intact membrane: An observational study. *Journal of Maternal and Fetal Neonatal Medicine, 23*, 1–4. https://doi.org/10.1080/14767058.2021.1918081

Contro, E., & Jauniaux, E. (2021). Amnioinfusion: from termination of pregnancy to therapy. *British Journal of Gynecology, 128*(2), 303. https://doi.org/10.1111/1471-0528.16484

Matson, S., & Smith, J. E. (2016). *Core curriculum for maternal-newborn nursing* (5th ed.). Elsevier.

Mol, B., Kempen, L., Teeffelen, A., Schuit, E., & Pajkrt, E. (2017). Does amnioinfusion improve perinatal outcome in midtrimester rupture of membranes? A randomized controlled trial. *Journal of Pediatric Child Health, 53*, 69–69. https://doi.org/10.1111/jpc.13494_203

Amputation Care 3420

Definition: Promotion of physical and psychological healing before and after amputation of a body part

Activities:

- Encourage the patient to participate in the decision to amputate, when possible
- Review informed consent with patient
- Provide information and support before and after surgery
- Facilitate use of a pressure-relieving mattress
- Position stump in proper body alignment
- Place a below-the-knee stump in an extended position
- Avoid putting stump in a dependent position to decrease edema and vascular stasis
- Avoid disturbing stump dressing immediately after surgery as long as there is no leakage or sign of infection
- Wrap the stump, as required
- Promote a smooth, conical-shaped stump through wrapping for a proper prosthesis fit
- Monitor amount of edema present in stump
- Monitor for phantom limb pain (i.e., check for burning, cramping, throbbing, crushing, or tingling pain where the limb was)
- Explain that phantom limb pain may start several weeks after surgery and may be triggered by pressure on other areas
- Administer pharmacological and nonpharmacological (e.g., TENS, phonophoresis, and massage) pain control, as needed
- Monitor for psychological concerns (e.g., depression and anxiety) and adjustment related to change in body image
- Monitor wound healing at incision site
- Place affected area in whirlpool bath, as appropriate
- Monitor tissue for skin integrity (e.g., fungal infection, contact dermatitis, and scar management)
- Instruct patient how to correctly perform postsurgical exercises (e.g., range of motion, endurance, and strengthening)
- Encourage patient to perform range-of-motion, endurance, and strengthening exercises after surgery, providing assistance, when necessary
- Instruct patient to avoid sitting for long periods
- Instruct in transfer techniques and assistive devices (e.g., trapeze)
- Assist patient with grieving process associated with the loss of the body part (e.g., accept initial need for concealment of stump)

- Provide gentle persuasion and support to view and handle altered body part
- Facilitate the identification of needed modifications in lifestyle and assistive devices (e.g., home and car)
- Identify modifications in clothing required
- Set mutual goals for progressive self-care
- Encourage patient to practice self-care of stump
- Provide appropriate education for self-care after discharge
- Instruct patient on signs and symptoms to be reported to health care provider (e.g., chronic pain, skin breakdown, tingling, absent peripheral pulse, cool skin temperature, and changes in functional needs or goals)
- Discuss potential long-term goals for rehabilitation (e.g., walking without a support device)
- Encourage and facilitate interaction with persons with similar amputations, as appropriate
- Supervise initial use and care of the prosthesis
- Cleanse the prosthesis
- Instruct patient and family how to care for and apply the prosthesis
- Assess prosthesis regularly for stability, ease of movement, energy efficiency, and gait appearance
- Remove prosthesis before surgery, as appropriate
- Secure prosthesis when not in use
- Refer to specialist for modification of prosthesis or treatment of complications related to its use

1st edition 1992; revised 2004, 2013

Background Evidence:

Bloomquist, T. (2001). Amputation and phantom limb pain: A pain-prevention model. *American Association of Nurse Anesthetists Journal, 69*(3), 211–217.

Bryant, G. (2001). Stump care. *AJN: American Journal of Nursing, 101*(2), 67–71.

Department of Veterans Affairs, Department of Defense. (2007). *VA/DoD Clinical practice guideline for rehabilitation of lower limb amputation.*

Esquenazi, A., & DiGiacomo, R. (2001). Rehabilitation after amputation. *Journal of the American Podiatric Association, 91*(1), 13–22.

Gibson, J. (2001). Lower limb amputation. *Nursing Standard, 15*(28), 47–52.

Perry, A. G., & Potter, P. A. (2010). *Clinical nursing skills and techniques* (pp. 1028–1032) (7th ed.). Mosby Elsevier.

Sjodahl, C., Jarnlo, G. B., & Persson, B. (2001). Gait improvement in unilateral transfemoral amputees by a combined psychological and physiotherapeutic treatment. *Journal of Rehabilitation Medicine, 33*(3), 114–118.

A

Analgesic Administration   2210

Definition: Use of pharmacologic agents to reduce or eliminate pain

Activities:

- Establish effective communication patterns among patient, family, and caregivers to achieve adequate pain management
- Ensure holistic approach to pain management (i.e., adequate consideration of physiological, social, spiritual, psychological, and cultural influences)
- Adapt pain monitoring techniques to accommodate patients with communication impairments (e.g., pediatric, elderly, cognitively impaired, psychotic, critically ill, non-English speaking, dementia)
- Determine pain onset, location, duration, characteristics, quality, intensity, pattern, relief measures, contributing symptoms, effects on patient, and severity before medicating patient
- Determine patient's current level of comfort and desired level of comfort, using an appropriate pain rating scale
- Document all pain monitoring findings
- Check medical order for drug, dose, and frequency of analgesic prescribed
- Determine patient's previous response to analgesics (e.g., if non-opioid medication as effective as opioid)
- Determine patient's previous doses and routes of analgesic administration to avoid undertreatment or overtreatment
- Check history for drug allergies
- Involve patient in selection of analgesic, route, and dose, as appropriate
- Choose the appropriate analgesic or combination of analgesics when more than one is prescribed
- Determine analgesic selections (narcotic, nonnarcotic, or NSAID), based on type and severity of pain
- Assure that patient is not at risk for NSAID use (e.g., history of GI bleeding or renal insufficiency)
- Assure that patient is not at risk for opioid use (e.g., history of obstructive or central sleep apnea)
- Determine the preferred analgesic, route of administration, and dosage to achieve optimal analgesia
- Choose the IV route, rather than IM, for frequent pain medication injections, when possible
- Avoid IM route in older adults
- Assure accurate 24-hour dosage is maintained (e.g., no more than 4000 mg acetaminophen and acetylsalicylic acid [ASA]; 3200 mg for ibuprofen)
- Assure appropriateness of opioid dosage (e.g., large doses acceptable in opioid-tolerant patients but not opioid-naïve patients)
- Titrate opioid to desired effect or to uncontrollable side effects (e.g., comfort versus respiratory depression)
- Adjust dosages for children and older adults, as appropriate
- Account for narcotics and other restricted drugs, according to agency protocol
- Monitor vital signs before and after administering narcotic analgesics with first-time dose or if unusual signs are noted
- Record pain level using appropriate pain scale before and after administering analgesics
- Attend to comfort needs and other activities that assist relaxation to facilitate response to analgesia
- Assist patient in selecting nonpharmacological activities that have relieved pain in the past (e.g., distraction, music, simple relaxation therapy)
- Administer analgesics around the clock to prevent peaks and troughs of analgesia, especially with severe pain, as appropriate
- Give analgesics before pain-producing procedures or activities
- Set positive expectations regarding the effectiveness of analgesics to optimize patient response
- Administer adjuvant analgesics and medications to potentiate analgesia, when needed
- Consider use of continuous infusion, either alone or in conjunction with bolus opioids, to maintain serum levels
- Institute safety precautions for those receiving narcotic analgesics, as appropriate
- Instruct to request PRN pain medication before the pain is severe
- Inform the individual that with narcotic administration, drowsiness sometimes occurs during the first 2 to 3 days and then subsides
- Correct misconceptions and myths patient or family members may hold regarding analgesics, particularly opioids (e.g., addiction and risks of overdose)
- Implement measures to reduce noxious stimuli in patient environment (i.e., keep patients clean, dry, correctly positioned, and turned regularly; prevent constipation and urinary retention; loosen constrictive bandages or clothing, as indicated; tighten and smooth wrinkled bed linens)
- Evaluate the effectiveness of analgesic at regular, frequent intervals after each administration, but especially after the initial doses
- Implement actions to decrease untoward effects of analgesics (e.g., respiratory depression, nausea and vomiting, dry mouth, constipation, gastric irritation)
- Document response to analgesic and any untoward effects
- Evaluate and document level of sedation for patients receiving opioids
- Administer opioid reversal agents (e.g., naloxone) for respiratory depression or undesirable sedation, if indicated
- Collaborate with the physician if drug, dose, route of administration, or interval changes are indicated, making specific recommendations based on equianalgesic principles
- Instruct patient and family about the use of analgesics, strategies to decrease side effects, and expectations for involvement in decisions about pain relief
- Involve family/significant other(s) in pain control measures such as simple massage or heat/cold application techniques

1st edition 1992; revised 1996, 2018

A

Background Evidence:

American Society for Pain Management Nursing. (2010). In B. St. Marie (Ed.), *Core curriculum for pain management nursing* (2nd ed.). Kendall Hunt.

Herr, K. (2010). Pain in the older adult. *Pain Management Nursing, 11*(Suppl. 2), S1–S10.

Herr, K., Coyne, P., Key, T., Manworren, R., McCaffery, M., Merkel, S., Pelosi-Kelly, J., & Wild, L. (2006). Pain assessment in the nonverbal patient: Position statement with clinical practice recommendations. *Pain Management Nursing, 7*(2), 44–52.

Pasero, C., & McCaffery, M. (2011). *Pain assessment and pharmacologic management.* Elsevier Mosby.

Perry, A., Potter, P., & Ostendorf, W. (Eds.). (2014). *Clinical nursing skills and techniques* (8th ed.). Elsevier Mosby.

Analgesic Administration: Intraspinal   2214

Definition: Administration of pharmacologic agents into the epidural or intrathecal space to reduce or eliminate pain

Activities:

- Instruct patient and significant others about the procedure
- Check patency and function of intraspinal catheter, port, or pump
- Ensure that IV access is in place at all times during therapy
- Label the intraspinal catheter and secure it appropriately
- Ensure catheter site is visible and covered with a transparent dressing for monitoring purposes
- Ensure that edges of site dressing are window-paned to prevent rolling of the dressing
- Monitor catheter site and dressings to check for a loose catheter or wet dressing and notify appropriate personnel per agency protocol
- Label tubing and site "Intraspinal Catheter—Do not Inject"
- Administer catheter site care according to agency protocol
- Avoid the use of alcohol on the catheter or connectors (i.e., alcohol is neurotoxic)
- Secure needle in place with tape and apply appropriate dressing according to agency protocol
- Ensure that the proper formulation of the drug is used (e.g., high concentrating and preservative free)
- Ensure narcotic antagonist availability for emergency administration and administer per physician order, as necessary
- Start continuous infusion of analgesic agent after correct catheter placement has been verified and monitor rate to ensure delivery of prescribed dosage of medication
- Monitor effectiveness of pain medication
- Monitor temperature, blood pressure, respirations, pulse, and level of consciousness at appropriate intervals and record on flow sheet
- Monitor respiratory status every hour for first 24 hours after catheter insertion, when patient is at highest risk for respiratory depression
- Monitor level of sensory blockade at appropriate intervals and record on flow sheet
- Determine sensation every 2 hours using cold sensation with ice
- Apply ice up from the toe and note where coldness is detected by the patient
- Document numbness, tingling or normal sensation, and motor block using appropriate dermatomes
- Determine the level of block to see if it is changing
- Notify physician of sensation or motor block higher than the initial documented level
- Identify weakness and sensation level for comparison (i.e., weakness should be correlated to the level of sensation)
- Monitor for adverse reactions, including respiratory depression, urinary retention, undue somnolence, itching, seizures, nausea, and vomiting
- Monitor orthostatic blood pressure and pulse before the first attempt at ambulation
- Instruct patient to report side effects, alterations in pain relief, numbness of extremities, and need for assistance with ambulation if weak
- Monitor intake and output
- Monitor for urinary retention
- Follow institutional policies for injection of intermittent analgesic agents into the injection port
- Provide adjunct medications for pain relief (e.g., antidepressants, anticonvulsants, and nonsteroidal anti-inflammatory agents), as appropriate
- Increase intraspinal dose, based on pain intensity score
- Instruct and guide patient through nonpharmalogical measures (e.g., relaxation therapy, guided imagery, and biofeedback) to enhance pharmacological effectiveness
- Instruct patient about proper home care for external or implanted delivery systems, as appropriate
- Remove or assist with removal of catheter according to agency protocol

2nd edition 1996; revised 2018

Background Evidence:

Coyne, P., Smith, T., Laird, J., Hansen, L., & Drake, D. (2005). Effectively starting and titrating intrathecal analgesic therapy in patients with refractory cancer pain. *Clinical Journal of Oncology Nursing, 9*(5), 581–583.

Hinkle, J., & Cheever, K. (2014). *Brunner & Suddarth's textbook of medical surgical nursing* (13th ed.). Lippincott Williams & Wilkins.

Pasero, C., Eksterowicz, N., Primeau, M., & Cowley, C. (2007). Registered nurse management and monitoring of analgesia by catheter techniques: Position statement. *Pain Management Nursing, 8*(2), 48–54.

Stearns, L., Boortz-Marx, R., Du Pen, S., Friehs, G., Gordon, M., Halyard, M., Herbst, L., & Kiser, J. (2005). Intrathecal drug delivery for the management of cancer pain: A multidisciplinary consensus of best clinical practice. *Journal of Supportive Oncology, 3*(6), 399–408.

Anaphylaxis Management 6412

Definition: Promotion of adequate ventilation and tissue perfusion for an individual with a severe allergic reaction

Activities:
- Perform rapid evaluation of airway, breathing, circulation, and mental status
- Establish and maintain patent airway
- Identify and remove source of allergen, if possible
- Administer solution of epinephrine, 1:1000, intramuscular (preferred) or subcutaneously, dosing appropriate for age
- Provide continuous monitoring of mental status, vital signs, and medication administration
- Place in position of comfort (may need to elevate lower extremities, depending on vital signs)
- Administer high-flow supplemental oxygen (6–8 L/min) via facemask
- Establish IV access using 0.9% (isotonic) saline
- Reassure individual and family members
- Monitor for signs of shock (e.g., respiratory difficulty, cardiac arrhythmias, seizures, hypotension)
- Administer IV fluids rapidly (e.g., 1000 mL/hr) to support blood pressure, per health care provider order or protocol
- Administer secondary medications (e.g., beta-2 adrenergic agonists, antihistamines, corticosteroids), as indicated if urticaria, angioedema, or bronchospasm present
- Consult with other health care providers and refer, as needed
- Instruct on medication management (e.g., epinephrine injection pen, antihistamine, corticosteroids)
- Instruct on prevention of future episodes (e.g., allergen testing)
- Instruct on importance of medical identification
- Include family in instruction, as appropriate
- Use teach-back to ensure understanding

3rd edition 2000; revised 2004, 2024

Background Evidence:

Curry, S. (2021). Managing anaphylaxis in adults. *British Journal of Nursing*, *30*(19), 1118–1122. https://doi.org/10.12968/bjon.2021.30.19.1118

Emergency Nurses Association. (2017). *Emergency nursing core curriculum* (7th ed.). Elsevier.

Long, B., & Gottlieb, M. (2021). Emergency medicine updates: Anaphylaxis. *American Journal of Emergency Medicine*, *49*, 35–39. https://doi.org/10.1016/j.ajem.2021.05.006

Sweet, V., & Foley, A. (2020). *Sheehy's emergency nursing: Principles and practice*. Elsevier.

Tanno, L., Alvarez-Perea, A., & Pouessel, G. (2019). Therapeutic approach of anaphylaxis. *Current Opinion in Allergy & Clinical Immunology*, *19*(4), 393–401. https://doi.org/10.1097/ACI.0000000000000539h

Anesthesia Administration 2840

Definition: Preparation for and administration of anesthetic agents and monitoring of patient responsiveness during administration

Activities:
- Evaluate patient preoperatively in advance of the scheduled surgical procedure, preferably one or more days before procedure
- Verify that the information provided by the patient is the same as the information in the identification device (e.g., wristbands, bed tag, fingerprint recognition software, palm vein scanner) and medical record
- Examine patient and the patient's record to determine preexisting conditions, allergies, and contraindications for specific anesthetic agents or techniques
- Document patient's readiness for anesthesia (e.g., preoperative fasting, medication regime, absence of upper respiratory tract infections, airway history)
- Document patient's weight
- Request appropriate consultations, including diagnostic and laboratory studies, based on the patient's health status and proposed surgery
- Implement indicated preoperative activities to prepare patient physiologically for surgery and anesthesia
- Develop and document an anesthetic plan appropriate for the patient and procedure
- Collaborate with involved health care providers throughout all phases of anesthesia care
- Inform the patient what to expect from anesthesia, answering any questions and concerns
- Obtain informed consent
- Perform a safety check on all anesthesia equipment before each anesthetic is administered
- Ensure availability of essential emergency and resuscitation equipment
- Start appropriate intravenous and invasive monitoring lines and initiate noninvasive monitoring modalities, per the American Society of Anesthesiologists Standards for Basic Anesthetic Monitoring
- Administer appropriate preanesthetic medications and fluids
- Assist in the transfer of the patient from the stretcher to the operating room table
- Ensure positioning of patient to prevent peripheral nerve damage and pressure injuries
- Ensure proper placement of safety strap and continuous patient safety throughout all phases of anesthesia care
- Deliver anesthetic consistent with each patient's physiological needs, patient's requests, clinical judgment, and the American Association of Nurse Anesthetists Scope and Standards for Nurse Anesthesia Practice
- Maintain an adequate airway, ensuring adequate oxygenation during all phases of anesthesia care
- Determine acceptable blood loss and administer blood, if needed
- Calculate appropriate fluid needs and administer intravenous fluids, as indicated
- Monitor vital signs, respiratory and circulatory adequacy, response to anesthesia, and other physiological parameters
- Measure and evaluate appropriate laboratory values
- Administer adjunct drugs and fluids necessary to manage the anesthetic, maintain physiological homeostasis, and correct adverse or unfavorable responses to anesthesia and surgery

A

- Provide eye protection
- Manage emergence from anesthesia by administering indicated medications, fluids, and ventilatory support
- Accompany patient to the postanesthesia or intensive care unit with appropriate monitoring and oxygen therapy
- Provide comprehensive patient report to nursing staff on arrival in unit
- Manage postoperative pain and anesthetic side effects
- Ascertain patient recovery and stability in the immediate postoperative period before transfer of care
- Provide postanesthesia follow-up evaluation and care related to anesthesia side effects and complications after discharge from postanesthesia care area

1st edition 1992; revised 1996, 2018

Background Evidence:

American Association of Nurse Anesthetists (AANA). (2013). *Professional practice manual for the certified registered nurse anesthetist.*

American Society for Anesthesiologists (ASA). (2011). *Standards for basic anesthetic monitoring.* https://www.asahq.org/

Naglehaut, J., & Plaus, K. (2014). *Nurse anesthesia* (5th ed.). Elsevier Saunders.

Perry, A., Potter, P., & Ostendorf, W. (Eds.). (2014). *Clinical nursing skills and techniques* (8th ed.). Elsevier Mosby.

Rothrock, J. C. (Ed.). (2015). *Alexander's care of the patient in surgery* (15th ed.). Elsevier Mosby.

Anger Control Assistance

4640

Definition: Facilitation of the expression of anger in an adaptive, nonviolent manner

Activities:

- Establish basic trust and rapport with patient
- Use a calm, reassuring approach
- Determine appropriate behavioral expectations for expression of anger, given patient's level of cognitive and physical functioning
- Limit access to frustrating situations until patient is able to express anger in an adaptive manner
- Encourage patient to seek assistance of nursing staff or responsible others during periods of increasing tension
- Monitor potential for inappropriate aggression and intervene before its expression
- Prevent physical harm if anger is directed at self or others (e.g., restrain and remove potential weapons)
- Discourage intense activities (e.g., punching bag, pacing, excessive exercise)
- Educate on methods to modulate experience of intense emotion (e.g., assertiveness training, relaxation techniques, writing in a journal, distraction)
- Provide reassurance to patient that nursing staff will intervene to prevent patient from losing control
- Encourage use of collaboration to solve problems
- Offer PRN medications, as appropriate
- Use external controls (e.g., physical or manual restraint, time outs, and seclusion) to calm patient who is expressing anger in a maladaptive manner, as needed (as last resort)
- Provide feedback on behavior to help patient identify anger
- Assist patient in identifying the source of anger
- Identify the function that anger, frustration, and rage serve for the patient
- Identify consequences of inappropriate expression of anger
- Assist patient in planning strategies to prevent the inappropriate expression of anger
- Identify with patient the benefits of expressing anger in an adaptive, nonviolent manner
- Establish expectation that patient can control his/her behavior
- Instruct on use of calming measures (e.g., time outs and deep breaths)
- Assist in developing appropriate methods of expressing anger to others (e.g., assertiveness and use of feeling statements)
- Provide role models who express anger appropriately
- Support patient in implementing anger control strategies and in the appropriate expression of anger
- Provide reinforcement for appropriate expression of anger

1st edition 1992; revised 2008

Background Evidence:

Bushman, B. J. (2002). Does venting anger feed or extinguish the flame? Catharsis, rumination, distraction, and aggressive responding. *Personality and Social Psychology Bulletin, 28*(6), 724–731.

Carpenito, L. J. (2004). *Nursing diagnosis: Application to clinical practice* (10th ed.). Lippincott Williams & Wilkins.

Harris, D., & Morrison, E. F. (1995). Managing violence without coercion. *Archives of Psychiatric Nursing, 9*(4), 203–210.

Kanak, M. F. (1992). Interventions related to safety. *Nursing Clinics of North America, 27*(2), 371–395.

Morrison, E. F. (1993). Toward a better understanding of violence in psychiatric settings: Debunking the Myths. *Archives of Psychiatric Nursing, 7*(6), 328–335.

Schultz, J. M., & Videbeck, S. L. (2005). *Lippincott's manual of psychiatric nursing care plans* (7th ed.). Lippincott Williams & Wilkins.

Stuart, G., & Laraia, M. T. (2005). *Principles and practice of psychiatric nursing* (8th ed.). Mosby.

Animal-Assisted Therapy   4320

A

Definition: Purposeful use of animals to provide comfort and emotional support, and to control anxiety and improve mood

Activities:
- Determine person's acceptance of animals as therapeutic agents
- Determine if any allergies to animals
- Explain purpose and rationale for having animals in care environment
- Enforce standards for screening, training, health maintenance, and grooming of animals in therapy program
- Fulfill health department regulations concerning animals in institution
- Develop policy or protocol that outlines appropriate response to accident or injury as result of animal contact
- Provide therapy animals as needed
- Wash hands before and after handling pet
- Avoid animal visits with unpredictable or violent persons
- Monitor animal visits with persons with special conditions (e.g., open wounds, delicate skin, multiple IV lines, other equipment)
- Facilitate person's holding and petting therapy animals
- Encourage interactions with therapy animal (e.g., petting, feeding, grooming)
- Note response to interactions with therapy animals
- Provide opportunity to reminisce and share previous experiences with pets or other animals

1st edition 1992; revised 2000, 2024

Background Evidence:

Aarskog, N., Hunskår, I., & Bruvik, F. (2019). Animal-Assisted interventions with dogs and robotic animals for residents with dementia in nursing homes: A systematic review. *Physical & Occupational Therapy in Geriatrics, 37*(2), 77–93. https://doi.org/10.1080/02703181.2019.1613466

Cooley, L. F., & Barker, S. B. (2018). Canine-assisted therapy as an adjunct tool in the care of the surgical patient: A literature review and opportunity for research. *Alternative Therapies in Health and Medicine, 24*(3), 48–51.

Lobato Rincón, L. L., Rivera Martín, B., Medina Sánchez, M. Á., Villafaina, S., Merellano-Navarro, E., & Collado-Mateo, D. (2021). Effects of dog-assisted education on physical and communicative skills in children with severe and multiple disabilities: A pilot study. *Animals: An Open Access Journal from MDPI, 11*(6). https://doi.org/10.3390/ani11061741

Miller, J. (2020). Animal-assisted interventions: Impact on patient outcomes and satisfaction. *Nursing Management, 51*(4), 16–23. https://doi.org/10.1097/01.NUMA.0000657240.17744.1b

Uglow, L. S. (2019). The benefits of an animal-assisted intervention service to patients and staff at a children's hospital. *British Journal of Nursing (Mark Allen Publishing), 28*(8), 509–515. https://doi.org/10.12968/bjon.2019.28.8.509

Anticipatory Guidance   5210

Definition: Preparation of patient for an anticipated developmental or situational crisis

Activities:
- Assist the patient to identify possible upcoming, developmental, or situational crisis and the effects the crisis may have on personal and family life
- Instruct about normal development and behavior, as appropriate
- Provide information on realistic expectations related to the patient's behavior
- Determine the patient's usual methods of problem solving
- Assist the patient to decide how the problem will be solved
- Assist the patient to decide who will solve the problem
- Use case examples to enhance the patient's problem-solving skills, as appropriate
- Assist the patient to identify available resources and options for course of action, as appropriate
- Rehearse techniques needed to cope with upcoming developmental milestone or situational crisis with the patient, as appropriate
- Assist the patient to adapt to anticipated role changes
- Provide a ready reference for the patient (e.g., educational materials, pamphlets), as appropriate
- Suggest printed literature and electronic sources for the patient to read, as appropriate
- Refer the patient to community agencies, as appropriate
- Schedule visits at strategic developmental or situational points
- Schedule extra visits for patient with concerns or difficulties
- Schedule follow-up phone calls to evaluate success or reinforcement needs
- Provide the patient with a phone number to call for assistance, if necessary
- Include the family and significant others, when possible

1st edition 1992; revised 2013

Background Evidence:

Craft-Rosenberg, M., & Krajicek, M. (Eds.). (2006). *Nursing excellence for children and families.* Springer.

Hagan, J., Shaw, J., & Duncan, P. (Eds.). (2007). *Bright futures: Guidelines for health supervision of infants, children, and adolescents* (3rd ed.). American Academy of Pediatrics.

Rancour, P. (2008). Using archetypes and transitions theory to help patients move from active treatment to survivorship. *Clinical Journal of Oncology Nursing, 12*(6), 935–940.

Rosen, L. (2008). Infant sleep and feeding. *Journal of Obstetric, Gynecologic, & Neonatal Nursing, 37*(6), 706–714.

Sattler, B., & Davis, A. (2008). Nurses' role in children's environmental health protection. *Pediatric Nursing, 34*(4), 329–339.

Skybo, T., & Policka, B. (2007). Health promotion model for childhood violence prevention and exposure. *Journal of Clinical Nursing, 16*(1), 38–45.

A

Anxiety Reduction   5820

Definition: Minimizing apprehension, dread, foreboding, or uneasiness related to an unidentified source of anticipated danger

Activities:
- Identify verbal and nonverbal signs of anxiety
- Use calm, reassuring approach
- Clearly state expectations for behavior
- Explain all procedures, including sensations likely to be experienced during procedures
- Seek to understand person's perspective of stressful situations
- Provide information concerning diagnosis, treatment, and prognosis
- Stay with person to promote safety and reduce anxiety
- Encourage family to stay with person, as appropriate
- Provide objects that symbolize safeness
- Administer back and neck massage, as appropriate
- Encourage noncompetitive activities, as appropriate
- Keep treatment equipment out of sight
- Listen attentively
- Reinforce behavior, as appropriate
- Create atmosphere to facilitate trust
- Encourage verbalization of feelings, perceptions, and fears
- Identify when level of anxiety changes
- Provide diversional activities geared toward reduction of tension
- Guide in taking slow deep breaths
- Help identify situations that precipitate anxiety
- Manage stimuli as appropriate for needs
- Support use of appropriate psychological defense mechanisms
- Assist to articulate realistic description of upcoming event
- Determine decision-making ability

- Instruct on use of relaxation techniques (e.g., guided imagery, music, massage, aroma therapy, art therapy, yoga, Tai Chi)
- Suggest use of phone apps and virtual immerse reality technology that promotes relaxation
- Administer medications to reduce anxiety, as appropriate

1st edition 1992; revised 2004; 2024

Background Evidence:

Boyer, P. J., Yell, J. A., Andrews, J. G., & Seckeler, M. D. (2020). Anxiety reduction after pre-procedure meetings in persons with CHD. *Cardiology in the Young, 30*(7), 991–994. https://doi.org/10.1017/S1047951120001407

Brandt, C. P., Paulus, D. J., Lopez-Gamundi, P., Green, C., Lemaire, C., & Zvolensky, M. J. (2019). HIV Anxiety Reduction/Management Program (HAMRT): Pilot randomized controlled trial. *AIDS Care, 31*(12), 1527–1532. https://doi.org/10.1080/09540121.2019.1597962

Keptner, K. M., Fitzgibbon, C., & O'Sullivan, J. (2021). Effectiveness of anxiety reduction interventions on test anxiety: A comparison of four techniques incorporating sensory modulation. *British Journal of Occupational Therapy, 84*(5), 289–297. https://doi.org/10.1177/0308022620935061

Sridhar, A., Shiliang, Z., Woodson, R., & Kwan, L. (2020). Non-pharmacological anxiety reduction with immersive virtual reality for first-trimester dilation and curettage: A pilot study. *European Journal of Contraception & Reproductive Health Care, 25*(6), 480–483. https://doi.org/10.1080/1362 5187.2020.1836146

Area Restriction   6420

Definition: Use of least restrictive limitation of patient mobility to a specified area for purposes of safety or behavior management

Activities:
- Establish that the least restrictive measure is being initiated (if a lower level was used, establish that it was deemed ineffective before advancing to the next level of restriction)
- Obtain a licensed independent practitioner (LIP) order as required by selection of measure based on institutional policy and state, federal, and regulatory agencies (e.g., Centers for Medicare & Medicaid Services, The Joint Commission)
- Identify for patient and significant others those behaviors that necessitated the intervention
- Explain the procedure, purpose, and time period of the intervention to patient and significant others in understandable and nonpunitive terms
- Identify for the patient and significant others the appropriate behaviors necessary for termination of the intervention, repeat as needed
- Restrict to designated area that is appropriate

- Modulate human and environmental sensory stimuli (e.g., visiting sessions, sights, sounds, lighting, temperature, etc.) in the designated area, as needed
- Use protective devices and measures (e.g., motion detectors, alarms, fences, gates, side rails, mitts, closed chairs, locked doors, restraints)
- Provide appropriate level of supervision/surveillance to monitor patient and allow for therapeutic actions, as needed
- Administer PRN medications (e.g., anxiolytics, antipsychotics, sedatives), as appropriate
- Monitor patient's response to the procedure
- Provide for the patient's physical needs and safety (e.g., cardiovascular, respiratory, neurological, elimination, and nutrition, and skin integrity), as appropriate
- Provide for the patient's psychological comfort and safety
- Offer structured activities within the designated area, as appropriate

- Give immediate feedback about inappropriate behavior the patient can control and that contributes to need for continued restrictive measure
- Provide verbal reminders to remain in designated area, as necessary
- Assist patient to modify inappropriate behavior, when possible
- Provide positive reinforcement for appropriate behavior
- Monitor the need for changes (e.g., lower/higher level measure, continue, or discontinue) to the restrictive measure at regular intervals
- Involve patient in decision to change a restrictive measure (e.g., lower/higher level measure, continue, or discontinue), when appropriate
- Hold a debriefing session (e.g., covering behaviors leading to the measures, and patient concerns about the intervention) with patient and staff after termination of the intervention
- Document (e.g., rationale for the restrictive measure, patient's physical and psychological condition, nursing care provided, and the rationale for terminating the intervention) at appropriate points in care according to institutional policy, state, federal, and/or regulatory agency requirements

1st edition 1992; revised 2008

Background Evidence:

American Psychiatric Nurses Association. (2000). *Position statement on the use of seclusion and restraint.*

Clark, M. A. (2005). Involuntary admission and the medical inpatient: Judicious use of physical restraint. *Medsurg Nursing, 14*(4), 213–218.

Gillies, J., Moriarty, H., Short, T., Pesnell, P., Fox, C., & Cooney, A. (2005). An innovative model for restraint use at the Philadelphia Veterans Affairs Medical Center. *Nursing Administration Quarterly, 29*(1), 45–56.

Harper-Jaques, S., & Reimer, M. (2005). Management of aggression and violence. In M. A. Boyd (Ed.), *Psychiatric nursing: Contemporary practice* (3rd ed., pp. 802–822). Lippincott Williams & Wilkins.

McCloskey, R. M. (2004). Caring for patients with dementia in an acute care environment. *Geriatric Nursing, 25*(3), 139–144.

Park, M., Hsiao-Chen, T. J., & Ledford, L. (2005). *Changing the practice of physical restraint use in acute care.* The University of Iowa, College of Nursing, Gerontological Nursing Interventions Research Center.

Rickelman, B. L. (2006). The client who displays angry, aggressive, or violent behavior. In W. K. Mohr (Ed.), *Psychiatric mental health nursing* (6th ed., pp. 659–686). Lippincott Williams & Wilkins.

Aromatherapy   1330

Definition: Administration of essential oils through massage, topical ointments or lotions, baths, inhalation, douches, or compresses (hot or cold) to calm and soothe, provide pain relief, and enhance relaxation and comfort

Activities:

- Obtain consent for use of aromatherapy
- Select appropriate essential oil or blend of essential oils to obtain desired outcome
- Administer essential oil using appropriate methods (e.g., topical, inhalation)
- Determine individual response to selected aroma before use
- Instruct in use of essential oils, mode of action, and any contraindications
- Monitor individual for discomfort and nausea before and after administration
- Dilute essential oils with appropriate carrier oils before topical use, as needed
- Avoid prolonged use of same essential oil or repeated topical application to same site
- Ensure adequate ventilation when using essential oils
- Instruct on purposes and application of aromatherapy, as appropriate
- Monitor baseline and follow-up vital signs, as appropriate
- Monitor for level of stress, mood, and anxiety before and after aromatherapy
- Evaluate response to aromatherapy
- Document responses to aromatherapy
- Use teach-back to ensure understanding

4th edition 2004; revised 2024

Background Evidence:

Allard, M. E., & Katseres, J. (2018). Using essential oils to enhance nursing practice and for self-care. *Nurse Practitioner, 43*(5), 39–46. https://doi.org/10.1097/01.NPR.0000531915.69268.8f

Dilek, B., & Necmiye, C. (2020). Usage of aromatherapy in symptom management in cancer patients: A systematic review. *International Journal of Caring Sciences, 13*(1), 537–546.

Es-haghee, S., Shabani, F., Hawkins, J., Zareian, M. A., Nejatbakhsh, F., Qaraaty, M., & Tabarrai, M. (2020). The effects of aromatherapy on premenstrual syndrome symptoms: A systematic review and meta-analysis of randomized clinical trials. *Evidence-Based Complementary & Alternative Medicine (ECAM), 2020,* 1–13.

Hui Zhao, Weiwei Gu, & Zhang, Min (2020). Massage therapy in nursing as nonpharmacological intervention to control agitation and stress in patients with dementia. *Alternative Therapies in Health & Medicine, 26*(6), 29–33.

Safajou, F., Soltani, N., Taghizadeh, M., Amouzeshi, Z., & Sandrous, M. (2020). The effect of combined inhalation aromatherapy with lemon and peppermint on nausea and vomiting of pregnancy: A double-blind, randomized clinical trial. *Iranian Journal of Nursing & Midwifery Research, 25*(5), 401–406. https://doi.org/10.4103/ijnmr.IJNMR_11_19

Wu, C-Y., Lee, H-F., Chang, C. W., Chiang, H-C., Tsai, Y-H., & Liu, H-E. (2020). The immediate effects of lavender aromatherapy massage versus massage in work stress, burnout, and HRV parameters: A randomized controlled trial. *Evidence-Based Complementary & Alternative Medicine (ECAM), 2020,* 1–10. https://doi.org/10.1155/2020/8830083

Art Therapy   4330

Definition: Facilitation of communication through drawings or other art forms

Activities:
- Identify form of art-based activity (e.g., preexisting, impromptu, directed, spontaneous)
- Identify art medium to be used, such as drawings (e.g., self-portrait, human figure drawings, family kinetic drawings), photos and other media (e.g., photo journal, media journal), graphics (e.g., timeline, body maps), or artifacts (e.g., masks, sculpture)
- Discuss with patient what to make, using direct or nondirect approach, as appropriate
- Provide art supplies appropriate for developmental level and goals for therapy
- Provide a quiet environment that is free from interruptions
- Monitor patient's engagement during the art-making process, including verbal comments and behaviors
- Encourage patient to describe drawing or artistic creation
- Discuss description of drawing or artistic creation with patient
- Record patient interpretation of drawings or artistic creation
- Identify themes in artwork collected over a period of time
- Copy patient's artwork for files, as needed and as appropriate
- Use human figure drawings to determine patient's self-concept
- Use drawings to determine the effects of stress events (e.g., hospitalization, divorce, or abuse) on patient
- Encourage patient to describe and talk about the art product and the art-making process
- Incorporate patient's description and interpretation of the art activity into patient assessment data

- Compare art product and art-making process to patient's developmental level and prior art making activities
- Interpret meaning of significant aspects of the drawings, incorporating patient assessment data and literature on art therapy
- Avoid reading meaning into drawings before having a complete history, baseline drawings, and a collection of drawings done over a period
- Provide referral (e.g., social work, art therapy), as indicated

1st edition 1992; revised 2013

Background Evidence:

Cox, M. (2005). *The pictorial world of the child.* Cambridge University Press.

Darley, S., & Health, W. (2008). *The expressive arts activity book: A resource for professionals.* Jessica Kingsley.

Dixon, S. D., & Stein, M. T. (2006). *Encounters with children: Pediatric behavior and development* (4th ed.). Mosby Elsevier.

Driessnack, M. (2006). Draw-and-tell conversations with children. *Qualitative Health Research, 16*(10), 1414–1435.

Driessnack, M. (2009). Using the Colored Eco-Genetic Relationship Map (CEGRM) with children. *Nursing Research, 58*(5), 304–311.

Malchiodi, C. A. (2002). *The soul's palette: Drawing on art's transformative power.* Shambhala.

McNiff, S. (2004). *Art heals: How creativity cures the soul.* Shambhala.

Seiden, D. (2001). *Mind over matter: The uses of materials in art, education, and therapy.* Magnolia Street Pub.

Artificial Airway Management   3180

Definition: Maintenance of endotracheal and tracheostomy tubes and prevention of complications associated with their use

Activities:
- Perform hand hygiene
- Use universal precautions
- Use personal protective equipment (e.g., gloves, goggles, and mask), as appropriate
- Provide an oropharyngeal airway or bite block to prevent biting on the endotracheal tube, as appropriate
- Provide 100% humidification of inspired air, oxygen, or gas
- Provide adequate systemic hydration via oral or intravenous fluid administration
- Inflate endotracheal/tracheostomy cuff using minimal occlusive volume (MOV) technique or minimal leak technique (MLT)
- Maintain inflation of the endotracheal/tracheostomy cuff at 15 to 25 mm Hg during mechanical ventilation and during and after feeding
- Monitor cuff pressures every 4 to 8 hours during expiration using a three-way stopcock, calibrated syringe, and manometer
- Check cuff pressure immediately after delivery of any general anesthesia or manipulation of endotracheal tube
- Institute endotracheal suctioning, as appropriate
- Suction the oropharynx and secretions from the top of the tube cuff before deflating the cuff
- Change endotracheal tapes/ties every 24 hours, inspect the skin and oral mucosa, and reposition ET to the other side of the mouth

- Loosen commercial endotracheal tube holders at least once a day and provide skin care
- Auscultate for presence of lung sounds bilaterally after insertion and after changing endotracheal/tracheostomy ties
- Note the centimeter reference marking on endotracheal tube to monitor for possible displacement
- Assist with chest x-ray examination to monitor position of tube, as needed
- Minimize leverage and traction on the artificial airway by suspending ventilator tubing from overhead supports, using flexible catheter mounts and swivels, and supporting tubes during turning, suctioning, and ventilator disconnection and reconnection
- Monitor for presence of crackles and rhonchi over large airways
- Monitor secretions color, amount, and consistency
- Perform oral care (e.g., use toothbrush, swabs, mouth and lip moisturizer), as needed
- Monitor for decrease in exhale volume and increase in inspiratory pressure in patients receiving mechanical ventilation
- Institute measures to prevent spontaneous decannulation (e.g., secure artificial airway with tape or ties, administer sedation and muscle paralyzing agent, use arm restraints), as appropriate
- Provide additional intubation equipment and ambu bag in a readily available location

- Provide trachea care every 4 to 8 hours, as appropriate: clean the inner cannula, clean and dry the area around the stoma, and change tracheostomy ties
- Inspect skin around tracheal stoma for drainage, redness, irritation, and bleeding
- Inspect and palpate for air under skin every 8 hours
- Monitor for presence of pain
- Maintain sterile technique when suctioning and providing tracheostomy care
- Shield the tracheostomy from water
- Tape the tracheostomy obturator to head of bed
- Tape a second tracheostomy (same type and size) and forceps to head of bed
- Institute chest physiotherapy, as appropriate
- Ensure that endotracheal/tracheostomy cuff is inflated during feedings, as appropriate
- Elevate head of the bed equal to or greater than 30 degrees or assist patient to a sitting position in a chair during feedings, as appropriate

1st edition 1992; revised 2013

Background Evidence:

Chulay, M. (2005). Suctioning: Endotracheal or tracheostomy tube. In D. Wiegand & K. Carlson (Eds.), *AACN procedure manual for critical care* (5th ed., pp. 63–70). Elsevier Saunders.

Evans-Smith, P. (2005). *Taylor's clinical nursing skills: A nursing process approach.* Lippincott Williams & Wilkins.

Schleder, B., Stott, K., & Lloyd, R. (2002). The effect of a comprehensive oral care protocol on patients at risk for ventilator-associated pneumonia. *Journal of Advocate Health Care, 4*(1), 27–30.

Simmons-Trau, D., Cenek, P., Counterman, J., Hockenbury, D., & Litwiller, L. (2004). Reducing VAP with 6 Sigma. *Nurse Manager, 35*(6), 41–45.

Skillings, K. N., & Curtis, B. L. (2005). Tracheal tube cuff care. In D. Wieland & K. Carlson (Eds.), *AACN procedure manual for critical care* (5th ed., pp. 71–86). Saunders.

Sole, M. L., Byers, J. F., Ludy, J. E., Zhang, Y., Banta, C. M., & Brummel, K. (2003). A multisite survey of suctioning techniques and airway management practices. *American Journal of Critical Care, 12*(3), 220–230.

Tablan, O., Anderson, L., Besser, R., Bridges, C., & Hajjeh, R. (2004). Guidelines for preventing health-care–associated pneumonia, 2003. *Morbidity & Mortality Weekly Report, 53*(RR-3), 1–36.

Aspiration Precautions   3200

Definition: Prevention or minimization of risk factors in the patient at risk for aspiration

Activities:

- Monitor level of consciousness, cough reflex, gag reflex, and swallowing ability
- Screen for dysphagia, as appropriate
- Maintain an airway
- Minimize use of narcotics and sedatives
- Minimize use of medications known to delay gastric emptying, as appropriate
- Monitor pulmonary status
- Monitor bowel care needs
- Position upright equal to or greater than 30 (NG feedings) to 90 degrees or as far as possible
- Keep head of bed elevated 30 to 45 minutes after feeding
- Keep tracheal cuff inflated, as appropriate
- Keep suction setup available
- Supervise eating or assist, as necessary
- Feed in small amounts
- Check NG or gastrostomy placement before feeding
- Check NG or gastrostomy residual before feeding
- Avoid feeding, if residuals are high (e.g., greater than 250 cc for feeding tubes or greater than 100 cc PEG tubes)
- Use continuous NG pump feedings in place of gravity or bolus, if appropriate
- Use prokinetic agents, as appropriate
- Avoid liquids or use thickening agent
- Offer foods or liquids that can be formed into a bolus before swallowing
- Cut food into small pieces
- Request medication in elixir form
- Break or crush pills before administration
- Inspect oral cavity for retained food or medications
- Provide oral care
- Suggest speech pathology consult, as appropriate
- Suggest barium cookie swallow or video fluoroscopy, as appropriate

1st edition 1992; revised 2013

Background Evidence:

Bowman, A., Greiner, J. E., Doerschug, K. C., Little, S. B., Bombei, C. L., & Comried, L. M. (2005). Implementation of an evidence-based feeding protocol and aspiration risk reduction algorithm. *Critical Care Nursing Quarterly, 28*(4), 324–333.

Eisenstadt, E. S. (2010). Dysphagia and aspiration pneumonia in older adults. *Journal of the American Academy of Nurse Practitioners, 22*(1), 17–22.

Evans-Smith, P. (2005). *Taylor's clinical nursing skills: A nursing process approach.* Lippincott Williams & Wilkins.

Maas, M., Buckwalter, K., Hardy, M., Tripp-Reimer, T., Titler, M., & Specht, J. (Eds.). (2001). *Nursing care of older adults: Diagnoses, outcomes, and interventions* (pp. 167–168). Mosby.

Perry, L., & Love, C. P. (2001). Screening for dysphagia and aspiration in acute stroke: A systematic review. *Dysphagia, 16*(1), 7–18.

A

Assertiveness Training 4340

Definition: Assistance with the effective expression of feelings, needs, and ideas while respecting the rights of others

Activities:
- Determine barriers to assertiveness (e.g., developmental stage, chronic medical or psychiatric condition, lack of knowledge, and female socialization)
- Help patient recognize and reduce cognitive distortions that block assertion
- Differentiate between assertive, aggressive, passive, and passive-aggressive behaviors
- Help to identify personal rights, responsibilities, and conflicting norms
- Help clarify problem areas in interpersonal relationships
- Promote expression of thoughts and feelings, both positive and negative
- Help identify self-defeating thoughts
- Assist patient to distinguish between thought and reality
- Instruct patient in the different ways to act assertively
- Instruct patient about strategies for practicing assertive behavior (e.g., making requests, saying no to unreasonable requests, and initiating and concluding conversation)
- Facilitate practice opportunities, using discussion, modeling, and role playing
- Help practice conversational and social skills (e.g., use of "I" statements, nonverbal behaviors, openness, and accepting compliments)
- Help to identify nonverbal communication (e.g., smiling, eye contact, tone and volume of voice) that will assist or hinder assertiveness
- Help to build communication skills that will enable the patient to accurately articulate information
- Praise efforts to express feelings and ideas
- Monitor anxiety level and discomfort related to behavioral change

1st edition 1992; revised 1996, 2018

Background Evidence:

Chitty, K. K. (2004). Mood disorders. In C. R. Kneisl, H. S. Wilson, & E. Trigoboff (Eds.), *Contemporary psychiatric-mental health nursing* (pp. 334–365). Pearson Prentice Hall.

McCabe, C., & Timmins, F. (2003). Teaching assertiveness to undergraduate nursing students. *Nurse Education in Practice, 3*(1), 30–42.

Prochaska, J. O., & Norcross, J. C. (2010). *Systems of psychotherapy: A transtheoretical analysis* (pp. 252–254) (7th ed.). Brooks/Cole.

Sadock, B. J., & Sadock, V. A. (2007). *Kaplan & Sadock's synopsis of psychiatry: Behavioral sciences/clinical psychiatry* (p. 955) (10th ed.). Wolters Kluwer Health/Lippincott, Williams, & Wilkins.

Stuart, G. W. (Ed.). (2013). *Principles and practice of psychiatric nursing* (10th ed., pp. 580–581). Elsevier Mosby.

Vanel, S., & Morris, B. (2010). Staff's perceptions of voluntary assertiveness skills training. *Journal for Nurses in Staff Development, 26*(6), 256–259.

Wheeler, K. (2008). *Psychotherapy for the advanced practice psychiatric nurse* (p. 185). Mosby Elsevier.

Asthma Management 3210

Definition: Identification, treatment, and prevention of reactions to inflammation or constriction in the airway passages

Activities:
- Determine baseline respiratory status
- Document baseline measurements in clinical record
- Compare current status with previous status to detect changes in respiratory status
- Obtain spirometry measurements (e.g., FEV_1, FVC, FEV_1/FVC ratio) at diagnosis, initially with use of short-acting bronchodilator, and as needed
- Monitor peak expiratory flow rate (PERF), as appropriate
- Educate on use of PERF meter at home
- Monitor for asthmatic reactions
- Note onset, characteristics, and duration of cough
- Observe chest movement, including symmetry, use of accessory muscles, and supraclavicular and intercostal muscle retractions
- Auscultate breath sounds, noting areas of decreased or absent ventilation and adventitious sounds
- Administer medication, as appropriate and per policy and procedural guidelines
- Auscultate breath sounds after treatment to determine results
- Offer warm fluids to drink, as appropriate
- Instruct on breathing and relaxation techniques
- Use calm, reassuring approach during asthma attack
- Determine understanding of condition and management
- Encourage good hand hygiene
- Recommend annual influenza vaccine
- Instruct on anti-inflammatory and bronchodilator medications and their appropriate usage
- Instruct on proper techniques for using medication and equipment (e.g., inhaler, nebulizer, peak flow meter, spacer)
- Instruct on proper cleaning of medication administration equipment
- Determine concordance with prescribed treatments
- Encourage verbalization of feelings about diagnosis, treatment, and effect on lifestyle
- Review coping strategies for enhanced self-management and care decision making
- Identify possible triggers (e.g., environmental allergens, animals, medication, food, exercise, temperature, emotions, other medical conditions) and usual reaction
- Instruct to identify and avoid triggers, as possible
- Avoid exposure to tobacco smoke
- Establish written asthma treatment plan with person for managing exacerbations and encourage to distribute to additional caregivers (e.g., day care, school nurse, athletic coach) as appropriate
- Assist in recognition of signs or symptoms of impending asthmatic reaction and implementation of appropriate response measures
- Identify symptoms that may indicate need for change in therapy

- Educate on when to seek emergency care
- Inform person and family about policy and procedures for carrying and administration of asthma medications at school
- Inform parent and guardian when child has needed or used PRN medication in school, as appropriate
- Establish regular schedule of follow-up care
- Instruct and monitor pertinent school staff in emergency procedures
- Prescribe and renew asthma medications, as appropriate
- Foster self-management of asthma as child increases in age and maturity
- Use teach-back to ensure understanding

4th edition 2004; revised 2024

Background Evidence:

Cloutier, M. M., Dixon, A. E., Krishnan, J. A., Lemanske, R. F., Jr., Pace, W., & Schatz, M. (2020). Managing asthma in adolescents and adults: 2020 Asthma guideline update from the National Asthma Education and Prevention Program. *JAMA, 324*(22), 2301–2317. https://doi.org/10.1001/jama.2020.21974

Garzon Maaks, D. L., Barber Starr, N., Brady, M. A., Gaylord, N. M., & Driessnack, M. (2021). and Karen Duderstadt: *Burns' pediatric primary care* (7th ed.). Elsevier.

Perry, S. E., Hockenberry, M. J., Lowdermilk, D. L., & Wilson, D. (2018). *Maternal child nursing care* (6th ed.). Elsevier.

Attachment Promotion   6710

Definition: Facilitating the development of an affective, enduring relationship between infant and parent

Activities:

- Discuss with patient culture-based expressions of attachment before and after birth
- Discuss patient's reaction to pregnancy
- Determine patient's image of unborn child
- Discuss patient's experience of hearing fetal heart tones
- Discuss patient's experience of viewing fetal ultrasound image
- Discuss patient's experience of fetal movements
- Encourage patient to attend prenatal classes
- Instruct patient's partner on ways to participate during labor and delivery
- Place newborn skin-to-skin with parent immediately after birth
- Provide opportunity for parent to see, hold, and examine newborn immediately after birth (i.e., delay unnecessary procedures and provide privacy)
- Facilitate eye contact between parent and newborn immediately after birth (i.e., demonstrate en face positioning; dim room lights; and provide a quiet, private environment)
- Complete maternal and newborn assessments while allowing parent to hold newborn
- Share information gained from physical assessments of infant with parent
- Inform parent of care being given to infant
- Provide pain relief to mother
- Encourage mother to breastfeed, if appropriate
- Provide adequate breastfeeding education and support, if appropriate
- Instruct parent on infant cues for feeding (e.g., rooting, sucking on fingers, crying)
- Instruct parent on importance of feeding as nurturing activity, as it provides opportunity for extended eye contact and physical closeness
- Assist parent in identifying infant's need when crying (e.g., hunger, pain, fatigue, fussiness)
- Encourage consistent, prompt response to infant crying
- Demonstrate infant soothing techniques to parent
- Discuss infant behavioral characteristics with parent
- Point out infant cues that show responsiveness to parent
- Instruct parent on signs of overstimulation
- Encourage frequent, sustained physical closeness between infant and parent (e.g., skin-to-skin contact, breastfeeding, child carrying, and sleeping in close proximity to infant)
- Instruct parent on various ways of providing skin-to-skin contact (e.g., kangaroo care, massaging, and cobathing)
- Instruct parent on infant cares (e.g., diaper changing, feeding, holding, massaging)
- Encourage use of family members and friends for infant caregiving
- Reinforce caregiver role behaviors
- Encourage parent to identify family characteristics observed in infant
- Provide assistance in self-care to maximize focus on infant
- Assist parent of multiples in recognizing individuality of each infant
- Facilitate parent's complete access to and care of hospitalized infant
- Explain equipment used to monitor hospitalized infant
- Instruct parent how to transfer infant from incubator, warmer bed, or bassinet while managing equipment and tubing
- Demonstrate ways to touch infant confined to isolette
- Provide visual objects depicting infant (e.g., photograph of infant, infant footprint) to parent of hospitalized infant
- Update parent frequently on status of hospitalized infant
- Instruct parent on attachment development, emphasizing its complexity, ongoing nature, and opportunities
- Provide anticipatory guidance on developmental milestones that will occur
- Determine how family is coping with transitions
- Provide opportunity for parent to discuss topics of concern (e.g., fears, questions pertaining to infant care, feelings of exhaustion, pain management, and ways to interact with and respond to infant)
- Monitor factors that may interfere with optimal attachment (e.g., mental health disturbance in parent, financial strain, parent and child separation due to medical or surgical intervention, difficulties with breastfeeding, providing foster care, and adopting)
- Provide referral to services (e.g., financial, pastoral care, and counseling), if appropriate

1st edition 1992; revised 2013

Background Evidence:

Denehy, J. A. (1992). Interventions related to parent-infant attachment. *Nursing Clinics of North America, 27*(2), 425–443.

Gribble, K. D. (2007). A model for caregiving of adopted children after institutionalization. *Journal of Child & Adolescent Psychiatric Nursing, 20*(1), 14–26.

Moore, E. R., Anderson, G. C., & Bergman, N. (2007). Early skin-to-skin contact for mothers and their healthy newborn infants. *Cochrane Database of Systematic Reviews, 2007*(3). https://doi.org/10.1002/14651858.CD003519.pub2

Murphy, N. L. (2009). Facilitating attachment after international adoption. *MCN: The American Journal of Maternal/Child Nursing, 34*(4), 210–215.

Ward, S. L., & Hisley, S. M. (2009). *Maternal-child nursing care: Optimizing outcomes for mothers, children, & families.* F.A. Davis.

Wheeler, B., & Wilson, D. (2007). Health promotion of the newborn and family. In M. J. Hockenberry & D. Wilson (Eds.), *Wong's nursing care of infants and children* (8th ed., pp. 257–309). Mosby Elsevier.

Autogenic Training 5840

Definition: Assisting with self-suggestions about feelings of heaviness and warmth for the purpose of inducing relaxation

Activities:
- Choose a quiet, comfortable setting
- Prepare a quiet environment
- Take precautions to prevent interruptions
- Instruct patient on purpose for the intervention
- Seat patient in a reclining chair or place in recumbent position
- Have patient wear comfortable, unrestricted clothing
- Read a prepared script to patient, pausing for enough time for the statement to be internally repeated
- Use statements in the script, which elicit feelings of heaviness, lightness, or floating of specific body parts
- Instruct patient to repeat statements to self and to elicit the feeling within the body part being directed
- Rehearse with the script for about 15 to 20 minutes
- Encourage patient to remain relaxed for another 15 to 20 minutes
- Proceed to elicit feelings of warmth after heaviness sensations have been mastered
- Follow the procedure for eliciting heaviness using a prepared script or audiotape for eliciting warmth
- Provide home instructions with a script or audiotape for patient to use
- Encourage patient to practice session three times a day
- Instruct patient to keep a diary to document progress made with each session

1st edition 1992; revised 2008

Background Evidence:
Crowther, D. (2001). Autogenic therapy. In D. Rankin-Box (Ed.), *The nurse's handbook of complementary therapies* (2nd ed., pp. 139–144). Bailliere Tindall.

Kanji, N., & Ernst, E. (2000). Autogenic training for stress and anxiety: A systematic review. *Complementary Therapies in Medicine, 8*(2), 106–110.

Linden, W. (1990). *Autogenic training: A clinical guide.* Guilford.

Linden, W. (1994). Autogenic training: A narrative and quantitative review of clinical outcome. *Biofeedback and Self-Regulation, 19*(3), 227–264.

Autotransfusion 2860

Definition: Collecting and reinfusing blood that has been lost intraoperatively or postoperatively from clean wounds

Activities:
- Adhere to institutional policy for qualifications, training, and procedures to perform salvage and autotransfusion
- Assure proper personnel are available before initiation of procedure
- Screen for appropriateness of salvage (i.e., contraindications include sepsis, infection, tumor at the site, blood containing an irrigant that is not injectable, hemostatic agents, or microcrystalline collagen)
- Obtain patient's informed consent
- Instruct patient regarding procedure
- Use appropriate blood retrieval system per institutional policy
- Label collection device with the patient's name, hospital number, date, and time that collection was begun
- Monitor patient and blood retrieval system frequently during retrieval
- Maintain integrity of the blood retrieval system before, during, and after blood retrieval
- Screen blood for appropriateness of reinfusion (i.e., contraindications include contaminants, pharmacologic agents, malignancy, hematologic disorders)
- Maintain integrity of blood between salvage and reinfusion
- Prepare blood for reinfusion
- Document time of initiation of collecting, condition of blood, type and amount of anticoagulants, and retrieval volume
- Reinfuse transfusion within 6 hours of retrieval
- Maintain universal precautions

2nd edition 1996; revised 2008, 2018

Background Evidence:
American Association of Blood Banks. (2014). *Standards for perioperative autologous blood collection and administration* (6th ed.).

Conner, R., Spruce, L., & Burlingame, B. (2013). *Perioperative standards and recommended practices.* Association of periOperative Registered Nurses.

Esper, S. A., & Waters, J. H. (2011). Intraoperative cell salvage: A fresh look at the indications and contraindications. *Blood Transfusion, 9*(2), 139–147.

Rothrock, J. C. (Ed.). (2015). *Alexander's care of the patient in surgery* (15th ed.). Elsevier Mosby.

Waters, J., Dyga, R., & Yazer, M. (2010). Guidelines for blood recovery and reinfusion in surgery and trauma. American Association of Blood Banks.

Bathing   1610

Definition: Cleaning of the body for the purposes of relaxation, cleanliness, and healing

Activities:
- Consider culture and age when promoting bathing activities
- Determine amount and type of assistance needed (e.g., complete bed bath, partial bath, bag bath, towel bath, tub bath, shower)
- Explain process of using warmed, packaged no-rinse cleanser or antimicrobial cleanser as indicated
- Provide desired personal articles (e.g., towel, deodorant, bath soap, shampoo, lotion, aromatherapy products)
- Provide therapeutic environment by ensuring warm, relaxing, private, and personalized experience
- Assist with chair shower, tub bath, bedside bath, standing shower, or sitz bath, as appropriate or desired
- Use safety strips in tub, and rubber bathmats or towels on floor to prevent slippage
- Cover all intravenous catheters or wound dressings with plastic, as indicated
- Assist with cleansing back, lower legs, and feet as indicated
- Cleanse from clean areas to dirty areas (i.e., chest to perineal area)
- Wash and comb hair and shave, as needed and desired
- Bathe in water of comfortable temperature
- Encourage parent or family participation in usual bedtime rituals, as appropriate
- Use fun bathing techniques with children (e.g., wash dolls or toys; pretend boat is submarine; punch holes in bottom of plastic cup, fill with water, and let it "rain" on child)
- Facilitate maintenance of usual bedtime routines, pre-sleep cues or props, and familiar objects (e.g., for children, a favorite blanket or toy, rocking, pacifier, or story; for adults, book to read or pillow from home), as appropriate
- Assist with perineal care, as needed
- Assist with hygiene measures (e.g., use of deodorant or perfume)
- Administer foot soaks, as needed

- Monitor skin condition when bathing
- Apply lubricating lotion and cream to dry skin areas
- Apply drying powders to deep skin folds sparingly to avoid caking and respiratory irritation
- Monitor functional ability when bathing
- Assist with entering or exiting tub or shower, as needed
- Promote psychosocial well-being by conversing during bathing
- Offer hand washing after toileting and before meals
- Facilitate bathing self, shaving and washing or combing hair, as appropriate
- Monitor cleaning of nails, according to self-care ability
- Provide assistance until fully able to assume self-care
- Facilitate assistance of a barber or beautician, as needed
- Document tolerance of procedure, as indicated

1st edition 1992; revised 2000, 2024

Background Evidence:
Berman, A., Snyder, S. J., & Frandsen, G. (2021). Hygiene. In *Kozier and Erb's fundamentals of nursing: Concepts, process and practice* (pp. 669–685) (11th ed.). Pearson.

Craven, R. F., Hirnle, C. J., & Henshaw, C. M. (2021). Hygiene and self-care: *Fundamentals of nursing: Human health and function* (pp. 604–634) (8th ed.). Wolters-Kluwer.

Hockenberry, M. J., Rodgers, C. C., & Wilson, D. (2022). *Wong's essentials of pediatric nursing* (11th ed.). Elsevier.

Perry, A. G., Potter, P. A., Ostendorf, W. R., & LaPlante, N. (2021). *Clinical nursing skills and technique* (10th ed.). Mosby.

Potter, P. A., Perry, A. G., Stockert, P. A., & Hall, A. M. (2021). *Fundamentals of Nursing* (10th ed.). Elsevier.

Williams, P. (2020). *Basic geriatric nursing* (7th ed). Elsevier.

Bed Rest Care   0740

Definition: Promotion of comfort and safety and prevention of complications for a patient unable to get out of bed

Activities:
- Explain reasons for requiring bed rest
- Place on an appropriate therapeutic mattress or bed
- Position in proper body alignment
- Avoid using rough-textured bed linens
- Keep bed linen clean, dry, and wrinkle free
- Apply a footboard to the bed
- Use devices on the bed that protect the patient
- Apply appliances to prevent foot drop
- Raise side rails, as appropriate
- Place bed-positioning switch within easy reach
- Place the call light within reach
- Place bedside table within patient's reach
- Attach trapeze to the bed, as appropriate
- Turn, as indicated by skin condition
- Turn the immobilized patient at least every 2 hours, according to a specific schedule
- Monitor skin condition
- Teach bed exercises, as appropriate

- Facilitate small shifts of body weight
- Perform passive and active range-of-motion exercises
- Assist with hygiene measures (e.g., use of deodorant or perfume)
- Assist with activities of daily living
- Apply antiembolism stockings
- Monitor for complications of bed rest (e.g., loss of muscle tone, back pain, constipation, increased stress, depression, confusion, sleep cycle changes, urinary tract infections, difficulty with urination, pneumonia)
- Place in upright posture intermittently for patients unable to be out of bed every day to protect against orthostatic intolerance

1st edition 1992; revised 2013

Background Evidence:
Cheng, K. (2010). Prolonged bed rest duration after percutaneous coronary intervention. *CONNECT: The World of Critical Care Nursing, 7*(2), 111–114.

Dunn, L. L., Handley, M. C., & Carter, M. R. (2006). Antepartal bed rest: Conflicts, costs, controversies, and ethical considerations. *Online Journal of Health Ethics*, 3(1). https://doi.org/10.18785//ojhe.0301.04

Fox, M. T., Sidani, S., & Brooks, D. (2010). The relationship between bed rest and sitting orthostatic intolerance in adults residing in chronic care facilities. *Journal of Nursing and Healthcare of Chronic Illness*, 2(3), 187–196.

Norton, L., Coutts, P., Fraser, C., Nicholson, T., & Sibbald, R. G. (2007). Is bed rest an effective treatment modality for pressure ulcers?. In D. L. Kesner, G. Rodeheaver, & R. G. Sibbald (Eds.), *Chronic wound care: A clinical source book for healthcare professionals* (4th ed., pp. 99–110). HMP Communications.

Sprague, A. E. (2004). The evolution of bed rest as a clinical intervention. *Journal of Obstetric, Gynecologic, & Neonatal Nursing*, 33(5), 542–549.

Behavior Contracting   4420

Definition: Negotiating an agreement with an individual that reinforces a specific behavior change

Activities:

- Assist in identifying behavior and desire to change
- Determine mental and cognitive ability
- Assist to identify own strengths and abilities
- Avoid focusing on diagnosis or disease process when assisting in identifying goals
- Foster an open, accepting environment for creation of contract
- Assist in identifying realistic, attainable goals
- Assist in identifying appropriate short-term and long-term goals, in easily observed behaviors and positive terms
- Encourage to write down goals, if possible
- Clarify roles of health care provider and individual respectively
- Explore resources and methods to achieve goals
- Assist in identifying and overcoming barriers
- Explore methods for evaluating accomplishment of goals
- Facilitate involvement of significant others in contracting process if desired by individual
- Facilitate making written contract, including all agreed-upon elements
- Assist in setting time or frequency requirements for performance of behaviors and actions
- Assist in setting realistic time limits
- Identify target date for termination of contract
- Coordinate opportunities for review of contract and goals
- Facilitate renegotiation of contract terms, if necessary
- Assist in discussing feelings about contract
- Observe for signs of incongruence and lack of commitment to fulfilling contract
- Identify consequences or sanctions for not fulfilling contract, if desired
- Have contract signed by all involved parties
- Provide copy of signed and dated contract
- Encourage to identify appropriate, meaningful reinforcers or rewards
- Encourage to choose reinforcer or reward that sustains behavior
- Specify timing of delivery of reinforcers or rewards
- Instruct on various methods of observing and recording behaviors
- Assist in developing flowchart to assist in tracking progress toward goals
- Use teach-back to ensure understanding

1st edition 1992; revised 2004, 2024

Background Evidence:

Bargmann, A. L., & Brundrett, S. M. (2020). Implementation of a multicomponent fall prevention program: Contracting with patients for fall safety. *Military Medicine*, 185, 28–34. https://doi.org/10.1093/milmed/usz411

Call, C. C., Schumacher, L. M., Rosenbaum, D. L., Convertino, A. D., Zhang, F., & Butryn, M. L. (2019). Participant and interventionist perceptions of challenges during behavioral weight loss treatment. *Journal of Behavioral Medicine*, 42(2), 353–364. https://doi.org/10.1007/s10865-018-9965-0

Fisher, E., Bromberg, M. H., Tai, G., & Palermo, T. M. (2017). Adolescent and parent treatment goals in an internet-delivered chronic pain self-management program: Does agreement of treatment goals matter?. *Journal of Pediatric Psychology*, 42(6), 657–666. https://doi.org/10.1093/jpepsy/jsw098

McAuliffe Staehler, T. M., & Palombi, L. C. (2020). Beneficial opioid management strategies: A review of the evidence for the use of opioid treatment agreements. *Substance Abuse*, 41(2), 208–215. https://doi.org/10.1080/08897077.2019.1692122

Rager, J. B., & Schwartz, P. H. (2017). Defending opioid treatment agreements: Disclosure, Not promises. *Hastings Center Report*, 47(3), 24–33.

Wickenbergh, E., Nilsson, L., Bladh, M., Kjølhede, P., & Wodlin, N. B. (2020). Agreements on perceived use of principles for Enhanced Recovery After Surgery between patients and nursing staff in a gynecological ward. *European Journal of Obstetrics & Gynecology & Reproductive Biology*, 250, 216–223. https://doi.org/10.1016/j.ejogrb.2020.04.014

Behavior Management   4350

Definition: Helping an individual to manage negative behavior

Activities:

- Identify undesired negative behavior
- Consult with family to establish individual's pattern of undesired behaviors
- Determine why, when, and how undesired behavior occurring
- Identify events that trigger or maintain problem behavior
- Hold individual responsible for behavior
- Praise efforts at self-control
- Set limits on negative behavior with individual
- Refrain from arguing or bargaining about established limits
- Develop behavior management plan
- Communicate expectation that individual will retain control
- Develop specific sequence of steps associated with instruction
- Provide positive reinforcement as meets each specific expectation

B

- Use positive reinforcement to increase desired behavior
- Consider using shaping strategies (i.e., gradually foster development of new behavior by repetitively reinforcing minor improvements or steps toward desired behaviors)
- Create situations for individual to imitate modeled behavior
- Provide positive reinforcement if models desired behavior
- Refrain from giving positive reinforcement if does not model desired behavior
- Establish routines
- Establish consistency in environment and care routines
- Use consistent repetition of health routines as means of establishing routines
- Avoid interruptions
- Increase physical activity, as appropriate
- Limit number of caregivers
- Utilize soft, low speaking voice
- Avoid cornering individual
- Redirect attention away from agitation source
- Avoid projecting threatening image
- Ignore inappropriate behavior
- Discourage passive-aggressive behavior
- Medicate, as prescribed

- Apply restraints to prevent self-harm or harm to others, per agency protocol

1st edition 1992; revised 2000, 2024

Background Evidence:

de la Fuente, M., Schoenfisch, A., Wadsworth, B., & Foresman-Capuzzi, J. (2019). Impact of behavior management training on nurses' confidence in managing patient aggression. *Journal of Nursing Administration, 49*(2), 73–78. https://doi.org/10.1097/NNA.0000000000000713

Hasani, S. M., Askary, P., Heidari, A., & Zadeh, P. E. (2020). The comparative effectiveness of parental behavior management training and schema therapy on aggression and oppositional defiant in adolescents. *Journal of Nursing & Midwifery Sciences, 7*(3), 146–152. https://doi.org/10.4103/JNMS.JNMS_6_20

Maag, J. W. (2018). *Behavior management: From theoretical implications to practice application* (3rd ed). Cengage Learning.

Martin, G., & Pear, J. J. (2019). *Behavior modification: What it is and how to do it* (11th ed.). Routledge.

Tuyen, L. T. T., & Gunawan, J. (2018). Behavior management in the field of nursing: A concept analysis. *Nursing Forum, 53*(4), 481–488. https://doi.org/10.1111/nuf.12275

Behavior Management: Inattention and Hyperactivity   4352

Definition: Provision of therapeutic strategies that safely accommodate inattention and hyperactivity while promoting optimal function

Activities:

- Identify undesired inattentive or hyperactive behavior
- Consult with family to establish individual's pattern of inattentive or hyperactive behavior
- Determine factors that trigger or maintain undesired inattentive and hyperactive behavior
- Identify factors that de-escalate inattentive and hyperactive behavior
- Determine appropriate behavioral expectations and consequences, given individual's level of cognitive functioning and capacity for self-control
- Provide structured and physically safe environment
- Use calm, matter-of-fact, reassuring approach
- Develop evidence-based behavioral management plan carried out consistently by all care providers
- Communicate rules, behavioral expectations, and consequences using simple language with visual cues, as necessary
- Refrain from arguing or bargaining about established limits
- Provide reassurance that staff will assist individual with managing behavior, as necessary
- Praise desired behaviors and efforts at self-control
- Provide consistent consequences for both desired and undesired behaviors
- Obtain individual's attention before initiating verbal interactions (e.g., call by name, obtain eye contact)
- Give any instructions or explanations slowly, using simple, concrete language
- Ask individual to repeat instructions before beginning activities
- Divide multiple-step instructions into simple steps
- Allow individual to carry out one step before being given another
- Provide assistance to complete activities, as necessary
- Provide positive feedback for completion of each step

- Provide aids to increase environmental structure, concentration, and attention to activities (e.g., watches, calendars, signs, step-by-step written instructions)
- Decrease or withdraw verbal and physical cues, as they become unnecessary
- Monitor and regulate level of activity and stimulation in environment
- Maintain routine schedule that includes balance of structured time (e.g., physical and nonphysical activities) and quiet time
- Limit choices, as necessary
- Redirect or remove from source of overstimulation (e.g., peer, problem situation)
- Use external controls to calm individual (e.g., time out, seclusion, physical restraint), when necessary
- Monitor physical status of hyperactive individual (e.g., body weight, hydration, condition of feet in individual who paces)
- Monitor fluid and nutritional intake
- Provide high-protein, high-calorie finger foods and fluids that can be consumed "on the run"
- Limit excessive intake of food and fluids
- Limit intake of caffeinated food and fluids
- Instruct in problem-solving skills
- Encourage expression of feelings in appropriate manner
- Demonstrate and reinforce appropriate social skills
- Set limits on intrusive, interruptive behavior(s)
- Provide information about illness (e.g., attention deficit disorder, hyperactivity, mania, schizophrenia) to individual and significant others, as appropriate
- Administer medications (e.g., stimulants, antipsychotics) to promote desired behavior changes
- Monitor individual for medication side effects and desired behavioral outcomes

- Provide medication instruction to individual and significant others
- Use alternative therapies to promote desired behaviors, as appropriate
- Facilitate reasonable behavioral expectations for individual with family and significant others
- Demonstrate behavioral management techniques to significant others
- Assist individual and involved others (e.g., family, employers, teachers) to adapt home, work, or school environments to accommodate limitations imposed by chronic inattention and hyperactivity
- Facilitate family coping through support groups, respite care, and family counseling, as appropriate
- Collaborate with providers in schools and others in community to enhance treatment management
- Use teach-back to ensure understanding

2nd edition 1996; revised 2018, 2024

Background Evidence:

Carbray, J. A. (2018). Attention-deficit/hyperactivity disorder in children and adolescents. *Journal of Psychosocial Nursing and Mental Health Services*, 56(12), 7–10. https://doi.org/10.3928/02793695-20181112-02

Caye, A., Swanson, J. M., Coghill, D., & Rohde, L. A. (2019). Treatment strategies for ADHD: An evidence-based guide to select optimal treatment. *Molecular Psychiatry*, 24(3), 390–408.

Nicholson, T. (2019). A nurse's introduction to attention deficit hyperactivity disorder. *British Journal of Nursing*, 28(11), 678–680. https://doi.org/10.12968/bjon.2019.28.11.678

Oliva, F., Malandrone, F., di Girolamo, G., Mirabella, S., Colombi, N., Carletto, S., & Ostacoli, L. (2021). The efficacy of mindfulness-based interventions in attention-deficit/hyperactivity disorder beyond core symptoms: A systematic review, meta-analysis, and meta-regression. *Journal of Affective Disorders*, 292, 475–486. https://doi.org/10.1016/j.jad.2021.05.068

Padilha, S. C. O. S., Tonin, F. S., Borba, H. H. L., Virtuoso, S., & Pontarolo, R. (2018). Efficacy and safety of drugs for attention deficit hyperactivity disorder in children and adolescents: A network meta-analysis. *European Child & Adolescent Psychiatry*, 27(10), 1335–1345. https://doi.org/10.1007/s00787-018-1125-0

Vaag, J. R., Lara-Cabrera, M. L., Hjemdal, O., Gjervan, B., & Torgersen, T. (2019). Psychoeducational groups versus waitlist in treatment of attention-deficit hyperactivity/impulsivity disorder (ADHD) in adults: A protocol for a pilot randomized waitlist-controlled multicenter trial. *Pilot and Feasibility Studies*, 5, 17. https://doi.org/10.1186/s40814-019-0401-1

Behavior Management: Self-Harm   4354

Definition: Assisting to decrease or eliminate self-mutilating or self-abusive behaviors

Activities:

- Determine motive, reason, or underlying dynamics for behaviors
- Identify previous history of self-mutilating behaviors or self-abusive behaviors
- Develop appropriate behavioral expectations and consequences based on level of cognitive functioning and capacity for self-control
- Communicate behavioral expectations and consequences to person
- Remove dangerous items from environment
- Apply mitts, splints, helmets, or restraints to limit mobility and ability to initiate self-harm, if necessary
- Monitor for self-harmful impulses that may progress to suicidal thoughts or gestures
- Communicate risk for self-harm to other care providers
- Identify cues that precede self-mutilating behavior
- Anticipate trigger situations that may prompt self-harm and intervene to prevent these
- Use calm, nonpunitive approach when dealing with self-harmful behaviors
- Assist to identify situations and feelings that may prompt self-harm or that prompted self-harmful behavior
- Assist to identify more appropriate coping strategies and consequences
- Contract for "no self-harm" to enable person to stay physically safe
- Provide ongoing surveillance of person and environment
- Provide close one-to-one observation of person when necessary to maintain safety
- Encourage to seek out care providers to talk as urge to harm self occurs
- Explain and reinforce effective coping behaviors and appropriate expression of feelings
- Formulate plan of care with person including goals for preventing undesired self-harm behaviors
- Suggest alternative behaviors, such as seeking interpersonal support or engaging in adaptive anxiety-reducing activity
- Instruct about coping strategies (e.g., assertiveness training, impulse control training, progressive muscle relaxation), as appropriate
- Use behavior management techniques (e.g., differential reinforcement, extinction, response interruption, redirection), as appropriate
- Use appropriate strategies of dialectical behavior therapy [DBT] (e.g., psychological education, problem solving, training in social skills, exercises in monitoring moods, modeling by therapist, homework assignments, meditation)
- Involve in individual and group therapies, as appropriate
- Administer medications to decrease anxiety, stabilize mood, and decrease self-stimulation, as appropriate
- Monitor for medication side effects and desired outcomes
- Provide medication instructions to person and significant others
- Provide predetermined consequences if engaging in self-harmful behaviors
- Place in more protective environment (e.g., area restriction, seclusion) if self-harmful impulses and behaviors escalate
- Assist to assume responsibility for consequences of behavior (e.g., dress own self-inflicted wound)
- Avoid giving positive reinforcement to self-harmful behaviors
- Provide care for wounds in neutral, matter of fact manner by refraining from punitive or overly sympathetic response, or providing additional attention
- Provide family or significant others with guidelines to manage self-harmful behavior outside care environment

- Provide illness teaching to person or significant others if self-harmful behavior is illness-based (e.g., borderline personality disorder, autism)
- Reinforce positive behaviors that decrease or eliminate self-mutilating or self-abusive behaviors
- Develop plan for safety with person to effectively deal with precursors to undesired behavior when in home environment

2nd edition 1996; revised 2018, 2024

Background Evidence:

Griffin, E., Bonner, B., O'Hagan, D., Kavalidou, K., & Corcoran, P. (2019). Hospital-presenting self-harm and ideation: Comparison of incidence, profile and risk of repetition. *General Hospital Psychiatry, 61*, 76–81. https://doi.org/10.1016/j.genhosppsych.2019.10.009

Iyengar, U., Snowden, N., Asarnow, J. R., Moran, P., Tranah, T., & Ougrin, D. (2018). A further look at therapeutic interventions for suicide attempts and self-harm in adolescents: an updated systematic review of randomized controlled trials. *Frontiers in Psychiatry, 9*, 583. https://doi.org/10.3389/fpsyt.2018.00583

Morrissey, J., Doyle, L., & Higgins, A. (2018). Self-harm: from risk management to relational and recovery-oriented care. *Journal of Mental Health Training, Education & Practice, 13*(1), 34–43. https://doi.org/10.1108/JMHTEP-03-2017-0017

Stewart, A., Hughes, N. D., Simkin, S., Locock, L., Ferrey, A., Kapur, N., Gunnell, D., & Hawton, K. (2018). Navigating an unfamiliar world: how parents of young people who self-harm experience support and treatment. *Child & Adolescent Mental Health, 23*(2), 78–84. https://doi.org/10.1111/camh.12205

Wand, A. P. F., Draper, B., Brodaty, H., & Peisah, C. (2019). Self-harm in the very old one year later: has anything changed? *International Psychogeriatrics, 31*(11), 1559–1568. https://doi.org/10.1017/S1041610219000632

Behavior Management: Sexual   4356

Definition: Delineation and prevention of socially unacceptable sexual behaviors

Activities:

- Identify sexual behaviors that are unacceptable given particular setting and population (e.g., inappropriate remarks in public places, inappropriate statements to people they know; unwanted advances; touches, hugs, or kisses another more than appropriate; attempts to have sexual intercourse with others; exposes self or masturbates in public)
- Specify explicit expectations (based on developmental stage, level of cognitive functioning, and capacity for self-control) related to sexual behavior or verbalizations that might be directed toward others or objects in environment
- Discuss consequences of socially unacceptable sexual behavior and verbalizations
- Provide parents information about age-appropriate sexual behavior
- Discuss with parents and children importance of internet safety and prevention of access to sexual material
- Encourage parents not to punish or admonish children for normative sexual behaviors
- Instruct parents to use gentle distraction such as asking child to hold hands with them to redirect behavior
- Discuss, based on developmental and cognitive ability, negative impact that socially unacceptable sexual behavior may have on others, as appropriate
- Avoid assigning roommates with communication difficulties, history of inappropriate sexual activity, or heightened vulnerabilities
- Assign to private room if assessed to be high risk for socially unacceptable sexual behavior
- Limit physical mobility to decrease opportunity for socially unacceptable sexual behaviors, as needed
- Communicate risk to other care providers
- Provide appropriate level of supervision to monitor person
- Use calm, matter-of-fact approach when responding to socially unacceptable sexual remarks and behavior
- Redirect from any socially unacceptable sexual behaviors or verbalizations
- Discuss why sexual behavior or verbalization unacceptable
- Explore intentions behind each behavior to address cognitive distortions, and negative conditioning techniques
- Provide predetermined consequences for undesirable sexual behavior
- Reinforce appropriate social skills
- Provide sex education, as appropriate to developmental level
- Discuss acceptable ways to fulfill individual sexual needs in privacy
- Discourage initiation of sexual or intimate relationships while under severe stress
- Encourage appropriate expression of feelings about past situational or traumatic crises
- Provide counseling for persons who have been sexually abused, as needed
- Consider pharmacologic treatment, as needed
- Assist family with understanding of and management of unacceptable sexual behaviors
- Provide opportunities for staff to process feelings about socially unacceptable sexual behavior
- Use teach-back to ensure understanding

2nd edition 1996; revised 2018, 2024

Background Evidence:

Cranbourne, R. M., Campbell, M., Pilkington, L., & Carthy, N. (2020). The role of presence when working with children and young people demonstrating harmful sexual behaviour. *Counselling & Psychotherapy Research, 20*(4), 580–590. https://doi.org/10.1002/capr.12338

Falligant, J. M., & Pence, S. T. (2020). Interventions for inappropriate sexual behavior in individuals with intellectual and developmental disabilities: A brief review. *Journal of applied behavior analysis, 53*(3), 1316–1320.

Keltner, N. L., & Steele, D. (2019). *Psychiatric nursing* (8th ed.). Elsevier.

Resnick, B., Galik, E., Kolanowski, A., VanHaitsma, K., Boltz, M., Zhu, S., Ellis, J., Behrens, L., & Eshraghi, K. (2021). Gender differences in presentation and management of behavioral and psychological symptoms associated with dementia among nursing home residents with moderate to severe dementia. *Journal of Women & Aging, 33*(6), 635–652. https://doi.org/10.1080/08952841.2020.1735925

Pritchard, D., Penney, H., & Mace, F. C. (2018). The ACHIEVE! program: A point and level system for reducing severe problem behavior. *Behavioral Interventions, 33*(1), 41–55.

Varcarolis, E. M., & Fosbre, C. D. (2021). *Essentials of psychiatric-mental health nursing* (4th ed.). Elsevier.

Behavior Modification 4360

Definition: Promotion of a behavior change

Activities:

- Determine motivation to change
- Assist to identify strengths, and reinforce these
- Identify problem in behavioral terms
- Identify behavior to be changed (target behavior) in specific, concrete terms
- Separate behaviors to be changed into smaller, measurable units of behavior (e.g., stopping smoking; number of cigarettes smoked)
- Use specific time periods when measuring units of behavior (e.g., number of cigarettes smoked per day)
- Determine whether identified target behavior needs to be increased, decreased, or learned
- Consider that it is easier to increase behavior than to decrease behavior
- Establish behavioral objectives in written form
- Develop behavior change program
- Establish baseline occurrence of behavior before initiating change
- Develop method (e.g., graph or chart) for recording behavior and changes
- Encourage substitution of undesirable habits with desirable habits
- Introduce to persons and groups who have successfully undergone same experience
- Promote learning of desired behavior by using modeling techniques
- Ensure consistency implementing strategies for change by all staff
- Reinforce constructive decisions concerning health needs
- Provide feedback when free of symptoms and looks relaxed
- Avoid showing rejection or belittlement during struggles with changing behavior
- Offer positive reinforcement for independently made decisions
- Encourage to examine own behavior
- Assist in identifying even small successes
- Encourage to participate in monitoring and recording behaviors
- Discuss behavior modification process with all involved persons
- Facilitate involvement of other health care providers in modification process, as appropriate
- Facilitate family involvement in modification process, as appropriate
- Develop treatment contract to support implementation of token or point system
- Foster skills acquisition by systematically reinforcing simple components of skill or task
- Administer positive reinforcers on predetermined schedule (continuous or intermittent) for desired behaviors
- Withdraw positive reinforcers from undesired behaviors, and attach reinforcers to more desirable replacement behavior
- Encourage to participate in selection of meaningful reinforcers
- Choose reinforcers that can be controlled (e.g., used only when behavior to be changed occurs)
- Coordinate token or point system of reinforcement for complex or multiple behaviors
- Determine changes in behavior by comparing baseline occurrences with postintervention occurrences of behavior
- Document and communicate modification process to treatment team, as necessary
- Follow up reinforcement over longer term by phone or personal contact
- Use teach-back to ensure understanding

1st edition 1992; revised 2013, 2024

Background Evidence:

Gonzalez, T. M., Katic, B. J., Torres-Págán, L., Divney, A., & Echeverria, S. E. (2020). Report of health behavior modification among Latinos diagnosed with multiple cardiovascular risk factors. *Medical Care, 58*(1), 59–64.

Hooker, S. A., Punjabi, A., Justesen, K., Boyle, L., & Sherman, M. D. (2018). Encouraging health behavior change: Eight evidence-based strategies: Using these brief interventions, you can help your patients make healthy behavior changes. *Family Practice Management, 25*(2), 31–36.

Martin, G., & Pear, J. (2019). *Behavior modification: What it is and how to do it.* Taylor and Francis.

Oral, A. (2020). Are environmental and behavioural modifications useful for improving food and liquid intake in individuals with dementia? A Cochrane Review summary with commentary. *Australasian Journal on Ageing, 39*(3), 313–316.

Piatkowski, C., Faulkner, G. E., Guhn, M., & Mâsse, L. C. (2020). User characteristics and parenting practices associated with adolescents' initial use of a lifestyle behavior modification intervention. *Childhood Obesity, 16*(6), 367–378.

Townsend, M. C., & Morgan, K. L. (2018). *Psychiatric mental health nursing: Concepts of care in evidence-based practice* (9th ed.). F.A. Davis.

Videbeck, S. L. (2020). *Psychiatric-mental health nursing* (8th ed.). Wolters Kluwer.

Behavior Modification: Social Skills 4362

Definition: Using behavioral strategies to develop or improve interpersonal social skills

Activities:

- Approach with genuine concern
- Ask to tell their story related to interpersonal behavioral problems
- Help identify behavioral problems that results from the way a person relates to others
- Use behavioral evidence-based interpersonal skills training program
- Encourage sharing of feelings (negative and positive) that occur related to these interpersonal problems
- Assist to identify desired outcomes or goals for problematic interpersonal relationships or situations

B

- Assist to determine if desired goals are realistic and attainable, or if better goals are needed
- Assist to identify possible courses of action and their social or interpersonal consequences, including changes they are likely to experience because of new relationship goals
- Help identify changes a person is willing to make to meet new interpersonal goals
- Identify specific social skills using guided discussion and examples that will be focus of training
- Assist to identify behavioral steps for targeted social skills that include changes person willing to make
- Provide methods (e.g., role play, video presentation) demonstrating behavioral steps in context of situations that are meaningful
- Assist to role play behavioral steps if comfortable in role play
- Involve significant others in social skills training sessions (e.g., role play), as appropriate
- Provide feedback (e.g., praise or rewards) about performance of targeted social skills
- Educate significant others (e.g., family, peers, employers) about purpose and process of social skills training, as appropriate
- Provide feedback about appropriateness of social responses in training situations
- Provide educational materials to assist understanding of interpersonal changes that will help meet goals, including educational material using role playing, videos, or written information
- Encourage to self-evaluate outcomes of social interactions, self-reward for positive outcomes, and problem-solve less desirable outcomes
- Use teach-back to ensure understanding

2nd edition 1996; revised 2018, 2024

Background Evidence:

Clarke, J., Sanatkar, S., Baldwin, P. A., Fletcher, S., Gunn, J., Wilhelm, K., Campbell, L., Zwar, N., Harris, M., Lapsley, H., Hadzi-Pavlovic, D., Christensen, H., & Proudfoot, J. (2019). A web-based cognitive behavior therapy intervention to improve social and occupational functioning in adults with type 2 diabetes (The Springboard Trial): Randomized Controlled Trial. *Journal of Medical Internet Research, 21*(5), e12246.

Gates, J. A., Kang, E., & Lerner, M. D. (2017). Efficacy of group social skills interventions for youth with autism spectrum disorder: A systematic review and meta-analysis. *Clinical Psychology Review, 52*, 164–181.

Mikami, A. Y., Smit, S., & Khalis, A. (2017). Social skills training and ADHD-what works? *Current Psychiatry Reports, 19*(12), 93.

Savarithmuthu, D. (2020). The potential role of nurses in leading positive behavior support. *British Journal of Nursing, 29*(7), 414–418.

Turner, D. T., McGlanaghy, E., Cuijpers, P., van der Gaag, M., Karyotaki, E., & MacBeth, A. (2018). A meta-analysis of social skills training and related interventions for psychosis. *Schizophrenia Bulletin, 44*(3), 475–491.

Varcarolic, E. M., & Halter, M. J. (2018). *Foundations of psychiatric mental health nursing.* Saunders/Elsevier.

Bereavement Care 5215

Definition: Providing care and support to those who are experiencing emotional and practical problems with the loss of a loved one

Activities:
- Determine willingness to discuss loss
- Facilitate spiritual support for family and significant others, as appropriate
- Promote open, trusting relationships
- Create supportive therapeutic environment
- Accept values in nonjudgmental manner
- Respect specific care requests
- Respect need for privacy
- Encourage sharing and expressing feelings and emotions
- Encourage sharing favorite memories
- Provide anticipatory guidance for feelings of grief and loss
- Assist to identify shared meaning of loss
- Foster realistic hope
- Support individual family members through personal stages of grief
- Encourage implementation of cultural, religious, and social customs
- Accept culturally diverse grief responses
- Offer to facilitate discussion of memorial arrangements (e.g., military honor, contacting religious leader)
- Assist with referral to bereavement services
- Express condolence in appropriate manner (e.g., sending card, attending memorial service, telephone call)

8th edition 2024

Background Evidence:

Blackburn, P., & Dwyer, K. (2017). A bereavement common assessment framework in palliative care: Informing practice, transforming care. *American Journal of Hospice and Palliative Medicine, 34*(7), 677–684. https://doi.org/10.1177/1049909116647403

Egerod, I., Kaldan, G., Albarran, J., Coombs, M., Mitchell, M., & Latour, J. M. (2019). Elements of intensive care bereavement follow-up services: A European survey. *Nursing in Critical Care, 24*(4), 201–208. https://doi.org/10.1111/nicc.12459

Erikson, A., Puntillo, K., & McAdam, J. (2019). Family members' opinions about bereavement care after cardiac intensive care unit patients' deaths. *Nursing in Critical Care, 24*(4), 209–221. https://doi.org/10.1111/nicc.12439

Jensen, J., Weng, C., & Spraker-Perlman, H. L. (2017). A provider-based survey to assess bereavement care knowledge, attitudes, and practices in pediatric oncologists. *Journal of Palliative Medicine, 20*(3), 266–272. https://doi.org/10.1089/jpm.2015.0430

Bibliotherapy 4680

Definition: Therapeutic use of literature to enhance expression of feelings, active problem solving, coping, or insight

Activities:
- Identify the patient's emotional, cognitive, developmental, and situational needs
- Determine ability for reading independently
- Set therapy goals (e.g., emotional change; personality development; learn new values and attitudes)
- Consult with a librarian who is skilled in book finding
- Consult sources to recommend literature for therapy
- Make selections appropriate for reading level
- Select stories, poems, essays, articles, self-help books, or novels that reflect the situation or feelings the patient is experiencing
- Read aloud, if needed or feasible
- Use pictures and illustrations
- Encourage reading and rereading
- Assist in helping the patient identify with the characters and emotional content in the literature
- Examine and talk about the feelings expressed by the characters
- Facilitate dialogue to help the patient compare and contrast the image, character, situation, or concept in the literature with his/her situation
- Assist in helping the patient recognize how the situation in the literature can help with making desired changes
- Follow up reading sessions with play sessions or role modeling work, either individually or in therapy groups
- Evaluate goal attainment

1st edition 1992; revised 2008

Background Evidence:
Abdullah, M.H. (2002). *Bibliotherapy.* Bloomington, IN: ERIC Digest: Education Resources Information Center Clearing House on Reading English and Communication.

Cohen, L. J. (1992). Bibliotherapy: The therapeutic use of books for women. *Journal of Nurse-Midwifery, 37*(2), 91–95.

Cohen, L. J. (1993). Discover the healing power of books. *American Journal of Nursing, 93*(10), 70–74.

Hynes, A. M., & Hynes-Berry, M. (1986). *Bibliotherapy the interactive process: A handbook.* Westview Press.

Marrs, R. W. (1995). A meta-analysis of bibliotherapy studies. *American Journal of Community Psychology, 23*(6), 843–870.

McArdle, S., & Byrt, R. (2001). Fiction, poetry and mental health: Expressive and therapeutic uses of literature. *Journal of Psychiatric and Mental Health Nursing, 8*(6), 517–524.

Silverberg, L. I. (2003). Bibliotherapy: The therapeutic use of didactic and literary texts in treatment, diagnosis, prevention, and training. *Journal of the American Osteopathic Association, 103*(3), 131–135.

Biofeedback 5860

Definition: Assisting the patient to gain voluntary control over physiological responses using feedback from electronic equipment that monitors physiologic processes

Activities:
- Interview patient to obtain a health history
- Analyze nature of the specific health condition to be treated
- Determine abilities and willingness for using the biobehavioral treatment
- Discuss rationale for using biofeedback and type of feedback
- Determine patient's acceptance of this type of treatment
- Decide on the specific monitoring device to be used (e.g., thermal feedback; electrodermal response or galvanic skin response; electromyography feedback; finger pulse feedback; breathing biofeedback; electroencephalograph biofeedback)
- Construct treatment plan to treat the problem
- Explain the procedure concerning the specific monitoring equipment used
- Arrange therapy room so that patient cannot touch any conductive object
- Connect patient to the instrumentation device, as needed
- Operate the biofeedback device according to instructions
- Establish an appropriate baseline against which to compare treatment effect
- Assist patient to learn to modify bodily responses to equipment cues
- Instruct patient to check instrumentation before use to ensure proper functioning
- Answer fears and concerns related to the instrumentation
- Discuss timing, frequency, length, and setting for sessions with patient/family
- Identify appropriate criteria for reinforcement of patient's responses
- Provide feedback of progress after each session
- Set conditions with patient to evaluate therapeutic outcome

1st edition 1992; revised 2008

Background Evidence:
Andrasik, F., & Lords, A. O. (2004). Biofeedback. In L. Freeman (Ed.), *Mosby's complementary & alternative medicine: A research-based approach* (2nd ed., pp. 207–235). Mosby.

Anselmo, J. (2005). Relaxation: The first step to restore, renew, and self-heal. In B. M. Dossey, L. Keegan, & C. E. Guzzetta (Eds.), *Holistic nursing: A handbook for practice* (4th ed., pp. 523–566). Jones and Bartlett.

Bray, D. (2001). Biofeedback. In D. Rankin-Box (Ed.), *The nurse's handbook of complementary therapies* (pp. 145–152). Bailliere Tindall.

Fontaine, K. L. (2005). *Complementary & alternative therapies for nursing practice* (2nd ed.). Pearson: Prentice Hall.

Good, M. (2006). Biofeedback. In M. Snyder & R. Lindquist (Eds.), *Complementary/alternative therapies in nursing* (5th ed., pp. 117–128). Springer.

Micozzi, M. S. (2006). *Fundamentals of complementary and integrative medicine* (3rd ed.). W. B. Saunders.

Bioterrorism Preparedness 8810

Definition: Preparing for an effective response to bioterrorism events or disaster

Activities:

- Develop response plan for types of chemical and biological agents that are likely terrorism agents (e.g., nerve agents, mustard agents, cyanide, anthrax, smallpox, botulism, plague)
- Identify notification priorities for each type of potential agent
- Ensure access to required contact numbers (e.g., internal infection control personnel, epidemiologist, healthcare facility administration, local, state, federal health agencies, federal and local police, disease control agency, medical emergency services)
- Ensure response plan include details for management of both types of potential scenarios (e.g., covert event bioterrorism outbreak, announced bioterrorism events or threats)
- Seek assistance of government health officials to determine type of event
- Follow instructions regarding screening persons during bioterrorism event, using pre-designed syndrome-based criteria to identify potential outbreaks
- Use epidemiologic principles to determine unusual outbreak versus endemic disease (e.g., clusters of persons arriving from single locale, rapidly increasing disease incidence, large numbers of rapidly fatal cases)
- Integrate biological and chemical terrorism into agency disaster preparedness planning and evaluation
- Identify all community medical, emergency, and social agency resources available (e.g., World Health Organization [WHO], Federal Emergency Management Agency [FEMA], National Disaster Medical System [NDMS], Centers for Disease Control and Prevention [CDC], state and local public health agencies)
- Use current WHO and CDC recommended strategies to contain natural or deliberate disease and chemical events
- Ensure personnel are familiar with signs, symptoms, and common onset presentations of persons exposed to bioterrorism agents
- Modify initial assessment questions and history to be inclusive of exposure risk and physical symptoms of exposure
- Monitor persons with vague yet possibly significant symptoms (e.g., flu-like)
- Report suspicious symptoms to appropriate triage officers and health agencies
- Consult appropriate epidemiology and infection control professionals, as necessary
- Consider reliability of information, especially in emergencies, potential disasters, or mass exposures
- Ensure regular staff training for protective equipment, protective procedures, and isolation techniques
- Ensure that protective equipment (e.g., hazmat suits, headgear, gloves, respirators) available and in good working order
- Ensure all staff are familiar with and follow all decontamination policies, procedures, and protocols
- Provide continuing staff education to maintain up-to-date knowledge
- Ensure regular training including simulations for all staff
- Use teach-back to ensure understanding

4th edition 2004; revised 2024

Background Evidence:

Centers for Disease Control and Prevention. (2018). Epidemic information exchange (Epi-X). *Centers for Disease Control and Prevention.* Accessed at. https://emergency.cdc.gov/epix/index.asp

Centers for Disease Control and Prevention. (2018). Preparation and planning for bioterrorism emergencies. *National Center for Emerging and Zoonotic Infectious Diseases (NCEZID).* https://emergency.cdc.gov/bioterrorism/prep.asp

Federal Emergency Management Agency (FEMA). (2021). Bioterrorism. *Ready site, official website of United States government.* Accessed at. https://www.ready.gov/Bioterrorism

Kako, M., Hammad, K., Mitani, S., & Arbon, P. (2018). Existing approaches to chemical, biological, radiological, and nuclear (CBRN) education and training for health professionals: Findings from an integrative literature review. *Prehospital & Disaster Medicine, 33*(2), 182–190. https://doi.org/10.1017/S1049023X18000043

Rebmann, T., & Carrico, R. (2017). Consistent infection prevention: Vital during routine and emerging infectious diseases care. *Online Journal of Issues in Nursing, 22*(1), 1. https://doi.org/10.3912/OJIN.Vol22No01Man01

Sharma, M., Dixon, J. K., Carter, E. J., & McCorkle, R. (2019). Essential evidence-based introductory bioterrorism content for practicing nurses. *Nurse Education in Practice, 34,* 104–110. https://doi.org/10.1016/j.nepr.2018.10.006

Veenema, T. G. (2019). *Disaster nursing and emergency preparedness: For chemical, biological, and radiological terrorism and other hazards* (4th ed.). Springer.

Birthing 6720

Definition: Delivery of a baby

Activities:

- Provide anticipatory guidance for delivery
- Include support person(s) in birth experience, as appropriate
- Perform vaginal examination to determine fetal position and station
- Maintain patient modesty and privacy in a quiet environment during delivery
- Adhere to patient's requests for management of delivery, when these requests are consistent with standards of perinatal care
- Obtain permission of patient and partner when other health care personnel enter delivery area
- Assist patient with position for delivery
- Inform patient about the need for an episiotomy
- Administer local anesthetic before delivery or episiotomy, as indicated
- Perform episiotomy, as appropriate
- Instruct patient on shallow breathing (e.g., "panting") with delivery of head

- Deliver fetal head slowly, maintaining flexion until parietal bones are born
- Support perineum during delivery
- Check for the presence of a nuchal cord
- Reduce nuchal cord (e.g., clamp and cut cord or slip over the head), as appropriate
- Suction secretions from nares and mouth of infant with a bulb syringe after delivery of head
- Suction for meconium-stained fluid, as appropriate
- Assist delivery of shoulders
- Use maneuvers to release shoulder dystocia (e.g., suprapubic pressure or McRobert's maneuver), as appropriate
- Deliver the body of infant slowly
- Support infant body
- Clamp and cut umbilical cord after pulsations have ceased, when not contraindicated
- Obtain cord blood if Rh negative or as needed for cord blood gas evaluation
- Anticipate spontaneous expulsion of the placenta
- Assign the 1-minute Apgar score
- Apply controlled umbilical cord traction while guarding the fundus of uterus
- Inspect cervix for lacerations after delivery of placenta
- Administer local anesthetic before surgical repair, when indicated
- Suture episiotomy or lacerations, as appropriate
- Perform rectal examination to ensure tissue integrity
- Inspect placenta, membranes, and cord after delivery
- Estimate blood loss after parturition
- Cleanse perineum
- Apply perineal pad
- Praise maternal and support person efforts
- Provide information about infant's appearance and condition
- Encourage verbalization of questions or concerns about birth experience and newborn
- Consult with attending physician about indicators of actual or potential complications
- Document events of birth
- Sign birth certificate, as appropriate

1st edition 1992; revised 1996, 2018

Background Evidence:

Aasheim, V., Nilsen, A., Lukasse, M., & Reiner, L. (2011). Perineal techniques during the second stage of labour for reducing perineal trauma. *Cochrane Database of Systematic Reviews, 2011*(12). https://doi.org/10.1002/14651858.CD006672.pub2

Davidson, M., London, M., & Ladewig, P. (2012). *Old's maternal-newborn nursing and women's health across the lifespan* (9th ed.). Pearson.

Minnesota Midwives Guild. (2013). *The Minnesota Midwives' Guild standards of care.*

Romano, A., Emesis, C., Bailey, J., Robuck, E., & Rothman, M. (2014). *Promoting physiological birth: Putting birthTOOLS.org into action.* Paper presented at the Midwifery Works! Conference October 17 in Chicago, IL. http://www.midwife.org/acnm/files/ccLibraryFiles/Filename/000000004513/BirthTOOLSforMidwiferyWorks.pdf

---

Bladder Irrigation   0550

Definition: Instillation of a solution into the bladder to provide cleansing or medication

Activities:

- Instruct patient and significant others about procedure
- Maintain privacy and assure uninterrupted time during procedure
- Determine whether the irrigation will be continuous or intermittent
- Observe universal precautions
- Set up sterile irrigating supplies, maintaining sterile technique per agency protocol
- Position patient in comfortable, lying, semirecumbent posture
- Cleanse site of entry or end of Y-connector with alcohol wipe before and after procedure
- Instill irrigating fluids, per agency protocol
- Keep patient fully informed of each irrigation, if repetition is necessary
- Monitor patient level of comfort and ease of irrigation with each instillation, if repetition is necessary
- Discontinue irrigations if procedure becomes too difficult or if it appears the catheter is obstructed
- Notify physician if catheter is obstructed
- Monitor and maintain correct flow rate with continuous infusions
- Connect catheter to new drainage bag at end of irrigation
- Record amount of fluid used, characteristics of fluid, amount returned, and patient responsiveness, according to agency protocol
- Assure patient comfort at end of procedure

2nd edition 1996; revised 2018

Background Evidence:

Cutts, B. (2005). Developing and implementing a new bladder irrigation chart. *Nursing Standard, 20*(8), 48–52.

Lynn, P. (2011). *Taylor's clinical nursing skills: A nursing process approach* (3rd ed.). Wolters Kluwer Health/Lippincott Williams & Wilkins.

Potter, P., Perry, A., Stockert, P., & Hall, A. (Eds.). (2013). *Fundamentals of nursing* (8th ed.). Elsevier Mosby.

Rew, M. (2005). Caring for catheterized patients: Urinary catheter maintenance. *British Journal of Nursing, 14*(2), 87–91.

Bleeding Precautions 4010

Definition: Reduction of stimuli that may induce bleeding or hemorrhage in at-risk patients

Activities:

- Review patient history for specific risk factors (e.g., surgery, trauma, ulcers, hemophilia, poor clotting function, clotting inhibition from medication regime)
- Monitor the patient closely for signs and symptoms of internal and external hemorrhage (e.g., distension or swelling of affected body part, change in type or amount of drainage from a surgical drain, bloody saturation of dressings, pooling of blood beneath patient)
- Note hemoglobin and hematocrit levels before and after blood loss, as indicated
- Monitor for signs and symptoms of persistent bleeding (e.g., hypotension, weak and rapid pulse, cool and clammy skin, rapid breathing, restlessness, reduced urine output)
- Maintain careful intake and output
- Maintain IV access, as appropriate
- Monitor coagulation studies, including prothrombin time, partial thromboplastin time, fibrinogen, fibrin degradation and split products, and platelet counts, as appropriate
- Monitor orthostatic vital signs
- Maintain bed rest during active bleeding
- Administer blood products (e.g., platelets and fresh frozen plasma), as appropriate
- Protect the patient from trauma, which may cause bleeding
- Avoid injections (IM or SQ), as appropriate
- Avoid administering medications that will further compromise clotting times (e.g., clopidogrel, heparin, warfarin, or nonsteroidal anti-inflammatory drugs [NSAIDs] such as aspirin)
- Instruct patient to avoid medications that will further compromise clotting times (e.g., clopidogrel, heparin, warfarin, or nonsteroidal anti-inflammatory drugs [NSAIDs] such as aspirin), as appropriate
- Instruct the ambulating patient to wear shoes

- Use soft toothbrush or toothettes for oral care
- Use electric razor, instead of straight edge, for shaving
- Instruct patient to avoid invasive procedures; if they are necessary, monitor closely for bleeding
- Coordinate timing of invasive procedures with platelet or fresh frozen plasma transfusions, if appropriate
- Refrain from inserting objects into a bleeding orifice
- Avoid taking rectal temperatures
- Instruct patient to avoid lifting heavy objects
- Administer medications (e.g., antacids), as appropriate
- Instruct patient to increase intake of foods rich in vitamin K (e.g., dark green leafy vegetables such as spinach and cabbage, cauliflower, broccoli, and soybeans), as appropriate
- Use therapeutic mattress to minimize skin trauma
- Instruct patient to avoid constipation (e.g., encourage fluid intake and stool softeners), as appropriate
- Instruct the patient and family on signs of bleeding (e.g., easy bruising, nosebleeds, bleeding gums, blood in the urine or stool, or extremely heavy menstrual periods) and appropriate actions (e.g., notify the nurse) should bleeding occur

1st edition 1992; revised 1996, 2018

Background Evidence:

Brown, C. G. (2010). *A guide to oncology symptom management.* Oncology Nursing Society.

Malli, S. (2005). Keep a close eye on vacuum-assisted wound closure. *Nursing, 35*(7), 25.

Nix, D. (2012). Skin and wound inspection and assessment. In R. Bryant & D. Nix (Eds.), *Acute and chronic wounds: Current management concepts* (4th ed.). Elsevier Mosby.

Potter, P., Perry, A., Stockert, P., & Hall, A. (Eds.). (2013). *Fundamentals of nursing* (8th ed.). Elsevier Mosby.

Bleeding Reduction 4020

Definition: Limitation of the loss of blood volume during an episode of bleeding

Activities:

- Identify the cause of the bleeding
- Monitor the patient closely for hemorrhage
- Apply direct pressure or pressure dressing, if appropriate
- Apply ice pack to affected area, as appropriate
- Monitor the amount and nature of blood loss
- Monitor size and character of hematoma, if present
- Note hemoglobin/hematocrit levels before and after blood loss
- Monitor trends in blood pressure and hemodynamic parameters, if available (e.g., central venous pressure and pulmonary capillary/artery wedge pressure)
- Monitor fluid status, including intake and output
- Monitor coagulation studies, including prothrombin time (PT), partial thromboplastin time (PTT), fibrinogen, fibrin degradation/split products, and platelet counts, as appropriate

- Monitor determinants of tissue oxygen delivery (e.g., PaO_2, SaO_2, and hemoglobin levels and cardiac output), if available
- Monitor neurological functioning
- Inspect for bleeding from mucous membranes, bruising after minimal trauma, oozing from puncture sites, and presence of petechiae
- Monitor for signs and symptoms of persistent bleeding (i.e., check all secretions for frank or occult blood)
- Arrange availability of blood products for transfusion, if necessary
- Maintain patent IV access
- Administer blood products (e.g., platelets and fresh frozen plasma), as appropriate
- Hematest all excretions and observe for blood in emesis, sputum, feces, urine, NG drainage, and wound drainage, as appropriate

- Perform proper precautions in handling blood products or bloody secretions
- Evaluate patient's psychological response to hemorrhage and perception of events
- Instruct the patient and family on signs of bleeding and appropriate actions (i.e., notify the nurse), should further bleeding occur
- Instruct the patient on activity restrictions
- Instruct patient and family on severity of blood loss and appropriate actions being performed

1st edition 1992; revised 2008, 2013

Background Evidence:
American Association of Critical-Care Nurses. (2006). In J. G. Alspach (Ed.), *Core curriculum for critical care nursing* (6th ed.). Saunders Elsevier.
Berman, A., Snyder, S., Kozier, B., & Erb, G. (2008). *Kozier & Erb's fundamentals of nursing: Concepts, processes, and practice* (8th ed.). Prentice Hall.
Monahan, F., Sands, J., Neighbors, M., Marek, J., & Green, C. (2007). *Phipps' medical-surgical nursing: Health and illness perspectives* (8th ed.). Mosby.
Smeltzer, S. C., Bare, B. G., Hinkle, J. L., & Cheever, K. H. (2010). Emergency nursing. In *Brunner & Suddarth's textbook of medical-surgical nursing* (pp. 2153–2190) (12th ed.). Lippincott Williams & Wilkins.

Bleeding Reduction: Antepartum Uterus   4021

Definition: Limitation of the amount of blood loss from the pregnant uterus during third trimester of pregnancy

Activities:

- Obtain client history of vaginal bleeding (e.g., onset, amount, frequency of changing peri pads, color of bleeding, presence and location of pain, and presence of clots)
- Review for risk factors related to late pregnancy bleeding (e.g., abruptio placentae, smoking, cocaine use, hypertension, diabetes, multiparity, previous cesarean birth, prior and current placenta previa, infertility treatment, multiple gestations, short interval between pregnancies, greater than 35 years of age)
- Obtain an accurate estimate of fetal age by last menstrual period report, prior ultrasound dating reports, or obstetrical history, if available
- Inspect perineum, clothing, sheets or pads for amount and characteristic of bleeding
- Weigh blood-soaked materials and clots to quantify blood loss
- Continually monitor characteristic and amount of bleeding
- Monitor maternal vital signs frequently
- Initiate continuous electronic fetal monitoring
- Palpate for uterine contractions or increased uterine tone
- Monitor electronic fetal tracing for evidence of uteroplacental insufficiency (e.g., late decelerations, decreased long-term variability, and absent accelerations)
- Monitor for rupture of membranes
- Report client status and any changes in amount and frequency of bleeding, as appropriate
- Initiate fetal resuscitation for abnormal (non-reassuring) signs of uteroplacental insufficiency
- Delay digital cervical examination until location of placenta has been verified by ultrasound
- Assist with fetal surveillance tests
- Perform or assist with speculum examination to visualize blood loss and cervical status
- Initiate IV access for fluid replacement
- Administer oxygen, as ordered
- Obtain diagnostic blood studies (e.g., CBC, clotting studies, Rh, type and cross match, Kleihauer-Betke test), as ordered
- Monitor intake and output
- Elevate lower extremities to increase perfusion to vital organs and fetus
- Administer blood products, as appropriate
- Initiate safety measures (e.g., strict bed rest and lateral position)
- Instruct patient to report increases in vaginal bleeding (e.g., gushes, clots, and trickles) during hospitalization
- Provide empathy, understanding and emotional support
- Provide information on procedures, diagnostic tests, and treatments
- Instruct woman to differentiate between old and fresh bleeding
- Inform woman to monitor fetal movement to evaluate fetal well-being
- Instruct client on life-style changes to reduce the chance of further bleeding (e.g., smoking cessation assistance, sexual abstinence, bed rest care, constipation management, nutrition management, and coping enhancement), as appropriate
- Provide discharge planning, including referral to home care nurses
- Schedule follow-up antepartum fetal surveillance
- Discuss reasons to return to the hospital
- Discuss use of emergency medical system for transportation, as appropriate

2nd edition 1996; revised 2018

Background Evidence:
Ladewig, P., London, M., & Davidson, M. (2014). *Contemporary maternal-newborn nursing care* (pp. 423–427) (8th ed.). Boston, MA: Pearson.
Quantification of blood loss: AWHONN Practice Brief Number 1. (2015). *Journal of Obstetric, Gynecologic, & Neonatal Nursing, 44*(1), 158–160.
Rhynders, P., Sayers, C., Presley, R., & Thierry, J. (2014). Providing young women with credible health information about bleeding disorders. *American Journal of Preventative Medicine, 47*(5), 674–680.
Ricci, S. (2013). *Essentials of maternity, newborn, & women's health nursing* (pp. 616–624) (3rd ed.). Wolters Kluwer Health/Lippincott Williams & Wilkins.

Bleeding Reduction: Gastrointestinal 4022

Definition: Limitation of the amount of blood loss from the upper and lower gastrointestinal tract and related complications

Activities:

- Evaluate patient's psychological response to hemorrhage and perception of events
- Maintain a patent airway, if necessary
- Monitor determinants of tissue oxygen delivery (e.g., PaO_2, SaO_2, and hemoglobin levels and cardiac output), if available
- Monitor for signs and symptoms of persistent bleeding (e.g., check all secretions for frank or occult blood)
- Monitor fluid status, including intake and output, as appropriate
- Administer IV fluids, as appropriate
- Monitor for signs of hypovolemic shock (e.g., decreased blood pressure; rapid, thready pulse; increased respiratory rate; diaphoresis; restlessness; cool, clammy skin)
- Measure abdominal girth, as appropriate
- Hematest all excretions and observe for blood in emesis, sputum, feces, urine, NG drainage, and wound drainage, as appropriate
- Document color, amount, and character of stools
- Monitor coagulation studies and complete blood count (CBC) with WBC differential, as appropriate
- Avoid administration of anticoagulants
- Monitor coagulation studies, including prothrombin time (PT), partial thromboplastin time (PTT), fibrinogen, fibrin degradation/split products, and platelet counts, as appropriate
- Administer medications (e.g., lactulose or vasopressin), as appropriate
- Avoid extremes in gastric pH level by administration of appropriate medication (e.g., antacids or histamine-2 blocking agent), as appropriate
- Insert nasogastric tube to suction and monitor secretions, if appropriate
- Maintain pressure in cuffed/balloon nasogastric tube, if appropriate
- Perform nasogastric lavage, as appropriate
- Promote stress reduction
- Assess the patient's nutritional status
- Establish a supportive relationship with the patient and family
- Instruct the patient and family on activity restriction and progression
- Instruct the patient and/or family on procedures (e.g., endoscopy, sclerosis, and surgery), if appropriate
- Instruct the patient and/or family on the need for blood replacement, as appropriate
- Instruct the patient and/or family to avoid the use of anti-inflammatory medications (e.g., aspirin and ibuprofen)
- Coordinate counseling for the patient and/or family (e.g., clergy, Alcoholics Anonymous), if appropriate

1st edition 1992; revised 2008

Background Evidence:

Cullen, L. (1992). Interventions related to circulatory care. *Nursing Clinics of North America, 27*(2), 445–476.

DeLaune, S., & Ladner, P. (2006). *Fundamentals of nursing: Standards & practice* (3rd ed.). Thomson Delmar Learning.

Kozier, B., Erb, G., Berman, A., & Snyder, S. (2004). *Fundamentals of nursing: Concepts, process, and practice* (7th ed.). Prentice Hall.

Monahan, F., Sands, J., Neighbors, M., Marek, J., & Green, C. (2007). *Phipps' medical-surgical nursing: Health and illness perspectives* (8th ed.). Mosby.

Bleeding Reduction: Nasal 4024

Definition: Limitation of the amount of blood loss from the nasal cavity

Activities:

- Apply manual pressure over the bridge of the nose
- Identify the cause of the bleeding
- Monitor the amount and nature of blood loss
- Monitor the amount of bleeding into the oropharynx
- Apply ice pack to affected area
- Place packing in nasal cavity, if appropriate
- Administer blood products (e.g., platelets and fresh frozen plasma), as appropriate
- Note hemoglobin/hematocrit levels before and after blood loss, as indicated
- Promote stress reduction
- Provide pain relief/comfort measures
- Maintain a patent airway
- Assist patient with oral care, as appropriate
- Administer humidified oxygen, if appropriate
- Monitor vital signs, as appropriate
- Place patient in mid-Fowler's position, as appropriate
- Instruct the patient on activity restrictions, if appropriate
- Instruct patient to avoid traumatizing nares (e.g., avoid scratching, blowing, or touching nose)
- Instruct the patient and/or family on signs of bleeding and appropriate actions (e.g., notify the nurse), should further bleeding occur

1st edition 1992; revised 2008

Background Evidence:

American Association of Critical-Care Nurses. (2006). In J. G. Alspach (Ed.), *Core curriculum for critical care nursing* (6th ed.). Saunders Elsevier.

Cullen, L. (1992). Interventions related to circulatory care. *Nursing Clinics of North America, 27*(2), 445–476.

Kozier, B., Erb, G., Berman, A., & Snyder, S. (2004). *Fundamentals of nursing: Concepts, process, and practice* (7th ed.). Prentice Hall.

Monahan, F., Sands, J., Neighbors, M., Marek, J., & Green, C. (2007). *Phipps' medical-surgical nursing: Health and illness perspectives* (8th ed.). Mosby.

B

Bleeding Reduction: Postpartum Uterus 4026

Definition: Limitation of the amount of blood loss from the postpartum uterus

Activities:

- Review obstetrical history and labor record for risk factors for postpartum hemorrhage (e.g., prior history of postpartum hemorrhage, overdistention of the uterus, rapid labor, prolonged third stage, uterine infection, lacerations, retained placenta, labor, induction, use of anesthesia, preeclampsia, prolonged second stage, assistive birth, cesarean birth, or precipitous birth)
- Perform fundal massage to ensure firm consistency
- Increase frequency of fundal massage until the uterus becomes firm
- Check episiotomy for blood loss
- Apply ice to perineum
- Inspect placenta for intactness and missing fragments
- Evaluate for bladder distention
- Encourage voiding or catheterize distended bladder
- Observe characteristics of lochia (e.g., color, clots, and volume)
- Quantify amount of blood loss
- Notify primary practitioner of excessive blood loss
- Request additional nurses to help with emergency procedures and to assume care for newborn
- Elevate legs
- Initiate IV infusion with needles suitable for blood transfusion
- Start second IV line, as appropriate
- Administer a uterotonic drug, per protocol or order
- Monitor maternal vital signs every 15 minutes or more frequently, as appropriate
- Cover with warm blankets
- Monitor maternal color, level of consciousness, pain, and anxiety level
- Initiate oxygen therapy at 6 to 8 L per face mask
- Insert Foley catheter with urometer to monitor urine output, as appropriate
- Order emergency laboratory tests or units of blood
- Administer blood products, as appropriate
- Identify mother's beliefs about blood transfusions
- Assist primary practitioner with packing uterus, evacuating hematoma, or suturing lacerations, as appropriate
- Keep patient and family informed of clinical condition and management
- Provide perineal care, as needed
- Prepare the woman for transfer to the operating room for surgical intervention
- Discuss events with nursing team for provision of adequate postpartum surveillance of maternal status

2nd edition 1996; revised 2018

Background Evidence:

Bringham, D. (2012). Eliminating preventable, hemorrhage-related maternal mortality and morbidity. *Journal of Obstetric, Gynecologic, & Neonatal Nursing, 41*(4), 529–530.

Guidelines for oxytocin administration after birth: AWHONN Practice Brief Number 2. (2015). *Journal of Obstetric, Gynecologic, & Neonatal Nursing, 44*(1), 161–163.

Ladewig, P., London, M., & Davidson, M. (2014). *Contemporary maternal-newborn nursing care* (pp. 734–741) (8th ed.). Pearson.

Quantification of blood loss: AWHONN Practice Brief Number 1. (2015). *Journal of Obstetric, Gynecologic, & Neonatal Nursing, 44*(1), 158–160.

Ricci, S. (2013). *Essentials of maternity, newborn, & women's health nursing* (pp. 746–755) (3rd ed.). Wolters Kluwer Health/Lippincott Williams & Wilkins.

Bleeding Reduction: Wound 4028

Definition: Limitation of the blood loss from a wound that may be a result of trauma, incisions, or placement of a tube or catheter

Activities:

- Apply manual pressure over the bleeding or the potential bleeding area
- Apply ice pack to affected area
- Apply pressure dressing to site of bleeding
- Use mechanical device (e.g., C-type clamp) for applying pressure for longer periods, if appropriate
- Replace or reinforce pressure dressing, as appropriate
- Monitor vital signs, as appropriate
- Monitor accurate intake and output
- Place bleeding extremity in an elevated position
- Maintain continuous bladder irrigation, if appropriate
- Monitor size and character of hematoma, if present
- Monitor pulses distal to bleeding site
- Instruct patient to apply pressure to site when sneezing, coughing, and so on
- Instruct the patient on activity restrictions, if appropriate
- Instruct the patient and/or family on signs of bleeding and appropriate actions (e.g., notify the nurse) should further bleeding occur

1st edition 1992; revised 2008

Background Evidence:

American Association of Critical-Care Nurses. (2006). In J. G. Alspach (Ed.), *Core curriculum for critical care nursing* (6th ed.). Saunders Elsevier.

Cullen, L. (1992). Interventions related to circulatory care. *Nursing Clinics of North America, 27*(2), 445–476.

Kozier, B., Erb, G., Berman, A., & Snyder, S. (2004). *Fundamentals of nursing: Concepts, process, and practice* (7th ed.). Prentice Hall.

Monahan, F., Sands, J., Neighbors, M., Marek, J., & Green, C. (2007). *Phipps' medical-surgical nursing: Health and illness perspectives* (8th ed.). Mosby.

Blood Products Administration   4030

Definition: Administration of blood or blood products and monitoring response

Activities:

- Verify health care provider orders
- Obtain transfusion history
- Assure identification band present
- Obtain or verify informed consent
- Verify that blood product has been prepared, typed, and cross-matched (if applicable)
- Verify correct person, blood type, Rh type, unit number, and expiration date with two licensed personnel
- Record verification per agency protocol
- Instruct related to risks, benefits, and alternatives to transfusion
- Instruct about signs and symptoms of transfusion reactions (e.g., dizziness, chest pain, pruritus, papules, skin rash, dyspnea, choking sensation, abdominal pain, back pain, hematuria)
- Premedicate if indicated
- Ensure ready to start transfusion
- Ensure good venous access before obtaining blood products
- Provide dedicated IV line and adequate gauge IV catheter for blood infusion
- Assemble administration system with filter appropriate for blood product and recipient's immune status
- Prime administration system with isotonic saline
- Prepare IV pump approved for blood product administration, if indicated
- Maintain strict aseptic technique
- Initiate blood transfusion no later than 30 minutes after removal from blood bank
- Avoid transfusion of more than one unit of blood, blood component, or blood product at a time, unless necessitated by recipient's condition
- Monitor IV site for signs and symptoms of infiltration, phlebitis, and local infection
- Monitor condition and vital signs (e.g., baseline, throughout and after transfusion)
- Monitor for transfusion reactions (e.g., fever, chills, tremors, increase of 1°C from initial temperature)
- Monitor for fluid overload
- Monitor and regulate flow rate during transfusion
- Refrain from administering IV medications or fluids, other than isotonic saline, into blood or blood product lines
- Refrain from transfusing blood product removed from controlled refrigeration over more than 4 hours.
- Change filter and administration set at least every 4 hours
- Administer saline when transfusion complete
- Document time frame of transfusion
- Document volume infused
- Stop transfusion if blood reaction occurs, keeping veins open with saline
- Obtain blood sample and first voided urine specimen after transfusion reaction
- Coordinate return of blood container and tubing to laboratory after blood reaction
- Notify laboratory immediately in event of blood reaction
- Document transfusion reaction and condition of recipient per agency policy

1st edition 1992; revised 1996, 2004, 2024

Background Evidence:

Akyol, A. (2019). Evaluating nurses' knowledge of blood transfusion in Turkey. *International Journal of Caring Sciences, 12*(1), 521–528.

American Association of Blood Banks (AABB). (2018). *Standards for blood banks and transfusion services* (31st ed.). American Association of Blood Banks.

Bezerra, C. M., Cardoso, M. V. L. M. L., Silva, G. R. F. D., & Rodrigues, E. D. C. (2018). Creation and validation of a checklist for blood transfusion in children. *Brazilian Nursing Journal, 71*(6), 3020–3026.

Infusion Nursing Society. (2021). *Policies and procedures for infusion therapy: Acute care* (6th ed.).

Infusion Nursing Society. (2021). *Standards of practice* (8th ed.).

Mirzaei, S. (2019). Association between adverse clinical outcomes after coronary artery bypass grafting and perioperative blood transfusions. *Critical Care Nurse, 39*(1), 26–35.

Perry, A. G., & Potter, P. A. (2020). *Fundamentals of nursing* (10th ed.). Elsevier.

Perry, A. G., Potter, P. A., Ostendorf, W., & LaPlante, N. (2021). *Clinical nursing skills and techniques* (10th ed.). Elsevier.

Body Image Enhancement   5220

Definition: Improving conscious and unconscious perceptions and attitudes toward physical self

Activities:

- Determine body image expectations based on developmental stage
- Use anticipatory guidance to prepare for predictable changes in body image
- Determine whether perceived dislike for certain physical characteristics creates dysfunctional social paralysis for teenagers and other high-risk groups
- Assist to discuss changes caused by illness or surgery, as appropriate
- Help determine extent of actual changes in body or level of functioning
- Determine whether recent physical change has been incorporated into body image
- Assist to separate physical appearance from feelings of personal worth, as appropriate
- Discuss changes caused by puberty, as appropriate
- Discuss cognitions (e.g., irrational beliefs, dichotomous thinking, automatic thoughts, cognitive errors) and role in feelings and behaviors related to body image
- Discuss changes caused by normal pregnancy, as appropriate
- Discuss changes caused by aging, as appropriate
- Determine person's and family's perceptions of alteration in body image versus reality

B

- Instruct about normal changes in body associated with various stages of aging, as appropriate
- Determine whether change in body image has contributed to increased social isolation
- Discuss stressors affecting body image due to congenital condition, injury, disease, or surgery
- Identify effects of culture, religion, race, sex, gender, and age in terms of body image
- Monitor frequency of statements of self-criticism
- Monitor whether person can look at changed body part
- Discuss how negative body image expressed in various behaviors (e.g., body checking, weighing, measuring, pinching, mirror checking), body avoidance (e.g., avoiding mirrors, wearing baggy clothing) or appearance preoccupation (i.e., time-consuming efforts to groom, manage, or alter appearance)
- Instruct how to self-monitor and restructure thoughts using log, journal, or diary
- Instruct how to change and improve use of negative body image language to describe body (e.g., "I have a disgusting belly") to non-judgmental and fact-based statements like "I have a round belly"
- Instruct to focus attention less on disliked body parts toward more attention on other body parts and on seeing body as a whole
- Conduct guided imagery exercises designed to focus and direct imagination to relive important event that influenced body image
- Discuss eating disorders and related behaviors and cognitions, including risk factors for developing eating disorder, unhealthy eating patterns (e.g., binging, fasting, dietary restraint, excessive exercising)
- Use exposure exercises with goal of gradually extinguishing negative body image reactions and situations (i.e., mirror exposure to expose participants to own body)
- Create and agree on verbal or written contract with specific tasks
- Identify barriers to performing specific behavior and plan ways of overcoming them
- Provide feedback about behaviors or performance on task
- Provide encouragement regarding continued performance of cognitive or behavioral exercises designed to improve body image perceptions
- Discuss concept of stress, what stress is (e.g., healthy vs. unhealthy forms), what causes stress, and consequences of stress for health and well-being
- Use stress management techniques that do not target body image cognition and behaviors but seek to reduce anxiety and stress (e.g., progressive muscle relaxation, deep breathing)
- Provide information about alternative help resources (e.g., self-help books, websites, social media, support group)
- Discuss causes for negative body image (e.g., media influence, receiving specific negative remarks or teasing about one's weight, internal need for perfectionism)
- Provide media literacy training to help decipher media messages that set unrealistic images of beauty critical of body types
- Discuss stereotypes, prejudice, and discrimination related to gender or appearance (e.g., stereotypes about women or men, thin or overweight people, impact of prejudice and discrimination on body image)
- Assist in use of strategies designed to resist impact of media (e.g., avoid negative sources)

- Provide alternative empowering images of women or men that go against current beauty ideal
- Discuss concept of self-esteem, how self-esteem formed, what factors influence self-esteem, how self-esteem relates to well-being
- Provide self-esteem enhancement exercises designed to enhance positive self-regard. (i.e., write list of talents and positive personality traits)
- Discuss physical activity and its role in promoting healthy body image
- Discuss interpersonal relations that impact on body images (e.g., peer pressure, social rejection, unacceptability, and impact of appearance-based teasing, effects of fat talk)
- Instruct on use of interpersonal skills designed to enhance communication with others (e.g., express opinions, how to resolve interpersonal conflicts)
- Provide mindfulness exercises designed to promote positive body image (e.g., deep breathing, body scan, meditation, mindful eating)
- Discuss psychological consequences of negative body image, such as development of eating disorder, depression, low self-esteem, social anxiety
- Identify coping strategies used by parents in response to changes in child's appearance
- Determine how child responds to parent's reactions, as appropriate
- Instruct on importance of child's responses to body changes and future adjustment, as appropriate
- Assist to identify feelings before intervening with child, as appropriate
- Assist in identifying parts of body that have positive perceptions associated with them
- Identify means of reducing effect of any disfigurement through clothing, wigs, or cosmetics, as appropriate
- Assist to identify actions that will enhance appearance
- Assist hospitalized person to apply cosmetics before seeing visitors, as appropriate
- Use teach-back to ensure understanding

1st edition 1992; revised 2000, 2024

Background Evidence:

Aboody, D., Siev, J., & Doron, G. (2020). Building resilience to body image triggers using brief cognitive training on a mobile application: A randomized controlled trial. *Behaviour Research and Therapy, 134*, 103723. https://doi.org/10.1016/j.brat.2020.103723

Johnson, S., Egan, S. J., Andersson, G., Carlbring, P., Shafran, R., & Wade, T. D. (2019). Internet-delivered cognitive behavioural therapy for perfectionism: Targeting dysmorphic concern. *Body Image, 30*, 44–55.

Morgan, K. I., & Townsend, M. C. (2021). *Davis Advantage for psychiatric mental health nursing* (10th ed.). F.A. Davis.

Sattler, F. A., Eickmeyer, S., & Eisenkolb, J. (2020). Body image disturbance in children and adolescents with anorexia nervosa and bulimia nervosa: A systematic review. *Eating and Weight Disorders: EWD, 25*(4), 857–865.

Varcarolis, E. M., & Fosbre, C. D. (2021). *Essentials of psychiatric mental health nursing: A communication approach to evidence-based care* (4th ed.). Elsevier.

B

Body Mechanics Promotion 0140

Definition: Facilitating the use of posture and movement in daily activities to prevent fatigue and musculoskeletal strain or injury

Activities:
- Determine patient's commitment to learning and using correct posture
- Collaborate with physical therapy in developing a body mechanics promotion plan, as indicated
- Determine patient's understanding of body mechanics and exercises (e.g., return demonstration of correct techniques when performing activities/exercises)
- Instruct patient on structure and function of spine and optimal posture for moving and using the body
- Instruct patient about need for correct posture to prevent fatigue, strain, or injury
- Instruct patient how to use posture and body mechanics to prevent injury when performing any physical activities
- Determine patient awareness of own musculoskeletal abnormalities and the potential effects of posture and muscle tissue
- Instruct to use a firm mattress/chair or pillow, if appropriate
- Instruct to avoid sleeping prone
- Assist to demonstrate appropriate sleeping positions
- Assist to avoid sitting in the same position for prolonged periods
- Demonstrate how to shift weight from one foot to another when standing
- Instruct patient to move feet first and then body when turning to walk from a standing position
- Use the principles of body mechanics in conjunction with safe patient handling and movement aids
- Assist patient/family to identify appropriate posture exercises
- Assist patient to select warm-up activities before beginning exercise or work not done routinely
- Assist patient to perform flexion exercises to facilitate back mobility, as indicated
- Instruct patient/family regarding frequency and number of repetitions for each exercise
- Monitor improvement in patient's posture/body mechanics
- Provide information about possible positional causes of muscle or joint pain

1st edition 1992; revised 2008

Background Evidence:
Kozier, B., Erb, G., Berman, A., & Snyder, S. (2004). *Fundamentals of nursing: Concepts, process, and practice* (7th ed.). Prentice Hall.
Patient Safety Center of Inquiry, Veterans Health Administration and Department of Defense. (2005). *Patient care ergonomics resource guide: Safe patient handling and movement.* http://www.visn8.va.gov/visn8/patientsafetycenter/resguide/ErgoGuidePtOne.pdf
Perry, A. G., & Potter, P. A. (2006). *Clinical nursing skills and techniques* (6th ed.). Elsevier Mosby.
Smith, S. F., Duell, D. J., & Martin, B. C. (2004). *Clinical nursing skills: Basic to advanced skills* (6th ed.). Prentice Hall.

Body Search 6425

Definition: Inspection of clothing, personal belongings, and external body for items that are deemed a safety concern

Activities:
- Determine reason for search (e.g., harm to self, harm to others, possession of unlawful substances)
- Follow agency policies that permit conducting body searches (e.g., have health care provider order, documented need for search)
- Create list of unsafe items not allowed on unit or care area and ensure list accessible to all persons and visitors entering care area (e.g., signs)
- Provide knowledge of rights and responsibilities when admitted, including possibility of body search
- Ask person if in possession of any items not allowed in care area and to give items to personnel
- Inform of legal rights before initiating search
- Inform of pattern of search as well as what will be examined during search
- Obtain consent from person or guardian
- Provide information about search in language and format that allows adequate comprehension
- Provide interpreter, if needed
- Determine when to conduct search (e.g., at the time of admission, upon return from leaves of absence, when deemed necessary)
- Use PPE and safety equipment during search, when necessary
- Establish pattern of search (i.e., search clothing first, followed by personal belongings and ending with external body)
- Conduct search with trained staff
- Observe for inappropriate bulges or areas person reluctant to reveal
- Avoid conversation or distracting activities during search
- Provide for adequate comfort and privacy during search (i.e., provide for person of same gender to be present or perform search)
- Remove all contraband obtained during searches for safekeeping according to agency policy
- Ask visitors to give prohibited items to personnel for safekeeping
- Review each situation individually, ensuring body searches conducted only when necessary
- Document searches in detail, including need for search and items found
- Document placement or storage of any items retrieved during search

8th edition 2024

Background Evidence:

Abela-Dimech, F. & Johnston, K. (2017). Safe searches. *Journal for Nurses in Professional Development, 33*(5), 247–254. https://doi.org/10.1097/NND.0000000000000385

Abela-Dimech, F., & Johnston, K. (2017). Safe searches. *Journal for Nurses in Professional Development, 33*(5), 247–254. https://doi.org/10.1097/NND.0000000000000385

Abela-Dimech, F., Johnston, K., & Strudwick, G. (2017). Development and pilot implementation of a search protocol to improve patient safety on a psychiatric inpatient unit. *Clinical Nurse Specialist, 31*(2), 104–114. https://doi.org/10.1097/NUR.0000000000000281

Frauenfelder, F. (2019). Psychiatric adult inpatient nursing described in the NANDA-I and NIC: A systematic evaluation of nursing classifications [Doctoral dissertation. Radbound University] Radbound Repository. https://repository.ubn.ru.nl/handle/2066/203856

American Psychiatric Nurses Association. (2014). *Psychiatric-mental health nursing: Scope and standards of practice* (2nd ed.).

Keltner, N. L., & Steele, D. (2019). *Psychiatric nursing* (8th ed.). Elsevier.

Rebar, C. R., Gersch, C., & Heimgartner, N. M. (2020). *Psychiatric nursing made incredibly easy* (3rd ed.). Wolters Kluwer.

University of Iowa Hospitals and Clinics. (2018). Patient search. *Policy and Procedure Manual.*

Varcarolis, E. M., & Fosbre, C. D. (2021). *Essentials of psychiatric-mental health nursing* (4th ed.). Elsevier.

Bottle Feeding 1052

Definition: Preparation and administration of fluids to an infant via a bottle

Activities:

- Determine infant sleep and wakefulness patterns before initiating feeding
- Warm fluid to room temperature before feeding
- Position infant with support in semi-Fowler's position for feeding
- Burp infant frequently during and after feeding
- Place nipple on top of tongue
- Control intake by regulating softness of nipple and size of hole and bottle
- Increase infant alertness by loosening infant's clothes, rubbing hands and feet, or talking to infant
- Encourage sucking by stimulating rooting reflex, if appropriate
- Increase effectiveness of suck by compressing cheeks in unison with suck, if appropriate
- Provide chin support to decrease leaking of fluid and improve lip closure
- Monitor fluid intake
- Monitor and evaluate suck reflex during feeding
- Monitor infant weight, as appropriate
- Boil unpasteurized milk
- Boil water used for preparing formula, if indicated
- Instruct on sterilization techniques for feeding equipment
- Instruct on proper dilution of concentrated formula
- Instruct on proper storage of formula
- Instruct on proper storage of breast milk
- Instruct on not forcing termination of liquid intake
- Determine fluoride content of water used to dilute concentrated or powdered formula and refer for fluoride supplementation, if indicated
- Caution about using microwave oven to warm formula
- Demonstrate oral hygiene techniques appropriate to infant's dentition to be used after each feeding
- Discuss alternatives to bedtime bottle to prevent bottle caries
- Use teach-back to ensure understanding

1st edition 1992; revised 2000, 2024

Background Evidence:

Appleton, J., Russell, C. G., Laws, R., Fowler, C., Campbell, K., & Denney-Wilson, E. (2018). Infant formula feeding practices associated with rapid weight gain: A systematic review. *Maternal Child Nutrition, 14*, e12602. https://doi.org/10.1111/mcn.12602

Hockenberry, M. J., Rodgers, C. C., & Wilson, D. (2022). *Wong's essentials of pediatric nursing.* Elsevier.

Kotowski, J., Fowler, C., Hourigan, C., & Orr, F. (2020). Bottle-feeding an infant feeding modality: An integrative literature review. *Maternal & Child Nutrition, 16*(2), e12939. https://doi.org/10.1111/mcn.12939

Matson, S., & Smith, J. E. (2016). *Core curriculum for maternal-newborn nursing.* Elsevier.

Savage, J. S., Hohman, E. E., Marini, M. E., Shelly, A., Paul, I. M., & Birch, L. L. (2018). INSIGHT responsive parenting intervention and infant feeding practices: Randomized clinical trial. *The International Journal of Behavioral Nutrition and Physical Activity, 15*(1), 64. https://doi.org/10.1186/s12966-018-0700-6

Bowel Incontinence Care 0410

Definition: Promotion of bowel continence and skin integrity

Activities:

- Review health history including diagnoses, surgeries, and bowel habits
- Identify factors that affect bowel habits (e.g., medications, exercise, sleep, stress, smoking, diet, toilet access)
- Note pre-existing bowel problems, bowel routine, and use of laxatives and enemas
- Monitor bowel movements including frequency, consistency, volume, and color, as appropriate
- Determine physical, cognitive, and psychological cause of fecal incontinence
- Explain etiology of problem and rationale for actions
- Eliminate cause of incontinence (e.g., medication, diet, infection, fecal impaction), if possible
- Develop bowel management program (e.g., procedure, outcomes)
- Instruct to record fecal output, as appropriate
- Monitor perineal skin for redness, itching, pain, pressure injury, and infection

- Wash perianal area and dry thoroughly after each stool (e.g., soap and water, nonionic detergent)
- Protect skin from excess moisture with barrier cream (e.g., lanolin, dimethicone), as prescribed
- Avoid powder and creams on perineal area unless prescribed
- Keep bed and clothing clean and dry
- Monitor diet and fluid requirements
- Instruct to avoid foods that cause diarrhea
- Administer prescribed medication for diarrhea (e.g., loperamide, atropine)
- Use rectal tube, anal plug device, or fecal collection device, per protocol
- Provide incontinent pants and pads as needed
- Implement bowel training program, as appropriate
- Use teach-back to ensure understanding

1st edition 1992; revised 2013, 2024

B

Background Evidence:

Axelrod, M. I., & Fontanini-Axelrod, A. (2021). Treating functional nonretentive fecal incontinence using a comprehensive behavioral treatment across settings. *Clinical Practice in Pediatric Psychology*. https://doi.org/10.1037/cpp0000425

Barrie, M. (2018). Nursing management of patients with faecal incontinence. *Nursing Standard, 33*(2), 69. https://doi.org/10.7748/ns.2018.e11167

Craven, R. F., Hirnle, C. J., & Henshaw, C. J. (2021). *Fundamentals of nursing: Human health and function* (8th ed.). Wolters-Kluwer.

Devendorf, A. R., Bradley, S. E., Barks, L., Klanchar, A., Orozco, T., & Cowan, L. (2021). Stigma among veterans with urinary and fecal incontinence. *Stigma and Health, 6*(3), 335–343. https://doi.org/10.31234/osf.io/3wv2u

Williams, P. (2020). *Basic geriatric nursing* (7th ed.). Elsevier.

Yates, A. (2018). Preventing skin damage and incontinence-associated dermatitis in older people. *British Journal of Nursing, 27*(2), 76–77. https://doi.org/10.12968/bjon.2018.27.2.76

Bowel Incontinence Care: Encopresis   0412

Definition: Promotion of bowel continence in children

Activities:

- Gather information about toilet training history, duration of encopresis, and attempts made to eliminate the problem
- Determine cause of soiling (e.g., constipation and fecal impaction), as appropriate
- Order tests for physical causes (e.g., endoscopy, radiographic procedures, and stool analysis)
- Prepare child and family for diagnostic tests
- Perform rectal examination, as appropriate
- Instruct family about physiology of normal defecation and toilet training
- Formulate a bowel retraining plan with the family (e.g., mineral oil, high fiber diet, regular toileting routine)
- Encourage child to sit on toilet 10 to 15 minutes after meals for intervals of 10 minutes
- Place a footstool below the feet to relax the abdomen
- Provide positive reinforcement (e.g., stickers, praise, special activities) to encourage the child to participate in the bowel regime
- Conduct family psychosocial assessment, including responses of caregivers and self-esteem of child
- Discuss psychosocial dynamics of encopresis with parents (e.g., familial patterns, family disruption, self-esteem issues, and self-limiting characteristic)

- Use play therapy to assist the child with working through feelings
- Investigate family communication patterns, strengths, and coping abilities
- Encourage parents to foster security by removing anxiety associated with toileting
- Encourage parents to demonstrate love and acceptance at home to counteract peer ridicule
- Refer for family therapy, as appropriate

2nd edition 1996; revised 2018

Background Evidence:

American Academy of Pediatrics. (2015). *Soiling (encopresis)*. http://www.healthychildren.org/English/health-issues/conditions/emotional-problems/Pages/Soiling-Encopresis.aspx

Coughlin, E. C. (2003). Assessment and management of pediatric constipation in primary care. *Pediatric Nursing, 29*(4), 296–301.

Hockenberry, M. J., & Wilson, D. (2011). *Wong's nursing care of infants and children* (pp. 722–723) (9th ed.). Elsevier Mosby.

Montgomery, D. F., & Navarro, F. (2008). Management of constipation and encopresis in children. *Journal of Pediatric Health Care, 22*(3), 199–204.

Bowel Management   0430

Definition: Establishment and maintenance of a regular pattern of bowel elimination

Activities:

- Review health history including diagnoses, surgeries, and bowel habits
- Identify factors that affect bowel habits (e.g., medications, exercise, sleep, stress, smoking, diet)
- Note pre-existing bowel problems, bowel routine, and use of laxatives and enemas
- Monitor bowel movements including date, frequency, consistency, volume, shape, and color, as appropriate

- Monitor for signs and symptoms of diarrhea, constipation, and impaction (e.g., quality of bowel sounds, frequency and consistency of stools)
- Evaluate medication profile for gastrointestinal side effects
- Evaluate for fecal incontinence, as necessary
- Instruct about specific foods that are assistive in promoting bowel regularity
- Consult dietitian as needed
- Instruct to record frequency, consistency, volume, shape, and color of stools

B

- Use rectal suppository, enema, or digital rectal dilatation as appropriate
- Initiate individualized bowel training program, as appropriate
- Instruct on principles of bowel training
- Initiate uninterrupted, consistent scheduled time for defecation
- Ensure privacy
- Modify bowel program, as needed
- Instruct on health bowel habits (e.g., avoid straining, proper positioning on toilet)
- Use biofeedback, as prescribed
- Encourage decreased gas-forming food intake, as appropriate
- Instruct on foods high in fiber, as appropriate
- Give warm liquids after meals, as appropriate
- Use teach-back to ensure understanding

1st edition 1992; revised 2000, 2024

Background Evidence:

Beierwaltes, P., Church, P., Gordon, T., Ambartsumyan, L., Brei, T., Castillo, H., & Castillo, J. (2020). Bowel function and care: Guidelines for the care of people with spina bifida. *Journal of Pediatric Rehabilitation Medicine, 13*(4), 491–498. https://doi.org/10.3233/PRM-200724

Craven, R. F., Hirnle, C. J., & Henshaw, C. J. (2021). *Fundamentals of nursing: Human health and function* (8th ed.). Wolters-Kluwer.

Dietz, N., Sarpong, K., Ugiliweneza, B., Wang, D., Aslan, S. S., Castillo, C., Boakye, M., & Herrity, A. N. (2021). Longitudinal trends and prevalence of bowel management in individuals with spinal cord injury. *Topics in Spinal Cord Injury Rehabilitation, 27*(4), 53–67. https://doi.org/10.46292/sci21-00008

Patton, V. (2021). Nurse-initiated bowel management strategies for first-line management of faecal incontinence. *Journal of Stomal Therapy Australia, 41*. (4), 14–17. https://doi.org/10.33235/jsta.41.4.14–17

Potter, P. A., Perry, A. G., Stockert, P. A. & Hall, A. M. (2021). *Fundamentals of Nursing* (10th ed.). Elsevier.

Williams, P. (2020). *Basic geriatric nursing* (7th ed.). Elsevier.

Breast Examination 6522

Definition: Inspection and palpation of the breasts and related areas

Activities:

- Explore possible risk factors for development of breast cancer (e.g., current age, age at first pregnancy, age at menarche, age at menopause, family history, history of breast disease, parity status, history of breastfeeding)
- Determine if pain, lump, thickening, or tenderness; discharge, distortion, retraction, or scaling of nipple is present
- Assist to positions of comfort as examination proceeds, allowing privacy and sensitivity
- Explain each specific step of examination
- Conduct examination in upright then supine position
- Instruct to remove gown or chest covering
- Inspect breasts for size, shape, changes in skin texture or color, including any redness, dimpling, puckering, scaling, or retraction of skin
- Note symmetry and contour of breasts and position of nipples bilaterally, for deviation or abnormality
- Instruct to utilize four different positions for visual inspection (e.g., arms at side, hands at waist and push inward toward hips, hands behind the head, and arms across waist with chest falling forward)
- Check for nipple discharge by gently squeezing each nipple
- Inspect and palpate lymph node chains, including supraclavicular, infraclavicular, lateral, central, subscapular, and anterior nodes, for abnormalities
- Note number, size, location, consistency, and mobility of nodes
- Place small pillow or towel under shoulder blade of breast to be examined, abduct arm on same side of breast, and place person's hand behind her head
- Using systematic approach, palpate breast tissue with palmar surface of first three fingers of examiner's dominant hand
- Move in rotary fashion and compress breast tissue against chest wall
- Examine all four quadrants of breast, including axillary tail
- Check for masses, including location, shape, size (in cm), tenderness, mobility, and consistency
- Observe mastectomy scar site for presence of rash, edema, thickening, or erythema, as appropriate
- Repeat same process with other breast
- Document all findings
- Report abnormalities to health care provider or nurse, as appropriate
- Encourage to demonstrate self-palpation during and after clinical breast examination
- Instruct about importance of regular breast self-examination, need to be familiar with how own breasts normally look and feel, and report any changes to health care provider
- Advise regular mammograms as appropriate for age, condition, history, ethnicity, race, diet, activity, and presence of risk factors

3rd edition 2000; revised 2024

Background Evidence:

Cadet, M. J. (2019). Comparing the various breast cancer screening guidelines. *Journal for Nurse Practitioners, 15*(8), 574–578.

Fenske, C., Watkins, K. D., Saunders, T., D'Amico, D. T., & Barbarito, C. (2019). *Health & Physical Assessment in Nursing* (4th ed.). Pearson.

Li, C., Liu, Y., Xue, D., & Chan, C. (2020). Effects of nurse-led interventions on early detection of cancer: A systematic review and meta-analysis. *International Journal of Nursing Studies, 110*, 103684.

Muhrer, J. C. (2017). Improving breast cancer screening in a federally qualified health center with a team of nursing leaders. *Nurse Practitioner, 42*(1), 12–16.

Schub, T., Holle, M. N., & Pravikoff, D. (2018, December 7). Breast cancer screening: Women at high risk. *CINAHL Nursing Guide: Evidence Based Care Sheet*

Weston, C., Akinlotan, M., Lichorad, A., McClellan, D., Helduser, J., Ojinnaka, C., Holland, B., & Bolin, J. N. (2018). The impact of interprofessional education on family nurse practitioner students' and family medicine residents' knowledge and confidence in screening for breast and cervical cancer. *Journal of the American Association of Nurse Practitioners, 30*(9), 511–518.

Calming Technique   5880

Definition: Reducing anxiety in a patient experiencing acute distress

Activities:
- Maintain calm, deliberate manner
- Maintain eye contact with patient
- Reduce or eliminate stimuli creating fear or anxiety
- Stay with patient
- Reassure patient of personal safety or security
- Identify significant others whose presence can assist patient
- Hold and comfort an infant or child
- Rock an infant, as appropriate
- Speak softly or sing to an infant or child
- Offer pacifier to infant, as appropriate
- Instruct patient on techniques to use to calm an infant (e.g., speak to infant, hand on belly, restraining arms, picking up, and holding and rocking)
- Provide time and space to be alone, as appropriate
- Sit and talk with patient
- Facilitate the patient's expression of anger in a constructive manner
- Rub forehead, as appropriate
- Offer warm fluids or milk
- Offer back rub, as appropriate
- Offer warm bath or shower
- Instruct patient on methods to decrease anxiety (e.g., slow breathing techniques, distraction, visualization, meditation, progressive muscle relaxation, listening to soothing music), as appropriate
- Provide antianxiety medications, as needed

1st edition 1992; revised 2013

Background Evidence:

Badger, J. M. (1994). Calming the anxious patient. *American Journal of Nursing, 94*(5), 46–50.

Hopkins, G. (2005). Calming presence. *Community Care, 1596*, 42–43.

Kneisl, C. R., Wilson, H. S., & Trigoboff, E. (2004). *Contemporary psychiatric-mental health nursing.* Prentice Hall.

Miller, T. (2003). Treating anxiety: A calming influence. *Healthcare Traveler, 11*(5), 42–47.

Stuart, G. W. (Ed.). (2009). Anxiety responses and anxiety disorders. In *Principles and practice of psychiatric nursing* (9th ed., pp. 218–240). Mosby Elsevier.

Ward, S.L., & Hisley, S.M. (2009). *Maternal-child nursing care: Optimizing outcomes for mothers, children, & families.* F.A. Davis.

Capillary Blood Sample   4035

Definition: Obtaining an arteriovenous sample from a peripheral body site, such as the heel, finger, or other transcutaneous site

Activities:
- Verify correct identification
- Minimize anxiety using age-appropriate procedures
- Maintain standard precautions
- Select puncture site (e.g., outer lower aspect of heel, sides of distal phalanges of fingers or toes, alternative sites such as forearm)
- Offer pain relief measure before venipuncture or capillary heel-pricks
- Warm site for approximately 5 minutes if arterialized sample, per agency protocol
- Use aseptic technique during skin puncture, per agency protocol
- Select length of lancet according to age (e.g., 0.85 mm for infants or young child, 2.2 mm for older child or adults)
- Puncture outer aspect of heel no deeper than 1.5 mm for child over 6 months but below 8 years, and up to 2.4 mm for child over 8 years
- Puncture skin with one quick, continuous, and deliberate stroke, with lancet or approved penetration device, per manufacturer's specifications
- Wipe off first drop of blood with dry gauze
- Collect blood in manner appropriate to test being performed (e.g., allow drop of blood to fall onto manufacturer's specified area of filter paper or test strips, draw blood into tubes by capillary action as droplets form)
- Apply intermittent pressure as far away from puncture site as possible to promote blood flow
- Avoid hemolysis caused by excessive squeezing or "milking" of puncture site
- Follow manufacturer's guidelines regarding timing on tests and preservation of blood sample (e.g., sealing blood tubes), as necessary
- Label specimen per agency protocol
- Send specimen to laboratory, as necessary
- Bandage site, as necessary
- Instruct and monitor for self-sampling capillary blood, as appropriate
- Dispose of equipment properly
- Document completion of capillary blood sampling

4th edition 2004; revised 2024

Background Evidence:

Glasgow-Roberts, N. (2021). Best practices in capillary blood collection. *MLO: Medical Laboratory Observer, 53*(2), 36–38.

Merter, O. S., & Bolişik, Z. B. (2021). The effects of manual and automatic lancets on neonatal capillary heel blood sampling pain: A prospective randomized controlled trial. *Journal of Pediatric Nursing, 58*, e8–e12.

Serafin, A., Malinowski, M., & Prażmowska-Wilanowska, A. (2020). Blood volume and pain perception during finger prick capillary blood sampling: Are all safety lancets equal? *Postgraduate Medicine, 132*(3), 288–295.

Wong, D. L., Perry, S. E., & Hockenberry, M. J. (2018). *Maternal child nursing care* (6th ed.). Mosby.

Yassin, D. F., & Al-Abbadi, M. A. (2017). Benefits of an instrument-compatible capillary blood collection microtube. *MLO: Medical Laboratory Observer, 49*(11), 50–52.

C

C

Cardiac Care 4040

Definition: Limitation of complications resulting from an imbalance between myocardial oxygen supply and demand for a patient with symptoms of impaired cardiac function

Activities:

- Monitor patient physically and psychologically per agency policy
- Ensure activity level that does not compromise cardiac output or provoke cardiac events
- Encourage gradual increase in activity when condition stabilized (i.e., encourage slower paced activities or shorter periods of activity with frequent rest periods after exercise)
- Instruct the patient on the importance of immediately reporting any chest discomfort
- Evaluate any episodes of chest pain (e.g., intensity, location, radiation, duration, and precipitating and alleviating factors)
- Monitor ECG for ST segment changes, as appropriate
- Perform a comprehensive appraisal of peripheral circulation (i.e., check peripheral pulses, edema, capillary refill, color, and temperature of extremity) per agency policy
- Monitor vital signs frequently
- Monitor cardiovascular status
- Monitor for cardiac dysrhythmias, including disturbances of both rhythm and conduction
- Document cardiac dysrhythmias
- Note signs and symptoms of decreased cardiac output
- Monitor respiratory status for symptoms of heart failure
- Monitor abdomen for indications of decreased perfusion
- Monitor fluid balance (e.g., intake/output and daily weight)
- Monitor appropriate laboratory values (e.g., cardiac enzymes, electrolyte levels)
- Monitor pacemaker functioning, if appropriate
- Evaluate blood pressure alterations
- Evaluate the patient's response to ectopy or dysrhythmias
- Provide antiarrhythmic therapy according to unit policy (e.g., antiarrhythmic medication, cardioversion, or defibrillation), as appropriate
- Monitor patient's response to antiarrhythmic medications
- Instruct the patient and family on treatment modalities, activity restriction and progression
- Arrange exercise and rest periods to avoid fatigue
- Restrict smoking
- Monitor the patient's activity tolerance
- Monitor for dyspnea, fatigue, tachypnea, and orthopnea
- Establish a supportive relationship with the patient and family
- Identify the patient's methods of handling stress
- Promote effective techniques for reducing stress
- Perform relaxation therapy, if appropriate
- Recognize psychological effects of underlying condition
- Screen patients for anxiety and depression, encouraging treatment with suitable antidepressants, as indicated
- Encourage noncompetitive activities for patients at risk for impaired cardiac function
- Discuss modifications in sexual activity with patient and significant other, if appropriate
- Instruct patient and family on the aims of care and how progress will be measured
- Ensure that all staff are aware of these goals and are working together to provide consistent care
- Refer to heart failure program or cardiac rehabilitation program for education, evaluation, and guided support to increase activity and rebuild life, as appropriate
- Offer spiritual support to the patient and family (e.g., contact a member of the clergy), as appropriate

1st edition 1992; revised 2000, 2013

Background Evidence:

American Association of Critical-Care Nurses. (2006). In J. G. Alspach (Ed.), *Core curriculum for critical care nursing* (6th ed.). Saunders Elsevier.

Chummun, H., Gopaul, K., & Lutchman, A. (2009). Current guidance on the management of acute coronary syndrome. *British Journal of Nursing*, *18*(21), 1292–1298.

Clancy, J., McVicar, A., & Hubbard, J. (2011). Homeostasis 4: Nurses as agents of control in myocardial infarction. *British Journal of Nursing*, *20*(6), 373–378.

LeMone, P., Burke, K., & Bauldoff, G. (2011). Nursing care of patient with coronary heart disease. In *Medical-surgical nursing: Critical thinking in patient care*, (pp. 908–969) (5th ed.). Pearson.

Marshall, K. (2011). Acute coronary syndrome: Diagnosis, risk assessment, and management. *Nursing Standard*, *25*(23), 47–57.

Smith, S., Jr., Allen, J., Blair, S., Bonow, R., Brass, L., Fonarow, G., Grundy, S. M., Hiratzuka, L., Jones, D., Krumholtz, H. M., Mosca, L., Pasternak, R. C., Person, T., Pfeffer, M. A., & Taubert, K. A. (2006). AHA/ACC guidelines for secondary prevention for patients with coronary and other atherosclerotic vascular disease: 2006 Update. *Circulation*, *113*(19), 2363–2372.

Thomas, S. A., Chapa, D. W., Friedmann, E., Durden, C., Ross, A., Lee, M. C., & Lee, H. (2008). Depression in patients with heart failure: Prevalence, pathophysiological mechanisms, and treatment. *Critical Care Nurse*, *28*(2), 40–55.

Cardiac Care: Acute 4044

Definition: Limitation of complications for a patient recently experiencing an episode of an imbalance between myocardial oxygen supply and demand resulting in impaired cardiac function

Activities:

- Evaluate chest pain (e.g., intensity, location, radiation, duration, and precipitating and alleviating factors)
- Instruct the patient on the importance of immediately reporting any chest discomfort
- Provide immediate and continuous means to summon nurse and let the patient and family know calls will be answered immediately
- Monitor ECG for ST segment changes, as appropriate
- Perform a comprehensive appraisal of cardiac status including peripheral circulation

- Monitor cardiac rhythm and rate
- Auscultate heart sounds
- Recognize the frustration and fright caused by inability to communicate and exposure to strange machinery and environment
- Auscultate lungs for crackles or other adventitious sounds
- Monitor the effectiveness of oxygen therapy, if appropriate
- Monitor determinants of oxygen delivery (e.g., PaO_2 and hemoglobin levels and cardiac output), if appropriate
- Monitor neurological status
- Monitor intake and output, urine output, and daily weight, as appropriate
- Select best EKG lead for continuous monitoring, as appropriate
- Obtain 12-lead EKG, as appropriate
- Draw serum, CK, LDH, and AST levels, as appropriate
- Monitor renal function (e.g., BUN and Cr levels), as appropriate
- Monitor liver function tests, if appropriate
- Monitor laboratory values for electrolytes that may increase the risk of dysrhythmias (e.g., serum potassium and magnesium), as appropriate
- Obtain chest x-ray, as appropriate
- Monitor trends in blood pressure and hemodynamic parameters, if available (e.g., central venous pressure and pulmonary capillary or artery wedge pressure)
- Provide small, frequent meals
- Provide appropriate cardiac diet (i.e., limit intake of caffeine, sodium, cholesterol, and food high in fat)
- Refrain from giving oral stimulants
- Substitute artificial salt, if appropriate
- Limit environmental stimuli
- Maintain an environment conducive to rest and healing
- Avoid causing intense emotional situations
- Identify the patient's methods of handling stress
- Promote effective techniques for reducing stress
- Perform relaxation therapy, if appropriate
- Refrain from arguing
- Discourage decision making when the patient is under severe stress
- Avoid overheating or chilling the patient
- Refrain from inserting a rectal tube
- Refrain from taking rectal temperatures
- Refrain from doing a rectal or vaginal examination
- Delay bathing, if appropriate
- Instruct the patient to avoid activities that result in the Valsalva maneuver (e.g., straining during bowel movement)
- Administer medications that will prevent episodes of the Valsalva maneuver (e.g., stool softeners, antiemetics), as appropriate

- Prevent peripheral thrombus formation (i.e., turn every 2 hours and administer low-dose anticoagulants)
- Administer medications to relieve or prevent pain and ischemia, as needed
- Monitor effectiveness of medication
- Instruct patient and family on the aims of care and how progress will be measured
- Ensure that all staff are aware of these goals and are working together to provide consistent care
- Offer spiritual support to the patient and family (e.g., contact a member of the clergy), as appropriate

1st edition 1992; revised 2000, 2013

Background Evidence:

American Association of Critical-Care Nurses. (2006). In J. G. Alspach (Ed.), *Core curriculum for critical care nursing* (6th ed.). Saunders Elsevier.

Chummun, H., Gopaul, K., & Lutchman, A. (2009). Current guidance on the management of acute coronary syndrome. *British Journal of Nursing, 18*(21), 1292–1298.

Clancy, J., McVicar, A., & Hubbard, J. (2011). Homeostasis 4: Nurses as agents of control in myocardial infarction. *British Journal of Nursing, 20*(6), 373–378.

Kushner, F., Hand, M., Smith, S., King, S., Jr., Anderson, J., III., Antman, E., Bailey, S. R., Bates, E. R., Blankenship, J. C., Casey, D. E., Green, L. A., Hochman, J. S., Jacobs, A. K., Krumholz, H. M., Morrison, D. A., Ornato, J. P., Pearles, D. L., Peterson, E. D., Sloan, M. A., Whitlow, P. L., & Williams, D. O. (2009). 2009 focused updates: ACC/AHA guidelines for the management of patients with ST-elevation myocardial infarction (updating the 2004 guideline and 2007 focused update) and ACC/AHA/SCAI guidelines on percutaneous coronary intervention (updating the 2005 guideline and 2007 focused update). *Journal of the American College of Cardiology, 54*(23), 2205–2241.

LeMone, P., Burke, K., & Bauldoff, G. (2011). Nursing care of patient with coronary heart disease. In *Medical-surgical nursing: Critical thinking in patient care,* (pp. 908–969) (5th ed.). Pearson.

Marshall, K. (2011). Acute coronary syndrome: Diagnosis, risk assessment, and management. *Nursing Standard, 25*(23), 47–57.

Wright, R., Anderson, J., Adams, C., Bridges, C., Casey, D., Jr., Ettinger, S., Fesmire, F. M., Ganias, T. G., Jneld, H., Lincoff, A. M., Peterson, E. D., Phillipides, G. J., Theroux, P., Wenger, N. K., & Zidar, J. P. (2011). 2011 ACCF/AHA focused update of the guidelines for the management of patients with unstable angina/non–ST-elevation myocardial infarction (updating the 2007 guideline). *Journal of the American College of Cardiology, 57*(19), 1920–1959.

Cardiac Care: Rehabilitative   4046

Definition: Promotion of maximum functional activity level for a patient who has experienced an episode of impaired cardiac function that resulted from an imbalance between myocardial oxygen supply and demand

Activities:

- Monitor the patient's activity tolerance
- Maintain ambulation schedule, as tolerated
- Encourage realistic expectations for the patient and family
- Instruct the patient and family on appropriate prescribed and over-the-counter medications
- Instruct the patient and family on cardiac risk factor modification (e.g., smoking cessation, diet, and exercise), as appropriate

- Instruct the patient on self-care of chest pain (i.e., take sublingual nitroglycerine every 5 minutes three times; if chest pain is unrelieved, seek emergency medical care)
- Instruct the patient and family on the exercise regimen, including warm up, endurance, and cool down, as appropriate
- Instruct the patient and family on any lifting/pushing weight limitations, if appropriate

- Instruct the patient and family on any special considerations with activities of daily living (e.g., isolate activities and allow rest periods), if appropriate
- Instruct the patient and family on wound care and precautions (e.g., sternal incision or catheterization site), if appropriate
- Instruct the patient and family on follow-up care
- Coordinate patient referrals (e.g., dietary, social services, and physical therapy)
- Instruct the patient and family on access of emergency services available in their community, as appropriate
- Screen patient for anxiety and depression, as appropriate

1st edition 1992; revised 2000, 2013

Background Evidence:

LeMone, P., Burke, K., & Bauldoff, G. (2011). Nursing care of patient with coronary heart disease. In *Medical-surgical nursing: Critical thinking in patient care,* (pp. 908–969) (5th ed.). Pearson.

Nazarko, L. (2008). Cardiology: Cardiac rehabilitation. *Nursing & Residential Care, 10*(9), 439–442.

Smith, S., Jr., Allen, J., Blair, S., Bonow, R., Brass, L., Fonarow, G., Grundy, S. M., Hiratzuka, L., Jones, D., Krumholtz, H. M., Mosca, L., Pasternak, R. C., Person, T., Pfeffer, M. A., & Taubert, K. A. (2006). AHA/ACC guidelines for secondary prevention for patients with coronary and other atherosclerotic vascular disease: 2006 Update. *Circulation, 113*(19), 2363–2372.

Thomas, S., Chapa, D., Friedmann, E., Durden, C., Ross, A., Lee, M., & Lee, H. (2008). Depression in patients with heart failure: Prevalence, pathophysiological mechanisms, and treatment. *Critical Care Nurse, 28*(2), 40–55.

Cardiac Risk Management   4050

Definition: Prevention of an acute episode of impaired cardiac function by minimizing contributing events and risk behaviors

Activities:

- Screen patient for risk behaviors associated with adverse cardiac events (e.g., smoking, obesity, sedentary lifestyle, high blood pressure, history of previous cardiac events, family history of cardiac events)
- Identify patient's readiness to learn lifestyle modification (e.g., diet, smoking, alcohol intake, exercise, and cholesterol levels)
- Instruct patient and family on signs and symptoms of early cardiac disease and worsening cardiac disease, as appropriate
- Instruct patient and family on cardiac risk factor modification, as appropriate
- Prioritize areas for risk reduction in collaboration with patient and family
- Instruct patient and family to monitor blood pressure and heart rate routinely and with exercise, as appropriate
- Encourage exercise, as indicated by patient cardiac risk factor
- Instruct the patient on regular and progressive exercise, as appropriate
- Encourage 30 minutes of exercise daily, as appropriate
- Instruct patient on need to achieve exercise goals in incremental periods of 10 minutes multiple times daily, if intolerant to sustained 30-minute activities
- Instruct patient and family on symptoms of cardiac compromise indicating need for rest
- Instruct patient and family on strategies for restricting or eliminating smoking
- Instruct patient and family on strategies for a heart healthy diet (e.g., low sodium, low fat, low cholesterol, high fiber, adequate fluid, appropriate caloric intake)
- Encourage patient to keep caloric intake at a level that achieves desired weight
- Instruct patient and family on therapies to reduce cardiac risk (e.g., medication therapies, blood pressure monitoring, fluid restrictions, alcohol restrictions, cardiac rehabilitation)
- Provide both verbal and written information to patient, family, and caregivers for all pertinent cares, as indicated
- Focus care and treatment goals to enable the patient to maintain weight control, to remain a nonsmoker, and to remain as active as possible
- Refer to heart failure program or cardiac rehabilitation program for lifestyle changes, as appropriate
- Alleviate patient's anxieties by providing accurate information and correcting any misconceptions
- Screen patient for anxiety and depression, as appropriate
- Identify the patient's methods of handling stress
- Promote effective techniques for reducing stress
- Perform relaxation therapy, if appropriate
- Monitor patient's progress at regular intervals

1st edition 1992; revised 2013

Background Evidence:

American Association of Critical-Care Nurses. (2006). In J. G. Alspach (Ed.), *Core curriculum for critical care nursing* (6th ed.). Saunders Elsevier.

Chummun, H., Gopaul, K., & Lutchman, A. (2009). Current guidance on the management of acute coronary syndrome. *British Journal of Nursing, 18*(21), 1292–1298.

Greenland, P., Alpert, J., Beller, G., Benjamin, E., Budoff, M., Fayad, Z., Foster, E., Hlatky, M. A., Hodgson, J. M., Kushner, F. G., Lauer, M. S., Shaw, L. J., Smith, S. C., Jr., Taylor, A. J., Weintraub, W. S., & Wenger, N. K. (2010). 2010 ACCF/AHA guideline for assessment of cardiovascular risk in asymptomatic adults: A report of the American College of Cardiology Foundation/American Heart Association Task Force on Practice Guidelines. *Journal of the American College of Cardiology, 56*(25), e50–e103.

LeMone, P., Burke, K., & Bauldoff, G. (2011). Nursing care of patient with coronary heart disease. In *Medical-surgical nursing: Critical thinking in patient care,* (pp. 908–969) (5th ed.). Pearson.

Nazarko, L. (2008). Cardiology: Cardiac rehabilitation. *Nursing & Residential Care, 10*(9), 439–442.

Smith, S., Jr., Allen, J., Blair, S., Bonow, R., Brass, L., Fonarow, G., Grundy, S. M., Hiratzuka, L., Jones, D., Krumholtz, H. M., Mosca, L., Pasternak, R. C., Person, T., Pfeffer, M. A., & Taubert, K. A. (2006). AHA/ACC guidelines for secondary prevention for patients with coronary and other atherosclerotic vascular disease: 2006 Update. *Circulation, 113*(19), 2363–2372.

Thomas, S., Chapa, D., Friedmann, E., Durden, C., Ross, A., Lee, M. C., & Lee, H. (2008). Depression in patients with heart failure: Prevalence, pathophysiological mechanisms, and treatment. *Critical Care Nurse, 28*(2), 40–55.

Caregiver Support   7040

Definition: Provision of necessary information, advocacy, and support to facilitate care by someone other than a health care professional

Activities:
- Determine caregiver's acceptance of role
- Determine amount of assistance needed
- Determine level of knowledge, capability, and limitations
- Accept expressions of negative emotions
- Acknowledge difficulties of caregiving role
- Make positive statements about caregiver's efforts
- Provide support for decisions made by caregiver
- Monitor interactions related to care
- Provide information about condition, treatment, and care in accordance with care recipient preferences
- Monitor stress and encourage coping strategies
- Instruct on stress management techniques and health care maintenance strategies
- Support caregiver in setting limits and taking care of self
- Educate about grieving process
- Support through grieving process
- Encourage participation in support groups, social networking, community, and online resources
- Encourage respite care as needed
- Offer to provide care for short periods, if experiencing difficulties or increased stress

1st edition 1992; revised 2004, 2024

Background Evidence:
Adashek, J. J., & Subbiah, I. M. (2020). Caring for the caregiver: A systematic review characterizing the experience of caregivers of older adults with advanced cancers. *ESMO open, 5*(5), e000862.

Bruening, R., Sperber, N., Miller, K., Andrews, S., Steinhauser, K., Wieland, G. D., Lindquist, J., Shepherd-Banigan, M., Ramos, K., Henius, J., Kabat, M., & Van Houtven, C. (2020). Connecting caregivers to support: Lessons learned from the VA Caregiver Support Program. *Journal of Applied Gerontology: The Official Journal of the Southern Gerontological Society, 39*(4), 368–376.

Egan, K. J., Pinto-Bruno, Á. C., Bighelli, I., Berg-Weger, M., van Straten, A., Albanese, E., & Pot, A. M. (2018). Online training and support programs designed to improve mental health and reduce burden among caregivers of people with dementia: A systematic review. *Journal of the American Medical Directors Association, 19*(3), 200–206.e1.

Parmar, J., Anderson, S., Duggleby, W., Holroyd, L. J., Pollard, C., & Brémault, P. S. (2021). Developing person-centered care competencies for the healthcare workforce to support family caregivers: Caregiver centered care. *Health & Social Care in the Community, 29*(5), 1327–1338.

Zebrak, K. A., & Campione, J. R. (2021). The effect of National Family Caregiver Support Program services on caregiver burden. *Journal of Applied Gerontology, 40*(9), 963–971.

Caring Interaction Development   5000

Definition: Establishing a helping relationship based on compassionate interaction, communication, respect for ethical values, acceptance, and empathy

Activities:
- Identify attitude and personal feelings toward person and situation
- Determine ethical boundaries of relationship
- Provide for physical comfort before interactions
- Provide privacy and confidentiality
- Create climate of warmth, caring, and unconditional acceptance
- Convey interest in concerns
- Use self-disclosure, as appropriate
- Discuss responsibilities in relationship and set limits of acceptable behavior, as appropriate
- Establish mutually acceptable agreement on time and length of meetings, as appropriate
- Build relationship of equality
- Return at established time to demonstrate trustworthiness and interest
- Establish open body posture, physical distance, and appropriate nonverbal expressions
- Monitor person's nonverbal communication
- Respond to nonverbal messages, as appropriate
- Identify readiness to explore identified problems and develop strategies for change
- Reflect main ideas and return conversation to main subject, as needed
- Encourage introspection and behavioral change
- Encourage to take time needed to express self
- Assist to identify feelings that impede ability to interact with others (e.g., anger, anxiety, hostility, sadness)
- Develop alternative ways of communicating (e.g., images, other words), as needed
- Listen actively to concerns and discussions
- Assist to identify areas of need to be addressed during meetings
- Convey recognition of accomplishments during relationship
- Support efforts to interact with others in positive manner
- Facilitate attempts to review therapeutic relationship experiences
- Summarize conversation at end of discussion
- Use summary as starting point for future conversations
- Establish time of next interaction before ending meeting each time
- Prepare for termination of relationship, as appropriate

2nd edition 1996; revised 2004, 2008, 2024

Background Evidence:
Allande, R. (2019). *Construcción y validación de una escala de evaluación del nivel de competencia en la interacción de cuidado para estudiantes de Grado en Enfermería [Development and validation of a scale to assess the level of caring interaction competence of nursing students]* [Doctoral Dissertation, University of Seville].

Allande-Cussó, R., Fernández-Garcia, E., & Porcel-Gálvez, A. M. (2021). Defining and characterizing the nurse–patient relationship: A concept analysis. *Nursing Ethics, 29*(2), 462–484. https://doi.org/10.1177/09697330211046651

Allande-Cussó, R., Gómez-Salgado, J., Fenández-García, E., & Porcel-Gálvez, A. M. (2022). Understanding the nurse-patient relationship: A predictive approach to caring interaction. *Collegian, 29*(5), 663–670. https://doi.org/10.1016/j.colegn.2022.04.003

Allande-Cussó, R., Gómez-Salgado, J., Macías-Seda, J., & Porcel-Gálvez, A. M. (2021). Assessment of the nurse-patient interaction competence in undergraduate nursing students. *Nurse Education Today, 96*, 104627. https://doi.org/10.1016/j.nedt.2020.104627

Allande-Cussó, R., Macías Seda, J., & Porcel Gálvez, A. M. (2020). La relación enfermera-paciente: identidad histórica, metodológica y terapéutica en los cuidados de enfermería [The nurse-patient relationship: Historical, methodological and therapeutic identity in nursing cares]. *Cultura De Los Cuidados*, (55), 78–84. http://ciberindex.com/c/cc/55078cc

Allande-Cussó, R., Siles, J., Ayuso, D., & Gómez, J. (2020). A new conceptualization of the nurse–patient relationship construct as caring interaction. *Nursing Philosophy. 22*(2), e12335. https://doi.org/10.1111/nup.12335

Egan, G., & Reese, R. J. (2019). *The skilled helper: A problem-management and opportunity-management approach to helping.* Cengage.

Salehian, M., Heydari, A., Aghebati, N., & Karimi Moonaghi, H. (2017). Faculty-student caring interaction in nursing education: An integrative review. *Journal of Caring Sciences, 6*(3), 257–267. https://doi.org/10.15171/jcs.2017.025

Case Management   7320

Definition: Advocating, planning, implementing, monitoring, and evaluating care for persons and families within and across settings

Activities:

- Identify individuals or populations who would benefit from case management (e.g., high cost, high volume, high risk)
- Explain case manager role
- Explain cost of service before providing care
- Identify payment source for case management service
- Obtain permission to be enrolled in case management program, as indicated
- Develop relationships with person, family, and other health care providers, as needed
- Use effective communication skills
- Treat with dignity and respect
- Maintain privacy and confidentiality
- Evaluate physical health status, mental status, functional capability, formal and informal support systems, financial resources, and home environment, as needed
- Individualize treatment plan and intended outcomes with input from person and family
- Explain plan of care to person and family
- Validate desired outcomes with person and family
- Discuss plan of care and intended outcomes with health care provider
- Integrate care management information and revised interventions into handoff report and group practice meetings, as needed
- Evaluate progress toward established goals
- Revise interventions and goals to meet needs, as necessary
- Coordinate provision of needed resources or services
- Coordinate care with other pertinent health care providers (e.g., primary care providers, nurses, advanced practice nurses, physicians, social workers, pharmacists, physical therapists, third-party payers)
- Educate on importance of self-care
- Encourage appropriate decision-making activities
- Document all case management activities
- Monitor plan of care for quality, quantity, timeliness, and effectiveness of services
- Assist with access to health care delivery system
- Guide through health care delivery system
- Assist in making informed decisions regarding health care
- Advocate as necessary
- Include clinical and financial concerns in decision-making
- Notify of change in service, termination of service, or discharge from case management program
- Promote efficient use of resources
- Monitor cost effectiveness of care
- Modify care to reduce cost, as indicated
- Establish quality improvement program to evaluate case management activities
- Document cost effectiveness of case management
- Report outcomes to insurers and other third-party payers
- Market case management services to individuals, families, insurers, and employers

3rd edition 2000; revised 2024

Background Evidence:

Joo, J. Y., & Liu, M. F. (2017). Case management effectiveness in reducing hospital use: a systematic review. *International Nursing Review, 64*(2), 296–308.

Joo, J. Y., & Liu, M. F. (2018). Experiences of case management with chronic illnesses: a qualitative systematic review. *International Nursing Review, 65*(1), 102–113.

Joo, J. Y., & Liu, M. F. (2019). Effectiveness of Nurse-Led Case Management in Cancer Care: Systematic Review. *Clinical Nursing Research, 28*(8), 968–991.

Joo, J. Y., & Huber, D. L. (2019). Case management effectiveness on health care utilization outcomes: A systematic review of reviews. *Western Journal of Nursing Research, 41*(1), 111–133.

Powell, S. K., & Tahan, H. M. (2019). *Case management: A practical guide for education and practice.* (4th ed.). Wolters Kluwer.

Tahan, H. M., & Treiger, T. M. (2017). CMSA Core curriculum for case management (3rd ed.). Wolters Kluwer.

Cast Care: Maintenance   0762

Definition: Care of a cast after the drying period

Activities:

- Monitor for signs of infection (foul-smelling cast, erythema, fever)
- Monitor for signs of cast impairment of circulation or neurological function (e.g., pain, pallor, pulselessness, paresthesias, paralysis, and pressure) on affected extremity
- Monitor circulation and neurological function of tissues above and below cast
- Address compromised circulation and pain symptoms immediately (e.g., reposition cast, perform ROM to extremity, immediate cast pressure-relieving action)
- Inspect cast for signs of drainage from wounds under the cast
- Mark the circumference of any drainage as a gauge for future assessments
- Protect the cast if close to groin
- Instruct patient not to scratch skin under the cast with any objects
- Offer alternatives to scratching (e.g., cold air from a hair dryer)
- Avoid getting a plaster cast wet (e.g., use appropriate protection for bathing or toileting, protective socks or gloves)
- Position cast on pillows to lessen strain on other body parts with cast heel off pillow

- Apply ice for first 24 to 36 hours to reduce swelling or inflammation
- Elevate casted extremity at or higher than heart level to reduce swelling or inflammation
- Check for cracking or breaks in the cast
- Apply an arm sling for support, if appropriate
- Pad rough cast edges and traction connections
- Teach patient and family care of cast
- Document cast care instructions given to patient and family
- Document observations of patient ability to perform cast care

1st edition 1992; revised 2008

Background Evidence:

McCance, K. L., & Huether, S. E. (2006). *Pathophysiology: The biologic basis for disease in adults and children* (5th ed.). Mosby.

Perry, A. G., & Potter, P. A. (2006). *Clinical nursing skills and techniques* (6th ed.). Elsevier Mosby.

Potter, P. A., & Perry, A. G. (2005). *Fundamentals of nursing* (6th ed.). Mosby.

Smeltzer, S. C., & Bare, B. G. (2004). *Brunner & Suddarth's textbook of medical-surgical nursing* (10th ed.). Lippincott Williams & Wilkins.

Cast Care: Wet   0764

Definition: Care of a new cast during the drying period

Activities:

- Monitor for signs of cast impairment of circulation or neurological function (e.g., pain, pallor, pulselessness, paresthesias, paralysis, and pressure) on affected extremity
- Monitor circulation and neurological function of tissues above and below cast
- Address compromised circulation and pain symptoms immediately, to avoid permanent damage in neurovascular status (e.g., reposition cast, report unresolved symptoms as needing immediate cast pressure relieving action)
- Support the cast with pillows during the drying period
- Handle the casted extremity with palms only until the cast is dry to avoid causing finger indentations that can lead to pressure sores
- Inform the patient that the cast will feel warm as the cast dries
- Protect cast if close to groin
- Maintain the angles of the cast during the drying period
- Inspect cast for signs of drainage from wounds under the cast
- Mark the circumference of any drainage as a gauge for future assessments
- Explain the need for limited activity as cast dries

- Identify any change in sensation or increased pain at the fracture site
- Apply ice for first 24 to 35 hours to reduce swelling or inflammation, as indicated
- Elevate casted extremity at or higher than heart level to reduce swelling or inflammation, as indicated
- Teach patient and family care of cast
- Document cast care instructions given to patient and family

1st edition 1992; revised 2008

Background Evidence:

Perry, A. G., & Potter, P. A. (2006). *Clinical nursing skills and techniques* (6th ed.). Elsevier Mosby.

Potter, P. A., & Perry, A. G. (2005). *Fundamentals of nursing* (6th ed.). Mosby.

Smeltzer, S. C., & Bare, B. G. (2004). *Brunner & Suddarth's textbook of medical-surgical nursing* (10th ed.). Lippincott Williams & Wilkins.

Smith, S. F., & Duell, D. J. (1992). *Clinical nursing skills: Nursing process model, basics to advanced skills* (3rd ed.). Appleton & Lange.

C

Central Venous Access Management: Central Insertion   4054

Definition: Care of persons with a device inserted into the central circulation via the jugular or subclavian vein

Activities:

- Determine location of catheter
- Determine agency guidelines, protocols, policies, and procedures
- Determine understanding of purpose, care, and maintenance of catheter
- Provide information related to catheter (e.g., indications, functions, type of device to be used, care of device, potential complications, insertion procedure)
- Avoid use until confirmation of tip placement post-implantation with baseline chest x-ray
- Employ strict aseptic technique whenever catheter handled, accessed, or used to administer medications, to reduce potential for central line associated blood stream infections (CLABSIs)
- Adapt care to type of catheter
- Check patency immediately before administering prescribed medications or infusions, per agency protocol
- Employ actions to ensure patency per agency protocol for occluded devices
- Flush lines per agency protocol
- Use smaller gauge silastic catheters to administer medications
- Use self-adhesive anchoring devices, when appropriate or per agency policy
- Change clear fluid administration sets per agency policy
- Record site care and fluid administration
- Avoid catheter insertion near stoma or areas such as diapers where contact with fecal material may occur
- Cleanse site and apply dressing per agency protocol
- Obtain chest x-ray immediately in event of suspected line infiltration, compromise, or migration
- Monitor for arm swelling or increased warmth on side ipsilateral to implanted device
- Monitor for complications (e.g., pneumothorax, cardiac tamponade, arterial puncture, hemorrhage, hemothorax, hydrothorax, air embolus, brachial nerve plexus injury, thoracic duct injury, infection, misplacement)
- Inspect entry site daily for redness, pain, tenderness, warmth, or swelling
- Report signs of inflammation, leakage, or discharge to health care provider
- Remove catheter per agency protocol
- Apply firm pressure and appropriate dressing to puncture site after removing catheter, per agency protocol
- Ensure documentation of manufacturer, model number, serial number, and implant date
- Report adverse signs and symptoms (e.g., tachycardia, hypotension, dyspnea, agitation, independent filling of access needle with fluid or blood, shoulder or back pain, cardiac arrest)
- Instruct to wear medical alert bracelet or necklace that identifies device
- Use teach-back to ensure understanding

6th edition 2013, revised 2024

Background Evidence:

Arvaniti, K. (2017). Preventing central venous line related bloodstream infections in adult ICUs: Start from the basics and bundle. *Intensive & Critical Care Nursing, 43*, 3–5. https://doi.org/10.1016/j.iccn.2017.08.007

Gorski, L. A. (2017). The 2016 Infusion Therapy Standards of Practice. *Home Healthcare Now, 35*(1), 10–18. https://doi.org/10.1097/NHH.0000000000000481

Infusion Nursing Society. (2021). *Policies and procedures for infusion therapy: Acute care* (6th ed.).

Infusion Nursing Society. (2021). Standards of practice (8th ed.).

Jarding, E. K., & Flynn Makic, M. B. (2021). Central line care and management: Adopting evidence-based nursing interventions. *Journal of PeriAnesthesia Nursing, 36*(4), 328–333. https://doi.org/10.1016/j.jopan.2020.10.010

Levett-Jones, T. (2019). Heparin vs. normal saline locking for prevention of catheter occlusion. *AJN American Journal of Nursing, 119*(9), 63. https://doi.org/10.1097/01.NAJ.0000580288.71902.d1

Urden, L. D., Stacy, K. M., & Lough, M. E. (2022). *Critical care nursing: Diagnosis and management* (pp. 502–503) (9th ed.). Elsevier.

Wiegand, D. (2017). *AACN procedural manual for high acuity, progressive, and critical care* (7th ed.). Elsevier.

Central Venous Access Management: Peripheral Insertion   4220

Definition: Care of persons with a device inserted into the central circulation via a peripheral vessel

Activities:

- Identify intended use of catheter to determine type needed (i.e., central or midline catheter)
- Explain purpose, benefits, and risks associated with use
- Obtain consent for insertion procedure
- Select appropriate size and type of catheter to meet needs
- Select most accessible and least used vein available, usually basilic or cephalic vein of dominant arm
- Position supine for insertion with arm at 90-degree angle to body
- Measure circumference of upper arm
- Measure distance for catheter insertion
- Prep site for insertion, according to agency protocol
- Insert catheter, using sterile technique and according to manufacturer's instructions and agency protocol
- Connect extension tubing and aspirate for blood return
- Obtain blood sample if indicated
- Flush with prepared heparin and saline, as appropriate and per agency protocol
- Secure catheter and apply sterile transparent dressing, per agency protocol
- Write date and time on dressing
- Verify catheter tip placement by ultrasound or x-ray examination, as appropriate and per agency protocol
- Avoid use of affected arm for blood pressure measurement and phlebotomy

- Monitor for immediate complications such as bleeding, nerve or tendon damage, cardiac decompression, respiratory distress, or catheter embolism
- Monitor for signs of phlebitis (e.g., pain, redness, warm skin, edema)
- Use sterile technique to change insertion-site dressing, according to agency protocol
- Instruct on dressing change technique, as appropriate
- Flush line after each use with appropriate solution per agency protocol
- Maintain line patency according to agency protocol, as appropriate
- Instruct about line flushes and medication administration techniques, as appropriate
- Remove catheter according to manufacturer's instructions and per agency protocol
- Document reason for removal and condition of catheter tip
- Instruct to report signs of infection (e.g., fever, chills, drainage from insertion site)
- Use teach-back to ensure understanding

1st edition 1992; revised 2004, 2013, 2024

Background Evidence:

DeVries, M., Lee, J., & Hoffman, L. (2019). Infection free midline catheter implementation at a community hospital (2 years). *American Journal of Infection Control, 47*(9), 1118–1121. https://doi.org/10.1016/j.ajic.2019.03.001

Gorski, L. A. (2017). The 2016 Infusion Therapy Standards of Practice. *Home Healthcare Now, 35*(1), 10–18. https://doi.org/10.1097/NHH.0000000000000481

Infusion Nursing Society. (2021). *Policies and procedures for infusion therapy: Acute care* (6th ed.).

Infusion Nursing Society. (2021). Standards of practice (8th ed.).

Nickel, B. (2019). Peripheral intravenous access: Applying infusion therapy standards of practice to improve patient safety. *Critical Care Nurse, 39*(1), 61–71. https://doi.org/10.4037/ccn2019790

Ureden, L. D., Stacy, K. M., & Lough, M. E. (2022). *Critical care nursing: Diagnosis and management* (pp. 502–503) (9th ed.). Elsevier.

Wiegand, D. (2017). *AACN procedural manual for high acuity, progressive, and critical care* (7th ed.). Elsevier.

Zhang, X., Lu, Z., Hu, Y., Xue, M., & Dai, H. (2017). Evidence-based implementation of peripherally inserted central catheters (PICCS) insertion at a vascular access care outpatient clinic. *Worldviews on Evidence-Based Nursing, 14*(2), 163–167. https://doi.org/10.1111/wvn.12203

Cerebral Edema Management　　　　2540

Definition: Limitation of secondary cerebral injury resulting from swelling of brain tissue

Activities:

- Monitor for confusion, changes in mentation, complaints of dizziness, syncope
- Monitor neurologic status closely and compare to baseline
- Monitor vital signs
- Monitor CSF drainage characteristics: color, clarity, consistency
- Record CSF drainage
- Monitor CVP, PAWP, and PAP, as appropriate
- Monitor ICP and CPP
- Analyze ICP waveform
- Monitor respiratory status: rate, rhythm, depth of respirations; PaO_2, PCO_2, pH, bicarbonate
- Allow ICP to return to baseline between nursing activities
- Monitor patient's ICP and neurologic response to care activities
- Decrease stimuli in patient's environment
- Plan nursing care to provide rest periods
- Give sedation, as needed
- Note patient's change in response to stimuli
- Screen conversation within patient's hearing
- Administer anticonvulsants, as appropriate
- Avoid neck flexion or extreme hip/knee flexion
- Avoid Valsalva maneuvers
- Administer stool softeners
- Position with head of bed up 30 degrees or greater
- Avoid use of PEEP
- Administer paralyzing agent, as appropriate
- Encourage family/significant other(s) to talk to patient
- Restrict fluids
- Avoid hypotonic IV fluids
- Adjust ventilator settings to keep $PaCO_2$ at prescribed level
- Limit suction passes to less than 15 seconds
- Monitor laboratory values: serum and urine osmolality, sodium, potassium
- Monitor volume pressure indices
- Perform passive range-of-motion exercises
- Monitor intake and output
- Maintain normothermia
- Administer loop-active or osmotic diuretics
- Implement seizure precautions
- Titrate barbiturate to achieve suppression or burst suppression of EEG as ordered
- Establish means of communication: ask yes or no questions; provide magic slate, paper and pencil, picture board, flashcards, VOCAID device

1st edition 1992; revised 2004

Background Evidence:

American Academy of Pediatrics. (1999). The management of minor closed head injury in children. *Pediatrics, 104*(6), 1407–1415.

American Association of Critical-Care Nurses. (1998). *Core curriculum for critical care nursing* (5th ed.). W. B. Saunders.

Orfanelli, L. (2001). Neurologic examination of the toddler: How to assess for increased intracranial pressure following head trauma. *American Journal of Nursing, 101*(12), 24CC–24FF.

Yanko, J. R., & Mitcho, K. (2001). Acute care management of severe traumatic brain injuries. *Critical Care Nursing Quarterly, 23*(4), 1–23.

C

Cerebral Perfusion Promotion 2550

Definition: Promotion of adequate perfusion and limitation of complications for a patient experiencing or at risk for inadequate cerebral perfusion

Activities:

- Consult with physician to determine hemodynamic parameters
- Administer and titrate vasoactive drugs, as prescribed, to maintain hemodynamic parameters
- Induce hypertension with volume expansion or inotropic or vasoconstrictive agents, as prescribed, to maintain hemodynamic parameters and maintain or optimize CPP
- Monitor patient's PT and PTT to keep one to two times normal, as appropriate
- Monitor for anticoagulant therapy side effects (e.g., test stool and NG drainage for blood)
- Administer rheologic agents (e.g., low-dose mannitol or low molecular weight dextrans), as prescribed
- Draw blood to monitor hematocrit level, electrolytes, and blood glucose
- Maintain hematocrit level for hypervolemic hemodilution therapy per protocol
- Monitor for seizures
- Consult with physician to determine optimal head of bed (HOB) placement (e.g., 0, 15, or 30 degrees) and monitor patient's responses to head positioning
- Avoid neck flexion or extreme hip or knee flexion
- Keep PCO_2 level at 25 mm Hg or greater
- Administer calcium channel blockers and vasopressors, as prescribed
- Administer and monitor effects of osmotic and loop-active diuretics and corticosteroids
- Administer pain medication, as appropriate
- Administer anticoagulant, antiplatelet, and thrombolytic medication, as prescribed
- Monitor neurological status
- Calculate and monitor CPP
- Monitor patient's ICP and neurologic response to care activities
- Monitor MAP
- Monitor CVP
- Monitor PAWP and PAP
- Monitor laboratory values for changes in oxygenation or acid-base balance, as appropriate
- Monitor respiratory status (e.g., rate, rhythm, and depth of respirations; partial oxygen pressure, PCO_2, pH, and bicarbonate levels)
- Monitor determinants of tissue oxygen delivery (e.g., $PaCO_2$, SaO_2, and hemoglobin levels and cardiac output), if available
- Auscultate lung sounds for crackles or other adventitious sounds
- Monitor for signs of fluid overload (e.g., rhonchi, JVD, edema, and increase in pulmonary secretions)
- Monitor intake and output

2nd edition 1996; revised 2018

Background Evidence:

Cecil, S., Chen, P., Callaway, S., Rowland, S., Adler, D., & Chen, J. (2011). Traumatic brain injury: Advanced multimodal neuromonitoring from theory to clinical practice. *Critical Care Nurse, 31*(2), 25–36.

Lang, S. S., Kofke, W. A., & Stiefel, M. F. (2012). Monitoring and intraoperative management of elevated intracranial pressure and decompressive craniectomy. *Anesthesiology Clinics, 30*(2), 289–310.

Smeltzer, S., Bare, B., Hinkle, J., & Cheever, K. (2010). (12th ed.) *Brunner & Suddarth's textbook of medical surgical nursing* (Vol. 2). Lippincott Williams & Wilkins.

Treggiari, M. M. (2011). Hemodynamic management of subarachnoid hemorrhage. *Neurocritical Care, 15*(2), 329–335.

Wijayatilake, D. S., Shepherd, S. J., & Sherren, P. B. (2012). Updates in the management of intracranial pressure in traumatic brain injury. *Current Opinion Anaesthesiology, 25*(5), 540–547.

Woodrow, P. (2012). *Intensive care nursing: A framework for practice* (3rd ed.). Routledge.

Cesarean Birth Care 6750

Definition: Provision of care to a patient delivering a baby through an abdominal incision into the uterus

Activities:

- Orient patient to unit
- Review prenatal history
- Explain reasons for surgery
- Discuss feelings, questions, and concerns patient has about surgery
- Obtain or confirm informed consent
- Obtain necessary blood work and document results
- Monitor vital signs
- Monitor fetal heart rate
- Prepare abdomen for surgery
- Place intravenous line
- Insert indwelling urinary catheter
- Administer medications
- Encourage intimate partner or support person to be present during delivery
- Give information about events taking place and sensations patient may be experiencing during surgery
- Give information about infant
- Transfer patient to recovery room or labor room
- Monitor physiological aspects of recovery (e.g., pain, uterine changes, airway patency, and lochia)
- Inspect condition of surgical incision and dressing
- Assist in performing leg exercises, turning, coughing, and deep breathing
- Encourage mother to breastfeed, if appropriate
- Provide adequate breastfeeding education and support, if appropriate (i.e., demonstrate infant positioning adaptations according to mobility limitations)
- Facilitate family bonding and attachment by minimizing maternal-infant separation (e.g., present infant en face to mother, provide unobstructed view of infant, facilitate skin-to-skin contact, and transfer mother and infant together)

1st edition 1992; revised 2013

Background Evidence:

Chertok, I. R. (2006). Breast-feeding initiation among post-caesarean women of the Negev, Israel. *British Journal of Nursing, 15*(4), 205–208.

Nolan, A., & Lawrence, C. (2009). A pilot study of a nursing intervention protocol to minimize maternal-infant separation after cesarean birth. *Journal of Obstetric, Gynecologic, & Neonatal Nursing, 38*(4), 430–442.

Ward, S. L., & Hisley, S. M. (2009). Caring for the woman experiencing complications during labor and birth. In *Maternal-child nursing care: Optimizing outcomes for mothers, children, & families* (pp. 427–465). F.A. Davis.

C

Chemical Restraint   6430

Definition: Administration and monitoring of the temporary use of psychotropic, hypnotics, or anxiolytics agents used to control behavior or movements

Activities:

- Identify behaviors that necessitate intervention (e.g., agitation, violence)
- Implement alternative interventions to attempt to eliminate need for restraint
- Provide distraction activities before use of restraints (e.g., television, visitors)
- Explain procedure, purpose, and duration of intervention in understandable terms
- Obtain consent as appropriate
- Follow six rights of medication administration
- Note medical history and allergies
- Monitor response to medications
- Monitor level of consciousness
- Monitor sedation, agitation, and mental status using validated tools, as appropriate
- Monitor vital signs (e.g., respiratory rate, oxygen saturation, temperature, blood pressure, end-tidal CO_2 level)
- Provide appropriate level of supervision or surveillance to allow for therapeutic actions, as needed
- Provide physical, psychological, and psychosocial comfort, as needed
- Monitor skin color, temperature, sensation, and condition
- Provide for movement and exercise, according to level of self-control, condition, and abilities
- Position for comfort, prevention of aspiration, and skin breakdown
- Assist with needs related to nutrition, elimination, hydration, and personal hygiene
- Evaluate need for continued restrictive intervention at regular intervals
- Involve person in making decisions to move to less restrictive form of intervention, when appropriate
- Record response to medications per agency protocol

4th edition 2004; revised 2024

Background Evidence:

Hupé, C., Larue, C., Gazemar, V., Pépin, C., & Contandriopoulos, D. (2020). Quality standards of nursing care for the use of chemical restraints. *Journal of Nursing Care Quality, 35*(3), 270–275. https://doi.org/10.1097/NCQ.0000000000000453

Jessop, T., & Peisah, C. (2021). Human rights and empowerment in aged care: Restraint, consent and dying with dignity. *International Journal of Environmental Research and Public Health, 18*(15). https://doi.org/10.3390/ijerph18157899

Muir, C. E., Oster, C., & Grimmer, K. (2020). International research into 22 years of use of chemical restraint: An evidence overview. *Journal of Evaluation in Clinical Practice, 26*(3), 927–956. https://doi.org/10.1111/jep.13232

Robins, L. M., Lee, D.-C. A., Bell, J. S., Srikanth, V., Möhler, R., Hill, K. D., & Haines, T. P. (2021). Definition and measurement of physical and chemical restraint in long-term care: A systematic review. *International Journal of Environmental Research and Public Health, 18*(7). https://www.mdpi.com/1660-4601/18/7/3639

Chemotherapy Management   2240

Definition: Assisting the patient and family to understand the action and minimize side effects of antineoplastic agents

Activities:

- Monitor pretreatment screening workups for patients at risk for earlier onset, longer duration, and more distressing side effects
- Promote activities to modify the identified risk factors
- Monitor for side effects and toxic effects of treatment
- Provide information to patient and family on antineoplastic drug effect on malignant cells
- Teach patient and family about the effects of therapy on bone marrow functioning
- Instruct patient and family on ways to prevent infection, such as avoiding crowds, using good hygiene, and handwashing techniques
- Instruct patient to promptly report fevers, chills, nosebleeds, excessive bruising, and tarry stools
- Instruct patient and family to avoid the use of aspirin products
- Institute neutropenic and bleeding precautions
- Determine the patient's previous experience with chemotherapy-related nausea and vomiting
- Administer medications to control side effects (e.g., antiemetics for nausea and vomiting), as needed
- Minimize stimuli from noises, light, and odors (especially food odors)
- Teach the patient relaxation and imagery techniques to use before, during, and after treatments, as appropriate
- Offer the patient a bland and easily digested diet
- Administer chemotherapeutic drugs in the late evening so the patient may sleep at the time emetic effects are greatest

C

- Ensure adequate fluid intake to prevent dehydration and electrolyte imbalance
- Monitor the effectiveness of measures to control nausea and vomiting
- Offer six small feedings daily, as tolerated
- Instruct patient to avoid hot, spicy foods
- Provide nutritious, appetizing foods of patient's choice
- Monitor nutritional status and weight
- Monitor for indications of infection of oral mucous membranes
- Encourage good oral hygiene with use of dental cleansing devices, such as unwaxed, non-shredding floss, sonic toothbrushes or water pik, as appropriate
- Initiate oral health restoration activities, such as use of artificial saliva, saliva stimulants, nonalcohol-based mouth sprays, sugarless mints, and fluoride treatments, as appropriate
- Teach patient on self-assessment of oral cavity, including signs and symptoms to report for further evaluation (e.g., burning, pain, tenderness)
- Teach patient need for frequent dental follow-up care as dental caries form rapidly
- Teach patient to use oral nystatin suspension to control fungal infection, as appropriate
- Teach patient to avoid temperature extremes and chemical treatments of the hair when receiving treatment
- Inform patient that hair loss is expected, as determined by type of therapy
- Assist patient in planning for hair loss, as appropriate, by teaching about available alternatives such as wigs, scarves, hats, and turbans
- Teach patient to gently wash and comb hair and to sleep on a silk pillowcase to prevent further hair loss, as appropriate
- Reassure patient that hair will grow back after treatment is terminated, as appropriate
- Teach patient and family to monitor for organ toxicity, as determined by type of therapy
- Discuss potential aspects of sexual dysfunction, as appropriate
- Teach implications of therapy on sexual function, including the time frame for contraceptive use, as appropriate
- Monitor fatigue level by soliciting the patient's description of fatigue

- Teach patient and family techniques of energy management, as appropriate
- Assist patient in managing fatigue by planning frequent rest periods, spacing of activities, and limiting daily demands, as appropriate
- Facilitate expression of fears about prognosis or success of treatments
- Provide concrete objective information related to the effects of therapy to reduce patient uncertainty, fear, and anxiety about treatment-related symptoms
- Instruct long-term survivors and their families of the possibility of second malignancies and the importance of reporting increased susceptibility to infection, fatigue, or bleeding
- Follow recommended guidelines for safe handling of parenteral antineoplastic drugs during drug preparation and administration

1st edition, 1992; revised 2008

Background Evidence:

Barsevick, A. M., Whitmer, K., Sweeney, C., & Nail, L. M. (2002). A pilot study examining energy conservation for cancer treatment-related fatigue. *Cancer Nursing, 25*(5), 333–341.

Brant, J. M., & Wickham, R. S. (Eds.). (2004). *Statement on the scope and standards of oncology nursing practice.* Pittsburgh, PA: Oncology Nursing Society.

Brown, K., Esper, P., Kelleher, L., O'Neill, J., Polovich, M., & White, J. (Eds.). (2001). *Chemotherapy and biotherapy guidelines and recommendations for practice.* Pittsburgh, PA: Oncology Nursing Society.

LeMone, P., & Burke, K. M. (2000). *Medical-surgical nursing: Critical thinking in client care* (pp. 338–344) (2nd ed.). Prentice Hall.

Nail, L. M. (2002). Fatigue in patients with cancer. *Oncology Nursing Forum, 29*(3), 537–546.

Oncology Nursing Society. (2005). In J. K. Itano & K. Taoka (Eds.), *Core curriculum for oncology nursing* (4th ed.). Elsevier Saunders.

Wegenka, M. H. (1999). Chemotherapy management. In G. Bulechek & J. McCloskey (Eds.), *Nursing interventions: Effective nursing treatments* (3rd ed., pp. 285–296). W.B. Saunders.

Yarbro, C. H., Frogge, M. H., & Goodman, M. (2005). *Cancer nursing: Principles and practice* (6th ed.). Jones & Bartlett.

Chest Physiotherapy 3230

Definition: Assisting the patient to mobilize airway secretions via percussion, vibration, and postural drainage

Activities:

- Determine presence of contraindications for use of chest physiotherapy (e.g., acute exacerbation of COPD, pneumonia without evidence of excess sputum production, osteoporosis, lung cancer, and cerebral edema)
- Perform chest physiotherapy at least 2 hours after eating
- Explain purpose and procedures used during chest physiotherapy to patient
- Position any necessary equipment nearby (e.g., suctioning equipment, sputum container, and tissues)
- Monitor respiratory and cardiac status (e.g., rate, rhythm, breath sounds, and depth of breath)
- Monitor amount and character of secretions
- Determine lung segment(s) containing excessive secretions

- Position patient with the lung segment to be drained in uppermost position, making modifications for patients unable to tolerate prescribed position (i.e., avoid placing patient with COPD, acute head injury, and cardiac problems in Trendelenburg position as it can increase shortness of breath, intracranial pressure, and stress, respectively)
- Use pillows to support patient in designated position
- Strike chest rhythmically and in rapid succession using cupped hands over area(s) to be drained for 3 to 5 minutes, avoiding percussion over spine, kidneys, female breasts, incisions, and broken ribs
- Apply pneumatic, acoustical, or electrical chest percussors

- Rapidly and vigorously vibrate hands, keeping shoulders and arms straight and wrists stiff, on area(s) to be drained while patient exhales or coughs 3 to 4 times
- Instruct patient to expectorate loosened secretions via deep breathing
- Encourage coughing during and after procedure
- Suction loosened secretions
- Monitor patient tolerance during and after procedure (e.g., pulse oximetry, vital signs, and reported comfort level)

1st edition 1992; revised 2013

Background Evidence:

Cantin, A. M., Bacon, M., & Berthiaume, Y. (2006). Mechanical airway clearance using the frequencer electro-acoustical transducer in cystic fibrosis. *Clinical & Investigative Medicine, 29*(3), 159–165.

Craven, R. F., & Hirnle, C. J. (2009). Oxygenation: Respiratory function. In *Fundamentals of nursing: Human health and function* (pp. 816–876) (6th ed.). Lippincott Williams & Wilkins.

Nelson, D. M. (1992). Interventions related to respiratory care. *Nursing Clinics of North America, 27*(2), 301–323.

Smith, S. F., Duell, D. J., & Martin, B. C. (2008). Respiratory function. In *Clinical nursing skills: Basic to advanced skills* (pp. 939–1002) (7th ed.). Pearson Prentice Hall.

Workman, M. L. (2010). Care of patients with noninfectious lower respiratory problems. In D. D. Ignatavicius & M. L. Workman (Eds.), *Medical-surgical nursing: Patient-centered collaborative care* (6th ed., pp. 609–652). Saunders Elsevier.

Yang, M., Yan, Y., Yin, X., Wang, B. Y., Wu, T., Liu, G. J., & Don, B. R. (2010). Chest physiotherapy for pneumonia in adults. *Cochrane Database of Systematic Reviews*, (2), CD006338. https://doi.org/10.1002/14651858.CD006338.pub2

Child Care   8274

Definition: Facilitating developmentally appropriate care to support physical, cognitive, social, and emotional growth

Activities:

- Build trusting, therapeutic relationship with child and caregivers
- Establish one-to-one interaction with child
- Assist each child to become aware of importance as individual
- Identify special needs of child and adaptations required, as appropriate
- Encourage shared decision making and self-care during illness and chronic disease management
- Model activities that promote development to caregivers
- Facilitate caregiver's contact with community resources, as appropriate
- Facilitate caregiver participation in child's care, as appropriate
- Facilitate family-professional collaboration in child's care plan
- Refer caregivers to support group for child and family, as appropriate
- Ensure body language agrees with verbal communication
- Provide opportunity for child to engage with peers, as appropriate
- Encourage child to express self through positive rewards or feedback for attempts
- Hold or rock and comfort child, especially when upset
- Create safe, well-defined space for child to explore and learn
- Instruct how to seek help from others, when needed
- Encourage dreaming or fantasy, when appropriate
- Offer age-appropriate toys or materials
- Help child perform and master self-help skills (e.g., feeding, toileting, brushing teeth, washing hands, dressing)
- Talk, sing, or dance with child
- Be consistent and structured with behavior management or modification strategies
- Redirect attention, when needed
- Have misbehaving child "take breaks" or "time outs", as appropriate
- Provide opportunity and materials for creative expression (e.g., building, drawing, clay modeling, painting, glue, cutting, coloring)
- Provide opportunities to complete schoolwork or developmentally appropriate educational activities
- Provide opportunities for and encourage exercise
- Provide opportunity to play on playground, as appropriate
- Go on walks with child
- Monitor prescribed medication regime, as appropriate
- Assure that medical tests and treatments are done in timely manner, as appropriate
- Provide honest, developmentally appropriate information
- Review immunization status, reinforce importance, and administer as needed
- Reinforce importance of handwashing
- Encourage annual dental visit
- Encourage healthy eating habits
- Encourage oral hygiene using soft bristled toothbrush and pea sized amount of fluoridated toothpaste
- Administer screening tools at regular intervals to evaluate child growth and development
- Evaluate hearing and vision screenings annually

3rd edition 2000; revised 2024

Background Evidence:

Garzon Maaks, D. L., Barber Starr, N., Brady, M. A., Gaylord, N. M., Driessnack, M., & Duderstadt, K. (2021). *Burns' pediatric primary care.* (7th ed.). Elsevier.

Hagan, J. F., Shaw, J. S., & Duncan, P. M. (2017). *Bright futures: Guidelines for health supervision of infants, children, and* (4th ed.). American Academy of Pediatrics.

Hockenberry, M. J., Wilson, D., & Rodgers, C. (2019). *Wong's nursing care of infants and children.* (11th ed.). Elsevier.

Perry, S. E., Hockenberry, M. J., Lowdermilk, D. L., & Wilson, D. (2018). *Maternal child nursing care.* (6th ed.). Elsevier.

Richardson, B. (2020). *Pediatric primary care: Practice guidelines for nurses* (4th ed.) Jones & Bartlett Learning.

Childbirth Preparation 6760

Definition: Providing information and support to facilitate childbirth and to enhance the ability of an individual to develop and perform the parental role

Activities:

- Teach the mother and partner about the physiology of labor and delivery
- Explore childbirth plan for labor and delivery (e.g., the birthing environment, who will assist mother, who will be in attendance, what technology will be used, who will cut the cord, feeding preferences, and discharge plans)
- Educate mother and partner about signs of labor
- Inform mother about when to come to the hospital in preparation for delivery
- Discuss pain control options with mother
- Instruct mother on steps to be taken if desire is to avoid episiotomy, such as perineal massage, Kegel's exercises, optimal nutrition, and prompt treatment of vaginitis
- Inform mother about delivery options if complications arise
- Explain routine monitoring that may occur during labor and delivery
- Teach mother and partner breathing and relaxation techniques to be used during labor and delivery
- Teach partner measures to comfort mother during labor (e.g., back rub, back pressure, and positioning)
- Prepare partner to coach mother during labor and delivery
- Review American Academy of Pediatrics recommendations for breastfeeding
- Discuss advantages and disadvantages of breastfeeding and bottle feeding
- Instruct mother to prepare nipples for breastfeeding, as indicated
- Encourage mother to put the infant to breast after delivery
- Provide opportunity for mother to be in close proximity to infant during postpartum hospitalization to facilitate bonding and breastfeeding

- Determine parent's knowledge and attitudes about parenting
- Promote parent's self-efficacy in taking on parental role
- Provide anticipatory guidance for parenthood
- Discuss arrangements for sibling care during hospitalization
- Determine how parent(s) prepared sibling(s) for coming of new baby, as appropriate
- Assist parent(s) in planning strategies to prepare siblings for newborn
- Refer parent(s) to sibling preparation class
- Assist parent to select a physician or clinic to receive child health supervision for newborn
- Encourage mother to obtain an approved infant car safety seat to transport newborn home from hospital

1st edition 1992; revised 2008

Background Evidence:

American Academy of Pediatrics. (2005). Policy statement: Breastfeeding and the use of human milk. *Pediatrics, 115*(2), 496–506.

Bradley, L., Horan, M. J., & Molloy, P. (2004). Pregnancy and childbearing. In M. C. Condon (Ed.), *Women's health: Body, mind, sprit: An integrated approach to wellness and illness* (pp. 463–499). Prentice Hall.

Institute for Clinical Systems Improvement (ICSI). (2005). *Health care guideline: Routine prenatal care.*

Kirkham, C., Harris, S., & Grzybowski, S. (2005). Evidence-based prenatal care: Part l. General prenatal care and counseling issues. *American Family Physician, 71*(7), 1307–1316.

Littleton, L. Y., & Engebertson, J. C. (2002). *Maternal, neonatal, and women's health nursing* (pp. 477–489). Delmar.

Wong, D. L., Perry, S. E., & Hockenberry, M. J. (2002). *Maternal child nursing care* (2nd ed.). Mosby.

Circulatory Care: Arterial Insufficiency 4062

Definition: Promotion of arterial circulation

Activities:

- Perform comprehensive appraisal of peripheral circulation (i.e., check all peripheral pulses, edema, capillary refill, color, and temperature)
- Conduct complete evaluation of clinical history and physical examination
- Perform palpation of carotid pulses
- Determine ankle-brachial index (ABI), as appropriate
- Measure blood pressure in both arms
- Inspect skin for arterial ulcers or tissue breakdown, especially poorly healing or nonhealing wounds
- Monitor degree of discomfort, fatigue, or pain with exercise or rest
- Provide pain relief with analgesic agents, hanging foot over side of bed, or sleeping in chair, as appropriate
- Monitor pain at regular intervals
- Use support surfaces to reduce pressure
- Evaluate leg symptoms with exertion, as may indicate claudication

- Place extremity in dependent position, as appropriate
- Administer statin therapy, antihypertensive, antiplatelet, or anticoagulant medications, as prescribed
- Change position at least every 2 hours, as appropriate
- Encourage to exercise, as tolerated
- Encourage consumption of healthy diet and weight loss, as appropriate
- Evaluate presence of risk factors for arterial disease (e.g., advanced age, tobacco use, diabetes, smoking, dyslipidemia, hypertension, obesity, hyperhomocysteinemia)
- Recommend smoking cessation, as appropriate
- Encourage vaccination
- Protect extremity from injury (e.g., sheepskin under feet and lower legs, footboard or bed cradle at foot of bed, well-fitted shoes)
- Provide warmth (e.g., additional bed clothes, increasing room temperature), as appropriate
- Elevate head of bed 15 to 30 degrees

- Protect extremities from cold, heat, and trauma
- Maintain adequate hydration to decrease blood viscosity
- Monitor nutrition and fluid status, including intake and output
- Implement gentle wound care and cleaning, as appropriate
- Restore cutaneous blood flow in arterial ulcers, as appropriate, to control possible infections
- Promote adequate oxygen delivery to wound
- Instruct on factors that interfere with circulation (e.g., restrictive clothing, exposure to cold temperatures, crossing of legs and feet)
- Instruct on proper foot care
- Use teach-back to ensure understanding

3rd edition 2000; revised 2004, 2024

Background Evidence:

Arnett, D. K., Blumenthal, R. S., Albert, M. A., Buroker, A. B., Goldberger, Z. D., Hahn, E. J., Himmelfarb, C. D., Khera, A., Lloyd-Jones, D., McEvoy, J. W., Michos, E. D., Miedema, M. D., Muñoz, D., Smith, S. C., Virani, S. S., Jr, Williams, K. A. , Sr, Yeboah, J., & Ziaeian, B. (2019). 2019 ACC/AHA Guideline on the primary prevention of cardiovascular disease: A report of the American College of Cardiology/American Heart Association task force on clinical practice guidelines. *Circulation, 140*(11), e596–e646.

Gerhard-Herman, M. D., Gornik, H. L., Barrett, C., Barshes, N. R., Corriere, M. A., Drachman, D. E., Fleisher, L. A., Fowkes, F. G., Hamburg, N. M., Kinlay, S., Lookstein, R., Misra, S., Mureebe, L., Olin, J. W., Patel, R. A., Regensteiner, J. G., Schanzer, A., Shishehbor, M. H., Stewart, K. J., Treat-Jacobson, D., & Walsh, M. E. (2017). 2016 AHA/ACC Guideline on the management of patients with lower extremity peripheral artery disease: A report of the American College of Cardiology/American Heart Association task force on clinical practice guidelines. *Circulation, 135*(12), e726–e779.

Lim, S., Chung, R., Holloway, S., & Harding, K. G. (2021). Modified compression therapy in mixed arterial–venous leg ulcers: An integrative review. *International Wound Journal, 18*(6), 822–842.

Logan, J. G., Kim, S., & Mijung, M. (2018).). Effects of static stretching exercise on lumbar flexibility and central arterial stiffness. *The Journal of Cardiovascular Nursing, 33*(4), 322–328.

Perpetua, E., & Keegan, P. (2020). *Cardiac nursing* (7th ed.). Wolters Kluwer.

Circulatory Care: Mechanical Assist Device   **4064**

Definition: Temporary support of circulation by managing use of mechanical devices or pumps

Activities:

- Determine peripheral circulation status (e.g., check peripheral pulses, edema, capillary refill, color, temperature)
- Monitor sensorium and cognitive abilities
- Monitor degree of chest discomfort or pain
- Evaluate pulmonary artery pressures, systemic pressures, cardiac output, and systemic vascular resistance, as indicated
- Match device indications and contraindications to ensure device coincides with condition
- Assist with insertion or implantation of device
- Coordinate waveforms with inflation and deflation of device, as indicated
- Observe for hemolysis (e.g., blood in urine, hemolyzed blood specimens, increase in daily serum hemoglobin, frank bleeding, hyperkalemia, kidney failure)
- Observe cannulas for kinks or disconnections
- Determine activated clotting times every hour, as appropriate
- Administer anticoagulants or anti-thrombolytics, as prescribed
- Monitor device regularly to ensure proper functioning (e.g., waveforms, alarm notes, catheter position information)
- Ensure back-up equipment available at all times
- Administer positive inotropic agents, as appropriate
- Monitor coagulation profiles every 6 hours, as appropriate
- Administer blood products, as appropriate
- Monitor vital signs and urine output every hour
- Monitor electrolytes, BUN, and creatinine daily
- Monitor, intake and output every hour, as prescribed
- Monitor daily weight daily
- Monitor peripheral circulation every hour with femoral or axillary device placements
- Obtain chest x-ray, as prescribed
- Use strict aseptic technique for dressings changing
- Administer prophylactic antibiotics as ordered
- Monitor for fever and leukocytosis
- Collect blood, urine, sputum, and wound cultures if febrile, as prescribed
- Administer antifungal oral solutions
- Administer total parenteral nutrition, as appropriate
- Administer analgesics, as needed
- Plan for early ambulation with axillary device implantations
- Instruct about device
- Provide emotional support
- Provide education related to purpose and care of device
- Use teach-back to determine understanding

2nd edition 1996; revised 2000, 2024

Background Evidence:

Asber, S. R., Shanahan, K. P., Lussier, L., Didomenico, D., Davis, M., Eaton, J., Esposito, M., & Kapur, N. K. (2020). Nursing management of patients requiring acute mechanical circulatory support devices. *Critical Care Nurse, 40*(1), e1–e11. https://doi.org/10.4037/ccn2020764

Hyotala, M. (2018). Caring for pediatric heart failure patients with long-term mechanical circulatory support. *Critical Care Nurse, 38*(5), 44–56. https://doi.org/10.4037/ccn2018313

Runyan, C., Marshall, C., Aronow, H., Vongkavivathanakul, S., Daniels, L., Currey, J., & Coleman, B. (2021). Evaluation of team-based learning to increase nurses' knowledge of the ventricular assist device. *Journal of Continuing Education in Nursing, 52*(1), 13–20. https://doi.org/10.3928/00220124-20201215-06

Urden, L. D., Stacy, K. M., & Lough, M. E. (2022). Pulmonary therapeutic management. *In Critical care nursing: Diagnosis and management* (pp. 502–503) (9th ed.). Elsevier.

Wiegand, D. (2017). *AACN procedural manual for high acuity, progressive, and critical care* (7th ed.). Elsevier.

Circulatory Care: Venous Insufficiency 4066

Definition: Promotion of venous circulation

Activities:
- Evaluate peripheral circulation (e.g., pulses, edema, capillary refill, color, temperature)
- Inspect skin for stasis ulcers and tissue breakdown
- Review history of comorbidities (e.g., hypertension, heart failure, peripheral vascular disease, asthma, obstructive airway disease, inflammatory bowel disease, present or past history of cancer, anemia, malnutrition, lack of mobility)
- Identify risk factors for venous ulcers (e.g., varicose veins, deep vein thrombosis, chronic venous insufficiency, poor calf muscle function, arteriovenous fistulae, obesity, history of leg fracture)
- Consider diet modifications, nutritional supplements, smoking cessation, weight reduction, avoidance of immobility, and maintenance of healthy cardiac status, as appropriate
- Examine physical, emotional, and lifestyle conditions that may contribute to venous stasis conditions
- Determine ability to conduct preventative self-care measures, including consistent management of leg edema
- Outline plan of care for self-care, using person and family input
- Promote psychosocial, economic, and health care system support, as appropriate
- Optimize local wound environment through cleansing, debriding, managing bacterial balance and managing moisture balance, as appropriate
- Irrigate ulcers with warmed saline solution, as needed
- Apply dressing appropriate for wound size and type, as indicated
- Administer antiplatelet or anticoagulant medications, as prescribed
- Protect affected extremity from injury (e.g., sheepskin under feet and lower legs, footboard or bed cradle at foot of bed, well-fitted shoes)
- Maintain adequate hydration to decrease blood viscosity
- Monitor fluid and nutritional status, including intake and output
- Monitor for signs of infection, cellulitis, deep vein thrombosis, and joint contractures
- Monitor degree of discomfort or pain
- Implement pain relief measures (e.g., compression therapy, exercise, leg elevation, analgesia)
- Apply compression therapy modalities (e.g., short-stretch or long-stretch bandages), as appropriate
- Instruct to remove compression and seek advice if any side effects (e.g., numbness, tingling, pain, discolored toes)
- Elevate affected limb 20 degrees or greater, to be higher than level of heart, as appropriate
- Change position at least every 2 hours, as appropriate
- Encourage passive or active range-of-motion exercises especially of lower extremities during bed rest
- Encourage to remain active wearing some form of compression system
- Instruct on importance of compression therapy, daily leg elevation and need for lifelong compression
- Instruct on proper foot care
- Instruct regarding care and application of compression stockings, including need to replace stockings every 6 months if worn daily
- Instruct to eliminate restrictive clothing, sit without legs crossed and avoid sitting or standing for long periods to reduce constriction of the blood vessels
- Instruct regarding measures to prevent injury
- Use teach-back to ensure understanding

3rd edition 2000; revised 2004, 2024

Background Evidence:
Atkln, L. (2019). Venous leg ulcer prevention 3: Supporting patients to self-manage. *Nursing Times, 115*(8), 23.

Clarke, C. (2019). Improving venous leg ulcer care in community services. *Nursing Times, 115*(9), 24.

Evans, R., Kuhnke, J.L., Burrows, C., Kayssi, A., Labreque, C., O'Sullivan-Drombolis, D., & Houghton, P. (2019). *Best practice recommendations for the prevention and management of venous leg ulcers.* In: Foundations of Best Practice for Skin and Wound Management. A supplement of Wound Care Canada. https://www.woundscanada.ca/docman/public/health-care-professional/bpr-workshop/1521-wc-bpr-prevention-and-management-of-venous-leg-ulcers-1874e-final/file

Guest, J. F., Fuller, G. W., & Vowden, P. (2018). Venous leg ulcer management in clinical practice in the UK: Costs and outcomes. *International Wound Journal, 15*(1), 29–37.

Love, S., White, J. R., & Vestal, B. (2021). Using compression therapy in a primary care setting to treat complications of chronic venous insufficiency. *Journal of the American Association of Nurse Practitioners, 33*(6), 484–490.

Perpetua, E., & Keegan, P. (2020). *Cardiac nursing* (7th ed.). Wolters Kluwer.

Todd, M. (2018). Assessment and management of older people with venous leg ulcers. *Nursing Older People, 30*(5), 39–48.

Trivellato, M., Kolchraiber, F., Frederico, G., Morales, D., Silva, A., & Gamba, M. (2018). Advanced practices in comprehensive nursing care for people with skin ulcers. *Acta Paulista de Enfermagem, 31*(6), 600–608.

Circulatory Precautions 4070

Definition: Protection of a localized area with limited perfusion

Activities:
- Perform a comprehensive appraisal of peripheral circulation (i.e., check peripheral pulses, edema, capillary refill, color, temperature of extremity, and ankle brachial index, if indicated)
- Target at-risk patients (e.g., diabetics, smokers, elderly, hypertensive patients and those with elevated cholesterols levels) for comprehensive peripheral assessments and modification of risk factors
- Do not start an IV or draw blood in the affected extremity
- Refrain from taking blood pressure in affected extremity
- Refrain from applying pressure or tourniquet to affected extremity
- Maintain adequate hydration to prevent increased blood viscosity
- Avoid injury to affected area
- Prevent infection in wounds

- Instruct the patient to test bath water before entering to avoid burning skin
- Instruct patient on foot and nail care
- Instruct patient and family on protection from injury of affected area
- Encourage smoking cessation and regular exercise in patients with claudication
- Encourage walking to the point of claudication and a little bit more each time to assist in the development of collateral circulation in the lower extremities
- Instruct patient and family on medication therapies for blood pressure control, anticoagulation, and reduction of cholesterol levels
- Instruct patient on avoidance of beta blockers for blood pressure control, as they cause constriction of peripheral vessels and worsens claudication
- Instruct patient on diet measures to improve circulation (e.g., diet low in saturated fat and good intake of omega 3 fish oils)
- Instruct diabetic patients on the need for proper management of blood sugar
- Instruct patient on proper skin care (e.g., moisturizing dry skin on legs, prompt attention to wounds and potential ulcers)
- Provide patient and family with smoking cessation information, if applicable
- Monitor extremities for areas of heat, redness, pain, or swelling

- Instruct patient on signs and symptoms indicating a need for emergent care (e.g., pain that does not go away upon rest, wound complications, loss of feeling)
- Encourage patient participation in vascular rehabilitation programs

1st edition 1992; revised 2013

Background Evidence:

Bonham, P. A., Flemister, B. G., Goldberg, M., Crawford, P. E., Johnson, J. J., & Varnado, M. F. (2009). What's new in lower-extremity arterial disease? WOCN's 2008 clinical practice guideline. *Journal of Wound, Ostomy & Continence Nursing, 36*(1), 37–44.

Conen, D., Everett, B., Kurth, T., Creager, M., Buring, J., Ridker, P., & Pradhan, A. (2011). Smoking, smoking status, and risk for symptomatic peripheral artery disease in women: A cohort study. *Annals of Internal Medicine, 154*(11), 719–726.

Lawson, G. (2005). The importance of obtaining ankle-brachial indexes in older adults: The other vital sign. *Journal of Vascular Nursing, 23*(2), 46–51.

Selby, M. (2008). Peripheral arterial disease. *Practice Nurse, 36*(7), 33–34, 36–37.

Sieggreen, M. (2008). Understanding critical limb ischemia. *Nursing, 38*(10), 50–56.

Ward, C. (2010). Peripheral arterial disease. *MEDSURG Nursing, 19*(4), 247–248.

Circumcision Care   3000

Definition: Pre- and post-procedural support to person undergoing circumcision

Activities:

- Verify surgical consent signed
- Verify correct identification
- Administer pain control approximately 1 hour before procedure (e.g., acetaminophen)
- Position in comfortable position during procedure
- Use padded circumcision seat for infants
- Use radiant warmer to maintain body temperature during procedure
- Shield eyes from direct light
- Use pacifier dipped in sucrose 24% during procedure and until next feeding with permission from parent or guardian, as indicated
- Swaddle infant's upper body during circumcision
- Play soft, appropriate music during procedure
- Monitor vital signs
- Administer topical local analgesia agent (e.g., eutectic mixture of local anesthetics [EMLA]), as ordered
- Assist with dorsal penile nerve block, as appropriate
- Apply white petroleum jelly or dressing, as appropriate
- Monitor for bleeding every 30 minutes for at least 2 hours post procedure
- Provide postprocedure pain control every 4 to 6 hours for 24 hours (e.g., acetaminophen)
- Instruct on signs and symptoms to report to health care provider (e.g., increased temperature, bleeding, swelling, inability to urinate)
- Instruct to follow up in 3 to 5 days with health care provider

- Instruct to apply dressing with each diaper change or after urinating until healing is complete or until plastic ring falls off, as indicated
- Arrange for cultural accommodations

4th edition 2004; revised 2024

Background Evidence:

Hockenberry, M. J., Rodgers, C. C., & Wilson, D. (2022). *Wong's essentials of pediatric nursing.* Elsevier.

Labban, M., Menhem, Z., Bandali, T., Hneiny, L., & Zaghal, A. (2021). Pain control in neonatal male circumcision: A best evidence review. *Journal of Pediatric Urology, 17*(1), 3–8. https://doi.org/10.1016/j.jpurol.2020.09.017

Matson, S., & Smith, J. E. (2016). *Core curriculum for maternal-newborn nursing.* Elsevier.

Omole, F., Smith, W., & Carter-Wicker, K. (2020). Newborn circumcision techniques. *American Family Physician, 101*(11), 680–685.

Prabhakaran, S., Ljuhar, D., Coleman, R., & Nataraja, R. M. (2018). Circumcision in the pediatric patient: A review of indications, technique and complications. *Journal of Pediatric Child Health, 54*(12), 1299–1307. https://doi.org/10.1111/jpc.14206

C

Code Management 6140

Definition: Coordination of emergency measures to sustain life

Activities:

- Evaluate patient's responsiveness to determine appropriate action
- Call for help if no breathing or no normal breathing and no response
- Call a code according to agency standard when obtaining the automated external defibrillator (AED) or assuring that someone is obtaining the automated external defibrillator
- Assure patient's airway is open
- Perform cardiopulmonary resuscitation that focuses on chest compressions in adults and compressions with breathing efforts for children, as appropriate
- Deliver cardioversion or defibrillation as soon as possible
- Minimize the interval between stopping chest compressions and delivering a shock, if indicated
- Bring the code cart to the bedside
- Monitor the quality of CPR provided
- Attach the cardiac monitor and determine the rhythm, assuring defibrillations will not be interrupted
- Assure that someone is oxygenating the patient and assisting with intubation, as indicated
- Initiate an IV line and administer IV fluids, as indicated
- Ensure that someone is: (1) setting up medications; (2) delivering medications; (3) interpreting EKG and delivering cardioversion/defibrillation, as needed; and (4) documenting care
- Remind personnel of current Advanced Cardiac Life Support protocols, as appropriate
- Ensure that special resuscitation protocols (e.g., asthma, anaphylaxis, pregnancy, morbid obesity, pulmonary embolism, electrolyte imbalance, ingestion of toxic substances, trauma, accidental hypothermia, avalanche, drowning, electric shock or lightning strikes, percutaneous coronary interventions, cardiac tamponade, cardiac surgery) are instituted, when appropriate
- Offer family members and significant other(s) opportunities to be present during resuscitation when in the best interests of the patient
- Support family members who are present during resuscitation (i.e., ensure safe environment, provide explanations and commentary, allow appropriate communication with patient, continually assess needs, provide opportunities to reflect on resuscitation efforts after event)
- Ensure that someone is coordinating care of other patients on the nursing unit
- Terminate code by patient condition, as indicated
- Assure organized post cardiac arrest care (e.g., cardiopulmonary and neurological support, therapeutic hypothermia, tapering of inspired oxygen concentration to avoid harmful hyperoxia, avoidance of hyperventilation)
- Implement appropriate procedures for possible tissue and organ donation that are timely, effective, and supportive of the family members' and patient's desires
- Review actions after code to identify areas of strength and those which need to be improved
- Provide opportunities for team members to be involved in team debriefings or reflect on resuscitation efforts after event
- Perform emergency cart check per agency protocol

1st edition 1992; revised 2008, 2013

Background Evidence:

American Association of Critical Care Nurses. (2006). In J. G. Alspach (Ed.), *Core curriculum for critical care nursing* (6th ed.). Saunders.

Boucher, M. (2010). Family witnessed resuscitation. *Emergency Nurse, 18*(5), 10–14.

Carlson, K. (Ed.). (2009). *AACN Advanced critical care nursing.* Saunders Elsevier.

Field, J., Hazinski, M., Sayre, M., Chameides, L., Schexnayder, S., Hemphill, R., Samson, R. A., Kattwinkel, J., Berg, R. A., Bhanji, F., Cave, D. M., Jauch, E. C., Kudenchuk, P. J., Neumar, R. W., Peberdy, M. A., Perlman, J. M., Sinz, E., Travers, A. H., berg, M. D., Billi, J. E., & Hoek, T. (2010). Part 1: Executive summary: 2010 American Heart Association guidelines for cardiopulmonary resuscitation and emergency cardiovascular care. *Circulation, 122*(18 Suppl. 3), S640–S656.

Hazinski, M. F. (Ed.). (2010). *Highlights of the 2010 American Heart Association guidelines for CPR and ECC.* American Heart Association.

Urden, L., Stacy, K. M., & Lough, M. E. (2010). *Critical care nursing: Diagnosis and management* (6th ed.). Mosby Elsevier.

Wiegand, D. (Ed.). (2011). *AACN procedure manual for critical care* (6th ed.). Elsevier Saunders.

Cognitive Restructuring 4700

Definition: Use of therapeutic techniques designed to assist a person to alter distorted thought patterns and view self and the world more realistically

Activities:

- Introduce self and ensure comfort, privacy, and confidentiality
- Convey authenticity, warmth, genuineness, interest, and unconditional caring
- Determine purpose, goals, and agenda for session
- Mutually establish goals
- Develop and understand concerns, problems, and difficulties
- Determine how problems may interfere with daily life
- Identify what thoughts are associated with problem
- Determine how long problem has persisted
- Identify any pattern of events that may be associated with problem
- Assist in accepting that self-statements mediate emotional arousal
- Assist in understanding irrational self-statements cause inability to attain desirable behaviors
- Assist in identifying styles of dysfunctional thinking (e.g., polarized thinking, overgeneralization, magnification, personalization)
- Encourage identification and naming of painful emotions (e.g., anger, anxiety, hopelessness)

- Assist in identifying perceived stressors (e.g., situations, events, interactions with other people) that contributed to stress
- Assist to identify faulty interpretations about perceived stressors
- Assist in recognizing irrationality of certain beliefs compared with actual reality
- Assist in changing irrational self-statements to rational self-statements
- Assist in replacing faulty interpretations with more reality-based interpretations of stressful situations, events, interactions
- Apply therapeutic techniques and strategies to facilitate changing thought patterns (e.g., Socratic questioning, life event visualization, feeling focusing, summary and reframing, thought records, de-catastrophizing or "what if" technique, positive belief records)
- Make statements and ask questions that challenge perception and behavior, as appropriate
- Make statements that describe alternative way of looking at situation
- Assist to identify belief system that affects health status
- Use belief systems to see situation in a different way

- Reinforce learning and use of new thought patterns
- Evaluate for progress toward achieving desired goals
- Prepare for ending of therapeutic session

1st edition 1992; revised 2000, 2004, 2024

Background Evidence:

Chrétien, M., Giroux, I., Goulet, A., Jacques, C., & Bouchard, S. (2017). Cognitive restructuring of gambling-related thoughts: A systematic review. *Addictive Behaviors, 75*, 108–121.

Pardo Cebrián, R., & Calero Elvira, A. (2019). Applying cognitive restructuring in therapy: The clinical reality in Spain. *Psychotherapy Research, 29*(2), 198–212.

van Teffelen, M. W., Voncken, M. J., Peeters, F., Mollema, E. D., & Lobbestael, J. (2021). The efficacy of incorporating mental imagery in cognitive restructuring techniques on reducing hostility: A randomized controlled trial. *Journal of Behavior Therapy & Experimental Psychiatry, 73*, 101677. https://doi.org/10.1016/j.jbtep.2021.101677

Cognitive Stimulation   4720

Definition: Promotion of awareness and comprehension of surroundings by utilization of planned stimuli

Activities:

- Consult with family to establish patient's cognitive baseline
- Inform patient of recent nonthreatening news events
- Offer environmental stimulation through contact with varied personnel
- Present change gradually
- Provide a calendar
- Stimulate memory by repeating patient's last expressed thought
- Orient to time, place, and person
- Talk to patient
- Demonstrate caregiver sensitivity by responding promptly and appropriately to cues
- Stimulate development by engaging in activities to enhance achievement and learning by being attuned to the patent's needs
- Offer cognitive stimulation at work, such as training opportunities, cognitive richness to work content, opportunities for growth, and multitasking
- Encourage cognitive stimulation outside of work, such as reading or active participation in cultural and artistic activities
- Encourage the use of a multi-stimulation program (e.g., singing and listening to music, creative activities, exercise, conversation, social interactions, problem solving) to promote and protect cognitive capacity
- Ask for opinions and views rather than factual answers
- Provide planned sensory stimulation
- Use television, radio, or music as part of planned stimuli program
- Allow for rest periods
- Place familiar objects and photographs in patient's environment
- Use repetition to present new material
- Vary methods of presentation of material
- Use memory aids: checklists, schedules, and reminder notices
- Reinforce or repeat information

- Present information in small, concrete portions
- Ask patient to repeat information
- Use touch purposefully, as appropriate
- Provide verbal and written instructions

1st edition 1992; revised 2013

Background Evidence:

Albers, E. M., Riksen-Walraven, J. M., & Weerth, C. D. (2010). Developmental stimulation in child care centers contributes to young infants' *cognitive development. Infant Behavior and Development, 33*(4), 401–408.

Karatay, G., & Akkus, Y. (2011). The effectiveness of a stimulation program on cognitive capacity among individuals older than 60. *Western Journal of Nursing Research, 33*(1), 26–44.

Livingston, G., Johnston, K., Katona, C., Paton, J., & Lyketsos, C. G. (2005). Systematic review of psychological approaches to the management of neuropsychiatric symptoms of dementia. *American Journal of Psychiatry, 162*(11), 1996–2021.

Marquié, J. C., Duarte, L. R., Bessières, P., Dalm, C., Gentil, C., & Ruidavets, J. B. (2010). Higher mental stimulation at work is associated with improved cognitive functioning in both young and older workers. *Ergonomics, 53*(11), 1287–1301.

Niu, Y., Tan, J., Guan, J., Zhang, Z., & Wang, L. (2010). Cognitive stimulation therapy in the treatment of neuropsychiatric symptoms of Alzheimer's disease: A randomized controlled trial. *Clinical Rehabilitation, 24*(12), 1102–1111.

Pearson, G. (2006). Psychopharmacology. In W. K. Mohr (Ed.), *Psychiatric-mental health nursing* (6th ed., pp. 243–285). Lippincott Williams & Wilkins.

Spector, A., Orrell, M., & Woods, B. (2010). Cognitive stimulation therapy (CST): Effects on different areas of cognitive function for people with dementia. *International Journal of Geriatric Psychiatry, 25*(12), 1253–1258.

C

Collaboration Enhancement 7615

Definition: Improving cooperation between disciplines and health providers

Activities:

- Seek input and respect the contributions of others
- Build teams of approximately 5 to 9 members
- Design group work spaces that easily support 5 to 9 people with everyone having equal access to digital and analog information displays and being able to see each other eye to eye
- Ensure that work spaces have easy projection and teleconferencing capabilities
- Encourage group members to switch where they sit on a regular basis to build stronger networks
- Provide individual workstations for private focused work with visual eyesight to others and a place for a visitor to sit (e.g., bench)
- Provide a social space in which individuals can talk casually
- Enable workers to have choice and control of where they work by providing a range of settings
- Support programs of interdisciplinary education including interprofessional orientation days and social events, joint faculty appointments, and interdisciplinary coursework and clinic activities
- Provide web-based tools (e.g., calendar, agendas, committee assignments, appropriate forms and documents) to help workers coordinate and communicate
- Include the patient as a teammate, as appropriate
- Use communication tools (e.g., daily huddles; repeat back; Situation, Background, Assessment, Recommendation [SBAR]; opportunity for questions), as needed
- Continue dialogue of legal and ethical matters as they apply to the situation
- Address misconceptions and stereotypes among team members
- Use negotiation as a strategy for conflict resolution
- Value the enhanced benefits of the collaborative efforts of the team

7th edition 2018

Background Evidence:

Freshman, B., Rubino, L., & Chassiakos, Y. R. (Eds.). (2010). *Collaboration across the disciplines in health care.* Jones and Bartlett.

Interprofessional Education Collaborative Expert Panel. (2011). *Core competencies for interprofessional collaborative practice: Report of an expert panel.*

The Joint Commission. (2012). *Improving patient and worker safety: Opportunities for synergy, collaboration and innovation.*

MacDonald, M., Bally, J., Ferguson, L., Murray, B., Fowler-Kerry, S., & Anonson, J. (2010). Knowledge of the professional role of others: A key interprofessional competency. *Nurse Education in Practice, 10*(4), 238–242.

Steelcase WorkSpace Futures. (2010). How the workplace can improve collaboration. http://www.steelcase.com/content/uploads/2015/01/three sixty-collaboration-white-paper-v2.6.pdf

Comfort Management 6482

Definition: Establishing and maintaining optimal comfort

Activities:

- Determine goals for management of environment and optimum comfort
- Ease transition by warmly welcoming to new environment
- Give consideration to placement of persons in multiple-bedded rooms (i.e., roommates with similar environmental concerns when possible)
- Provide single room if preference and need for quiet and rest, if possible
- Provide prompt attention to call bells that should always be within reach
- Prevent unnecessary interruptions and allow for rest period
- Provide safe, clean, calm, and airy environment
- Provide choice whenever possible for social activities and visitation
- Determine sources of discomfort, such as damp dressings, positioning of tubing, constrictive dressings, wrinkled bed linens, and environmental irritants
- Adjust room temperature to that most comfortable for individual, if possible
- Provide or remove blankets to regulate temperature, as indicated
- Avoid unnecessary exposure, drafts, overheating, or chilling
- Adjust lighting to meet needs of activities, avoiding direct light in eyes
- Facilitate hygiene measures (e.g., wiping brow; applying skin creams; cleaning body, hair, and oral cavity)
- Position to facilitate comfort (e.g., using principles of body alignment, support with pillows, support joints during movement, splint over incisions, immobilize painful body part)
- Encourage non-pharmacological actions to increase comfort (e.g., music therapy, massage therapy)
- Encourage self-comforting strategies
- Monitor skin, especially over bony prominences, for signs of pressure or irritation
- Avoid exposing skin or mucous membranes to irritants (e.g., diarrheal stool, wound drainage)
- Provide relevant and useful educational resources concerning management of illnesses and injuries
- Document actions taken for comfort

1st edition 1992; revised 2008, 2024

Background Evidence:

Perry, A. G., Potter, P. A., Ostendorf, W. R., & LaPlante, N. (2021). *Clinical nursing skills and technique* (10th ed.). Mosby.

Wensley, C., Botti, M., McKillop, A., & Merry, A. F. (2020). Maximizing comfort: How do patients describe the care that matters? A two-stage qualitative descriptive study to develop a quality improvement framework for comfort-related care in inpatient settings. *BMJ Open, 10*(5), e033336.

Williams, P. (2020). *Basic geriatric nursing* (7th ed.). Elsevier.

You, W. Y., Yeh, T. P., Lee, K. C., & Ma, W. F. (2020). A preliminary study of the comfort in patients with leukemia staying in a positive pressure isolation room. *International Journal of Environmental Research, 17*(10), 3655.

Commendation   **4364**

Definition: Offering statements of praise and admiration to identify and emphasize the strengths and capabilities evident in the individual, family, or community

Activities:

- Recognize resourcefulness in coping with present situation
- Assist individuals to realize their personal strengths, potential, and capacity
- Demonstrate your valuing of individual or family
- Build collaborative relationship with individual or family
- Support and encourage learning
- Recognize individual's strength in modifying behavior to address the situation
- Provide positive feedback to encourage and sustain new behavior
- Acknowledge the capacity to live with chronic, long-term health issue or illness, as appropriate
- Congratulate one in achieving improved outcome
- Reinforce a behavior or outcome to increase the probability that it will be sustained
- Facilitate motivation to continue with improved behavioral changes to attain the main goal
- Apply strategies to reinforce learning and promote confidence and worth in learner
- Write up statements of praise and send to individual or other persons (e.g., supervisor, award program), as appropriate

Background Evidence:

Abualrub, R. F., & Al-Zaree, I. M. (2008). Job stress, recognition, job performance, and intention to stay at work among Jordanian hospital nurses. *Journal of Nursing Administration, 16*(3), 227–236.

Day, R. A., Paul, P., Williams, B., Smeltzer, S. C., & Bare, B. (2010). *Brunner and Suddarth's textbook of Canadian medical-surgical nursing* (2nd ed.). Lippincott Williams & Wilkins.

Kozier, B., Erb, G., Berman, A., Snyder, S. J., Bouchal, S. R., Hirst, S., Yiu, L., Stamler, L. L., & Buck, M. (2010). *Fundamentals of Canadian nursing: Concepts, process and practice* (2nd ed.). Toronto: Pearson Education Canada.

McElheran, N. G., & Harper-Jacques, S. R. (1994). Commendations: A resource intervention for clinical practice. *Clinical Nurse Specialist, 8*(1), 7–10.

Psychological Associates and DAISY Foundation. (2009). *Literature review on meaningful recognition in nursing.* Psychological Associates.

Stone, C. L., & Rowles, C. J. (2002). What rewards do clinical preceptors in nursing think are important? *Journal for Nurses in Staff Development, 18*(3), 162–166.

Tourangeau, A. E., & Cranley, L. A. (2006). Nurse intention to remain employed: Understanding and strengthening determinants. *Journal of Advanced Nursing, 55*(4), 497–509.

6th edition 2013

Communicable Disease Management   **8820**

Definition: Working with a community to decrease and manage the incidence and prevalence of contagious diseases

Activities:

- Analyze infection data routinely in healthcare settings and community to make evidence-based decisions
- Identify individuals who are potentially contagious
- Isolate potentially contagious individuals if indicated, quickly and appropriately
- Require use of standard precautions with all person-to-person contact
- Promote frequent handwashing or cleansing with antimicrobial hand sanitizer
- Promote use of personal protective equipment (PPE) where indicated
- Create triage areas in affected healthcare settings where isolation is possible, during known outbreaks
- Create specific isolation areas for affected individuals during known outbreaks
- Monitor at-risk populations for compliance with prevention and treatment regimen
- Ensure provision of strengthened forms of support, including social and emotional support, to prevent adverse effects when source isolation or other forms of constraints are in use
- Monitor adequate continuation of immunization in targeted populations
- Ensure community workers and at-risk health care workers receive relevant and up-to-date vaccinations
- Provide vaccine to targeted populations, as available
- Ensure regular educational programs related to benefits of vaccinations within community
- Monitor incidence of exposure to communicable diseases during known outbreak
- Encourage persons to avoid crowded settings during known outbreaks
- Provide information related to respiratory hygiene and cough etiquette
- Instruct persons to stay away from work or school when having active symptoms of infection
- Monitor sanitation
- Promote use of disinfectants in institutions and schools
- Monitor environmental factors that influence the transmission of communicable diseases
- Use available technological advancements to monitor communicable diseases in communities (e.g., wastewater-based epidemiology, water fingerprinting)
- Provide information about adequate preparation and storage of food, as needed
- Provide information about adequate control of vectors and animal reservoir hosts, as needed
- Inform the public regarding disease and activities associated with management, as needed

C

- Encourage proper prescribing and use of antibiotics to avoid superinfections
- Provide information about antibiotic use and need to finish complete dosage, as prescribed
- Promote access to adequate, regular health care treatment and health education related to prevention and treatment of communicable diseases and prevention of recurrence (e.g., safe sex practices, proper food handling, handwashing, avoidance of intravenous drug use)
- Promote harm-reduction services for persons who inject drugs, such as medication-assisted treatment and syringe service programs (SSPs), to reduce risk of blood borne infectious disease acquisition (e.g., hepatitis C, HIV)
- Improve surveillance systems for communicable diseases, as needed
- Promote legislation that ensures appropriate monitoring and treatment for communicable diseases
- Report activities to appropriate agencies, as required
- Ensure regular interactions with media to keep public properly informed of risks and proper actions to avoid spread of communicable diseases

3rd edition 2000, revised 2024

Background Evidence:

Fraser, H., Vellozzi, C., Hoerger, T., Evans, J., Kral, A., Havens, J., Young, A., Stone, J., Handanagic, S., Hariri, S., Barbosa, C., Hickman, M., Leib, A., Martin, N., Nerlander, L., Raymond, H., Page, K., Zibbell, J., Ward, J., & Vickerman, P. (2019). Scaling up hepatitis C prevention and treatment interventions for achieving elimination in the United States. *American Journal of Epidemiology*, 188(8), 1539–1551. https://doi.org/10.1093/aje/kwz097

Gammon, J., & Hunt, J. (2018). Source isolation and patient wellbeing in healthcare settings. *British Journal of Nursing*, 27(2), 88–91. https://doi.org/10.12968/bjon.2018.27.2.88

Hawker, J., Begg, N., Reintjes, R., Ekdahl, K., Edeghere, O., & van Steenbergen, J. (2019). *Communicable disease control and health protection handbook*. Wiley Blackwell.

Rebmann, T., & Carrico, R. (2017). Consistent infection prevention: Vital during routine and emerging infectious diseases care. *OJIN: The Online Journal of Issues in Nursing*, 22(1). https://doi.org/10.3912/OJIN.Vol22No01Man01. Manuscript 1.

Sims, N., & Kasprzyk-Hordern, B. (2020). Future perspectives of wastewater-based epidemiology: Monitoring infectious disease spread and resistance to the community level. *Environment International*, 139, 105689.

Sakamoto, S., Terashita, D., & Balter, S. (2020). Liaison public health nurse project: Innovative public health approach to combat infectious disease in hospitals. *Journal of Public Health Management and Practice*, 26(6), 557–561. https://doi.org/10.1097/PHH.0000000000001068

Communication Enhancement: Hearing Deficit   4974

Definition: Use of strategies augmenting communication capabilities for a person with diminished hearing

Activities:

- Perform or arrange for routine hearing assessments and screenings
- Monitor for excessive accumulation of cerumen
- Instruct patient not to use foreign objects smaller than patient's fingertip (e.g., cotton-tipped applicators, bobby pins, toothpicks, and other sharp objects) for cerumen removal
- Remove excessive cerumen with twisted end of washcloth while pulling down the auricle
- Consider ear irrigation for the removal of excessive cerumen if watchful waiting, manual removal, and ceruminolytic agents are ineffective
- Note and document patient's preferred method of communication (e.g., verbal, written, lip reading, or American Sign Language) in plan of care
- Gain patient's attention before speaking (e.g., obtain attention through touch)
- Avoid noisy backgrounds when communicating
- Avoid communicating more than 2 to 3 feet from patient
- Use gestures, when necessary
- Listen attentively, allowing patient adequate time to process communication and respond
- Refrain from shouting at patient
- Facilitate lip reading by facing patient directly in good lighting
- Ask patient to suggest strategies for improved communication (e.g., speaking toward better ear and moving to well-lit area)
- Face the patient directly, establishing eye contact, and avoid turning away midsentence
- Simplify language (i.e., do not use slang and use short, simple sentences), as appropriate
- Use a lower, deeper voice when speaking
- Avoid "baby talk" and exaggerated expressions

- Avoid smoking, chewing food or gum, and covering mouth when speaking
- Verify what was said or written using patient's response before continuing
- Facilitate use of hearing aids and assistive listening devices (e.g., phone amplifier, hardwire device, personal frequency modulation, and computers)
- Remove and insert hearing aid properly
- Remove hearing aid battery when hearing aid is not in use for several days
- Clean detachable earmold using a mild soapy solution, removing moisture or debris with soft cloth, and avoiding isopropyl alcohol, solvents, and oil
- Clean nondetachable earmold using a damp cloth, removing moisture or debris with soft cloth, and avoiding isopropyl alcohol, solvents, and oil
- Check hearing aid batteries routinely, replacing, when necessary
- Refer to manufacturer's guidelines on proper use of, care for, and maintenance of hearing aids and assistive listening devices
- Instruct patient, nursing personnel, and family on use of, care for, and maintenance of hearing aids and assistive listening devices
- Assist patient or family in acquiring hearing aid and assistive listening device
- Refer to primary care provider or specialist for evaluation, treatment, and hearing rehabilitation

1st edition 1992; revised 2000, 2013

Background Evidence:

Adams-Wendling, L., & Pimple, C. (2008). Nursing management of hearing impairment in nursing facility residents [S. Adams & M. G. Titler, Eds.]. *Journal of Gerontological Nursing*, 34(11), 9–17.

Lindblade, D., & McDonald, M. (1995). Removing communication barriers for the hearing-impaired elderly. *MedSurg Nursing, 4*(5), 377–385.

Maas, M., Buckwalter, K., Hardy, M., Tripp-Reimer, T., Titler, M., & Specht, J. (Eds.). (2001). *Nursing care of older adults: Diagnoses, outcomes, & interventions,* (pp. 485). Mosby.

Smeltzer, S. C., & Bare, B. G. (2004). (10th ed.) *Brunner & Suddarth's textbook of medical surgical nursing* (Vol. 2). Lippincott Williams & Wilkins.

Communication Enhancement: Speech Deficit   4976

Definition: Use of strategies augmenting communication capabilities for a person with impaired speech

Activities:

- Monitor speech speed, pressure, pace, quantity, volume, and diction
- Monitor cognitive, anatomical, and physiological processes associated with speech capabilities (e.g., memory, hearing, and language)
- Instruct patient or family on cognitive, anatomical, and physiological processes involved in speech capabilities
- Monitor patient for frustration, anger, depression, or other responses to impaired speech capabilities
- Recognize emotional and physical behaviors as forms of communication
- Provide alternative methods of speech communication (e.g., writing tablet, flash cards, eye blinking, communication board with pictures and letters, hand signals or other gestures, and computer)
- Provide alternative methods of writing or reading, as appropriate
- Adjust communication style to meet needs of client (i.e., stand in front of patient when speaking; listen attentively; present one idea or thought at a time; speak slowly but avoid shouting; use written communication; or solicit family's assistance in understanding patient's speech)
- Maintain structured environment and routines (i.e., ensure consistent daily schedules; provide frequent reminders; and provide calendars and other environmental cues)
- Modify environment to minimize excess noise and decrease emotional distress (i.e., limit visitors and excessive equipment noise)
- Ensure call light is within reach and central call light system is marked to indicate patient cannot speak
- Repeat what patient said to ensure accuracy
- Instruct patient to speak slowly
- Phrase questions so patient can answer using a simple "yes" or "no," being aware that patient with expressive aphasia may provide automatic responses that are incorrect
- Collaborate with family and speech language pathologist or therapist to develop a plan for effective communication
- Provide one-way valve for patient with tracheostomy, replacing need for finger occlusion over tube
- Instruct patient or family on use of speech aids after laryngectomy (e.g., esophageal speech, electrolarynges, tracheoesophageal fistulas)
- Allow patient to hear spoken language frequently, as appropriate
- Provide positive reinforcement, as appropriate
- Use interpreter, as necessary
- Refer patient to community support systems (e.g., The International Association of Laryngectomees and American Cancer Society)
- Provide referral to speech language pathologist or therapist
- Coordinate rehabilitation team activities

2nd edition 1996; revised 2013

Background Evidence:

Craven, R., & Hirnle, C. (2009). Cognitive processes. In *Fundamentals of nursing: Human health and function,* (pp. 1237–1268) (6th ed.). Lippincott Williams & Wilkins.

Ignatavicius, D. D., & Workman, M. L. (2010). *Medical-surgical nursing: Patient-centered collaborative care* (6th ed.). Saunders Elsevier.

Kelly, H., Brady, M. C., & Enderby, P. (2010). Speech and language therapy for aphasia following stroke. *Cochrane Database of Systematic Reviews, 2010*(5). https://doi.org/10.1002/14651858.CD000425.pub2

Law, J., Garrett, Z., & Nye, C. (2003). Speech and language therapy interventions for children with primary speech and language delay or disorder. *Cochrane Database of Systematic Reviews, 2003*(3). https://doi.org/10.1002/14651858.CD004110

Communication Enhancement: Visual Deficit   4978

Definition: Use of strategies augmenting communication capabilities for a person with diminished vision

Activities:

- Perform or arrange for routine vision assessments and screenings
- Monitor functional implications of diminished vision (e.g., risk of injury, depression, anxiety, and ability to perform activities of daily living and valued activities)
- Identify yourself when entering the patient's space
- Assist patient in enhancing stimulation of other senses (e.g., savoring aroma, taste, and texture of food)
- Ensure that patient's eyeglasses or contact lens have current prescription, are cleaned, and stored properly when not in use
- Provide adequate room lighting
- Minimize glare (i.e., offer sunglasses or draw window covering)
- Provide literature with large print
- Describe environment to patient
- Maintain uncluttered environment
- Avoid rearranging items in patient's environment without notifying patient
- Provide daily living aids (e.g., clock and telephone with large numbers)
- Apply labels to distinguish frequently used items (i.e., color-code dials on appliances, mark medication bottles using high-contrasting colors or rubber bands, and safety-pin labels on similar-colored clothing)

C

- Use bright, contrasting colors in environment
- Read mail, newspaper, and other pertinent information to patient
- Identify items on food tray in relation to numbers on a clock
- Fold paper money in different ways for easy identification
- Provide magnifying devices (e.g., handheld, stand, and video magnifier)
- Provide sight substitutes (e.g., Braille materials, audio books, talking watches, and tactile markers)
- Assist parents, family, educators, and caretakers involved with a child with diminished vision in meeting informational needs (e.g., how to teach child, anticipatory guidance, and developmental considerations)
- Instruct parents, family, educators, and caretakers to recognize and respond to nontraditional expressive forms of communication (e.g., movements and facial expressions)
- Assist parents, family, educators, and caretakers in developing reliable, functional communication systems (e.g., microswitches or speech-output devices)
- Assist patient or family in identifying available resources for vision rehabilitation
- Provide referral for the patient in need of surgical or other medical treatment
- Provide referral for supportive services (e.g., social, occupational, and psychological)

1st edition 1992; revised 2013

Background Evidence:

American Academy of Ophthalmology Vision Rehabilitation Committee. (2007). *Preferred practice pattern guidelines: Vision rehabilitation for adults.*

Craven, R., & Hirnle, C. (2009). *Fundamentals of nursing: Human health and function* (6th ed.). Lippincott Williams & Wilkins.

Maas, M., Buckwalter, K., Hardy, M., Tripp-Reimer, T., Titler, M., & Specht, J. (Eds.). (2001). *Nursing care of older adults: Diagnoses, outcomes, & interventions* (pp. 483–485). Mosby.

Parker, A. T., Grimmett, E. S., & Summers, S. (2008). Evidence-based communication practices for children with visual impairments and additional disabilities: An examination of single-subject design studies. *Journal of Visual Impairment & Blindness, 102*(9), 540–552.

Community Disaster Preparedness 8840

Definition: Preparing for an effective response to a large-scale disaster

Activities:

- Identify potential types of disasters for area (e.g., industrial, environmental)
- Identify all community medical and social agency resources available to respond to disasters
- Work with other agencies in planning for disasters (e.g., EMS services, local, state, and government agencies)
- Build disaster leadership team with prearranged roles, adequate availability, and designated command center
- Develop plans for specific types of disasters (e.g., multiple-casualty incident, bomb, tornado, hurricane, flood, chemical spill), as appropriate
- Develop disaster notification network to alert personnel
- Develop triage procedures
- Identify rendezvous site for assisting disaster victims
- Identify alternate rendezvous sites for health care personnel
- Ensure adequate personnel
- Establish housing for personnel to remain on site if needed
- Know where disaster equipment and supplies are stored
- Develop internal (e.g., place of business, home) and external (e.g., city, county, state) evacuation routes for various disaster scenarios (e.g., earthquake, hurricane, flood, terrorist)
- Encourage regular review of internal and external evacuation routes throughout community
- Encourage posting of evacuation plans in all buildings
- Create shelters for displaced persons (e.g., bomb shelter, flood shelter) and signage to locate shelters
- Conduct periodic equipment checks
- Check and restock shelter supplies routinely
- Develop community preparations for disaster events
- Assist to prepare shelters and emergency aid stations
- Educate community members on safety, self-help, location of shelters, evacuation routes, and first aid measures
- Encourage community members to have personal preparedness plan (e.g., emergency telephone numbers, battery-operated radio, working flashlight, first aid kit, medical information, health care provider information, persons to be notified in an emergency, personal medications)
- Educate health care personnel on disaster plans on routine basis
- Conduct mock disaster drills annually or as appropriate
- Evaluate performance of disaster personnel after disaster or mock disaster drill
- Identify mechanism for debriefing for health care personnel after disaster
- Sensitize health care personnel to potential psychological effects (e.g., depression, sadness, fear, anger, phobias, guilt, irritability, anxiety) of disaster
- Identify post-disaster referral resources (e.g., rehabilitation, convalescence, counseling)
- Identify post-disaster needs (e.g., ongoing disaster-related health care needs, collection of epidemiological data, assessment of cause of disaster, steps for prevention of reoccurrence)
- Update disaster plans, as needed

3rd edition 2000; revised 2024

Background Evidence:

Federal Emergency Management Agency (FEMA). (2021). *Developing and maintaining emergency operations plans: Comprehensive preparedness guide (CPG)* 101 (ver. 3). https://www.fema.gov/sites/default/files/documents/fema_cpg-101-v3-developing-maintaining-eops.pdf

Smith, S. F., Duell, D. J., Martin, B. C., Aebersold, M. L., & Gonzales, L. (2017). *Clinical nursing skills: Basic to advanced skills* (9th ed.). Pearson.

United States Department of Health and Human Services, Center for Disease Control. (2021, January 25). Public health emergency preparedness and response capabilities: National standards for state, local, tribal, and territorial public health. https://www.cdc.gov/cpr/readiness/capabilities.htm

Veenema, T. G. (2019). *Disaster nursing and emergency preparedness.* (4th ed.) Springer.

Community Health Advocacy   8510

Definition: Developing public support to change the ideas and attitudes about specific health care matters

Activities:
- Define the objectives of the advocacy and the specific community to be assisted
- Assist community members to navigate the health care system (e.g., to access low-cost or free care, to solve billing issues, to understand patient rights
- Provide access to translation services, when needed
- Work with lay community health workers and community leaders to identify needs and provide services
- Assist community leaders to conduct a needs assessment whereby needs can be prioritized and activities to be identified
- Understand the cultural health beliefs and practices of the identified community members
- Help to mobilize resources in a community that will assist in achieving goals
- Seek consultation, training, and support for community advocacy efforts to build coalitions
- Participate in media campaigns to increase public awareness
- Attend school board meetings to share the negative effect of not having enough school nurses to monitor students' health statuses
- Attend and speak at public forums about the positive effect of proposed health care services, projects, and legislation
- Provide appropriate health care information and education to the public and legislators
- Assist in the introduction and passage of health care legislation by finding sponsors and persuading potential cosponsors to sign on with their support
- Use real-life examples from clinical practice to illustrate the needs of patients and the outcomes of public policy on patient care
- Identify obstacles that prevent success and implement strategies to reduce barriers

7th edition 2018

Background Evidence:

Center for Healthy Communities. (2015). *Community health advocate program.* https://medicine.wright.edu/center-for-healthy-communities/community-health-advocate-program

Loue, S. (2006). Community health advocacy. *Journal of Epidemiology & Community Health, 60*(6), 458–463.

Maryland, M. A., & Gonzalez, R. I. (2012). Patient advocacy in the community and legislative arena. *Online Journal of Issues in Nursing, 17*(1). https://doi.org/10.3912/OJIN.Vol12N001Man02

Porter-O'Grady, T., & Malloch, K. (2011). *Quantum leadership advancing innovation transforming healthcare* (3rd ed.). Jones & Bartlett Learning.

Community Health Development   8500

Definition: Assisting members of a community to identify health concerns, mobilize resources, and implement solutions

Activities:
- Identify health concerns, strengths, and priorities with community partners
- Provide opportunities for participation by members in community
- Assist in raising awareness of health problems and concerns
- Dialogue with community to clarify health concern priorities
- Collaboratively develop strategic initiatives with community members
- Facilitate implementation and revision of community plans
- Assist community members with resource development and procurement
- Enhance community support networks
- Develop potential community leaders
- Maintain open communication with community members and agencies
- Strengthen contacts between groups to discuss common and competing interests
- Provide organizational framework to enhance communication and negotiation skills
- Cultivate environment that provides safe expressions of views
- Develop strategies for managing conflict
- Unify community members behind common mission
- Ensure that community members maintain control of decision making
- Build commitment to community by demonstrating how participation will influence individual lives and improve outcomes
- Develop mechanisms for involvement in local, state, and national activities related to community health concerns
- Facilitate access to community health centers with free to low-cost health care provision
- Provide educational programs related to community health needs

3rd edition 2000; revised 2024

Background Evidence:

Davis, S. M., Jones, A., Jaynes, M. E., Woodrum, K. N., Canaday, M., Allen, L., & Mallow, J. A. (2020). Designing a multifaceted telehealth intervention for a rural population using a model for developing complex interventions in nursing. *BMC Nursing, 19*(1), 1–9. https://doi.org/10.1186/s12912-020-0400-9

Han, E., Quek, R. Y. C., Tan, S. M., Singh, S. R., Shiraz, F., Gea-Sánchez, M., & Legido-Quigley, H. (2019). The role of community-based nursing interventions in improving outcomes for individuals with cardiovascular disease: A systematic review. *International Journal of Nursing Studies, 100*, 103415. https://doi.org/10.1016/j.ijnurstu.2019.103415

Layton, H., Bendo, D., Amani, B., Bieling, P. J., & Van Lieshout, R. J. (2020). Public health nurses' experiences learning and delivering a group cognitive behavioral therapy intervention for postpartum depression. *Public Health Nursing, 37*(6), 863–870. https://doi.org/10.1111/phn.12807

Macduff, C., Marie Rafferty, A., Prendiville, A., Currie, K., Castro-Sanchez, E., King, C., Carvalho, F., & Iedema, R. (2020). Fostering nursing innovation to prevent and control antimicrobial resistance using approaches from the arts and humanities. *Journal of Research in Nursing, 25*(3), 189–207. https://doi.org/10.1177/1744987120914718

C

Palm, R., & Hochmuth, A. (2020). What works, for whom and under what circumstances? Using realist methodology to evaluate complex interventions in nursing: A scoping review. *International Journal of Nursing Studies, 109,* 103601. https://doi.org/10.1016/j.ijnurstu.2020.103601

Nies, M. A., & McEwan, M. (2022). *Community and Public Health Nursing: Promoting the health of populations* (7th ed.). Elsevier.

Stanhope, M., & Lancaster, J. (2022). *Foundations for population health in Community/Public Health Nursing* (5th ed.). Elsevier.

C

Competency Management 7850

Definition: Developing, enriching, and monitoring knowledge and skill level

Activities:
- Identify learning needs (e.g., new or change in policy and procedures, transition to practice, equipment)
- Identify learner characteristics (e.g., literacy, language, educational background, previous experience, age, motivation, attitude)
- Identify performance problems (e.g., knowledge deficit, skill deficit, motivational deficit), as appropriate
- Identify instructional goals, objectives, and learning activities
- Identify resources to support instruction (e.g., expert consultation, learning materials, time, fiscal resources)
- Develop instructional content
- Design methods of pre- and post-assessment
- Provide instructional program (e.g., self-directed learning packets, classroom, online, simulation)
- Evaluate effectiveness of instruction
- Provide feedback on results of staff development instruction to appropriate individuals
- Determine frequency of knowledge and skill evaluation
- Provide financial assistance and time off to attend educational programs as required by job

Background Evidence:

Barton, G., Bruce, A., & Schreiber, R. (2018). Teaching nurses teamwork: Integrative review of competency-based team training in nursing education. *Nurse Education in Practice, 32,* 129–137. https://doi.org/10.1016/j.nepr.2017.11.019

Chen, T., Hsiao, Chia-Chi Hsiao, Tsui-Ping Chu, Chen, S., Mei-Nan, Liao, & Chang-Chiao, H. (2021). Exploring core competencies of clinical nurse preceptors: A nominal group technique study. *Nurse Education in Practice, 56,* 03200. https://doi.org/10.1016/j.nepr.2021.103200

Konrad, S., Fitzgerald, A., & Deckers, C. (2021). Nursing fundamentals – supporting clinical competency online during the COVID-19 pandemic. *Teaching and Learning in Nursing: Official Journal of the National Organization for Associate Degree Nursing, 16*(1), 53–56. https://doi.org/10.1016/j.teln.2020.07.005

Potter, P. A., Perry, A. G., Stockert, P. A., & Hall, A. M. (2021). *Fundamentals of nursing* (10th ed.). Elsevier.

Rees, S., Farley, H., & Moloney, C. (2021). How registered nurses balance limited resources in order to maintain competence: a grounded theory study. *BMC Nursing, 20*(1), 1–10. https://doi.org/10.1186/s12912-021-00672-6

Song, Y., & McCreary, L. L. (2020). New graduate nurses' self-assessed competencies: An integrative review. *Nurse Education in Practice, 45,* 102801. https://doi.org/10.1016/j.nepr.2020.102801

3rd edition 2000; revised 2024

Conflict Mediation 5020

Definition: Facilitation of constructive dialogue between opposing parties to resolve disputes in a mutually acceptable manner

Activities:
- Provide private, neutral setting for conversation
- Allow parties to voice personal concerns
- Offer guidance through process
- Create and maintain non-threatening environment
- Maintain neutrality throughout process
- Employ variety of communication techniques (e.g., active listening, establish common ground, clarify meaning, reframing, paraphrasing, reflecting)
- Facilitate defining issues
- Assist parties to identify possible solutions to issues
- Facilitate search for acceptable outcomes
- Support efforts of participants to foster resolution
- Monitor mediation process

Background Evidence:

American Psychiatric Nurses Association. (2014). *Psychiatric-mental health nursing: Scope and standards of practice* (2nd ed.).

Benedikt, A., Susło, R., Paplicki, M., & Drobnik, J. (2020). Mediation as an alternative method of conflict resolution: A practical approach. *Family Medicine & Primary Care Review, 22*(3), 235–239. https://doi.org/10.5114/fmpcr.2020.98252

Keltner, N. L., & Steele, D. (2019). *Psychiatric nursing* (8th ed.). Elsevier.

Rebar, C. R., Gersch, C., & Heimgartner, N. M. (2020). *Psychiatric nursing made incredibly easy* (3rd ed.). Wolters Kluwer.

Sbordoni, E. C., Madaloni, P. N., Oliveria, G. S., Fogliano, R. R. F., Neves, V. R., & Balsanelli, A. P. (2020). Strategies used by nurses for conflict mediation. *Revista Brazileiria Enfermagen, 73*(suppl 5), e20190894. https://doi.org/10.1590/0034-7167-2019-0894

Varcarolis, E. M., & Fosbre, C. D. (2021). *Essentials of psychiatric-mental health nursing.* (4th ed.). Elsevier.

3rd edition 2000; revised 2024

Constipation Management 0450

Definition: Prevention and alleviation of infrequent bowel movements

Activities:
- Review health history including diagnoses, surgeries, and bowel habits
- Identify factors that may cause or contribute to constipation (e.g., medications, exercise, sleep, stress, diet)
- Monitor for signs and symptoms of constipation (e.g., bloating, pain, nausea, absent bowel sounds)
- Monitor for signs and symptoms of impaction
- Monitor bowel movements, including frequency, consistency, shape, volume, and color, as appropriate
- Consult with health care provider about frequency of bowel movements
- Explain etiology of problem and rationale for care
- Institute toileting schedule, as appropriate
- Use abdominal massage, as tolerated
- Remove fecal impaction manually, if necessary
- Inform of procedure for manual removal of stool, if necessary
- Administer enema or irrigation, as appropriate
- Weigh regularly
- Encourage increased fluid intake, unless contraindicated
- Evaluate medication profile for gastrointestinal side effects
- Instruct to record color, volume, frequency, and consistency of stools
- Instruct on how to keep a food diary
- Instruct on high-fiber diet, as appropriate
- Consult dietitian, as needed
- Instruct on appropriate use of laxatives, stool softeners, and enemas
- Instruct on importance of diet, exercise, fluid intake, and sleep
- Instruct about time frame for resolution of constipation
- Use teach-back to ensure understanding

1st edition 1992; revised 2000, 2004, 2024

Background Evidence:
Berman, A., Snyder, S. J., & Frandsen, G. (2018). *Kozier and Erb's fundamentals of nursing: Concepts, process and practice.* (10th ed.). Pearson.

Choi, Y. I., Kim, K. O., Chung, J. W., Kwon, K. A., Kim, Y. J., Kim, J. H., & Park, D. K. (2021). Effects of automatic abdominal massage device in treatment of chronic constipation patients: A prospective study. *Digestive Diseases and Sciences, 66*(9), 3105–3112. https://doi.org/10.1007/s10620-020-06626-3

Cochrane, D. J. (2021). Care planning, diagnosis and management in paediatric functional constipation. *The New Zealand Medical Journal, 134*(1536), 113–143.

Craven, R.F., Hirnle, C.J., & Henshaw, C.J. (2021). *Fundamentals of nursing: Human health and function* (8th ed.). Wolters-Kluwer.

Potter, P. A., Perry, A. G., Stockert, P. A., & Hall, A. M. (2021). *Fundamentals of nursing* (10th ed.). Elsevier.

Robertson, J., Baines, S., Emerson, E., & Hatton, C. (2018). Constipation management in people with intellectual disability: A systematic review. *Journal of Applied Research in Intellectual Disabilities, 31*(5), 709–724. https://doi.org/10.1111/jar.12426

Rodriguez, G., Muter, P., Inglese, G., Goldstine, J. V., & Neil, N. (2021). Evolving evidence supporting use of rectal irrigation in the management of bowel dysfunction: An integrative literature review. *Journal of Wound, Ostomy, and Continence Nursing: Official Publication of The Wound, Ostomy and Continence Nurses Society, 48*(6), 553–559. https://doi.org/10.1097/WON.0000000000000816

Trads, M., Deutch, S. R., & Pedersen, P. U. (2018). Supporting patients in reducing postoperative constipation: Fundamental nursing care – a quasi-experimental study. *Scandinavian Journal of Caring Sciences, 32*(2), 824–832. https://doi.org/10.1111/scs.12513

Wang, Q.-S., Liu, Y., Zou, X.-N., Ma, Y.-L., & Liu, G.-L. (2020). Evaluating the efficacy of massage intervention for the treatment of poststroke constipation: A meta-analysis. *Evidence-Based Complementary & Alternative Medicine (ECAM), 2020,* 1–8. https://doi.org/10.1155/2020/8934751

Williams, P. (2020). *Basic geriatric nursing* (7th ed.). Elsevier.

Consultation 7910

Definition: Using expert knowledge to enable individuals, families, groups, or agencies to achieve identified goals

Activities:
- Identify the purpose for consultation
- Determine preferred communication method (e.g., in person, telephone, video, web-based)
- Consider culture, ethnicity, and context when developing consultative relationships
- Collect data to identify nature of problem
- Identify and clarify expectations of all parties involved
- Identify accountability structure
- Determine appropriate model of consultation to be used (e.g., purchase of expertise model, process consultation model)
- Identify fee expectations, as appropriate
- Mutually identify desired outcomes aimed to solve problem
- Develop written contract to define agreement and avoid misunderstandings
- Promote progress with self-direction and responsibility
- Provide expert knowledge for those seeking help
- Involve those who are seeking help throughout consulting process
- Develop plan of agreed upon actions and strategies designed to achieve desired outcomes
- Respond professionally to acceptance or rejection of ideas
- Obtain commitment from decision makers to carry out agreed-upon actions
- Prepare final report of recommendations

3rd edition 2000; revised 2024

Background Evidence:
Arvelos Mendes, D. I., & Clemente Ferrito, C. R. (2021). Preoperative nursing consultations: Implementation and evaluation. *Revista de Enfermagem Referência, 8,* 1–8. https://doi.org/10.12707/RV20216

da Silva Emiliano, M., da Costa Lindolpho, M., Cavalcanti Valente, G. S., Marinho Chrizóstimo, M., Chaves Sá, S. P., & Moraes da Rocha, I. da C. (2017).

Perception of nursing consultation by elderly people and their caregivers. *Journal of Nursing UFPE / Revista de Enfermagem UFPE*, 11(5), 1791–1797. https://doi.org/10.5205/reuol.11077-98857-1-SM.1105201706

de Castro Júnior, A. R., de Abreu, L. D. P., de Lima, L. L., de Araújo, A. F., Martins Torres, R. A., & Ferreira da Silva, M. R. (2019). Nursing consultation in the outpatient care of youths. *Journal of Nursing UFPE / Revista de Enfermagem UFPE*, 13(4), 1157–1166. https://doi.org/10.5205/1981-8963-v13i04a239115p1157-1166-2019

Elwyn, G., Durand, M. A., Song, J., Aarts, J., Barr, P. J., Berger, Z., Cochran, N., Frosch, D., Galasiński, D., Gulbrandsen, P., Han, P., Härter, M., Kinnersley, P., Lloyd, A., Mishra, M., Perestelo-Perez, L., Scholl, I., Tomori, K., Trevena, L., Witteman, H. O., & Van der Weijden, T. (2017). A three-talk model for shared decision making: Multistage consultation process. *British Medical Association (Clinical Research ed.)*, 359, j4891.

Gomes da Rocha, C. G., Buss Heidemann, I. T. S., Fernandes Rumor, P. C., Oliveira Antonini, F., Kuntz Durand, M., & Bitencourt Magagnin, A. (2019). Social determinants of health in prenatal nursing consultation. *Journal of Nursing UFPE / Revista de Enfermagem UFPE*, 13, 944–950. https://doi.org/10.5205/1981-8963.2019.241571

Vasconcelos Sobral, M., Mendes de Paula Pessoa, V., Sampaio Florêncio, R., Alves Braga Solon, A., de Castro Bento, J., Ribeiro Feitosa Cestari, V., & de Menezes, L. (2018). Essential elements of the child and adolescent nursing consultation. *Journal of Nursing UFPE / Revista de Enfermagem UFPE*, 12(12), 3464–3475.

Contact Lens Care 1620

Definition: Assisting patient in the proper use of contact lenses

Activities:
- Monitor eyes and surrounding area for open lesions and ecchymosis
- Determine patient's understanding of required lens care
- Determine patient's physical and emotional capability to learn and perform required lens care
- Instruct patient to perform hand hygiene before touching lenses
- Instruct patient on proper care of contact lenses depending on type (e.g., hard or soft)
- Instruct patient to remove lenses at appropriate interval (e.g., remove daily wear lenses at night and do not wear disposable lenses more than once)
- Instruct patient wearing extended-wear contacts of increased risks (e.g., corneal ulcers and infection-caused eruptions)
- Instruct patient wearing hard contacts of increased risks (e.g., corneal edema and corneal abrasions)
- Instruct patient on symptoms to report to health care professional (e.g., eye and conjunctiva redness, discomfort or pain, excessive tearing, and visual changes)
- Instruct patient to use recommended solutions to clean, moisten, rinse, and disinfect lenses
- Instruct patient to rub and rinse lenses with recommended solution before and after storage
- Instruct patient on importance of monitoring for and discontinuing use of recalled contact lens care products
- Instruct patient not to use saliva, tap water, or sterile saline found in health care agencies for rinsing or storing lenses
- Instruct patient to avoid exposing eyes to tap water, swimming pool water, or spa water when wearing lenses
- Instruct patient to store lenses in lens container with recommended solution
- Instruct on care of lens container (e.g., clean daily, leave open to air, and replace regularly)
- Instruct patient how to examine lenses for damage
- Instruct the patient who wears eye cosmetics to use caution in their selection and application (i.e., choose cosmetics without irritating properties and apply before lens insertion)
- Instruct patient to avoid exposure to or use of damaging or irritating environmental contaminants (e.g., dust, smoke, soaps, lotions, creams, and sprays)
- Instruct patient to carry appropriate identification on type and care for lenses
- Provide lens care for the patient unable to do so for self (e.g., removal, cleaning, storing, and insertion)
- Make referral to eye specialist, as appropriate

1st edition 1992; revised 2013

Background Evidence:

Craven, R. F., & Hirnle, C. J. (2009). Self-care and hygiene. In *Fundamentals of nursing: Human health and function* (pp. 703–755) (6th ed.). Lippincott Williams & Wilkins.

Craven, R. F., & Hirnle, C. J. (2009). Sensory perception. In *Fundamentals of nursing: Human health and function* (pp. 1216–1236) (6th ed.). Lippincott Williams & Wilkins.

Smith, S. F., Duell, D. J., & Martin, B. C. (2008). Personal hygiene. In *Clinical nursing skills: Basic to advanced skills* (pp. 208–248) (7th ed.). Pearson: Prentice Hall.

Sweeney, D., Holden, B., Evans, K., Ng, V., & Cho, P. (2009). Best practice contact lens care: A review of the Asia Pacific Contact Lens Care Summit. *Clinical & Experimental Optometry*, 92(2), 78–89.

Workman, M. L. (2010). Care of patients with eye and vision problems. In D. D. Ignatavicius & M. L. Workman (Eds.), *Medical-surgical nursing: Patient-centered collaborative care* (6th ed., pp. 1084–1108). Saunders Elsevier.

Controlled Substance Checking 7620

Definition: Promoting appropriate use and maintaining security of controlled substances

Activities:
- Account for access to controlled substances at all times
- Follow agency protocol for dispensing and administering controlled substances
- Count all controlled substances with an RN on opposite shift
- Inspect packaging of controlled substances for signs of tampering
- Report discrepancies immediately, per agency policy
- Follow agency protocol for resolving discrepancies
- Lock controlled substances cabinet after count is finished

- Document accuracy of count on appropriate form
- Count controlled substances received from pharmacy
- Return controlled substances not in routine use to pharmacy
- Document wasting of controlled substances
- Keep abreast of federal and state regulations regarding the use of controlled substances
- Monitor for evidence of misadministration or diversion of controlled substances (e.g., provider arriving early, staying late, coming to work on day off; volunteering to give medication to other's patients; frequent bathroom breaks; patients reporting unrelieved pain despite adequate prescription of pain medication)
- Review computer reports, when available, to identify outliers regarding individual practitioner's use of controlled agents

- Report suspected misadministration or diversion of controlled substances, according to agency policy

2nd edition 1996; revised 2018

Background Evidence:

Bryson, E. O., & Silverstein, J. H. (2008). Addiction and substance abuse in anesthesiology. *Anesthesiology, 109*(5), 905–917.

Karch, A. M. (2013). Introduction to drugs. In *Focus on nursing pharmacology* (pp. 3–17) (6th ed.). Wolters Kluwer/Lippincott Williams & Wilkins.

Maher, B. P. (2007). Addiction: An occupational hazard in nursing. *American Journal of Nursing, 107*(8), 78–79.

Noort, J. M. (2007). The nursing role in controlled substance prescribing compliance: A legal perspective. *PainReporter, 1*(3), 1–4.

Coping Enhancement   5230

Definition: Facilitation of cognitive and behavioral efforts to manage perceived stressors, changes, or threats that interfere with meeting life demands and roles

Activities:

- Assist the patient in identifying appropriate short-term and long-term goals
- Assist the patient in examining available resources to meet the goals
- Assist the patient in breaking down complex goals into small, manageable steps
- Encourage relationships with persons who have common interests and goals
- Assist the patient to solve problems in a constructive manner
- Appraise a patient's adjustment to changes in body image, as indicated
- Appraise the effect of the patient's life situation on roles and relationships
- Encourage patient to identify a realistic description of change in role
- Appraise the patient's understanding of the disease process
- Appraise and discuss alternative responses to situation
- Use a calm, reassuring approach
- Provide an atmosphere of acceptance
- Assist the patient in developing an objective appraisal of the event
- Help patient to identify the information he/she is most interested in obtaining
- Provide factual information concerning diagnosis, treatment, and prognosis
- Provide the patient with realistic choices about certain aspects of care
- Encourage an attitude of realistic hope as a way of dealing with feelings of helplessness
- Evaluate the patient's decision-making ability
- Seek to understand the patient's perspective of a stressful situation
- Discourage decision making when the patient is under severe stress
- Encourage gradual mastery of the situation
- Encourage patience in developing relationships
- Encourage social and community activities
- Encourage the acceptance of limitations of others
- Acknowledge the patient's spiritual/cultural background
- Encourage the use of spiritual resources, if desired
- Explore patient's previous achievements

- Explore patient's reasons for self-criticism
- Confront patient's ambivalent (angry or depressed) feelings
- Foster constructive outlets for anger and hostility
- Arrange situations that encourage patient's autonomy
- Assist patient in identifying positive responses from others
- Encourage the identification of specific life values
- Explore with the patient previous methods of dealing with life problems
- Introduce patient to persons (or groups) who have successfully undergone the same experience
- Support the use of appropriate defense mechanisms
- Encourage verbalization of feelings, perceptions, and fears
- Discuss consequences of not dealing with guilt and shame
- Encourage the patient to identify own strengths and abilities
- Reduce stimuli in the environment that could be misinterpreted as threatening
- Appraise patient needs/desires for social support
- Assist the patient to identify available support systems
- Determine the risk of the patient's inflicting self-harm
- Encourage family involvement, as appropriate
- Encourage the family to verbalize feelings about ill family member
- Provide appropriate social skills training
- Assist the patient to identify positive strategies to deal with limitations and manage needed lifestyle or role changes
- Instruct the patient on the use of relaxation techniques, as needed
- Assist the patient to grieve and work through the losses of chronic illness and/or disability, if appropriate
- Assist the patient to clarify misconceptions
- Encourage the patient to evaluate own behavior

1st edition 1992; revised 2013

Background Evidence:

Boyd, M. A. (Ed.). (2008). *Psychiatric nursing: Contemporary practice* (4th ed.). Lippincott Williams & Wilkins.

Carroll-Johnson, R., Gorman, L., & Bush, N. (Eds.). (2006). *Psychosocial nursing care along the cancer continuum* (2nd ed.). Pittsburgh, PA: Oncology Nursing Society.

Clarke, P., & Black, S. E. (2005). Quality of life following stroke: Negotiating disability, identity, and resources. *Journal of Applied Gerontology, 24*(4), 319–336.

Garcia, C. (2009). Conceptualization and measurement of coping during adolescence: A review of the literature. *Journal of Nursing Scholarship, 42*(2), 166–185.

Lorenz, R. (2010). Coping with preclinical disability: Older women's experiences of everyday activities. *Journal of Nursing Scholarship, 42*(4), 439–447.

Meadus, R. J. (2007). Adolescents coping with mood disorder: A grounded theory study. *Journal of Psychiatric and Mental Health Nursing, 14*(2), 209–217.

Pavlish, C., & Ceronsky, L. (2009). Oncology nurses' perceptions of nursing roles and professional attributes in palliative care. *Clinical Journal of Oncology Nursing, 13*(4), 404–412.

Peek, G., & Melnyk, B. (2010). Coping interventions for parents of children newly diagnosed with cancer: An evidence review with implications for clinical practice and future research. *Pediatric Nursing, 36*(6), 306–313.

Stuart, G. W. (Ed.). (2009). *Principles and practice of psychiatric nursing* (9th ed.). Mosby Elsevier.

C

Cost Containment 7630

Definition: Management and facilitation of efficient and effective use of resources

Activities:

- Use supplies and equipment efficiently and effectively
- Document current or previously used resources
- Determine appropriate health care setting needed to provide services (e.g., home care, urgent care, emergency department, clinic, acute care, long-term care)
- Assign personnel within budget according to acuity needs
- Apply technology to assist with budgeting and cost containment (e.g., staffing programs, product tracking, supply prediction programs)
- Communicate and coordinate care needs with other departments so care delivered in timely manner
- Evaluate necessity of health care (e.g., procedures, laboratory tests, specialty care)
- Negotiate with interprofessional team members to prevent unnecessary or duplicative tests and procedures
- Discharge when care no longer required
- Investigate competitive prices for supplies and equipment routinely
- Determine whether supplies should be disposable or reusable, purchased or leased
- Secure supplies and equipment at competitive prices
- Use standardized documentation to contain costs and maintain quality
- Collaborate with interprofessional team members to contain costs and maintain quality
- Use quality improvement programs to monitor delivery of quality care in cost-effective manner
- Evaluate services and programs for cost effectiveness on ongoing basis
- Identify mechanisms to reduce costs
- Inform of cost and alternatives of when and where to acquire health care services
- Inform of cost, time, and alternatives involved in specific test or procedure
- Encourage to ask questions about services and charges
- Discuss financial situation as appropriate
- Explore creative options to secure needed resources
- Use teach-back to ensure understanding

3rd edition 2000; revised 2024

Background Evidence:

Brydges, G., Krepper, R., Nibert, A., Young, A., & Luquire, R. (2019). Assessing executive nurse leaders' financial literacy level: A mixed-methods study. *JONA: The Journal of Nursing Administration, 49*(12), 596–603. https://doi.org/10.1097/NNA.0000000000000822

Conley, P. (2019). Certified and advanced degree critical care nurses improve patient outcomes. *Dimensions of Critical Care Nursing, 38*(2), 108–112. https://doi.org/10.1097/DCC.0000000000000342

Huber, D. L., & Joseph, M. L. (2021). *Leadership and nursing care management* (7th ed.). Elsevier.

Kelly, P., & Porr, C. (2018). Ethical nursing care versus cost containment: Considerations to enhance RN practice. *Online Journal of Issues in Nursing, 23*(1), 3. https://doi.org/10.3912/OJIN.Vol23No01Man06

Marquis, B. L., & Huston, C. J. (2021). *Leadership roles and management functions in nursing: Theory and applications.* (10th ed.). Wolters Kluwer.

Stadhouders, N., Kruse, F., Tanke, M., Koolman, X., & Jeurissen, P. (2019). Effective healthcare cost-containment policies: A systematic review. *Health Policy, 123*(1), 71–79. https://doi.org/10.1016/j.healthpol.2018.10.015

Ultimate Kronos Group. (2021). Unleashing the power of healthcare workforce data. *Healthcare Financial Management, 75*(3), 16–19.

Welch, T. D., & Smith, T. (2020). Understanding FTEs and nursing hours per patient day. *Nurse Leader, 18*(2), 157–162. https://doi.org/10.1016/j.mnl.2019.10.003

Young, C., White, M., & Dorrington, M. (2018). Nurse staffing improvements through interprofessional strategic workforce action planning. *Nursing Economic$, 36*(4), 163–194.

Cough Enhancement 3250

Definition: Promotion of deep inhalation with subsequent generation of high intrathoracic pressures and compression of underlying lung parenchyma for the forceful expulsion of air

Activities:

- Assist to sitting position with head slightly flexed, shoulders relaxed, and knees flexed
- Encourage to take several deep breaths
- Encourage to take deep breath, hold for 2 seconds, and cough two or three times in succession

- Use varied techniques to assist with effective coughing (e.g., huff cough, quad cough, manually assisted cough, diaphragmatic breathing)
- Instruct to inhale deeply, bend forward slightly, and perform three or four huffs against open glottis
- Instruct to inhale deeply several times, to exhale slowly, and to cough at end of exhalation
- Initiate lateral chest wall rib spring techniques during expiration phase of cough maneuver, as appropriate
- Compress abdomen below xiphoid with flat hand while assisting to flex forward while coughing
- Instruct to follow coughing with several maximal inhalation breaths
- Encourage use of incentive spirometry, as appropriate
- Promote systemic fluid hydration, as appropriate
- Encourage ambulation, as appropriate
- Offer support devices (e.g., folded blanket, pillow, palmed hands) to splint incisions for pain minimization during directed coughing
- Assist to use pillow or rolled blanket as splint against incision when coughing
- Evaluate effectiveness of coughing
- Encourage persons with respiratory infections or chronic pulmonary diseases to deep breathe and cough every 2 hours while awake
- Encourage persons with large amounts of sputum production to deep breathe and cough every hour while awake

- Monitor results of pulmonary function tests, particularly vital capacity, maximal inspiratory force, forced expiratory volume in 1 second (FEV_1), and FEV_1/FVC, as appropriate

---

1st edition 1992; revised 2004, 2024

Background Evidence:

Boon, C. J. W. (2021). Oxygenation. In P. A., Potter, A. G., Perry, P. A., Stockert, & A. M. Hall, (Eds.), *Fundamentals of nursing* (10th ed., pp. 930–935). Elsevier.

Bryant, R. (2022). The child with respiratory dysfunction. In Hockenberry, Rodgers & Wilson (Eds.), *Wong's essentials of pediatric nursing* (11th ed., pp. 619–677). Elsevier.

Jett, K. (2020). Respiratory health and illness. In K. Jett & T. A. Touhy, (Eds.), *Toward healthy aging* (10th ed., pp. 315–320). Elsevier.

Slang, R., Finsrud, L. T., & Olsen, B. F. (2020). Nursing interventions in intensive care unit patients with breathing difficulties: A scoping review of the evidence. *Nordic Journal of Nursing Research*, *40*(4), 176–187. https://doi.org/10.1177/2057158520948834

Stacy, K. (2022). Pulmonary therapeutic management. In L. D. Urden, K. M., Stacy, & M. E. Lough, (Eds.), *Critical care nursing: Diagnosis and management* (9th ed., pp. 499–532). Elsevier.

Williams, P. (2020). Activity and exercise: *Basic geriatric nursing* (pp. 310–332) (7th ed.). Elsevier.

C

Counseling   5240

Definition: Providing assistance and guidance toward resolving personal, social, or psychological problems and difficulties

Activities:
- Provide privacy and confidentiality
- Convey authenticity, warmth, genuineness, interest, and unconditional caring
- Introduce self and ensure person is comfortable
- Invite social conversation to ease anxiety
- Invite to describe reasons for seeking counseling
- Determine purpose, goals, and agenda for counseling sessions
- Establish therapeutic relationship based on trust, empathy, compassion, and respect
- Establish length of counseling sessions and length of counseling relationship
- Mutually establish goals
- Develop understanding of concerns, problems, and difficulties
- Assist to identify problem or situation causing distress
- Determine how problems may interfere with daily life
- Identify what thoughts, feelings, and behaviors are associated with problem
- Determine how long problem has persisted
- Identify any pattern of events that may be associated with problem
- Determine how family behavior may be affecting person
- Determine what strategies previously used to manage problem
- Assist to list and prioritize all possible alternatives to problem
- Identify any differences between person's and health care team's view of situation
- Verbalize discrepancy between feelings and behaviors
- Maintain awareness of nonverbal behaviors as signs of emotional state

- Provide factual information, as necessary and appropriate
- Encourage expression of feelings
- Allow time to respond
- Use techniques of reflection and clarification to facilitate expression of concern
- Ask person and significant others to identify what they can and cannot do about what is happening
- Use tools to help increase self-awareness and knowledge of situation (e.g., paper and pencil measures, audiotape, videotape, interactional exercises with other people), as appropriate
- Discourage decision-making when under severe stress, when possible
- Reveal selected aspects of own experiences or personality to foster genuineness and trust, as appropriate
- Use established therapeutic approach to guide counseling sessions (e.g., psychodynamic, behavioral, cognitive, humanistic, integrative-holistic)
- Assist to identify strengths, and reinforce them
- Encourage new skill development, as appropriate
- Encourage substitution of undesirable habits with desirable habits
- Reinforce new skills
- Evaluate for achievement of established goals and for resolution of presenting problem
- Prepare for ending of therapeutic relationship
- Arrange for follow-up or referral

1st edition 1992; revised 2000, 2024

Background Evidence:

Egan, G., & Reese, R. J. (2019). *The skilled helper: A problem management and opportunity development approach to helping.* (11th ed.). Cengage.

Rosenthal, H. (2017). *Encyclopedia of counseling: Master review and tutorial for the national counselor examination, state counseling exams, and the counselor preparation comprehensive examination.* (4th ed.). Routledge.

Sommers-Flanagan, J., & Sommers-Flanagen, R. (2018). *Counseling and psychotherapy theories in context and practice: Skills, strategies, and techniques* (3rd ed.). Wiley.

Sue, D. W., Sue, D., Neville, H. A., & Smith, L. (2019). *Counseling the culturally diverse: Theory and practice.* (8th ed.). Wiley.

Wong, D. W., Hall, K. R., & Hernandez, L. W. (2021). *Counseling individuals through the lifespan.* (2nd ed.). Sage.

Crisis Intervention 6160

Definition: Use of short-term strategies to facilitate management of a situation of intense difficulty, trouble, or danger

Activities:

- Provide safe and supportive atmosphere
- Establish therapeutic relationship
- Determine if safety risk to self or others
- Initiate necessary precautions to safeguard person or others
- Use active, acute crisis management approach, as needed
- Support person to feel safe and less anxious
- Promote person's sense of control and self-efficacy to regain control as soon as possible
- Focus on interaction by eliminating prejudices, presumptions, personal worries, and other distractions
- Listen with full attention using communication techniques (e.g., eye contact, rapport, frequent responses to verify and transmit understanding, summarizing what person saying)
- Avoid giving false reassurances
- Encourage expression of feelings in nondestructive manner
- Encourage to use own resources to make changes
- Recognize type of crisis (e.g., maturational, situational, adventitious) to help develop person-centered plan of care, as appropriate
- Monitor cognitive, emotional, and behavioral reactions to adjust interventions accordingly
- Assist in identification of precipitants and dynamics of crisis
- Encourage to focus on present and immediate situation ("here and now") and not anticipating future events
- Identify if previously agreed to a crisis plan and whether it is applicable in current situation
- Develop crisis prevention plan to outline preferred ways of managing and preventing future crisis (e.g., information on early warning signs of crisis, medications, supports that help manage crisis, preferences for care, contact details for family members, information about 24-hour services), as necessary
- Identify cultural beliefs or spiritual practices that should be addressed in assessing and intervening in crisis
- Develop awareness of meaning of crisis from person's point of view
- Recognize and understand impact of trauma histories of people experiencing crisis
- Involve in identifying realistic and suitable interventions
- Encourage to focus on one implication at a time
- Assist in identification of personal strengths and abilities to use in resolving crisis
- Assist in identification of past and present coping skills and effectiveness
- Assist in development of new coping and problem-solving skills, as needed
- Explore and enable educational needs of person and family, as appropriate
- Instruct on specific coping skills (e.g., decision-making, problem solving, assertiveness, meditation, relaxation), as necessary
- Provide social skills training, as needed
- Assist in identification of alternative courses of action to resolve crisis
- Assist in evaluation of possible consequences of various courses of action
- Assist to decide on particular course of action
- Assist in formulating time frame for implementation of chosen course of action
- Evaluate with person whether crisis has been resolved by chosen course of action
- Plan with person how adaptive coping skills can be used to deal with future crises
- Assist in identification of available support systems
- Link person and family with community resources, as needed
- Provide guidance to develop and maintain support systems
- Introduce to people or groups who have successfully undergone same experience
- Identify social supports available to family (e.g., groups; education about disease, treatment, prognosis, drugs; community supports for family; community supports for person to reach optimal functioning)
- Provide information or refer person and family to additional support or services as needed
- Facilitate access to community-based outreach support, appropriate health care providers, peer support workers, and mental health and substance use services
- Plan regular follow-up (e.g., phone calls, clinic visits, home visits)
- Document progress
- Evaluate and refer to rehabilitation program, as necessary
- Encourage use of telecommunication- and technology-based solutions (e.g., psycho-education, online skills, online tools) for receiving emergency assessment, triage, and support, or for support with coping and self-management, as appropriate
- Use teach-back to ensure understanding

1ˢᵗ Edition 1992; revised 2008, 2024

Background Evidence:

Cavaiola, A. A., & Colford, J. E. (2018). *Crisis intervention: A practical guide.* Sage.

Christiansen, K. (2017). *The crisis intervention manual.* (3rd Ed.). Empathy Works.

Halter, M. J. (2022). *Varcarolis' foundations of psychiatric-mental health nursing: A Clinical approach* (9th Ed). Elsevier.

Nizum, N., Yoon, R., Ferreira-Legere, L., Poole, N., & Lulat, Z. (2020). Nursing interventions for adults following a mental health crisis: A systematic review guided by trauma-informed principles. *International Journal of Mental Health Nursing, 29*(3), 348–363. https://doi.org/10.1111/inm.12691

Registered Nurses' Association of Ontario. (2017). *Crisis intervention for adults using a trauma-informed approach: Initial four weeks of management* (3rd ed.).

Zalaquett, P., & Muñoz, E. (2017). Intervención en crisis para pacientes hospitalizados. *Revista Médica Clínica Las Condes, 28*(6), 835–840. https://doi.org/10.1016/j.rmclc.2017.11.008

Critical Path Development   7640

Definition: Constructing and using a timed sequence of patient care activities to enhance desired patient outcomes in a cost-efficient manner

Activities:

- Conduct chart audit to determine current patterns of care for patient population
- Review current standards of practice related to patient population
- Collaborate with other health professionals to develop the critical path
- Identify appropriate intermediate and final outcomes with time frames
- Identify appropriate interventions with time frames
- Place relevant variables (e.g., outcomes, interventions, laboratory and diagnostic tests, consultations, patient and family education) sequentially on a decision tree
- Keep the decision tree as simple as possible, even when the clinical events are complex (i.e., provide important details but minimize wordiness and length)
- Include key decision points in which provider judgment is critical
- Share critical path with patient and family, as appropriate
- Evaluate patient progress toward identified outcomes at defined intervals
- Calculate variances and report through appropriate channels
- Document patient progress toward identified outcomes, per agency policy
- Document reason for variances from planned interventions and expected outcomes
- Implement corrective action(s) for variance(s), as appropriate
- Revise critical path, as appropriate

2nd edition 1996; revised 2018

Background Evidence:

Abrams, M.N., Hage, D., & Abrams, E.R. (2011, November 29). Engaging physicians in predictive care paths. *Hospitals and Health Networks Daily.* http://www.hhnmag.com/articles/4784-engaging-physicians-in-predictive-care-paths

Evans-Lacko, S., Jarrett, M., McCrone, P., & Thronicroft, G. (2010). Facilitators and barriers to implementing clinical care pathways. *BMC Health Services Research, 10*, 182. https://doi.org/10.1186/1472-6963-10-182

Huber, D. L. (2014). *Leadership and nursing care management* (5th ed.). Elsevier Saunders.

Kinsman, R. T., Machotta, J. E., Willis, G. H., Snow, P., & Kugler, J. (2010). Clinical pathways: Effects on professional practice, patient outcomes, length of stay and hospital costs. *Cochrane Database of Systematic Reviews, 2010*(3). https://doi.org/10.1002/14651858.CD006632.pub2

Vanhaect, K., Panella, M., van Zelm, R., & Sermeus, W. (2010). An overview on the history and concept of care pathways as complex interventions. *International Journal of Care Pathways, 14*(3), 117–123.

Culture Care Negotiation   7330

Definition: Assisting, accommodating, facilitating, or enabling actions that promote culturally congruent, safe, and effective care

Activities:

- Determine understanding of health condition using exploratory questions (e.g., how is this illness affecting you? What do you think the cause of the illness might be?)
- Use cultural assessment tools if needed to determine areas of agreement and disagreement with health care practices or health care provider recommendations (e.g., ABCD Cultural Assessment Tool, LEARN Model of Cross-Cultural Communication)
- Promote open discussion of cultural beliefs
- Acknowledge commonalities between provider and person
- Resolve gaps in communication
- Identify cultural practices that may negatively affect health
- Discuss and clarify discrepancies openly
- Negotiate, when issues cannot be resolved, acceptable compromise of treatment based on biomedical knowledge, knowledge of belief systems, and ethical standards
- Recommend plan of care that involves person and family, and includes culturally appropriate and relevant strategies compatible with provider recommendations
- Allow more than usual time to process information and work through decisions
- Appear relaxed and unhurried in interactions
- Use nontechnical language
- Arrange for cultural accommodation
- Provide information to health care team about cultural preferences
- Include family in plan for prescribed regimen, when appropriate
- Select final plan with involvement of provider and person
- Accommodate involvement of family to give support or direct care
- Facilitate intercultural communication between all providers (e.g., use of translator, bilingual written materials or media, accurate nonverbal communication, avoid stereotyping)

- Provide information about health care system
- Assist other health care providers to understand and accept person's reasons for nonadherence
- Provide caregivers who share life experiences or language with persons where possible
- Alter therapeutic environment by incorporating appropriate cultural elements
- Treat every encounter with persons from culturally diverse backgrounds as unique experiences
- Modify typical interventions (e.g., teaching) in culturally congruent ways

1st edition 1992; revised 2000, 2024

Background Evidence:

Ali, P. A., & Watson, R. (2018). Language barriers and their impact on provision of care to patients with limited English proficiency: Nurses' perspectives. *Journal of Clinical Nursing, 27*(5-6), e1152–e1160.

American Nurses Association (ANA). (2021). *Nursing: Scope and standards of practice* (4th ed.), Nursesbooks.

Berman, A., Snyder, S. J., & Frandsen, G. (2018). *Kozier and Erb's fundamentals of nursing: Concepts, process and practice* (10th ed.). Pearson.

Mikell, M. J., & Snethen, J. (2020). Perceptions of health promotion and maintenance among latinos in faith communities. *Journal of Christian Nursing, 37*, 100–107. https://doi.org/10.1097/CNJ.0000000000000709

Perry, A. G., Potter, P. A., Ostendorf, W. R., & LaPlante, N. (2021). *Clinical nursing skills and technique* (10th ed.). Mosby.

Persaud, S. (2021). Culturally congruent care in radiology nursing. *Journal of Radiology Nursing, 40*(3), 227–231.

Potter, P. A., Perry, A. G., Stockert, P. A., & Hall, A. M. (2021). *Fundamentals of nursing* (10th ed.). Elsevier.

Wehbe-Alamah, H. B. (2020). Madeleine Leininger's Theory of Cultural Care Diversity and Universality. In *M. C. Smith Nursing theories and nursing practice* (5th ed.). F.A. Davis.

Williams, P. (2020). *Basic geriatric nursing* (7th ed.). Elsevier.

Cup Feeding: Newborn 8240

Definition: Preparation and administration of fluid to a newborn using a cup

Activities:

- Determine newborn state before initiating feeding
- Use clean cup without lid, spout, or lip
- Pour expressed milk at room temperature or formula into cup
- Hold swaddled newborn upright or semi-upright while supporting newborn's back, neck, and head
- Hold cup to newborn's lip, resting slightly on the lower lip with cup's edges touching outer parts of upper lip
- Monitor for newborn signs of feeding readiness (e.g., increased alertness, open mouth and eyes, movements with mouth and face)
- Tip cup so that milk touches newborn's lips
- Avoid pouring milk too fast
- Monitor newborn's intake mechanism (i.e., preterm/low birth weight newborn tends to lap milk, whereas full-term/older infant tends to sip or suck milk)
- Monitor milk flow
- Burp the newborn frequently during and after the feeding
- Monitor for newborn signs of fullness (e.g., closing mouth, not taking in more milk, change in infant state, infant not responding to verbal or tactile stimulation)
- Discontinue feeding upon newborn sign of distress or infant sign of fullness
- Measure newborn's milk intake over 24 hours
- Instruct parent on cup feeding procedures
- Instruct parent about feeding readiness, distress, and feeding termination signs

6th edition 2013

Background Evidence:

Abouelfettoh, A. M., Dowling, D. A., Dabash, S. A., Elguindy, S. R., & Seoud, I. A. (2008). Cup versus bottle feeding for hospitalized late preterm infants in Egypt: A quasi-experimental study. *International Breastfeeding Journal, 3*(27), 11.

Collins, C. T., Makrides, M., Gillis, J., & McPhee, A. J. (2008). Avoidance of bottles during the establishment of breast feeds in preterm infants. *Cochrane Database of Systematic Reviews, 2008*(4). https://doi.org/10.1002/14651858.CD005252.pub2

Dowling, D. A., Meier, P. P., DiFiore, J. M., Blatz, M. A., & Martin, R. J. (2002). Cup-feeding for preterm infants: Mechanics and safety. *Journal of Human Lactation, 18*(1), 13–20.

Howard, C. R., de Blieck, E. A., ten Hoopen, C. B., Howard, F. M., Lanphear, B. P., & Lawrence, R. A. (1999). Physiologic stability of newborns during cup- and bottle-feeding. *Pediatrics, 104*(Suppl. 6), 1204–1207.

Lang, S., Lawrence, C., & Orme, R. (1994). Cup feeding: An alternative method of infant feeding. *Archives of Disease in Childhood, 71*(4), 365–369.

Marinelli, K. A., Burke, G. S., & Dodd, V. L. (2001). A comparison of the safety of cupfeedings and bottlefeedings in premature infants whose mothers intend to breastfeed. *Journal of Perinatology, 21*(6), 350–355.

Rocha, N. M., Martinez, F. E., & Jorge, S. M. (2002). Cup or bottle for preterm infants: Effects on oxygen saturation, weight gain and breastfeeding. *Journal of Human Lactation, 18*(2), 132–138.

World Health Organization. (1993). *Breastfeeding counseling: A training course.*

Cutaneous Stimulation 1340

Definition: Stimulation of the skin and underlying tissues for the purpose of decreasing undesirable signs and symptoms such as pain, muscle spasm, inflammation, or nausea

Activities:

- Discuss various methods of skin stimulation, their effects on sensation, and expectations of patient during activity
- Select a specific cutaneous stimulation strategy based on the individual's willingness to participate, ability to participate, preference, support of significant others, and contraindications
- Select the most appropriate type of cutaneous stimulation for the patient and the condition (e.g., massage, cold, ice, heat, menthol, vibration, or TENS)
- Instruct on indications for, frequency of, and procedure for application
- Select stimulation site, considering alternate sites when direct application is not possible (e.g., adjacent to, distal to, between affected areas and the brain)
- Consider acupressure points as sites of stimulation, as appropriate
- Determine the duration and frequency of stimulation, based on method chosen
- Ensure that the electrical stimulation device is in good working order, as appropriate
- Apply stimulation directly on or around the affected site, as appropriate
- Encourage the use of an intermittent method of stimulation, as appropriate
- Allow the family to participate, as much as possible
- Select alternate method or site of stimulation, if altered sensation is not achieved
- Discontinue stimulation, if increased pain or skin irritation occurs
- Evaluate and document response to stimulation

1st edition 1992; revised 2013

Background Evidence:

Konno, R. (2010). Cochrane review summary for cancer nursing: Acupuncture-point stimulation for chemotherapy-induced nausea or vomiting. *Cancer Nursing, 33*(6), 479–480.

Kubsch, S. M., Neveau, T., & Vandertie, K. (2001). Effect of cutaneous stimulation on pain reduction in emergency department patients. *Accident and Emergency Nursing, 9*(3), 143–151.

Smith, T. J., Coyne, P. J., Parker, G. L., Dodson, P., & Ramakrishnan, V. (2010). Pilot trial of a patient-specific cutaneous electrostimulation device (MC5-A Calmare) for chemotherapy-induced peripheral neuropathy. *Journal of Pain and Symptom Management, 40*(6), 883–891.

Timby, B. K., & Smith, N. E. (2007). Caring for clients with pain. In *Introductory medical-surgical nursing* (pp. 175–188) (9th ed.). Lippincott Williams & Wilkins.

C

D

Dance Therapy 4367

Definition: The use of body movements in concert with the beat of a musical rhythm to facilitate a specific therapeutic physical, mental, emotional, or spiritual change

Activities:

- Determine the individual's interest in the dance therapy
- Inform the individual about purpose of the dance experience
- Discuss with individual the desired goals (e.g., relaxation, stimulation, concentration, pain reduction)
- Determine the individual's capabilities for movement
- Identify preferences for the type of music and dance related to desired goals
- Determine the duration of the session
- Determine the time intervals between each session
- Recommend the wearing of comfortable and appropriate clothing and shoes for dancing
- Limit distracting visual and auditory stimuli
- Select a suitable place and the necessary equipment (e.g., sound equipment, music selections, mirrors, chairs), as applicable
- Plan sessions according to progress in the execution of movements
- Encourage the expression of emotions
- Allow time for pauses and breaks, if applicable
- Instruct the individual to perform the dance therapy at home, if applicable
- Incorporate family participation in the sessions, if applicable
- Monitor continuously the achievement of the objectives and targets

Background Evidence:

Bradt, J., Goodill, S. W., & Dileo, C. (2011). Dance/movement therapy for improving psychological and physical outcomes in cancer patients (review). *Cochrane Database of Systematic Reviews, 2011*(10). https://doi.org/10.1002/14651858.CD007103.pub2

Lane, M. (2005). Creativity and spirituality in nursing: Implementing art in healing. *Holistic Nursing Practice, 19*(3), 122–125.

Payne, H. (Ed.). (2006). *Dance movement therapy: Theory, research, and practice* (2nd ed.). Routledge.

Picard, C. (1994). The healing expression of dance. In D. Gaut & A. Boykin (Eds.), *Caring as healing: Renewal through hope* (pp. 146–149). National League for Nursing.

Strassel, J. K., Cherkin, D. C., Steuten, L., Sherman, K. J., & Vrijhoef, H. J. (2011). A systematic review of the evidence for the effectiveness of dance therapy. *Alternative Therapies in Health & Medicine, 17*(3), 50–59.

Winther, H., Grøntved, S., Gravesen, E., & Ilkjaer, I. (2015). The dancing nurses and the language of the body. *Journal of Holistic Nursing, 33*(3), 182–192.

7th edition 2018

Decision-Making Support 5250

Definition: Providing information and support for a patient who is making a decision regarding health care

Activities:

- Determine whether there are differences between the patient's view of own condition and the view of health care providers
- Assist patient to clarify values and expectations that may assist in making critical life choices
- Inform patient of alternative views or solutions in a clear and supportive manner
- Help patient identify the advantages and disadvantages of each alternative
- Establish communication with patient early in admission
- Facilitate patient's articulation of goals for care
- Obtain informed consent, when appropriate
- Facilitate collaborative decision making
- Be familiar with institution's policies and procedures
- Respect patient's right to receive or not to receive information
- Provide information requested by patient
- Help patient explain decision to others, as needed
- Serve as a liaison between patient and family
- Serve as a liaison between patient and other health care providers
- Use interactive computer software or web-based decision aides as an adjunct to professional support
- Refer to legal aid, as appropriate
- Refer to support groups, as appropriate

Background Evidence:

Donahue, M. (1985). . Advocacy. In G. M. Bulechek & J. C. McCloskey (Eds.), *Nursing interventions: Treatments for nursing diagnosis* (pp. 338–351). W.B. Saunders.

Edwards, A., & Elwyn, G. (2001). *Evidence-based patient choice: Inevitable or impossible?* Oxford University Press.

Edwards, A., Evans, R., & Elwyn, G. (2003). Manufactured but not imported: New directions for research in shared decision making support and skills. *Patient Education and Counseling, 50*(1), 33–38.

Marcus, P. E. (2004). Anxiety and related disorders. In K. M. Fortinash & P. A. Holoday-Worret (Eds.), *Psychiatric mental health nursing* (pp. 171–194). Mosby.

Moeller, M. D. (2005). Neurobiological responses and schizophrenia and psychotic disorders. In G. W. Stuart & M. T. Laraia (Eds.), *Principles and practice of psychiatric nursing* (8th ed., pp. 390–391). Mosby.

Sime, M. (1992). Decisional control. In M. Snyder (Ed.), *Independent nursing interventions* (2nd ed., pp. 110–114). Delmar.

1st edition 1992; revised 2008

De-Escalation Management 6170

Definition: Use of non-physical interpersonal and communication skills to prevent a potentially dangerous situation from becoming a violent episode

Activities:

- Examine entire situation, including person and environment, determining level of agitation and potential for violence
- Ensure safety of person, self, staff, and bystanders, removing bystanders if possible
- Recruit other staff for assistance, employing teamwork (i.e., one staff interacting with person while other staff manage environmental safety for all)
- Keep all interacting persons in an open space
- Establish ability of person to communicate verbally, using person's preferred name
- Identify self verbally, noting why person there (i.e., in psychiatric unit for counseling or medication review)
- Approach using a calm, soft, clear voice when speaking, keeping sentences short and simple
- Determine what person wants and its level of urgency, identifying actual and potential stressors
- Provide clearly stated options and choices whenever possible, avoiding opinions on issues and grievances beyond staff control
- Offer reassurance and help when setting boundaries while avoiding judgmental attitudes
- Demonstrate control of situation without becoming demanding or authoritative
- Avoid overreacting to situation
- Listen to concerns with empathetic, genuine, non-confrontational approach at all times
- Use silence and listening to encourage expression of thoughts, feelings, and concerns
- Use non-threatening verbal and nonverbal communication patterns, avoiding excessive stimulation, aggressive postures and prolonged eye contact (i.e., relax shoulders with arms down and hands open outwards)
- Avoid invading personal space
- Avoid mirroring any negative body language
- Avoid smiles or grimaces when person delusional or hallucinating
- Avoid making sudden movements and threatening postures (e.g., gesticulation, pointing, crossing arms, putting hands on hips)
- Administer calming medication to enhance communication ability, if indicated and as needed
- Allow for choice in type or route of medication administration, if possible
- Reassess person and environment for safety concerns frequently
- Address medical issues, especially pain and discomfort
- Provide appropriate level of care for person once situation under control (e.g., seclusion, restraint, return to room)
- Promote engagement with social and support network, if appropriate
- Ensure effective communication related to episode with other health care providers
- Document episode following agency guidelines

8th edition 2024

Background Evidence:

Adams, J. (2017). Assessing the effectiveness of clinical education to reduce the frequency and recurrence of workplace violence. *Australian Journal of Advanced Nursing, 34*(3), 6–15. https://doi.org/10.3316/informit.9466 27915561528

Frauenfelder, F. (2019). *Psychiatric adult inpatient nursing described in the NANDA-I and NIC: A systematic evaluation of nursing classifications* [Doctoral dissertation. Radbound University] Radbound Repository. https://repository.ubn.ru.nl/handle/2066/203856

Halter, M. J. (2019). *Manual of care plans in psychiatric nursing: An interprofessional approach.* Elsevier.

Halter, M. J. (2022). *Varcarolis' foundations of psychiatric mental health nursing: A clinical approach* (9th ed.). Elsevier.

Nizum, N., Yoon, R., Ferreira-Legere, L., Poole, N., & Lulat, Z. (2020). Nursing interventions for adults following a mental health crisis: A systematic review guided by trauma-informed principles. *International Journal of Mental Health Nursing, 29*(3), 348–363. https://doi.org/10.1111/inm.12691

Patel, M.X., Sethi, F.N., Barnes, T.R. E., Dix, R., Dratcu, L., Fox, B., Garriga, M., Haste, J., C., Kahl, G., Lingford-Hughes, A., McAllister-Williams, H., O'Brien, A., Parker, C., Paterson, B., Paton, C., Posporelis, S., Taylor, D.M., Vieta, E., Völlm, B., Wilson-Jones, C., & Woods, L. (2018). Joint BAP NAPICU evidence-based consensus guidelines for the clinical management of acute disturbance: De-escalation and rapid tranquillization. Journal of Psychiatric Intensive Care, 14(2), 8 9–132. https://doi.org/10.20299/jpi.2018.008

Defibrillator Management: External 4095

Definition: Care of the person receiving defibrillation for termination of life-threatening cardiac rhythm disturbances

Activities:

- Initiate cardiopulmonary resuscitation, as indicated
- Prepare for immediate defibrillation of pulseless, unresponsive patient in conjunction with cardiopulmonary resuscitation
- Maintain cardiopulmonary resuscitation when not administering external defibrillation
- Determine type and operation techniques for available defibrillator
- Apply pads or paddles according to machine recommendations (e.g., paddles need conduction agent; pads are ready-made with conduction agent)
- Place appropriate monitoring devices on patients (automated external defibrillator pads or monitor leads)
- Place paddles or pads to avoid clothing or bed linens, as appropriate
- Determine need for shock per defibrillator instructions or interpretation of arrhythmia
- Charge machine to appropriate joules
- Use safety precautions before discharging (e.g., call "clear" three times; ensure no one is touching the patient including self)
- Monitor results and repeat, as indicated

- Minimize interruptions to chest compressions in unresponsive patients
- Record events appropriately
- Assist in patient recovery (e.g., activate emergency medical systems when out of hospital for transport of patient to emergency care institution; arrange for transport within hospital to appropriate nursing unit for intensive cardiac care) as indicated
- Instruct new nursing staff on type and operation techniques for available defibrillator
- Assist in education of public related to proper use and indications of external defibrillation in cardiopulmonary arrest

5th edition 2008

Background Evidence:

American Association of Critical-Care Nurses. (2006). In J. G. Alspach (Ed.), *Core curriculum for critical care nursing* (6th ed.). Saunders Elsevier.

American College of Cardiology Foundation and the American Heart Association. (2002). *Guideline update for implantation of cardiac pacemakers and antiarrhythmia devices.*

American Heart Association. (2005). 2005 American Heart Association guidelines for cardiopulmonary resuscitation and emergency cardiovascular care. *Circulation, 112*(Suppl. 24), IV-1–IV-211.

American Heart Association. (2005). Electric therapies: Automated external defibrillators, defibrillation, cardioversion, and pacing. *Circulation, 112*(Suppl. 24), IV-35–IV-46.

Smeltzer, S. C., & Bare, B. G. (2004). (10th ed.) *Brunner & Suddarth's textbook of medical-surgical nursing* (Vol. 1). Lippincott Williams & Wilkins.

Urden, L. D., Stacy, K. M., & Lough, M. E. (2006). *Thelan's critical care nursing: Diagnosis and management* (5th ed.). Mosby Elsevier.

Wiegand, D., & Carlson, K. (Eds.). (2005). *AACN procedure manual for critical care* (5th ed.). Elsevier Saunders.

Defibrillator Management: Internal 4096

Definition: Care of the person receiving permanent detection and termination of life-threatening cardiac rhythm disturbances through the insertion and use of an internal cardiac defibrillator

Activities:

- Provide information to patient and family related to defibrillator implantation (e.g., indications, functions, cardioversion experience, required lifestyle changes, potential complications)
- Provide concrete, objective information related to the effects of defibrillator therapy to reduce patient uncertainty, fear, and anxiety about treatment-related symptoms
- Document pertinent data in patient's permanent record regarding initial insertion of defibrillator (e.g., manufacturer, model number, serial number, implant date, mode of operation, capability for pacing and/or shock delivery, delivery system for shocks, upper and lower rate limits for rate-responsive devices)
- Confirm defibrillator placement postimplantation with baseline chest x-ray
- Monitor for potential complications associated with defibrillator insertion (e.g., pneumothorax, hemothorax, myocardial perforation, cardiac tamponade, hematoma, PVCs, infections, hiccups, muscle twitches)
- Observe for changes in cardiac or hemodynamic status, which indicate a need for modifications of defibrillator parameters
- Monitor for conditions that potentially influence sensing (e.g., fluid status changes, pericardial effusion, electrolyte or metabolic abnormalities, certain medications, tissue inflammation, tissue fibrosis, tissue necrosis)
- Monitor for arm swelling or increased warmth on side ipsilateral to implanted device and leads
- Monitor for redness or swelling at the device site
- Instruct patient to avoid tight or restrictive clothing that might cause friction at insertion site
- Instruct patient on activity restrictions (e.g., initial arm movement restrictions for pectoral implantations, avoidance of heavy lifting, avoid contact sports, adhere to driving restrictions)
- Monitor for symptoms of arrhythmias, ischemia, or heart failure (e.g., dizziness, syncope, palpitations, chest pain, shortness of breath) particularly with each outpatient contact
- Instruct patient and family member(s) regarding symptoms to report (e.g., dizziness, fainting, prolonged weakness, nausea, palpitations, chest pain, difficulty breathing, discomfort at insertion or external electrode site, electrical shocks)
- Instruct patient about emergent symptoms and what to do if symptoms occur (e.g., call emergency responders if dizzy)
- Monitor drug and electrolyte levels for patients receiving concurrent antiarrhythmic medications
- Monitor for metabolic conditions with adverse effects on defibrillators (acid-base disturbances, myocardial ischemia, hyperkalemia, severe hyperglycemia [greater than 600 mg/dL], renal failure, hypothyroidism)
- Instruct patient about potential defibrillator complications from electromagnetic interference (inappropriate discharges, potential proarrhythmic effects of defibrillator, decreased defibrillator generator life, cardiac arrhythmia and arrest)
- Instruct patient about basic safety in avoidance of electromagnetic interference (e.g., keep at least 6 inches away from sources of interference; do not leave cell phones in the "on" mode in a shirt pocket over the defibrillator)
- Instruct patient about sources of highest electromagnetic interference (e.g., arc welding equipment, electronic muscle stimulators, radio transmitters, concert speakers, large motor-generator systems, electric drills, handheld metal detectors, magnetic resonance imaging, radiation treatments)
- Instruct patient regarding special considerations at airport or government building security gates (e.g., always inform security guard of implantable defibrillator; walk through security gates; DO NOT allow handheld metal detectors near the device site; always walk quickly through metal detection devices or ask to be searched by hand; do not lean on or stand near detection devices for long periods)
- Instruct patient that handheld metal detectors contain magnets that can reset the defibrillator and cause malfunction
- Instruct patient to check manufacturer warnings when in doubt about household appliances

- Instruct patient to carry manufacturer identification card at all times
- Instruct patient to wear a medical alert bracelet or necklace that identifies defibrillator
- Instruct patient about the need for regular checkups with primary cardiologist
- Monitor for defibrillator problems that have occurred between scheduled checkup visits (e.g., inappropriate discharges, frequent discharges)
- Instruct patient to keep a detailed log of all discharges (e.g., time, location, and activity of patient when discharge occurred; physical symptoms before and after discharge) to review with the physician
- Instruct patient to consult primary cardiologist for all changes in medications
- Instruct patient with new defibrillator to refrain from operating motor vehicles until permitted per primary cardiologist (usually 3–6 months after the last symptomatic arrhythmic event)
- Instruct patient about the need for regular interrogation of defibrillator by cardiologist for routine maintenance
- Instruct patient about the need to obtain chest x-ray annually for defibrillator placement confirmation
- Avoid frightening family or friends about unexpected shocks
- Instruct patient's family (particularly sexual partners) that no harm comes to a person touching a patient who is receiving a defibrillator discharge (e.g., may feel the shock, but it is not harmful)
- Teach patient and family member(s) precautions and restrictions required
- Explore psychological responses (e.g., changes in self-image, depression due to driving restrictions, fear of shocks, increased anxiety, concerns related to sexual activities, changes in partner relationships)

- Encourage patient and family members to attend CPR classes
- Encourage attendance at support group meetings

5th edition 2008

Background Evidence:

American Association of Critical-Care Nurses. (2006). In J. G. Alspach (Ed.), *Core curriculum for critical care nursing* (6th ed.). Saunders Elsevier.

American College of Cardiology Foundation and the American Heart Association. (2002). *Guideline update for implantation of cardiac pacemakers and antiarrhythmia devices.*

Burke, L. J. (1996). Securing life through technology acceptance: The first six months after transvenous internal cardioverter defibrillator implantation. *Heart & Lung, 25*(5), 352–366.

Dougherty, C. M., Benoliel, J. Q., & Bellin, C. (2000). Domains of nursing intervention after sudden cardiac arrest and automatic internal cardioverter defibrillator implantation. *Heart & Lung, 29*(2), 79–86.

Finch, N. J., Sneed, N. V., Leman, R. B., & Watson, J. (1997). Driving with an internal defibrillator: Legal, ethical, and quality of life issues. *Journal of Cardiovascular Nursing, 11*(2), 58–67.

James, J. E. (1997). The psychological and emotional impact of living with an automatic internal cardioverter defibrillator (AICD): How can nurses help? *Intensive and Critical Care Nursing, 13*(6), 316–323.

Overbay, D., & Criddle, L. (2004). Mastering temporary invasive cardiac pacing. *Critical Care Nurse, 24*(3), 25–32.

Smeltzer, S. C., & Bare, B. G. (2004). *Brunner & Suddarth's textbook of medical-surgical nursing* (10th ed.). Lippincott Williams & Wilkins.

Wiegand, D., & Carlson, K. (Eds.). (2005). *AACN procedure manual for critical care* (5th ed.). Elsevier Saunders.

Yeo, T. P., & Berg, N. C. (2005). Counseling patients with implanted cardiac devices. *The Nurse Practitioner, 29*(12), 58–65.

Delegation 7650

Definition: Transfer of responsibility for the performance of patient care while retaining accountability for the outcome

Activities:

- Determine the patient care that needs to be completed
- Identify the potential for harm
- Evaluate the complexity of the care to be delegated
- Determine the problem-solving and innovative skills required
- Consider the predictability of the outcome
- Estimate the effect on the nurse's time with the patient and subsequent development of a trusting relationship
- Evaluate the competency and training of the health care worker
- Be familiar with the defined scope of practice, as outlined by state law and facility guidelines, of the health care provider that will assume the tasks, as appropriate
- Explain the task to the health care worker
- Ask questions to learn and clarify the other's understanding of the care to be provided
- Determine the level of supervision needed for the specific delegated intervention or activity (e.g., physically present or immediately available)
- Institute controls, so that the nurse can review the interventions or activities of the health care worker and intervene, as necessary
- Follow up with health care workers on a regular basis to evaluate their progress in completing the specific tasks

- Evaluate the outcome of the delegated intervention or activity and the performance of the health care worker
- Monitor patient's and family's satisfaction with care

2nd edition 1996; revised 2018

Background Evidence:

Cipriano, P. (2010). Overview and summary: Delegation dilemmas: Standards and skills for practice. *OJIN: The Online Journal of Issues in Nursing, 15*(2). https://doi.org/10.3912/OJIN.Vol15No02ManOS

Huber, D. L. (2014). *Leadership and nursing care management* (5th ed.). Elsevier Saunders.

Resnick, M. E., Bakerjian, A. J., Hertz, J., Gardner, W., Rapp, M. P., Reinhard, S., Young, H., & Mezey, M. (2010). Nursing delegation and medication administration in assisted living. *Nursing Administration Quarterly, 34*(2), 162–171.

Weydt, A. (2010). Developing delegation skills. *OJIN: The Online Journal of Issues in Nursing, 15*(2). https://doi.org/10.3912/OJIN.Vol15No02Man01

Whitman, M. M. (2005). Return and report: Establishing accountability in delegation. *American Journal of Nursing, 105*(3), 97.

Delirium Management 6440

Definition: Provision of a safe and therapeutic environment for the patient who is experiencing an acute confusional state

Activities:

- Identify etiological factors causing delirium (e.g., check hemoglobin oxygen saturation)
- Initiate therapies to reduce or eliminate factors causing the delirium
- Recognize and document the motor subtype of the delirium (e.g., hypoactive, hyperactive, and mixed)
- Monitor neurological status on an ongoing basis
- Increase surveillance with a delirium rating scale universally understood by nursing staff when confusion first appears so that acute changes can be easily tracked
- Use family members or friendly hospital volunteers for surveillance of agitated patients instead of restraints
- Acknowledge the patient's fears and feelings
- Provide optimistic but realistic reassurance
- Allow the patient to maintain rituals that limit anxiety
- Provide patient with information about what is happening and what can be expected to occur in the future
- Avoid demands for abstract thinking if patient can think only in concrete terms
- Limit need for decision making if frustrating or confusing to patient
- Administer PRN medications for anxiety or agitation, but limit those with anticholinergic side effects
- Reduce sedation in general, but do control pain with analgesics, as indicated
- Encourage visitation by significant others, as appropriate
- Do not validate a delirium patient's misperceptions or inaccurate interpretations of reality (e.g., hallucinations or delusions)
- State your perception in a calm, reassuring, and nonargumentative manner
- Respond to the tone, rather than the content, of the hallucination or delusion
- Remove stimuli that create excessive sensory stimuli (e.g., television or broadcast intercom announcements), when possible
- Maintain a well-lit environment that reduces sharp contrasts and shadows
- Assist with needs related to nutrition, elimination, hydration, and personal hygiene
- Maintain a hazard-free environment
- Place identification bracelet on patient
- Provide appropriate level of supervision and surveillance to monitor patient and to allow for therapeutic actions, as needed
- Use physical restraints, as needed
- Avoid frustrating patient by quizzing with orientation questions that cannot be answered
- Inform patient of person, place, and time, as needed
- Provide a consistent physical environment and daily routine
- Provide caregivers who are familiar to the patient
- Use environmental cues (e.g., signs, pictures, clocks, calendars, and color coding of environment) to stimulate memory, reorient, and promote appropriate behavior
- Provide a low-stimulation environment for patient in whom disorientation is increased by overstimulation
- Encourage use of aids that increase sensory input (e.g., eyeglasses, hearing aids, and dentures)
- Approach patient slowly and from the front
- Address the patient by name when initiating interaction
- Reorient the patient to the health care provider with each contact
- Communicate with simple, direct, descriptive statements
- Prepare patient for upcoming changes in usual routine and environment before their occurrence
- Provide new information slowly and in small doses, with frequent rest periods
- Focus interpersonal interactions on what is familiar and meaningful to the patient

1st edition 1992; revised 2013

Background Evidence:

Culp, K. R., & Cacchione, P. Z. (2008). Nutritional status and delirium in long-term care elderly individuals. *Applied Nursing Research, 21*(2), 66–74.

Lemiengre, J., Nelis, T., Joosten, E., Braes, T., Foreman, M., Gastmans, C., & Milisen, K. (2006). Detection of delirium by bedside nurses using the confusion assessment method. *Journal of the American Geriatric Society, 54*(4), 685–689.

McCaffrey, R. (2009). The effect of music on acute confusion in older adults after hip or knee surgery. *Applied Nursing Research, 22*(2), 107–112.

Meagher, D. (2009). Motor subtypes of delirium: Past, present, and future. *International Review of Psychiatry, 21*(1), 59–73.

Moyer, D. D. (2011). Review article: Terminal delirium in geriatric patients with cancer at end of life. *American Journal of Hospice and Palliative Medicine, 28*(1), 44–51.

Nelson, L. S. (2009). Teaching staff nurses the CAM-ICU for delirium screening. *Critical Care Nursing Quarterly, 32*(2), 137–143.

Wang, J., & Mentes, J. C. (2009). Factors determining nurses' clinical judgments about hospitalized elderly patients with acute confusion. *Issues in Mental Health Nursing, 30*(6), 399–405.

Yang, F. M., Marcantonio, E. R., Inouye, S. K., Kiely, D. K., Rudolph, J. L., Fearing, M. A., & Jones, R. N. (2009). Phenomenological subtypes of delirium in older persons: Patterns, prevalence, and prognosis. *Psychosomatics, 50*(3), 248–254.

Delusion Management 6450

Definition: Promoting the comfort, safety, and reality orientation of a patient experiencing false, fixed beliefs that have little or no basis in reality

Activities:

- Establish a trusting, interpersonal relationship with patient
- Convey unconditional acceptance and support
- Provide patient with opportunities to discuss delusions with caregivers
- Avoid arguing about false beliefs

- State doubt matter-of-factly
- Avoid reinforcing delusional ideas
- Focus discussion on the underlying feelings, rather than the content of the delusion ("It appears as if you may be feeling frightened.")
- Respond to the patient's delusions with calm, realistic statements
- Provide comfort and reassurance
- Encourage patient to validate delusional beliefs with trusted others (e.g., reality testing)
- Encourage patient to verbalize delusions to caregivers before acting on them
- Assist patient to identify situations in which it is socially unacceptable to discuss delusions
- Encourage discussion of fears, anxiety, and anger without assuming that the delusion is right or wrong
- Provide recreational, diversional activities that require attention or skill
- Monitor self-care ability
- Assist with self-care, as needed
- Monitor physical status of patient
- Provide for adequate rest and nutrition
- Monitor delusions for presence of content that is self-harmful or violent
- Protect the patient and others from delusional behaviors that might be harmful
- Maintain a safe environment
- Provide appropriate level of surveillance and supervision to monitor patient
- Reassure the patient of safety
- Provide for the safety and comfort of patient and others when patient is unable to control behavior (e.g., limit setting, area restriction, physical restraint, or seclusion)

- Decrease excessive environmental stimuli, as needed
- Assist patient to avoid or eliminate stressors that precipitate delusions
- Maintain a consistent daily routine
- Assign consistent caregivers on a daily basis
- Administer antipsychotic and antianxiety medications on a routine and as needed basis
- Provide medication teaching to patient and significant others
- Monitor patient for medication side effects and desired therapeutic effects
- Educate family and significant others about ways to deal with patient who is experiencing delusions
- Provide illness teaching to patient and significant others, if delusions are illness-based (e.g., delirium, schizophrenia, or depression)

2nd edition 1996; revised 2018

Background Evidence:

Fortinash, K., & Worret, P. (2012). *Psychiatric mental health nursing* (5th ed.). Mosby Elsevier.

Kneisl, C., & Trigoboff, E. (2012). *Contemporary psychiatric-mental health nursing* (3rd ed.). Prentice Hall.

Mohr, W. K. (2012). *Psychiatric-mental health nursing: Evidence-based concepts, skills, and practices* (8th ed.). Wolters Kluwer Health/Lippincott Williams & Wilkins.

Stuart, G. W. (Ed.). (2013). *Principles and practice of psychiatric nursing* (10th ed.). Elsevier Mosby.

D

Dementia Management   6460

Definition: Provision of a modified environment for the person who is experiencing a chronic confusion

Activities:

- Understand person's values, beliefs, interests, abilities, likes and dislikes
- Include family members in planning, providing, and evaluating care, to extent desired
- Identify usual patterns of behavior for such activities as sleep, medication use, elimination, food intake, and self-care
- Determine physical, social, and psychological history, usual habits, and routines
- Understand and accept person's reality
- Treat with dignity and respect
- Determine behavioral expectations appropriate for cognitive status
- Use standardized assessments to determine functional and cognitive ability
- Monitor environment to avoid over- and under-stimulation
- Identify and remove potential dangers in environment
- Place identification bracelet on person
- Provide consistent physical environment and daily routine
- Prepare for interaction with eye contact and touch, as culturally appropriate
- Introduce self when initiating contact
- Address distinctly by name when initiating interaction
- Ensure physical, psychological, emotional, and social needs are met

- Modify factors (e.g., unmet needs), caregiver factors (e.g., communication), and environmental factors (e.g., over- or under-stimulation) when managing behavior
- Avoid patronizing and infantilizing communication
- Use distraction or redirection rather than confrontation to manage behavior
- Provide caregivers that are familiar (e.g., avoid frequent rotations of staff assignments)
- Avoid unfamiliar situations, when possible (e.g., room changes and appointments without familiar people present)
- Provide rest periods to prevent fatigue and reduce stress
- Monitor nutrition and weight
- Provide support for eating (e.g., homelike atmosphere, adaptive food and utensils, culturally appropriate foods, proper oral health)
- Provide support for toileting (e.g., scheduled bathroom visits, continence promotion)
- Provide safe space for pacing and wandering
- Avoid agitating by quizzing with orientation questions that cannot be answered
- Decrease noise levels by avoiding paging systems and call lights that ring or buzz
- Provide opportunities for meaningful interaction
- Select activities geared to cognitive abilities and interests
- Label familiar photos with names of individuals in photos

- Discuss with family members and friends how best to interact with person
- Provide choices rather than open-ended questions
- Use symbols, other than written signs, to assist person to locate room, bathroom, or other areas
- Monitor carefully for physiological causes of increased confusion that may be acute and reversible
- Discuss home safety issues and interventions (e.g., access to weapons or chemicals, elopement)
- Encourage use of eyeglasses or hearing aids if needed
- Encourage advance care planning
- Provide opportunities for music and reminisce therapy

2nd edition 1996; revised 2004, 2024

Background Evidence:

Fazio, S., Pace, D., Maslow, K., Zimmerman, S., & Kallmyer, B. (2018). Alzheimer's Association dementia care practice recommendations. *The Gerontologist*, *58*(S1), S1–S9.

Lee, K. H., Lee, J. Y., & Kim, B. (2021). Person-centered care in persons living with dementia: A systematic review and meta-analysis. *The Gerontologist*, *62*(4), e253–e264. https://doi.org/10.1093/geront/gnaa207

Halter, M. J. (2022). *Varcarolis' Foundations of psychiatric mental health nursing: A clinical approach.* Elsevier.

Powers, L., & Smith-East, M. (2021). *Handbook of Geropsychiatry for the Advanced Practice Nurse: Mental Health Care for the Older Adult.* Springer.

Williams, P. (2020). *Basic geriatric nursing.* (7th ed.). Elsevier.

Dementia Management: Bathing   6462

Definition: Reduction of responsive behaviors during cleaning of the body

Activities:

- Personalize bath according to person's usual bathing preferences or cultural preferences (e.g., assistance from family, cover body parts as requested)
- View as whole person by focusing on person rather than task
- Determine preferences for bathing (e.g., soaking bath, shower, towel bath, bag-bath with no-rinse soap, disposable wipes with no-rinse soap)
- Determine preferences for time of day, use of products, location, and frequency of bathing
- Maintain privacy by using location that allows for uninterrupted bathing
- Maintain warmth of environment (e.g., radiant heat panels, infrared heat lamps, heated floors)
- Maintain warmth of bathing supplies (e.g., warming cabinet for towels or towelettes, ensure water appropriate temperature)
- Maintain warmth of person (i.e., keep covered with bath blanket)
- Reduce extraneous environmental noise (e.g., place acoustic panels in bathroom)
- Create relaxing environment with preferred music (i.e., individualized bathing playlist)
- Socialize with person prior to initiating bathing
- Seek input from other caregivers related to preferences and successful or unsuccessful bathing strategies
- Invite family caregivers into bathing process
- Prepare all bathing supplies prior to approaching person
- Use familiar or preferred bath products
- Order body parts being washed from least sensitive to most sensitive
- Encourage person to assist with bath as able
- Support flexible bathing times and approach person when calm
- Give pain medication before bath if movement is painful
- Assess for cues that indicate discomfort
- Provide choices (e.g., "would you like me to wash your hand or arm next?")
- Ask permission before touching person
- Use gentle touch
- Announce tasks and describe actions
- Speak in soft, relaxing, non-patronizing tone
- Respond accordingly to person's perceptions (e.g., temperature, pain, fear of drowning)
- Use distraction
- Identify antecedents or "triggers" if responsive behavior occurs
- Do not use physical restraints and avoid chemical restraints (e.g., psychoactive medications)
- Monitor for verbal and nonverbal warning signs of increasing rejection of care
- Accept negative comments and accept refusals
- Validate person's feelings (i.e., do not contradict)
- Complete towel or bag bath in person preferred location (e.g., bed, recliner)
- Assure family when giving towel or bag bath that washing without water improves skin condition compared to traditional bed bath and that there are no differences in skin or hygienic outcomes when comparing washing without water compared to traditional bath or shower
- Introduce bath or shower slowly when giving traditional bath or shower by first letting water trickle on hand
- Perform gentle massage during bathing or with lotion after bathing
- Use no rinse shampoo product or have hair stylist shampoo hair, as needed
- Use bathing equipment that is comfortable for person
- Use proper ergonomic equipment and techniques to ensure health provider and person safety
- Attempt other methods of bathing for future hygienic care if rejection of care occurs
- Provide evidenced-based and person-centered education about bathing for health providers, as appropriate

4th edition 2004; revised 2024

Background Evidence:

Backhouse, T., Dudzinski, E., Killett, A., & Mioshi, E. (2020). Strategies and interventions to reduce or manage refusals in personal care in dementia: A systematic review. *International Journal of Nursing Studies*, *109*, 103640. https://doi.org/10.1016/j.ijnurstu.2020.103640

Foster, S., Balmer, D., Gott, M., Frey, R., Robinson, J., & Boyd, M. (2019). Patient-centered care training needs of health care assistants who provide care for people with dementia. *Health & Social Care in the Community*, *27*(4), 917–925. https://doi.org/10.1111/hsc.12709

Groven, F., Zwakhalen, S., Odekerken-Schröder, G., Joosten, E., & Hamers, J. (2017). How does washing without water perform compared to the traditional bed bath: A systematic review. *BMC Geriatrics*, *17*(1), 31–31. https://doi.org/10.1186/s12877-017-0425-4

Gutman, G., Karbakhsh, M., Vashisht, A., Kaur, T., Churchill, R., & Moztarzadeh, A. (2021). Feasibility study of a digital screen-based calming device (MindfulGarden) for bathing-related agitation among LTC residents with dementia. *Gerontechnology*, *20*(2), 1–8. https://doi.org/10.4017/gt.2021.20.2.439.04

Yous, M. L., Ploeg, J., Kaasalainen, S., & Martin, L. S. (2019). Nurses' experiences in caring for older adults with responsive behaviors of dementia in acute care Jan-Dec. *SAGE Open Nursing*, *5*. https://doi.org/10.1177/2377960819834127. 2377960819834127.

D

Dementia Management: Wandering 6466

Definition: Provision of care for a person experiencing pacing patterns, elopement attempts, or getting lost unless accompanied

Activities:

- Include family members in planning, providing, and evaluating care to extent desired
- Identify usual patterns of wandering behavior
- Support safer walking by providing secure and safe place for wandering
- Identify and remove potential dangers in environment
- Provide appropriate supervision (i.e., place in room that allows for maximum surveillance, conduct regular checks, use volunteer or specialized personnel)
- Modify unsafe aspects of environment (e.g., throw rugs, adequate lighting)
- Alert neighbors about wandering behavior
- Alert police and have current pictures of person taken
- Provide person with medical alert bracelet or necklace
- Use technology strategies such as pressure pads, locating devices, door alarms, surveillance, and wandering detection devices for elopement concerns
- Use locating strategies such as radio frequency identification devices (RFID), global positioning system (GPS) devices, or electronic tagging
- Use visual exiting barriers such as cloth coverings over doorknobs, mirrors in front of exit doors, and tape on floors in front of exit doors for elopement concerns
- Reduce environmental triggers for wandering (e.g., avoid placing in rooms near areas of high traffic or noise, avoid rooms near elevators, exit signs or stairs, position bed with best visibility of bathroom)
- Determine causes of wandering (e.g., searching for loved ones, going to work)
- Adapt strategies to causes of wandering
- Provide assurances of safety and belonging
- Provide card with information (e.g., address, phone number)
- Monitor carefully for physiological causes of increased confusion that may be acute and reversible
- Monitor nutrition, hydration, and weight
- Use symbols, other than written signs, to assist person to locate room, bathroom, or other areas
- Provide rest periods to prevent fatigue and reduce stress
- Use distraction or redirection, rather than confrontation, to manage behavior
- Provide meaningful activities for person including but not limited to music, art, doll therapy, exercise programing, and aromatherapy
- Increase social interactions and engagement in activities
- Reduce noise, draw shades at sundown to reduce shadows, play soothing music, and use non-glare lighting, which may also help decrease agitation that can lead to wandering
- Accommodate bedtime and sleep rituals to prevent insomnia and nighttime wandering
- Follow organizational protocols for lost persons

6th edition 2013; revised 2024

Background Evidence:

Eliopoulos, C. (2022). *Gerontological nursing* (10th ed.). Wolters Kluwer.

MacAndrew, M., Brooks, D., & Beattie, E. (2017). Nonpharmacological interventions for managing wandering in the community: A narrative review to the evidence base. *Health and Social Care, 27,*(30) 6–319.

Neubauer, N. A., Azad-Khaneghah, P., Miguel-Cruz, A., & Liu, L. (2018). What do we know about strategies to manage dementia-related wandering? A scoping review. *Alzheimer's & Dementia, 10*, 615–628.

Silverstein, N. M., & Flaherty, G. (2018). Wandering in hospitalized older adults. *Try This: Best Practices in Nursing Care for Older Adults with Dementia*, D6, 1–2.

Varcarolic, E. M., & Halter, M. J. (2018). *Foundations of psychiatric mental health nursing*. Saunders/Elsevier.

Williams, P. (2020). *Basic geriatric nursing*. (7th ed.). Elsevier.

Deposition 7930

Definition: Provision of recorded sworn testimony for legal proceedings based upon knowledge of the case

Activities:

- Contact employer and malpractice carrier when notice of deposition or subpoena for testimony received
- Prepare thoroughly
- Retain attorney, as necessary
- Discuss case only with attorney representing self at deposition
- Avoid discussing case with co-workers, health care providers, and others involved without attorney present
- Request that attorney explain deposition process
- Prepare by reviewing clinical chart and reading or rereading any documents to be presented during deposition
- Keep all documents in safe and secure place
- Review documents prior to deposition
- Listen carefully to entire question to understand it before attempting to answer
- Ask for clarification if question is unclear

D

- Answer questions directly and truthfully
- Avoid second guessing questions
- Avoid interrupting or interjecting words when questions asked
- Answer only questions pertaining to personal experience and role; do not speculate on role and duties of others
- Answer "I do not remember" or "I don't recall" if not able to remember a fact
- Follow directions of attorney in providing answers
- Testify only about documents read
- Clarify facts if misstated
- Be respectful, courteous, and polite
- Speak calmly, clearly, and with confidence
- Spell unusual words after clearly enunciating them, if requested
- Avoid using acronyms
- Ask to talk with attorney privately, if needed

- Communicate with opposing counsel or opposing party only with attorney present
- If tired, ask to get up to take break

4th edition 2004; revised 2024

Background Evidence:

American Nurses Association. (2015). *Code of ethics for nurses with interpretive statements.*

American Nurses Association. (2021). *Nursing: Scope and standards of practice* (4th ed.).

Flanagan, M. (2020). Deposition 101: Tips for success. *Journal of Legal Nurse Consulting*, 31(2), 18–21.

Guido, G. W. (2020). *Legal and ethical issues in nursing.* (7th ed.). Pearson.

Keltner, N. L., & Steele, D. (2019). *Psychiatric nursing.* (8th ed.). Elsevier.

Lee Lockeretz, M. (2018). Tales from the court: Experienced LNCs at trial and deposition. *Journal of Legal Nurse Consulting*, 29(3), 24–28.

Developmental Enhancement: Infant 8278

Definition: Facilitating optimal physical, cognitive, social, and emotional growth of child under 1 year of age

Activities:

- Instruct parent on what constitutes appropriate infant nutrition and nutritional habits
- Discuss and support decision to breastfeed or bottle feed
- Instruct on proper storage, preparation, and handling of breast milk or prepared infant formula
- Introduce solid foods at approximately 6 months of age, instructing parent on the selection and preparation of foods, methods of introduction, and food storage
- Instruct parent to avoid offering the infant a bottle containing juice or milk when in bed
- Provide anticipatory guidance for infant weaning, including signs of readiness
- Encourage establishment of bedtime rituals that reduce or eliminate disturbances in sleep-wake cycle
- Assisting parent in identifying presence of sleep disturbance or disorder
- Determine appropriate management technique for sleep disturbance or disorder
- Discuss the risks and benefits of infant and caregiver co-sleeping
- Provide visual, auditory, tactile, and kinetic stimulation during play
- Structure play and care around infant's behavioral style and temperament patterns
- Provide developmentally appropriate, safe toys and activities
- Explain the need for fluoride supplementation beginning at 6 months of age
- Instruct parent to begin cleaning infant's oral cavity with damp cloth upon eruption of first tooth
- Use soft-bristled toothbrush with water or non-fluoridated toothpaste once several teeth have erupted
- Determine appropriate scheduling for initial and subsequent dental examinations
- Perform recommended screenings (e.g., anemia, lead exposure, and vision)
- Provide accurate information pertaining to risks, benefits, contraindications, and side effects of scheduled immunizations
- Identify need for additional immunizations for selected groups of children

- Provide anticipatory guidance concerning discipline, dependency, increased mobility, and safety
- Discuss timeout versus corporal punishment strategies for discipline, encouraging the former
- Instruct parent on injury prevention strategies tailored to child's specific developmental stage and curiosity level
- Encourage provision of safe space for infant exploration
- Discuss injury prevention strategies for fire and electrical burns, suffocation and aspiration, poisoning, falls, bodily injury, drowning, and motor vehicle injury
- Instruct parent on prevention strategies for sudden infant death syndrome (SIDS)
- Instruct parent about child temperament and its association with infant's interaction type with others
- Promote and facilitate family bonding and attachment with infant
- Support and praise parent skills and efforts
- Discuss parent return to work and childcare options
- Identify and address presence of family strife, lack of support, and pathology
- Provide information to parent about child development and child rearing
- Refer for parenting education, as needed

6th edition 2013

Background Evidence:

Ball, J. W., & Bindler, R. C. (2008). Health promotion and health maintenance for the newborn and infant. In *Pediatric nursing: Caring for children* (pp. 281–308) (4th ed.). Pearson: Prentice Hall.

Levine, D. A. (2006). Evaluation of the well child. In R. M. Kliegman, K. J. Marcdante, H. B. Jenson, & R. E. Behrman (Eds.), *Nelson essentials of pediatrics* (5th ed., pp. 34–43). Elsevier Saunders.

Wilson, D. (2007). Health promotion of the infant and family. In M. J. Hockenberry & D. Wilson (Eds.), *Wong's nursing care of infants and children* (8th ed., pp. 499–565). Mosby Elsevier.

Wong, D. L., Hockenberry, M. J., Wilson, D., Perry, S. E., & Lowdermilk, D. L. (2006). The infant and family. In *Maternal child nursing care* (pp. 1027–1088) (3rd ed.). Elsevier.

Dialysis Access Maintenance 4240

Definition: Preservation of vascular (arterial-venous) access sites

D

Activities:
- Monitor catheter exit site for migration
- Monitor access site for redness, edema, heat, drainage, bleeding hematoma, and decreased sensation
- Apply sterile gauze, ointment, and dressing to central venous dialysis catheter site with each treatment
- Monitor for AV fistula patency at frequent intervals (e.g., palpate for thrill and auscultate for bruit)
- Heparinize newly inserted central venous dialysis catheters
- Reheparinize central venous dialysis catheters after dialysis or every 72 hours
- Avoid mechanical compression of peripheral access sites
- Avoid mechanical compression of patient's limbs near central dialysis catheter
- Teach patient to avoid mechanical compression of peripheral access site
- Teach patient about how to care for dialysis access site
- Avoid venipuncture and blood pressures in peripheral access extremity

4th edition 2004

Background Evidence:

Eisenbud, M.D. (1996). The handbook of dialysis access. Anadem.

Gutch, C. F., Stoner, M. H., & Corea, A. L. (1993). *Review of hemodialysis for nurses and dialysis personnel* (5th ed.). St. Louis: Mosby.

Lancaster, L.E. (Ed.). (1995). ANNA's core curriculum for nephrology nurses (3rd ed., Section X). American Nephrology Nurses.

Levine, D. Z. (1997). *Caring for the renal patient* (3rd ed.). W. B. Saunders.

Diarrhea Management 0460

Definition: Management and alleviation of loose frequent, bowel movements

Activities:
- Review health history including diagnoses, surgeries, and bowel habits
- Identify factors that may cause or contribute to diarrhea (e.g., medications, exercise, sleep, stress, diet)
- Determine history of diarrhea (e.g., acute, persistent, chronic)
- Obtain stool for culture and sensitivity if diarrhea continues, as prescribed
- Evaluate medication profile for gastrointestinal side effects
- Monitor bowel movements including frequency, consistency, volume, and color
- Instruct on appropriate use of antidiarrheal medications
- Instruct to record frequency, consistency, volume, and color of stools
- Explain etiology of problem and rationale for actions
- Evaluate recorded intake for nutritional content
- Observe skin turgor and other signs of dehydration (e.g., sunken eyes, dry mucous membranes)
- Monitor skin in perianal area for irritation and ulceration
- Weigh regularly
- Encourage frequent, small, bland food feedings, adding bulk gradually
- Instruct to eliminate lactose, spicy or fatty foods, and caffeine
- Identify factors that may cause or contribute to diarrhea (e.g., medications, bacteria, tube feedings)
- Consult health care provider if signs and symptoms of diarrhea persist
- Instruct in low-fiber, high-protein, high-calorie diet, as appropriate
- Consult dietitian as needed
- Instruct in avoidance of laxatives
- Instruct how to keep food diary
- Instruct on stress-reduction techniques, as appropriate
- Monitor safe food preparation and sanitation
- Perform actions to rest bowel (e.g., NPO, liquid diet)
- Use teach-back to ensure understanding

1st edition 1992; revised 2000, 2004, 2024

Background Evidence:

Craven, R. F., Hirnle, C. J., & Henshaw, C. J. (2021). *Fundamentals of nursing: Human health and function* (8th ed.). Wolters-Kluwer.

Guarino, A., Lo Vecchio, A., Dias, J. A., Berkley, J. A., Boey, C., Bruzzese, D., Cohen, M. B., Cruchet, S., Liguoro, I., Salazar-Lindo, E., Sandhu, B., Sherman, P. M., & Shimizu, T. (2018). Universal recommendations for the management of acute diarrhea in nonmalnourished children. *Journal of Pediatric Gastroenterology and Nutrition, 67*(5), 586–593. https://doi.org/10.1097/MPG.0000000000002053

Motamedi, H., Fathollahi, M., Abiri, R., Kadivarian, S., Rostamian, M., & Alvandi, A. (2021). A worldwide systematic review and meta-analysis of bacteria related to antibiotic-associated diarrhea in hospitalized patients. *PloS One, 16*(12), e0260667. https://doi.org/10.1371/journal.pone.0260667

Potter, P. A., Perry, A. G., Stockert, P. A., & Hall, A. M. (2021). *Fundamentals of nursing* (10th ed.). Elsevier.

Thabit, A. K., Alsolami, M. H., Baghlaf, N. A., Alsharekh, R. M., Almazmumi, H. A., Alselami, A. S., & Alsubhi, F. A. (2019). Comparison of three current Clostridioides difficile infection guidelines: IDSA/SHEA, ESCMID, and ACG guidelines. *Infection, 47*(6), 899–909. https://doi.org/10.1007/s15010-019-01348-9

van Erp, L. W., Roosenboom, B., Komdeur, P., Dijkstra-Heida, W., Wisse, J., Horjus Talabur Horje, C. S., Liem, C. S., van Cingel, R. E. H., Wahab, P., & Groenen, M. J. M. (2021). Improvement of fatigue and quality of life in patients with quiescent inflammatory bowel disease following a personalized exercise program. *Digestive Diseases and Sciences, 66*(2), 597–604. https://doi.org/10.1007/s10620-020-06222-5

D

Diet Staging 1020

Definition: Instituting required diet restrictions with subsequent progression of diet as tolerated

Activities:

- Determine presence of bowel sounds
- Institute NPO, as needed
- Clamp nasogastric tube and monitor tolerance, as appropriate
- Monitor for alertness and presence of gag reflex, as appropriate
- Monitor tolerance to ingestion of ice chips and water
- Determine whether patient is passing flatus
- Collaborate with other health care team members to progress diet as rapidly as possible without complications
- Progress diet from clear liquid, full liquid, soft, to regular or special diet, as tolerated, for adults and children
- Progress from glucose water or oral electrolyte solution, half-strength formula, to full-strength formula for babies
- Monitor tolerance to diet progression
- Offer six small feedings, rather than three meals, as appropriate
- Find ways to include patient preferences in the prescribed diet
- Make the environment in which the meal is offered as pleasant as possible
- Post the diet restrictions at bedside, on chart, and in care plan

1st edition 1992; revised 2013

Background Evidence:

Dudek, S. G. (2007). Feeding patients: Hospital food and enteral and parenteral nutrition. In *Nutrition essentials for nursing practice* (pp. 417–456) (5th rev. ed.). Lippincott Williams & Wilkins.

Holloway, N. M. (2004). *Medical-surgical care planning* (pp. 689) (4th ed.). Lippincott, Williams & Wilkins.

Nyberg, M., & Olsen, T. D. (2010). Meals at work: Integrating social and architectural aspects. *International Journal of Workplace Health Management*, 3(3), 222–232.

Stanfield, P., & Hui, Y. H. (2010). *Nutrition and diet therapy: Self-instructional approaches* (pp. 266) (5th ed.). Jones & Bartlett.

Diet Staging: Weight Loss Surgery 1024

Definition: Instituting required diet changes in progressive phases following bariatric surgery

Activities:

- Institute NPO or sips of water only for the first 24 to 48 hours after surgery, according to agency policy
- Administer solutions of dextrose, saline, or lactated Ringer's to provide adequate nutrition in first 24 hours and until patient can tolerate a full liquid diet
- Progress to a liquid diet that lasts 2 to 3 weeks
- Instruct patient to sip room-temperature liquids (e.g., broth, unsweetened juice, milk) slowly, consuming between two to three ounces at a time
- Instruct patients to carry with them sugar-free beverages and drink often
- Incorporate pureed foods (e.g., broth blended with well-cooked beans, fish, or ground meats; yogurt; blended fruits) in diet once the patient's body has adjusted to liquids
- Add mashed solid foods (e.g., finely diced meats, canned fruits, oatmeal, eggs) between 6 to 8 weeks post-surgery
- Instruct patient to eat the protein foods on the plate first
- Progress to firmer foods that are low in sugar, low in saturated and trans-fat, and contain high-quality protein, maintaining this diet for life
- Encourage patients to eat breakfast and at least four to five small meals daily
- Instruct patients to take small bites, eat slowly, and chew solids that are well-cooked
- Instruct patients to incorporate fresh fruits and vegetables in their fluid and food intake
- Monitor for lactose intolerance as a possible postsurgical complication
- Work with a dietitian after surgery to ensure that protein nutrition is optimal and to modify the diet as required
- Find ways to include patient preferences in the prescribed diet
- Make the environment in which the meal is offered as pleasant as possible
- Post the diet restrictions at bedside, on chart, and in care plan
- Instruct patient to avoid foods and beverages with large amounts of sugar (e.g., soda, juice drinks, milk shakes, regular ice cream) as these may cause a dumping syndrome
- Instruct patient to avoid drinking approximately half an hour before eating, during the meal, and half an hour after the meal to reduce vomiting and diarrhea
- Instruct patient about need to take an adult strength multivitamin with iron, a B-complex supplement, and added calcium
- Monitor tolerance to diet progression
- Encourage patients to keep a record of types and quantities of foods that cause discomfort, distress, or intolerance
- Encourage patients to do at least 35 minutes of daily aerobic exercise with strength training three times per week to maintain a good metabolic rate
- Encourage attendance at a support group for several months post-surgery

6th edition 2013

Background Evidence:

Dowd, J. (2005). Nutrition management after gastric bypass surgery. *Diabetes Spectrum*, 18(2), 82–84.

Elliot, K. (2003). Nutritional considerations after bariatric surgery. *Critical Care Nursing Quarterly*, 26(2), 133–138.

Farraye, F. A., & Forse, R. A. (Eds.). (2006). *Bariatric surgery: A primer for your medical practice* (pp. 148–153). Slack.

Strohmayer, E., Via, M. A., & Yanagisawa, R. (2010). Metabolic management following bariatric surgery. *Mount Sinai Journal of Medicine*, 77(5), 431–445.

Discharge Follow-Up 8190

Definition: Providing test results, confirming understanding plan of care, and evaluating satisfaction with care

Activities:
- Confirm speaking to correct person
- Obtain permission to give personal information if speaking with someone other than person
- Identify self with name, credentials, and organization
- Use intermediary services for communication as indicated
- Inform about call process and obtain consent
- Advise if call being recorded (e.g., for quality monitoring)
- Review current health condition
- Notify test results, as indicated
- Assist with prescription refills, according to established guidelines
- Ensure all questions are answered
- Determine satisfaction with care episodes using organizational guidelines
- Document satisfaction using organizational guidelines
- Review information from previous treatment, examination or testing to ensure adequate comprehension and adequate home care obtained or followed
- Provide information about community resources, educational programs, support groups, and self-help groups, as indicated
- Establish date and time for follow-up care or referral appointment
- Provide information about current treatment regimen and resultant self-care responsibilities according to scope of practice and established guidelines, as necessary
- Inform when to seek additional care
- Maintain confidentiality
- Do not leave follow-up messages on voice mail
- Document any assessments, advice, instructions, or other information given according to specified guidelines
- Determine how person or family member can be reached for return telephone call, as appropriate
- Document permission for return call and identify persons able to receive call
- Use teach-back to ensure understanding

3rd edition 2000; revised 2024

Background Evidence:

American Academy of Ambulatory Care Nursing. (2017). *Scope and standards of practice for professional ambulatory care nursing* (9th ed.).

American Academy of Ambulatory Care Nursing. (2018). *Scope and standards of practice for professional telehealth nursing* (6th ed.).

Berdal, G., Bø, I., Dager, T. N., Dingsør, A., Eppeland, S. G., Hagfors, J., Hamnes, B., Mowinckel, P., Nielsen, M., Sand, S. A., Slungaard, B., Wigers, S. H., Hagen, K. B., Dagfinrud, H. S., Kjeken, I., & Sand-Svartrud, A.-L. (2018). Structured goal planning and supportive telephone follow-up in rheumatology care: Results from a pragmatic, stepped-wedge, cluster-randomized trial. *Arthritis Care & Research, 70*(11), 1576–1586.

Jackson, A., Curtin, E., Giddins, E., Read-Allsopp, C., & Joseph, A. (2021). Connecting with trauma patients after discharge: A phone call follow-up study. *Journal of Trauma Nursing, 28*(3), 179–185.

Nasser, L., & Stratton, T. (2019). BET 1: Follow-up phone calls and compliance with discharge instructions in elderly patients discharged from the emergency department. *Emergency Medicine Journal, 36*(2), 126–127.

Rutledge, C. M., Kott, K., Schweickert, P. A., Poston, R., Fowler, C., & Haney, T. S. (2017). Telehealth and eHealth in nurse practitioner training: Current perspectives. *Advances in Medical Education and Practice, 8*, 399–409.

Woods, C. E., Jones, R., O'Shea, E., Grist, E., Wiggers, J., & Usher, K. (2019). Nurse-led post-discharge telephone follow-up calls: A mixed study systematic review. *Journal of Clinical Nursing, 28*, 3386–3399.

Discharge Planning 7370

Definition: Preparation for moving a person from one level of care to another within or outside the current health care agency

Activities:
- Gather data related to discharge needs upon admission and ongoing
- Determine preferred languages for in-person oral communication, phone communication, and written materials
- Observe for impaired health literacy cues (e.g., failing to complete written forms, inability to identify medications or reasons for taking them, deferment to family members for information about health condition)
- Arrange for a qualified health care interpreter, including translation of written materials, as indicated
- Elicit person's goals for discharge
- Provide ongoing instruction to person, family and caregivers related to hospital stay (e.g., cause for admission, treatments, care needed)
- Ensure person, family, and caregivers are active participants in care
- Determine home resources, challenges, and family or caregiver availability
- Assist in planning for supportive environment to provide post-hospital care
- Develop discharge plan that considers health literacy, health care, social, cultural, and financial needs
- Formulate plan for post-discharge follow-up with person, family, and caregiver involvement
- Ensure that dietary advice is consistent with religious or cultural practices
- Ensure ability to obtain required medications and take as prescribed
- Monitor readiness for discharge
- Assist to prepare for discharge as indicated
- Instruct on required after-hospital follow-up care (e.g., medicines, diet, exercise, herbal supplements)
- Review any areas of poor understanding during instructions

D

- Communicate discharge plans to interprofessional team, as appropriate
- Ensure that adequate communication with primary care providers is ongoing
- Coordinate efforts of interprofessional team to ensure timely discharge
- Report any areas of concern related to discharge teaching or planning, prior to discharge
- Provide copies of all information in preferred language
- Expedite transmission of discharge summary to clinicians accepting care of person
- Inform post-discharge caregivers of preferred language and cultural needs
- Place discharge instructions in electronic portal for easy access, if appropriate
- Provide contact information with discharge instructions
- Schedule appointments for follow-up care (e.g., appointments, post-discharge tests or labs)
- Arrange for post-discharge evaluation, as appropriate
- Plan for follow-up results from lab tests or labs that are pending at discharge
- Organize post-discharge outpatient services and health care equipment
- Provide reinforcement of discharge plan within 48 hours of discharge (e.g., via telephone, text messages, video chat, home visit)
- Coordinate with home health agencies to increase discharge information, follow-up, and after-hospital care received, as indicated
- Arrange for caregiver support, as appropriate
- Document discharge plans
- Use teach-back to ensure understanding

1st edition 1992; revised 2008, 2024

Background Evidence:

Agency for Healthcare Research and Quality [AHRQ]. (2019). Re-Engineered Discharge (RED) Toolkit. http://www.ahrq.gov/professionals/systems/hospital/red/toolkit/index.html

Brooks, K. L. (2020). Start your discharge planning early. *New Mexico Nurse*, 65(2), 4–5.

Glasper, A. (2019). Ensuring smooth transition of frail elderly patients from hospital to community. *British Journal of Nursing*, 28(20), 133 8–1339.

Sexson, K., Lindauer, A., & Harvath, T. (2017). Discharge planning and teaching. *American Journal of Nursing*, 117(5), 58–60.

Seigert, L. (2021). Improving discharge procedures to reduce hospital readmissions. *AJN, American Journal of Nursing*, 121(12), 12. https://doi.org/10.1097/01.NAJ.0000803148.45426.39

Wrotny, C. (2021). Back so soon? A community hospital creates new ways to prevent readmission. *Professional Case Management*, 26(4), 177–185. https://doi.org/10.1097/NCM.0000000000000475

Wrotny, C., Bradley, D., & Brulé, M. (2021). Back so soon? Part 2: Use of the 5 "Whys" process in unplanned hospital readmissions. *Professional Case Management*, 26(4), 186–193. https://doi.org/10.1097/NCM.0000000000000505

Discharge Planning: Home Preparation   6485

Definition: Preparing the home for safe and effective delivery of care

Activities:

- Determine at-home needs based on current health (e.g., comorbidities, cognitive or motor deficits)
- Review home environment with person or family to determine problem areas
- Consult with person and family concerning preparation for care delivery at home
- Order and validate operation of any equipment needed
- Order and confirm delivery of medications and supplies, as needed
- Arrange scheduling of support personnel
- Confirm that emergency plans are in place
- Confirm date and time of transfer to home
- Confirm arrangements for transportation to home with accompanying escort, as needed
- Encourage transition of care, with special attention to strengthening bond between person and family and new team or service
- Follow up to assure that plans were feasible and carried out
- Provide written materials regarding medications, supplies, and assistive devices as guides for caregivers, as needed
- Instruct family or caregiver about health-disease process that person experiences
- Provide guidance on organization of airy, light, and clean environment
- Instruct family about situations requiring return to hospital
- Prepare teaching plans for use in home to coincide with any earlier teaching already accomplished
- Provide documentation to meet agency guidelines
- Document person's health status upon arrival at home

3rd edition 2000; revised 2024

Background Evidence:

Backman, C., Chartrand, J., Dingwall, O., & Shea, B. (2017). Effectiveness of person- and family-centered care transition interventions: A systematic review protocol. *Systematic Reviews*, 6(1), 158. https://doi.org/10.1186/s13643-017-0554-z

Berman, A., Snyder, S. J., & Frandsen, G. (2018). *Kozier and Erb's Fundamentals of Nursing: Concepts, process and practice* (10th ed.). Pearson.

Craven, R. F., Hirnle, C. J., & Henshaw, C. J. (2021). *Fundamentals of nursing: Human health and function* (8th ed.). Wolters-Kluwer.

de Abreu Moniz, M., Vago Daher, D., Sabóia, V. M., & Batista Ribeiro, C. R. (2020). Environmental health: Emancipatory care challenges and possibilities by the nurse. *Revista Brasileira de Enfermagem*, 73(3), 1–5.

Næss, G., Kirkevold, M., Hammer, W., Straand, J., & Wyller, T. B. (2017). Nursing care needs and services utilised by home-dwelling elderly with complex health problems: observational study. *BMC Health Services Research*. 17(1), 645.

Perry, A. G., Potter, P. A., Ostendorf, W. R., & Laplante, N. (2022). *Clinical Nursing Skills and Techniques* (10th ed.). Elsevier.

Ridwan, E. S., Hadi, H., Wu, Y. L., & Tsai, P. S. (2019). Effects of transitional care on hospital readmission and mortality rate in subjects with COPD: A systematic review and meta-analysis. *Respiratory care*. 64(9), 1146–1156.

Ugur, H. G., & Erci, B. (2019). The effect of home care for stroke patients and education of caregivers on the caregiver burden and quality of life. *Acta Clinica Croatica. 58*(2), 321–332.

Valatka, R., Krizo, J., & Mallat, A. (2021). A survey-based assessment of "matter of balance" participant fall-related experience. *Journal of Trauma Nursing, 28*(5), 304–309.

Williams, P. (2020). *Basic geriatric nursing* (7th ed.). Elsevier.

Yamaguchi, Y., Greiner, C., Ryuno, H., & Fukuda, A. (2019). Dementia nursing competency in acute care settings: A concept analysis. *International Journal of Nursing Practice, 25*(3), 1–5.

Distraction 5900

D

Definition: Purposeful diverting of attention or temporarily suppressing negative emotions and thoughts away from undesirable sensations

Activities:

- Encourage the individual to choose the distraction technique(s) desired (e.g., music, engaging in conversation or telling a detailed account of event or story, recalling positive event, focusing on photo or neutral object, guided imagery, humor, or deep breathing exercises)
- Instruct the patient on the benefits of stimulating a variety of senses (e.g., music, counting, television, reading, video/hand-held games, or virtual reality)
- Use distraction techniques for children (e.g., play, activity therapy, reading stories, singing songs, or rhythm activities) that are novel, appeal to more than one sense, and do not require literacy or thinking ability
- Suggest techniques consistent with energy level, ability, age appropriateness, developmental level, and effective use in the past
- Identify with the patient a list of pleasurable activities (e.g., exercise, going for walks, bubble baths, talking to friends or family)
- Individualize the content of the distraction technique, based on those used successfully in the past and age or developmental level
- Advise patient to practice the distraction technique before the time needed, if possible
- Instruct patient how to engage in the distraction (e.g., prompting neutral word, equipment, or materials) before the time needed, if possible
- Encourage participation of family and significant others and provide teaching, as necessary
- Use distraction alone or in conjunction with other measures or distractions, as appropriate
- Evaluate and document response to distraction

1st edition 1992; revised 2013

Background Evidence:

Huffziger, S., & Kuehner, C. (2008). Rumination, distraction, and mindful self-focus in depressed patients. *Behaviour Research and Therapy, 47*(3), 224–230.

Kleiber, C. (2001). Distraction. In M. Craft-Rosenberg & J. Denehy (Eds.), *Nursing interventions for infants, children, and families* (pp. 315–328). Sage.

Kleiber, C., McCarthy, A. M., Hanrahan, K., Myers, L., & Weathers, N. (2007). Development of the distraction coaching index. *Children's Health Care, 36*(3), 219–235.

Lemoult, J., Hertel, P. T., & Joormann, J. (2010). Training the forgetting of negative words: The role of direct suppression and the relation to stress reactivity. *Applied Cognitive Psychology, 24*(3), 365–375.

Malloy, K. M., & Milling, L. S. (2010). The effectiveness of virtual reality distraction for pain reduction: A systematic review. *Clinical Psychology Review, 30*(8), 1011–1018.

Masuda, A., Feinstein, A. B., Wendell, J. W., & Sheehan, S. T. (2010). Cognitive defusion versus thought distraction: A clinical rationale, training, and experiential exercise in altering psychological impacts of negative self-referential thoughts. *Behavior Modification, 34*(6), 520–538.

Schneider, S. M., & Workman, M. L. (2000). Virtual reality as a distraction intervention for older children receiving chemotherapy. *Pediatric Nursing, 26*(6), 593–597.

Documentation 7920

Definition: Written or electronic recording of pertinent data in a health care record

Activities:

- Ensure correct record prior to documentation
- Record initial and ongoing assessment findings
- Include nursing assessments, nursing diagnoses, nursing interventions, and outcomes of care provided
- Use principles for documentation (e.g., factual, accurate, complete, timely)
- Use standardized, systematic, and prescribed documentation policy required by facility
- Use vendor and agency specific forms and flowsheets as indicated (e.g., Braden scale, fall risk)
- Record all entries as promptly as possible
- Avoid duplication of information
- Use approved abbreviations
- Ensure accurate date and time of all events
- Describe behaviors objectively and accurately using quotations, as needed
- Record response to nursing interventions
- Record when provider was notified of change in status
- Include deviations from expected outcomes, as appropriate
- Record use of safety measures, as appropriate
- Include photos per facility policy
- Record involvement of significant others, as appropriate
- Record observations of home environment, as appropriate
- Record status of identified problems
- Ensure that record complete at discharge
- Sign record, using legal signature, credentials, and title
- Maintain privacy and confidentiality of record

- Document and report situations, as mandated by law

2nd edition 1996; revised 2000, 2024

Background Evidence:

Ali, R., Syed, S., Sastry, R. A., Abdulrazeq, H., Shao, B., Roye, G. D., Doberstein, C. E., Oyelese, A., Niu, T., Gokaslan, Z. L., & Telfeian, A. (2021). Toward more accurate documentation in neurosurgical care. *Neurosurgical Focus, 51*(5), E11. https://doi.org/10.3171/2021.8.FOCUS21387

Berman, A., Snyder, S. J., & Frandsen, G. (2018). *Kozier and Erb's fundamentals of nursing: Concepts, process and practice.* (10th ed.). Pearson.

Craven, R. F., Hirnle, C. J., & Henshaw, C. J. (2021). *Fundamentals of nursing: Human health and function* (8th ed.). Wolters-Kluwer.

Limandri, B. J. (2021). Efficient and effective documentation in nursing care. *Oregon State Board of Nursing Sentinel, 40*(3), 4–7.

Potter, P. A., Perry, A. G., Stockert, P. A., & Hall, A. M. (2021). *Fundamentals of nursing* (10th ed.). Elsevier.

Shiells, K., Holmerova, I., Steffl, M., & Stepankova, O. (2019). Electronic patient records as a tool to facilitate care provision in nursing homes: An integrative review. *Informatics for Health & Social Care, 44*(3), 262–277. https://doi:10.1080/17538157.2018.1496091

Sievers, V., & Faugno, D. (2021). Best practice forensic photo-documentation: Show me the injuries! *Journal of Legal Nurse Consulting, 32*(4), 26–31.

Steinkamp, J., Kantrowitz, J., Sharma, A., & Bala, W. (2021). Beyond notes: Why it is time to abandon an outdated documentation paradigm. *Journal of Medical Internet Research, 23*(4), e24179. https://doi.org/10.2196/24179

Documentation: Meetings 7926

Definition: Recording the minutes of workplace committees or professional meetings to create a formal record of proceedings

Activities:

- Take minutes with a laptop or tablet in addition to any recording device used
- Ensure that any electronic devices and media are connected and working well
- Sit close to the officiating officer so you can easily ask questions and get clarification
- Circulate an attendance list labeled with the meeting's name and date
- Take advantage of name tags or placards if participants' names are unfamiliar
- Begin the document with the name of the facility or organization committee as well as the meeting's location, time, place, and date
- List names of those who are present and possibly the names of those absent or excused
- Identify the purpose of the meeting and the officiating officer
- Use the agenda as a structure for the minutes, but record the minutes to reflect the actual sequence of events (e.g., approval of minutes of previous meetings, approval of agenda, unfinished business, new business)
- Record all motions and the outcomes of all votes
- Include key discussion items and actions that have been agreed upon including assignments and timelines
- Record any additional items, including announcements and adjournment of the meeting
- Create an attachments list of any reports distributed for the meeting
- Keep the writing clear, objective, and succinct
- Finish the minutes as soon as possible while the details are fresh in mind
- Include your name at the end as the minute's recorder
- Proofread the document and send to the chair for approval
- Distribute the minutes to the membership before the next meeting
- File approved minutes according to organizational policy
- Consult the most current edition of Robert's Rules of Order for information on meeting protocol and taking minutes

7th edition 2018

Background Evidence:

Manion, J., & Huber, D. L. (2014). Team building and working with effective groups. In D. L. Huber (Ed.), *Leadership and nursing care management* (5th ed., pp. 138–142). Elsevier Saunders.

Robert, H., III., Honemann, D. H., & Balch, T. (2011). *Robert's rules of order newly revised* (11th ed.). Da Capo Press.

Schirling, J. (2011). Effective meeting management. In C. A. Gassiot, V. L. Searcy, & C. W. Giles (Eds.), *The medical staff services handbook: Fundamentals and beyond* (2nd ed., pp. 325–354). Jones & Bartlett.

Dressing 1630

Definition: Assisting in choosing, applying, and removing clothes for a person who is unable to dress self

Activities:

- Consider culture and age when promoting dressing activities
- Schedule dressing or undressing at time when not fatigued, often with bathing
- Provide analgesia, if needed
- Allow enough time to provide care
- Preserve person's modesty by not undressing unnecessarily
- Close door or draw curtains when undressing person
- Keep room warm for comfort
- Identify areas in which person can dress independently
- Encourage to do as much as possible to increase independence and boost morale, as appropriate
- Talk to person during process to allay anxieties and embarrassment
- Use clear simple instructions for persons with cognitive deficits
- Do not rush through procedure

- Inform of available clothing for selection, providing personal clothing as appropriate
- Encourage participation in selection of clothing
- Provide clothes in accessible area (e.g., at bedside)
- Lay clothes out in order and place within easy reach
- Be available for assistance in dressing as necessary
- Identify areas in which needs assistance in dressing
- Monitor ability to dress self
- Dress after personal hygiene completed
- Encourage use of devices and simple dressing aids (e.g., dressing stick, long handled shoehorn, long handled reaching apparatus), as appropriate
- Dress most disabled extremity first, as appropriate
- Place shirt sleeve as high as possible on shoulder of affected arm to facilitate dressing or undressing
- Dress in nonrestrictive, comfortable, loose-fitting clothing, as appropriate
- Be gentle in movements and pull clothes, not person
- Encourage to wear type of clothes normally worn (i.e., pajamas in bed, underwear and outerwear when up), as appropriate
- Select shoes or slippers conducive to walking and safe ambulation
- Avoid back fastenings and tight-fitting garments if limited movement of arms
- Provide clothes with front pocket as more accessible when sitting down
- Use front-fastening bras for woman with arthritic hands or recuperating after stroke
- Use cotton clothes where possible to absorb perspiration better
- Help with laces, buttons, and zippers, as needed
- Use extension equipment for pulling on clothing if appropriate
- Place removed clothing in laundry
- Offer to hang up clothing or place in dresser
- Offer to rinse special garments, such as nylons
- Reinforce efforts to dress self
- Give assistance until fully able to assume responsibility for dressing self

1st edition 1992; revised 2000, 2024

Background Evidence:

Craven, R. F., Hirnle, C. J., & Henshaw, C. J. (2021). Self-care and hygiene. In *Fundamentals of nursing: Human health and function* (8th ed.). Wolters-Kluwer.

Esmail, A., Poncet, F., Auger, C., Rochette, A., Dahan-Oliel, N., Labbé, D., Kehayia, E., Billebaud, C., de Guise, É., Lessard, I., Ducharme, I., Vermeersch, O., & Swaine, B. (2020). The role of clothing on participation of persons with a physical disability: A scoping review. *Applied Ergonomics*, 85, 103058.

Hawkins, B., Ventresco, C., Cummings, M., McCaffrey, K., Willwerth, A. J., Blume, E. D., & VanderPluym, C. (2022). Design and pilot testing of therapeutic clothing for hospitalized children. *Journal for Specialists in Pediatric Nursing*, 27(2), 1–8.

Hou, Y.-J., Zeng, S.-Y., Lin, C.-C., Yang, C.-T., Huang, H.-L., Chen, M.-C., Tsai, H.-H., Liang, J., & Shyu, Y.-I. L. (2022). Smart clothes-assisted home-nursing care program for family caregivers of older persons with dementia and hip fracture: a mixed-methods study. *BMC Geriatrics*, 22(1), 1–10.

Keane, J. M., Franklin, N. F., & Vaughan, B. (2020). Simulation to educate healthcare providers working within residential age care settings: A scoping review. *Nurse Education Today*, 85, 104228.

Perry, A. G., Potter, P. A., Ostendorf, W. R., & LaPlante, N. (2021). *Clinical nursing skills and technique* (10th ed.). Mosby.

Dry Eye Prevention   1350

Definition: Prevention and early detection of dry eye in an individual at risk

Activities:

- Monitor signs and symptoms (e.g., redness, burning, itching, drainage, pain around and in the eye, difficulty in opening eyes on waking and moving lids, blurred vision) of dry eye
- Identify personal characteristics (e.g., age, gender, hormones, autoimmune diseases, chemical burn) and environmental factors (e.g., dry air, air conditioning, sunlight) that may increase potential of dry eye
- Monitor blink reflex
- Identify eyelid position
- Monitor amount of tearing using tear strips
- Screen the corneal epithelial damage using a standard test
- Monitor patient's ability to wear, remove, and clean contact lenses, as appropriate
- Instruct patient to avoid prolonged reading and lengthy computer use
- Ensure the endotracheal bandages are not too tight in patients ventilated through an endotracheal tube
- Monitor the mode and the pressure of the ventilator in mechanically ventilated patients
- Identify the frequency and the type of the care according to the eyelid position in lagophthalmos (e.g., in comatose, under deep sedation and neuromuscular blockage, facial paralysis, Bell's palsy, thyrotoxic exophthalmos, paralytic ectropion)
- Administer eye care at least twice a day, as appropriate
- Apply lubricants (e.g., eye drops, ointments) to support tear production, as appropriate
- Cover the eyes with effective devices (e.g., polyethylene cover, polyacrylamide gel, hypoallergenic tape), as appropriate
- Ensure the eyelids are closed
- Prepare the patient for a tarsorrhaphy to protect the cornea
- Inspect ocular surface and the cornea for effects of care and prophylactic treatment
- Report abnormal signs and symptoms to the physician

6th edition 2013

Background Evidence:

Germano, E. M., Mello, M. J., Sena, D. F., Correia, J. B., & Amorim, M. M. (2009). Incidence and risk factors of corneal epithelial defects in mechanically ventilated children. *Critical Care Medicine*, 37(3), 1097–1100.

Kanski, J. J. (2007). *Clinical ophthalmology: A systemic approach* (6th ed.). Oxford: Butterworth-Heinemann.

Latkany, R. (2008). Dry eyes: Etiology and management. *Current Opinion in Ophthalmology*, 19(4), 287–291.

Rosenberg, J. B., & Eisen, L. A. (2008). Eye care in the intensive care unit: Narrative review and meta-analysis. *Critical Care Medicine*, 36(12), 3151–3155.

Stollery, R., Shaw, M., & Lee, A. (2005). *Ophthalmic nursing* (3rd ed.). Oxford: Blackwell.

D

Dying Care 5260

Definition: Promotion of physical comfort and psychological peace in the final phase of life

Activities:

- Identify the patient's care priorities
- Communicate willingness to discuss death
- Encourage patient and family to share feelings about death
- Assist patient and family to identify a shared meaning of death
- Seek to understand patient's actions, feelings, and attitudes
- Monitor patient for anxiety
- Stay physically close to frightened patient
- Monitor deterioration of physical and/or mental capabilities
- Reduce demand for cognitive functioning when patient is ill or fatigued
- Monitor mood changes
- Respect the patient's and family's specific care requests
- Include the family in care decisions and activities, as desired
- Support patient and family through stages of grief
- Monitor pain
- Minimize discomfort, when possible
- Medicate by alternate route when swallowing problems develop
- Postpone feeding when patient is fatigued
- Offer fluids and soft foods frequently
- Offer culturally appropriate foods
- Provide frequent rest periods
- Assist with basic care, as needed
- Respect the need for privacy
- Modify the environment, based on patient's needs and desires
- Support the family's efforts to remain at the bedside
- Facilitate obtaining spiritual support for patient and family
- Facilitate care by others, as appropriate
- Facilitate referral to hospice, as desired
- Facilitate discussion of funeral arrangements

1st edition 1992; revised 2013

Background Evidence:

Adams, C. (2010). Dying with dignity in America: The transformational leadership of Florence Wald. *Journal of Professional Nursing, 26*(2), 125–132.

Cartwright, J. C., Miller, L., & Volpin, M. (2009). Hospice in assisted living: Promoting good quality care at end of life. *The Gerontologist, 49*(4), 508–516.

Klossner, N. J., & Hatfield, N. (2005). The dying child. In *Introductory maternity and pediatric nursing* (pp. 754–771). Lippincott Williams & Wilkins.

Law, R. (2009). Bridging worlds: Meeting the emotional needs of dying patients. *Journal of Advanced Nursing, 65*(12), 2630–2641.

LeGrand, S., & Walsh, D. (2010). Comfort measures: Practical care of the dying cancer patient. *American Journal of Hospice & Palliative Medicine, 27*(7), 488–493.

Timby, B. K., & Smith, N. E. (2006). Caring for dying clients. In *Introductory medical-surgical nursing* (pp. 102–111) (9th ed.). Lippincott Williams & Wilkins.

Dysreflexia Management 2560

Definition: Prevention and elimination of stimuli, which cause hyperactive reflexes and inappropriate autonomic responses in a patient with a cervical or high thoracic cord lesion

Activities:

- Identify and minimize stimuli that may precipitate dysreflexia (e.g., bladder distention, renal calculi, infection, fecal impaction, rectal examination, suppository insertion, skin breakdown, and constrictive clothing or bed linen)
- Monitor for signs and symptoms of autonomic dysreflexia (e.g., paroxysmal hypertension, bradycardia, tachycardia, diaphoresis higher than the level of injury, facial flushing, pallor lower than the level of injury, headache, nasal congestion, engorgement of temporal and neck vessels, conjunctival congestion, chills without fever, pilomotor erection, and chest pain)
- Investigate and remove offending cause (e.g., distended bladder, fecal impaction, skin lesions, constricting bed clothes, supportive stockings, and abdominal binders)
- Place head of bed in upright position to decrease blood pressure and promote cerebral venous return, as appropriate
- Stay with patient and monitor status every 3 to 5 minutes if hyperreflexia occurs
- Administer antihypertensive agents intravenously, as ordered
- Instruct patient and family about causes, symptoms, treatment, and prevention of dysreflexia

1st edition 1992; revised 2008

Background Evidence:

McCance, K. L., & Huether, S. E. (2006). *Pathophysiology: The biologic basis for disease in adults and children* (5th ed.). Mosby.

Smeltzer, S. C., & Bare, B. G. (2004). (10th ed.) *Brunner & Suddarth's textbook of medical-surgical nursing* (Vol. 2). Lippincott Williams & Wilkins.

Urden, L. D., Stacy, K. M., & Lough, M. E. (2006). *Thelan's critical care nursing: Diagnosis and management* (5th ed.). Mosby Elsevier.

Dysrhythmia Management   4090

Definition: Preventing, recognizing, and facilitating treatment of abnormal cardiac rhythms

Activities:

- Ascertain patient and family history of heart disease and dysrhythmias
- Monitor for and correct oxygen deficits, acid-base imbalances, and electrolyte imbalances, which may precipitate dysrhythmias
- Apply electrocardiographic (ECG) "wireless" telemetry or "hardwired" electrodes and connect to a cardiac monitor, as indicated
- Ensure appropriate lead selection in relation to patient needs
- Ensure proper lead placement, and signal quality
- Set alarm parameters on the ECG monitor
- Ensure ongoing monitoring of bedside ECG by qualified individuals
- Monitor ECG changes that increase risk of dysrhythmia development (e.g., arrhythmia, ST-segment, ischemia, and QT-interval monitoring)
- Facilitate acquisition of a 12-lead ECG, as appropriate
- Note activities associated with the onset of dysrhythmias
- Note frequency and duration of dysrhythmia
- Monitor hemodynamic response to the dysrhythmia
- Determine whether patient has chest pain or syncope associated with the dysrhythmia
- Ensure ready access of emergency dysrhythmia medications
- Initiate and maintain IV access, as appropriate
- Administer basic or advanced cardiac life support, if indicated
- Administer prescribed IV fluids and vasoconstrictor agents, as indicated, to facilitate tissue perfusion
- Assist with insertion of temporary transvenous or external pacemaker, as appropriate
- Instruct patient and family about the risks associated with the dysrhythmia(s)
- Prepare patient and family for diagnostic studies (e.g., cardiac catheterization or electrical physiological studies)
- Assist patient and family in understanding treatment options
- Instruct patient and family about actions and side effects of prescribed medications
- Instruct patient and family about self-care behaviors associated with use of permanent pacemakers and AICD devices, as indicated
- Instruct patient and family about measures to decrease the risk of recurrence of the dysrhythmia(s)
- Instruct patient and family about how to access the emergency medical system
- Instruct a family member in CPR, as appropriate

1st edition 1992; revised 2013

Background Evidence:

American Association of Critical-Care Nurses. (2006). In J. G. Alspach (Ed.), *Core curriculum for critical care nursing* (6th ed.). Saunders Elsevier.

American Heart Association. (2005). 2005 American Heart Association guidelines for cardiopulmonary resuscitation and emergency cardiovascular care. *Circulation, 112*(Suppl. 24), IV-1–IV-211.

American Heart Association. (2005). Electric therapies: Automated external defibrillators, defibrillation, cardioversion, and pacing. *Circulation, 112*(Suppl. 24), IV-35–IV-46.

Drew, B., Califf, R., Funk, M., Kaufman, E., Krucoff, M., Laks, M., Macfarlane, P. W., Sommargren, C., Swiryn, S., & Van Hare, G. F. (2004). Practice standards for electrocardiographic monitoring in hospital settings: An American Heart Association Scientific Statement from the Councils on Cardiovascular Nursing, Clinical Cardiology and Cardiovascular Disease in the Young. *Circulation, 110*(17), 2721–2746.

Funk, M., Winkler, C. G., May, J. L., Stephens, K., Fennie, K. P., Rose, L. L., et al. (2010). Unnecessary arrhythmia monitoring and underutilization of ischemia and QT interval monitoring in current clinical practice: Baseline results of the practical use of the latest standards for electrocardiography trial. *Journal of Electrocardiology, 43*(6), 542–547.

McKinley, M. G. (2011). Electrocardiographic leads and cardiac monitoring. In D. Wiegand (Ed.), *AACN procedure manual for critical care* (6th ed., pp. 490–501). Elsevier Saunders.

Urden, L. D., Stacy, K. M., & Lough, M. E. (2006). *Thelan's critical care nursing: Diagnosis and management* (5th ed.). Mosby Elsevier.

D

Ear Care 1640

Definition: Prevention or minimization of threats to ear or hearing

Activities:

- Monitor auditory function
- Monitor anatomical structures for signs and symptoms of infection (e.g., inflamed tissue and drainage)
- Instruct patient on the ear's anatomical structures and their function
- Monitor for patient-reported signs and symptoms of dysfunction (e.g., pain, tenderness, itching, change in hearing, tinnitus, and vertigo)
- Monitor episodes of chronic otitis media (i.e., ensure appropriate preventative measures and treatments are employed)
- Instruct parent how to observe for signs and symptoms of auditory dysfunction or infection in child
- Administer hearing test, as appropriate
- Instruct patient on importance of annual hearing testing
- Instruct women of childbearing age on importance of prenatal care (e.g., avoidance of ototoxic medications, adequate dietary intake, and strict control of alcoholism)
- Inform parent about vaccinations, which eliminate the possibility of sensorineural hearing loss (e.g., vaccination against rubella, measles, and mumps)
- Cleanse external ear using washcloth-covered finger
- Instruct patient how to cleanse ears
- Monitor for an excessive accumulation of cerumen
- Instruct patient not to use foreign objects smaller than patient's fingertip (e.g., cotton-tipped applicators, bobby pins, toothpicks, and other sharp objects) for cerumen removal
- Remove excessive cerumen with twisted end of washcloth while pulling down the auricle
- Consider ear irrigation for the removal of excessive cerumen if watchful waiting, manual removal, and ceruminolytic agents are ineffective
- Instruct parent to ensure child does not place foreign objects into ear
- Administer eardrops, as needed
- Instruct patient on proper eardrop administration
- Instruct patient how to monitor for persistent exposure to loud noise
- Instruct patient on importance of hearing protection during persistent exposure to loud noise
- Instruct parent to avoid bottle-feeding or allowing infant to bottle-feed when in supine position
- Instruct patient with pierced ears how to avoid infection at the insertion site
- Encourage use of earplugs for swimming if patient is susceptible to ear infections
- Instruct patient on appropriate use of and care for assistive devices or treatments (e.g., hearing aids, medication regimen, and ear tubes)
- Instruct patient on signs and symptoms warranting reporting to health care provider
- Refer patient to ear care specialist, as needed

1st edition 1992; revised 2013

Background Evidence:

Bryant, R. (2007). The child with cognitive, sensory, or communication impairment. In M. J. Hockenberry & D. Wilson (Eds.), *Wong's nursing care of infants and children* (8th ed., pp. 989–1027). Mosby Elsevier.

Craven, R., & Hirnle, C. (2009). *Fundamentals of nursing: Human health and function* (6th ed.). Lippincott Williams & Wilkins.

Russek, J. A. (2010). Care of patients with ear and hearing problems. In D. D. Ignatavicius & M. L. Workman (Eds.), *Medical-surgical nursing: Patient-centered collaborative care* (6th ed., pp. 1120–1137). Elsevier Saunders.

Ear Irrigation 1645

Definition: Flushing the ear to cleanse the external ear canal of wax or debris

Activities:

- Check accuracy and completeness of each medication administration record (MAR) prior to giving any medications, if indicated
- Follow six rights of medication administration
- Identify using at least two identifiers (e.g., name, birthday)
- Note medical history and allergies, if indicated
- Determine knowledge of medication and method of administration or treatment
- Perform necessary pre-medication or pre-procedure assessments (e.g., blood pressure, pulse)
- Position lying on side or sitting with head tilted toward affected ear
- Place absorbent pads under head, neck, and shoulders
- Place basin under ear to catch draining
- Cleanse pinna of ear and meatus of ear canal
- Warm irrigation solution
- Explain that feeling of fullness common during procedure
- Instruct there may be discomfort when solution reaches tympanic membrane
- Fill syringe with warmed solution
- Straighten ear canal and insert tip of syringe into auditory meatus
- Direct solution gently upward against top of canal
- Continue instilling fluid until all solution used or until canal cleansed
- Avoid blocking outward flow of solution with syringe
- Hang irrigating container and run solution through tubing with nozzle if not using syringe method, assuring no air in tubing prior to instilling in ear
- Assist to side-lying position on affected side when irrigation completed, to drain excess fluid
- Place cotton ball in auditory meatus to absorb excess fluid, as indicated
- Monitor response to irrigation as indicated
- Document character and amount of discharge, appearance of canal, discomfort immediately after instillation and again when medication, if used, expected to act
- Inspect cotton ball for drainage when removed, if used

- Document medication administration and responsiveness according to agency protocol

---

8th edition 2024

Background Evidence:

Berman, A., Snyder, S., & Frandsen, G. (2021). Otic medications. In *Kozier and Erb's Fundamentals of nursing: Concepts, process and practice* (pp. 902–904) (11th ed.). Pearson.

Kirby, N. (2021). Medication administration. In R. F. Craven, C. J. Hirnle, & C. J. Henshaw, (Eds.), *Fundamentals of nursing: Human health and function* (8th ed., pp. 410–471). Wolters-Kluwer.

Perry, A. G. (2018). Administering ear medications. In A. G. Perry, P. A. Potter, W. R. Ostendorf, & N. Laplante (Eds.), *Clinical nursing skills and techniques* (9th ed., pp. 547–550). Mosby.

Sanoski, C. A., & Vallerand, A. H. (2021). *Davis's drug guide for nurses* (17th ed.). F.A. Davis.

E

Eating Disorders Management   1030

Definition: Prevention and treatment of severe diet restriction, binging and purging of food and fluids, and overexercising

Activities:

- Determine health status, support systems, and goals for treatment
- Collaborate with other members of health care team to develop treatment plan
- Involve person and significant others, as appropriate
- Confer with team and person to set target weight if not within recommended weight range for age and body frame
- Establish amount of daily weight gain desired
- Confer with dietitian to determine daily caloric intake necessary to attain and maintain target weight
- Instruct and reinforce concepts of good nutrition, as needed
- Encourage to discuss food preferences with dietitian
- Respect, when possible, dietary lifestyle choices (e.g., vegetarian, vegan, pollotarian)
- Develop supportive relationship
- Regularly use hope engendering comments and actions to encourage efforts toward recovery
- Monitor physiological parameters (e.g., vital signs, electrolytes), as needed
- Weigh on routine basis (i.e., at same time of day and after voiding)
- Attempt to control variables that may alter weight (e.g., different clothes, hidden objects within clothes)
- Monitor intake and output of fluids, as appropriate
- Monitor daily caloric food intake
- Encourage self-monitoring of daily food intake, weight gain, and weight maintenance, as appropriate
- Monitor for suicidal or self-harm behaviors
- Establish expectations for appropriate behaviors (e.g., intake of food and fluid, amount of physical activity)
- Use behavioral contracting to elicit desired weight gain or maintenance behaviors
- Restrict food availability to scheduled, pre-served meals, and snacks
- Observe during and after meals or snacks to ensure that adequate intake achieved and maintained
- Accompany to bathroom during designated observation times after meals or snacks
- Limit time spent in bathroom during periods when not under observation
- Monitor for behaviors related to eating, weight loss, and weight gain
- Use behavior modification techniques to promote behaviors that contribute to weight gain and to limit weight loss behaviors, as appropriate
- Provide reinforcement for weight gain and behaviors that promote weight gain

- Provide remedial consequences in response to weight loss, weight loss behaviors, or lack of weight gain
- Provide support (e.g., relaxation therapy, desensitization exercises, opportunities to talk about feelings) as integrates new eating behaviors, changing body image, and lifestyle changes
- Encourage use of daily logs to record feelings and circumstances surrounding urge to purge, vomit, and overexercise
- Limit physical activity as needed to promote weight gain
- Provide supervised exercise program, when appropriate
- Allow opportunity to make limited choices about eating and exercise as weight gain progresses in desirable manner
- Assist person and significant others to examine and resolve personal issues that may contribute to eating disorder, as needed
- Assist to develop self-esteem compatible with healthy body weight
- Confer with health care team on routine basis about progress
- Initiate maintenance phase of treatment when target weight achieved and has consistently shown desired eating behaviors for designated period of time
- Monitor weight on routine basis
- Determine acceptable range of weight variation in relation to target range
- Place responsibility for choices about eating and physical activity with person, as appropriate
- Provide support and guidance, as needed
- Assist to evaluate appropriateness and consequences of choices about eating and physical activity
- Reinstitute weight gain protocol if unable to remain in target weight range
- Institute treatment program and follow-up care (e.g., medical, counseling) for home management

---

1st edition 1992; revised 2000, 2024

Background Evidence:

Dudek, S. G. (2021). Obesity and eating disorders. In *Nutrition essentials for nursing practice* (9th ed). Lippincott Williams & Wilkins.

Halter, M. J. (2019). *Manual of care plans in psychiatric nursing: An interprofessional approach.* Elsevier.

Halter, M. J. (2022). *Varcarolis' Foundations of psychiatric mental health nursing: A clinical approach* (9th ed.). Elsevier.

Hovde, K., Markovchick, T., Netzky, J., Sandberg, H., & Mehler, P. S. (2021). Care of the hospitalized patient with severe anorexia nervosa or avoidant restrictive food intake disorder. *MEDSURG Nursing, 30*(3), 197–211.

Smith, A. R., Ortiz, S. N., Forrest, L. N., Velkoff, E. A., & Dodd, D. R. (2018). Which comes first? An examination of associations and shared risk factors for eating disorders and suicidality. *Current Psychiatry Reports, 20*(9), 77.

Stavarski, D. H., Alexander, R. K., Ortiz, S. N., & Wasser, T. (2019). Exploring nurses' and patients' perceptions of hope and hope-engendering nurse interventions in an eating disorder facility: A descriptive cross-sectional study. *Journal of Psychiatric and Mental Health Nursing, 26*(1-2), 29–38.

Videbeck, S. H. (Ed.), (2020). *Psychiatric-mental health nursing* (8th ed.). Lippincott Williams & Wilkins.

Electroconvulsive Therapy (ECT) Management   2570

Definition: Assisting with the safe and efficient provision of electroconvulsive therapy (ECT) in the treatment of psychiatric illness

Activities:

- Explore current knowledge and beliefs about ECT including rationale for treatment
- Instruct about treatment where needed to clarify knowledge gaps
- Encourage to express feelings regarding prospect of electroconvulsive therapy (ECT) treatment
- Provide emotional support, as needed
- Review pretreatment orders and complete pretreatment checklist to ensure readiness for treatment and anesthesia (e.g., fasting, medication holds)
- Verify identify by using at least two personal identifiers
- Ensure person (or legal designee if person unable to give informed consent) has adequate understanding of ECT when obtaining informed consent
- Confirm written order and signed informed consent for ECT treatment
- Record height and weight in health care record
- Discontinue or taper medications contraindicated for ECT as recommended
- Review medication instructions before ECT treatment
- Inform health care provider of any laboratory abnormalities
- Confirm NPO status and medication instructions have been followed
- Assist to dress in loose fitting clothing that can be opened in front to allow placement of monitoring equipment
- Perform routine pre-procedure preparation (e.g., removal of dentures, jewelry, glasses, contact lenses; obtain vital signs; emptying bladder)
- Ensure hair clean, dry, and devoid of hair ornaments in preparation for electrode placement
- Obtain fasting blood glucose reading pre- and post-procedure if insulin-dependent
- Administer medications before and throughout treatment
- Verbally communicate unusual vital signs, physical complaints or symptoms, or unusual occurrences during handoff
- Assist in placing leads for various monitors (e.g., EEG, ECG) and monitoring equipment (e.g., pulse oximeter, blood pressure cuff, peripheral nerve stimulator)
- Place bite block in mouth and support chin to allow for airway patency during delivery of electrical stimulus
- Position on side with side rails raised when unconscious
- Perform routine postprocedural assessments (e.g., monitor vital signs, mental status, pulse oximeter, ECG)
- Administer oxygen, as prescribed
- Suction oropharyngeal secretions, as needed
- Administer intravenous fluids, as prescribed
- Provide supportive care and behavior management for postictal disorientation and agitation
- Notify anesthesia provider or attending provider if unstable
- Observe in recovery area until fully awake, oriented to time and place, and independently able to perform self-care activities
- Assist to return to inpatient unit or another recovery area, when adequately alert, oriented, and physically stable
- Provide report on treatment and response when transitioning care
- Determine level of observation needed upon return to unit or recovery area
- Provide determined level of observation upon transfer from treatment area
- Place on fall precautions, as needed
- Observe first attempt to ambulate independently to ensure full muscle control has returned after receiving muscle relaxant during ECT treatment
- Ensure gag reflex has returned before offering oral medications, food, or fluids
- Monitor for potential side effects of ECT (e.g., muscle soreness, headache, nausea, confusion, disorientation)
- Administer medications (e.g., analgesics, antiemetics) as ordered for side effects
- Treat disorientation by restricting environmental stimulation and frequently reorienting
- Encourage to verbalize feelings about experience
- Remind of amnesia effect of ECT treatment
- Provide emotional support, as needed
- Reinforce teaching on ECT, as appropriate
- Update significant others on status, as appropriate
- Discharge outpatient recipient of ECT to responsible adult when adequately recovered from treatment, as per agency protocol
- Collaborate with treatment team to evaluate effectiveness of ECT (e.g., mood, cognitive status) and modify treatment plan, as needed
- Document pretreatment preparation, procedure details, treatment, and responses

4th edition 2004; revised 2024

Background Evidence:

American Psychiatric Nurses Association. (2014). *Scope and standards of psychiatric-mental health nursing.* (2nd ed.).

American Psychological Association. (2020). Electroconvulsive therapy as an essential procedure.

da Silva Guimarães, J. C., Dos Santos, B. L., de Souza Aperibense, P. G. G., Martins, G. D. C. S., de Almeida Peres, M. A., & Santos, T. C. F. (2018). Electroconvulsive therapy: Historical construction of nursing care (1989–2002). *Revista Brasileira De Enfermagem, 71* https://doi.org/10.1590/0034-7167-2018-0168. 2743–2450

Keltner, N. L., & Steele, D. (2019). *Psychiatric nursing.* (8th ed.). Elsevier.

Livingston, R., Wu, C., Mu, K., & Coffey, M. J. (2018). Regulation of electroconvulsive therapy: A systematic review of U.S. State laws. *Journal of ECT, 34*(1), 60–68.

Rebar, C. R., Gersch, C., & Heimgartner, N. M. (2020). *Psychiatric nursing made incredibly easy.* (3rd ed.). Wolters Kluwer.

Varcarolis, E. M., & Fosbre, C. D. (2021). *Essentials of psychiatric-mental health nursing.* (4th ed.). Elsevier.

Electrolyte Management   2000

Definition: Promotion of electrolyte balance and prevention of complications resulting from abnormal or undesired serum electrolyte levels

Activities:

- Monitor for abnormal serum electrolytes, as available
- Monitor for manifestations of electrolyte imbalance
- Maintain patent IV access
- Administer fluids as prescribed, if appropriate
- Maintain accurate intake and output record
- Maintain intravenous solution containing electrolyte(s) at constant flow rate, as appropriate
- Administer supplemental electrolytes (e.g., oral, NG, and IV) as prescribed, if appropriate
- Consult physician on administration of electrolyte-sparing medications (e.g., spironolactone), as appropriate
- Administer electrolyte-binding or electrolyte-excreting resins (e.g., sodium polystyrene sulfonate [Kayexalate]) as prescribed, if appropriate
- Obtain ordered specimens for laboratory analysis of electrolyte levels (e.g., ABG, urine, and serum levels), as appropriate
- Monitor for loss of electrolyte-rich fluids (e.g., nasogastric suction, ileostomy drainage, diarrhea, wound drainage, and diaphoresis)
- Institute measures to control excessive electrolyte loss (e.g., by resting the gut, changing type of diuretic, or administering antipyretics), as appropriate
- Irrigate nasogastric tubes with normal saline
- Minimize the amount of ice chips or oral intake consumed by patients with gastric tubes connected to suction
- Provide diet appropriate for patient's electrolyte imbalance (e.g., potassium-rich, low-sodium, and low-carbohydrate foods)
- Instruct the patient and/or family on specific dietary modifications, as appropriate
- Provide a safe environment for the patient with neurological and/or neuromuscular manifestations of electrolyte imbalance
- Promote orientation
- Teach patient and family about the type, cause, and treatments for electrolyte imbalance, as appropriate
- Consult physician if signs and symptoms of fluid and/or electrolyte imbalance persist or worsen
- Monitor patient's response to prescribed electrolyte therapy
- Monitor for side effects of prescribed supplemental electrolytes (e.g., GI irritation)
- Monitor closely the serum potassium levels of patients taking digitalis and diuretics
- Place on cardiac monitor, as appropriate
- Treat cardiac arrhythmias, according to policy
- Prepare patient for dialysis (e.g., assist with catheter placement for dialysis), as appropriate

1st edition 1992; revised 2008

Background Evidence:

American Association of Critical-Care Nurses. (2006). In J. G. Alspach (Ed.), *Core curriculum for critical care nursing* (6th ed.). Saunders Elsevier.

Banker, D., Whittier, G. C., & Rutecki, G. (2003). Acid-base disturbances: 5 rules that can simplify diagnosis. *Consultant, 43*(3), 381–384, 399–400.

McCance, K. L., & Huether, S. E. (2002). *Pathophysiology: The biologic basis for disease in adults and children.* Mosby.

Price, S. A., & Wilson, L. M. (2003). *Pathophysiology: Clinical concepts of disease processes* (6th ed.). Mosby.

Electrolyte Management: Hypercalcemia   2001

Definition: Promotion of calcium balance and prevention of complications resulting from serum calcium levels higher than desired

Activities:

- Monitor trends in serum levels of calcium (e.g., ionized calcium) in at risk populations (e.g., patients with malignancies, hyperparathyroidism, prolonged immobilization in severe or multiple fractures or spinal cord injuries)
- Estimate the concentration of the ionized fraction of calcium when total calcium levels only are reported (e.g., use serum albumin and appropriate formulas)
- Monitor patients receiving medication therapies that contribute to continued calcium elevation (e.g., thiazide diuretics, milk-alkali syndrome in peptic ulcer patients, Vitamin A and D intoxication, lithium)
- Monitor intake and output
- Monitor renal function (e.g., BUN and Cr levels)
- Monitor for digitalis toxicity (e.g., report serum levels higher than therapeutic range, monitor heart rate and rhythm before administering dose, and monitor for side effects)
- Observe for clinical manifestations of hypercalcemia (e.g., excessive urination, excessive thirst, muscle weakness, poor coordination, anorexia, intractable nausea [late sign], abdominal cramps, obstipation [late sign], confusion)
- Monitor for psychosocial manifestations of hypercalcemia (e.g., confusion, impaired memory, slurred speech, lethargy, acute psychotic behavior, coma, depression, and personality changes)
- Monitor for cardiovascular manifestations of hypercalcemia (e.g., dysrhythmias, prolonged PR interval, shortening of QT interval and ST segments, cone-shaped T wave, sinus bradycardia, heart blocks, hypertension, and cardiac arrest)
- Monitor for GI manifestations of hypercalcemia (e.g., anorexia, nausea, vomiting, constipation, peptic ulcer symptoms, abdominal pain, abdominal distention, paralytic ileus)
- Monitor for neuromuscular manifestations of hypercalcemia (e.g., weakness, malaise, paresthesias, myalgia, headache, hypotonia, decreased deep tendon reflexes, and poor coordination)
- Monitor for bone pain
- Monitor for electrolyte imbalances associated with hypercalcemia (e.g., hypophosphatemia or hyperphosphatemia, hyperchloremic acidosis, and hypokalemia from diuresis), as appropriate

- Provide therapies to promote renal excretion of calcium and limit further buildup of excess calcium (e.g., IV fluid hydration with normal saline or half-normal saline and diuretics; mobilizing the patient; restricting dietary calcium intake), as appropriate
- Administer prescribed medications to reduce serum ionized calcium levels (e.g., calcitonin, indomethacin, plicamycin, phosphate, sodium bicarbonate, and glucocorticoids), as appropriate
- Monitor for systemic allergic reactions to calcitonin
- Monitor for fluid overload resulting from hydration therapy (e.g., daily weight, urine output, jugular vein distention, lung sounds, and right atrial pressure), as appropriate
- Avoid administration of vitamin D (e.g., calcifediol or ergocalciferol), which facilitates GI absorption of calcium, as appropriate
- Discourage intake of calcium (e.g., dairy products, seafood, nuts, broccoli, spinach, and supplements), as appropriate
- Avoid medications that prevent renal calcium excretion (e.g., lithium carbonate and thiazide diuretics), as appropriate
- Monitor for indications of kidney stone formation (e.g., intermittent pain, nausea, vomiting, and hematuria) resulting from calcium accumulation, as appropriate
- Encourage diet rich in fruits (e.g., cranberries, prunes, or plums) to increase urine acidity and reduce the risk of calcium stone formation, as appropriate
- Monitor for causes of increasing calcium levels (e.g., indications of severe dehydration and renal failure), as appropriate
- Encourage mobilization to prevent bone resorption

- Instruct patient and/or family about medications to avoid in hypercalcemia (e.g., certain antacids)
- Instruct the patient and/or family on measures instituted to treat the hypercalcemia
- Monitor for rebound hypocalcemia resulting from aggressive treatment of hypercalcemia
- Monitor for recurring hypercalcemia 1 to 3 days after cessation of therapeutic measures

1st edition 1992; revised 2008

Background Evidence:

American Association of Critical-Care Nurses. (2006). In J. G. Alspach (Ed.), *Core curriculum for critical care nursing* (6th ed.). Saunders Elsevier.

American Heart Association. (2002). *Advanced cardiovascular life support (ACLS) provider manual.*

American Nephrology Nurses' Association. (2005). *Nephrology nursing standards of practice and guidelines for care* [S. Burrows-Hudson & B. Prowant, Eds.].

Cullen, L. (1992). Interventions related to fluid and electrolyte balance. *Nursing Clinics of North America, 27*(2), 569–597.

Oncology Nursing Societ. (1996). *Statement on the scope and standards of oncology nursing practice.* American Nurses Association.

Parker, J. (1998). *Contemporary nephrology nursing.* American Nephrology Nurses' Association.

Smeltzer, S. C., & Bare, B. G. (2004). *Brunner & Suddarth's textbook of medical-surgical nursing* (10th ed.). Lippincott Williams & Wilkins.

Springhouse Corporation. (2004). *Just the facts: Fluids and electrolytes.* Lippincott Williams & Wilkins.

Electrolyte Management: Hyperkalemia   2002

Definition: Promotion of potassium balance and prevention of complications resulting from serum potassium levels higher than desired

Activities:

- Obtain specimens for laboratory analysis of potassium levels and associated electrolyte imbalances (e.g., ABG, urine, and serum levels), as appropriate
- Avoid false reports of hyperkalemia resulting from improper collection methodology (e.g., prolonged use of tourniquets during venous access; unusual exercise of extremity before venous access; delay in delivery of sample to laboratory)
- Verify all highly abnormal elevations of potassium
- Monitor cause(s) of increasing serum potassium levels (e.g., renal failure, excessive intake, and acidosis), as appropriate
- Monitor neurological manifestations of hyperkalemia (e.g., muscle weakness, reduced sensation, hyporeflexia, and paresthesias)
- Monitor cardiac manifestations of hyperkalemia (e.g., decreased cardiac output, heart blocks, peaked T waves, fibrillation, or asystole)
- Monitor gastrointestinal manifestations of hyperkalemia (e.g., nausea, intestinal colic)
- Monitor for hyperkalemia associated with a blood reaction, if appropriate
- Monitor laboratory values for changes in oxygenation or acid-base balance, as appropriate
- Monitor for symptoms of inadequate tissue oxygenation (e.g., pallor, cyanosis, and sluggish capillary refill)
- Administer electrolyte-binding and electrolyte-excreting resins (e.g., sodium polystyrene sulfonate [Kayexalate]) as prescribed, if appropriate

- Administer prescribed medications to shift potassium into the cell (e.g., 50% dextrose and insulin, sodium bicarbonate, calcium chloride, and calcium gluconate), as appropriate
- Insert rectal catheter for administration of cation-exchanging or binding resins (e.g., sodium polystyrene sulfonate [Kayexalate] per rectum), as appropriate
- Maintain potassium restrictions
- Maintain IV access
- Administer prescribed diuretics, as appropriate
- Avoid potassium-sparing diuretics (e.g., spironolactone [Aldactone] and triamterene [Dyrenium]), as appropriate
- Monitor for therapeutic effect of diuretic (e.g., increased urine output, decreased CVP/PCWP, and decreased adventitious breath sounds)
- Monitor renal function (e.g., BUN and Cr levels), if appropriate
- Monitor fluid status (e.g., intake and output, weight, adventitious breath sounds, shortness of breath), as appropriate
- Insert urinary catheter, if appropriate
- Prepare patient for dialysis (e.g., assist with catheter placement for dialysis), as appropriate
- Monitor patient's hemodynamic response to dialysis, as appropriate
- Monitor infused and returned volume of peritoneal dialysate, as appropriate
- Encourage adherence to dietary regimens (e.g., avoiding high-potassium foods, meeting dietary needs with salt substitutes and low-potassium foods), as appropriate

- Monitor for digitalis toxicity (e.g., report serum levels higher than therapeutic range; monitor heart rate and rhythm before administering dose; and monitor for side effects), as appropriate
- Monitor for unintentional potassium intake (e.g., penicillin G potassium or dietary), as appropriate
- Monitor potassium levels after therapeutic interventions (e.g., diuresis, dialysis, electrolyte-binding and electrolyte-excreting resins)
- Monitor for rebound hypokalemia (e.g., excessive diuresis, excessive use of cation-exchanging resins, and postdialysis)
- Monitor for cardiac instability and/or arrest and be prepared to institute ACLS, as appropriate
- Instruct patient about the rationale for use of diuretic therapy
- Instruct patient and/or family on measures instituted to treat the hyperkalemia

1st edition 1992; revised 2008

Background Evidence:

American Association of Critical-Care Nurses. (2006). In J. G. Alspach (Ed.), *Core curriculum for critical care nursing* (6th ed.). Saunders Elsevier.

American Heart Association. (2002). *Advanced cardiovascular life support (ACLS) provider manual.*

American Nephrology Nurses' Association. (2005). *Nephrology nursing standards of practice and guidelines for care* [S. Burrows-Hudson & B. Prowant, Eds.].

Cullen, L. (1992). Interventions related to fluid and electrolyte balance. *Nursing Clinics of North America*, 27(2), 569–597.

Oncology Nursing Society. (1996). *Statement on the scope and standards of oncology nursing practice.* American Nurses Association.

Parker, J. (Ed.). (1998). *Contemporary nephrology nursing.* American Nephrology Nurses' Association.

Smeltzer, S. C., & Bare, B. G. (2004). *Brunner & Suddarth's textbook of medical-surgical nursing* (10th ed.). Lippincott Williams & Wilkins.

Springhouse Corporation. (2004). *Just the facts: Fluids and electrolytes.* Lippincott Williams & Wilkins.

E

Electrolyte Management: Hypermagnesemia   2003

Definition: Promotion of magnesium balance and prevention of complications resulting from serum magnesium levels higher than desired

Activities:

- Obtain specimens for laboratory analysis of magnesium level, as appropriate
- Monitor trends in magnesium levels, as available
- Monitor for electrolyte imbalances associated with hypermagnesemia (e.g., elevated BUN and Cr levels), as appropriate
- Assess dietary and pharmaceutical intake of magnesium
- Monitor for causes of increased magnesium levels (e.g., magnesium infusions, parenteral nutrition, magnesium rich dialysate solutions, antacids, laxatives, frequent magnesium sulfate enemas, lithium therapy, renal insufficiency or failure)
- Monitor for causes of impaired magnesium excretion (e.g., renal insufficiency, advanced age)
- Monitor urinary output in patients on magnesium therapy
- Monitor for cardiovascular manifestations of hypermagnesemia (e.g., hypotension, flushing, bradycardia, heart blocks, widened QRS, prolonged QT, and peaked T waves)
- Monitor for CNS manifestations of hypermagnesemia (e.g., drowsiness, lethargy, confusion, and coma)
- Monitor for neuromuscular manifestations of hypermagnesemia (e.g., weak-to-absent deep tendon reflexes, muscle paralysis, and respiratory depression)
- Administer prescribed calcium chloride or calcium gluconate IV to antagonize neuromuscular effects of hypermagnesemia, as appropriate
- Increase fluid intake to promote dilution of serum magnesium levels and urine output, as indicated
- Maintain bed rest and limit activities, as appropriate
- Position patient to facilitate ventilation, as indicated
- Prepare patient for dialysis (e.g., assist with catheter placement for dialysis), as indicated
- Instruct patient and/or family on measures instituted to treat the hypermagnesemia

1st edition 1992; revised 2008

Background Evidence:

American Association of Critical-Care Nurses. (2006). In J. G. Alspach (Ed.), *Core curriculum for critical care nursing* (6th ed.). Saunders Elsevier.

Cullen, L. (1992). Interventions related to fluid and electrolyte balance. *Nursing Clinics of North America*, 27(2), 569–597.

Luckey, A., & Parsa, C. (2003). Fluid and electrolytes in the aged. *Archives of Surgery*, 138(10), 1055–1060.

Metheny, N. M. (2000). *Fluid and electrolyte balance nursing considerations* (4th ed.). J. B. Lippincott.

Springhouse Corporation. (2004). *Just the facts: Fluids and electrolytes.* Lippincott Williams & Wilkins.

Topf, J. M., & Murray, P. T. (2003). Hypomagnesemia and hypermagnesemia. *Reviews in Endocrine & Metabolic Disorders*, 4(2), 195–206.

Electrolyte Management: Hypernatremia   2004

Definition: Promotion of sodium balance and prevention of complications resulting from serum sodium levels higher than desired

Activities:

- Monitor trends in serum levels of sodium in at-risk populations (e.g., unconscious patients, very old or very young patients, cognitively impaired patients, patients receiving hypertonic intravenous infusions)
- Monitor sodium levels closely in the patient experiencing conditions with escalating effects on sodium levels (e.g., diabetes insipidus, ADH deficiency, heatstroke, near drowning in sea water, dialysis)
- Monitor for neurological or musculoskeletal manifestations of hypernatremia (e.g., restlessness, irritability, weakness,

disorientation, delusions, hallucinations, increased muscle tone or rigidity, tremors and hyperreflexia, seizures, coma [late signs])
- Monitor for cardiovascular manifestations of hypernatremia (e.g., orthostatic hypotension, flushed skin, peripheral and pulmonary edema, mild elevations in body temperature, tachycardia, flat neck veins)
- Monitor for GI manifestations of hypernatremia (e.g., dry swollen tongue and sticky mucous membranes)
- Obtain appropriate laboratory specimens for analysis of altered sodium levels (e.g., serum and urine sodium, serum and urine chloride, urine osmolality, and urine specific gravity)
- Monitor for electrolyte imbalances associated with hypernatremia (e.g., hyperchloremia and hyperglycemia), as appropriate
- Monitor for indications of dehydration (e.g., decreased sweating, decreased urine, decreased skin turgor, and dry mucous membranes)
- Monitor for insensible fluid loss (e.g., diaphoresis and respiratory infection)
- Monitor intake and output
- Weigh daily and monitor trends
- Maintain patent IV access
- Offer fluids at regular intervals for debilitated patients
- Administer adequate water intake for patients receiving enteral feeding therapy
- Collaborate for alternate routes of intake when oral intake is inadequate
- Administer isotonic (0.9%) saline, hypotonic (0.45% or 0.3%) saline, hypotonic (5%) dextrose, or diuretics based on fluid status and urine osmolality
- Administer prescribed antidiuretic agents (e.g., desmopressin [DDAVP] or vasopressin [Pitressin]) in the presence of diabetes insipidus
- Avoid administration/intake of high-sodium medications (e.g., sodium polystyrene sulfonate [Kayexalate], sodium bicarbonate, hypertonic saline)
- Maintain sodium restrictions, including monitoring medications with high-sodium content
- Administer prescribed diuretics in conjunction with hypertonic fluids for hypernatremia associated with hypervolemia
- Monitor for side effects resulting from rapid or overcorrections of hypernatremia (e.g., cerebral edema and seizures)

- Monitor renal function (e.g., BUN and Cr levels), if appropriate
- Monitor hemodynamic status, including CVP, MAP, PAP, and PCWP, if available
- Provide frequent oral hygiene
- Provide comfort measures to decrease thirst
- Promote skin integrity (e.g., monitor areas at risk for breakdown, promote frequent weight shifts, prevent shearing, and promote adequate nutrition), as appropriate
- Instruct patient on appropriate use of salt substitutes, as appropriate
- Instruct the patient/family about foods and over-the-counter medications that are high in sodium (e.g., canned foods and selected antacids)
- Institute seizure precautions in severe cases of hypernatremia, if indicated
- Instruct the patient and/or family on measures instituted to treat the hypernatremia
- Instruct the family or significant other on signs and symptoms of hypovolemia (if hypernatremia is related to abnormal fluid intake or output)

1st edition 1992; revised 2008

Background Evidence:

American Association of Critical-Care Nurses. (2006). In J. G. Alspach (Ed.), *Core curriculum for critical care nursing* (6th ed.). Saunders Elsevier.

American Heart Association. (2002). *Advanced cardiovascular life support (ACLS) provider manual.*

American Nephrology Nurses' Association. (2005). *Nephrology nursing standards of practice and guidelines for care* [S. Burrows-Hudson & B. Prowant, Eds.].

Cullen, L. (1992). Interventions related to fluid and electrolyte balance. *Nursing Clinics of North America, 27*(2), 569–597.

Oncology Nursing Society. (1996). *Statement on the scope and standards of oncology nursing practice.* American Nurses Association.

Parker, J. (Ed.). (1998). *Contemporary nephrology nursing.* American Nephrology Nurses' Association.

Smeltzer, S. C., & Bare, B. G. (2004). *Brunner & Suddarth's textbook of medical-surgical nursing* (10th ed.). Lippincott Williams & Wilkins.

Springhouse Corporation. (2004). *Just the facts: Fluids and electrolytes.* Lippincott Williams & Wilkins.

Electrolyte Management: Hyperphosphatemia   2005

Definition: Promotion of phosphate balance and prevention of complications resulting from serum phosphate levels higher than desired

Activities:
- Monitor trends in serum levels of phosphorus (e.g., inorganic phosphorus) in at-risk-populations (e.g., patients receiving chemotherapy, patients with high phosphate intake, patients with high vitamin D intake)
- Monitor phosphate levels closely in the patient experiencing conditions with escalating effects on phosphate levels (e.g., acute and chronic renal failure, hypoparathyroidism, diabetic ketoacidosis, respiratory acidosis, profound muscle necrosis, rhabdomyolysis)
- Obtain specimens for laboratory analysis of phosphate and associated electrolyte levels (e.g., ABG, urine, and serum levels), as appropriate

- Monitor for electrolyte imbalances associated with hyperphosphatemia
- Monitor for manifestations of hyperphosphatemia (e.g., tingling sensations in fingertips and around mouth, anorexia, nausea, vomiting, muscle weakness, hyperreflexia, tetany, tachycardia)
- Monitor for symptoms of soft tissue, joint, and artery calcifications (e.g., decreased urine output, impaired vision, palpitations)
- Administer prescribed phosphate-binding and diuretic medications with food to decrease absorption of dietary phosphate
- Provide comfort measures for the GI effects of hyperphosphatemia
- Prevent constipation resulting from phosphate-binding medications
- Avoid laxatives and enemas that contain phosphate

- Administer prescribed calcium and vitamin D supplements to reduce phosphate levels
- Avoid phosphate-rich foods (e.g., dairy products, whole grain cereal, nuts, dried fruits or vegetables, and organ meats)
- Prepare patient for dialysis (e.g., assist with catheter placement for dialysis), as appropriate
- Institute seizure precautions
- Instruct the patient and/or family on measures instituted to treat the hyperphosphatemia
- Instruct patient and/or family on signs and symptoms of impending hypocalcemia (e.g., changes in urine output)

1st edition 1992; revised 2008

Background Evidence:

American Association of Critical-Care Nurses. (2006). In J. G. Alspach (Ed.), *Core curriculum for critical care nursing* (6th ed.). Saunders Elsevier.

American Heart Association. (2002). *Advanced cardiovascular life support (ACLS) provider manual.*

American Nephrology Nurses' Association. (2005). *Nephrology nursing standards of practice and guidelines for care* [S. Burrows-Hudson & B. Prowant, Eds.].

Cullen, L. (1992). Interventions related to fluid and electrolyte balance. *Nursing Clinics of North America, 27*(2), 569–597.

Oncology Nursing Society. (1996). *Statement on the scope and standards of oncology nursing practice.* American Nurses Association.

Parker, J. (Ed.). (1998). *Contemporary nephrology nursing.* American Nephrology Nurses' Association.

Smeltzer, S. C., & Bare, B. G. (2004). *Brunner & Suddarth's textbook of medical-surgical nursing* (10th ed.). Lippincott Williams & Wilkins.

Springhouse Corporation. (2004). *Just the facts: Fluids and electrolytes.* Lippincott Williams & Wilkins.

E

Electrolyte Management: Hypocalcemia   2006

Definition: Promotion of calcium balance and prevention of complications resulting from serum calcium levels lower than desired

Activities:

- Monitor trends in serum levels of calcium (e.g., ionized calcium) in at-risk populations (e.g., primary or surgically induced hypoparathyroidism; radical neck dissection [particularly first 24 to 48 hours postoperatively]; any thyroid or parathyroid surgery; patients receiving massive transfusions of citrated blood; cardiopulmonary bypass)
- Monitor calcium levels closely in the patient experiencing conditions with depleting effects on calcium levels (e.g., osteoporosis, pancreatitis, renal failure, inadequate vitamin D consumption, hemodilution, chronic diarrhea, small bowel disease, medullary thyroid cancer, low serum albumin, alcohol abuse, renal tubular dysfunction, severe burns or infections, prolonged bed rest)
- Estimate the concentration of the ionized fraction of calcium when total calcium levels only are reported (e.g., use serum albumin and appropriate formulas)
- Observe for clinical manifestations of hypocalcemia (e.g., tetany [classic sign]; tingling in tips of fingers, feet, or mouth; spasms of muscles in face or extremities; Trousseau's sign; Chvostek's sign; altered deep tendon reflexes; seizures [late sign])
- Monitor for psychosocial manifestations of hypocalcemia (e.g., personality disturbances, impaired memory, confusion, anxiety, irritability, depression, delirium, hallucinations, and psychosis)
- Monitor for cardiovascular manifestations of hypocalcemia (e.g., decreased contractility, decreased cardiac output, hypotension, lengthened ST segment, prolonged QT interval, torsades de pointes)
- Monitor for GI manifestations of hypocalcemia (e.g., nausea, vomiting, constipation, and abdominal pain from muscle spasm)
- Monitor for integument manifestations of hypocalcemia (e.g., scaling, eczema, alopecia, and hyperpigmentation)
- Monitor for electrolyte imbalances associated with hypocalcemia (e.g., hyperphosphatemia, hypomagnesemia, and alkalosis)
- Monitor patients receiving medications that contribute to continued calcium loss (e.g., loop diuretics, aluminum-containing antacids, aminoglycosides, caffeine, cisplatin, corticosteroids, mithramycin, phosphates, isoniazid)
- Monitor fluid status, including intake and output
- Monitor renal function (e.g., BUN and Cr levels)
- Maintain patent IV access
- Administer appropriate prescribed calcium salt (e.g., calcium carbonate, calcium chloride, and calcium gluconate) using only calcium diluted in D_5W, administered slowly with a volumetric infusion pump, as indicated
- Maintain bed rest for patients receiving parenteral calcium replacement therapy to control side effect of postural hypotension
- Monitor blood pressure in patients receiving parenteral calcium replacement therapy
- Monitor infusions of calcium chloride closely for adverse effects (higher incidence of tissue sloughing with IV infiltration; not usually initial medication of choice in treatment plans)
- Monitor for side effects of IV administration of ionized calcium (e.g., calcium chloride), such as increased effects of digitalis, digitalis toxicity, bradycardia, postural hypotension, cardiac arrest, thrombophlebitis, soft tissue damage with extravasation, clotting, and thrombus formation, as appropriate
- Avoid administration of medications that decrease serum ionized calcium (e.g., bicarbonate and citrated blood), as appropriate
- Avoid administration of calcium salts with phosphates or bicarbonates to prevent precipitation
- Monitor for acute laryngeal spasm and tetany requiring emergency airway management
- Monitor for exacerbation of tetany resulting from hyperventilation or pressure on efferent nerves (e.g., by crossing legs), as appropriate
- Initiate seizure precautions in patients with severe hypocalcemia
- Initiate safety precautions in patients with potentially harmful psychosocial manifestations (e.g., confusion)
- Encourage increased oral intake of calcium (e.g., at least 1000 to 1500 mg/day from dairy products, canned salmon, sardines, fresh oysters, nuts, broccoli, spinach, and supplements), as appropriate

- Provide adequate intake of vitamin D (e.g., vitamin supplement and organ meats) to facilitate GI absorption of calcium, as appropriate
- Administer phosphate-decreasing medications (e.g., aluminum hydroxide, calcium acetate, or calcium carbonate) as indicated in chronic renal failure patients
- Provide pain relief/comfort measures
- Monitor for overcorrection and hypercalcemia
- Instruct the patient and/or family on measures instituted to treat hypocalcemia
- Instruct the patient on need for life-style changes to control hypocalcemia (regular weight-bearing exercises, decreased alcohol and caffeine intake, decreased cigarette smoking, strategies to reduce risks for falls)
- Instruct patient on medications that decrease the rate of bone loss (e.g., calcitonin, alendronate, raloxifene, risedronate)

1st edition 1992; revised 2008

Background Evidence:

American Association of Critical-Care Nurses. (2006). In J. G. Alspach (Ed.), *Core curriculum for critical care nursing* (6th ed.). Saunders Elsevier.

American Heart Association. (2002). *Advanced cardiovascular life support (ACLS) provider manual.* Dallas, TX: Author.

American Nephrology Nurses' Association. (2005). *Nephrology nursing standards of practice and guidelines for care* [S. Burrows-Hudson & B. Prowant, Eds.].

Cullen, L. (1992). Interventions related to fluid and electrolyte balance. *Nursing Clinics of North America, 27*(2), 569–597.

Oncology Nursing Society. (1996). *Statement on the scope and standards of oncology nursing practice.* American Nurses Association.

Parker, J. (Ed.). (1998). *Contemporary nephrology nursing.* American Nephrology Nurses' Association.

Smeltzer, S. C., & Bare, B. G. (2004). *Brunner & Suddarth's textbook of medical-surgical nursing* (10th ed.). Lippincott Williams & Wilkins.

Springhouse Corporation. (2004). *Just the facts: Fluids and electrolytes.* Lippincott Williams & Wilkins.

Electrolyte Management: Hypokalemia   2007

Definition: Promotion of potassium balance and prevention of complications resulting from serum potassium levels lower than desired

Activities:

- Obtain specimens for laboratory analysis of potassium levels and associated electrolyte imbalances (e.g., ABG, urine, and serum levels), as appropriate
- Monitor for early presence of hypokalemia to prevent life-threatening sequelae in at-risk patients (e.g., fatigue, anorexia, muscle weakness, decreased bowel motility, paresthesias, dysrhythmias)
- Monitor laboratory values associated with hypokalemia (e.g., elevated glucose, metabolic alkalosis, reduced urine osmolality, urine potassium, hypochloremia, and hypocalcemia), as appropriate
- Monitor intracellular shifts causing decreasing serum potassium levels (e.g., metabolic alkalosis; dietary [especially carbohydrate] intake; and administration of insulin), as appropriate
- Monitor renal cause(s) of decreasing serum potassium levels (e.g., diuretics, diuresis, metabolic alkalosis, and potassium-losing nephritis), as appropriate
- Monitor GI cause(s) of decreasing serum potassium levels (e.g., diarrhea, fistulas, vomiting, and continuous NG suction), as appropriate
- Monitor dilutional cause(s) of decreasing serum potassium levels (e.g., administration of hypotonic solutions and increased water retention, secondary to inappropriate ADH), as appropriate
- Administer supplemental potassium, as prescribed
- Collaborate with physician and pharmacist for appropriate potassium preparations when supplementing potassium (e.g., IV potassium supplements only for severe or symptomatic hypokalemia or when the GI tract cannot be used)
- Monitor renal functions, EKG, and serum potassium levels during replacement, as appropriate
- Prevent/reduce irritation from oral potassium supplement (e.g., administer PO or NG potassium supplements during or after meals to minimize GI irritation; controlled-release microencapsulated tablets are preferred to decrease GI irritation and erosion; divide larger daily oral doses)
- Prevent/reduce irritation from intravenous potassium supplement (e.g., consider infusion via central line for concentrations greater than 10 mEq/L; dilute IV potassium adequately; administer IV supplement slowly; apply topical anesthetic to IV site), as appropriate
- Maintain patent IV access
- Provide continuous cardiac monitoring if potassium replacement rate exceeds 10 mEq/hour
- Administer potassium-sparing diuretics (e.g., spironolactone [Aldactone] or triamterene [Dyrenium]), as appropriate
- Monitor for digitalis toxicity (e.g., report serum levels higher than therapeutic range; monitor heart rate and rhythm before administering dose; and monitor for side effects), as appropriate
- Avoid administration of alkaline substances (e.g., IV sodium bicarbonate and PO or NG antacids), as appropriate
- Monitor neurological manifestations of hypokalemia (e.g., muscle weakness, altered level of consciousness, drowsiness, apathy, lethargy, confusion, and depression)
- Monitor cardiac manifestations of hypokalemia (e.g., hypotension, T wave flattening, T wave inversion, presence of U wave, ectopy, tachycardia, and weak pulse)
- Monitor renal manifestations of hypokalemia (e.g., acidic urine, reduced urine osmolality, nocturia, polyuria, and polydipsia)
- Monitor GI manifestations of hypokalemia (e.g., anorexia, nausea, cramps, constipation, distention, and paralytic ileus)
- Monitor pulmonary manifestations of hypokalemia (e.g., hypoventilation and respiratory muscle weakness)
- Position patient to facilitate ventilation
- Monitor for symptoms of respiratory failure (e.g., low PaO_2 and elevated $PaCO_2$ levels; respiratory muscle fatigue)
- Monitor for rebound hyperkalemia
- Monitor for excessive diuresis
- Monitor fluid status, including intake and output, as appropriate
- Provide foods rich in potassium (e.g., salt substitutes, dried fruits, bananas, green vegetables, tomatoes, yellow vegetables, chocolate, and dairy products), as appropriate
- Instruct patient and/or family on measures instituted to treat the hypokalemia
- Provide patient education related to hypokalemia resulting from laxative or diuretic abuse

1st edition 1992; revised 2008

Background Evidence:

American Association of Critical-Care Nurses. (2006). In J. G. Alspach (Ed.), *Core curriculum for critical care nursing* (6th ed.). Saunders Elsevier.

American Heart Association. (2002). *Advanced cardiovascular life support (ACLS) provider manual*. Dallas, TX: Author.

American Nephrology Nurses' Association. (2005). *Nephrology nursing standards of practice and guidelines for care* [S. Burrows-Hudson & B. Prowant, Eds.].

Cullen, L. (1992). Interventions related to fluid and electrolyte balance. *Nursing Clinics of North America, 27*(2), 569–597.

Infusion Nursing Society. (2006). Infusion nursing standards of practice. *Journal of Infusion Nursing, 29*(Suppl. 1), S1–S90.

Kraft, M., Btaiche, I., Sacks, G., & Kudsk, K. (2005). Treatment of electrolyte disorders in adult patients in the intensive care unit. *American Journal Health-System Pharmacists, 62*(16), 1663–1682.

Oncology Nursing Society. (1996). *Statement on the scope and standards of oncology nursing practice*. American Nurses Association.

Parker, J. (Ed.). (1998). *Contemporary nephrology nursing*. American Nephrology Nurses' Association.

Pestana, C. (2000). *Fluids and electrolytes in the surgical patient* (5th ed.). Lippincott Williams & Wilkins.

Smeltzer, S. C., & Bare, B. G. (2004). *Brunner & Suddarth's textbook of medical-surgical nursing* (10th ed.). Lippincott Williams & Wilkins.

Springhouse Corporation. (2002). *Fluids & electrolytes made incredibly easy* (2nd ed.). Lippincott Williams & Wilkins.

Springhouse Corporation. (2004). *Just the facts: Fluids and electrolytes*. Lippincott Williams & Wilkins.

E

Electrolyte Management: Hypomagnesemia   2008

Definition: Promotion of magnesium balance and prevention of complications resulting from serum magnesium levels lower than desired

Activities:

- Obtain specimens for laboratory analysis of magnesium level, as appropriate
- Monitor trends in magnesium levels, as available
- Monitor for electrolyte imbalances associated with hypomagnesemia (e.g., hypokalemia, hypocalcemia), as appropriate
- Monitor for reduced intake due to malnutrition, prolonged IV fluid therapy, or, use of enteral or parenteral nutrition containing insufficient amounts of magnesium, as appropriate
- Monitor for decreased levels of magnesium resulting from inadequate absorption of magnesium (e.g., surgical resection of bowel, pancreatic insufficiency, inflammatory bowel disease, and excess dietary intake of calcium), as appropriate
- Monitor for increased urinary excretion of magnesium (e.g., diuretics, renal disorders, renal excretion after transplant, diabetic ketoacidosis, hyperparathyroidism, hypoparathyroidism), as appropriate
- Monitor for increased GI loss of magnesium (e.g., NG suctioning, diarrhea, fistula drainage, acute pancreatitis), as appropriate
- Monitor renal sufficiency in patients receiving magnesium replacement
- Offer foods rich in magnesium (e.g., unmilled grains, green leafy vegetables, nuts, and legumes), as appropriate
- Administer prescribed oral supplements as indicated, continuing for several days after magnesium level returns to normal
- Administer prescribed IV magnesium for symptomatic hypomagnesemia, as appropriate
- Monitor for side effects of IV magnesium replacement (e.g., flushing, sweating, sensation of heat, and hypocalcemia), as appropriate
- Keep calcium gluconate available during rapid magnesium replacement in case of associated hypocalcemic tetany or apnea, as appropriate
- Avoid administration of magnesium-depleting medications (e.g., loop and thiazide diuretics, aminoglycoside antibiotics, amphotericin B, digoxin, and cisplatin), as appropriate
- Monitor for CNS manifestations of hypomagnesemia (e.g., lethargy, insomnia, auditory and visual hallucinations, agitation, and personality change)
- Monitor for neuromuscular manifestations of hypomagnesemia (e.g., weakness, muscle twitching, foot or leg cramps, paresthesias, hyperactive deep tendon reflexes, Chvostek's sign, Trousseau's sign, dysphagia, nystagmus, seizures, and tetany)
- Monitor for GI manifestations of hypomagnesemia (e.g., nausea, vomiting, anorexia, diarrhea, and abdominal distention)
- Monitor for cardiovascular manifestations of hypomagnesemia (e.g., widened QRS complexes, torsades de pointes, ventricular tachycardia; flattened T waves; depressed ST segments; prolonged QT; ectopy; tachycardia; elevated serum digoxin level)
- Instruct patient and/or family on measures instituted to treat the hypomagnesemia

1st edition 1992; revised 2008

Background Evidence:

American Association of Critical-Care Nurses. (2006). In J. G. Alspach (Ed.), *Core curriculum for critical care nursing* (6th ed.). Saunders Elsevier.

Cullen, L. (1992). Interventions related to fluid and electrolyte balance. *Nursing Clinics of North America, 27*(2), 569–597.

Luckey, A., & Parsa, C. (2003). Fluid and electrolytes in the aged. *Archives of Surgery, 138*(10), 1055–1060.

Metheny, N. M. (2000). *Fluid and electrolyte balance: Nursing considerations* (4th ed.). Lippincott Williams & Wilkins.

Saris, N., Mervaala, E., Karppanen, H., Khawaja, J., & Lewenstam, A. (2000). Magnesium: An update on physiological, clinical, and analytical aspects. *Clinica Chimica Acta, 294*(1–2), 1–26.

Springhouse Corporation. (2004). *Just the facts: Fluids and electrolytes*. Lippincott Williams & Wilkins.

Topf, J. M., & Murray, P. T. (2003). Hypomagnesemia and hypermagnesemia. *Reviews in Endocrine & Metabolic Disorders, 4*(2), 195–206.

E

Electrolyte Management: Hyponatremia   2009

Definition: Promotion of sodium balance and prevention of complications resulting from serum sodium levels lower than desired

Activities:

- Monitor trends in serum levels of sodium in at-risk populations (e.g., confused elderly, patients on low-salt diet or diuretics)
- Monitor sodium levels closely in the patient experiencing conditions with depleting effects on sodium levels (e.g., oat-cell lung cancer; aldosterone deficiency; adrenal insufficiency; syndrome of inappropriate antidiuretic hormone [SIADH]; hyperglycemia; vomiting; diarrhea; water intoxication; fistulas; excessive sweating)
- Monitor for neurological or musculoskeletal manifestations of hyponatremia (e.g., lethargy; increased ICP; altered mental status; headache; apprehension; fatigue; tremors; muscle weakness or cramping; hyperreflexia; seizures; coma [late signs])
- Monitor for cardiovascular manifestations of hyponatremia (e.g., orthostatic hypotension, elevated blood pressure, cold and clammy skin, poor skin turgor, hypovolemia, hypervolemia)
- Monitor for GI manifestations of hyponatremia (e.g., dry mucosa, decreased saliva production, anorexia, nausea, vomiting, abdominal cramps, and diarrhea)
- Obtain appropriate laboratory specimens for analysis of altered sodium levels (e.g., serum and urine sodium, serum and urine chloride, urine osmolality, and urine specific gravity)
- Monitor for electrolyte imbalances associated with hyponatremia (e.g., hypokalemia, metabolic acidosis, and hyperglycemia)
- Monitor for renal loss of sodium (oliguria)
- Monitor renal function (e.g., BUN and Cr levels)
- Monitor intake and output
- Weigh daily and monitor trends
- Monitor for indications of fluid overload/retention (e.g., crackles; elevated CVP or pulmonary capillary wedge pressure; edema; neck vein distention; and ascites), as appropriate
- Monitor hemodynamic status, including CVP, MAP, PAP, and PCWP, as available
- Restrict water intake as safest first line treatment of hyponatremia in patients with normal or excess fluid volume (800 mL/24 hours)
- Maintain fluid restriction, as appropriate
- Encourage foods/fluids high in sodium, as appropriate
- Monitor all parenteral fluids for sodium content
- Administer hypertonic (3% to 5%) saline at 3 mL/kg/hr or per policy for cautious correction of hyponatremia in intensive care settings under close observation only, as appropriate
- Prevent rapid or overcorrection of hyponatremia (e.g., serum Na level of greater than 125 mEq/L and hypokalemia)
- Administer plasma expanders cautiously and only in the presence of hypovolemia
- Avoid excessive administration of hypotonic IV fluids, especially in the presence of SIADH
- Administer diuretics (e.g., thiazides, loop diuretics similar to furosemide, or ethacrynic acid), only as indicated
- Limit patient activities to conserve energy, as appropriate
- Institute seizure precautions if indicated in severe cases of hyponatremia
- Instruct the patient and/or family on all therapies instituted to treat the hyponatremia

1st edition 1992; revised 2008

Background Evidence:

American Association of Critical-Care Nurses. (2006). In J. G. Alspach (Ed.), *Core curriculum for critical care nursing* (6th ed.). Saunders Elsevier.

American Heart Association. (2002). *Advanced cardiovascular life support (ACLS) provider manual.*

American Nephrology Nurses' Association. (2005). *Nephrology nursing standards of practice and guidelines for care* [S. Burrows-Hudson & B. Prowant, Eds.].

Cullen, L. (1992). Interventions related to fluid and electrolyte balance. *Nursing Clinics of North America, 27*(2), 569–597.

Oncology Nursing Society. (1996). *Statement on the scope and standards of oncology nursing practice.* American Nurses Association.

Parker, J. (1998). *Contemporary nephrology nursing.* American Nephrology Nurses' Association.

Smeltzer, S. C., & Bare, B. G. (2004). *Brunner & Suddarth's textbook of medical-surgical nursing* (10th ed.). Lippincott Williams & Wilkins.

Springhouse Corporation. (2004). *Just the facts: Fluids and electrolytes.* Lippincott Williams & Wilkins.

Electrolyte Management: Hypophosphatemia   2010

Definition: Promotion of phosphate balance and prevention of complications resulting from serum phosphate levels lower than desired

Activities:

- Monitor trends in serum levels of inorganic phosphorus in at-risk populations (e.g., alcoholics, anorexia nervosa patients, severely debilitated elderly)
- Monitor phosphate levels closely in the patient experiencing conditions with depleting effects on phosphate levels (e.g., hyperparathyroidism; diabetic ketoacidosis; major thermal burns; prolonged intense hyperventilation; overzealous administration of simple carbohydrates in severe protein-calorie malnutrition)
- Obtain specimens for laboratory analysis of phosphate and associated electrolyte levels (e.g., ABG, urine, and serum levels), as appropriate
- Monitor for electrolyte imbalances associated with hypophosphatemia (e.g., hypokalemia; hypomagnesemia; respiratory alkalosis; metabolic acidosis)
- Monitor for decreasing levels of phosphate resulting from reduced intake and absorption (e.g., starvation; hyperalimentation without phosphate; vomiting; small bowel or pancreatic disease; diarrhea; and ingestion of aluminum or magnesium hydroxide antacids)

- Monitor for decreasing phosphate levels resulting from renal loss (e.g., hypokalemia; hypomagnesemia; heavy metal poisoning; alcohol; hemodialysis with phosphate-poor dialysate; thiazide diuretics; and vitamin D deficiency)
- Monitor for decreasing phosphate levels resulting from extracellular to intracellular shifts (e.g., glucose administration, insulin administration, alkalosis, and hyperalimentation)
- Monitor for neuromuscular manifestations of hypophosphatemia (e.g., weakness, lassitude, malaise, tremors, paresthesias, ataxia, muscle pain, increased creatinine phosphokinase, abnormal EMG, and rhabdomyolysis)
- Monitor for CNS manifestations of hypophosphatemia (e.g., irritability, fatigue, memory loss, reduced attention span, confusion, convulsions, coma, abnormal EEG, numbness, decreased reflexes, impaired sensory function, and cranial nerve palsies)
- Monitor for skeletal manifestations of hypophosphatemia (e.g., aching bone pain, fractures, and joint stiffness)
- Monitor for cardiovascular manifestations of hypophosphatemia (e.g., decreased contractility, decreased cardiac output, heart failure, and ectopy)
- Monitor for pulmonary manifestations of hypophosphatemia (e.g., rapid, shallow respirations; decreased tidal volume; and decreased minute ventilation)
- Monitor for GI manifestations of hypophosphatemia (e.g., nausea, vomiting, anorexia, impaired liver function, and portal hypertension)
- Monitor for hematological manifestations of hypophosphatemia (e.g., anemia; increased hemoglobin affinity with oxygen leading to increased SaO_2; increased risk of infection resulting from impaired WBC functioning; thrombocytopenia; bruising and hemorrhage resulting from platelet dysfunction)
- Administer prescribed phosphate supplements IV (replacement rate not to exceed 10 mEq/hr), as appropriate
- Administer PO phosphate replacement therapy when possible (preferred route)
- Monitor IV sites carefully for extravasation as tissue sloughing and necrosis occur with infiltration of phosphate supplements

- Monitor for rapid or overcorrection of hypophosphatemia (e.g., hyperphosphatemia, hypocalcemia, hypotension, hyperkalemia, hypernatremia, tetany, metastatic calcifications)
- Monitor renal function during parental phosphate supplementations, as appropriate
- Avoid phosphate-binding and diuretic medications (e.g., Amphojel, PhosLo cookie, and Basaljel)
- Encourage increased oral intake of phosphate (e.g., dairy products, whole grain cereal, nuts, dried fruits or vegetables, and organ meats), as appropriate
- Conserve muscle strength (e.g., assist with passive or active range-of-motion exercises)
- Institute preventive care for infection avoidance as hypophosphatemia causes severe depletion of granulocytes
- Instruct the patient and/or family on all measures instituted to treat the hypophosphatemia

1st edition 1992; revised 2008

Background Evidence:

American Association of Critical-Care Nurses. (2006). In J. G. Alspach (Ed.), *Core curriculum for critical care nursing* (6th ed.). Saunders Elsevier.

American Heart Association. (2002). *Advanced cardiovascular life support (ACLS) provider manual.*

American Nephrology Nurses' Association. (2005). *Nephrology nursing standards of practice and guidelines for care* [S. Burrows-Hudson & B. Prowant, Eds.].

Cullen, L. (1992). Interventions related to fluid and electrolyte balance. *Nursing Clinics of North America, 27*(2), 569–597.

Oncology Nursing Society. (1996). *Statement on the scope and standards of oncology nursing practice.* American Nurses Association.

Parker, J. (Ed.). (1998). *Contemporary nephrology nursing.* American Nephrology Nurses' Association.

Smeltzer, S. C., & Bare, B. G. (2004). (10th ed.) *Brunner & Suddarth's textbook of medical-surgical nursing* (Vol. 1). Lippincott Williams & Wilkins.

Springhouse Corporation. (2004). *Just the facts: Fluids and electrolytes.* Lippincott Williams & Wilkins.

Electrolyte Monitoring   2020

Definition: Collection and analysis of patient data to regulate electrolyte balance

Activities:

- Monitor the serum level of electrolytes
- Monitor serum albumin and total protein levels, as indicated
- Monitor for associated acid-base imbalances
- Identify possible causes of electrolyte imbalances
- Recognize and report presence of electrolyte imbalances
- Monitor for fluid loss and associated loss of electrolytes, as appropriate
- Monitor for Chvostek's and/or Trousseau's sign
- Monitor for neurological manifestation of electrolyte imbalance (e.g., altered sensorium and weakness)
- Monitor adequacy of ventilation
- Monitor serum and urine osmolality levels
- Monitor EKG tracings for changes related to abnormal potassium, calcium, and magnesium levels
- Note changes such as numbness and tremors in peripheral sensation
- Note muscle strength
- Monitor for nausea, vomiting, and diarrhea

- Identify treatments that can alter electrolyte status, such as GI suctioning, diuretics, antihypertensives, and calcium channel blockers
- Monitor for underlying medical disease that can lead to electrolyte imbalance
- Monitor for signs and symptoms of hypokalemia: muscular weakness; cardiac irregularities (PVC); prolonged QT interval; flattened or depressed T wave; depressed ST segment; presence of U wave; fatigue; paresthesia; decreased reflexes; anorexia; constipation; decreased GI motility; dizziness; confusion; increased sensitivity to digitalis; and depressed respirations
- Monitor for signs/symptoms of hyperkalemia: irritability; restlessness; anxiety; nausea; vomiting; abdominal cramps; weakness; flaccid paralysis; circumoral numbness and tingling; tachycardia progressing to bradycardia; ventricular tachycardia/fibrillation; tall peaked T waves; flattened P wave; broad slurred QRS complex; and heart block progressing to asystole
- Monitor for signs/symptoms of hyponatremia: disorientation; muscle twitching; nausea and vomiting; abdominal cramps;

E

headaches; personality changes; seizures; lethargy; fatigue; withdrawal; and coma

- Monitor for signs and symptoms of hypernatremia: extreme thirst; fever; dry, sticky mucous membranes; tachycardia, hypotension, lethargy, confusion, altered mentation; and seizures
- Monitor for signs and symptoms of hypocalcemia: irritability; muscle tetany; Chvostek's sign (facial muscle spasm); Trousseau's sign (carpal spasm); peripheral numbness and tingling; muscle cramps; decreased cardiac output; prolonged ST segment and QT interval; bleeding; and fractures
- Monitor for signs and symptoms of hypercalcemia: deep bone pain; excessive thirst; anorexia; lethargy; weakened muscles; shortened QT segment; wide T wave; widened QRS complex; and prolonged P-R interval
- Monitor for signs and symptoms of hypomagnesemia: respiratory muscle depression; mental apathy; Chvostek's sign (facial muscle spasm); Trousseau's sign (carpal spasm); confusion; facial tics; spasticity; and cardiac dysrhythmias
- Monitor for signs and symptoms of hypermagnesemia: muscle weakness; inability to swallow; hyporeflexia; hypotension; bradycardia; CNS depression; respiratory depression; lethargy; coma; and depression
- Monitor for signs and symptoms of hypophosphatemia: bleeding tendencies; muscular weakness; paresthesia; hemolytic anemia; depressed white cell function; nausea; vomiting; anorexia; and bone demineralization
- Monitor for signs and symptoms of hyperphosphatemia: tachycardia; nausea; diarrhea; abdominal cramps; muscle weakness; flaccid paralysis; and increased reflexes

- Monitor for signs and symptoms of hypochloremia: hyperirritability; tetany; muscular excitability; slow respirations; and hypotension
- Monitor for signs and symptoms of hyperchloremia: weakness; lethargy; deep, rapid breathing; and coma
- Administer prescribed supplemental electrolytes, as appropriate
- Provide diet appropriate for patient's electrolyte imbalance (e.g., potassium-rich foods or low-sodium diet)
- Teach patient ways to prevent or minimize electrolyte imbalance
- Instruct patient and family on specific dietary modifications, as appropriate
- Consult physician if signs and symptoms of fluid and/or electrolyte imbalance persist or worsen

1st edition1992; revised 2008

Background Evidence:

American Association of Critical-Care Nurses. (2006). In J. G. Alspach (Ed.), *Core curriculum for critical care nursing* (6th ed.). Saunders Elsevier.

Elgart, H. N. (2004). Assessment of fluids and electrolytes. *AACN Clinical Issues, 15*(4), 607–621.

McCance, K. L., & Huether, S. E. (2002). *Pathophysiology: The biologic basis for disease in adults and children.* Mosby.

Price, S. A., & Wilson, L. M. (2003). *Pathophysiology: Clinical concepts of disease processes* (6th ed.). Mosby.

Sheppard, M. (2000). Monitoring fluid balance in acutely ill patients. *Nursing Times, 96*(21), 39–40.

Electronic Fetal Monitoring: Antepartum   6771

Definition: Electronic evaluation of fetal heart rate response to movement, external stimuli, or uterine contractions during antepartal testing

Activities:

- Review obstetrical history, if available, to determine obstetrical or medical risk factors requiring antepartum testing of fetal status
- Determine patient knowledge about reasons for antepartum testing
- Monitor maternal vital signs
- Provide written patient and family education material for antepartum tests (e.g., nonstress, oxytocin challenge, biophysical profile tests), as well as electronic fetal monitor
- Inquire about oral intake, including diet, cigarette smoking, and medication use
- Label monitor strip per protocol
- Review prior antepartum tests
- Verify maternal and fetal heart rates before initiation of electronic fetal monitoring
- Instruct patient about the reason for electronic monitoring, as well as the types of information obtainable
- Encourage the mother to empty the bladder
- Perform Leopold maneuver to determine fetal position, as appropriate
- Ensure that the mother is in a comfortable position
- Apply toco transducer snugly at the fundus to observe contraction frequency and duration
- Apply ultrasound transducer to area of uterus in which fetal heart sounds are audible and trace clearly

- Differentiate among multiple fetuses by documenting on the tracing when simultaneous tracings are conducted, using one electronic fetal monitor
- Distinguish among multiple fetuses by comparing data when simultaneous tracings are conducted, using two different fetal monitors
- Discuss appearance of rhythm strip with mother and support person
- Reassure about normal fetal heart rate signs, including such typical features as artifact, loss of signal with fetal movement, high rate, and irregular appearance
- Adjust monitors to achieve and maintain clarity of the tracing
- Obtain baseline tracing of fetal heart rate per protocol for specific testing procedure
- Interpret electronic monitor strip for baseline heart rate, long-term variability, and presence of spontaneous accelerations, decelerations, or contractions
- Provide vibroacoustic stimulation, per protocol or physician or midwife order
- Initiate IV infusion per protocol to begin oxytocin challenge test, as appropriate, per physician or midwife order
- Increase oxytocin infusion, per protocol, until the appropriate number of contractions are achieved (i.e., usually three contractions in 10 minutes)
- Observe monitor strip for the presence or absence of late decelerations

- Interpret tracing based on protocol for nonstress or oxytocin challenge test criteria
- Perform ultrasound for biophysical profile testing, per protocol or physician or midwife order
- Score ultrasound based on protocol for biophysical profile criteria
- Communicate test results to primary practitioner or midwife
- Provide anticipatory guidance for abnormal test results (e.g., non-reassuring, nonstress test; positive oxytocin challenge test; or low biophysical profile score)
- Reschedule antepartum testing, per protocol or physician or midwife order
- Provide written discharge instructions to remind patient of future testing times and other reasons to return for care (e.g., labor onset, spontaneous leaking of the bag of waters, bleeding, decreased fetal movement)
- Clean equipment, including abdominal belts

2nd edition 1996; revised 2018

Background Evidence:

O'Neill, E., & Thorp, J. (2012). Antepartum evaluation of the fetus and fetal well-being. *Clinical Obstetrics and Gynecology, 55*(3), 722–730.

Perry, S., Hockenberry, M., Lowdermilk, D., & Wilson, D. (Eds.). (2014). *Maternal child nursing care* (5th ed.). Elsevier Mosby.

Pillitteri, A. (2014). *Maternal & child health nursing: Care of the childbearing & childrearing family* (7th ed.). Lippincott Williams & Wilkins.

E

Electronic Fetal Monitoring: Intrapartum   6772

Definition: Electronic evaluation of fetal heart rate response to uterine contractions during intrapartal care

Activities:

- Verify maternal and fetal heart rates before initiation of electronic fetal monitoring
- Instruct woman and support person about the reason for electronic monitoring, as well as information to be obtained
- Perform Leopold maneuver to determine fetal positions
- Apply toco transducer snugly at the fundus to observe contraction frequency, intensity, and duration
- Apply ultrasound transducer to area of uterus in which fetal heart sounds are audible and trace clearly
- Differentiate among multiple fetuses by documenting on the tracing when simultaneous tracings are conducted, using one electronic fetal monitor (e.g., baby A, baby B)
- Distinguish among multiple fetuses by comparing data when simultaneous tracings are conducted, using two separate fetal monitors
- Discuss appearance of rhythm strip with mother and support person
- Reassure about normal fetal heart rate signs, including such typical features as artifact, loss of signal with fetal movement, high rate, and irregular appearance
- Adjust monitors to achieve and maintain clarity of the tracing
- Evaluate the strip every 30 minutes in the first stage and every 15 minutes during second stage
- Document elements of the external tracing (e.g., baseline heart rate, oscillatory patterns, long-term variability, accelerations, decelerations, contraction frequency and duration)
- Document relevant intrapartal care (e.g., vaginal examinations, medication administration, maternal vital signs) directly on the monitor strip, as appropriate
- Remove electronic monitors before ambulation, after verifying that the tracing is normal
- Use intermittent or telemetry fetal monitoring, if available, to facilitate maternal ambulation and comfort
- Initiate fetal resuscitation interventions to treat non-reassuring (abnormal) fetal heart patterns, as appropriate
- Document changes in fetal heart patterns after resuscitation
- Calibrate equipment, as appropriate, for internal monitoring with a spiral electrode and/or intrauterine pressure catheter
- Use universal precautions
- Apply internal fetal electrode after rupture of membranes for reducing artifact or for evaluation of short-term variability, when necessary
- Apply internal uterine pressure catheter after rupture of membranes for obtaining pressure data for uterine contractions and resting tone, when necessary
- Document maternal response to application of internal monitors, including degree of discomfort or pain, appearance of amniotic fluid, and presence of bleeding
- Document fetal response to internal monitor placement, including short-term variability and accelerations or decelerations of the fetal heart rate
- Keep physician informed of pertinent changes in the fetal heart rate, interventions for non-reassuring patterns, subsequent fetal response, labor progress, and maternal response to labor
- Continue electronic monitoring through second-stage labor or up to the time of cesarean delivery
- Remove internal monitors before cesarean delivery to prevent maternal infection
- Document monitor interpretation, according to institutional policy
- Provide safekeeping of intrapartal strip as part of the permanent patient record

2nd edition 1996; revised 2018

Background Evidence:

American College of Nurse-Midwives. (2010). ACNM Clinical Bulletin No. 11. Intermittent auscultation for intrapartum fetal heart rate surveillance. *Journal of Midwifery & Women's Health, 55*(4), 397–403.

Bailey, R. E. (2009). Intrapartum fetal monitoring. *American Family Physician, 80*(12), 1388–1396.

National Institute for Health and Clinical Excellence. (2014). *Intrapartum care for healthy women and babies [NICE Clinical Guidelines 190]*. London, England: National Collaborating Centre for Women's and Children's Health.

Perry, S., Hockenberry, M., Lowdermilk, D., & Wilson, D. (2014). *Maternal child nursing care* (5th ed.). Elsevier Mosby.

Pillitteri, A. (2014). *Maternal & child health nursing: Care of the childbearing & childrearing family* (7th ed.). Lippincott Williams & Wilkins.

E

Electronic Health Record Access Assistance 8070

Definition: Facilitating electronic access to personal health information and communication with health care providers

Activities:

- Determine experience and comfort with portal before attempting to present and promote
- Collaborate with providers, person, and family members in initiating portal access and providing desired information
- Implement portals using systematic process with accommodation for visual and physical limitations
- Determine level of ability related to electronic device to be used for personal portal access
- Tailor portal to individual health condition and level of activity
- Provide kiosk, laptop, or tablet to orient to uses and importance of portal, where possible
- Provide user-friendly instructions that highlight portal benefits (e.g., access to medications, laboratory results, diagnostic testing results, person-specific education resources, timely access to health information, reminders for preventive and follow-up care)
- Actively promote portal use (e.g., bulk enrollment, ensure all providers and staff refer to portal, add to all handouts, endorse benefits)
- Instruct about portal features and how to use each application
- Ensure that portal has proactive, engaging portal features (e.g., problem-solving orientation, interactive decision tools, personalized messages and tools)
- Ensure that portal operates in real time for current condition or activities (e.g., current medications with last dose and next dose times, current laboratory and diagnostic workup reports)
- Offer guidance about effective communication with providers
- Consider portals with gaming features as stress reduction measure or incentive system for select persons
- Gather regular feedback related to portal use to facilitate refinements

8th edition 2024

Background Evidence:

Ammenwerth, E., Hoerbst, A., Lannig, S., Mueller, G., Siebert, U., & Schnell-Inderst, P. (2019). Effects of adult patient portals on patient empowerment and health-related outcomes: A systematic review. *Studies in Health Technology and Informatics, 264*, 1106–1110.

Centers for Medicare and Medicaid Services. (2020). *Medicare promoting interoperability program eligible hospitals, critical access hospitals, and dual-eligible hospitals attesting to CMS Objectives and Measures for 2020. Promoting Interoperability.* https://www.cms.gov/files/document/medicare-eh-2020-provide-patients-electronic-access-their-health-information.pdf

Elkind, E., & Higgins, K. M. (2018). Patient portal considerations. *Nursing Management, 49*(3), 9–11.

Gerber, D. E., Beg, M. S., Duncan, T., Gill, M., & Lee, S. J. C. (2017). Oncology nursing perceptions of patient electronic portal use: A qualitative analysis. *Oncology Nursing Forum, 44*(2), 165–170.

Irizarry, T., Shoemaker, J., Nilsen, M. L., Czaja, S., Beach, S., & DeVito Dabbs, A. (2017). Patient portals as a tool for health care engagement: A mixed-method study of older adults with varying levels of health literacy and prior patient portal use. *Journal of Medical Internet Research, 19*(3), 99.

Mayhew, C., Strudwick, G., & Waddell, J. (2018). Clinical Nurse Specialists' perceptions of a mental health patient portal. *Clinical Nurse Specialist: The Journal for Advanced Nursing Practice, 32*(6), 313–322.

Sadasivaiah, S., Lyles, C. R., Kiyoi, S., Wong, P., & Ratanawongsa, N. (2019). Disparities in patient-reported interest in web-based patient portals: Survey at an urban academic safety-net hospital. *Journal of Medical Internet Research, 21*(3), e1.

Elopement Precautions 6470

Definition: Minimizing the risk of a patient leaving a treatment setting without authorization when departure presents a threat to the safety of patient or others

Activities:

- Monitor patient's mental status (e.g., dementia, delirium, developmental disabilities, altered mental status due to brain injury or illness, psychosis, depression)
- Monitor patient for indicators of elopement potential (e.g., verbal indicators, loitering near exits, multiple layers of clothing, packing belongings, disorientation, separation anxiety, homesickness, suicidal ideation)
- Clarify the legal status of patient (e.g., minor or adult and voluntary or court-ordered treatment)
- Communicate risk to other care providers
- Familiarize patient with environment and routine to decrease anxiety
- Limit patient to a physically secure environment (e.g., locked or alarmed doors at exits, locked windows), as needed
- Provide adaptive devices to increase safety (e.g., side rails, cribs, gates, camouflaged exits, physical restraint) while always maintaining the least restrictive environment
- Provide appropriate level of supervision to monitor patient
- Increase supervision when patient is outside secure environment (e.g., hold hands, increase staff-to-patient ratio)
- Provide adaptive devices that monitor patient's physical location (e.g., electronic sensors placed on patient that trigger alarms or locks)
- Record physical description (e.g., height; weight; eye, hair, skin color; any distinguishing characteristics) for reference, should patient elope
- Provide patient with identification band
- Maintain consistent daily routine and caregivers
- Implement an exercise program to setting, as appropriate
- Engage the patient in structured activities (e.g., music therapy, reading, painting, drawing, supervised outdoor activities), as appropriate for setting
- Encourage patient to seek care providers for assistance when experiencing feelings (e.g., anxiety, anger, fear) that may lead to elopement

- Provide reassurance and comfort
- Discuss with patient why he/she desires to leave the treatment setting
- Identify with patient the positive and negative consequences of leaving treatment, as appropriate
- Identify with patient any variables that may be altered to make the patient feel more comfortable with remaining in the treatment setting, when possible
- Encourage patient to make a commitment to continue treatment, as appropriate

2nd edition 1996; revised 2018

Background Evidence:

Futrell, M., Melilo, K., & Remington, R. (2014). *Wandering.* Iowa City, IA: The University of Iowa College of Nursing Csomay Center for Gerontological Excellence.

Hodgkinson, B., Koch, S., Nay, R., & Lewis, M. (2007). Managing the wandering behaviour of people living in a residential aged care facility. *International Journal of Evidence-Based Healthcare, 5*(4), 406–436.

Moore, D., Algase, D., Powell-Cope, G., Applegarth, S., & Beattie, E. (2009). A framework for managing wandering and preventing elopement. *American Journal of Alzheimer's Disease and Other Dementias, 24*(3), 208–219.

Perese, E. F. (2012). *Psychiatric advanced practice nursing: A biopsychosocial foundation for practice.* F.A. Davis.

E

Embolus Care: Peripheral   4104

Definition: Management of a patient experiencing occlusion of peripheral circulation

Activities:

- Elicit a detailed patient health history in order to plan current and future preventative care
- Evaluate changes in respiratory and cardiac status (e.g., new-onset wheezing, hemoptysis, dyspnea, tachypnea, tachycardia, syncope) as patients who experience DVT are at a higher risk of recurrence and PE
- Evaluate all chest, shoulder, back, or pleuritic pain (i.e., check for intensity, location, radiation, duration, and precipitating and alleviating factors)
- Perform a comprehensive appraisal of peripheral circulation (i.e., check peripheral pulses, edema, capillary refill, color, and temperature of extremity)
- Monitor for pain in affected area
- Monitor for signs of decreased venous circulation in affected extremity (e.g., increased extremity circumference; painful swelling and tenderness; pain worsening in dependent position; pain persisting with extremity use; palpable hard vein; enlargement of the superficial veins; severe cramping; redness and warmth; numbness and tingling; discoloration of skin; fever)
- Administer anticoagulant medication
- Elevate any suspected affected limb 20 degrees or greater, higher than the level of the heart, to improve venous return
- Apply the Wells Prediction Rule to assist with diagnosing DVT
- Instruct the patient and family regarding diagnostic procedures (e.g., plethysmography; computerized strain gauze; venography; d-dimer assay; multidetector spiral computerized tomography; magnetic resonance imaging; ultrasonographies), as appropriate
- Apply graduated elastic compression stockings or sleeves to reduce the risk of postthrombotic syndrome or recurrence of DVT
- Remove graduated elastic compression stockings or sleeves for 15 to 20 minutes every 8 hours or per organizational policy and protocol
- Avoid antecubital intravenous access and instruct radiology and laboratory personnel to limit access of antecubital veins for tests, if possible
- Administer intravenous promethazine only in a 25 cc to 50 cc saline solution at a slow rate and avoid giving in less than 10 cc saline dilution
- Assist patient with passive or active range of motion, as appropriate
- Maintain patient on bed rest and change position every 2 hours

- Provide for early ambulation and exercise under the direction and supervision of a physiotherapist
- Monitor neurological status
- Provide pain relief and comfort measures
- Elevate bed sheets by using bed cradle over the affected extremity, if appropriate
- Refrain from massaging or compressing affected limb muscles
- Instruct the patient not to massage or compress the affected area
- Monitor patient's prothrombin time (PT) and partial thromboplastin time (PTT) to keep one to two times normal, as appropriate
- Monitor for side effects from anticoagulant medications
- Keep protamine sulfate and vitamin K available in case of emergency
- Administer antacids and analgesics, as appropriate
- Instruct patient not to cross legs and to avoid sitting for long periods with legs dependent
- Instruct the patient to avoid activities that result in the Valsalva maneuver (e.g., straining during bowel movement)
- Administer medications that will prevent episodes of the Valsalva maneuver (e.g., stool softeners and antiemetics), as appropriate
- Instruct the patient and family on appropriate precautions (e.g., walking; drinking plenty of fluids; avoiding alcohol; avoiding long periods of immobility, especially with legs dependently positioned such as in air travel or long automobile trips)
- Instruct the patient and family on all prophylactic, low-dose anticoagulant and/or antiplatelet medication
- Instruct the patient to report excessive bleeding (e.g., unusual nosebleeds; vomiting blood; blood in the urine; bleeding gums; unexpected vaginal bleeding; unusually heavy menstrual bleeding; bloody or tarry bowel movements), unusual bruising, unusual pain or swelling, blue or purple color of the toes, pain in the toes, ulcers or white spots in the mouth or throat
- Instruct the patient to wear a medical-alert bracelet
- Instruct patient to maintain a consistent diet (i.e., eat a consistent amount of green leafy vegetables that are high in vitamin K and can interfere with anticoagulants as the medication dosage will be adjusted to dietary intake)
- Administer prophylactic, low-dose anticoagulant and/or antiplatelet medication (e.g., heparin, clopidogrel, warfarin, aspirin, dipyridamole, dextran) per organizational policy and protocol
- Instruct patient to take anticoagulant medication at the same time each day and not to double up the next day if a dose is missed

- Instruct patient to check with health care provider: before taking any medication or herbal preparations, including over-the-counter products; before changing brands of medication; and before discontinuing a medication
- Instruct the patient and family on graduated elastic compression stockings
- Encourage smoking cessation

1st edition 1992; revised 2013

Background Evidence:

Agnelli, G., & Becattini, C. (2008). Treatment of DVT: How long is enough and how do you predict recurrence. *Journal of Thrombosis and Thrombolysis, 25*(1), 37–44.

American Association of Critical-Care Nurses. (2006). In J. G. Alspach (Ed.), *Core curriculum for critical care nursing* (6th ed.). Saunders Elsevier.

Fekrazad, M. H., Lopes, R. D., Stashenko, G. J., Alexander, J. H., & Garcia, D. (2009). Treatment of venous thromboembolism: Guidelines translated for the clinician. *Journal of Thrombosis and Thrombolysis, 28*(3), 270–275.

Findlay, J., Keogh, M., & Cooper, L. (2010). Venous thromboembolism prophylaxis: The role of the nurse. *British Journal of Nursing (BJN), 19*(16), 1028–1032.

Fitzgerald, J. (2010). Venous thromboembolism: Have we made headway? *Orthopaedic Nursing, 29*(4), 226–234.

Kearon, C., Kahn, S. R., Agnelli, G., Goldhaber, S., Raskob, G. E., & Comerota, A. J. (2008). Antithrombotic therapy for venous thromboembolic disease: American College of Chest Physicians evidence-based clinical practice guidelines (8th ed.). *Chest, 133*(Suppl. 6), 454S–545S.

Lancaster, S., Owens, A., Bryant, A., Ramey, L., Nicholson, J., Gossett, K., Forni, J., & Padgett, T. (2010). Emergency: Upper-extremity deep vein thrombosis. *AJN: American Journal of Nursing, 110*(5), 48–52.

Lankshear, A., Harden, J., & Simms, J. (2010). Safe practice for patients receiving anticoagulant therapy. *Nursing Standard, 24*(20), 47–56.

Meetoo, D. (2010). In too deep: Understanding, detecting and managing DVT. *British Journal of Nursing (BJN), 19*(16), 1021–1022, 1024–1027.

Embolus Care: Pulmonary 4106

Definition: Management of a patient experiencing occlusion of pulmonary circulation

Activities:

- Prepare for thrombolytic therapy (e.g., streptokinase, urokinase, activase), as indicated
- Elicit a detailed patient health history in order to plan current and future preventative care
- Evaluate changes in respiratory and cardiac status (e.g., new-onset wheezing, hemoptysis, dyspnea, tachypnea, tachycardia, syncope) as patients who experience PE or DVT are at a higher risk of recurrence
- Evaluate all chest, shoulder, back, or pleuritic pain (i.e., check for intensity, location, radiation, duration, and precipitating and alleviating factors)
- Assist with diagnostic tests and assessments to rule out conditions with similar signs and symptoms (e.g., acute myocardial infarction; pericarditis; aortic dissection; pneumonia; pneumothorax; anxiety with hyperventilation; asthma; heart failure; pericardial tamponade; and gastrointestinal abnormalities such as peptic ulcer, esophageal rupture, gastritis)
- Instruct the patient and/or family regarding diagnostic procedures (e.g., V/Q scan, d-dimer assay, multidetector spiral CT, ultrasonographies), as appropriate
- Auscultate lung sounds for crackles or other adventitious sounds
- Obtain arterial blood gas levels, as indicated
- Monitor determinants of tissue oxygen delivery (e.g., PaO_2, SaO_2, hemoglobin levels, and cardiac output)
- Monitor for symptoms of inadequate tissue oxygenation (e.g., pallor, cyanosis, and sluggish capillary refill)
- Monitor for symptoms of respiratory failure (e.g., low PaO_2 and elevated $PaCO_2$ levels and respiratory muscle fatigue)
- Initiate appropriate thromboprophylaxis regimen immediately per organizational policy and protocol
- Administer prophylactic, low-dose anticoagulant and/or antiplatelet medication (e.g., heparin, clopidogrel, warfarin, aspirin, dipyridamole, dextran) per organizational policy and protocol
- Elevate any suspected affected limb 20 degrees or greater, higher than the level of the heart, to improve venous return
- Apply graduated elastic compression stockings or sleeves (GECS) to reduce the risk of DVT or recurrence of DVT per organizational policy and protocol
- Maintain graduated elastic compression stockings or sleeves to avoid development of postthrombotic syndrome (PTS)
- Apply intermittent pneumatic compression device stockings per organizational policy and protocol
- Remove graduated elastic compression stockings or sleeves and intermittent pneumatic compression device stockings for 15 to 20 minutes every 8 hours or per organizational policy and protocol
- Avoid antecubital intravenous access and instruct radiology and laboratory personnel to limit access of antecubital veins for tests, if possible
- Assist patient with passive or active range of motion, as appropriate
- Encourage flexion and extension of feet and legs at least 10 times every hour
- Change patient position every 2 hours, encourage early mobilization, or ambulate as tolerated
- Encourage good ventilation (e.g., incentive spirometry, cough and deep breath every 2 hours)
- Monitor laboratory values for changes in oxygenation or acid-base balance, as appropriate
- Instruct the patient and/or family regarding any planned treatments to remove the embolus (e.g., fibrinolysis, catheter embolectomy, or surgical pulmonary embolectomy)
- Encourage the patient to relax
- Monitor side effects of anticoagulant medications
- Avoid overwedging of pulmonary artery catheter to prevent pulmonary artery rupture, if appropriate
- Monitor pulmonary artery tracing for spontaneous wedge of catheter, if appropriate
- Reposition spontaneously wedged pulmonary artery catheter, if appropriate
- Maintain thromboprophylaxis after an embolus
- Instruct patient and family on need for anticoagulation after an embolus for a minimum of 3 months

- Provide detailed education for patient and family related to prevention of future emboli and thrombi

1st edition 1992; revised 2013

Background Evidence:

American Association of Critical-Care Nurses. (2006). In J. G. Alspach (Ed.), *Core curriculum for critical care nursing* (6th ed.). Saunders Elsevier.

Findlay, J., Keogh, M., & Cooper, L. (2010). Venous thromboembolism prophylaxis: The role of the nurse. *British Journal of Nursing (BJN), 19*(16), 1028–1032.

Fitzgerald, J. (2010). Venous thromboembolism: Have we made headway? *Orthopaedic Nursing, 29*(4), 226–234.

Headley, C. M., & Melander, S. (2011). When it may be a pulmonary embolism. *Nephrology Nursing Journal, 38*(2), 127–152.

Lancaster, S., Owens, A., Bryant, A., Ramey, L., Nicholson, J., Gossett, K., Forni, J., & Padgett, T. (2010). Emergency: Upper-extremity deep vein thrombosis. *AJN: American Journal of Nursing, 110*(5), 48–52.

Lankshear, A., Harden, J., & Simms, J. (2010). Safe practice for patients receiving anticoagulant therapy. *Nursing Standard, 24*(20), 47–56.

Meetoo, D. (2010). In too deep: understanding, detecting and managing DVT. *British Journal of Nursing (BJN), 19*(16), 1021–1022, 1024–1027.

Shaughnessy, K. (2007). Massive pulmonary embolism. *Critical Care Nurse, 27*(1), 39–40, 42–51.

Yee, C. A. (2010). Conquering pulmonary embolism. *OR Nurse, 4*(5), 18–24.

E

Embolus Precautions   4110

Definition: Reduction of the risk of an embolus in a patient with thrombi or at risk for thrombus formation

Activities:

- Elicit a detailed patient health history to determine risk level of patient (e.g., recent surgery, bone fractures, current cancer treatment, pregnancy, postpartum, immobility, paralysis, edematous extremities, COPD, stroke, CVAD, history of previous DVT or PE, or obesity put patients at high risk)
- Implement agency protocol for patients who are found at risk
- Critically evaluate any reports of: new-onset wheezing, hemoptysis, or pain with inspiration; chest, shoulder, back, or pleuritic pain; dyspnea, tachypnea, tachycardia, or syncope
- Evaluate for the presence of Virchow's triad: venous stasis, hypercoagulability, and trauma resulting in intimal damage
- Perform a comprehensive appraisal of pulmonary status
- Perform a comprehensive appraisal of peripheral circulation (i.e., check peripheral pulses, edema, capillary refill, color, presence of pain in the affected extremity, and temperature of extremity)
- Initiate appropriate thromboprophylaxis regimen in at risk patients immediately per organizational policy and protocol
- Administer prophylactic low-dose anticoagulant and/or antiplatelet medication (e.g., heparin, clopidogrel, warfarin, aspirin, dipyridamole, dextran) per organizational policy and protocol
- Elevate any suspected affected limb 20 degrees or greater, higher than the level of the heart, to improve venous return
- Apply graduated elastic compression stockings or sleeves (GECS) to reduce the risk of DVT or recurrence of DVT per organizational policy and protocol
- Maintain graduated elastic compression stockings or sleeves to avoid development of postthrombotic syndrome (PTS), which is precipitated by long-term clots in the affected extremity and poor venous flow
- Apply intermittent pneumatic compression device stockings per organizational policy and protocol
- Remove graduated elastic compression stockings or sleeves and intermittent pneumatic compression device stockings for 15 to 20 minutes every 8 hours or per organizational policy and protocol
- Avoid antecubital intravenous access and instruct radiology and laboratory personnel to limit access of antecubital veins for tests, if possible
- Administer intravenous promethazine in a 25 cc to 50 cc saline solution at a slow rate and avoid giving in less than 10 cc saline dilution
- Assist patient with passive or active range of motion, as appropriate
- Encourage flexion and extension of feet and legs at least 10 times every hour
- Change patient position every 2 hours, encourage early mobilization or ambulate as tolerated
- Prevent injury to vessel lumen by preventing local pressure, trauma, infection, or sepsis
- Refrain from massaging or compressing affected limb muscles
- Instruct patient not to cross legs and to avoid sitting for long periods with legs dependent
- Instruct the patient to avoid activities that result in the Valsalva maneuver (e.g., straining during bowel movement)
- Administer medications that will prevent episodes of the Valsalva maneuver (e.g., stool softeners, antiemetics), as appropriate
- Instruct the patient and/or family on appropriate precautions (e.g., walking; drinking plenty of fluids; avoiding alcohol; avoiding long periods of immobility, especially with legs dependently positioned such as in air travel or long automobile trips)
- Instruct the patient and/or family on all prophylactic low-dose anticoagulant and/or antiplatelet medication new
- Instruct the patient to report excessive bleeding (e.g., unusual nosebleeds; vomiting blood; blood in the urine; bleeding gums; unexpected vaginal bleeding; unusually heavy menstrual bleeding; bloody or tarry bowel movements), unusual bruising, unusual pain or swelling, blue or purple color of the toes, pain in the toes, ulcers or white spots in the mouth or throat
- Instruct the patient to wear a medical-alert bracelet
- Instruct patient to maintain a consistent diet (i.e., eat a consistent amount of green leafy vegetables that are high in vitamin K and can interfere with anticoagulants as the medication dosage will be adjusted to dietary intake)
- Instruct patient to take anticoagulant medication at the same time each day and not to double up the next day if a dose is missed
- Instruct patient to check with health care provider: before taking any medication or herbal preparations, including over-the-counter products; before changing brands of medication; and before discontinuing a medication
- Instruct the patient and family on graduated elastic compression stockings
- Encourage smoking cessation

1st edition 1992; revised 2013

Background Evidence:

American Association of Critical-Care Nurses. (2006). *Core curriculum for critical care nursing.* In J. G. Alspach (Ed.), (6th ed.). Saunders Elsevier.

Findlay, J., Keogh, M., & Cooper, L. (2010). Venous thromboembolism prophylaxis: The role of the nurse. *British Journal of Nursing (BJN)*, 19(16), 1028–1032.

Fitzgerald, J. (2010). Venous thromboembolism: Have we made headway? *Orthopaedic Nursing*, 29(4), 226–234.

Headley, C. M., & Melander, S. (2011). When it may be a pulmonary embolism. *Nephrology Nursing Journal*, 38(2), 127–152.

Lancaster, S., Owens, A., Bryant, A., Ramey, L., Nicholson, J., Gossett, K., Forni, J., & Padgett, T. (2010). Emergency: Upper-extremity deep vein thrombosis. *AJN: American Journal of Nursing*, 110(5), 48–52.

Lankshear, A., Harden, J., & Simms, J. (2010). Safe practice for patients receiving anticoagulant therapy. *Nursing Standard*, 24(20), 47–56.

Meetoo, D. (2010). In too deep: Understanding, detecting, and managing DVT. *British Journal of Nursing (BJN)*, 19(16), 1021–1022, 1024–1027.

Shaughnessy, K. (2007). Massive pulmonary embolism. *Critical Care Nurse*, 27(1), 39–40, 42–51.

Yee, C. A. (2010). Conquering pulmonary embolism. *OR Nurse*, 4(5), 18–24.

E

Emergency Care 6200

Definition: Providing evaluation and treatment measures in urgent situations

Activities:

- Activate the emergency medical system
- Obtain the automated external defibrillator (AED) or assure that someone is obtaining the automated external defibrillator, if possible and appropriate
- Initiate rescue actions to the most critically ill patients in the case of multiple victims
- Evaluate any unresponsive patient to determine appropriate action
- Check for signs and symptoms of cardiac arrest
- Call for help if no breathing or no normal breathing and no response
- Instruct others to call for help, if needed
- Employ precautionary measures to reduce risk of infection when giving care
- Attach the AED and implement specified actions, as appropriate
- Assure rapid defibrillation, as appropriate
- Perform cardiopulmonary resuscitation that focuses on chest compressions in adults and compressions with breathing efforts for children, as appropriate
- Initiate 30 chest compressions at specified rate and depth, allowing for complete chest recoil between compressions, minimizing interruptions in compressions, and avoiding excessive ventilation, as appropriate
- Minimize the interval between stopping chest compressions and delivering a shock, if indicated
- Tailor rescue actions to the most likely cause of arrest (e.g., cardiac or respiratory)
- Create or maintain an open airway
- Check for signs and symptoms of severely compromised breathing (e.g., pneumothorax or flailing chest)
- Provide two rescue breaths after initial 30 chest compressions completed, as appropriate
- Perform the Heimlich maneuver, as appropriate
- Provide age-appropriate care for elderly and children
- Check for signs and symptoms of severely compromised hemodynamic status (e.g., arterial trauma or rupture)
- Institute measures (e.g., pressure, pressure dressing, positioning) to reduce or minimize bleeding
- Institute measures for management of shock (e.g., positioning for optimal perfusion, MAST trousers), as needed
- Monitor the amount and nature of blood loss
- Monitor vital signs, if possible and appropriate
- Check for signs and symptoms of compromised neurological status (e.g., paralysis, paresthesia, bowel or bladder incontinence)
- Immobilize patient with suspected head or spine injury using appropriate devices and techniques (i.e., apply cervical collar, move patient as a unit, and transport patient in supine position on backboard)
- Position patient's body part or body-as-unit in appropriate position (e.g., body part affected with insect sting lower than heart level, and left-side lying for poison ingestion or alcohol and drug intoxication)
- Immobilize fractures, large wounds, and any injured part
- Move patient only using appropriate technique and body mechanics, when necessary
- Monitor for signs and symptoms of hypoglycemia (e.g., shakiness, tachycardia, chills, clamminess, drowsiness, dizziness, blurred vision, confusion)
- Monitor level of consciousness
- Remove patient from cold environment
- Remove patient's wet clothing
- Remove overheated patient from direct sunlight and heat source
- Fan the patient and give cool oral fluids, as needed
- Check for medical alert tags
- Administer medication (e.g., nitroglycerin, bronchodilator, activated charcoal, insulin, epinephrine, and antivenin), as needed
- Determine the history of the accident from the patient or others in the area
- Determine type of motor vehicle accident and use of restraining devices, if appropriate
- Determine the exact nature of trauma involved, if appropriate
- Determine whether an overdose of a drug or other substance is involved
- Determine whether toxic or poisonous substances are involved
- Send suspected drugs involved with patient to treatment facility, as appropriate
- Contact poison control center, proceeding with treatment as directed
- Do not leave suicidal patient alone
- Provide reassurance and emotional support to patient or family
- Assist with ongoing treatment, providing pertinent information surrounding life-threatening situation to other health care providers
- Coordinate medical transport, as appropriate
- Transport using a back board, as appropriate

1st edition 1992; revised 2013

Background Evidence:

Carlson, K. (2009). *Advanced critical care nursing.* Saunders Elsevier.

Emergency Nurses Association. (2005). *Sheehy's manual of emergency care* (6th ed.). Mosby Elsevier.

Emergency Nurses Association. (2007). *Emergency nursing core curriculum* (6th ed.). Saunders Elsevier.

Field, J., Hazinski, M., Sayre, M., Chameides, L., Schexnayder, S., Hemphill, R., Samson, R. A., Kattwinkel, J., Berg, R. A., Bhanji, F., Cave, D. M., Jauch, E. C., Kedenchuk, P. J., Newmar, R. W., Peberdy, M. A., Perlma, J. M., Sinz, E., Travers, A. H., Berg, M. D., Billi, J. B., & Hoek, T. (2010). Part 1: Executive summary: 2010 American Heart Association guidelines for cardiopulmonary resuscitation and emergency cardiovascular care. *Circulation, 122*(18 Suppl. 3), S640–S656.

Hazinski, M. F. (2010). *Highlights of the 2010 American Heart Association guidelines for CPR and ECC.* American Heart Association.

Hickey, J. (2009). *The clinical practice of neurological and neurosurgical nursing* (6th ed.). Lippincott Williams & Wilkins.

McQuillan, K. A., Makic, M. B., & Whalen, E. (2009). *Trauma nursing: From resuscitation through rehabilitation* (4th ed.). Saunders Elsevier.

Wiegand, D. (2011). *AACN procedure manual for critical care* (6th ed.). Elsevier Saunders.

Emergency Cart Checking   7660

Definition: Systematic review and maintenance of the contents of an emergency cart at established time intervals

Activities:

- Ensure ease of usability of equipment and supplies per proper cart design and location of supplies during initial cart setup and with all checks
- Compare equipment on cart with list of designated equipment
- Locate all designated equipment and supplies on cart
- Replace missing or outdated supplies and equipment
- Ensure that latex-free products are stocked when available, per agency protocol
- Ensure that equipment is operational via trial run (i.e., assemble laryngoscope and check light bulb function), as indicated
- Ensure that defibrillator remains plugged in and charging between all uses
- Test defibrillator per machine and agency protocol, including a trial discharge of low energy joules (less than 200)
- Clean equipment, as needed
- Verify current expiration date on all supplies and medications
- Document cart check, per agency policy
- Replace equipment, supplies, and medications as technology and guidelines are updated
- Ensure safeguarding of cart supplies, equipment, and patient information per agency protocol and governmental regulations (e.g., Health Insurance Portability and Accountability Act [HIPAA])
- Instruct new nursing staff on proper emergency cart checking procedures

Background Evidence:

American Association of Critical-Care Nurses. (2006). *Core curriculum for critical care nursing.* In J. G. Alspach (Ed.), (6th ed.). Saunders Elsevier.

American Heart Association. (2005). 2005 American Heart Association guidelines for cardiopulmonary resuscitation and emergency cardiovascular care. *Circulation, 112*(24 Suppl. 1), IV-1–IV-211.

American Heart Association. (2005). Electric therapies: Automated external defibrillators, defibrillation, cardioversion, and pacing. *Circulation, 112*(24 Suppl.), IV-35–IV-46.

Bernstein, M. L. (1998). Latex-safe emergency cart products list. *Journal of Emergency Nursing, 24*(1), 58–61.

DeVita, M. A., Schaefer, J., Lutz, J., Dongilli, T., & Wang, H. (2004). Improving medical crisis team performance. *Critical Care Medicine, 32*(2 Suppl.), S61–S65.

McLaughlin, R. C. (2003). Redesigning the crash cart: Usability testing improves one facility's medication drawers. *American Journal of Nursing, 103*(4). Hospital Extra: 64A, 64D, 64G–H.

Misko, L., & Molle, E. (2003). Beyond the classroom: Teaching staff to manage cardiac arrest situations. *Journal for Nurses in Staff Development, 19*(6), 292–296.

Shanaberger, C. J. (1988). Equipment failure is often human failure. *Journal of Emergency Medical Services, 13*(1), 124–125.

Wiegand, D., & Carlson, K. (Eds.). (2005). *AACN procedure manual for critical care* (5th ed.). Elsevier Saunders.

2nd edition 1996; revised 2008

Emotional Support   5270

Definition: Provision of reassurance, acceptance, and encouragement during times of stress

Activities:

- Convey authenticity, warmth, genuineness, interest, and unconditional caring
- Provide privacy and ensure confidentiality
- Introduce self and ensure person comfortable
- Use open-ended questions to help guide conversation and stir discussion (e.g., what happened, how did that make you feel, what will you do next?)
- Listen attentively to concerns, thoughts, feelings, and beliefs
- Refrain from making judgments about experiences
- Focus on understanding experiences
- Explore what triggered emotions
- Make supportive or empathetic statements
- Restate concerns to seek understanding and convey empathy (e.g., It sounds like you are saying…; or What I'm hearing is…)
- Use touch to support emotionally, if appropriate
- Encourage to express feelings of anxiety, anger, or sadness
- Empathize and validate experience (e.g., That's a lot to deal with; I'm sorry that this is happening; It sounds like that really hurt you; I understand; That would make me angry too)
- Facilitate identification of usual response pattern in coping with fears
- Explore actions to deal with situation
- Provide assistance in decision making

- Discuss possible consequences of not dealing with feelings of guilt and shame
- Provide support during denial, anger, bargaining, and acceptance phases of grieving
- Identify function that anger, frustration, and rage can serve
- Encourage talking or crying as means to express and release emotional responses
- Stay with person and provide assurance of safety and security during periods of anxiety
- Reduce demand for cognitive functioning when ill or fatigued
- Refer for counseling, as appropriate

1st edition 1992; revised 2004, 2024

Background Evidence:

Arnold, J. L., & Baker, C. (2018). The role of mental health nurses in supporting young people's mental health: A review of the literature. *Mental Health Review Journal, 23*(3), 197–220. https://doi.org/10.1108/MHRJ-09-2017-0039

Cole, E. (2019). "Many nurses don't know what to say to someone in distress." *Nursing Standard, 34*(1), 40–42. https://doi.org/10.7748/ns.34.1.40.s18

Duarte Bard, N., Olizsewski Feijó, I., Ramires Ipuchima, J., Aparecida Paz, A., & da Costa Linch, G. F. (2020). Nursing diagnoses and interventions in mental health used in hospital admissions units: Integrative review. *Revista de Pesquisa: Cuidado e Fundamental, 12*(1), 1165–1171. https://doi.org/10.9789/2175-5361.rpcfo.v12.8029

Joo, S., Chai, H. W., Jun, H. J., & Almeida, D. M. (2020). Daily stressors facilitate giving and receiving of emotional support in adulthood. *Stress & Health: Journal of the International Society for the Investigation of Stress, 36*(3), 330–337. https://doi.org/10.1002/smi.2927

Levy-Storms, L., & Chen, L. (2020). Communicating emotional support: family caregivers' visits with residents living with dementia in nursing homes. *Journal of Women & Aging, 32*(4), 389–401. https://doi.org/10.1080/08952841.2020.1787787

Endotracheal Extubation   3270

Definition: Purposeful removal of the endotracheal tube from the nasopharyngeal or oropharyngeal airway

Activities:

- Instruct patient and significant others about the procedure
- Assure that the patient has the device removed at the earliest appropriate time
- Assure that the patient is capable of maintaining a patent airway and adequate spontaneous ventilation and does not require high levels of positive airway pressure to maintain normal arterial blood oxygenation
- Assure that extubation readiness criteria are met (e.g., stability in hemodynamic status, respiratory status, vital capacity, peak expiratory flow; respiratory frequency to tidal volume; maximal expiratory pressure)
- Assure that patient is a candidate for problem-free extubation (e.g., breathing spontaneously, well oxygenated, CO_2 normal, awake and responsive, following commands, adequate cough strength to clear secretions, adequate laryngeal function, adequate nutritional status, clearance of sedative and neuromuscular blocking effects)
- Evaluate for known risk factors for extubation failure (e.g., age less than 70 or less than 24; Hgb less than 10 mg/dL; use of continuous IV sedation; longer duration of mechanical sedation; presence of a syndrome or chronic medical condition; known medical or surgical airway condition; frequent pulmonary toilet; loss of airway protective reflexes)
- Provide environment in which patient can be physiologically monitored and in which emergency equipment and appropriately trained health care providers with airway management skills are immediately available
- Provide equipment to assure patient oxygenation during extubation (e.g., oxygen source; devices to deliver oxygen; high volume suction source and catheters for tracheal and pharyngeal suctioning; appropriately sized face masks; intubation equipment such as laryngoscope blades, handles, batteries)
- Provide equipment for emergency surgical airway procedures during extubation (e.g., scalpel, lidocaine, emergency surgical airway)
- Provide equipment for adequate patient monitoring during extubation (e.g., pulse oximeter, cardiac monitor, supplies for ABGs)
- Provide for patient comfort during extubation (e.g., medications for sedation, proper positioning)
- Position the patient for best use of ventilatory muscles, usually with the head of the bed elevated 75 degrees
- Hyper-oxygenate the patient and suction the endotracheal airway
- Suction the oral airway
- Deflate the endotracheal cuff and remove the endotracheal tube
- Encourage the patient to cough and expectorate sputum
- Administer oxygen as ordered
- Encourage coughing and deep breathing
- Suction the airway, as needed
- Provide for measures to prevent aspiration post-extubation, as indicated
- Monitor airway protective reflexes for depression immediately after extubation and for some time after extubation to avoid aspiration complications (i.e., high risk period immediately after extubation)
- Monitor the post-extubation period, including ensuring the equipment, personnel, and medications are readily available in the event of emergent, post-extubation phenomena
- Monitor for respiratory distress, including frequent respiratory evaluation that includes vital signs, assessment of neurological status, patency of airway, auscultatory findings, work of breathing, and hemodynamic status
- Observe for signs of airway occlusion
- Monitor vital signs
- Encourage voice rest for 4 to 8 hours, as appropriate
- Monitor ability to swallow and talk
- Exercise standard precautions for all patients, using the Centers for Disease Control and Prevention recommendations for control of exposure to tuberculosis and droplet nuclei
- Institute appropriate precautions empirically for airborne, droplet, and contact agents ending confirmation of diagnosis in patients suspected of having serious infections
- Interact with patient and family to determine needs for home care

2nd edition 1996; revised 2018

Background Evidence:

American Association of Critical Care Nurses. (2006). Core curriculum for critical care nursing. In J. G. Alspach (Ed.), (6th ed.). W.B. Saunders.

American Association of Respiratory Care. (2007). AARC clinical practice guidelines: Removal of the endotracheal tube – 2007 revision & update. *Respiratory Care, 52*(1) 81–93.

Dawkins, S. (2011). A literature review and guidance for nurse-led patient extubation in the recovery room/post anesthetic care unit: Endotracheal tubes. *Journal of Perioperative Practice, 21*(10), 352–355.

Endotracheal Extubation: Palliative — 1360

Definition: Purposeful removal of endotracheal tube and mechanical ventilation with knowledge that natural death may result

Activities:
- Determine appropriateness of extubation based on person and family's wishes
- Involve interprofessional team in decision-making process
- Review records to ensure wishes regarding discontinuation of ventilator support are documented
- Prepare family on what to expect (e.g., episodes of abnormal breathing or involuntary movements, discontinuation of interventions that do not provide comfort)
- Provide spiritual support as desired
- Discontinue neuromuscular blocking agents at appropriate interval before extubation, as prescribed
- Maintain intravenous or subcutaneous access as indicated
- Raise head of bed to 35–45 degrees
- Encourage family to spend time with person prior to extubation
- Remove unnecessary equipment from bedside
- Remove soft ties, mitts, and other devices that hinder contact between person and family
- Decrease or turn off sound of monitoring equipment and electronic devices (e.g., alarm settings, television, radios, phones, computers) except when requested otherwise by family
- Premedicate prior to extubation for comfort, as prescribed
- Proceed with steps of extubation (e.g., deflate cuff, remove tube)
- Maintain cannula for person with tracheostomy or significant airway edema
- Suction residual secretions, as needed
- Administer medication to alleviate respiratory distress, pain, or anxiety, as prescribed
- Provide family support as indicated
- Document process, medications, and outcomes (e.g., instability, stability, death)

8th edition 2024

Background Evidence:

Coradazzi, A. L., Inhaia, C. L., Santana, M. T. E. A., Sala, A. D., Ricardo, C. P., & Suadicani, C. O. (2019). Palliative withdrawal ventilation: Why, when and how to do it? *Hospice & Palliative Medicine International Journal, 3,* 10–14.

Faircloth, A. C. (2017). Anesthesia involvement in palliative care. *Annual Review of Nursing Research, 35,* 135–158.

Haas, N. L., Larabell, P., Schaeffer, W., Hoch, V., Arribas, M., Melvin, A. C., Laurinec, S. L., & Bassin, B. S. (2020). Descriptive analysis of extubations performed in an Emergency Department-based Intensive Care Unit. *The Western Journal of Emergency Medicine, 21*(3), 532–537. https://doi.org/10.5811/westjem.2020.4.47475

Potter, J., Shields, S., & Breen, R. (2021). Palliative sedation, compassionate extubation, and the principle of double effect: An ethical analysis. *American Journal of Hospice & Palliative Medicine, 38*(12), 1536–1540. https://doi.org/10.1177/1049909121998630

White, D.B. (2019). Withholding and withdrawing ventilatory support in adults in the intensive care unit. In I. Finlay, G. (Ed.), *UpToDate.* https://www.uptodate-com.proxy.lib.uiowa.edu/contents/withholding-and-withdrawing-ventilatory-support-in-adults-in-the-intensive-care-unit

---

Enema Administration — 0466

Definition: Instillation of a solution into the lower gastrointestinal tract

Activities:
- Determine reason for enema (e.g., gastrointestinal cleansing; medication administration; distention reduction)
- Verify practitioner order for enema and absence of any contraindications (e.g., glaucoma and increased intracranial pressure)
- Explain procedure to patient or family, including expected sensations during and after procedure (e.g., distention and urge to defecate)
- Gather and assemble equipment specific to type of enema
- Provide privacy
- Assist patient into appropriate position (e.g., left side-lying position with right knee flexed for adults and dorsal recumbent for children)
- Place waterproof or absorbent pad under hips and buttocks
- Cover patient with bath blanket leaving only rectal area uncovered
- Ascertain appropriate temperature of irrigating solution
- Instruct patient to exhale before inserting solution
- Insert lubricated tip of solution container or tubing into rectum, angling tip toward umbilicus and inserting appropriate length based on patient's age
- Squeeze bottle until all solution has entered rectum and colon
- Determine appropriate height of enema bag, solution volume, instillation rate, and handling of tubing
- Encourage patient to retain fluid until urge to defecate, assisting by squeezing buttocks, if necessary
- Provide bedpan, commode, or easy access to toilet
- Monitor character of feces and solution (e.g., color, amount, and appearance)

- Monitor patient response to procedure, including signs of intolerance (e.g., rectal bleeding, distention, and abdominal pain), diarrhea, constipation, and impaction
- Assist patient in perineal cleansing
- Provide instruction to patient, caregiver, or unlicensed assistive personnel on enema administration
- Instruct on signs that warrant ending the procedure and reporting to health care practitioner (e.g., palpitations, diaphoresis, pallor, and shortness of breath)

Background Evidence:

Craven, R., & Hirnle, C. (2009). Bowel elimination. In *Fundamentals of nursing: Human health and function* (pp. 1116–1158) (6th ed.). Lippincott Williams & Wilkins.

Smith, S. F., Duell, D. J., & Martin, B. C. (2008). Bowel elimination. In *Clinical nursing skills: Basic to advanced skills* (pp. 811–847) (7th ed.). Pearson: Prentice Hall.

Wood, T. (2007). Assisting with elimination. In M. K. Elkin, A. G. Perry, & P. A. Potter (Eds.), *Nursing interventions & clinical skills* (4th ed., pp. 176–198). Mosby Elsevier.

6th edition 2013

Energy Management

0180

Definition: Regulating energy use to treat or prevent fatigue and optimize function

Activities:

- Assess patient's physiological status for deficits resulting in fatigue within the context of age and development
- Encourage verbalization of feelings about limitations
- Use valid instruments to measure fatigue, as indicated
- Determine patient's/significant other's perception of causes of fatigue
- Correct physiological status deficits (e.g., chemotherapy-induced anemia) as priority items
- Select interventions for fatigue reduction using combinations of pharmacological and nonpharmacological categories, as appropriate
- Determine what and how much activity is required to build endurance
- Monitor nutritional intake to ensure adequate energy resources
- Consult with dietitian about ways to increase intake of high-energy foods
- Negotiate desired mealtimes, which may or may not coincide with standard hospital schedules
- Monitor patient for evidence of excess physical and emotional fatigue
- Monitor cardiorespiratory response to activity (e.g., tachycardia, other dysrhythmias, dyspnea, diaphoresis, pallor, hemodynamic pressures, respiratory rate)
- Encourage aerobic workouts, as tolerated
- Monitor/record patient's sleep pattern and number of sleep hours
- Monitor location and nature of discomfort or pain during movement/activity
- Reduce physical discomforts that could interfere with cognitive function and self-monitoring/regulation of activity
- Set limits with hyperactivity when it interferes with others or with the patient
- Assist the patient to understand energy conservation principles (e.g., the requirement for restricted activity or bed rest)
- Teach activity organization and time management techniques to prevent fatigue
- Assist the patient in assigning priority to activities to accommodate energy levels
- Assist the patient/significant other to establish realistic activity goals
- Assist the patient to identify preferences for activity
- Encourage the patient to choose activities that gradually build endurance
- Assist the patient to identify tasks that family and friends can perform in the home to prevent/relieve fatigue
- Consider electronic communication (e.g., e-mail or instant messaging) to maintain contact with friends when visits are not practical or advisable
- Assist the patient to limit daytime sleep by providing activity that promotes wakefulness, as appropriate
- Limit environmental stimuli (e.g., light and noise) to facilitate relaxation
- Limit number of and interruptions by visitors, as appropriate
- Promote bed rest/activity limitation (e.g., increase number of rest periods) with protected rest times of choice
- Encourage alternate rest and activity periods
- Arrange physical activities to reduce competition for oxygen supply to vital body functions (e.g., avoid activity immediately after meals)
- Use passive and/or active range-of-motion exercises to relieve muscle tension
- Provide calming diversional activities to promote relaxation
- Offer aids to promote sleep (e.g., music or medications)
- Encourage an afternoon nap, if appropriate
- Assist patient to schedule rest periods
- Avoid care activities during scheduled rest periods
- Plan activities for periods when the patient has the most energy
- Assist patient to sit on side of bed ("dangle"), if unable to transfer or walk
- Assist with regular physical activities (e.g., ambulation, transfers, turning, and personal care), as needed
- Monitor administration and effect of stimulants and depressants
- Encourage physical activity (e.g., ambulation, performance of activities of daily living) consistent with patient's energy resources
- Evaluate programmed increases in levels of activities
- Monitor patient's oxygen response (e.g., pulse rate, cardiac rhythm, respiratory rate) to self-care or nursing activities
- Assist patient to self-monitor by developing and using a written record of calorie intake and energy expenditure, as appropriate
- Instruct the patient and/or significant other on fatigue, its common symptoms, and latent recurrences
- Instruct patient and significant other on techniques of self-care that will minimize oxygen consumption (e.g., self-monitoring and pacing techniques for performance of activities of daily living)
- Instruct patient/significant other to recognize signs and symptoms of fatigue that require reduction in activity
- Instruct the patient/significant other on stress and coping interventions to decrease fatigue

- Instruct patient/significant other to notify health care provider if signs and symptoms of fatigue persist

1st edition 1992; revised 2008

Background Evidence:

Erickson, J. M. (2004). Fatigue in adolescents with cancer: A review of the literature. *Clinical Journal of Oncology Nursing, 8*(2), 139–145.

Gelinas, C., & Fillion, L. (2004). Factors related to persistent fatigue following completion of breast cancer treatment. *Oncology Nursing Forum, 31*(2), 269–278.

Glick, O. J. (1992). Interventions related to activity and movement. *Nursing Clinics of North America, 27*(2), 541–568.

McFarland, G. K., & McFarlane, E. A. (1997). *Nursing diagnosis and intervention: Planning for patient care* (3rd ed.). Mosby.

Nail, L. M. (2002). Fatigue in patients with cancer. *Oncology Nursing Forum, 29*(3), 537–546.

Oncology Nursing Society. (2005). In J. K. Itano & K. Taoka (Eds.), *Core curriculum for oncology nursing* (4th ed.). Elsevier Saunders.

Piper, B. (1997). Measuring fatigue. In M. Frank-Stromborg & S. Olsen (Eds.), *Pathophysiological phenomena in nursing: Human response to illness* (pp. 219–234). W. B. Saunders.

E

Enteral Tube Feeding   1056

Definition: Delivering nutrients and fluid through a tube inserted in the gastrointestinal tract

Activities:

- Consult with dietitian in selecting type and strength of enteral feeding
- Verify correct formula, expiration date, and integrity of container
- Prepare formula for administration following manufacturer guidelines, assuring formula at room temperature
- Perform appropriate abdominal assessments prior to initiating feedings (e.g., bowel sounds, firmness on palpation, expanding girth)
- Monitor for proper placement of tube, according to agency protocol
- Avoid pH testing for confirmation of placement in persons receiving acid-suppression medications or on continuous feedings
- Mark tubing at point of exit to maintain proper placement and check regularly for movement, once placement confirmed by x-ray
- Confirm tube placement by x-ray examination before initial administration of feedings or medications via tube, per agency protocol
- Monitor reports of routine chest and abdominal radiographic films for reference to feeding tube location
- Obtain repeat x-ray film confirmation of placement if bedside assessments create any doubt regarding tube location
- Check tube placement immediately before each intermittent feeding or per agency protocol for continuous feedings
- Avoid IV syringes when administering feedings or solutions into tubes to decrease chance of inadvertently accessing IV lines
- Check residual per health care provider prescription or agency policy, prior to medication administration and changes in enteral feeding
- Wait to verify placement at least 1 hour after medication administration by tube or mouth
- Elevate head of bed 30 to 45 degrees during feedings
- Place in reverse Trendelenburg during feedings if person needs to remain supine
- Offer pacifier to infant during feeding, as appropriate
- Hold and talk to infant during feeding to simulate usual feeding activities
- Monitor for signs and symptoms of respiratory distress during feeding (e.g., coughing, choking, reduced oxygen saturation)
- Stop feedings if distress noted and obtain x-ray per agency protocol
- Discontinue feedings 30 to 60 minutes before lowering head of bed
- Turn off tube feeding 1 hour before procedure or transport if person needs to be positioned less than 30 degrees head elevation
- Irrigate tube every 4 to 6 hours during continuous feedings, before and after every intermittent feeding, after giving medications, and when disconnecting tube feedings, to prevent clogging of tube, per agency protocol
- Unclog feeding tubes using solution of meat tenderizer and water (i.e., 1 tablespoon in 30 mL of warm water) let sit for 5 minutes and then flush with warm water, per agency protocol
- Implement total free-water requirement per day per registered dietitian recommendation
- Use clean technique in administering tube feedings, with aseptic technique for tubing connections
- Avoid handling feeding system or touching can tops, container openings, spike or spike port to prevent bacterial growth
- Check gravity drip rate or pump rate every hour
- Use only pumps designated for tube feedings
- Label bag with tube feeding type, strength, amount, date, time, and initials
- Slow tube feeding rate or decrease strength to control diarrhea
- Monitor for sensation of fullness, nausea, and vomiting
- Keep open containers of enteral feeding refrigerated
- Change insertion site and infusion tubing according to agency protocol
- Wash skin around skin level device daily with mild soap and dry thoroughly
- Discard enteral feeding containers and administration sets every 24 hours
- Monitor for growth, height or weight changes monthly, as appropriate
- Monitor for signs of edema or dehydration
- Monitor for conditions that increase risk for tube migration or dislocation (e.g., vomiting, retching, nasotracheal suction, agitation)
- Monitor fluid intake and output
- Monitor calorie, fat, carbohydrate, vitamin, and mineral intake for adequacy (or refer to dietitian) two times weekly initially, decreasing to once per month
- Monitor for mood changes
- Prepare individual and family for home tube feedings, as appropriate

1st edition 1992; revised 1996, 2000, 2004, 2024

Background Evidence:

Berman, A., Snyder, S. J., & Frandsen, G. (2018). Nutrition. In *Kozier and Erb's fundamentals of nursing: Concepts, process and practice.* (pp. 1127–1167) (10th ed.). Pearson.

Miller, T. (2021). Nutrition. In A. Perry, P. Potter, P. Stockert, & A. Hall (Eds.), *Fundamentals of Nursing* (10th ed., pp. 1120–1147). Elsevier.

Potter, P. A., Ostendorf, W. R., & LaPlante, N. (2018). Enteral nutrition. In *Clinical nursing skills and techniques* (pp. 830–860) (9th ed.). St. Louis: Mosby.

Rebar, C. R. (2021). Concepts of care for patients with malnutrition: Undernutrition and obesity. In D. Ignativicius, M. L. Workman, C. R. Rebar, & N. M. Heimgaartner, (Eds.), *Medical-Surgical nursing: Concepts for interprofessional collaborative care.* (10th ed., pp. 1205–1208). Elsevier.

St. Onge, J. L. (2021). Nutrition. In R. F. Craven, C. J. Hirnle, & C. J. Henshaw (Eds.), *Fundamentals of nursing: Human health and function* (8th ed., pp. 410–471). Wolters-Kluwer.

Williams, P. (2020). Maintaining fluid balance and meeting nutritional needs. In *Basic geriatric nursing.* (pp. 104–130) (7th ed.). Elsevier.

Yang, G., Zheng, B., & Yu, Y. (2021). Risk assessment of intermittent and continuous nasogastric enteral feeding methods in adult inpatients: A meta-analysis. *Evidence-based Complementary & Alternative Medicine (eCAM),* *2021,* 1–10.

Environmental Management 6480

Definition: Establishing and maintaining surroundings for therapeutic benefit, sensory appeal, and psychological well-being

Activities:

- Identify safety needs, based on level of physical and cognitive function, and past history of behavior
- Remove environmental hazards (e.g., loose rugs, movable furniture)
- Remove harmful objects from environment
- Safeguard with side rails or side-rail padding, as appropriate
- Escort during off-unit activities, as appropriate
- Provide low-height bed, as appropriate
- Provide adaptive devices (e.g., step stools, handrails), as appropriate
- Place furniture in room in arrangement that best accommodates disabilities
- Provide sufficiently long tubing to allow freedom of movement, as appropriate
- Place frequently used objects within reach
- Provide single room, as indicated
- Consider aesthetics of environment when selecting roommates
- Provide clean, comfortable bed and environment
- Provide linens and gown in good repair, free of residual stains
- Place bed-positioning switch within easy reach
- Neatly arrange supplies and linens that must remain in view
- Block view of bathroom, commode, or other equipment used for elimination
- Remove materials used during dressing changes and elimination, as well as any residual odors before visitation and meals
- Reduce environmental stimuli, as appropriate
- Avoid unnecessary exposure, drafts, overheating, or chilling
- Avoid unnecessary interruptions that may wake person from rest periods
- Adjust environmental temperature to meet needs, if body temperature is altered
- Control or prevent undesirable or excessive noise, when possible
- Provide music of choice and device for private listening when music may disturb others
- Manipulate lighting and air for therapeutic benefit
- Provide attractively arranged meals and snacks
- Clean areas used for eating and drinking utensils before use
- Allow family to stay
- Limit visitors, if indicated
- Individualize visiting restrictions to meet needs
- Individualize daily routine to meet needs
- Bring familiar objects from home
- Facilitate use of personal items such as pajamas, robes, and toiletries
- Maintain consistency of staff assignment over time
- Provide immediate and continuous means to summon nurse
- Educate about changes and precautions, so no inadvertent disruption occurs
- Provide information about making home environment safe
- Promote fire safety, as appropriate
- Control environmental pests, as appropriate
- Provide room deodorizers, as needed
- Instruct in building safe and peaceful care environment at home
- Use teach-back to ensure understanding

1st edition 1992; revised 1996, 2000, 2004, 2024

Background Evidence:

Aziz, M. G. (2021). Hygiene and self-care. In R. F. Craven, C. J. Hirnle, & C. J. Henshaw (Eds.), *Fundamentals of nursing: Human health and function* (8th ed.). Wolters-Kluwer.

Berman, A., Snyder, S. J., & Frandsen, G. (2018). Hygiene. In *Kozier and Erb's Fundamentals of nursing: Concepts, process and practice* (pp. 684–688) (10th ed.). Pearson.

de Abreu Moniz, M., Vago Daher, D., Sabóia, V. M., & Batista Ribeiro, C. R. (2020). Environmental health: Emancipatory care challenges and possibilities by the nurse. *Revista Brasileira de Enfermagem, 73*(3), 1–5.

Perry, A. G., Potter, P. A., Ostendorf, W. R., & Laplante, N. (2022). *Clinical Nursing Skills and Techniques* (10th ed.). Elsevier.

Valatka, R., Krizo, J., & Mallat, A. (2021). A survey-based assessment of "matter of balance" participant fall-related experience. *Journal of Trauma Nursing, 28*(5), 304–309.

Williams, P. (2020). *Basic geriatric nursing* (7th ed.). Elsevier.

Yamaguchi, Y., Greiner, C., Ryuno, H., & Fukuda, A. (2019). Dementia nursing competency in acute care settings: A concept analysis. *International Journal of Nursing Practice, 25*(3), 1–5.

Environmental Management: Community 6484

Definition: Monitoring and modifying physical, social, cultural, economic, and political conditions that affect community health

Activities:

- Initiate screening for environmental health risks
- Participate in interprofessional teams to identify threats to safety in community
- Identify emerging at-risk populations
- Determine information about community culture in order to understand practices, beliefs, and values that affect health care
- Remove barriers to accessing health services
- Encourage relationships within community related to health promotion and disease prevention
- Monitor status of known health risks
- Participate in community programs to deal with known risks
- Collaborate in development of community action programs
- Promote governmental policy to reduce specified risks
- Encourage neighborhoods to become active participants in community safety
- Coordinate services to at-risk groups and communities
- Conduct educational programs for targeted risk groups
- Work with environmental groups to secure appropriate governmental regulations

2nd edition 1996; revised 2000, 2024

Background Evidence:

Jakubec, S. L., Szabo, J., Gleeson, J., Currie, G., & Flessati, S. (2021). Planting seeds of community-engaged pedagogy: Community health nursing practice in an intergenerational campus-community gardening program. *Nurse Education in Practice. 51*, 102980.

Potter, P. A., Perry, A. G., Stockert, P. A., & Hall, A. (2020). *Fundamentals of Nursing* (10th ed.). Elsevier.

Resnik, D. B., MacDougall, D. R., & Smith, E. M. (2018). Ethical dilemmas in protecting susceptible subpopulations from environmental health risks: Liberty, utility, fairness, and accountability for reasonableness. *American Journal of Bioethics, 18*(3), 29–41.

Sela-Vilensky, Y., Grinberg, K., & Nissanholtz-Gannot, R. (2020). Attracting Israeli nursing students to community nursing. *Israel Journal of Health Policy Research. 9*(1), 1–7.

Weaver, C. P., & Miller, C. A. (2019). A framework for climate change-related research to inform environmental protection. *Environmental Management, 64*(3), 245–257.

Environmental Management: Safety 6486

Definition: Establishing and maintaining the physical environment to promote safety

Activities:

- Determine safety needs, based on physical, emotional, and cognitive function
- Identify safety hazards in environment
- Remove hazards from environment
- Modify environment to minimize hazards and risk
- Provide adaptive devices (e.g., step stools, handrails) to increase safety of environment
- Use protective devices (e.g., restraints, side rails, locked doors, fences, gates) to physically limit mobility or access to harmful situations
- Provide information for emergency contacts
- Monitor environment for changes in safety status
- Assist in relocating to safer environment (e.g., referral for housing assistance)
- Initiate or conduct screening programs for environmental hazards (e.g., lead, radon)
- Instruct on need for air, light, and periodically cleaned environment
- Educate high-risk individuals and groups about environmental hazards
- Collaborate with agencies to improve environmental safety (e.g., health department, Emergency Medical Services [EMS], Department of Human Services [DHS])
- Notify agencies authorized to protect environment (e.g., health department, EMS, DHS)
- Document situations of danger to person safety and mitigation actions
- Encourage reporting of failures and adverse events to appropriate institutional department

1st edition 1992; revised 1996, 2000, 2024

Background Evidence:

Dehdashti, A., Fatemi, F., Jannati, M., Asadi, F., & Kangarloo, M. B. (2020). Applying health, safety, and environmental risk assessment at academic settings. *BMC Public Health, 20*(1), 1328.

Gualniera, P., Scurria, S., Sapienza, D., & Asmundo, A. (2021). Electrosurgical unit: Iatrogenic injuries and medico-legal aspect. Italian legal rules, experience and article review. *Annals of Medicine and Surgery, 62*, 26–30.

King, B., Pecanac, K., Krupp, A., Liebzeit, D., & Mahoney, J. (2018). Impact of fall prevention on nurses and care of fall risk patients. *Gerontologist, 58*(2), 331–340.

Potter, P. A., Perry, A. G., Stockert, P. A., & Hall, A. (2022). *Fundamentals of Nursing* (10 ed.). Elsevier.

Takano, H., & Inoue, K. I. (2017). Environmental pollution and allergies. *Journal of Toxicologic Pathology, 30*(3), 193–199.

Turner, S. L., Johnson, R. D., Weightman, A. L., Rodgers, S. E., Arthur, G., Bailey, R., & Lyons, R. A. (2017). Risk factors associated with unintentional house fire incidents, injuries and deaths in high-income countries: a systematic review. Injury prevention: journal of the *International Society for Child and Adolescent Injury Prevention. 23*(2), 131–137.

E

E

Environmental Management: Violence Prevention 6487

Definition: Monitoring and manipulation of the physical environment to decrease the potential for violent behavior directed toward self, others, or environment

Activities:

- Remove potential weapons from environment (e.g., sharp and ropelike objects such as guitar strings)
- Search environment routinely to maintain it as hazard-free
- Search patient and belongings for weapons/potential weapons during inpatient admission procedure, as appropriate
- Monitor the safety of items being brought to the environment by visitors
- Instruct visitors and other caregivers about relevant patient safety issues
- Limit patient use of potential weapons (e.g., sharp and ropelike objects)
- Monitor patient during use of potential weapons (e.g., razor)
- Place patient with potential for self-harm with a roommate to decrease isolation and opportunity to act on self-harm thoughts, as appropriate
- Assign single room to patient with potential for violence toward others
- Place patient in bedroom located near nursing station
- Limit access to windows, unless locked and shatterproof, as appropriate
- Lock utility and storage rooms
- Provide paper dishes and plastic utensils at meals
- Place patient in least restrictive environment that allows for necessary level of observation
- Provide ongoing surveillance of all patient access areas to maintain patient safety and therapeutically intervene, as needed
- Remove other individuals from the vicinity of a violent or potentially violent patient
- Maintain a designated safe area (e.g., seclusion room) for patient to be placed when violent
- Apply mitts, splints, helmets, or restraints to limit mobility and ability to initiate self-harm, as appropriate
- Provide plastic, rather than metal, clothes hangers, as appropriate

1st edition 1992; revised 2013

Background Evidence:

Bracken, M. I., Messing, J. T., Campbell, J. C., La Flair, L. N., & Kub, J. (2010). Intimate partner violence and abuse among female nurses and nursing personnel: Prevalence and risk factors. *Issues in Mental Health Nursing, 31*(2), 137–148.

Campbell, J. C., Webster, D. W., & Glass, N. (2009). The danger assessment: Validation of a lethality risk assessment instrument for intimate partner femicide. *Journal of Interpersonal Violence, 24*(4), 653–674.

Constantino, R. E., & Privitera, M. R. (2010). Prevention terminology: Primary, secondary, tertiary and an evolution of terms. In M. R. Privitera (Ed.), *Workplace violence in mental and general healthcare settings* (pp. 15–22). Jones and Bartlett.

Cutcliffe, J. R., & Barker, P. (2004). The Nurses' Global Assessment of Suicide Risk (NGASR): Developing a tool for clinical practice. *Journal of Psychiatric and Mental Health Nursing, 11*(4), 393–400.

Delaney, K. R., Esparza, D., Hinderliter, D., Lamb, K., & Mohr, W. K. (2006). Violence and abuse within the community. In W. K. Mohr (Ed.), *Psychiatric-mental health nursing* (6th ed., pp. 353–376). Lippincott Williams & Wilkins.

Larsson, P., Nilsson, S., Runeson, B., & Gustafsson, B. (2007). Psychiatric nursing care of suicidal patients described by the sympathy-acceptance-understanding-competence model for confirming nursing. *Archives of Psychiatric Nursing, 21*(4), 222–232.

Moracco, K., & Cole, T. (2009). Preventing intimate partner violence: Screening is not enough. *JAMA: Journal of the American Medical Association, 302*(5), 568–570.

Ramsay, J., Carter, Y., Davidson, L., Dunne, D., Eldridge, S., Hegarty, K., Rivas, C., Taft, A., Warburton, A., & Feder, G. (2009). Advocacy interventions to reduce or eliminate violence and promote the physical and psychosocial well-being of women who experience intimate partner abuse. *Cochrane Database of Systematic Reviews*, (3). https://doi.org/10.1002/14651858.CD005043.pub2. Article CD005043

Schmidt, H., III., & Ivanoff, A. (2007). Behavioral prescriptions for treating self-injurious and suicidal behaviors. In O. J. Thienhaus & M. Piasecki (Eds.), *Correctional psychiatry: Practice guidelines and strategies* (pp. 7/1–7/23). Civic Research Institute.

Environmental Management: Worker Safety 6489

Definition: Monitoring and manipulation of the worksite environment to promote safety and health of workers

Activities:

- Maintain confidential health records on employees
- Determine employee's fitness for work
- Identify worksite environmental hazards and stressors (e.g., physical, biological, psychological, chemical, ergonomic)
- Identify applicable OSHA standards and worksite compliance with standards
- Understand state and local regulations related to issues such as pharmaceutical and vaccine storage, workplace safety requirements, and medical waste
- Inform workers of their rights and responsibilities under OSHA (i.e., provide an OSHA poster, copies of Act, and copies of standards)
- Inform workers of hazardous substances to which they may be exposed
- Use labels or signs to warn workers of potential worksite hazards
- Maintain records of occupational injuries and illnesses on forms acceptable to OSHA and participate in OSHA inspections
- Keep log of occupational injuries and illnesses for workers
- Identify risk factors for occupational injuries and illnesses through reviewing records for patterns of injuries and illnesses
- Initiate modification of the environment to eliminate or minimize hazards (e.g., training programs to prevent back injuries or workplace violence)
- Initiate worksite screening programs for early detection of work-related and nonoccupational illnesses and injuries (e.g., blood pressure, hearing and vision, pulmonary function tests)
- Initiate worksite health promotion programs based on health risk assessments (e.g., smoking cessation, stress management, immunizations)

- Identify and treat acute conditions at worksite
- Develop emergency protocols and train selected employees on emergency care
- Coordinate follow-up care for work-related injuries and illnesses
- Bring unsafe working conditions to employer's attention, preserving worker confidentiality in discussions

2nd edition 1996; revised 2018

Background Evidence:

Fink, J. L. W. (2013). Keeping nurses safe: Nursing is one of the most dangerous professions. *Healthcare Traveler.* http://healthcaretraveler.modern medicine.com/healthcare-traveler/content/tags/american-nurses-association/keeping-nurses-safe-nursing-one-most-da

Geiger-Brown, J., & Lipscomb, J. (2010). The health care work environment and adverse health and safety consequences for nurses. *Annual Review of Nursing Research, 28*(1), 191–231.

Guzik, A. (2013). *Essentials for occupational health nursing.* Wiley Blackwell.

United States Department of Labor, Occupational Safety & Health Administration. (n.d.). *Clinicians.* https://www.osha.gov/dts/oom/clinicians/NIC 7e Part 3 D-G.doc

Zaidman, B. (2010). *Evaluation of the workplace safety consultation nursing home ergonomics services program.* Minnesota Department of Labor & Industry. http://www.dli.mn.gov/RS/PDF/nursinghome_ergo.pdf

E

Environmental Risk Protection   8880

Definition: Preventing and detecting disease and injury in populations at risk from environmental hazards

Activities:
- Examine environment for risk
- Analyze level of risk (e.g., living habits, work, atmosphere, water, housing, food, waste, radiation, violence)
- Use periodic exposure assessment for populations or at-risk locations
- Inform populations at risk about environmental hazards
- Monitor incidents of illness and injury related to environmental hazards
- Maintain knowledge associated with specific environmental standards (e.g., Environmental Protection Agency [EPA], Occupation Safety and Health Administration [OSHA])
- Collaborate with agencies to improve environmental safety
- Advocate for safer environmental designs, protection systems, and use of protective devices
- Support programs to disclose environmental hazards
- Screen populations at risk for evidence of exposure to environmental hazards
- Participate in data collection related to incidence and prevalence of exposure to environmental hazards
- Encourage appropriate resources to eliminate and reduce use or formation of harmful agents
- Ensure regular assessment and control measures are in place
- Instruct in identification of situations involving environmental risks
- Document populations, situations, and places at risk
- Notify agencies authorized to protect environment of known hazards

3rd edition 2000; revised 2024

Background Evidence:

Caplin, A., Ghandehari, M., Lim, C., Glimcher, P., & Thurston, G. (2019). Advancing environmental exposure assessment science to benefit society. *Nature Communications. 10*(1), 1236.

Holzemer, S., & Klainberg, M. (2021). *Community health nursing: An alliance for health,* (2nd ed.) McGraw-Hill.

Munnangi, S., & Boktor, S. W. (2021). Epidemiology of study design. In: *StatPearls [Internet]* (1st ed.) StatPearls.

Resnik, D. B., MacDougall, D. R., & Smith, E. M. (2018). Ethical dilemmas in protecting susceptible subpopulations from environmental health risks: Liberty, utility, fairness, and accountability for reasonableness. *American Journal of Bioethics, 18*(3), 29–41.

Weaver, C. P., & Miller, C. A. (2019). A framework for climate change-related research to inform environmental protection. *Environmental Management, 64*(3), 245–257.

Examination Assistance   7680

Definition: Providing assistance to the patient and another health care provider during a procedure or exam

Activities:
- Ensure consent is completed, as appropriate
- Explain the rationale for the procedure
- Provide sensory preparation information, as appropriate
- Use developmentally appropriate language when explaining procedures to children
- Ensure availability of emergency equipment and medications before procedure
- Assemble appropriate equipment
- Keep threatening equipment out of view, as appropriate
- Provide a private environment
- Include parent or significant other, as appropriate
- Alert physician to any abnormal findings (e.g., laboratory values, radiology results, patient and family concerns) away from the patient, as appropriate
- Position and drape patient, as appropriate
- Restrain patient, as appropriate
- Explain need for restraints, as appropriate
- Prepare procedure site, as appropriate
- Maintain universal precautions
- Maintain strict aseptic technique, as appropriate
- Explain each step of the procedure to patient
- Monitor patient status during procedure
- Provide patient with emotional support, as indicated
- Provide distraction during procedure, as appropriate
- Assist patient to maintain positioning during procedure
- Reinforce expected behavior during examination of a child
- Facilitate use of equipment, as appropriate
- Note amount and appearance of fluids removed, as appropriate
- Collect, label, and arrange for transport of specimens, as appropriate

- Provide site care and dressing, as appropriate
- Ensure that follow-up tests (e.g., x-ray examinations, laboratory work) are done
- Instruct patient on post-procedure care
- Monitor patient after procedure, as appropriate
- See that the examination room is cleaned and disinfected, as needed

2nd edition 1996; revised 2018

Background Evidence:

Comrie, R. (2013). Health assessment and physical examination. In P. Potter, A. Perry, P. Stockert, & A. Hall (Eds.), *Fundamentals of nursing* (8th ed., pp. 487–564). Elsevier Mosby.

Jarvis, C. (2012). *Student laboratory manual for physical examination and health assessment* (6th ed.). Elsevier Saunders.

Seidel, H., Ball, J., Dains, J., Flynn, J., Solomon, B., & Stewart, R. (2011). *Mosby's guide to physical examination* (7th ed.). Mosby Elsevier.

Exercise Promotion   0200

Definition: Facilitation of regular physical activity to maintain or advance to a higher level of fitness and health

Activities:

- Obtain health care provider approval for instituting exercise plan, as needed
- Appraise health beliefs and desires about physical exercise
- Explore prior exercise experiences
- Determine motivation to begin or continue exercise program
- Explore barriers to exercise
- Encourage verbalization of feelings about exercise or need for exercise
- Encourage to begin or continue exercise
- Assist in identifying positive role model for maintaining exercise program
- Assist to develop appropriate exercise program to meet needs
- Assist to set short-term and long-term goals for exercise program
- Assist to schedule regular periods for exercise program into weekly routine
- Advise to use comfortable clothing, shoes, and socks
- Instruct about water intake at least 2 hours before beginning of activity
- Perform exercise activities with individual, as appropriate
- Include family or caregivers in planning and maintaining exercise program
- Inform about health benefits and physiological effects of exercise
- Instruct about appropriate type of exercise for level of health, in collaboration with health care provider or exercise physiologist
- Instruct about desired frequency, duration, and intensity of exercise program
- Monitor adherence to exercise program or activity
- Assist to prepare and maintain progress graph or chart to motivate adherence to exercise program
- Instruct about conditions warranting cessation or alteration in exercise program
- Instruct on proper warm-up and cool-down exercises
- Instruct in techniques to avoid injury when exercising
- Instruct in proper breathing techniques to maximize oxygen uptake during physical exercise
- Provide reinforcement schedule to enhance motivation (e.g., increased endurance estimation, weekly weigh-in)
- Monitor response to exercise program
- Provide positive feedback
- Use teach-back to ensure understanding

1st edition 1992; revised 2000, 2004, 2024

Background Evidence:

Bertoncello, C., Sperotto, M., Bellio, S., Pistellato, I., Fonzo, M., Bigolaro, C., Ramon, R., Imoscopi, A., & Baldo, V. (2021). Effectiveness of individually tailored exercise on functional capacity and mobility in nursing home residents. *British Journal of Community Nursing, 26*(3), 144–149.

Simpson, R. J., Campbell, J. P., Gleeson, M., Krüger, K., Nieman, D. C., & Pyne, D. B. (2020). Can exercise affect immune function to increase susceptibility to infection? *Exercise immunology review, 26*, 8–22.

Dunleavy, K., & Slowik, A. K. (2018). *Therapeutic exercise prescription.* Elsevier.

Kisner, C., Colby, L. A., & Bortner, J. (2018). *Therapeutic exercise: Foundations and techniques* (7th ed.). F.A. Davis.

Exercise Promotion: Strength Training   0201

Definition: Facilitating regular resistive muscle training to maintain or increase muscle strength

Activities:

- Conduct pre-exercise health screening to identify risks for exercise using standardized physical activity readiness scales or health history and physical examination
- Obtain approval from health care provider for initiating strength-training program, as appropriate
- Assist to express own beliefs, values, and goals for muscle fitness and health
- Provide information about muscle function, exercise physiology, and consequences of disuse
- Determine muscle fitness levels using exercise field or laboratory tests (e.g., maximum lift, number of lifts per unit of time)
- Provide information about types of muscle resistance that can be used (e.g., free weights, weight machines, rubberized stretch bands, weighted objects, aquatic)
- Assist to set realistic short-term and long-term goals and to take ownership of exercise plan
- Assist to develop ways to minimize effects of procedural, emotional, attitudinal, financial, or comfort barriers to resistance muscle training

- Assist to obtain resources needed to engage in progressive muscle training
- Assist to develop home or work environment that facilitates engaging in exercise plan
- Instruct to wear clothing that prevents overheating or cooling and not restrictive
- Assist to develop strength training program consistent with muscle fitness level, musculoskeletal constraints, functional health goals, exercise equipment resources, personal preference, and social support
- Provide age and health condition-compatible strength training program
- Use standardized scales or instruments for functional assessment prior to strength training
- Specify level of resistance, number of repetitions, number of sets and frequency of "training" sessions according to fitness level and presence or absence of exercise risk factors
- Instruct to rest briefly after each set, as needed
- Specify type and duration of warm-up and cool-down activity (e.g., stretches, walking, calisthenics)
- Demonstrate proper body alignment, posture, and lift form for exercising each major muscle group
- Use reciprocal movements to avoid injury in selected exercises
- Assist to talk through and perform prescribed movement patterns without weights until correct form learned
- Modify movements and methods of applying resistance for chair-bound or bed-bound persons
- Instruct to recognize signs and symptoms of exercise tolerance or intolerance during and after exercise sessions (e.g., light-headedness; dyspnea; more than usual muscle, skeletal, or joint pain; weakness; extreme fatigue; angina; profuse sweating; palpitations)
- Instruct to conduct exercise sessions for specific muscle groups every other day to facilitate muscle adaptation to training
- Instruct to avoid strength training exercise during temperature extremes
- Assist to determine rate of progressively increasing muscle work (i.e., amount of resistance and number of repetitions and sets)
- Provide illustrated, take-home, written instructions for general guidelines and movement form for each muscle group
- Assist to develop record-keeping system that includes amount of resistance, along with number of repetitions and sets to monitor progress in muscle fitness
- Reevaluate muscle fitness levels monthly
- Establish follow-up schedule to maintain motivation, to assist in problem solving, and to monitor progress
- Assist to alter programs or develop other strategies to prevent boredom and dropout
- Collaborate with family and other health professionals (e.g., activity therapist, exercise physiologist, occupational therapist, recreational therapist, physical therapist) in planning, teaching, and monitoring muscle training program)
- Use teach-back to ensure understanding

3rd edition 2000; revised 2024

Background Evidence:

Brigatto, F. A., Braz, T. V., da Costa Zanini, T. C., Germano, M. D., Aoki, M. S., Schoenfeld, B. J., Marchetti, P. H., & Lopes, C. R. (2019). Effect of resistance training frequency on neuromuscular performance and muscle morphology after 8 weeks in trained men. *Journal Of Strength and Conditioning Research, 33*(8), 2104–2116.

Dunleavy, K., & Slowik, A. K. (2018). *Therapeutic exercise prescription.* Elsevier.

Kisner, C., Colby, L. A., & Bortner, J. (2018). *Therapeutic exercise: Foundations and techniques* (7th ed.). F.A. Davis.

Exercise Promotion: Stretching   0202

Definition: Facilitation of systematic, slow-stretch-hold muscle exercises

Activities:

- Obtain health care provider approval for instituting stretching exercise plan, as needed
- Assist to explore beliefs, motivation, and level of neuromusculoskeletal fitness
- Assist to develop realistic short-term and long-term goals, based on current fitness level and lifestyle
- Explain purposes for stretching (e.g., relaxation, muscle and joint prep for more vigorous exercise, flexibility, balance, functional independence)
- Provide information about age-related changes in neuromusculoskeletal structure and effects of disuse
- Provide information about options for sequence-specific stretching activities, place, and time
- Assist to develop schedule for exercise consistent with age, physical status, goals, motivation, and lifestyle
- Assist to develop exercise plan that incorporates orderly sequence of stretching movements, increments in duration of hold phase of movement, and increments in number of repetitions for each slow-stretch-hold movement, consistent with level of musculoskeletal fitness or presence of pathology
- Instruct to begin exercise routine in muscle or joint groups that are least stiff or sore and gradually move to more restricted muscle or joint groups
- Stretch major muscle groups, including hip extensors, knee extensors, ankle plantar flexors, biceps, triceps, shoulders, back extensor, and abdominal muscles
- Instruct to slowly extend muscle or joint to point of full stretch (or reasonable discomfort) and hold for specified time and slowly release stretched muscles
- Instruct to avoid quick, forceful, or bouncing movement to prevent overstimulation of myotatic reflex or excessive muscle soreness
- Instruct in ways to monitor own adherence to schedule and progress toward goals (e.g., increments in joint ROM; awareness of releasing muscle tension; increasing duration of "hold" phase and number of repetitions without pain and fatigue; increases in tolerance to vigorous exercise)
- Provide illustrated, take-home, written instructions for each movement component
- Monitor adherence to technique and schedule at specified follow-up time and place
- Monitor exercise tolerance (i.e., presence of breathlessness, rapid pulse, pallor, lightheadedness, joint or muscle pain, or swelling) during exercise
- Reevaluate exercise plan if symptoms of low exercise tolerance persist after cessation of exercise

- Collaborate with family members in planning, teaching, and monitoring exercise plan
- Use teach-back to ensure understanding

2nd edition 1996; revised 2018, 2024

Background Evidence:

Brigatto, F. A., Braz, T. V., da Costa Zanini, T. C., Germano, M. D., Aoki, M. S., Schoenfeld, B. J., Marchetti, P. H., & Lopes, C. R. (2019). Effect of resistance training frequency on neuromuscular performance and muscle morphology after 8 weeks in trained men. *Journal of Strength and Conditioning Research, 33*(8), 2104–2116.

Dunleavy, K., & Slowik, A. K. (2018). *Therapeutic exercise prescription.* Elsevier.

Kisner, C., Colby, L. A., & Bortner, J. (2018). *Therapeutic exercise: Foundations and techniques* (7th ed.). F.A. Davis.

Thomas, E., Bellafiore, M., Petrigna, L., Paoli, A., Palma, A., & Bianco, A. (2021). Peripheral nerve responses to muscle stretching: A systematic review. *Journal of Sports Science & Medicine, 20*(2), 258–267.

Wanderley, D., Lemos, A., Moretti, E., Barros, M. M. M. B., Valença, M. M., & de Oliveira, D. A. (2019). Efficacy of proprioceptive neuromuscular facilitation compared to other stretching modalities in range of motion gain in young healthy adults: A systematic review. *Physiotherapy Theory & Practice, 35*(2), 109–129.

Exercise Therapy: Ambulation   0221

Definition: Promotion and assistance with walking to maintain or restore autonomic and voluntary body functions during treatment and recovery from illness or injury

Activities:

- Obtain health care provider approval for instituting exercise plan, as needed
- Dress in nonrestrictive clothing
- Assist to use footwear that facilitates walking and prevents injury
- Provide low-height bed, as appropriate
- Monitor gait profile and clinical conditions before starting ambulation therapy
- Encourage to sit in bed, on side of bed, or in chair, as tolerated
- Consult physical therapist about ambulation plan, as needed
- Instruct in availability of assistive devices, if appropriate
- Instruct how to position self throughout transfer process
- Use gait belt to assist with transfer and ambulation, as needed
- Assist to transfer, as needed
- Ensure removal of environmental barriers along route
- Provide cueing cards at head of bed to facilitate learning to transfer
- Apply and provide assistive device (e.g., cane, walker, wheelchair) for ambulation, if unsteady
- Assist with initial ambulation and as needed
- Instruct about safe transfer and ambulation techniques
- Monitor use of crutches, canes, or other walking aids
- Assist to stand and ambulate specified distance and with specified number of staff
- Assist to establish realistic increments in distance for ambulation
- Encourage independent ambulation within safe limits
- Use teach-back to ensure understanding

1st edition 1992; revised 2000, 2024

Background Evidence:

Arrieta, H., Rezola-Pardo, C., Gil, S. M., Irazusta, J., & Rodriguez, L. (2018). Physical training maintains or improves gait ability in long-term nursing home residents: A systematic review of randomized controlled trials. *Maturitas, 109*, 45–52.

Chen, C. H., Lin, C. J., Chen, C. H., & Hu, F. W. (2020). Factors influencing the recovery of walking ability in older adults after hospital discharge. *Hu Li Za Zhi, 67*(2), 65–74. https://doi.org/10.6224/JN.202004_67(2).09. Chinese.

Dunleavy, K., & Slowik, A. K. (2018). *Therapeutic exercise prescription.* Elsevier.

Kisner, C., Colby, L. A., & Bortner, J. (2018). *Therapeutic exercise: Foundations and techniques* (7th ed.). F.A. Davis.

Exercise Therapy: Balance   0222

Definition: Use of specific activities, postures, and movements to maintain, enhance, or restore balance

Activities:

- Determine ability to participate in activities requiring balance
- Obtain health care provider approval for instituting exercise plan, as needed
- Collaborate with physical, occupational, and recreational therapists in developing and executing exercise program, as appropriate
- Evaluate sensory functions (e.g., vision, hearing, proprioception)
- Monitor motor functions through use of standardized instruments, as needed
- Monitor situations that promote loss of balance
- Provide opportunity to discuss factors that influence fear of falling
- Provide safe environment for practice of exercises
- Instruct on importance of exercise therapy in maintaining and improving balance

- Encourage low-intensity exercise programs with opportunities to share feelings
- Instruct on balance exercises such as standing on one leg, bending forward, stretching and resistance, as appropriate
- Assist with ankle strengthening and walking programs
- Provide information on alternative therapies such as yoga and Tai Chi
- Adjust environment to facilitate concentration
- Provide assistive devices (e.g., cane, walker, pillows, pads) to support in performing exercise
- Assist to formulate realistic, measurable goals
- Reinforce or provide instruction about how to position self and perform movements to maintain or improve balance during exercises or activities of daily living
- Assist to participate in stretching exercises when lying, sitting, or standing
- Assist to move to sitting position, stabilize trunk with arms placed at side on bed or chair, and rock trunk over supporting arms
- Assist to stand or sit and rock body from side to side to stimulate balance mechanisms
- Encourage to maintain wide base of support, if needed
- Assist to practice standing with eyes closed for short periods at regular intervals to stimulate proprioception
- Monitor response to balance exercises
- Conduct home assessment to identify existing environmental and behavioral hazards if applicable
- Provide resources for balance, exercise, or falls education programs
- Refer to physical and occupational therapy for vestibular habituation training exercises
- Use teach-back to ensure understanding

1st edition 1992; revised 2008, 2024

Background Evidence:

Azkia, Z., Setiyani, R., & Kusumawardani, L. H. (2021). Balance strategy exercise versus Lower Limb-ROM exercise for reducing the risk of falls among older people. *Nurse Media Journal of Nursing, 11*(1), 114–123.

Bushatsky, A., Alves, L. C., Duarte, Y. A. O., & Lebrão, M. L. (2019). Factors associated with balance disorders of elderly living in the city of São Paulo in 2006: evidence of the Health, Well-being and Aging (SABE) Study. *Revista Brasileira de Epidemiologia, 21*(02), 1–14.

Dunleavy, K., & Slowik, A. K. (2018). *Therapeutic exercise prescription.* Elsevier.

Kisner, C., Colby, L. A., & Bortner, J. (2018). *Therapeutic exercise: Foundations and techniques* (7th ed.). F.A. Davis.

While, A. E. (2020). Falls and older people: Preventative interventions. *British Journal of Community Nursing, 25*(6), 288–292.

Exercise Therapy: Joint Mobility   0224

Definition: Use of active or passive body movement to maintain or restore joint flexibility

Activities:

- Determine limitations of joint movement and effect on function
- Obtain health care provider approval for instituting exercise plan, as needed
- Collaborate with physical therapy in developing and executing exercise program
- Determine motivation level for maintaining or restoring joint movement
- Explain purpose and plan for joint exercises
- Monitor location and nature of discomfort or pain during movement or activity
- Monitor breathing pattern while performing exercise
- Initiate pain control measures before beginning joint exercise
- Dress in nonrestrictive clothing
- Protect from trauma during exercise
- Assist to optimal body position for passive and active joint movement
- Encourage active range-of-motion (ROM) exercises, according to regular, planned schedule
- Perform passive ROM exercises, as indicated
- Instruct how to systematically perform passive, assisted, or active ROM exercises
- Provide written instructions for exercise
- Assist to develop schedule for active ROM exercises
- Encourage to visualize body motion before beginning movement
- Assist with regular rhythmic joint motion within limits of pain, endurance, and joint mobility
- Encourage to sit in bed, on side of bed, or in chair, as tolerated
- Encourage ambulation, if appropriate
- Determine progress toward goal achievement
- Provide positive reinforcement for performing joint exercises
- Use teach-back to ensure understanding

1st edition 1992; revised 2000, 2024

Background Evidence:

Cruz-Díaz, D., Hita-Contreras, F., Martínez-Amat, A., Aibar-Almazán, A., & Kim, K. M. (2020). Ankle-joint self-mobilization and crossfit training in patients with chronic ankle instability: a randomized controlled trial. *Journal of Athletic Training, 55*(2), 159–168.

Ersoy, U., Kocak, U. Z., Unuvar, E., & Unver, B. (2019). The acute effect of talocrural joint mobilization on dorsiflexor muscle strength in healthy individuals: a randomized controlled single blind study. *Journal of Sport Rehabilitation, 28*(6), 601–605.

Racinais, S., Cocking, S., & Périard, J. D. (2017). Sports and environmental temperature: from warming-up to heating-up. *Temperature (Austin), 4*(3), 227–257.

Dunleavy, K., & Slowik, A. K. (2018). *Therapeutic exercise prescription.* Elsevier.

Kisner, C., Colby, L. A., & Bortner, J. (2018). *Therapeutic exercise: Foundations and technique* (7th ed.). F.A. Davis.

E

Exercise Therapy: Muscle Control   0226

Definition: Use of specific activity or exercise protocols to enhance or restore muscle control

Activities:

- Determine readiness to engage in activity or exercise protocol
- Obtain health care provider approval for instituting exercise plan, as needed
- Collaborate with physical, occupational, and recreational therapists in developing and executing exercise program, as appropriate
- Consult physical therapy to determine optimal position during exercise and number of repetitions for each movement pattern
- Evaluate sensory functions (e.g., vision, hearing, proprioception)
- Explain rationale for type of exercise and protocol
- Provide privacy for exercising, if desired
- Adjust lighting, room temperature, and noise level to enhance concentration for exercise activity
- Sequence daily care activities to enhance effects of specific exercise therapy
- Initiate pain control measures before beginning exercise or activity
- Dress in nonrestrictive clothing
- Assist to maintain trunk and proximal joint stability during motor activity
- Apply splints to achieve stability of proximal joints involved with fine motor skills, as prescribed
- Reevaluate need for assistive devices at regular intervals in collaboration with physical therapist, occupational therapist, or respiratory therapist
- Assist to sitting or standing position for exercise protocol, as appropriate
- Reinforce instructions about proper performance of exercises to minimize injury and maximize effectiveness
- Identify any misperceptions of body image
- Reorient to body awareness and movement functions of body
- Encourage to visually scan affected side of body when performing ADLs or exercises, if indicated
- Provide step-by-step cueing for each motor activity during exercise or ADLs
- Instruct to recite each movement as performed
- Use visual aids to facilitate learning methods to perform ADLs or exercise movements, as appropriate
- Provide restful environment after periods of exercise
- Assist to develop exercise protocol for strength, endurance, and flexibility
- Assist to formulate realistic, measurable goals
- Use motor activities that require attention to and use of both sides of body
- Incorporate ADLs into exercise protocol, if appropriate
- Encourage to practice exercises independently, as indicated
- Encourage to use warm-up and cool-down activities before and after exercise protocol
- Use tactile (e.g., tapping) stimuli to minimize muscle spasm
- Assist to prepare and maintain progress graph or chart for adherence with exercise protocol
- Monitor emotional, cardiovascular, and functional responses to exercise protocol
- Monitor self-exercise for correct performance
- Evaluate progress toward enhancement and restoration of body movement and function
- Provide positive reinforcement for efforts in exercise and physical activity
- Collaborate with home caregivers regarding exercise protocol and ADLs
- Assist to make prescribed revisions in home exercise plan, as indicated
- Use teach-back to ensure understanding

1st edition 1992; revised 2000, 2024

Background Evidence:

Cruz, A. G., de Oliveira Parola, V., Leiria Neves, H., Batista Cardoso, D. F., Alves Bernardes, R., & Diniz Parreira, P. (2021). Exercise programs for work-related musculoskeletal pain: A scoping review protocol. *Revista de Enfermagem Referência*, V(6), 1–7.

Dunleavy, K., & Slowik, A. K. (2018). *Therapeutic exercise prescription*. Elsevier.

Dzubur, E. K., & Poronsky, C. B. (2018). Exercise therapy benefits for Heart Failure. *The Journal for Nurse Practitioners*, 14(5), 396–401. https://doi.org/10.1016/j.nurpra.2018.01.019

Kerr, L., Jewell, V. D., & Jensen, L. (2020). Stretching and splinting interventions for poststroke spasticity, hand function, and functional tasks: A systematic review. *AJOT: American Journal of Occupational Therapy*, 74(5), 7405205050p1–7405205050p15.

Kisner, C., Colby, L. A., & Bortner, J. (2018). *Therapeutic exercise: Foundations and techniques* (7th ed.). F.A. Davis.

Extracorporeal Membrane Oxygenation Therapy   4115

Definition: Providing oxygenation and removing carbon dioxide from blood using an artificial lung machine

Activities:

- Determine hemodynamic status using multiple parameters to evaluate clinical status and appropriateness for extracorporeal membrane oxygenation therapy (ECMO) therapy (e.g., blood pressure, heart rate, pulses, jugular venous pressure, central venous pressure, right and left atrial and ventricular pressures, pulmonary artery pressure), as appropriate
- Draw pretreatment blood sample and review blood chemistries (e.g., blood urea nitrogen, serum creatinine, serum Na, K, PO_4 levels)
- Record baseline vital signs (e.g., temperature, pulse, respirations, blood pressure, weight)
- Explain ECMO procedure and obtain informed consent
- Determine type of ECMO needed (i.e., using a vein and an artery [VA ECMO] for problems with both heart and lungs, or

E

using one or more veins near heart [VV ECMO] for problems only in lungs)

- Check equipment and solutions, according to protocol
- Assist as needed with initiation of ECMO cannulation, assuring time out for procedure and presence of properly trained staff (e.g., respiratory therapist, surgical team, nurses)
- Ensure proper sedation, paralysis, anticoagulation and ventilation, as prescribed
- Obtain post-cannulation radiology studies (e.g., anterior posterior chest or abdomen or both)
- Initiate ECMO, according to protocol, increasing blood flow until respiratory and hemodynamic targets are met
- Maintain blood flow at set rate determined by achievement of respiratory and hemodynamic targets, while providing continuous venous oximetry
- Maintain anticoagulation with continuous IV infusion of unfractionated heparin or direct thrombin inhibitor to achieve an activated clotting time (ACT) of 180 to 210 seconds
- Reduce ACT target if bleeding occurs, as prescribed
- Monitor platelet counts and maintain level above 50,000/mL, per protocol
- Monitor hemoglobin and maintain level within normal range
- Adjust ventilator settings to prevent barotrauma, ventilator-induced lung injury, and oxygen toxicity, as prescribed
- Monitor urine output and laboratory values to determine adequacy of kidney function
- Monitor for signs of infection and poor perfusion such as increased lactic acid level, metabolic acidosis, decreased urine output, and increased liver enzymes
- Monitor lower limbs for signs of ischemia, coolness, or mottling of feet
- Conduct daily wakeup and hourly pupil checks to monitor neurological status
- Practice diligent repositioning to prevent skin breakdown
- Provide for care with two-member team (e.g., ECMO specialist, nurse)
- Ensure team includes ECMO specialist nurse providing 24-hour, 7-day ECMO care and supported by perfusionist backup for technical aspects of circuit management
- Ensure that ECMO order sets are available for machine priming, daily parameters, circuit settings, parameters for blood transfusions and orders for radiology (e.g., echocardiogram for symptoms)

- Ensure instructions available for all perfusionists or nurses in charge of ECMO machine
- Monitor daily and routine laboratory values per protocol
- Monitor anticoagulation status and adjust settings per protocol and order sets
- Ensure instructions available to alert ECMO health care providers, as needed
- Anchor connections and tubing securely
- Check person-circuit interactions per protocols and order sets (e.g., flow rate, pressure, temperature, pH level, conductivity, clots, air detector, negative pressure for ultrafiltration, blood sensor) to ensure safety
- Manage clinical needs through continuous surveillance and troubleshooting to prevent and manage circuit emergencies
- Monitor blood pressure, pulse, respirations, temperature, and response continuously during ECMO therapy
- Ensure interprofessional team is involved in plan of care (e.g., physical therapy, occupational therapy, nutritionist, case management)
- Discontinue ECMO, according to protocol
- Compare post-ECMO vitals and blood chemistries to pre-ECMO values
- Document tolerance of procedure and achievement of outcomes, as appropriate

8th edition 2024

Background Evidence:

Calhoun, A. (2018). ECMO: Nursing care of adult patients on ECMO. *Critical Care Nursing Quarterly, 41*(4), 394–398. https://doi.org/10.1097/CNQ.0000000000000226

McCallister, D., Pilon, L., Forrester, J., Alsaleem, S., Kotaru, C., Hanna, J., Hickey, G., Roberts, R., Douglass, E., Libby, M., & Firstenberg, M. S. (2019). Clinical and administrative steps to the ECMO program development. *Advances in Extracorporeal Membrane Oxygenation, vol. 3.* https://doi.org/10.5772/intechopen.84838

Naddour, M., Kalani, M., Ashraf, O., Patel, K., Bajwa, O., & Cheema, T. (2019). Extracorporeal membrane oxygenation in ARDS. *Critical Care Nursing Quarterly, 42*(4), 400–410. https://doi.org/10.1097/CNQ.0000000000000280

O'Connor, N., & Smith, J. (2018). An innovative ECMO staffing model to reduce harm. *The Journal of Perinatal & Neonatal Nursing, 32*(3), 204–205. https://doi.org/10.1097/jpn.0000000000000355

Eye Care   1650

Definition: Prevention or minimization of threats to eye or visual integrity

Activities:
- Explain procedures regardless of level of consciousness
- Monitor for redness, exudate, or ulceration
- Instruct not to touch eye
- Monitor corneal reflex and determine if pupils are equal, round, and reactive to light and accommodation (e.g., PERRLA)
- Observe symmetry of movement of eyes
- Place in supine position prior to any procedures
- Use clean warm washcloth or cotton balls moistened with warm water or saline to cleanse
- Remove contact lenses, as appropriate
- Apply eye shield and alternate as needed for vision, as appropriate
- Apply lubricating eye drops or ointments, as appropriate

- Tape eyelids shut, as appropriate
- Apply moisture chamber, as appropriate
- Keep movement from inner aspect or nasal area to outer aspect when cleansing eye
- Start with cleanest eye first when doing procedures to both eyes
- Ensure new separate swab, cotton ball, or corner of washcloth used for each eye
- Avoid sharing swabs or shields between eyes
- Perform eye care every 4 hours or as prescribed
- Adjust eye care frequency when receiving oxygen therapies that dry eyes
- Instruct on wearing sunglasses and hats to avoid or reduce ultraviolet sun exposure
- Instruct on proper eye care, as indicated

- Instruct on regular eye examinations (i.e., age 65 and older need comprehensive dilated eye exams every year)
- Document care and eye condition
- Use teach-back to ensure understanding

1st edition 1992; revised 2000, 2024

Background Evidence:

Fowler, S. B. (2020). Climate change and eye health. *Insight: The Journal of the American Society of Ophthalmic Registered Nurses, 45*(3), 31–41.

Perry, A., Potter, P. A., Ostendorf, W. R., & LaPlante, N. (2018). Care of the eye and ear. In *Clinical nursing skills and techniques* (pp. 485–491) (9th ed.). Mosby.

Ramke, J., Zwi, A. B., Silva, J. C., Nyawira, M., Rono, H., Gichangi, M., Qureshi, M. B., & Gilbert, C. E. (2018). Evidence for national universal eye health plans. *Bulletin of the World Health Organization, 96*(10), 695–704.

Watkinson, S., Williamson, S., & Seewoodhary, R. (2020). Coronavirus and ocular involvement: Promoting safe eye care. *Insight: The Journal of the American Society of Ophthalmic Registered Nurses, 45*(4), 29–33.

E

Eye Irrigation 1655

Definition: Flushing the eye to administer medications or remove particles or harmful chemicals

Activities:

- Check accuracy and completeness of each medication administration record (MAR) prior to giving any medications, if indicated
- Follow six rights of medication administration if medication administered
- Identify using at least two identifiers (e.g., name, birthdate)
- Note medical history and allergies, if indicated
- Determine knowledge of medication and understanding of method of administration or procedure
- Perform necessary pre-medication or pre-procedure assessments (e.g., blood pressure, pulse)
- Position lying on side with affected eye down
- Place absorbent pads under head, neck, and shoulders
- Place basin next to eye to catch drainage
- Expose lower conjunctival sac
- Prepare to expose upper and lower lids if irrigating in stages (i.e., first hold lower lid down, then hold upper lid up)
- Use slight pressure on bony prominences of eye orbits to keep eyelids in place and prevent reflexive blinking
- Hold eye irrigator 2.5 cm (1 inch) above eye to avoid excessive pressure while irrigating
- Irrigate eye directing solution onto conjunctival area from inner canthus to outer canthus
- Avoid irrigating toward nasal lacrimal duct
- Irrigate until solution leaving eye is clear, or as ordered for medication
- Instruct to close and move eye periodically during irrigation to enhance secretion or debris removal
- Clean and dry eye as needed when done
- Wipe eyelids from inner to outer canthus when cleansing
- Apply eye pad as indicated
- Monitor response to irrigation as indicated
- Document medication administration and responsiveness according to agency protocol

8th edition 2024

Background Evidence:

Berman, A., Snyder, S. J., & Frandsen, G. (2018). Medications: *Kozier and Erb's Fundamentals of nursing: Concepts, process and practice* (pp. 814–815) (10th ed.). Pearson. 823–824.

Kirby, N. (2021). Medication administration. In R. F. Craven, C. J. Hirnle, & C. J. Henshaw, C. J. (Eds.), *Fundamentals of nursing: Human health and function* (8th ed., pp. 410–471). Wolters-Kluwer.

Potter, P. A., Ostendorf, W. R., & LaPlante, N. (2018). Administering ophthalmic medications: In *Clinical nursing skills and techniques* (pp. 541–547) (9th ed.). Mosby.

Sanoski, C. A., & Vallerand, A. H. (2021). *Davis's drug guide for nurses* (17th ed.). F.A. Davis.

Fall Prevention   6490

Definition: Instituting precautions for persons at risk for falling

Activities:
- Identify cognitive or physical deficits that may increase risk of falling
- Identify behaviors and factors that affect risk of falls
- Review history of falls
- Identify characteristics of environment that increase potential for falls (e.g., slippery floors, rugs, open stairways)
- Institute fall safety guideline (e.g., signage, colored clothing, bracelet), per facility policy
- Assist with toileting at frequent, scheduled intervals
- Evaluate gait, balance, and fatigue level with ambulation
- Consult physical therapy as needed
- Assist unsteady individual with ambulation
- Encourage use of cane, walker, or gait belt as appropriate
- Instruct on use of cane, walker, or gait belt as appropriate
- Lock wheels of wheelchair, bed, or gurney during transfer
- Place articles within easy reach
- Instruct to call for assistance with movement, as appropriate
- Post signs to remind to call for help when getting out of bed, as appropriate
- Monitor ability to transfer from bed to chair and vice versa
- Provide elevated toilet seat for easy transfer, as needed
- Provide chairs of proper height with backrests and armrests for easy transfer
- Provide bed mattress with firm edges for easy transfer
- Place mechanical bed in lowest position
- Provide sleeping surface close to floor, as needed
- Use bed and chair alarms as appropriate
- Mark doorway thresholds and edges of steps, as needed
- Remove low-lying furniture (e.g., footstools, tables) and clutter on floor surface
- Provide adequate lighting for increased visibility
- Provide visible handrails and grab bars
- Provide nonslip surfaces in bathtub, shower, and floor surfaces
- Provide sturdy, nonslip step stools to facilitate easy reaches
- Provide heavy furniture that will not tip if used for support
- Avoid unnecessary rearrangement of physical environment
- Ensure shoes fit properly, fasten securely, and have non-skid soles
- Instruct to wear prescription glasses, as appropriate
- Educate about risk factors that contribute to falls and ways to decrease risks
- Suggest home adaptations to increase safety
- Instruct on importance of handrails for stairs, bathrooms, and walkways
- Assist in identifying and modifying hazards in home
- Instruct to avoid ice and other slippery outdoor surfaces
- Develop ways to participate safely in leisure activities
- Institute routine physical exercise program that includes walking
- Collaborate with interprofessional team to minimize side effects of medications that contribute to falling (e.g., orthostatic hypotension, unsteady gait)
- Provide close supervision and safety devices
- Institute fall safety agreement, as appropriate
- Maintain crib side rails in elevated position when caregiver not present, as appropriate
- Fasten latches securely on access panel of incubator when leaving bedside of infant in incubator
- Use teach-back to ensure understanding

1st edition 1992; revised 2000, 2004, 2024

Background Evidence:

Bargmann, A. L., & Brundrett, S. M. (2020). Implementation of a multicomponent fall prevention program: Contracting with patients for fall safety. *Military Medicine, 185*(Suppl. 2), 28–34. https://doi.org/10.1093/milmed/usz411

Garcia, A., Bjarnadottir, R. I., Keenan, G. M., & Macieira, T. R. (2021). Nurses' perceptions of recommended fall prevention strategies. *Journal of Nursing Care Quality, Publish Ahead of Print.* https://doi.org/10.1097/NCQ.0000000000000605

Gray-Miceli, D., Ratcliffe, S. J., Thomasson, A., Quigley, P., Li, K., & Craelius, W. (2020). Clinical risk factors for orthostatic hypotension: Results among elderly fallers in long-term care. *Journal of Patient Safety, 16*(3), e143–e147. https://doi.org/10.1097/PTS.0000000000000274

Kim, E.-J., Kim, G.-M., & Lim, J.-Y. (2021). A systematic review and meta-analysis of fall prevention programs for pediatric inpatients. *International Journal of Environmental Research and Public Health, 18*(11). https://doi.org/10.3390/ijerph18115853

Racey, M., Markle-Reid, M., Fitzpatrick-Lewis, D., Ali, M. U., Gagne, H., Hunter, S., Ploeg, J., Sztramko, R., Harrison, L., Lewis, R., Jovkovic, M., & Sherifali, D. (2021). Fall prevention in community-dwelling adults with mild to moderate cognitive impairment: A systematic review and meta-analysis. *BMC Geriatrics, 21*(1). https://doi.org/10.1186/s12877-021-02641-9

Usmani, S., Saboor, A., Haris, M., Khan, M. A., & Park, H. (2021). Latest research trends in fall detection and prevention using machine learning: A systematic review. *Sensors (Basel, Switzerland), 21*(15). https://doi.org/10.3390/s21155134

Wisler, H., Prado, G., & Cohn, T. (2021). Reducing unwitnessed falls on a medical-surgical unit. *MEDSURG Nursing, 30*(3), 208–211.

Zubkoff, L., Neily, J., Quigley, P., Delanko, V., Young-Xu, Y., Boar, S., & Mills, P. (2018). Preventing falls and fall-related injuries in state veterans homes. *Journal of Nursing Care Quality, 33*(4), 334–340. https://doi.org/10.1097/NCQ.0000000000000309

F

Family Integrity Promotion   7100

Definition: Promotion of family cohesion and unity

Activities:
- Be a listener for the family members
- Establish trusting relationship with family members
- Determine family understanding of condition
- Determine family feelings regarding their situation
- Assist family to resolve unrealistic feelings of guilt or responsibility, as warranted
- Determine typical family relationships for each family

- Monitor current family relationships
- Identify typical family coping mechanisms
- Identify conflicting priorities among family members
- Assist family with conflict resolution
- Counsel family members on additional effective coping skills for their own use
- Respect privacy of individual family members
- Provide for family privacy
- Tell family members that it is safe and acceptable to use typical expressions of affection when in a hospital setting
- Facilitate a tone of togetherness within/among the family
- Provide family members with information about the patient's condition regularly, according to patient preference
- Collaborate with family in problem solving and decision making
- Encourage family to maintain positive relationships
- Facilitate open communication among family members
- Provide for care of patient by family members, as appropriate
- Facilitate family visitation

- Refer family to support group of other families dealing with similar problems
- Refer for family therapy, as indicated

1st edition 1992; revised 2008

Background Evidence:

Keefe, M. R., Barbaos, G. A., Froese-Fretz, A., Kotzer, A. M., & Lobo, M. (2005). An intervention program for families with irritable infants. *MCN: American Journal of Maternal/Child Nursing, 30*(4), 230–236.

McBride, K. L., White, C. L., Sourial, R., & Mayo, N. (2004). Postdischarge nursing interventions for stroke survivors and their families. *Journal of Advanced Nursing, 47*(2), 192–200.

Mu, P., Kuo, H., & Chang, K. (2005). Boundary ambiguity, coping patterns, and depression in mothers caring for children with epilepsy in Taiwan. *International Journal of Nursing Studies, 42*(3), 273–282.

Family Integrity Promotion: Childbearing Family   7104

Definition: Facilitation of the growth of individuals or families who are adding an infant to the family unit

Activities:
- Establish trusting relationship with parent(s)
- Listen to family's concerns, feelings, and questions
- Respect and support family's cultural value system
- Identify family interaction patterns
- Assist family in identifying strengths and weaknesses
- Identify normal family coping mechanisms
- Assist family in developing adaptive coping mechanisms to deal with the transition to parenthood
- Monitor parent's adaptation to parenthood
- Prepare parent(s) for expected role changes involved in becoming a parent
- Educate parent(s) about potential role conflict and role overload
- Promote self-efficacy in carrying out parental role
- Prepare parent(s) for responsibilities of parenthood
- Encourage parents to articulate their values, beliefs, and expectations regarding parenthood
- Assist parents in having realistic role expectations about parenthood
- Assist parents in dealing with suggestions, criticisms, and concerns about parental role expectations and performance from others (e.g., parents, grandparents, co-workers, friends)
- Educate parents about the effects of sleep deprivation on family functioning
- Reinforce positive parenting behaviors
- Assist parents in gaining skills needed to perform tasks appropriate to family developmental stage
- Assist parents in balancing work, parental, and marital roles
- Assist mother in making plans for returning to work, as appropriate
- Provide parent(s) an opportunity to express their feelings about parenthood
- Identify effect of newborn on family dynamics and equilibrium

- Encourage parents to spend time together as a couple to maintain marital satisfaction
- Encourage parents to discuss household maintenance role responsibilities
- Encourage verbalization of feelings, perceptions, and concerns about the birth experience
- Explain causes and manifestations of postpartum depression
- Encourage parent(s) to maintain individual hobbies or outside interests
- Encourage family to attend sibling preparation classes, as appropriate
- Provide information about sibling preparation, as appropriate
- Give family information on sibling rivalry, as appropriate
- Discuss reaction of sibling(s) to newborn, as appropriate
- Assist family in identifying support systems
- Encourage family to use support systems, as appropriate
- Assist family in developing new support networks, as appropriate
- Offer to be an advocate for the family

1st edition 1992; revised 2008

Background Evidence:

Cowan, C. P., & Cowan, P. A. (1995). Interventions to ease the transition to parenthood: Why they are needed and what they can do. *Family Relations, 44*(4), 412–423.

Newman, B. M. (2000). The challenges of parenting infants and young children. In P. C. McKenry & S. J. Price (Eds.), *Families & change: Coping with stressful events and transitions* (2nd ed., pp. 43–70). Sage.

Swartz, M. K., & Knafl, K. (2006). Enhancement of family support systems. In M. Craft-Rosenberg & M. J. Krajicek (Eds.), *Nursing excellence for children & families* (pp. 77–95). Springer.

F

Family Involvement Promotion 7110

Definition: Facilitating participation of family members in the emotional and physical care of the patient

Activities:

- Establish a personal relationship with the patient and family members who will be involved in care
- Identify family members' capabilities for involvement in care of the patient
- Create a culture of flexibility for the family
- Determine physical, emotional, and educational resources of primary caregiver
- Identify patient's self-care deficits
- Identify family members' preferences for involvement with patient
- Identify family members' expectations for the patient
- Anticipate and identify family needs
- Encourage the family members and the patient to assist in the development of a plan of care, including expected outcomes, and implementation of the plan of care
- Encourage the family members and patient to be assertive in interactions with health care professionals
- Monitor family structure and roles
- Monitor involvement in patient's care by family members
- Encourage care by family members during hospitalization or care in a long-term care facility
- Provide crucial information to family members about the patient in accordance with patient preference
- Facilitate understanding of the medical aspects of the patient's condition for family members
- Provide the support needed for the family to make informed decisions
- Identify family members' perception of the situation, precipitating events, patient's feelings, and patients' behaviors
- Identify other situational stressors for family members
- Identify individual family members' physical symptoms related to stress (e.g., tearfulness, nausea, vomiting, distractibility)
- Determine level of patient dependence on family members for age or illness, as appropriate
- Encourage focus on any positive aspects of the patient's situation
- Identify and respect coping mechanisms used by family members
- Identify with family members the patient's coping difficulties
- Identify with family members the patient's strengths and abilities with family
- Inform family members of factors that may improve patient's condition
- Encourage family members to keep or maintain family relationships, as appropriate
- Discuss options for type of home care, such as group living, residential care, or respite care, as appropriate
- Facilitate management of the medical aspects of illness by family members

1st edition 1992; revised 2000, 2004, 2008

Background Evidence:

Gosline, M. B. (2003). Client participation to enhance socialization for frail elders. *Geriatric Nursing, 24*(5), 286–289.

Powaski, K. M. (2006). Nursing interventions in pediatric palliative care. *Child and Adolescent Psychiatric Clinics of North America, 15*(3), 717–737.

Schumacher, K., Koresawa, S., West, C., Hawkins, C., Johnson, C., Wais, E., Dodd, M., Paul, S. M., Tripathy, D., Koo, P., & Miaskowski, C. (2002). Putting cancer pain management regimens into practice at home. *Journal of Pain Symptom Management, 23*(5), 369–382.

Family Mobilization 7120

Definition: Utilization of family strengths to influence patient's health in a positive direction

Activities:

- Be a listener for family members
- Establish trusting relationships with family members
- View family members as potential experts in the care of the patient
- Identify strengths and resources within the family, in family members, and in their support system and community
- Determine the readiness and ability of family members to learn
- Provide information frequently to the family to assist them in identifying the patient's limitations, progress, and implications for care
- Foster mutual decision making with family members related to the patient's care plan
- Teach home caregivers about the patient's therapy, as appropriate
- Explain to family members the need for continuing of professional health care, as appropriate
- Collaborate with family members in planning and implementing patient therapies and lifestyle changes
- Support family activities in promoting patient health or management of condition, when appropriate
- Assist family members to identify health services and community resources that can be used to enhance the health status of the patient
- Monitor the current family situation
- Refer family members to support groups, as appropriate
- Determine expected patient outcome achievement systematically

1st edition 1992; revised 2004, 2008

Background Evidence:

Deatrick, J. A. (2006). Family partnerships in nursing care. In M. Craft-Rosenberg & M. Krajicek (Eds.), *Nursing excellence for children & families* (pp. 41–58). Springer.

Gerdner, L. A., Buckwalter, K. C., & Reed, D. (2002). Impact of a psychoeducational intervention of caregiver response to behavioral problems. *Nursing Research, 51*(6), 363–374.

Sylvain, H., & Talbot, L. R. (2002). Synergy towards health: A nursing intervention model for women living with fibromyalgia, and their spouses. *Journal of Advanced Nursing, 38*(3), 264–273.

Family Planning: Contraception   6784

Definition: Assisting patient in determining and providing method of pregnancy prevention

Activities:
- Appraise patient's knowledge and understanding of contraceptive choices
- Instruct patient on physiology of human reproduction, including both female and male reproductive systems, as needed
- Conduct relevant physical examination if indicated by patient history
- Determine ability and motivation for using a method
- Determine level of commitment to consistently use method
- Discuss religious, cultural, developmental, socioeconomical, and individual considerations pertaining to contraceptive choice
- Discuss methods of contraception (e.g., medication-free, barrier, hormonal, intrauterine device, and sterilization), including effectiveness, side effects, contraindications, and signs and symptoms that warrant reporting to a health care professional
- Assist adolescents to obtain contraceptive information in a confidential manner
- Assist female patient to determine ovulation through basal body temperature, changes in vaginal secretions, and other physiological indicators
- Provide contraception to patient, if indicated
- Discuss emergency contraception, as needed
- Provide emergency contraception (e.g., morning after pill, copper intrauterine device), as appropriate
- Instruct on safe sex activities, as indicated
- Refer patient to other health care professional or community resources (e.g., social worker and home health care professional), as needed
- Determine financial resources for contraception and refer, as appropriate

1st edition 1992; revised 2013

Background Evidence:

Cheng, L., Gulmezoglu, A., Piaggio, G., Ezcurra, E., & Van Look, P. (2008). Interventions for emergency contraception. *Cochrane Database of Systematic Reviews*, (2). https://doi.org/1002/14651858.CD001324.pub3

Lopez, L., Tolley, E., Grimes, D., & Chen-Mok, M. (2009). Theory-based interventions for contraception. *Cochrane Database of Systematic Reviews*, (1). https://doi.org/1002/14651858.CD007249.pub2

Oringanje, C., Meremikwu, M. M., Eko, H., Esu, E., Meremikwu, A., & Ehiri, J. E. (2009). Interventions for preventing unintended pregnancies among adolescents. *Cochrane Database of Systematic Reviews*, (4). https://doi.org/1002/14651858.CD005215.pub2

U.S. Department of Health and Human Services. (2000). Healthy People 2010: Understanding and improving health (2nd ed.).

Ward, S. L., & Hisley, S. M. (2009). *Maternal-child nursing care: Optimizing outcomes for mothers, children, & families*. F.A. Davis.

Family Planning: Infertility   6786

Definition: Management, education, and support of the patient and significant other undergoing evaluation and treatment for infertility

Activities:
- Support couple through infertility history and evaluation, acknowledging stress often experienced in obtaining detailed history and during lengthy evaluation and treatment process
- Explain types of infertility (e.g., primary or secondary, male or female)
- Explain female reproductive cycle to patient, as needed
- Assist female patient to determine ovulation through basal body temperature, changes in vaginal secretions, midluteal phase serum progesterone level, and other physiological indicators
- Prepare patient physically and psychologically for gynecological examination
- Explain purpose of procedure and sensations the patient might experience during the procedure
- Assist male partner to complete semen analysis and medical workup
- Determine couple's understanding of test results and recommended therapy
- Determine extent to which partners are able and willing to participate in complex infertility treatment
- Assist with expressions of grief and disappointment and feelings of failure
- Encourage expressions of feelings about sexuality, self-image, and self-esteem
- Assist individuals to redefine concepts of success and failure, as needed
- Refer to support group for infertile couples, as appropriate
- Assist with problem solving to help couple evaluate alternatives to biologic parenthood
- Determine effect of infertility on couple's relationship

1st edition 1992; revised 1996, 2018

Background Evidence:

Devine, K. (2003). Caring for the infertile woman. *MCN: The American Journal of Maternal/Child Nursing*, 28(2), 100–105.

Evaluation of the infertile couple Hoffman, B., Schorge, J., Schaffer, J., Halvorson, L., Bradshaw, K., & Cunningham, F. (Eds.), (2012). *Williams gynecology* (2nd ed., pp. 506–528). McGraw-Hill.

Lobo, R. (2012). Infertility. In G. Lentz, R. Lobo, D. Gershenson, & V. Katz (Eds.), *Comprehensive gynecology* (6th ed. pp. 869–895). Elsevier Mosby.

Onwere, C., & Vakharia, H. (2014). *Crash course: Obstetrics and gynaecology* (3rd ed.). Edinburgh, Scotland: Mosby Elsevier.

Family Planning: Unplanned Pregnancy   6788

Definition: Facilitation of decision-making regarding pregnancy outcome

Activities:

- Determine whether patient has made a choice about outcome of pregnancy
- Discuss with patient and significant other (if involved) the options regarding outcomes of pregnancy, including termination of pregnancy, keeping the infant, or relinquishing the infant for adoption
- Discuss factors related to unplanned pregnancy (e.g., multiple partners, substance abuse, intimate partner violence, likelihood of sexually transmitted disease)
- Assist patient in identifying support system
- Encourage patient to involve support system during decision-making process
- Support patient and significant other in decision about pregnancy outcome
- Clarify any misinformation about contraceptive use
- Refer to community agencies that have services that will support patient in acting on decision regarding pregnancy outcome, as well as other health concerns (e.g., sexually transmitted diseases, substance abuse, intimate partner violence)

1st edition 1992; revised 1996, 2018

Background Evidence:

Barry, M. (2011). Preconception care at the edges of the reproductive life-span. *Nursing for Women's Health, 15*(1), 68–74.

Jensen, J., & Mishell, D., Jr. (2012). Family planning. In G. Lentz, R. Lobo, D. Gershenson, & V. Katz (Eds.), *Comprehensive gynecology* (6th ed., pp. 215–272). Elsevier Mosby.

Kartoz, C. R. (2004). New options for teen pregnancy prevention. The *American Journal of Maternal Child Nursing, 29*(1), 30–35.

Simmonds, K., & Likis, F. (2011). Caring for women with unintended pregnancies. *Journal of Obstetric, Gynecologic, and Neonatal Nursing, 40*(6), 794–807.

Taylor, D., & James, E. (2011). An evidence-based guideline for unintended pregnancy prevention. *Journal of Obstetric, Gynecologic and Neonatal Nursing, 40*(6), 782–793.

Family Presence Facilitation   7170

Definition: Facilitation of the family's presence in support of an individual undergoing resuscitation and invasive procedures

Activities:

- Obtain consensus from interprofessional team for family's presence and timing of family's presence
- Appraise situation to determine when appropriate for family presence
- Minimize risk of physical presence by following appropriate infection control guidelines
- Communicate proactively so families are aware of any restrictions
- Provide specifically trained team members (e.g., chaplain, nurse, social worker) to be designated for family, who can handle difficult and exceptional family situations
- Clearly state compassionate exceptions to infection control or other restrictions
- Use shared decision-making approach to communicate risks and benefits in cases where family can be physically present
- Invite family presence during resuscitation, as appropriate
- Introduce self and other members of interprofessional team to family and person
- Determine suitability of physical location for family presence
- Ensure family has been informed about what to expect (e.g., what they will see, hear, smell, condition of person, equipment used)
- Inform family to report if they feel faint or ill
- Inform family of behavior expectations and limits
- Ensure family members are not left unattended
- Apprise interprofessional team of family's emotional reaction to person's condition, as appropriate
- Obtain information concerning person's status, response to treatment, identified needs
- Provide timely information and explanations to family of person's status, response to treatment and identified needs, in understandable terms
- Enlist family to assist in assuring other members abide by established safety protocols, if indicated
- Use person's name when speaking to family
- Determine person's and family's emotional, physical, psychosocial, and spiritual support needs and initiate measures to meet those needs, as needed
- Determine psychological burden of prognosis for family
- Foster realistic hope, as appropriate
- Advocate for family, as needed
- Accompany family to and from treatment or resuscitation area and announce their presence to treatment staff each time family enters treatment area
- Escort family from bedside if requested by staff providing direct care
- Provide opportunity for family to ask questions, to see, touch, or speak to person before transfers
- Assist person or family members in making telephone calls, as needed
- Enhance discharge education and follow-up to support successful transitions of care (e.g., hospice)
- Provide comfort measures and support, including appropriate referrals, as needed
- Participate in evaluation of staff emotional needs
- Assist in identifying need for critical incident stress debriefing and individual defusing of events

F

- Participate in, initiate, or coordinate family bereavement follow-up at established intervals, as appropriate

4th edition 2004; revised 2024

Background Evidence:

Afzali-Rubin, M., Svensson, T. L. G., Herling, S. F., Wirenfeldt-Klausen, T., Jabre, P., & Møller, A. M. (2020). Family presence during resuscitation. *Cochrane Database of Systematic Reviews*, (5). https://doi.org/10.1002/14651858.CD013619

Emergency Nurses Association. (2018). *Emergency Nurses Association position statement: Resuscitative decisions in the emergency care setting.*

Frampton, S., Agrawal, S., & Guastello, S. (2020). Guidelines for family presence policies during the COVID-19 Pandemic. *JAMA Health Forum, 1*(7), e200807. https://doi.org/10.1001/jamahealthforum.2020.0807

Powers, K., & Reeve, C. L. (2020). Family presence during resuscitation: Medical-surgical nurses' perceptions, self-confidence, and use of invitations. *American Journal of Nursing, 120*(11), 28–38.

Powers, K. A. (2018). Family presence during resuscitation: The education needs of critical care nurses. *Dimensions of Critical Care Nursing, 37*(4), 210–216. https://doi.org/10.1097/DCC.0000000000000304

Family Process Maintenance · 7130

F

Definition: Minimization of family process disruption effects

Activities:

- Determine typical family processes
- Determine disruption in typical family processes
- Identify effects of role changes on family process
- Encourage continued contact with family members, as appropriate
- Keep opportunities for visiting flexible to meet needs of family members and patient
- Discuss strategies for normalizing family life with family members
- Assist family members to implement normalizing strategies for their situation
- Discuss existing social support mechanisms for the family
- Assist family members to use existing support mechanisms
- Minimize family routine disruption by facilitating family routines and rituals, such as private meals together or family discussions for communication and decision-making
- Provide mechanisms for family members staying to communicate with other family members (e.g., telephones, e-mail messages, and pictures, tape recordings, photographs, and videotapes)
- Provide opportunities for ongoing parental care of hospitalized children, when the patient is a child
- Provide opportunities for adult family members to maintain ongoing commitments to their jobs if possible, or to use the Family Leave Act in the United States
- Assist family members to facilitate home visits by patient, when appropriate
- Identify home care needs and how these might be incorporated into family lifestyle
- Design schedules of home care activities that minimize disruption of family routine
- Teach family time management/organization skills when performing home care, as needed

1st edition 1992; revised 2008

Background Evidence:

Broome, M. E., & Huth, M. M. (2001). Preparation for hospitalization, surgery and procedures. In M. Craft-Rosenberg & J. Denehy (Eds.), *Nursing interventions for infants, children, and families* (pp. 281–298). Sage.

Daugherty, J., Saarmann, L., Riegel, B., Sornborger, K., & Moser, D. (2002). Can we talk? Developing a social support nursing intervention for couples. *Clinical Nurse Specialist, 16*(4), 211–218.

Drageset, J. (2004). The importance of activities of daily living and social contact for loneliness: A survey among residents in nursing homes. *Scandinavian Journal of Caring Sciences, 18*(1), 65–71.

Finfgeld-Connett, D. (2005). Clarification of social support. *Journal of Nursing Scholarship, 37*(1), 4–9.

Titler, M. G., Cohen, M. Z., & Craft, M. J. (1991). Impact of adult critical care hospitalization: Perceptions of patients, spouses, children, and nurses. *Heart & Lung, 20*(2), 174–182.

Family Support · 7140

Definition: Promotion of family values, interests, and goals

Activities:

- Appraise family's emotional reaction to patient's condition
- Determine the psychological burden of prognosis for family
- Foster realistic hope
- Promote open, trusting relationship with family
- Create a supportive therapeutic environment for family
- Accept the family's values in a nonjudgmental manner
- Answer all questions of family members or assist them to get answers
- Listen to family concerns, feelings, and questions
- Facilitate communication of concerns and feelings between patient and family or among family members
- Assist the family in prioritizing family health needs
- Orient family to the health care setting, such as hospital unit or clinic
- Provide assistance in meeting basic needs for family, such as shelter, food, and clothing
- Assist in organizing a network of resources designed to provide support services
- Identify congruence among patient, family, and health professional expectations
- Reduce discrepancies in patient, family, and health professional expectations through use of communication skills
- Assist family to identify family strengths and coping abilities
- Provide opportunities for family to apply coping strategies that may work in the current situation

- Respect and support adaptive coping mechanisms used by family
- Provide feedback for family regarding their coping
- Counsel family members on additional effective coping skills for their own use
- Provide spiritual resources for family, as appropriate
- Provide family with information about patient's progress frequently, according to patient preference
- Assist family members in identifying and resolving a conflict in values
- Instruct the medical and nursing plans of care to family
- Include family members with patient in decision making about care, when appropriate
- Encourage family decision making in planning long-term patient care affecting family structure and finances
- Acknowledge understanding of family decision about postdischarge care
- Assist family to acquire necessary knowledge, skills, and equipment to sustain their decision about patient care
- Advocate for family, as appropriate
- Foster family assertiveness in information seeking, as appropriate
- Consider using a communication and information technology support system as a means to provide in home family support
- Provide opportunities for visitation by extended family members, as appropriate
- Introduce family to other families undergoing similar experiences, as appropriate
- Give care to patient when family is unable to give care

- Initiate and coordinate referrals to social service, respite care, family therapy, financial counselors, support groups, home health care, and other community resource agencies, if indicated
- Provide opportunities for peer group support
- Inform family members how to reach the nurse
- Assist family members through the death and grief processes, as appropriate
- Support the family member's need for privacy

1st edition 1992; revised 1996, 2018

Background Evidence:

Davidson, J. E. (2009). Family-centered care: Meeting the needs of patients' families and helping families adapt to critical illness. *Critical Care Nurse, 29*(3), 28–35.

Hohashi, N., & Honda, J. (2012). Development and testing of the Survey of Family Environment (SFE): A novel instrument to measure family functioning and needs for family support. *Journal of Nursing Measurement, 20*(3), 212–229.

Lundberg, S. (2014). The results from a two-year case study of an information and communication technology support system for family caregivers. *Disability & Rehabilitation: Assistive Technology, 9*(4), 353–358.

Mattila, E., Kaunonen, M., Aalto, P., & Astedt-Kurki, P. (2014). The method of nursing support in hospital and patients' and family members' experiences of the effectiveness of the support. *Scandinavian Journal of Caring Sciences, 28*(2), 305–314.

Family Therapy   7150

Definition: Assisting family members to move their family toward a more productive way of living

Activities:
- Use family-history taking to encourage family discussion
- Determine family communication patterns
- Identify how family solves problems
- Determine how family makes decisions
- Determine whether abuse is occurring in the family
- Identify family strengths/resources
- Identify usual roles within the family system
- Identify specific disturbances related to role expectations
- Determine whether any family members are dealing with substance abuse
- Determine family alliances
- Identify areas of dissatisfaction and/or conflict
- Determine recent or impending events that have threatened the family
- Help family members communicate more effectively
- Facilitate family discussion
- Help members prioritize and select the most immediate family issue to address
- Help family members clarify what they need and expect from each other
- Facilitate strategies to reduce stress
- Provide education and information
- Help family enhance existing positive coping strategies
- Share therapy plan with family
- Ask family members to participate in homework assignments of experiential activities such as eating some of their meals together
- Provide challenges within family discussion to encourage new behavior
- Discuss hierarchical relationship of subsystem members

- Assist family members to change how they relate to other family members
- Facilitate restructuring family subsystems, as appropriate
- Help family set goals toward a more competent way of handling dysfunctional behavior
- Monitor family boundaries
- Monitor for adverse therapeutic responses
- Plan termination and evaluation strategies

1st edition 1992; revised 2008

Background Evidence:

Craft, M. J., & Willadsen, J. A. (1992). Interventions related to family. *Nursing Clinics of North America, 27*(2), 517–540.

Friedman, M. M., Bowden, V. R., & Jones, E. G. (2003). *Family nursing: Research, theory, and practice* (5th ed.). Prentice Hall.

Goldenberg, I., & Goldenberg, H. (2004). *Family therapy: An overview* (6th ed.). Thomson Learning.

Johnson, G., Kent, G., & Leather, J. (2005). Strengthening the parent-child relationship: A review of family interventions and their use in medical settings. *Child: Care Health & Development, 31*(1), 25–32.

Kelly, M., & Newstead, L. (2004). Family intervention in routine practice: It is possible! *Journal of Psychiatric & Mental Health Nursing, 11*(1), 64–72.

Minuchen, S., & Fishman, H. C. (1981). *Family therapy techniques.* Harvard University Press.

Rojano, R. (2004). The practice of community family therapy. *Family Practice, 43*(1), 59–77.

Walsh, F. (2003). Family resilience: A framework for clinical practice. *Family Process, 42*(1), 1–18.

Feeding   1050

Definition: Providing nutritional intake for person who is unable to feed self

Activities:
- Identify prescribed diet
- Set food tray and table attractively
- Determine food, cultural, or religious preferences and incorporate into feeding routines
- Create pleasant environment during mealtime, removing unnecessary equipment and supplies
- Provide adequate pain relief before meals, as appropriate
- Provide oral hygiene before meals, as needed
- Identify presence of swallowing reflex, if necessary
- Fix food on tray as prefers (e.g., cutting meat, opening packages)
- Avoid placing food on blind side
- Describe location of food on tray for person with vision impairment
- Place in comfortable eating position
- Offer opportunity to smell foods to stimulate appetite
- Ask preference for order of eating
- Sit down when feeding to convey pleasure and relaxation
- Maintain in upright position with head and neck flexed slightly forward during feeding
- Place food in unaffected side of mouth, as appropriate
- Place food within vision area if has visual-field defect
- Choose different-colored dishes to help distinguish items, if perceptual deficit
- Follow feedings with water, if needed
- Protect with bib, as appropriate
- Pace feeding to avoid fatigue
- Ask to indicate when finished, as appropriate
- Record intake, if appropriate
- Avoid disguising medications in food
- Avoid presenting drink or bite up to mouth when still chewing
- Provide drinking straw, as needed or desired
- Provide finger foods or preferred foods and drinks, as appropriate
- Provide foods at most appetizing temperature
- Avoid distracting during swallowing
- Feed unhurriedly and slowly
- Maintain attention to person while they are eating
- Postpone feeding if fatigued
- Check mouth for residue at end of meal
- Wash face and hands after meal
- Encourage parents or family to feed person
- Encourage to eat in dining room if available
- Provide social interaction, as appropriate
- Provide adaptive devices to facilitate feeding self (e.g., long handles, handle with large circumference, small strap on utensils) as needed
- Use cup with large handle if necessary
- Use unbreakable and weighted dishes and glasses as necessary
- Provide frequent cueing and close supervision, as appropriate
- Praise self-feeding attempts
- Monitor body weight, hydration status, and laboratory values, as appropriate
- Instruct person and family on methods to assist with feeding needs
- Use teach-back to ensure understanding
- Document feeding sessions as indicated

1st edition 1992; revised 2008, 2024

Background Evidence:

Berman, A., Snyder, S. J., & Frandsen, G. (2018). Nutrition. In *Kozier and Erb's fundamentals of nursing: Concepts, process and practice* (pp. 1152–1154) (10th ed.). Pearson.

Berta, J. W. (2022). Nutrition alterations and management. In L. D. Urden, K. M. Stacy, & M. E. Lough (Eds.), *Critical care nursing: Diagnosis and management* (9th ed., p. 95). Elsevier.

Miller, T. (2021). Nutrition. In P. A. Potter, A. G. Perry, P. A. Stockert, & A. M. Hall (Eds.), *Fundamentals of nursing* (10th ed., pp. 1120–1121). Elsevier.

Perry, A. G., Potter, P. A., Ostendorf, W. R., & LaPlante, N. (2021). Oral nutrition. In *Clinical nursing skills and technique* (pp. 826–831) (10th ed.). Mosby.

St. Onge, J. L. (2021). Nutrition. In R. F. Craven, C. J. Hirnle, & C. J. Henshaw (Eds.), *Fundamentals of nursing: Human health and function* (8th ed.). Wolters-Kluwer.

Touhy, T. (2020). Nutrition. In K. Jett & T. A. Touhy (Eds.), *Toward healthy aging* (10th ed., pp. 173–189). Elsevier.

Williams, P. (2020). Maintaining fluid balance and meeting nutritional needs. In *Basic geriatric nursing* (pp. 117–124) (7th ed.). Elsevier.

Fertility Preservation   7160

Definition: Providing information, counseling, and treatment that facilitate reproductive health and the ability to conceive

Activities:
- Discuss factors related to infertility (e.g., maternal age greater than 35, sexually transmitted diseases, chemotherapy, and radiation)
- Encourage conception before age 35, as appropriate
- Instruct patient how to prevent sexually transmitted diseases
- Inform patient of signs and symptoms of sexually transmitted diseases and importance of early, aggressive treatment
- Perform pelvic examination, as appropriate
- Obtain cervical cultures, as appropriate
- Prescribe treatment, as indicated for sexually transmitted disease or vaginal infection
- Advise patient to seek evaluation and treatment for sexually transmitted disease if partner exhibits any symptoms, even if patient experiences no symptoms
- Advise patient to have partner treated for sexually transmitted disease, if culture positive
- Report positive sexually transmitted disease cultures, as required by law
- Discuss effects of different contraceptive methods on future fertility
- Counsel patient about contraceptive use
- Advise patient to avoid use of intrauterine devices

- Inform patients about occupational and environmental hazards to fertility (e.g., radiation, chemicals, stress, infections, other environmental factors, and shift rotation)
- Inform patient about more conservative options that are likely to preserve fertility, when gynecological or abdominal surgery is indicated
- Refer patient for thorough physical examination for health problems affecting fertility (e.g., amenorrhea, diabetes, endometriosis, and thyroid disease)
- Encourage early, aggressive treatment for endometriosis
- Review lifestyle habits that may alter fertility (e.g., smoking, substance use, alcohol consumption, nutrition, exercise, and sexual behavior)
- Refer to wellness or lifestyle modification program, as appropriate
- Inform patient about the effects of alcohol, tobacco, drugs, and other factors on sperm production and male sexual function
- Refer patient with history indicative of possible fertility disorder for early diagnosis and treatment
- Assist patient in receiving occupational support for fertility treatment
- Inform patient to consider the potential or lack of potential reversibility of different methods of sterilization
- Advise patient considering sterilization to consider procedure irreversible

2nd edition 1996; revised 2018

Background Evidence:

Hoffman, B., Schorge, J., Schaffer, J., Halvorson, L., Bradshaw, K., & Cunningham, F. (2012). Treatment of the infertile couple. In *Williams gynecology* (pp. 529–553) (2nd ed.). McGraw-Hill.

Jensen, J., & Mishell, D., Jr. (2012). Family planning. In G. Lentz, R. Lobo, D. Gershenson, & V. Katz (Eds.), *Comprehensive gynecology* (6th ed., pp. 215–272). Elsevier Mosby.

Leyland, N., Casper, R., Laberge, P., & Singh, S. (2010). & Society of Obstetricians and Gynaecologists of Canada. *Endometriosis: Diagnosis and management. Journal of Obstetrics & Gynaecology Canada, 32*(Suppl. 2), S1–S32.

Onwere, C., & Vakharia, H. (2014). *Crash course: Obstetrics and gynaecology* (3rd ed.). Edinburgh, Scotland: Mosby Elsevier.

Shoupe, D. (Ed.). (2011). *Gynecology in practice: Contraception [A. Arici, series editor]*. Oxford: Wiley-Blackwell.

F

Financial Resource Assistance   7380

Definition: Assisting persons to secure and manage finances to meet health care needs

Activities:

- Determine current use of healthcare system and financial effect
- Assist to identify financial needs, including analysis of assets and liabilities
- Determine cognitive ability to read, fill out forms, manage money
- Determine daily living expenses
- Assist to develop plan to prioritize daily living needs
- Devise plan of care to encourage person or family to access appropriate levels of care in most cost-effective manner
- Inform of services available through state and federal programs
- Determine whether eligible for waiver programs
- Refer person who may be eligible for state or federally funded programs to appropriate individuals
- Inform of available resources and assist in accessing resources (e.g., medication assistance program, county relief program)
- Assist to develop budget or make referral to appropriate financial resource person (e.g., financial planner, estate planner, consumer counselor), as needed
- Assist to fill out applications for available resources, as needed
- Assist in long-term care placement planning, as needed
- Assist to assure money in secure place (e.g., bank), as needed
- Assist in obtaining burial fund, as appropriate
- Encourage family to be involved in financial management, as appropriate
- Represent economic needs at multidisciplinary conferences, as needed
- Collaborate with community agencies to provide needed services

3rd edition 2000; revised 2024

Background Evidence:

Brandow, C. L., Swarbrick, M., & Nemec, P. B. (2020). Rethinking the causes and consequences of financial wellness for people with serious mental illness. *Psychiatric Services, 71*, 89–91. https://doi.org/10.1176/appi.ps.20190032

Crawford, C. A. (2021). Studying social workers' roles in natural disasters during a global pandemic: What can we learn? *Qualitative Social Work, 20*(1/2), 456–462. https://doi.org/10.1177/1473325020973449

Lechuga-Peña, S., Becerra, D., Mitchell, F. M., Lopez, K., & Sangalang, C. C. (2019). Subsidized housing and low-income mother's school-based parent involvement: Findings from the fragile families and child wellbeing study wave five. *Child & Youth Care Forum, 48*(3), 323–338. https://doi.org/10.1007/s10566-018-9481-y

McMullen, L. (2019). Patient Assistance Programs: Easing the burden of financial toxicity during cancer treatment. *Clinical Journal of Oncology Nursing, 23*(5), 36–40. https://doi.org/10.1188/19.CJON.S2.36-40

Nedjat-Haiem, F. R., Cadet, T., Parada, H., Jr, Jones, T., Jimenez, E. E., Thompson, B., Wells, K. J., & Mishra, S. I. (2021). Financial hardship and health related quality of life among older Latinos with chronic diseases. *American Journal of Hospice & Palliative Medicine, 38*(8), 938–946.

Semin, J. N., Palm, D., Smith, L. M., & Ruttle, S. (2020). Understanding breast cancer survivors' financial burden and distress after financial assistance. *Supportive Care in Cancer, 28*(9), 4241–4248.

Shankaran, V., Linden, H., Steelquist, J., Watabayashi, K., Kreizenbeck, K., Leahy, T., & Overstreet, K. (2017). Development of a financial literacy course for patients with newly diagnosed cancer. *The American Journal of Managed Care, 23*(3 Suppl), S58–S64.

Spencer, J. C., Samuel, C. A., Wheeler, S. B., Rosenstein, D. L., Reeder-Hayes, K. E., Manning, M. L., & Sellers, J. B. (2018). Oncology navigators' perceptions of cancer-related financial burden and financial assistance resources. *Supportive Care in Cancer, 26*(4), 1315–1321.

Fire-Setting Precautions 6500

Definition: Prevention of fire-setting behaviors

Activities:

- Search patient for incendiary materials (e.g., matches or lighters) on admission and each time that patient returns to care environment (i.e., from a pass or a recreational activity)
- Search patient environment on routine basis to remove fire-setting materials
- Determine appropriate behavioral expectations and consequences, given the patient's level of cognitive functioning and capacity for self-control
- Communicate rules, behavioral expectations, and consequences to patient
- Communicate risk to other care providers
- Provide ongoing surveillance in an environment that is free of fire-setting materials
- Provide close supervision if patient is allowed to smoke
- Obtain verbal contract from patient to refrain from fire-setting activity
- Encourage the expression of feelings in an appropriate manner
- Assist patient with impulse control training, as appropriate
- Increase surveillance and security (e.g., area restriction or seclusion) if risk of fire-setting behavior increases

2nd edition 1996; revised 2018

Background Evidence:

Gannon, T. A., & Pina, A. (2010). Firesetting: Psychopathology, theory and treatment. *Aggression and Violent Behavior, 15*(3), 224–238.

Jones, J., Fitzpatrick, J., & Rogers, V. (2012). *Psychiatric-mental health nursing: An interpersonal approach.* Springer.

Lambie, I., Ioane, J., Randell, I., & Seymour, F. (2013). Offending behaviours of child and adolescent firesetters over a 10-year follow-up. *Journal of Child Psychology and Psychiatry and Allied Disciplines, 54*(12), 1295–1307.

Schultz, J. M., & Videbeck, S. L. (2013). *Lippincott's manual of psychiatric nursing care plans* (9th ed.). Lippincott Williams & Wilkins.

First Aid 6240

Definition: Providing immediate care for minor burns, injuries, poisoning, bites, and stings

Activities:

- Instruct others to call for help, if needed
- Employ precautionary measures to reduce risk of infection when giving care
- Monitor vital signs, as appropriate
- Note characteristics of the wound or burn including drainage, color, size, and odor
- Institute appropriate care of wound or burn
- Institute measures (e.g., pressure, pressure dressing, positioning) to reduce or minimize bleeding
- Use rest, ice, compression, and elevation (RICE) for extremity bone, joint, and muscle injuries
- Splint affected extremity
- Cleanse skin exposed to poison ivy, oak, or sumac (i.e., use water and soap or liberal amount of rubbing alcohol) and stinging nettle (i.e., use water and soap)
- Flush tissue exposed to chemicals (except lye or white phosphorous) with water
- Remove embedded stinger and venom sac from insect sting or tentacles from marine animal sting by scraping a hard object over site (e.g., fingernail, credit card, or comb)
- Remove tick from the skin using tweezers or specialized tick-removal tool
- Administer medication (e.g., prophylactic antibiotic, vaccination, antihistamine, anti-inflammatory, and analgesic), as appropriate
- Relieve itching (i.e., administer medication, apply calamine lotion or baking soda paste, and instruct patient to bathe in colloidal oatmeal)
- Report animal bites to appropriate authority (e.g., police or animal control)
- Provide instructions for necessary follow-up care
- Instruct patient on care of injury
- Coordinate medical transport, as needed

1st edition 1992; revised 2013

Background Evidence:

American Academy of Orthopaedic Surgeons. (2005). In A. A. Thygerson & B. Gulli (Eds.), *First aid, CPR, and AED* (4th ed.). Jones and Bartlett.

Boy Scouts of America. (2009). *The Boy Scout handbook* (12th ed.).

Pfeiffer, R. P., Thygerson, A., & Palmieri, N. F. (2009). In B. Gulli & E. W. Ossman, Medical (Eds.), *Sports first aid and injury prevention.* Jones and Bartlett.

Fiscal Resource Management 8550

Definition: Procuring and directing the use of financial resources

Activities:

- Develop business plan
- Develop cost-benefit analysis of programs and services
- Maintain budget appropriate to services provided
- Identify sources of financing services
- Generate grant applications
- Identify marketing efforts to enhance programs
- Solicit matched contributions that support programs and services

- Analyze economic viability of program based on trends
- Implement relevant policies and procedures to secure reimbursement
- Maximize potential reimbursement (e.g., program certification, qualified providers)
- Use appropriate accounting methods to ensure accurate and designated use of funds
- Use appropriate methods to address fiduciary responsibility
- Evaluate outcomes and cost effectiveness of program
- Make appropriate changes in financial management in response to evaluation

3rd edition 2000; revised 2024

Background Evidence:

Brydges, G., Krepper, R., Nibert, A., Young, A., & Luquire, R. (2019). Assessing executive nurse leaders' financial literacy level: A mixed-methods study. *JONA: The Journal of Nursing Administration, 49*(12), 596–603. https://doi.org/10.1097/NNA.0000000000000822

Dion, K. W., Oerther, D. B., & Davidson, P. M. (2021). Nurse leaders and financial literacy: Learning to become CFO of me. *Nursing Economic$, 39*(3), 151–155.

Dion, K. W., Oerther, D. B., & White, K. M. (2021). Mastering the health savings account. *Nursing Economic$, 39*(5), 255–259.

Huber, D. L., & Joseph, M. L. (2021). *Leadership and nursing care management* (7th ed.). Elsevier.

Marquis, B. L., & Huston, C. J. (2021). *Leadership roles and management functions in nursing: Theory and applications* (10th ed.). Wolters Kluwer.

McFarlan, S. (2020). An experiential educational intervention to improve nurse managers' knowledge and self-assessed competence with health care financial management. *Journal of Continuing Education in Nursing, 51*(4), 181–188. https://doi.org/10.3928/00220124-20200317-08

Raftery, C., Sassenberg, A.-M., & Bamford-Wade, A. (2021). Business acumen for nursing leaders, optional or essential in today's health system? A discussion paper. *Collegian, 28*(6), 610–615. https://doi.org/10.1016/j.colegn.2021.08.001

Welch, T. D., & Smith, T. B. (2022). Anatomy of a business case. *Nursing Administration Quarterly, 46*(1), 88–95. https://doi.org/10.1097/NAQ.0000000000000498

Flatulence Reduction 0470

Definition: Prevention of flatus formation and facilitation of passage of excessive gas

Activities:

- Inform patient how flatus is produced and methods for alleviation
- Inform patient that passing gas around 13 to 21 times a day is normal
- Instruct patient to avoid situations that cause excessive air swallowing (e.g., chewing gum, drinking carbonated beverages, eating rapidly, sucking through straws, chewing with mouth open, talking with mouth full, wearing loose fitting dentures)
- Instruct patient to avoid foods that cause flatulence (e.g., beans, cabbage, Brussels sprouts, radishes, onions, cauliflower, cucumbers, beer, prunes, pears, apples, whole wheat products)
- Discuss use of dairy products
- Advise to discontinue use of artificial sweeteners found in some sugar free goods, gums, and candies
- Advise to cut back on fried and fatty foods
- Discuss cutting back temporarily on high fiber foods and slowly adding these back to diet monitoring gas increase
- Advise to take fiber supplements with a glass of water and to drink plenty of liquids throughout the day
- Monitor for bloated feeling, abdominal distension, cramping pains, and excessive passage of gas from the mouth or anus
- Monitor bowel sounds
- Advise patient to keep a diary of food and drinks consumed and times of day that gas is passed
- Provide for adequate exercise (e.g., ambulate)
- Insert lubricated rectal tube into the rectum; tape in place; insert distal end of tube into a receptacle, as appropriate
- Administer a laxative, suppository, or enema, as appropriate
- Monitor side effects of medication administration
- Limit oral intake, if lower gastrointestinal system is inactive
- Position on left side with knees flexed, as appropriate
- Offer antiflatulence medications (e.g., Beano, Gas-X, Lactaid), as appropriate
- Discuss use of probiotic food (e.g., soy sauce, yogurt, pickled vegetables) and probiotics (e.g., PreScript-Assist, VSL#3) to lessen abnormal intestinal gas
- Notify physician if gas is accompanied by prolonged abdominal pain, bloody stools, weight loss, chest pain, or persistent nausea or vomiting

1st edition 1992; revised 1996, 2018

Background Evidence:

Mayo Clinic Staff. (2014). *Gas and gas pains.* http://www.mayoclinic.org/diseases-conditions/gas-and-gas-pains/basics/definition/con-20019271NIC 7e Part 3 D-G.doc

Morgan, M.E. (2014). *Review: The best probiotics for eliminating gas.* http://beneficialbacteria.net/the-best-probiotics-for-eliminating-gas/

National Institute of Diabetes and Digestive and Kidney Diseases. (2016). *Gas in the digestive tract.* http://digestive.niddk.nih.gov/ddiseases/pubs/gas/

Savino, F., Cordisco, L., Tarasco, V., Locatelli, E., Di Gioia, D., Oggero, R., & Matteuzzi, D. (2011). Antagonistic effect of Lactobacillus strains against gas-producing coliforms isolated from colicky infants. *BMC Microbiology, 11*(1), 157. https://doi.org/1186/1471-2180-11-157

Winham, D. M., & Hutchins, A. M. (2011). Perceptions of flatulence from bean consumption among adults in 3 feeding studies. *Online Nutrition Journal, 10*(128). https://doi.org/1186/1475-2891-10-128

Fluid/Electrolyte Management 2080

Definition: Regulation and prevention of complications from altered fluid and/or electrolyte levels

Activities:

- Monitor for abnormal serum electrolyte levels, as available
- Monitor for changes in pulmonary or cardiac status indicating fluid overload or dehydration
- Monitor for signs and symptoms of worsening overhydration or dehydration (e.g., moist crackles in lung sounds, polyuria or oliguria, behavior changes, seizures, frothy or thick viscous saliva, edematous or sunken eyes, rapid shallow breathing)
- Obtain laboratory specimens for monitoring of altered fluid or electrolyte levels (e.g., hematocrit, BUN, protein, sodium, and potassium levels), as appropriate
- Weigh daily and monitor trends
- Give fluids, as appropriate
- Promote oral intake (e.g., provide oral fluids that are the patient's preference, place in easy reach, provide a straw, and provide fresh water), as appropriate
- Administer prescribed nasogastric replacement based on output, as appropriate
- Irrigate nasogastric tubes with normal saline, per agency policy and as indicated
- Provide free water with tube feedings, per agency policy and as indicated
- Administer fiber as prescribed for the tube-fed patient to reduce fluid and electrolyte loss through diarrhea
- Minimize the number of ice chips consumed or amount of oral intake by patients with gastric tubes connected to suction
- Minimize intake of foods and drinks with diuretic or laxative effects (e.g., tea, coffee, prunes, herbal supplements)
- Maintain an appropriate intravenous infusion, blood transfusion, or enteral flow rate especially if not regulated by a pump
- Ensure that intravenous solution containing electrolytes is administered at a constant flow rate, as appropriate
- Monitor laboratory results relevant to fluid balance (e.g., hematocrit, BUN, albumin, total protein, serum osmolality, and urine specific gravity levels)
- Monitor laboratory results relevant to fluid retention (e.g., increased specific gravity, increased BUN, decreased hematocrit, and increased urine osmolality levels)
- Monitor hemodynamic status, including CVP, MAP, PAP, and PCWP levels, if available
- Keep an accurate record of intake and output
- Monitor for signs and symptoms of fluid retention
- Restrict free water intake in the presence of dilutional hyponatremia with serum Na level lower than 130 mEq per liter
- Institute fluid restriction, as appropriate
- Monitor vital signs, as appropriate
- Correct preoperative dehydration, as appropriate
- Monitor patient's response to prescribed electrolyte therapy
- Monitor for manifestations of electrolyte imbalance
- Provide prescribed diet appropriate for specific fluid or electrolyte imbalance (e.g., low-sodium, fluid-restricted, renal, and no added salt)
- Administer prescribed supplemental electrolytes, as appropriate
- Administer prescribed electrolyte binding or excreting resins, as appropriate
- Monitor for side effects (e.g., nausea, vomiting, diarrhea) of prescribed supplemental electrolytes
- Watch patient's buccal membranes, sclera, and skin for indications of altered fluid and electrolyte balance (e.g., dryness, cyanosis, and jaundice)
- Consult physician if signs and symptoms of fluid and/or electrolyte imbalance persist or worsen
- Institute measures to control excessive electrolyte loss (e.g., by resting the gut, changing type of diuretic, or administering antipyretics), as appropriate
- Institute measures to rest the bowel (i.e., restrict food or fluid intake and decrease intake of milk products), if appropriate
- Follow quick-acting glucose with long-acting carbohydrates and proteins for management of acute hypoglycemia, as appropriate
- Prepare patient for dialysis (e.g., by assisting with catheter placement for dialysis), as appropriate
- Monitor for fluid loss (e.g., bleeding, vomiting, diarrhea, perspiration, and tachypnea)
- Promote a positive body image and self-esteem if concerns are expressed as a result of excessive fluid retention, if appropriate
- Assist patients with impaired mental or physical conditions (e.g., dysphagia, cognitive impairment, mentally challenged, reduction in physical strength or coordination) to achieve adequate fluid balance
- Assist patients with undesirable sequelae from prescribed therapeutic regimen (e.g., patient with fear of urinary frequency or incontinence from diuretic limits own fluid intake) to achieve adequate fluid balance
- Instruct patient and family about rationale for fluid restrictions, hydration measures, or supplemental electrolyte administration, as indicated

1st edition 1992; revised 2013

Background Evidence:

Allsopp, K. (2010). Caring for patients with kidney failure. *Emergency Nurse*, 18(10), 12–16.

Harvey, S., & Jordan, S. (2010). Diuretic therapy: Implications for nursing practice. *Nursing Standard*, 24(43), 40–50.

Murch, P. (2005). Optimizing the fluid management of ventilated patients with suspected hypovolaemia. *Nursing in Critical Care*, 10(6), 279–288.

Ostendorf, W. R. (2011). Fluid, electrolyte, and acid-base balances. In P. A. Potter, A. G. Perry, P. Stockert, & A. Hall (Eds.), *Basic nursing* (7th ed., pp. 466–521). Mosby Elsevier.

Scales, K., & Pilsworth, J. (2008). The importance of fluid balance in clinical practice. *Nursing Standard*, 22(47), 50–58.

Tang, V., & Lee, E. (2010). Fluid balance chart: Do we understand it? *Clinical Risk*, 16(1), 10–13.

Welch, K. (2010). Fluid balance. *Learning Disability Practice*, 13(6), 33–38.

Young, E., Sherrard-Jacob, A., Knapp, K., Craddock, T. S., Kemper, C., Falvo, R., Hunter, S., Everson, C., & Giarrizzo-Wilson, S. (2009). Perioperative fluid management. *AORN Journal*, 89(1), 167–182.

Fluid Management 4120

Definition: Promotion of fluid balance and prevention of complications resulting from abnormal or undesired fluid levels

Activities:

- Determine baseline fluid status (e.g., overloaded, dehydrated, normovolemic)
- Monitor for changes in fluid status using regularly obtained data (e.g., weights, laboratory values, vital signs)
- Conduct medication reconciliation to determine medications influencing fluid balance
- Treat underlying cause of fluid imbalance where possible (e.g., overuse of diuretics, congestive heart failure, hyperglycemia)
- Maintain accurate intake (e.g., IV, oral) and output record (e.g., urinary void, urinary catheter, incontinence briefs, weighed diapers)
- Monitor hydration status (e.g., moist mucous membranes, adequacy of pulses, orthostatic blood pressure, fontanel appearance, skin turgor), as appropriate
- Monitor laboratory results relevant to fluid retention (e.g., increased specific gravity, increased BUN, decreased hematocrit, increased urine osmolality levels)
- Monitor vital signs and hemodynamic status
- Monitor for indications of fluid overload or retention (e.g., crackles, elevated CVP or pulmonary capillary wedge pressure, edema, neck vein distention, ascites), as appropriate
- Monitor for indications of dehydration (e.g., dry mucous membranes, weak peripheral pulses, flat neck or hand veins, decreased urine output, dizziness, syncope)
- Monitor weight
- Monitor location and extent of edema if present
- Monitor food and fluid ingested and calculate daily caloric intake, as appropriate
- Administer IV therapy at room temperature, as prescribed
- Monitor nutrition status
- Administer prescribed diuretics and fluid regulating medications (e.g., aldosterone, electrolytes, albumin), as appropriate
- Promote oral intake (e.g., provide drinking straw; offer fluids between meals; change ice water routinely; make freezer pops using child's favorite juice; cut gelatin into fun squares; use small medicine cups), as appropriate
- Provide fluids that observe prescribed dietary restrictions (e.g., sugar-free, low-sodium, thickened)
- Instruct on nothing by mouth (NPO) status, as appropriate
- Administer prescribed nasogastric replacement based on output, as appropriate
- Distribute fluid intake over 24 hours, as appropriate
- Encourage significant other to assist with feedings, as appropriate
- Restrict free water intake in presence of dilutional hyponatremia with serum Na level lower than 130 mEq per liter
- Monitor response to prescribed electrolyte therapy
- Consult health care provider if signs and symptoms of fluid volume excess persist or worsen
- Arrange availability of blood products for transfusion, if necessary
- Prepare for administration of blood products (i.e., check blood with identification and prepare infusion setup), as appropriate
- Administer blood products (e.g., platelets, fresh frozen plasma), as appropriate
- Monitor response to therapies at least every 2 hours
- Instruct related to fluid intake or restriction, medications influencing fluid balance and dietary intake for maintaining adequate fluid balance
- Instruct related to signs and symptoms of fluid imbalances
- Use teach-back to ensure understanding

1st edition 1992; revised 2000, 2024

Background Evidence:

Hockenberry, M. J., Rodgers, C. C., & Wilson, D. (2022). *Wong's essentials of pediatric nursing* (11th ed.). Elsevier.

Jett, K., & Touhy, T. A. (2020). *Toward healthy aging* (10th ed.). Elsevier.

Kear, T. M. (2017). Fluid and electrolyte management across the age continuum. *Nephrology Nursing Journal, 44*(6), 491–496.

Perry, A. G., & Potter, P. A. (2020). *Clinical nursing skills and techniques* (5th ed.). Mosby.

Roumelioti, M. E., Glew, R. H., Khitan, Z. J., Rondon-Berrios, H., Argyropoulos, C. P., Malhotra, D., Raj, D. S., Agaba, E. I., Rohrscheib, M., Murata, G. H., Shapiro, J. I., & Tzamaloukas, A. H. (2018). Fluid balance concepts in medicine: Principles and practice. *World Journal of Nephrology, 7*(1), 1–28.

Williams, P. (2020). *Basic geriatric nursing* (7th ed.). Elsevier.

Workman, M. L. (2021). Concepts of fluid and electrolyte balance. In D. D. Ignatavicius, M. L. Workman, C. R. Rebar, & N. M. Heimgartner (Eds.), *Medical-surgical nursing: Concepts for interprofessional collaborative care* (10th ed.). Elsevier.

Fluid Monitoring 4130

Definition: Collection and analysis of patient data to regulate fluid balance

Activities:

- Determine history of amount and type of fluid intake and elimination habits
- Determine possible risk factors for fluid imbalance (e.g., albumin loss state, burns, malnutrition, sepsis, nephrotic syndrome, hyperthermia, diuretic therapy, renal pathologies, cardiac failure, diaphoresis, liver dysfunction, strenuous exercise, heat exposure, infection, postoperative state, polyuria, vomiting, and diarrhea)
- Determine whether patient is experiencing thirst or symptoms of fluid changes (e.g., dizziness, change of mentation, lightheadedness, apprehension, irritability, nausea, twitching)
- Examine capillary refill by holding the patient's hand at the same level as their heart and pressing on the pad of their middle finger for 5 seconds, releasing pressure, and counting time until color returns (i.e., should be less than 2 seconds)
- Examine skin turgor by grasping tissue over a bony area such as the hand or shin, pinching the skin gently, holding it for a second and releasing (i.e., skin will fall back quickly if patient is well hydrated)
- Monitor weight
- Monitor intake and output
- Monitor serum and urine electrolyte values, as appropriate
- Monitor serum albumin and total protein levels

F

F

- Monitor serum and urine osmolality levels
- Monitor BP, heart rate, and respiratory status
- Monitor orthostatic blood pressure and change in cardiac rhythm, as appropriate
- Monitor invasive hemodynamic parameters, as appropriate
- Keep an accurate record of intake and output (e.g., oral intake, enteral intake, IV intake, antibiotics, fluids given with medications, NG tubes, drains, vomit, rectal tubes, colostomy drainage, and urine)
- Insure to measure all intake and output on all patients with intravenous therapy, subcutaneous infusions, enteral feedings, NG tubes, urinary catheters, vomiting, diarrhea, wound drains, chest drains, and medical conditions that affect fluid balance (e.g., heart failure, renal failure, malnutrition, burns, sepsis)
- Record incontinence episodes in patients requiring accurate intake and output
- Correct mechanical problems (e.g., kinked or blocked catheter) in patients experiencing sudden cessation of urine output
- Monitor mucous membranes, skin turgor, and thirst
- Monitor color, quantity, and specific gravity of urine
- Monitor for distended neck veins, crackles in the lungs, peripheral edema, and weight gain
- Monitor for signs and symptoms of ascites
- Note presence or absence of vertigo on rising
- Administer fluids, as appropriate
- Assure that all IV and enteral intake devices are operating at the correct rates, especially if not regulated by a pump
- Restrict and allocate fluid intake, as appropriate
- Consult physician for urine output less than 0.5 mL/kg/hr or adult fluid intake less than 2000 in 24 hours, as appropriate

- Administer pharmacological agents to increase urinary output, as appropriate
- Administer dialysis noting patient response, as appropriate
- Maintain accurate fluid container reference charts to assure standardization of container measurements
- Audit intake and output graphs periodically to ensure good practice patterns

1st edition 1992; revised 2013

Background Evidence:

Allsopp, K. (2010). Caring for patients with kidney failure. *Emergency Nurse*, 18(10), 12–16.

Harvey, S., & Jordan, S. (2010). Diuretic therapy: Implications for nursing practice. *Nursing Standard*, 24(43), 40–50.

Murch, P. (2005). Optimizing the fluid management of ventilated patients with suspected hypovolaemia. *Nursing in Critical Care*, 10(6), 279–288.

Ostendorf, W. R. (2011). Fluid, electrolyte, and acid-base balances. In P. A. Potter, A. G. Perry, P. Stockert, & A. Hall (Eds.), *Basic nursing* (7th ed., pp. 466–521). Mosby Elsevier.

Scales, K., & Pilsworth, J. (2008). The importance of fluid balance in clinical practice. *Nursing Standard*, 22(47), 50–58.

Tang, V. C. Y., & Lee, E. W. Y. (2010). Fluid balance chart: Do we understand it? *Clinical Risk*, 16(1), 10–13.

Welch, K. (2010). Fluid balance. *Learning Disability Practice*, 13(6), 33–38.

Young, E., Sherrard-Jacob, A., Knapp, K., Craddock, T. S., Kemper, C., Falvo, R., Hunter, S., Everson, C., & Giarrizzo-Wilson, S. (2009). Perioperative fluid management. *AORN Journal*, 89(1), 167–182.

Fluid Resuscitation 4140

Definition: Administering prescribed intravenous fluids rapidly

Activities:

- Obtain and maintain a large-bore IV
- Collaborate with physicians to ensure administration of both crystalloids (e.g., normal saline and lactated Ringer's) and colloids (e.g., Hesban and Plasmanate), as appropriate
- Administer IV fluids, as prescribed
- Obtain blood specimens for crossmatching, as appropriate
- Administer blood products, as prescribed
- Monitor hemodynamic response
- Monitor oxygen status
- Monitor for fluid overload
- Monitor output of various body fluids (e.g., urine, nasogastric drainage, and chest tube)

- Monitor BUN, creatinine, total protein, and albumin levels
- Monitor for pulmonary edema and third spacing

1st edition 1992; revised 2008

Background Evidence:

Urden, L. D., Stacy, K. M., & Lough, M. E. (2006). *Thelan's critical care nursing: Diagnosis and management* (5th ed.). Mosby Elsevier.

Thompson, J. M., Hirsch, J. E., Tucker, S. M., & McFarland, G. K. (2002). *Mosby's clinical nursing* (5th ed.). Mosby.

Foot Care 1660

Definition: Cleansing and inspecting the feet for the purposes of relaxation, cleanliness, and health

Activities:

- Determine current level of knowledge and skills related to foot care
- Determine current foot care practices and routines
- Inspect skin of feet, including ankles, for irritation, cracks, lesions, corns, calluses, deformities, or edema
- Inspect shoes for proper fit, noting areas of wear

- Monitor gait and weight distribution on feet
- Monitor cleanliness and general condition of shoes and stockings
- Monitor hydration level of feet, arterial insufficiency in lower legs, and lower extremity edema
- Wash feet or administer foot soaks, as needed
- Dry carefully between toes

- Apply lotion or moisture-absorbing powder, if indicated
- Inspect nails for thickness or discoloration
- Clean nails and cut normal thickness toenails when soft, using toenail clipper and using curve of toe as guide, following agency protocol for trimming nails
- Do not cut down into nail groove
- Use emery board to file nails to ensure smooth corners
- Instruct on importance of foot care
- Provide information related to level of risk for injury
- Determine capacity to carry out foot care, (e.g., visual acuity, physical mobility, judgment)
- Recommend assistance of significant other with foot care if vision impaired or if mobility problems
- Offer positive feedback about self-care foot activities
- Instruct to inspect inside of shoes for rough areas
- Instruct to monitor temperature of feet using back of hand
- Instruct in importance of regular inspection, especially when sensation diminished
- Assist in developing plan for daily foot assessment and care at home
- Recommend daily foot inspection over all surfaces and between toes, looking for redness, swelling, warmth, dryness, maceration, tenderness, or open areas
- Instruct to use mirror or assistance of another to carry out foot inspection, as needed
- Advise daily washing of feet using warm water and mild soap
- Advise thoroughly drying feet after washing them, especially between toes
- Instruct to hydrate skin daily by brief soaking, bathing in room-temperature water or application of emollient
- Provide information regarding relationship between neuropathy, injury, and vascular disease and risk for ulceration and lower extremity amputation in persons with diabetes
- Advise regarding when to contact health professional, including presence of nonhealing or infected lesions
- Advise regarding appropriate self-care measures for minor foot problems
- Caution about potential sources of injury to feet, (e.g., heat, cold, cutting corns or calluses, chemicals, strong antiseptics or astringents, adhesive tape, going barefoot or wearing thongs or open-toe shoes)
- Instruct on proper technique for toenail trimming, (i.e., cutting relatively straight across, following contour of toe, and filing sharp edges with emery board)
- Instruct on care of soft calluses, including gentle buffing with towel or pumice stone after bath
- Recommend specialist care for thick or ingrown toenails, corns, calluses, or bony deformities, as indicated
- Recommend appropriate shoes (i.e., low heeled with shoe shape that matches foot shape; adequate depth of toe box; soles made of material that will absorb shock; adjustable fit by lace or straps; uppers made of breathable, soft, and flexible materials; changes made for gait and limb-length disorders; and potential for modification, if necessary)
- Recommend appropriate socks, (i.e., absorbent and non-constricting)
- Recommend guidelines to follow when purchasing new shoes, including having feet properly measured and fitted at time of purchase
- Recommend wearing new shoes only few hours at a time for first 2 weeks
- Instruct to inspect inside shoes daily for foreign objects, nail points, torn linings, and rough areas
- Instruct to change shoes two times, (e.g., 12 noon and 5 p.m.) each day to avoid local repetitive pressure
- Explain necessity for prescriptive footwear or orthotics, as appropriate
- Caution about activities that cause pressure on nerves and blood vessels, including elastic bands on socks or crossing legs
- Advise to stop smoking, as appropriate
- Include family in instruction, as appropriate
- Reinforce information provided by other health professionals, as appropriate
- Provide written foot care guidelines
- Document instruction as indicated
- Use teach-back to ensure understanding

1st edition 1992; revised 2004, 2024

Background Evidence:

Aziz, M. G. (2021). Hygiene and self-care. In R. F. Craven, C. J. Hirnle, & C. J. Henshaw (Eds.), *Fundamentals of nursing: Human health and function* (8th ed.). Wolters-Kluwer.

Berman, A., Snyder, S. J., & Frandsen, G. (2018). Hygiene. In *Kozier and Erb's Fundamentals of nursing: Concepts, process and practice* (pp. 684–688) (10th ed.). Pearson.

Perry, A. G., Potter, P. A., Ostendorf, W. R., & Laplante, N. (2022). Personal hygiene and bedmaking. In *Clinical Nursing Skills and Techniques* (10th ed.). Elsevier.

Porter-O'Grady, T. (2021). Wound and foot care nursing on the streets of the city: A view from here. *Journal of Wound, Ostomy & Continence Nursing. 48*(1), 69–74.

Potter, P. A., Perry, A. G., Stockert, P. A., & Hall, A. M. (2021). *Fundamentals of Nursing*, (10th ed.). Elsevier.

Trelease, J., & Simmons, J. (2021). Getting ready for foot care certification: Intervention and treatment for dermatological conditions affecting the feet and lower extremities. *Journal of Wound, Ostomy & Continence Nursing, 48*(3), 262–264.

Williams, P. (2020). *Basic geriatric nursing* (7th ed.). Elsevier.

Forensic Data Collection   7940

Definition: Collection and recording of pertinent patient data for a forensic report

Activities:
- Establish rapport with the patient or significant other, as appropriate
- Establish collaborative working relationship with all additional examiners
- Complete all parts of the examination, including normals
- Record omissions in examinations, including rationale for omission
- Provide facts only (e.g., what was examined, what was normal [pertinent negatives], what was abnormal) as seen at the time of examination

F

- Describe physical injuries by size, color, type of injury, location (add depth and trajectory if indicated)
- Measure in inches and increments of inches, including the greatest perpendicular dimensions of irregular wounds
- Describe wounds simply and with basic colors as much as possible (e.g., red, blue, purple, maroon)
- Determine wound location in two dimensions (length and midline standpoint) with body divided into anterior midline and posterior midline, describing in terms of how far right or left of midline
- Measure consistently from center of the lesion being described
- Record all contusions immediately as marks will fade and be lost as evidence
- Record directionality in abrasions using piling up of skin cells on the side opposite of the force
- Differentiate lacerations from incised wounds and stab wounds
- Note the order of wounds and why each is known to be first, second, etc., if possible
- Avoid long lists of probable injurious instruments (implies uncertainty and incompetence with examination)
- Determine wound trajectory
- Describe gunshot wounds completely (e.g., sooting, stippling, abrasion ring, or absence of sooting, etc.)
- Describe gunshot wounds as the face of a clock and identify in the report where 12:00 is on the body
- Describe any surrounding bruising or discolorations to gunshot wounds, including any muzzle imprints
- Use body diagrams and photographs to supplement written report
- Adhere to rules about information that must be added to each body diagram (e.g., case number, victim name, examination date and time, time finished, names and identification numbers of those present during examination)
- Draw in all identifying features (e.g., scars, tattoos, nail polish, body piercings, skin lesions)
- Draw scars in their orientation on the body
- Take injury photos similarly to crime scene photography (e.g., victim as part of crime scene, case number in every photograph) assuring case number does not cover or shadow injuries
- Obtain initial photographs as overall entire body photographs before the injuries are cleaned
- Obtain next set of photos as midrange and closer up with identifiers or landmarks (e.g., nipple in a chest wound)
- Obtain final photos as close-up photos (injury fills nearly entire frame with small identifying number) before and after cleaning
- Ensure that two photographs are obtained in pointer shots (one with and one without pointer) assuring nothing covered in photo with pointer
- Ensure that photographs of injuries are taken perpendicular to the skin surface to prevent distortion
- Ensure that photographs include a measuring scale for perspective
- Ensure that color scales are added to photographs of colored injuries to avoid color distortion
- Wash injured areas and blot dry before photographing to avoid wetness glare and ensure jury use
- Describe clothing (e.g., brand, size), jewelry, and personal property
- Record where items found (e.g., yellow metal watch on the left wrist)
- Record pertinent information related to items (e.g., gunshot wound with soot on the shirt)
- Ensure all items are photographed
- Diagram all medical interventions (e.g., EKG pads, endotracheal tubes, IVs, Foleys)
- Collect and package all specimens in clearly labeled paper bags
- Record date, time, type, and collection method for all specimens
- Use correct chain-of-evidence protocol for all specimens
- Record additional information or events that unfold later as an addendum report
- Describe all responses to additional information or events that unfold later (e.g., sexual assault examination completed 24 hours later after evidence presented indicating a sexual assault occurred)
- Plan daily follow-up visits with victims to document developing injury patterns, if possible
- Prepare reports as customary for state legal evidence requirements (e.g., complete date; military time; black ink; no correction fluid; numbered pages, including all diagrams and worksheets; all pages initialed; no blanks)
- Follow hospital or medical examiner protocol for saving original reports; if self-employed, save own originals
- Provide log sheet on which all contact about case is recorded in file with case
- Generate a report entitled "Amended Report" for any report that needs to be rewritten or corrected due to an error, including date and time of new report, why generated, description of error in original report, and correction
- Obtain information from additional examiners (e.g., medical examiner, emergency room physician, emergency room nurse) when unable to obtain information per self (e.g., wound trajectory, wound depth)
- Document information, informant and title, date and time of data collection, when obtaining information from additional examiners
- Provide for appropriate counseling and follow-up care for victims and family, as indicated

5th edition 2008

Background Evidence:

Burgess, A. W., Brown, K., Bell, K., Ledray, L. E., & Poarch, J. C. (2005). Sexual abuse of older adults: Assessing for signs of a serious crime and reporting it. *American Journal of Nursing, 105*(10), 66–71.

Calianno, C., & Martin-Boyan, A. (2006). When is it appropriate to photograph a patient's wound? *Advances in Skin & Wound Care, 19*(6), 304–307.

Cohen, S. S. (2003). *Trauma nursing secrets.* Hanley & Belfus.

Hoyt, C. A. (2006). Integrating forensic science into nursing processes in the ICU. *Critical Care Nursing Quarterly, 29*(3), 259–270.

Lynch, V. A. (2006). *Forensic nursing.* Mosby.

Forgiveness Facilitation   5280

Definition: Assisting an individual's willingness to replace feelings of anger and resentment toward another, self, or higher power, with beneficence, empathy, and humility

Activities:
- Identify patient's beliefs that may hinder/help in "letting go" of an issue
- Acknowledge when anger and resentment are justifiable
- Identify source of anger and resentment, when possible
- Listen empathetically without moralizing or offering platitudes
- Explore forgiveness as a process
- Help the patient explore feelings of anger, bitterness, and resentment
- Use presence, touch, and empathy to facilitate the process, as appropriate
- Explore possibilities of making amends and reconciliation with self, others, and/or higher power
- Assist the patient to examine the health and healing dimension of forgiveness
- Assist patient to overcome blocks to healing by using spiritual practices (e.g., prayers of praise, guidance, and discernment; healing, touch, visualization of healing, and thanksgiving), as appropriate
- Teach the art of emotional release and relaxation
- Assist client to seek out arbitrator (objective party) to facilitate process of individual or group concern
- Invite use of faith tradition rituals, as appropriate (e.g., anointing, confession, reconciliation)
- Communicate God's/higher power's or inner self's forgiveness through prayer, scripture, other readings, as appropriate
- Communicate acceptance for the individual's level of progress

3rd edition 2000; revised 2008

Background Evidence:

Brush, B. L., McGee, E. M., Cavanaugh, B., & Woodward, M. (2001). Forgiveness: A concept analysis. *Journal of Holistic Nursing, 19*(1), 27–41.

Burkhardt, M. A., & Nagai-Jacobson, M. G. (2002). *Spirituality: Living our connectedness.* Albany, NY: Delmar.

Enright, R. D. (2001). *Forgiveness is a choice: A step-by-step process for resolving anger and restoring hope.* American Psychological Association.

Enright, R. D., & Fitzgibbons, R. P. (2000). *Helping clients to forgive: An empirical guide for resolving anger and restoring hope.* American Psychological Association.

Festa, L. M., & Tuck, I. (2000). A review of forgiveness literature and with implications for nursing practice. *Holistic Nursing Practice, 14*(4), 77–86.

Worthington, E. L., Jr. (1998). An empathy-humility-commitment model of forgiveness applied within family dyads. *Journal of Family Therapy, 20*(1), 59–76.

Functional Ability Enhancement   1665

Definition: Maximizing physical functioning to prevent a decline in activities of daily living

Activities:
- Establish realistic functional goals with a plan to achieve these
- Address risk factors that affect goal achievement (e.g., side effects of multiple medications, recent hospitalization visit, depression, impaired cognition, nutritional problems, fear of falling)
- Address disease processes (e.g., thyroid disease, infection, cardiac or pulmonary conditions, metabolic disturbances, anemia) that may be the cause of functional decline
- Determine need for glasses, hearing aids, and mobility devices (e.g., cane, walker)
- Ensure adequate lighting, nonglare flooring, nonslip carpets, and handrails, where needed
- Address problems in sleep-wake cycle (e.g., excessive daytime napping, nocturnal wakefulness), as needed
- Address use of alcohol, tobacco, and illicit drugs
- Modify tasks or environment, as needed
- Increase pulmonary function through aerobic exercises and muscle reconditioning, as needed
- Explore barriers to exercise
- Encourage individual to begin or continue exercise
- Assist individual to develop an appropriate exercise program to meet needs
- Include family and caregivers in planning and maintaining the exercise program
- Advise older adults about ways to optimize cognitive abilities in aging, including puzzles, word games, computer use
- Counsel patients on cognitive benefits of social engagement, balanced nutrition, and physical activities
- Educate older adults to promote understanding of age-related changes, appropriate lifestyle adjustments, and effective coping
- Assist in planning a well-balanced diet, if needed
- Encourage regularly scheduled visits with a health care provider
- Provide positive feedback for individual's efforts

7th edition 2018

Background Evidence:

Aldwin, C. M., & Gilmer, D. F. (2013). *Health, illness, and optimal aging: Biological and psychosocial perspectives* (2nd ed.). Springer.

Boltz, M., Resnik, B., & Galik, E. (2013). *Nursing standard of practice protocol: Function-focused care (FFC) interventions.* https://consultgeri.org/geriatric-topics/function-focused-care-ffc-interventions

Matzo, M., & Sherman, D. W. (2015). *Palliative care nursing: Quality care to the end of life* (4th ed.). Springer.

Potter, P. A., Perry, A. G., Stockert, P. A., & Hall, A. M. (2013). *Fundamentals of nursing* (8th ed.). Elsevier Mosby.

Williams, K., & Kemper, S. (2010). Exploring interventions to reduce cognitive decline in aging. *Journal of Psychosocial Nursing Mental Health Services, 48*(5), 42–51.

F

Gardening Therapy 4368

Definition: Using gardening to promote physical, psychological, social, or spiritual health and well-being

Activities:

- Determine desired change in social, physical, behavioral, spiritual, or group dynamics (e.g., relaxation, stimulation, concentration, stress reduction, physical activity)
- Describe purpose of gardening and skills needed for successful experience including pacing physical activity, observational skills and tasks needed for optimal plant growth, and time of activities
- Identify gardening preferences (e.g., indoor, outdoor, seasonal, location, time commitment)
- Choose plants (e.g., vegetables, flowers, herbs) and garden location (e.g., indoor, outdoor, raised beds) preferences
- Limit exposure to extraneous physical stress (e.g., excessive heat, cold, rain, lightning)
- Adapt gardening activities to endurance levels and abilities
- Make gardening equipment, fertilizer, and water available
- Provide ongoing gardening advice
- Provide educational materials at appropriate learning level
- Allow time for self-reflection, group interchange, and therapeutic evaluation
- Actively encourage participation with others to promote social interaction
- Monitor quality, transformation, and quantity of plants and produce
- Monitor physical, social, and therapeutic response
- Debrief regularly on challenges and benefits of gardening

8th edition 2024

Background Evidence:

Bassi, M., Rassiga, C., Fumagalli, N., & Senes, G. (2018). Quality of experience during horticultural activities: an experience sampling pilot study among older adults living in a nursing home. *Geriatric Nursing*, *39*(4), 457–464. https://doi.org/10.1016/j.gerinurse.2018.01.002

Brown, B., Dybdal, L., Noonan, C., Pedersen, M. G., Parker, M., & Corcoran, M. (2020). Group gardening in a Native American Community: A collaborative approach. *Health Promotion Practice*, *21*(4), 611–623. https://doi.org/10.1177/1524839919830930

Chalmin-Pui, L. S., Griffiths, A., Roe, J., Heaton, T., & Cameron, R. (2021). Why garden? – Attitudes and the perceived health benefits of home gardening, *Cities*, *112*, 103118. https://doi.org/10.1016/j.cities.2021.103118

Chu, H.-Y., Chen, M.-F., Tsai, C.-C., Chan, H.-S., & Wu, T.-L. (2019). Efficacy of a horticultural activity program for reducing depression and loneliness in older residents of nursing homes in Taiwan. *Geriatric Nursing*, *40*(4), 386–391. https://doi.org/10.1016/j.gerinurse.2018.12.012

Dahlkvist, E., Engström, M., & Nilsson, A. (2020). Residents' use and perceptions of residential care facility gardens: A behaviour mapping and conversation study. *International Journal of Older People Nursing*, *15*(1), e12283. https://doi.org/10.1111/opn.12283

Hardin-Fanning, F., Adegboyega, A. O., & Rayens, M. K. (2018). Adolescents' perceptions of a gardening activity at a juvenile justice center. *Journal of Holistic Nursing*, *36*(2), 170–178. https://doi.org/10.1177/0898010117707865

Lohr, A. M., Henry, N., Roe, D., Rodriguez, C., Romero, R., & Ingram, M. (2020). Evaluation of the impact of school garden exposure on youth outlook and behaviors toward vegetables in Southern Arizona. *Journal of School Health*, *90*(7), 572–581. https://doi.org/10.1111/josh.12905

Stowell, D. R., Owens, G. P., & Burnett, A. (2018). A pilot horticultural therapy program serving veterans with mental health issues: Feasibility and outcomes. *Complementary Therapies in Clinical Practice*, *32*, 74–78. https://doi.org/10.1016/j.ctcp.2018.05.007

Thompson, R. (2018). Gardening for health: a regular dose of gardening. *Clinical Medicine (London, England)*, *18*(3), 201–205.

White, P. C. L., Wyatt, J., Chalfont, G., Bland, J. M., Neale, C., Trepel, D., & Graham, H. (2018). Exposure to nature gardens has time-dependent associations with mood improvements for people with mid- and late-stage dementia: Innovative practice. *Dementia*, *17*(5), 627–634. https://doi.org/10.1177/1471301217723772

Genetic Counseling 5242

Definition: Use of a therapeutic communication process to help individual, family, or group to understand and cope with specific genetic condition

Activities:

- Ensure privacy and confidentiality
- Establish therapeutic relationship based on trust, empathy, compassion, and respect
- Determine knowledge base, myths, perceptions, and misperceptions related to genetic conditions
- Explore confirmed genetic risk factors to determine level of understanding
- Determine purpose, goals, and agenda for genetic counseling session
- Determine presence and quality of support systems and previous coping skills
- Explore estimates of risk, based upon phenotype (e.g., person characteristics), family history (e.g., pedigree analysis), calculated risk information, or genotype (e.g., genetic testing results)
- Provide estimates of occurrence or recurrence risk for person and at-risk family members
- Provide information on natural history of disease or condition, treatment and management strategies, prognostic information, and prevention strategies, if known
- Provide information about risks, benefits, and limitations of treatment or management options, as well as options for dealing with recurrence risk
- Provide decision-making support as persons consider their options
- Prioritize areas of risk reduction in collaboration with individual, family, or group
- Monitor response when person learns about own genetic risk factors
- Allow and stimulate expression of feelings

- Support coping process
- Institute crisis support skills, as needed
- Provide referral to genetic health care specialists, as necessary
- Provide referral to community resources, including genetic support groups, as needed
- Record summary of genetic counseling session, as indicated
- Use teach-back to ensure understanding

1st edition 1992; revised 2000, 2024

Background Evidence:

McEwen, A., & Jacobs, C. (2021). Who we are, what we do, and how we add value: The role of the genetic counseling 'philosophy of practice' statement in a changing time. *Journal of Genetic Counseling, 30*(1), 114–120. https://doi.org/10.1002/jgc4.1308

Mendes, Á., Metcalfe, A., Paneque, M., Sousa, L., Clarke, A. J., & Sequeiros, J. (2018). Communication of information about genetic risks: Putting families at the center. *Family Process, 57*(3), 836–846. https://doi.org/10.1111/famp.12306

Patch, C., & Middleton, A. (2018). Genetic counselling in the era of genomic medicine. *British Medical Bulletin, 126*(1), 27–36. https://doi.org/10.1093/bmb/ldy008

Sharma, S., Khanna, G., & Gangane, S. D. (2019). *Textbook of pathology and genetics for nurses* (2nd ed.). Elsevier.

G

Grief Work Facilitation 5290

Definition: Assistance with the resolution of a significant loss

Activities:

- Provide privacy and ensure confidentiality
- Convey authenticity, warmth, genuineness, interest, and unconditional caring
- Introduce self and ensure person comfortable
- Identify loss
- Assist in identifying nature of attachment to lost object or person
- Consider social context of person experiencing loss
- Assist to identify initial reaction to loss
- Encourage expression of feelings about loss
- Actively listen to expressions of grief
- Assist expression of feelings of guilt
- Encourage discussion of previous loss experiences
- Encourage expression of memories of loss, both past and current
- Assure that grief is natural reaction to experiencing loss
- Assure that everyone experiences grief in own unique way
- Make empathetic statements about grief
- Encourage identification of greatest fears concerning loss
- Explain phases of grieving process, as appropriate
- Support progression through personal grieving stages
- Include significant others in discussions and decisions, as appropriate
- Assist to identify personal coping strategies
- Encourage to implement cultural, religious, and social customs associated with loss
- Communicate acceptance of discussing loss
- Answer children's questions associated with loss
- Use clear words, such as "dead" or "died", rather than euphemisms
- Encourage children to discuss feelings
- Encourage expression of feelings in ways comfortable to child, such as writing, drawing, or playing
- Assist child to clarify misconceptions
- Identify sources of community support
- Recommend attending grief support group, if appropriate
- Support efforts to resolve previous conflict, as appropriate
- Reinforce progress made in grieving process
- Assist in identifying modifications needed in lifestyle

1st edition 1992; revised 2004, 2024

Background Evidence:

Harrop, E., Morgan, F., Longo, M., Semedo, L., Fitzgibbon, J., Pickett, S., Scott, H., Seddon, K., Sivell, S., Nelson, A., & Byrne, A. (2020). The impacts and effectiveness of support for people bereaved through advanced illness: A systematic review and thematic synthesis. *Palliative Medicine, 34*(7), 871–888.

Milman, E., Neimeyer, R. A., Fitzpatrick, M., MacKinnon, C. J., Muis, K. R., & Cohen, S. R. (2019). Prolonged grief and the disruption of meaning: Establishing a mediation model. *Journal of Counseling Psychology, 66*(6), 714–725.

Thacker, N. E., & Duran, A. (2020). Operationalizing intersectionality as a framework in qualitative grief research. *Death Studies,* 1–11.

Grief Work Facilitation: Perinatal Death 5294

Definition: Assistance with the resolution of a perinatal loss

Activities:

- Discuss what to expect with parents and family if the loss is impending or likely
- Encourage participation in decisions about discontinuing life support
- Assist in keeping infant alive until parents arrive
- Baptize the infant, as appropriate
- Encourage parents in holding infant while dying, as appropriate
- Support parents and family in whatever attachment they may or may not have to the pregnancy and fetus

- Determine how and when the fetal or infant death was diagnosed
- Discuss plans that have been made (e.g., burial, funeral, infant name)
- Discuss decisions that will need to be made about funeral arrangements, autopsy, genetic counseling, and family participation
- Describe mementos that will be obtained, including footprints, handprints, pictures, caps, gowns, blankets, diapers, and blood pressure cuffs, as appropriate
- Discuss available support groups, as appropriate
- Discuss differences between male and female patterns of grieving, as appropriate
- Obtain infant footprints, handprints, length, and weight, as needed
- Prepare infant for viewing by bathing and dressing, including parents in activities, as appropriate
- Encourage family members to view and hold infant for as long as desired
- Discuss appearance of infant based on gestational age and length of demise
- Focus on normal features of infant, while sensitively discussing anomalies
- Encourage family time alone with infant, as desired
- Provide referrals to chaplain, social service, grief counselor, and genetic counselor, as appropriate
- Create keepsakes and present to family before discharge, as appropriate
- Offer to complete a commemorative birth certificate if state law does not require one at the gestational age of delivery
- Discuss characteristics of normal and abnormal grieving, including triggers that precipitate feelings of sadness
- Notify laboratory or funeral home for disposition of body, as appropriate
- Transfer infant to morgue or prepare body to be transported by family to funeral home

2nd edition 1996; revised 2018

Background Evidence:

Broderick, S., & Cochraine, R. (2013). *Perinatal loss: A handbook for working with women and their families*. Radcliffe.

Hochberg, T. (2011). Moments held—photographing perinatal loss. *The Lancet, 377*(9774), 1310–1311.

Johnson, O., & Langford, R. W. (2010). Proof of life: A protocol for pregnant women who experience pre-20-week perinatal loss. *Critical Care Nursing Quarterly, 33*(3), 204–211.

Lang, A., Fleiszer, A., Duhamel, F., Sword, W., Gilbert, K., & Corsini-Munt, S. (2011). Perinatal loss and parental grief: The challenge of ambiguity and disenfranchised grief. *OMEGA-Journal of Death and Dying, 63*(2), 183–196.

Limbo, R., & Kobler, K. (2010). The tie that binds: Relationships in perinatal bereavement. *MCN: The American Journal of Maternal/Child Nursing, 35*(6), 316–321.

Musters, A., Taminiau-Bloem, E., van den Boogaard, E., van der Veen, F., & Goddijn, M. (2011). Supportive care for women with unexplained recurrent miscarriage: Patients' perspectives. *Human Reproduction, 26*(4), 873–877.

Guided Imagery   6000

Definition: Purposeful use of imagination to achieve a particular state, outcome, or action or to direct attention away from undesirable sensations

Activities:

- Screen for severe emotional problems, history of psychiatric illness, or hallucinations
- Screen for current decreased energy level, inability to concentrate, or other symptoms that may interfere with cognitive ability to create focus on mental images
- Describe the rationale for and the benefits, limitations, and types of guided imagery techniques available
- Elicit information on past coping experiences to determine whether guided imagery might be helpful
- Discuss ability to create vivid mental images and to experience them as if they were real
- Determine capability for doing non-nurse guided imagery (e.g., alone or with tape)
- Encourage the individual to choose from a variety of guided imagery techniques (e.g., nurse guided, taped)
- Suggest that the individual assume a comfortable position, with unrestricted clothing and eyes closed
- Provide comfortable environment without interruptions (e.g., using headphones), as possible
- Discuss an image the patient has experienced that is pleasurable and relaxing, such as lying on a beach, watching a new snowfall, floating on a raft, or watching the sun set
- Individualize the images chosen, considering religious or spiritual beliefs, artistic interest, or other individual preferences
- Described the scene using as many of the five senses as possible
- Make suggestions to induce relaxation (e.g., peaceful images, pleasant sensations, or rhythmic breathing), as appropriate
- Use modulated voice when guiding the imagery experience
- Have the patient travel mentally to the scene and assist in describing the setting in detail
- Use permissive directions and suggestions when leading the imagery, such as "perhaps," "if you wish," or "you might like"
- Have the patient slowly experience the scene: how does it look? smell? sound? feel? taste?
- Use words or phrases that convey pleasurable images, such as floating, melting, releasing, and so on
- Develop cleansing or clearing portion of imagery (e.g., all pain appears as red dust and washes downstream in a creek as you enter)
- Assist the patient to develop a method of ending the imagery technique, such as counting slowly while breathing deeply, slow movements, and thoughts of being relaxed, refreshed, and alert
- Encourage patient to express thoughts and feelings regarding the experience
- Prepare patient for unexpected (but often therapeutic) experiences, such as crying
- Instruct patient to practice the imagery, if possible
- Tape-record the imaged experience if useful
- Plan with patient an appropriate time to do guided imagery

- Use the imagery techniques preventively
- Plan follow-up to assess effects of imagery and any resultant changes in sensation and perception
- Use guided imagery as an adjuvant strategy to pain medications or in conjunction with other measures, as appropriate
- Evaluate and document response to guided imagery

1st edition 1992; revised 2008

Background Evidence:

Dossey, B. (1995). Using imagery to help heal your patient. *American Journal of Nursing, 95*(6), 41–46.

Eller, L. S. (1999). Guided imagery interventions for symptom management. In J. (1999). Fitzpatrick (Ed.), *Annual review of nursing research* (Vol. 17, pp. 57–84). Springer.

Herr, K. A., & Mobily, P. R. (1999). Pain management. In G. M. Bulechek & J. C. McCloskey (Eds.), *Nursing interventions: Effective nursing treatments* (3rd ed., pp. 149–171). W.B. Saunders.

Kwekkeboom, K., Kneip, J., & Pearson, L. (2003). A pilot study to predict success with guided imagery for cancer pain. *Pain Management Nursing, 4*(3), 112–123.

McCaffery, M., & Pasero, C. (1999). Practical nondrug approaches to pain. In M. McCaffery & C. Pasero (Eds.), *Pain: Clinical manual* (2nd ed., pp. 399–427). Mosby.

Post-White, J. (1998). Imagery. In M. Snyder & R. Lindquist (Eds.), *Complementary/Alternative therapies in nursing* (3rd ed., pp. 103–122). Springer.

Van Kuiken, D. (2004). A meta-analysis of the effect of guided imagery practice on outcomes. *Journal of Holistic Nursing, 22*(2), 164–179.

G

Guided Reflection   4730

Definition: Assisting a person to thoughtfully examine and explore an experience to achieve deeper insight, meaning, and understanding

Activities:

- Determine willingness to engage in reflection processes
- Determine if concern or experience appropriate for guided reflection process
- Select strategies for engaging in reflection activities (e.g., in person, internet, telehealth, written reflection)
- Establish therapeutic relationship based on trust and respect
- Demonstrate empathy, warmth, and genuineness
- Identify focus of guided reflection with person
- Determine agreeable time allowance
- Monitor feelings and emotions expressed during reflection
- Assist to describe what occurred (e.g., What, where and when did this happen? What did you do? In what order did things occur? What was the result?)
- Ask to describe what they were thinking and feeling about event (e.g., What was your initial reaction? What were you thinking or feeling during and after situation? What do you think about it now?)
- Support expression of thoughts and feelings through use of silence and active listening
- Encourage to think-aloud while examining experience to enhance clarity
- Avoid barriers to active listening (e.g., minimizing feelings, offering easy solutions, interrupting, talking about self, premature closure)
- Assist in evaluating experience (e.g., What went well? What were the challenges? Who or what was unhelpful? What needs improvement?)
- Assist in clarifying misinformation or inaccuracies, if indicated
- Assist in seeking needed information and resources
- Assist in finding meaning in situation (e.g., What similarities or differences are there between this experience and other experiences? What choices did you make and what effect did they have? What did you do well? What went wrong or did not turn out how it should have done?)
- Explore other actions or choices that could have been taken (e.g., What factors do you believe affected the outcome? What are some alternative actions or approaches?)
- Explore different choices for future occurrences of same situation (e.g., If similar situation or experience arose again, what would you do? What might you do to increase likelihood of positive outcomes and minimize likelihood of undesirable outcomes? What did you learn from this experience?)
- Explore progress toward resolution at appropriate intervals
- End session by encouraging reflection on discussion and what was learned, as appropriate
- Refer to counseling, support group, or other health care providers at end of session, if indicated
- Document as appropriate

8th edition 2024

Background Evidence:

Aaron, L., Hicks, J., McKnight, A., & Andary, J. (2021). Reflection as a tool for personal and professional development. *Radiologic Technology, 93*(2), 130–140.

Engbers, R. A. (2020). Students' perceptions of interventions designed to foster empathy: An integrative review. *Nurse Education Today, 86*, 104325. https://doi.org/10.1016/j.nedt.2019.104325

Fearon-Lynch, J. A., Sethares, K. A., Asselin, M. E., Batty, K., & Stover, C. M. (2019). The effects of guided reflection on diabetes self-care: A randomized controlled trial. *The Diabetes Educator, 45*(1), 66–79.

Frauenfelder, F. (2019). Psychiatric adult inpatient nursing described in the NANDA-I and NIC: A systematic evaluation of nursing classifications [Doctoral dissertation. Radbound University] Radbound Repository. https://repository.ubn.ru.nl/handle/2066/203856

Jobes, M. J., & Duncan, K. (2019). A guided reflection activity on sudden death. *Journal of Nursing Education, 58*(5), 313.

Johnson, R., & Richard-Eaglin, A. (2020). Combining SOAP notes with guided reflection to address implicit bias in health care. *Journal of Nursing Education, 59*(1), 59. https://doi.org/10.3928/01484834-20191223-16

Sethares, K. , A., & Asselin, M. E. (2017). The effect of guided reflection on heart failure self-care maintenance and management: A mixed methods study, *Heart Lung, 46*(3), 192–198.

Walsh, J. A., & Sethares, K. A. (2022). The use of guided reflection in simulation-based education with prelicensure nursing students: An integrative review. *Journal of Nursing Education, 61*(2), 73–79. https://doi.org/10.3928/01484834-20211213-01

Guilt Work Facilitation   5300

Definition: Helping another to cope with painful feelings of actual or perceived responsibility

Activities:

- Guide patient/family in identifying painful feelings of guilt
- Help patient/family identify and examine the situations in which these feelings are experienced or generated
- Assist patient/family members to identify their behaviors in the guilt situation
- Help patient/family understand that guilt is a common reaction to trauma, abuse, grief, catastrophic illness, or accidents
- Use reality testing to help the patient/family identify possible irrational beliefs
- Help patient/family to identify destructive displacement of feelings onto other individuals sharing responsibility in the situation
- Facilitate discussion of the effect of the situation on family relationships
- Facilitate genetic counseling, as appropriate
- Refer patient/family to the appropriate trauma, abuse, grief, illness, caregiver, or survivor group for education and support
- Facilitate spiritual support, as appropriate
- Teach patient to use thought stopping technique and thought substitution in conjunction with deliberate muscle relaxation when persistent thoughts of guilt enter the mind
- Guide the patient through steps of self-forgiveness when one's guilt is valid

- Assist the patient/family to identify options for prevention, restitution, atonement, and resolution, when appropriate

1st edition 1992; revised 2008

Background Evidence:

Antai-Otong, D. (2003). Crisis intervention management: The role of adaptation. In *Psychiatric nursing: Biological and behavioral concepts* (pp. 841–862). Thomson Delmar Learning.

Kemp, C. (2004). Grief and loss. In K. M. Fortinash & P. A. Holloday Worret (Eds.), *Psychiatric mental health nursing* (3rd ed., pp. 573–588). Mosby.

Stuart, G. (2005). Self-concept responses and dissociative disorders. In G. W. Stuart & M. T. Laraia (Eds.), *Principles and practice of psychiatric nursing* (8th ed., pp. 303–329). Mosby.

Sundeen, S. (2005). Psychiatric rehabilitation and recovery. In G. W. Stuart & M. T. Laraia (Eds.), *Principles and practice of psychiatric nursing* (8th ed., pp. 239–257). Mosby.

Veenema, T. G., & Schroeder-Bruce, K. (2002). The aftermath of violence: Children, disaster, and posttraumatic stress disorder. *Journal of Pediatric Health Care, 16*(5), 235–244.

G

Hair and Scalp Care   1670

Definition: Promotion of healthy, clean, and attractive hair and scalp

Activities:

- Monitor condition of hair and scalp, including abnormalities (e.g., dry, course, or brittle hair, pest infestation, dandruff, and nutritional deficiencies)
- Provide treatment for abnormalities or notify appropriate health care provider
- Prepare supplies for cleansing hair (e.g., basin, shampoo board, waterproof pad, towel, shampoo, and conditioner)
- Assist patient into comfortable position
- Use hydrogen peroxide or alcohol to dissolve matted blood, if present, before cleansing hair
- Place commercially prepared, disposable cleansing cap on patient's head and massage head to work solution through hair and scalp, being sure to use cap according to manufacturer's instructions
- Wash and condition hair, massaging shampoo and conditioner into scalp and hair
- Avoid chilling during cleansing (i.e., adjust room temperature and provide warmed towels)
- Dry hair with hair dryer on a low setting to avoid burning scalp
- Brush or comb hair, using wide-toothed comb or pick, as needed
- Apply small amount of oil to dry or flaking areas of scalp
- Style hair
- Monitor patient response to hair loss, providing support (i.e., assist in selecting a hat, wig, or scarf, refer to community agency, and discuss hair transplants and drugs to stimulate hair growth), if indicated
- Arrange for barber or hairdresser to cut hair
- Prepare supplies for shaving (e.g., shaving cream, towel, and safety or electric razor)
- Shave bodily hair using an electric razor for patients at-risk for excessive bleeding, if desired
- Perform hair removal procedures using scissors, hair clippers, or chemical depilatory agents before surgical procedure, being sure to refer to institutional policies and physician order
- Instruct patient or parent on hair care (e.g., cleansing infant scalp and hair and preventing pest infestation)
- Provide referral, as appropriate

1st edition 1992; revised 2008, 2013

Background Evidence:

Craven, R., & Hirnle, C. (2009). *Fundamentals of nursing: Human health and function* (6th ed.). Lippincott Williams & Wilkins.

Smith, S. F., Duell, D. J., & Martin, B. C. (2008). *Clinical nursing skills: Basic to advanced skills* (7th ed.). Pearson Prentice Hall.

Titler, M., Pettit, D., Bulechek, G., McCloskey, J., Craft, M., Cohen, M., Crossley, J. D., Denehy, J. A., Glick, O. J., Kruckeberg, T. W., Maas, M. L., Prophet, C. M., & Tripp-Reimer, T. (1991). Classification of nursing interventions for care of the integument. *Nursing Diagnosis, 2*(2), 45–56.

H

Hallucination Management   6510

Definition: Promoting the safety, comfort, and reality orientation of a patient experiencing hallucinations

Activities:

- Establish a trusting, interpersonal relationship with the patient
- Monitor and regulate the level of activity and stimulation in the environment
- Maintain a safe environment
- Provide appropriate level of supervision to monitor patient
- Record patient behaviors that indicate hallucinations
- Maintain a consistent routine
- Assign consistent caregivers on a daily basis
- Promote clear and open communication
- Use concrete statements rather than abstract statements when speaking to the patient
- Provide patient with opportunities to discuss hallucinations
- Encourage patient to express feelings appropriately
- Refocus patient to topic, if patient's communication is inappropriate to circumstances
- Monitor hallucinations for presence of content that is violent or self-harmful
- Encourage patient to develop control and responsibility over own behavior, if ability allows
- Encourage patient to discuss feelings and impulses, rather than acting on them
- Encourage patient to validate hallucinations with trusted others (e.g., reality testing)
- Point out, if asked, that you are not experiencing the same stimuli
- Avoid arguing with patient about the validity of the hallucinations
- Focus discussion upon the underlying feelings, rather than the content of the hallucinations (e.g., "It appears as if you are feeling frightened")
- Provide antipsychotic and antianxiety medications on a routine and PRN basis
- Provide medication information to patient and significant others
- Monitor patient for medication side effects and desired therapeutic effects
- Provide for safety and comfort of patient and others when patient is unable to control behavior (e.g., limit setting, area restriction, physical restraint, and seclusion)
- Discontinue or decrease medications (after consulting with prescribing caregiver) that may be causing hallucinations
- Provide illness information to patient and significant others if hallucinations are illness based (e.g., delirium, schizophrenia, depression)
- Educate family and significant others about ways to deal with patient who is experiencing hallucinations
- Monitor self-care ability
- Assist with self-care, as needed
- Monitor physical status of patient (e.g., body weight, hydration, soles of feet in patient who paces)
- Provide for adequate rest and nutrition
- Involve patient in reality-based activities that may distract from the hallucinations (e.g., listening to music)

1st edition 1992; revised 1996, 2018

Background Evidence:

Bostrum, A. C., & Boyd, M. A. (2005). Schizophrenia. In M. A. Boyd (Ed.), *Psychiatric nursing: Contemporary practice* (3rd ed., pp. 265–310). Lippincott Williams & Wilkins.

Fortinash, K., & Worret, P. (2012). Schizophrenia and other psychotic disorders. In *Psychiatric mental health nursing* (pp. 259–299) (5th ed.). Mosby Elsevier.

Moller, M. (2009). Neurobiological responses and schizophrenia and psychotic disorders. In G. W. Stuart (Ed.), *Principles and practice of psychiatric nursing* (9th ed., pp. 334–368). Mosby Elsevier.

Varcarolis, E. M. (2006). Schizophrenia and other psychotic disorders. In *Manual of psychiatric nursing care plans* (pp. 232–237) (3rd ed.). Saunders Elsevier.

Yang, C., Lee, T., Lo, S., & Beckstead, J. (2015). The effects of auditory hallucination symptom management programme for people with schizophrenia: A quasi-experimental design. *Journal of Advanced Nursing, 71*(12), 2886–2897.

Handoff Report   8140

Definition: Exchanging essential patient care information with other nursing staff at change of shift or change of care setting

Activities:

- Select the type of reporting (e.g., face to face, audiotape, at patient's bedside, walking rounds, electronic health record summary, team huddle) to use
- Introduce self to oncoming staff, as needed
- Review pertinent demographic data, including name, age, and room number
- Identify chief complaint, reason for admission, and recent surgeries, as appropriate
- Identify attending and consulting physicians
- Summarize significant past health history, as necessary
- Identify key medical and nursing diagnoses, as appropriate
- Identify resolved medical and nursing diagnoses, as appropriate
- Present information succinctly, focusing on recent and significant data needed by nursing staff assuming responsibility for care
- Encourage patient to contribute to report and to ask questions if it is given at bedside
- Use a standardized report format, tool, or mnemonic (e.g., SBAR: Situation, Background, Assessment, Recommendation)
- Describe treatment regimen, including diet, fluid therapy, medications, and exercise
- Review the tubes the patient has, where they are, when they were placed, and when containers need to be emptied, as appropriate
- Identify laboratory and diagnostic tests to be completed during the next 24 hours
- Review recent pertinent laboratory and diagnostic test results, as appropriate
- Describe health status data, including vital signs and signs and symptoms present during the recent care period
- Describe nursing interventions being implemented
- Describe patient and family response to nursing interventions
- Summarize progress toward goals
- Summarize discharge plans, as appropriate
- Train nurses new to the clinical setting in the handoff process
- Evaluate the handoff process periodically and revise, as indicated

2nd edition 1996; revised 2018

Background Evidence:

Agency for Healthcare Research and Quality. (2013). *Nurse bedside shift report: Implementation handbook.* http://www.ahrq.gov/professionals/systems/hospital/engagingfamilies/strategy3/index.html

Laws, D., & Amato, S. (2010). Incorporating bedside reporting into change-of-shift report. *Rehabilitation Nursing, 35*(2), 70–74.

Riesenberg, L. A., Leitzsch, J., & Cunningham, J. M. (2010). Nursing handoffs: A systematic review of the literature. *American Journal of Nursing, 110*(4), 24–34.

Staggers, N., & Jennings, B. M. (2009). The content and context of change of shift report on medical and surgical units. *Journal of Nursing Administration, 39*(9), 393–398.

Wakefield, D. S., Ragan, R., Brandt, J., & Tregnago, M. (2012). Making the transition to nursing bedside shift reports. *The Joint Commission Journal on Quality and Patient Safety, 38*(6), 243–253.

Healing Touch   1390

Definition: Providing a noninvasive, biofield therapy using touch and compassionate intentionality to influence the energy system of a person, affecting their physical, emotional, mental, and spiritual health and healing

Activities:

- Create a comfortable, private environment without distractions
- Determine willingness to have body touched
- Identify mutual goals for the session
- Advise the patient to ask questions whenever they arise
- Place patient in a comfortable and safe position that facilitates relaxation (e.g., chair, recliner, or massage table may be used if the body can be safely supported)
- Remove constricting items (e.g., eyeglasses, shoes, and belt)
- Keep the patient comfortably clothed
- Drape only to provide temperature comfort
- Center self by focusing awareness on inner self
- Ground self by attuning to earth's energy
- Attune to the patient's energy field
- Set intention to work for the patient's highest good
- Conduct an assessment of the patient's energy field (aura) and energy centers to determine whether clearing, balancing, or energizing techniques are to be used
- Determine the specific healing touch approach to promote healing (e.g., unruffling or smoothing the energy field, full body connection, Etheric Vitality, magnetic unruffled, magnetic pain drain, spiral meditation, pyramid technique)

- Use hands to clear, balance, and energize the patient's field
- Continue until the energy fields and energy centers feel balanced, smooth, connected, symmetrical, and flowing
- Repeat an energy assessment to identify what changes have occurred
- Instruct the patient to gently move his or her body and stretch before one gets up
- Touch the patient's body to help him or her ground or connect with the earth's energy if they experience dizziness when getting up
- Offer client a glass of water to replenish the water lost with the energy movement
- Provide feedback to the patient regarding the energetic work in terms he or she understands
- Ask the patient to describe what he or she experienced or noted during and after the session

- Record the characteristics of the energy work
- Record the physical, mental, and emotional responses to session

6th edition 2013

Background Evidence:

Hover-Kramer, D. (2002). *Healing touch: A guidebook for practitioners.* Delmar Thomson Learning.

Hutchison, C. P. (1999). Healing touch: An energetic approach. *American Journal of Nursing, 99*(4), 43–48.

Umbreit, A. (2006). Healing touch. In M. Snyder & R. Lindquist (Eds.), *Complementary/alternative therapies in nursing* (5th ed., pp. 203–223). Springer.

Wardell, D. W., & Weymouth, K. F. (2004). Review of studies of healing touch. *Journal of Nursing Scholarship, 36*(2), 147–154.

Health Care Information Exchange   7960

Definition: Providing patient care information to other health professionals

Activities:
- Identify yourself or other referring professional and location
- Obtain physician order for referral, if required
- Identify patient's essential demographic data
- Describe pertinent past health history
- Identify current nursing and medical diagnoses
- Identify resolved nursing and medical diagnoses, as appropriate
- Describe plan of care, including diet, medications, and exercise
- Describe nursing interventions being implemented
- Identify equipment and supplies necessary for care
- Summarize progress of patient toward goals
- Identify anticipated date of discharge or transfer, as appropriate
- Identify planned return appointment for follow-up care, as appropriate
- Discuss patient's strengths and resources
- Describe role of family in continuing care
- Identify other agencies providing care
- Request information from health professionals in other agencies
- Coordinate care with other health professionals
- Share concerns of patient or family with other health care providers
- Share information from other health professionals with patient and family, as appropriate
- Transfer information via electronic technology if available

- Participate in the development and improvement of electronic patient records
- Maintain education related to knowledge of health information technology

2nd edition 1996; revised 2004, 2018

Background Evidence:

Berman, A., & Snyder, S. (2012). *Kozier & Erb's fundamentals of nursing: Concepts, process, and practice* (9th ed.). Pearson Education.

Edwards, N., Davies, B., Ploeg, J., Virani, T., & Skelly, J. (2007). Implementing nursing best practice guidelines: Impact on patient referrals. *BMC Nursing, 6*(1), 1–9. https://doi.org/10.1186/1472-6955-6-4

Huston, C. (2013). The impact of emerging technology on nursing care: Warp speed ahead. *OJIN: The Online Journal of Issues in Nursing, 18*(2), Manuscript 1.

National Transitions of Care Coalition. (2010). *Improving transitions of care with health information technology.* http://www.ntocc.org/Portals/0/PDF/Resources/HITPaper.pdf

Vest, J. R., & Gamm, L. D. (2010). Health information exchange: Persistent challenges and new strategies. *Journal of the American Medical Informatics Association, 17*(3), 288–294.

Health Care Provider Collaboration   7685

Definition: Working interprofessionally to deliver quality health care

Activities:
- Establish working relationship with interprofessional team
- Participate in orientation of interprofessional team
- Assist health care providers to learn routines of care unit
- Participate in educational programs
- Encourage open, direct communication
- Follow-up important electronic messages (e.g., texts, e-mails) with verbal contact
- Encourage use of structured communication tool (e.g., Situation, Background, Assessment, Recommendation [SBAR]) to foster clear communication as needed

- Create and use system to inform interprofessional team of assigned caregivers
- Coach residents and health care providers through unfamiliar routines
- Alert interprofessional team to changes in scheduled procedures
- Discuss care concerns or practice-related issues directly with health care provider involved
- Encourage to voice concerns to interprofessional team
- Report changes in status, as appropriate
- Participate in bedside rounds and interprofessional care teams, as appropriate

H

- Participate on interprofessional committees to address clinical issues
- Use interprofessional projects and committees as forums
- Provide information to appropriate interprofessional team
- Follow up interprofessional team requests for new equipment or supplies
- Provide feedback to interprofessional team about changes in practice, equipment, and staffing
- Include interprofessional team on in-services for new equipment or practice changes
- Encourage interprofessional team to participate in collaborative education programs
- Support collaborative research and quality improvement activities

8th edition 2024

Background Evidence:

Abu Dalal, H. J., Ramoo, V., Chong, M. C., Danaee, M., & Aljeesh, Y. I. (2022). The impact of organizational communication satisfaction on health care professionals' work engagement. *Journal of Nursing Management, 30*(1), 214–225. https://doi.org/10.1111/jonm.13476

Berman, A., Snyder, S. J., & Frandsen, G. (2021). *Kozier and Erb's Fundamentals of nursing: Concepts, process and practice* (11th ed.). Pearson.

Craven, R. F., Hirnle, C. J., & Henshaw, C. J. (2021). *Fundamentals of nursing: Human health and function* (9th ed.). Wolters-Kluwer.

Galeno Rodrigues, M. E. N., da Costa Belarmino, A., Custódio, L. L., Verde Gomes, I. L., & Ferreira Júnior, A. R. (2020). Communication in health work during the COVID-19 pandemic. *Investigacion & Educacion En Enfermeria, 38*(3), 1–11. https://doi.org/10.17533/udea.iee.v38n3e09

Homeyer, S., Hoffmann, W., Hingst, P., Oppermann, R. F., & Dreier-Wolfgramm, A. (2018). Effects of interprofessional education for medical and nursing students: Enablers, barriers and expectations for optimizing future interprofessional collaboration—A qualitative study. *BMC Nursing, 17*(1), 1–10. https://doi.org/10.1186/s12912-018-0279-x

Michel, L. (2017). A failure to communicate? Doctors and nurses in American hospitals. *Journal of Health Politics, Policy & Law, 42*(4), 709–717. https://doi.org/10.1215/03616878-3856149

Potter, P. A., Ostendorf, W. R., & LaPlante, N. (2018). *Clinical nursing skills and techniques* (9th ed.). Mosby.

Williams, P. (2020). *Basic geriatric nursing* (7th ed.). Elsevier.

Health Coaching   5305

Definition: Helping individuals make choices and behavior changes that will promote their overall health and well-being

Activities:

- Create a relationship that promotes trust and intimacy
- Respect the individual as the authority on his own health and well-being
- Listen carefully and validate understanding of the individual's experience
- Review all aspects of the individual's life pertinent to health enhancement
- Refer the individual to other professionals and services, as appropriate
- Help the individual consider the stage of readiness for change (e.g., precontemplation, contemplation, preparation, action, maintenance)
- Help the individual to consider personal strengths, resources, and barriers to change
- Track the individual's concerns in a manner that leads to identification of goals that will be the focus of the coaching process
- Involve the individual in formulating goals that are specific, measurable, realistic, and time-lined
- Support the individual's inner wisdom, intuition, and innate ability for knowing what is best for self
- Assist the individual to identify strategies to attain goals
- Create with the individual an action plan with clearly defined steps and anticipated results
- Reinforce individual strengths and resources for the direction and action chosen
- Request that the individual commit to the plan and take action to move forward
- Provide support for new ideas, behaviors, and actions that involve risk taking or fear of failure
- Facilitate the individual to take action that will lead to achievement of desired goals and prevent relapse
- Assist the individual to evaluate the effectiveness of actions in relation to attainment of the expected goals
- Support autonomy by recognizing the individual is the determinant of progress and success
- Document evaluation of progress and attainment of coaching goals

7th edition 2018

Background Evidence:

Hayes, E., & Kalmakis, K. (2007). From the sidelines: Coaching as a nurse practitioner strategy for improving health outcomes. *Journal of the American Academy of Nurse Practitioner, 19*(11), 555–562.

Heinen, M., Bartholomew, L., Wensing, M., van de Kerkhof, P., & van Achterberg, T. (2006). Supporting adherence and healthy lifestyles in leg ulcer patients: Systematic development of the Lively Legs program for dermatology outpatient clinics. *Patient Education and Counseling, 61*(2), 279–291.

Hess, D., Dossey, B., Southard, M., Luck, S., Schalb, B., & Bark, L. (2013). *The art and science of nurse coaching: the provider's guide to coaching scope and competencies.* American Nurses Association.

Kreitzer, M. J., & Sierpina, V. (2008). Health coaching: Innovative education and clinical programs emerging. *Explore: The Journal of Science and Healing, 4*(2), 154–155.

H

Health Education   5510

Definition: Developing and providing instruction and learning experiences to facilitate voluntary changes in behavior conducive to health in individuals, families, groups, or communities

Activities:

- Target high-risk groups and age ranges that would benefit most from health education
- Target needs identified in United Nations' Sustainable Development Goals, Healthy People 2030: National Health Promotion and Disease Prevention Objectives, or other local, state, and national needs
- Identify internal or external individual, group or community factors that may enhance or reduce motivation for healthy behavior
- Determine type and focus of health education program (e.g., physical health, social health, emotional and mental health, spiritual health)
- Determine personal context and social-cultural history of health behavior
- Determine current health knowledge and lifestyle behaviors
- Assist in clarifying health beliefs and values
- Identify ethnic and cultural background, family and community support, social environment, accommodation, religion, spiritual beliefs and lifestyle factors
- Identify characteristics of target population that affect selection of learning strategies
- Prioritize individual learner needs based on person preference and needs, skills of nurse, resources available, and likelihood of successful goal attainment
- Formulate clear and achievable goals for health education program
- Identify resources (e.g., personnel, space, equipment, money) needed to conduct program
- Consider accessibility, consumer preference, and cost in program planning
- Strategically place attractive advertising to capture attention of target audience
- Use strategies to motivate people to change health or lifestyle behaviors
- Discuss group rules before starting health education group
- Emphasize immediate or short-term positive health benefits rather than long-term benefits or negative effects of noncompliance
- Determine model, methodology, modality (individual or group), and length of education session
- Design modules, number of sessions and schedule of health educational intervention considering needs of individuals, family or caregivers, community and health care professionals
- Use best available information (e.g., high quality research), understandable, adjusted to language and culture needs, using facilitative counseling and didactic teaching skills
- Incorporate strategies to enhance self-esteem of target audience
- Develop educational materials written at readability level appropriate to target audience
- Incorporate strategies for resisting unhealthy behavior or risk taking
- Facilitate dialogue, interaction, social learning, space for support and cooperation within group intervention
- Provide knowledge on specific illness (e.g., course of disease, etiological factors, effects and impact, common signs and symptoms, role of treatment in recovery, myths and misconceptions about specific illness), as necessary
- Instruct on medication management (e.g., teach about medications, compliance and adverse effects, when and how to seek treatment, answer questions, prepare for self-management), as necessary
- Provide knowledge related to relapse (e.g., identification and management of triggers, consequences, early signs and symptoms, early identification of impending relapse), as necessary
- Keep presentation focused and short, and begin and end on main point
- Encourage group activities to provide support and alleviate insecurities
- Use peer leaders, teachers, and support groups in implementing programs to groups less likely to listen to health professionals or adults (e.g., adolescents), as appropriate
- Encourage personal exchange of experiences
- Use lectures to convey maximum amount of information, when appropriate
- Use group discussions and role-playing to influence health beliefs, attitudes, and values
- Use demonstrations with return demonstrations, learner participation, and manipulation of materials when teaching psychomotor skills
- Use computer-assisted instruction, television, interactive video, and other technologies to convey information
- Use teleconferencing, telecommunications, and computer technologies for distance learning
- Involve in planning and implementing plans for lifestyle or health behavior modification
- Determine family, peer, and community support for behavior conducive to health
- Use social and family support systems to enhance effectiveness of lifestyle or health behavior modification
- Emphasize importance of healthy patterns of eating, sleeping, and exercising, to persons who model these values and behaviors to others, particularly children
- Use variety of strategies and intervention points in educational program
- Use teach-back to ensure understanding
- Plan long-term follow-up to reinforce health behavior or lifestyle changes
- Implement strategies to measure outcomes at regular intervals during and after completion of program
- Implement strategies to measure program and cost effectiveness of education, using data to improve effectiveness of subsequent programs
- Influence development of policy that guarantees health education as employee benefit
- Encourage policy in which insurance companies give consideration for premium reductions or benefits for healthful lifestyle practices

2nd edition 1996; revised 2000, 2024

Background Evidence:

Aşık, E., & Ünsal, G. (2020). An evaluation of a psychoeducation programme for emotion identification and expression in individuals diagnosed with schizophrenia. *International Journal of Mental Health Nursing, 29*(4), 693–702. https://doi.org/10.1111/inm.12703

H

Bastable, S. B. (2020). *Nurse as educator: Principles of teaching and learning for nursing practice* (5th ed.). Jones & Bartlett.

Iriarte-Roteta, A., Lopez-Dicastillo, O., Mujika, A., Ruiz-Zaldibar, C., Hernantes, N., Bermejo-Martins, E., & Pumar-Méndez, M. J. (2020). Nurses' role in health promotion and prevention: A critical interpretive synthesis. *Journal of Clinical Nursing, 29*(21–22), 3937–3949. https://doi.org/10.1111/jocn.15441

Magill, M., Martino, S., & Wampold, B. (2021). The principles and practices of psychoeducation with alcohol or other drug use disorders: A review and brief guide. *Journal of Substance Abuse Treatment, 126*, 108442. https://doi.org/10.1016/j.jsat.2021.108442

McElroy, K. G., Gilden, R., & Sattler, B. (2021). Environmental health nursing education: One school's journey. *Public Health Nursing, 38*(2), 258–265. https://doi.org/10.1111/phn.12815

Sarkhel, S., Singh, O. P., & Arora, M. (2020). Clinical practice guidelines for psychoeducation in psychiatric disorders general principles of psychoeducation. *Indian Journal of Psychiatry, 62*(Suppl 2), S319–323.

Sharpe, L., Jones, E., Ashton-James, C. E., Nicholas, M. K., & Refshauge, K. (2020). Necessary components of psychological treatment in pain management programs: A Delphi study. *European Journal of Pain, 24*(6), 1160–1168. https://doi.org/10.1002/ejp.1561

Ramos, C., Araruna, R., Lima, C., Santana, C., & Tanaka, L. H. (2018). Education practices: Research-action with nurses of Family Health Strategy. *Revista brasileira de enfermagem, 71*(3), 1144–1151. https://doi.org/10.1590/0034-7167-2017-0284

Ross, A., Yang, L., Wehrlen, L., Perez, A., Farmer, N., & Bevans, M. (2019). Nurses and health-promoting self-care: Do we practice what we preach? *Journal of Nursing Management, 27*(3), 599–608. https://doi.org/10.1111/jonm.12718

Whitehead, D. (2018). Exploring health promotion and health education in nursing. *Nursing Standard, 33*(8), 38–44. https://doi.org/10.7748/ns.2018.e11220

H

Health Literacy Enhancement 5515

Definition: Assisting individuals with limited ability to obtain, process, and understand information related to health and illness

Activities:

- Create a health care environment in which a patient with impaired literacy can seek help without feeling ashamed or stigmatized
- Use appropriate and clear communication
- Use plain language
- Simplify language whenever possible
- Use a slow speaking pace
- Avoid medical jargon and use of acronyms
- Communicate with consideration for culture, age, and gender suitability
- Determine patient's experience with the health care system, including health promotion, health protection, disease prevention, health care and maintenance, and health care system navigation
- Determine health literacy status at initiation of contact with the patient through informal and/or formal assessments
- Determine patient's learning style
- Observe for impaired health literacy cues (e.g., failing to complete written forms, missing appointments, not taking medications appropriately, inability to identify medications or describe reasons for taking them, deferring to family members for information about health condition, asking multiple questions about topics already covered in handouts and brochures, avoiding reading things in front of health care providers)
- Obtain interpreter services, as needed
- Provide essential written and oral information to a patient in his/her first language
- Determine what the patient already knows about his/her health condition or risks and relate new information to what is already known
- Provide one-to-one teaching or counseling whenever feasible
- Provide understandable written materials (i.e., use short sentences and common words with fewer syllables, highlight key points, use an active voice, use large print, have a user-friendly layout and design, group similar content into segments, emphasize behaviors and action that should be taken, use pictures or diagrams to clarify and decrease the reading burden)
- Use strategies to enhance understanding (i.e., start with the most important information first, focus on key messages and repeat, limit the amount of information presented at any one time, use examples to illustrate important points, relate to the individual's experience, use a storytelling style)
- Use multiple communication tools (e.g., audiotapes, videotapes, digital video devices, computers, pictograms, models, diagrams)
- Evaluate patient understanding by having patient repeat back in own words or demonstrate skill
- Encourage the individual to ask questions and seek clarification (e.g., What is my main problem? What do I need to do? Why is it important for me to do this?)
- Assist the individual in anticipating his or her experiences in the health care system (e.g., being asked questions, seeing different health professionals, needing to let providers know when information is not understood, getting the results from laboratory tests, making and keeping appointments)
- Encourage use of effective measures for coping with impaired health literacy (e.g., being persistent when asking for help, bringing a written list of questions or concerns to each health care encounter, depending on oral explanations or demonstrations of tasks, seeking the assistance of family or friends in getting health information)

5th edition 2008

Background Evidence:

Baker, D. W. (2006). The meaning and measure of health literacy. *Journal of General Internal Medicine, 21*(8), 878–883.

DeWalt, D. A., Berkman, N. D., Sheridan, S., Lohr, K. N., & Pignone, M. P. (2004). Literacy and health outcomes: A systematic review of the literature. *Journal of General Internal Medicine, 19*(12), 1228–1239.

Doak, C. C., Doak, L. G., & Root, J. H. (1996). *Teaching patients with low literacy skills* (2nd ed.). J.B. Lippincott.

Dubrow, J. (2004). *Adequate literacy and health literacy: Prerequisites for informed health care decision making.* AARP Public Policy Institute.

Institute of Medicine. (2004). In L. Nielsen-Bohlman, A. Panzer, & D. Kindig (Eds.), *Health literacy: A prescription to end confusion.* National Academies Press.

Osborne, H. (2005). *Health literacy from A to Z. Practical ways to communicate your health message.* Jones and Bartlett.

Schwartzberg, J. G., VanGeest, J. B., & Wang, C. (Eds.). (2005). *Understanding health literacy: Implications for medicine and public health.* American Medical Association.

Speros, C. (2005). Health literacy: Concept analysis. *Journal of Advanced Nursing, 50*(6), 633–640.

Weiss, B. D., Mays, M. Z., Martz, W., Castro, K. M., DeWalt, D. A., Pignone, M. P., Mockbee, J., & Hale, F. A. (2005). Quick assessment of literacy in primary care: The newest vital sign. . *Annals of Family Medicine, 3*(6), 514–522.

Health Policy Monitoring 7970

Definition: Surveillance and influence of government and organization regulations, rules, and standards that affect nursing systems and practices to ensure quality care of patients

Activities:

- Review proposed policies and standards in organizational, professional, and governmental literature, and in the popular media
- Monitor online relevant websites (e.g., Centers for Medicare and Medicaid Services, home state governmental policy websites) for ongoing policy changes that may affect patient care
- Compare requirements of new policies and standards with current practices
- Determine negative and positive effects of health policies and standards on nursing practice, patient, and cost outcomes
- Identify and resolve discrepancies between health policies and standards and current nursing practice
- Acquaint policy makers with implications of current and proposed policies and standards for patient welfare
- Lobby policy makers to make changes in health policies and standards to benefit patients
- Submit written comments on pending rules and actions related to health policy changes
- Testify in organizational, professional, and public forums to influence the formulation of health policies and standards that benefit patients
- Support and participate in the efforts of nursing organizations, such as the ANA, to respond to and influence national health policy
- Help elect nurses to key leadership positions on health care boards and committees
- Assist consumers of health care to be informed of current and proposed changes in health policies and standards and the implications for health outcomes

2nd edition 1996; revised 2018

Background Evidence:

Institute of Medicine. (2011). *The future of nursing: Leading change, advancing health.* The National Academies Press.

Mason, D. J., Leavitt, J. K., & Chaffee, M. W. (2007). *Policy and politics in nursing and health care* (5th ed.). Saunders Elsevier.

Stanhope, M., & Lancaster, J. (2012). *Public health nursing* (8th ed.). Elsevier Mosby.

H

Health Screening 6520

Definition: Detecting health risks or problems by means of history, examination, and other procedures

Activities:

- Determine target population for health screening
- Advertise health screening services to increase public awareness
- Provide detail on screening services to enhance attendance (e.g., special screening tools, presence of advanced practitioners)
- Provide easy access to screening services (e.g., time and place)
- Schedule appointments to enhance efficiency and individualized care
- Use valid, reliable health screening instruments appropriate for specific conditions (e.g., cardiovascular disease, immunization, health literacy, depression, malnutrition, obesity, drug and alcohol use, prenatal health, health-related quality of life, partner violence, risk assessment), as indicated
- Follow appropriate guidelines from relevant groups (e.g., government agency, specialty organization, clinical practice) for proper time frame and type of screenings
- Determine patient level of understanding before initiating screening
- Accommodate cultural diversity in screening interviews and interpretation of findings
- Instruct on rationale and purpose of health screenings and self-monitoring
- Obtain informed consent for health screening procedures, as appropriate
- Provide for privacy and confidentiality
- Provide for comfort during screening procedures
- Obtain detailed health history including description of health habits, risk factors, and medications, as appropriate
- Obtain family health history, as appropriate
- Measure blood pressure, height, weight, percent body fat, cholesterol and blood sugar levels, and urinalysis, as appropriate
- Perform (or refer for) Pap smear, mammography, prostate check, EKG, testicular examination, and vision check, as appropriate
- Obtain specimens for analysis by assessments, as indicated
- Complete appropriate Department of Health or other records for monitoring abnormal results, such as high blood pressure
- Provide appropriate self-monitoring information during screening
- Provide results of health screenings to patient
- Inform patient of limitations and margin of error of specific screening tests

- Counsel patient who has abnormal findings about treatment alternatives or need for further evaluation
- Refer patient to other health care providers, as necessary
- Provide follow-up contact for all patients

1st edition 1992; revised 1996, 2018

Background Evidence:

Comrie, R. (2013). Health assessment and physical examination. In P. Potter, A. Perry, P. Stockert, & A. Hall (Eds.), *Fundamentals of nursing* (8th ed., pp. 487–564). Elsevier Mosby.

Hinkle, J., & Cheever, K. (2014). Adult health and nutritional assessment (13th ed.) *Brunner & Suddarth's textbook of medical surgical nursing* (Vol. 1, pp. 56–73). Wolters Kluwer Health/Lippincott Williams & Wilkins.

Kauschinger, E., & Trybulski, J. (2013). Routine health screening and immunizations. In T. Buttaro, J. Trybulski, P. Bailey, & J. Sandberg-Cook (Eds.), *Primary care: A collaborative practice* (4th ed., pp. 142–158). Elsevier Mosby.

Perry, A., Potter, P., & Ostendorf, W. (Eds.). (2014). *Clinical nursing skills and techniques* (8th ed.). Elsevier Mosby.

Health System Guidance 7400

H

Definition: Facilitating use of appropriate health services based on location

Activities:

- Determine qualifying services available by location
- Determine current knowledge of health care system and health care needs
- Explain immediate health care services, how they work, and what to expect
- Assist to coordinate health care and communication
- Assist to choose appropriate health care professionals
- Instruct on what type of services to expect from each type of health care provider
- Inform about different types of health care facilities (e.g., general hospital, specialty hospital, teaching hospital, walk-in clinic, outpatient surgical clinic), as appropriate
- Inform of accreditation and state health department requirements for judging facility quality
- Inform of recognitions and awards for judging facility quality (e.g., Leapfrog Safety, Magnet, Pathway to Excellence)
- Inform of appropriate community resources and contact persons
- Encourage use of second opinion as appropriate
- Inform how to access emergency services, as appropriate
- Facilitate communication among health care providers and person, as appropriate
- Encourage consultation with other health care professionals, as appropriate
- Review and reinforce information given by other health care professionals
- Provide information on how to obtain equipment
- Coordinate or schedule time needed by each service to deliver care, as appropriate
- Inform about cost, time, alternatives, and risks involved in specific test or procedure
- Give written or printed instructions for purpose and location of posthospitalization or outpatient activities, as appropriate
- Give written or printed instructions for purpose and location of health care activities, as appropriate
- Discuss outcome of visit with other health care providers, as appropriate
- Facilitate transportation needs for obtainment of health care services
- Provide follow-up contact, as appropriate
- Monitor adequacy of current health care follow-up
- Provide report to posthospital caregivers, as appropriate
- Encourage to ask questions about services and charges
- Comply with regulations for third-party reimbursement
- Assist to complete forms for assistance (e.g., housing, financial aid), as needed
- Notify of scheduled appointments, as appropriate
- Provide written or printed instructions as appropriate
- Use teach-back to ensure understanding

1st edition 1992; revised 2000, 2004, 2024

Background Evidence:

Craven, R. F., Hirnle, C. J., & Henshaw, C. J. (2021). *Fundamentals of nursing: Concepts and competencies for practice* (9th ed.). Wolters-Kluwer.

De Looper, M., Damman, O., Smets, E., Timmermans, D., & Van Weert, J. (2020). Adapting online patient decision aids: effects of modality and narration style on patients' satisfaction, information recall and informed decision making. *Journal of Health Communication, 25*(9), 712–726.

Hota, S., Manning, P. G., Voo, T. C., & Chin, J. C. (2019). Overcoming professional and system barriers to achieving patient-centered informed consent. *The Journal of Hospital Ethics, 6*(1), 81–82.

Pedersen, H. F., Holsting, A., Frostholm, L., Rask, C., Jensen, J. S., Høeg, M. D., & Schröder, A. (2019). Understand your illness and your needs: Assessment-informed patient education for people with multiple functional somatic syndromes. *Patient Education and Counseling, 102*(9), 1662–1671. https://doi.org/10.1016/j.pec.2019.04.016

Potter, P. A., Perry, A. G., Stockert, P. A., & Hall, A. M. (2021). *Fundamentals of Nursing* (10th ed.). Elsevier.

Schaaf, M., Warthin, C., Freedman, L., & Topp, S. M. (2020). The community health worker as service extender, cultural broker and social change agent: A critical interpretive synthesis of roles, intent and accountability. *BMJ Global Health, 5*(6), e002296. https://doi.org/10.1136/bmjgh-2020-002296

Stoll, K., & Jackson, J. (2019). Supporting patient autonomy and informed decision-making in prenatal genetic testing. *Cold Spring Harbor Perspectives in Medicine*, a036509.

Heat/Cold Application   1380

Definition: Stimulation of the skin and underlying tissues with heat or cold for the purpose of decreasing pain, muscle spasms, or inflammation

Activities:
- Explain the use of heat or cold, the reason for the treatment, and how it will affect the patient's symptoms
- Screen for contraindications to cold or heat, such as decreased or absent sensation, decreased circulation, and decreased ability to communicate
- Select a method of stimulation that is convenient and readily available (e.g., waterproof plastic bags with melting ice; frozen gel packs; chemical ice envelope; ice immersion; cloth or towel in freezer for cold; hot water bottle; electric heating pad; hot, moist compresses; immersion in tub or whirlpool; paraffin wax; sitz bath; radiant bulb; or plastic wrap for heat)
- Determine availability and safe working condition of all equipment used for heat or cold application
- Determine condition of skin and identify any alterations requiring a change in procedure or contraindications to stimulation
- Select stimulation site, considering alternate sites when direct application is not possible (e.g., adjacent to, distal to, between affected areas and the brain, and contralateral)
- Wrap the heat or cold application device with a protective cloth, if appropriate
- Use a moist cloth next to the skin to increase the sensation of cold or heat, when appropriate
- Use ice after an ankle sprain to reduce edema, followed by rest, compression, and elevation
- Instruct how to avoid tissue damage associated with heat or cold
- Check the temperature of the application, especially when using heat
- Determine duration of application based on individual verbal, behavioral, and biological responses
- Time all applications carefully
- Apply cold or heat directly on or near the affected site, if possible
- Avoid using heat or cold on tissue that has been exposed to radiation therapy
- Inspect the site carefully for signs of skin irritation or tissue damage throughout the first 5 minutes and then frequently during the treatment
- Finish with a cold treatment to encourage vasoconstriction when alternating heat and cold applications for an injured athlete
- Evaluate general condition, safety, and comfort throughout the treatment
- Position to allow movement from the temperature source, if needed
- Instruct not to adjust temperature settings independently without prior instruction
- Change sites of cold or heat application or switch form of stimulation if relief is not achieved
- Instruct that cold application may be painful briefly, with numbness about 5 minutes after the initial stimulation
- Instruct on indications for, frequency of, and procedure for application
- Instruct to avoid injury to the skin after stimulation
- Evaluate and document response to heat and cold application

1st edition 1992; revised 2013

Background Evidence:

Berman, A., Snyder, S., Kozier, B., & Erb, G. (2008). Skin integrity and wound care. In *Kozier & Erb's Fundamentals of nursing: Concepts, processes, and practice* (pp. 902–938) (8th ed.). Prentice Hall.

Smeltzer, S. C., Bare, B. G., Hinkle, J. L., & Cheever, K. H. (2010). Pain management (12th ed.) *Brunner & Suddarth's textbook of medical surgical nursing* (Vol. 1, pp. 230–262). Lippincott Williams & Wilkins.

Thompson, C., Kelsberg, G., Anna, L., St, & Poddar, S. (2003). Heat or ice for acute ankle sprain. *Journal of Family Practice, 52*(8), 642–643.

White, L. (2005). *Foundations of nursing* (pp. 471) (2nd ed.). Thomson Delmar Learning.

H

Hemodialysis Therapy   2100

Definition: Management of extracorporeal passage of the patient's blood through a dialyzer

Activities:
- Draw blood sample and review blood chemistries (e.g., blood urea nitrogen, serum creatinine, serum Na, K, and PO_4 levels) pretreatment
- Record baseline vital signs: weight, temperature, pulse, respirations, and blood pressure
- Explain hemodialysis procedure and its purpose
- Check equipment and solutions, according to protocol
- Use sterile technique to initiate hemodialysis and for needle insertions and catheter connections
- Use gloves, eyeshield, and clothing to prevent direct contact with blood
- Initiate hemodialysis, according to protocol
- Anchor connections and tubing securely
- Check system monitors (e.g., flow rate, pressure, temperature, pH level, conductivity, clots, air detector, negative pressure for ultrafiltration, and blood sensor) to ensure patient safety
- Monitor blood pressure, pulse, respirations, temperature, and patient response during dialysis
- Administer heparin, according to protocol
- Monitor clotting times and adjust heparin administration appropriately
- Adjust filtration pressures to remove an appropriate amount of fluid
- Institute appropriate protocol if patient becomes hypotensive
- Discontinue hemodialysis, according to protocol
- Compare post-dialysis vitals and blood chemistries to pre-dialysis values
- Avoid taking blood pressure or doing intravenous punctures in arm with fistula
- Provide catheter or fistula care, according to protocol
- Work collaboratively with patient to adjust diet regulations, fluid limitations, and medications to regulate fluid and electrolyte shifts between treatments

- Teach patient to self-monitor signs and symptoms that indicate need for medical treatment (e.g., fever, bleeding, clotted fistula, thrombophlebitis, and irregular pulse)
- Work collaboratively with patient to relieve discomfort from side effects of the disease and treatment (e.g., cramping, fatigue, headaches, itching, anemia, bone demineralization, body image changes, and role disruption)
- Work collaboratively with patient to adjust length of dialysis, diet regulations, and pain and diversion needs to achieve optimal benefit of the treatment

1st edition 1992; revised 1996, 2004

Background Evidence:

Fearing, M. O., & Hart, L. K. (1992). Dialysis therapy. In G. M. Bulechek & J. C. McCloskey (Eds.), *Nursing interventions: Essential nursing treatments* (2nd ed., pp. 587–601). W.B. Saunders.

Smeltzer, S. C., & Bare, B. G. (2004). Management of patients with upper or lower urinary tract dysfunction (10th ed.) *Brunner & Suddarth's textbook of medical surgical nursing* (Vol. 2, pp. 1271–1308). Lippincott Williams & Wilkins.

Thompson, J. M., McFarland, G. K., Hirsch, J. E., & Tucker, S. M. (1998). *Mosby's clinical nursing* (4th ed.). Mosby.

Hemodynamic Regulation 4150

Definition: Optimization of heart rate, preload, afterload, and contractility

Activities:

- Perform a comprehensive appraisal of hemodynamic status (i.e., check blood pressure, heart rate, pulses, jugular venous pressure, central venous pressure, right and left atrial and ventricular pressures, and pulmonary artery pressure), as appropriate
- Use multiple parameters to determine patient's clinical status (i.e., proportional pulse pressure is considered the definitive parameter)
- Monitor and document proportional pulse pressure (i.e., systolic blood pressure minus diastolic blood divided by systolic blood pressure, resulting in a proportion or percentage)
- Provide frequent physical examination in at-risk populations (e.g., heart failure patients)
- Alleviate patient anxieties by providing accurate information and correcting any misconceptions
- Instruct patient and family on hemodynamic monitoring (e.g., medications, therapies, purposes of equipment)
- Explain the aims of care and how progress will be measured
- Recognize presence of early warning signs and symptoms of compromised hemodynamic system (e.g., dyspnea, decreased ability to exercise, orthopnea, profound fatigue, dizziness, lightheadedness, edema, palpitations, paroxysmal nocturnal dyspnea, sudden weight gain)
- Determine volume status (i.e., Is patient hypervolemic, hypovolemic, or in a balanced fluid level?)
- Monitor for signs and symptoms of volume status problems (e.g., neck vein distension, elevated pressure in the right internal jugular vein, positive abdominal jugular neck vein reflex, edema, ascites, crackles, dyspnea, orthopnea, paroxysmal nocturnal dyspnea)
- Determine perfusion status (i.e., Is patient cold, lukewarm, or warm?)
- Monitor for signs and symptoms of perfusion status problems (e.g., symptomatic hypotension; cool extremities, including arms and legs; mental obtundation or constant sleepiness; elevation in serum levels of creatinine and urea nitrogen; hyponatremia; narrow pulse pressure; and proportional pulse pressure of 25% or less)
- Auscultate lung sounds for crackles or other adventitious sounds
- Recognize that adventitious lung sounds are not the sole indicator of hemodynamic issues
- Auscultate heart sounds
- Monitor and document blood pressure, heart rate, rhythm, and pulses

- Monitor pacemaker functioning, if appropriate
- Monitor systemic and pulmonary vascular resistance, as appropriate
- Monitor cardiac output and cardiac index and left-ventricular stroke work index, as appropriate
- Administer positive inotropic and contractility medications
- Administer antiarrhythmic medications, as appropriate
- Monitor effects of medications
- Monitor peripheral pulses, capillary refill, and temperature and color of extremities
- Elevate the head of the bed, as appropriate
- Elevate foot of bed, as appropriate
- Monitor for peripheral edema; jugular vein distension; S_3 and S_4 heart sounds; dyspnea; gains in weight; and organ distension, especially in the lungs or liver
- Monitor pulmonary capillary and artery wedge pressure and central venous and right-atrial pressure, as appropriate
- Monitor electrolyte levels
- Maintain fluid balance by administering IV fluids or diuretics, as appropriate
- Administer vasodilator and vasoconstrictor medication, as appropriate
- Monitor intake and output, urine output, and patient weight, as appropriate
- Evaluate effects of fluid therapy
- Insert urinary catheter, if appropriate
- Minimize environmental stressors
- Collaborate with physician, as indicated

1st edition 1992; revised 2013

Background Evidence:

Albert, N., Trochelman, K., Li, J., & Lin, S. (2010). Signs and symptoms of heart failure: Are you asking the right questions? *American Journal of Critical Care, 19*(5), 443–453.

American Association of Critical-Care Nurses. (2006). In J. G. Alspach (Ed.), *Core curriculum for critical care nursing* (6th ed.). Saunders Elsevier.

Blissitt, P. (2006). Hemodynamic monitoring in the care of the critically ill neuroscience patient. *AACN Advanced Critical Care, 17*(3), 327–340.

Whitlock, A., & MacInnes, J. (2010). Acute heart failure: Patient assessment and management. *British Journal of Cardiac Nursing, 5*(11), 516–525.

Hemofiltration Therapy   2110

Definition: Cleansing of acutely ill patient's blood via a hemofilter controlled by the patient's hydrostatic pressure

Activities:

- Determine baseline vital signs and weight
- Draw blood sample and review blood chemistries (e.g., BUN, serum creatinine, serum Na, Ca, K, and PO_4 levels) before therapy
- Determine and record patient's hemodynamic function
- Explain procedure to patient and significant others, as appropriate
- Obtain written consent
- Adjust technology to account for patient's multiple system pathologies (e.g., place patient on rotating-airflow bed)
- Use sterile technique to flush and prime the arterial tubing, venous tubing, and hemofilter with heparinized saline, and to connect to other tubing as required
- Remove all air bubbles from hemofiltration system
- Administer heparin loading dose per protocol or physician order
- Use mask, glove, and apron to prevent contact with blood
- Use sterile technique to initiate venous and arterial access per protocol
- Anchor connections and tubing securely
- Apply restraints, as appropriate
- Monitor ultrafiltration rate, adjusting rate per protocol or physician's order
- Monitor hemofiltration system for leaks at connections and clotting of filter or tubing
- Monitor patient's multiple system parameters per protocol
- Monitor and care for access sites and lines, according to protocol
- Monitor for signs and symptoms of infection
- Instruct patient/family about precautions posttreatment

3rd edition 2000

Background Evidence:

Gutch, C., Stoner, M., & Corea, A. (1993). *Review of hemodialysis for nurses and dialysis personnel* (5th ed.). Mosby.

Holloway, N. (1988). *Nursing the critically ill adult* (3rd ed.). Addison-Wesley.

Kinney, M., Packa, D., & Dunbar, S. (1998). *AACN's reference for critical-care nursing* (4th ed.). Mosby.

Smeltzer, S. C., & Bare, B. G. (2004). Management of patients with upper or lower urinary tract dysfunction (10th ed.) *Brunner & Suddarth's textbook of medical surgical nursing* (Vol. 2, pp. 1271–1308). Lippincott Williams & Wilkins.

H

High-Risk Pregnancy Care   6800

Definition: Identification and management of a high-risk pregnancy to promote healthy outcomes for mother and baby

Activities:

- Determine the presence of medical factors that are related to poor pregnancy outcome (e.g., diabetes, thyroid disease, hypertension, obesity, thrombophilias or history of DVT, autoimmune conditions, herpes, hepatitis, HIV, cardiac conditions or history of cardiac surgery, chronic pain conditions managed with opioid analgesics, use of opioid substitution therapies, seizure disorder)
- Review obstetrical history for pregnancy-related risk factors (e.g., recurrent pregnancy loss, prematurity, postmaturity, preeclampsia, multifetal pregnancy, intrauterine growth retardation, placental abruption, placenta previa, hyperemesis, Rh sensitization, premature rupture of membranes, family history of genetic disorder)
- Recognize demographic and social factors related to poor pregnancy outcome (e.g., young or advanced maternal age, race, ethnicity, low socioeconomic status, late or no prenatal care, physical abuse, substance abuse)
- Determine patient's understanding of identified risk factors
- Encourage expression of feelings and fears about lifestyle changes of pregnancy and parenting, fetal well-being, financial changes, family functioning, and personal safety
- Provide educational materials that address the risk factors and usual surveillance tests and procedures
- Instruct patient in self-care techniques to increase the chance of a healthy outcome (e.g., hydration, diet, activity modifications, importance of regular prenatal check-ups, normalization of blood sugars, sexual precautions)
- Instruct about alternate methods of sexual gratification and intimacy
- Refer as appropriate for specific programs (e.g., smoking cessation, substance abuse treatment, diabetes education, preterm birth prevention education; abuse shelter, pain management providers, genetic counseling, sexually transmitted disease clinic)
- Instruct patient on use of prescribed medication (e.g., insulin, tocolytics, antihypertensives, antibiotics, anticoagulants, anticonvulsants)
- Instruct patient on self-monitoring skills (e.g., vital signs, blood glucose testing, uterine activity monitoring), as appropriate
- Provide written instructions for addressing signs and symptoms that require immediate medical attention (e.g., bright red vaginal bleeding, leaking of amniotic fluid, unusual vaginal discharge, decreased fetal movement, four or more contractions per hour before 37 weeks of gestation, headache, visual disturbances, epigastric pain, rapid weight gain with facial edema)
- Discuss fetal risks associated with preterm birth at various gestational ages
- Tour the neonatal intensive care unit if preterm birth is anticipated (e.g., multifetal pregnancy)
- Conduct tests to evaluate fetal status and placental function (e.g., nonstress, biophysical profiles, ultrasound tests)
- Obtain cervical samples, as appropriate
- Assist with fetal diagnostic procedures (e.g., blood draws, amniocentesis, chorionic villus sampling, percutaneous umbilical blood sampling, Doppler blood flow studies)
- Assist with fetal therapy procedures (e.g., fetal transfusions, fetal surgery, selective reduction, termination procedure)
- Interpret medical explanations for test and procedure results

- Administer Rh$_o$(D) immune globulin (e.g., RhoGAM or Gamulin Rh) to prevent Rh sensitization after invasive procedures, as appropriate
- Establish plan for clinic follow-up
- Provide anticipatory guidance for likely treatments during birth process
- Encourage early enrollment in prenatal classes or provide childbirth education materials for patients on bed rest
- Provide anticipatory guidance for common experiences that high-risk mothers have during the postpartum period (e.g., exhaustion, depression, chronic stress, disenchantment with childbearing, loss of income, partner discord, sexual dysfunction)
- Refer to high-risk mother support group, as needed
- Refer to home care agencies (e.g., specialized perinatal nursing services, perinatal case management, public health nursing)
- Monitor physical and psychosocial status closely throughout pregnancy
- Report deviations from normal in maternal and fetal status immediately to physician or nurse midwife
- Document patient education, laboratory results, fetal testing results, and client responses

2nd edition 1996; revised 2018

Background Evidence:

Bayrampour, H., Heaman, M., Duncan, K. A., & Tough, S. (2012). Advanced maternal age and risk perception: A qualitative study. *BMC Pregnancy and Childbirth, 12*(1), 100.

Gilbert, E. S. (2011). *Manual of high-risk pregnancy and delivery* (5th ed.). Mosby Elsevier.

Kellogg, A., Rose, C. H., Harms, R. H., & Watson, W. J. (2011). Current trends in narcotic use in pregnancy and neonatal outcomes. *American Journal of Obstetrics and Gynecology, 204*(3), 259.e1–259.e4.

Krans, E. E., & Davis, M. M. (2012). Preventing low birthweight: 25 years, prenatal risk, and the failure to reinvent prenatal care. *American Journal of Obstetrics and Gynecology, 206*(5), 398–403.

Nakamura, Y. (2010). Nursing intervention to enhance acceptance of pregnancy in first-time mothers: Focusing on the comfortable experiences of pregnant women. *Japan Journal of Nursing Science, 7*(1), 29–36.

Niebyl, J. R. (2010). Nausea and vomiting in pregnancy. *New England Journal of Medicine, 363*(16), 1544–1550.

Simpson, K. R., & Creehan, P. A. (2014). *Perinatal nursing* (4th ed.). Lippincott Williams & Wilkins.

Home Maintenance Assistance 7180

Definition: Facilitating continuance of clean and safe home environment

Activities:

- Determine home maintenance requirements
- Involve person in deciding home maintenance requirements
- Identify basic sanitation needs in place of residence
- Suggest necessary structural alterations to make home accessible
- Provide information on how to make home environment safe and clean
- Assist family members to develop realistic expectations in performance of their roles
- Advise alleviation of all offensive odors
- Suggest services for pest control as needed
- Facilitate cleaning of dirty laundry
- Suggest services for home repair as needed
- Discuss cost of needed maintenance and available resources
- Offer solutions to financial concerns
- Order homemaker services, as appropriate
- Help family use social support network
- Provide information on respite care as needed
- Instruct about basic home care
- Coordinate use of community resources

1st edition 1992; revised 2004, 2024

Background Evidence:

Hrybyk, R. L., Frankowski, A. C., Nemec, M., & Peeples, A. D. (2021). "It's a lot!" The universal worker model and dementia care in assisted living. *Geriatric Nursing, 42*(1), 233–239.

Keefe, J. M., Funk, L., Knight, L., Lobchuk, M., Macdonald, M., Mitchell, L., Rempel, J., Warner, G., & Stevens, S. (2020). Home care clients: A research protocol for studying their pathways. *BMC health services research, 20*(1), 535.

Perry, A. G., Potter, P. A., Ostendorf, W. R., & LaPlante, N. (2021). *Clinical nursing skills and technique* (10th ed.). Mosby.

Sorrell, J. M. (2020). Tidying up: Good for the aging brain. *Journal of Psychosocial Nursing & Mental Health Services, 58*(4), 16–18.

Williams, P. (2020). *Basic geriatric nursing* (7th ed.). Elsevier.

Hope Inspiration 5310

Definition: Enhancing the belief in one's capacity to initiate and sustain actions

Activities:

- Assist patient and family to identify areas of hope in life
- Inform the patient about whether the current situation is a temporary state
- Demonstrate hope by recognizing the patient's intrinsic worth and viewing the patient's illness as only one facet of the individual
- Expand the patient's repertoire of coping mechanisms
- Teach reality recognition by surveying the situation and making contingency plans
- Assist the patient to devise and revise goals related to the hope object
- Help the patient expand spiritual self
- Avoid masking the truth
- Facilitate the patient's incorporating a personal loss into his/her body image

- Facilitate the patient's/family's reliving and savoring past achievements and experiences
- Emphasize sustaining relationships, such as mentioning the names of loved ones to the unresponsive patient
- Employ guided life review and/or reminiscence, as appropriate
- Involve the patient actively in own care
- Develop a plan of care that involves degree of goal attainment, moving from simple to more complex goals
- Encourage therapeutic relationships with significant others
- Teach family about the positive aspects of hope (e.g., develop meaningful conversational themes that reflect love and need for the patient)
- Provide patient/family opportunity to be involved with support groups
- Create an environment that facilitates patient practicing religion, as appropriate

1st edition 1992; revised 2008

Background Evidence:

Brown, P. (1989). The concept of hope: Implications for care of the critically ill. *Critical Care Nurse, 9*(5), 97–105.

Forbes, S. B. (1994). Hope: An essential human need in the elderly. *Journal Gerontological Nursing, 20*(6), 5–10.

Herth, K. (1990). Fostering hope in terminally-ill people. *Journal of Advanced Nursing, 15*, 1250–1259.

Miller, J. F. (2000). Inspiring hope. In J. F. Miller (Ed.), *Coping with chronic illness: Overcoming powerlessness* (3rd ed., pp. 523–546). F.A. Davis.

Pilkington, F. B. (1999). The many facets of hope. In R. R. Parse (Ed.), *Hope: An international human becoming perspective* (pp. 9–44). Jones and Bartlett.

Poncar, P. J. (1994). Inspiring hope in the oncology patient. *Journal of Psychosocial Nursing and Mental Health Services, 32*(1), 33–38.

Snyder, C. R., Sympson, S. C., Ybasco, F. C., Borders, T. F., Babyak, M. A., & Higgins, R. L. (1996). Development and validation of the State Hope Scale. *Journal of Personality and Social Psychology, 70*(2), 321–335.

H

Hormone Replacement Therapy   2280

Definition: Facilitation of safe and effective use of hormone replacement therapy

Activities:

- Determine reason for choosing hormone replacement therapy
- Review alternatives to hormone replacement therapy
- Monitor for therapeutic and adverse effects
- Review knowledge regarding beneficial and adverse effects of different hormonal components (e.g., estrogen, progesterone, androgen)
- Review knowledge regarding interaction effects of adjunct therapies (e.g., calcium and vitamin D supplementation, exercise, thiazide use)
- Review knowledge regarding different methods and routes of administration (e.g., oral continuous combined, oral sequential, dermal, vaginal)
- Review diet and suggest limiting caffeine, saturated fats, and sugar
- Facilitate decision to continue or discontinue
- Facilitate changes in hormone replacement therapy with primary care provider, as appropriate
- Ensure dose and regimen of therapy are individualized, choosing lowest appropriate dose in relation to severity of symptoms and menopause onset age
- Recommend short-term annual decisions about continuation
- Adjust medications or medication dose, as appropriate
- Use teach-back to ensure understanding

4th edition 2004; revised 2024

Background Evidence:

Dilks, A., & Soos, E. (2019). Bioidentical hormone replacement therapy: Implications for practice. *Journal of Aesthetic Nursing, 8*(4), 166–171. https://doi.org/10.12968/joan.2019.8.4.166

Lobo, R. A. (2017). Hormone-replacement therapy: Current thinking. *Nature Reviews. Endocrinology, 13*(4), 220–231. https://doi.org/10.1038/nrendo.2016.164

Perry, M. (2019). Menopausal symptoms and hormone replacement therapy. *Journal of Community Nursing, 33*(3), 61–66.

Smeltzer, S. C., & Bare, B. G. (2021). Assessment and management of female physiologic processes (15th ed.) *Brunner & Suddarth's textbook of medical surgical nursing* (Vol. 2, pp. 1389–1412). Lippincott Williams & Wilkins.

Speroff, L., Glass, R., & Kase, N. (2019). *Clinical gynecologic endocrinology and infertility* (pp. 834–879) (9th ed.). Lippincott Williams & Wilkins.

Human Trafficking Detection   6525

Definition: Actions to identify and prevent acts of recruiting, harboring, transporting, providing, or obtaining a person through use of fraud, force, or coercion

Activities:

- Determine at-risk populations (e.g., people who endured emotional, physical and psychological trauma)
- Identify indicators of possible trafficking (e.g., bruises or wounds consistent with application of physical restraints; untreated infections; urinary difficulties, pregnancy, rectal trauma, malnourishment, lack of health care)
- Be alert for person accompanied by another person who is controlling, provides all information, or does all communicating
- Note unusual circumstances such as persons with no identification or fake identification, or controller has person's identification with them
- Identify persons who seem confused, submissive or fearful, refuse to make eye contact, seem afraid to speak in presence of others, or are reluctant to discuss injuries

- Be alert for persons who do not state an address, claim to just be visiting, or seem unable to identify their location
- Consider risk factors for possible trafficking (e.g., frequent truancy or runaway, recurrent sexually transmitted infections, reports high number of sex partners, far along in pregnancy with no prenatal care, inappropriately dressed, accompanied by someone who will not leave person alone or let person speak, improper dress for weather)
- Address any emergency regarding person's physical needs or immediate safety concerns (i.e., call authorities if indicated)
- Provide safe, non-judgmental environment
- Speak to person alone in appointment and address any concerns, in private room with closed doors
- Ask partner to fill out forms in separate lobby or firmly state need for private exam
- Communicate with person using professional interpreter and do not permit family member or accompanying partner to translate
- Make eye contact, practice active listening, and convey attitude of caring
- Provide with confidential questionnaire with human trafficking screening questions if indicated
- Determine potential danger and care needs
- Involve authorities when person is a minor, reports self or family in danger, trafficker present, or staff or other persons are in danger
- Respect limits of confidentiality, but explain legal requirements to report suspected abuse, neglect, or violence to external agencies, including mandated reporting obligations
- Do not violate Health Insurance Portability and Accountability Act (HIPAA) regulations
- Gain consent and permission from any adult patient before disclosing personal health information (PHI)
- Report PHI in known or suspected child abuse or neglect to public health authority or other appropriate government authority authorized by law to receive such reports
- Offer methods to seek help when ready, if unwilling to discuss captive situation, or if declines or denies need for assistance
- Use discreet methods of help to avoid further danger to person if abuser discovers (i.e., hide National Human Trafficking Hotline number on barcode of personal item, such as lipstick, soap, box of bandages)
- Document all findings and suspicions to create legal record for future reference
- Ensure yearly education for staff concerning red flags to identify possible trafficking victims and, if indicated, assist them to report
- Ensure ability to offer victims community supports and resources to meet needs revealed during health care encounter
- Work to develop policies and protocols within organizations to streamline screening, assessment, and response and ensure systematic approach to human trafficking identification and intervention
- Promote community health and wellness, child welfare, gender equality, and violence prevention with community leaders

8th edition 2024

Background Evidence:

Bauer, R., Brown, S., Cannon, E., & Southard, E. (2019). What health providers should know about human sex trafficking. *MedSurg Nursing, 28*(6), 347–351.

Byrne, M., Parsh, S., & Parsh, B. (2019). Human trafficking. *Nursing Management (Springhouse), 50*(8), 18–24. https://doi.org/10.1097/01.NUMA.0000575304.15432.07

McDow, J., & Dols, J. D. (2021). Implementation of a human trafficking screening protocol. *Journal for Nurse Practitioners, 17*(3), 339–343. https://doi.org/10.1016/j.nurpra.2020.10.031

Raker, K. A., & Hromadik, L. K. (2021). Human trafficking in the radiology setting. *Journal of Radiology Nursing, 40*(1), 69–74. https://doi.org/10.1016/j.jradnu.2020.10.002

Stevens, C., & Dinkel, S. (2021). From awareness to action: Assessing for human trafficking in primary care. *Journal for Nurse Practitioners, 17*, 492–496.

Washburn, J. (2018). What nurses need to know about human trafficking: Update. *Journal of Christian Nursing, 35*(1), 18–25. https://doi.org/10.1097/CNJ.0000000000000459

Yates, S. (2020). Be a voice for the voiceless: Human trafficking in Alaska. *Alaskan Nurse, 2020*, 12–15.

Humor   5320

Definition: Facilitating the patient to perceive, appreciate, and express what is funny, amusing, or ludicrous in order to establish relationships, relieve tension, release anger, facilitate learning, or cope with painful feelings

Activities:

- Determine the types of humor appreciated by the patient
- Determine the patient's typical response to humor (e.g., laughter or smiles)
- Determine the time of day that patient is most receptive
- Avoid content areas about which patient is sensitive
- Discuss advantages of laughter with patient
- Select humorous materials that create moderate arousal for the individual
- Make available a selection of humorous games, cartoons, jokes, videos, tapes, books, etc.
- Point out humorous incongruity in a situation
- Encourage visualization with humor (e.g., picture a forbidding authority figure dressed only in underwear)
- Encourage silliness and playfulness
- Remove environmental barriers that prevent or diminish the spontaneous occurrence of humor
- Monitor patient response and discontinue humor strategy if ineffective
- Avoid use with patient who is cognitively impaired
- Demonstrate an appreciative attitude about humor
- Respond positively to humor attempts made by patient

1st edition 1992; revised 2008

Background Evidence:

Buxman, K. (1991). Make room for laughter. *American Journal of Nursing, 91*(12), 46–51.

Kolkmeier, L. G. (1988). Play and laughter: Moving toward harmony. In B. M. Dosseyk, L. Keegan, C. E. Guzetta, & L. G. Kolkmeier (Eds.), *Holistic nursing: A handbook for practice* (pp. 289–304). Aspen.

Smith, K. (2006). Humor. In M. Snyder & R. Lindquist (Eds.), *Complimentary/alternative therapies in nursing* (5th ed., pp. 93–106). Springer.

Sullivan, J. L., & Deane, D. M. (1988). Humor and health. *Journal of Gerontological Nursing, 14*(1), 20–24.

Hyperglycemia Management   2120

Definition: Preventing and treating higher than normal blood glucose levels

Activities:

- Identify persons at risk for hyperglycemia
- Determine ability for recognition of hyperglycemia signs and symptoms
- Monitor blood glucose levels, as indicated
- Monitor for signs and symptoms of hyperglycemia (e.g., polyuria, polydipsia, polyphagia, weakness, lethargy, malaise, blurring of vision, headache)
- Monitor urine ketones, as indicated
- Monitor ABG, electrolyte, and glycated or glycosylated hemoglobin (A1C) levels, as indicated
- Monitor orthostatic blood pressure and pulse, as indicated
- Administer medications (e.g., insulin, oral hyperglycemic), as prescribed
- Encourage oral fluid intake
- Monitor fluid status including I&O, as appropriate
- Maintain IV access, as appropriate
- Administer IV fluids, as needed
- Administer IV electrolytes, as appropriate
- Consult health care provider if signs and symptoms of hyperglycemia persist or worsen
- Assist with ambulation if orthostatic hypotension is present
- Provide oral hygiene, if necessary
- Identify possible cause of hyperglycemia
- Anticipate situations in which insulin requirements will increase (e.g., stress, illness)
- Restrict exercise when blood glucose levels are greater than 250 mg/dL, especially if urine ketones are present
- Instruct person and significant others on prevention, recognition, and management of hyperglycemia
- Encourage self-monitoring of blood glucose levels
- Assist to interpret blood glucose levels and signs or symptoms of hyperglycemia
- Review blood glucose records with person and family
- Instruct on urine ketone testing, as appropriate
- Instruct on indications for and significance of urine ketone testing, if appropriate
- Instruct to report moderate or large urine ketone levels to health professional
- Instruct on diabetes management during illness and episodes of high stress (e.g., use of insulin and oral agents, monitoring fluid intake, carbohydrate replacement, when to seek health professional assistance)
- Provide assistance in adjusting regimen to prevent and treat hyperglycemia (e.g., increasing insulin or oral agent), as indicated
- Facilitate adherence to diet and exercise regimen
- Provide educational interventions on glucose awareness training
- Provide feedback regarding appropriateness of self-management of hyperglycemia
- Instruct on signs and symptoms, risk factors, and treatment of hyperglycemia
- Instruct to obtain and carry or wear appropriate emergency identification
- Determine educational needs about medication, supplies, and appointments
- Facilitate adherence to follow-up
- Facilitate resources and support
- Use teach-back to ensure understanding

1st edition 1992; revised 2004, 2024

Background Evidence:

American Diabetes Association. (2021). *Standards of medical care in diabetes.*

American Diabetes Association. (2021). *Blood sugar testing and control: Hyperglycemia (high blood glucose).* https://www.diabetes.org/healthy-living/medication-treatments/blood-glucose-testing-and-control/hyperglycemia

Bellary, S., Kyrou, I., Brown, J. E., & Bailey, C. J. (2021). Type 2 diabetes mellitus in older adults: clinical considerations and management. *National Review of Endocrinology, 17*(9), 534–548. https://doi.org/10.1038/s41574-021-00512-2

Perry, A. G., & Potter, P. A. (2020). *Fundamentals of nursing* (10th ed.). Elsevier.

Perry, A. G., Potter, P. A., Ostendorf, W., & LaPlante, N. (2021). *Clinical nursing skills and techniques* (10th ed.). Elsevier.

Peter, P. R., & Lupsa, B. C. (2019). Personalized management of type 2 diabetes. *Current Diabetes Reports, 19*(115). https://doi.org/10.1007/s11892-019-1244-0

Ryan, D., Burke, S. D., Lichtman, M. L., Bronich-Hall, L., Kolb, L., Rinker, J., & Yehl, K. (2020). Competencies for diabetes care and education specialists. *The Diabetes Educator, 46*(4), 384–397.

H

Hyperlipidemia Management

2125

Definition: Preventing and treating cholesterol and triglyceride blood levels higher than normal

Activities:

- Elicit a detailed patient health history to determine presence of hyperlipidemia or risk level of patient, including medication use and laboratory values
- Identify possible causes of hyperlipidemia (e.g., diet high in saturated fats, red meats, fried foods, dairy products, low in fiber; smoking; obesity; sedentary lifestyle; family history of high cholesterol levels), including metabolic conditions and drugs affecting lipid metabolism (e.g., hypothyroidism, liver or renal disease, anorexia nervosa, untreated diabetes, glucocorticoids, estrogens)
- Perform thorough physical examination, including vital signs, height, weight, waist-to-hip ratio, and body mass index (BMI)
- Determine at-risk patients (e.g., diet high in saturated fats, red meats, fried foods, dairy products and low in fiber; obesity; sedentary lifestyle; family history of high cholesterol levels; smoking or exposure to smoke)
- Use the National Cholesterol Education Expert Adult Treatment Panel III guidelines to determine risk categories and treatment options
- Determine level of patient risk
- Apply treatment guidelines to determine treatment goals (e.g., lifestyle changes as preventative measures versus lifestyle changes with medications)
- Advise at-risk patients to practice lifestyle modification to reduce risk of developing hyperlipidemia (e.g., increase exercise, decrease weight, modify diet, avoid or stop smoking, avoid overconsumption of alcohol)
- Advise at-risk patients to seek appropriate drug therapy if a trial of lifestyle modification fails to reduce hyperlipidemia from at-risk levels
- Assist patients with hyperlipidemia to practice lifestyle modifications and to use appropriate drug therapy, as indicated per treatment guidelines
- Monitor blood chemistry, including cholesterol, triglycerides, LDL and HDL, as indicated per treatment guidelines
- Monitor weight and waist-to-hip ratio
- Instruct at-risk patients to have regular preventative health screenings including cholesterol levels
- Encourage patient to follow the American Heart Association recommendation of cholesterol testing every 4 to 6 years starting at age 20
- Instruct related to healthy dietary pattern (e.g., calorie intake appropriate for height and weight; adequate fiber intake; no saturated fats; cook with vegetable oils; select lean cuts of meat; limit red meat intake; limit dairy products; moderate to low alcohol intake)
- Instruct related to proper weight, weight management, and relationship of weight to hyperlipidemia
- Instruct related to proper physical activity (e.g., moderate exercise 30–45 minutes a day)
- Instruct related to contributing lifestyle habits that should be avoided (e.g., use of tobacco in any form and overconsumption of alcohol)
- Provide information on possible changes in lifestyle necessary to avoid future complications and control the disease process
- Provide information related to the purpose and benefit of the lifestyle changes
- Instruct the patient on possible causes and sequelae of hyperlipidemia
- Educate about usual lack of symptoms and the need for long-term follow-up and therapy
- Instruct patient and family to take an active role in management of disease process
- Instruct patient and family on medication usage and indications, as appropriate
- Inform patient that hyperlipidemia is a major controllable risk factor for coronary artery disease and stroke
- Encourage patient and family to maintain a list of current medications and reconcile routinely at wellness checks, hospital visits, or hospital admissions

7th edition 2018

Background Evidence:

American Association of Critical Care Nurses. (2006). In J. G. Alspach (Ed.), *Core curriculum for critical care nursing* (6th ed.). W.B. Saunders.

Pease, D. (2013). Metabolic syndrome. In T. M. Buttaro, J. Trybulski, P. P. Bailey, & J. Sandberg-Cook (Eds.), *Primary care: A collaborative practice* (4th ed., pp. 1112–1117). . Elsevier Mosby.

Stanhope, M., & Lancaster, J. (2010). *Foundations of nursing in the community: Community-oriented practice* (3rd ed.). Mosby Elsevier.

Stone, N., Robinson, J., Lichtenstein, A., Merz, N., Blum, C., Eckel, R., goldberg, A. C., Gordon, D., Levy, D., Lloyd-Jones, D. M., McBride, P., Schwartz, J. S., Shero, S. T., Smith, S. C., Jr., Watson, K., & Wilson, P. W. F. (2014). 2013 ACC/AHA guideline on the treatment of blood cholesterol to reduce atherosclerotic cardiovascular risk in adults. *Circulation*, *129*(Suppl. 2), S1–S45.

Young, M. (2013). Lipid disorders. In T. M. Buttaro, J. Trybulski, P. P. Bailey, & J. Sandberg-Cook (Eds.), *Primary care: A collaborative practice* (4th ed., pp. 1101–1111). Elsevier Mosby.

Hypertension Management

4162

Definition: Preventing and treating blood pressure levels higher than normal

Activities:

- Elicit a detailed patient health history to determine risk level of patient, including medication use
- Identify possible causes of hypertension
- Evaluate for associated risk factors and contributing factors (e.g., diabetes mellitus, dyslipidemia, obesity, metabolic syndrome, age over 60 years, gender, race, smoking, hyperuremia, sedentary lifestyle, family history of hypertension, cardiovascular disease, history of stroke)
- Measure BP to determine presence of hypertension (e.g., normal, less than 120/80; elevated, 120 to 129/80 or less; hypertension stage 1, 130 to 139/80 to 89; hypertension stage 2, equal or greater than 140/90)

- Assure proper assessment of blood pressure (i.e., classification is based on the average of two or more properly measured, seated, BP readings on each of two or more office visits)
- Avoid measurement of blood pressure for classification when contributing factors are present (e.g., consumption of caffeine, migraine headache, insomnia, agitation)
- Implement proper nursing care for patients based on classification of hypertension
- Assist patients with prehypertensive classification to practice lifestyle modification in order to reduce their risk of developing hypertension in the future (e.g., increase exercise, decrease weight, modify diet, obtain adequate sleep)
- Advise patients with prehypertensive classification and comorbid conditions (e.g., heart failure, diabetes, kidney disease) to seek appropriate drug therapy if a trial of lifestyle modification fails to reduce BP to 130/80 mm Hg or less
- Assist patients with hypertensive stage 1 classification and no comorbid conditions (e.g., heart failure, diabetes, kidney disease) to practice lifestyle modifications and to use appropriate drug therapy (e.g., thiazide-type diuretics for most, possibly angiotensin-converting enzyme inhibitor; angiotensin receptor blocker; beta blocker; calcium channel blocker; or combinations of previous)
- Assist patients with hypertensive stage 2 classification and no comorbid conditions (e.g., heart failure, diabetes, kidney disease) to practice lifestyle modifications and to use appropriate drug therapy (e.g., combinations of angiotensin converting enzyme inhibitor, angiotensin receptor blocker, beta blocker, calcium channel blocker)
- Assist patients with hypertensive stage 1 or 2 classification and comorbid conditions (e.g., heart failure, diabetes, kidney disease) to practice lifestyle modifications as able and to follow recommended drug regime protocols for comorbid condition with hypertension
- Monitor at-risk patients for signs and symptoms of hypertension crisis (e.g., severe headache, dizziness, nausea or vomiting, pallor, sweating, cold skin, changes in vision, epistaxis, confusion, nervousness, restlessness, visual disturbances, altered level of consciousness, chest pain, seizures, cardiac arrest)
- Monitor vital signs such as heart rate, respiratory rate, oxygen saturation, temperature, and blood panels for early identification of complications
- Instruct at-risk patients to have regular preventative health screenings, including electrocardiogram, echocardiogram, electrolytes, urinalysis, as indicated
- Monitor patient for signs and symptoms of hypertension or hypotension after administering prescribed hypertension medication
- Instruct related to healthy dietary pattern
- Instruct related to proper physical activity (e.g., exercise 30 to 45 minutes a day)
- Instruct related to contributing lifestyle habits that should be avoided (e.g., use of tobacco in any form and alcohol)

- Instruct the patient on lifestyle modification related to sleep and rest patterns (e.g., 8 hours per night is recommended)
- Provide information on possible changes in lifestyle necessary to avoid future complications and control the disease process
- Provide information related to the purpose and benefit of the lifestyle changes
- Instruct related to self-blood pressure monitoring and to report abnormal findings
- Instruct the patient on possible causes of hypertension
- Instruct the patient and family to take an active role in the management of disease process, (e.g., medication indications and administration, maintaining proper diet, exercise and healthy habits, quitting smoking, reducing stress, reducing weight, reducing sodium intake, reducing alcohol consumption, increasing exercise, as indicated)
- Instruct the patient and family on medication usage and indications
- Encourage the patient and family to maintain a list of current medications and reconcile routinely at wellness checks, hospital visits, or hospital admissions
- Instruct the patient to recognize and avoid situations that can cause increased BP (e.g., stress or sudden discontinuation of drug treatment)

7th edition 2018

Background Evidence:

American Association of Critical Care Nurses. (2006). In J. G. Alspach (Ed.), *Core curriculum for critical care nursing* (6th ed.). W.B. Saunders.

Chummun, H. (2009). Hypertension: A contemporary approach to nursing care. *British Journal of Nursing*, 18(13), 784–789.

Hacihasanoğlu, R., & Gözüm, S. (2011). The effect of patient education and home monitoring on medication compliance, hypertension management, healthy lifestyle behaviors and BMI in a primary health care setting. *Journal of Clinical Nursing*, 20(5/6), 692–705.

Margolius, D., & Bodenheimer, T. (2010). Controlling hypertension requires a new primary care model. *The American Journal of Managed Care*, 16(9), 648–650.

U.S. Department of Health and Human Services, National Institutes of Health, National Heart, & Lung and Blood Institute. (2004). *Seventh report of the Joint National Committee on prevention, detection, evaluation and treatment of high blood pressure*. National Institute of Health.

Whelton, P. K., Carey, R. M., Aronow, W. S., Casey, D. E. Jr., Collins, K. J., Himmelfarb, C, D., DePalma, S. M., Gidding, S., Jameson, K. A., Jones, D. W., MacLaughlin, E. J., Munter, P., Ovbiagele, B., Smith, S. C., Jr., Spencer, C. C., Stanford, R. S., Taler, S. J., Thomas, R. J., Williams, K. A. Sr., Williamson, J. D., & Wright, J. T. Jr. (2017). ACC/AHA/AAPA/ABC/ACPM/AGS/APhA/ASH/ASPC/NMA/PCNA Guideline for the Prevention, Detection, Evaluation, and Management of High Blood Pressure in Adults. *Journal of the American College of Cardiology*, 71(19), e127–e248. https://doi.org/10.1016/j.jacc.2017.11.006

H

Hyperthermia Management   3786

Definition: Management of symptoms and related conditions associated with an increase in body temperature due to infection or prolonged exposure to excessive heat

Activities:

- Determine cause of increased body temperature (e.g., infection, heat stroke, dehydration, exposure to elements)
- Monitor fever response including body temperature, heart rate, respiratory rate, mental status, thermal comfort, and recently tested microbiology or immunologic lab tests

- Administer oral or IV medications (e.g., antipyretics, antibacterial agents, shiver prevention medications)
- Avoid administering aspirin to children
- Discontinue physical activity and remove from heat source to cooler environment
- Loosen or remove clothing

- Apply external cooling methods (e.g., cold packs to neck, chest, abdomen, scalp, armpits, and groin; hydrogel or air-circulating cooling blankets), as appropriate
- Apply water compresses or sponges in conjunction with antipyretics
- Use antipyretic and shiver prevention with physical cooling for increased efficacy
- Wet body surface and fan but avoid shivering
- Avoid alcohol sponge bath
- Apply internal cooling methods (e.g., iced gastric, bladder, peritoneal, or thoracic lavage), as appropriate
- Provide oral rehydrating solution (e.g., sports drink) or other cold fluid
- Moisturize dry lips and nasal mucosa
- Administer oxygen, as appropriate
- Increase air circulation
- Encourage fluid consumption
- Facilitate rest, applying activity restrictions, if needed
- Monitor for fever-related complications and signs and symptoms of fever-causing condition (e.g., seizure, decreased level of consciousness, abnormal electrolyte status, acid-base imbalance, cardiac arrhythmia)
- Ensure other signs of infection are monitored in elderly persons, as may not display fever during infection
- Ensure safety measures are in place if becomes restless or delirious
- Discontinue cooling activities when core body temperature reaches 39° C
- Monitor for complications (e.g., renal impairment, acid-base imbalance, coagulopathy, pulmonary edema, cerebral edema, multiple organ dysfunction syndrome)
- Instruct on risk factors for heat-related illness (e.g., high environmental temperature, high humidity, dehydration, physical exertion, extremes of age)

- Instruct on measures to prevent heat-related illness (e.g., prevent sun overexposure; ensure adequate fluid intake; seek settings in which air conditioning available; wear lightweight, light-colored, and loose-fitting clothing)
- Instruct on early signs and symptoms of heat-related illness and when to seek assistance from health care professional
- Use teach-back to ensure understanding

6th edition 2013; revised 2024

Background Evidence:

LaPierre, L., & Mondor, E. E. (2017). The ups and downs of fever: Where are we at with targeted temperature management in the ICU? *Canadian Journal of Critical Care Nursing, 28*(2), 39.

Moreda, M., Beacham, P. S., Reese, A., & Mulkey, M. A. (2021). Increasing the effectiveness of targeted temperature management. *Critical Care Nurse, 41*(5), 59–63. https://doi.org/10.4037/ccn2021637

Rodway, G. W., & Suether, S. E. (2019). Pain, temperature, sleep, and sensory function. In S. E. Huether & K. L. McCance (Eds.), *Understanding Pathophysiology.* Elsevier.

Schell-Chaple, H. (2018). Fever suppression in patients with infection. *Nursing Critical Care, 13*(5), 6–13. https://doi.org/10.1097/01.CCN.0000534921.93547.1a

Souza, M. V., Damião, E. B. C., Buchhorn, S. M. M., & Rossato, L. M. (2021). Non-pharmacological fever and hyperthermia management in children: An integrative review. *Acta Paul Enferm, 34*, eAPE00743.

Turan, N., Çulha, Y., Aydın, G. Ö., & Kaya, H. (2020). Persistent fever and nursing care in neurosurgical patients. *Journal of Neurological & Neurosurgical Nursing, 2*, 80–85. https://doi.org/10.15225/PNN.2020.9.2.6

Hypervolemia Management   4170

Definition: Reduction in extracellular and/or intracellular fluid volume and prevention of complications in a patient who is fluid overloaded

Activities:

- Weigh daily at consistent times (e.g., after voiding, before breakfast) and monitor trends
- Monitor hemodynamic status, including HR, BP, MAP, CVP, PAP, PCWP, CO, and CI, if available
- Monitor respiratory pattern for symptoms of pulmonary edema (e.g., anxiety, air hunger, orthopnea, dyspnea, tachypnea, cough, frothy sputum production, and shortness of breath)
- Monitor for adventitious lung sounds
- Monitor for adventitious heart sounds
- Monitor for jugular venous distention
- Monitor for peripheral edema
- Monitor for laboratory evidence of hemoconcentration (e.g., sodium, BUN, hematocrit; urine specific gravity), if available
- Monitor for laboratory evidence of the potential for increased plasma oncotic pressure (e.g., increased protein and albumin), if available
- Monitor for laboratory evidence of the underlying cause for hypervolemia (e.g., B-type natriuretic peptide for heart failure; BUN, Cr, and GFR for renal failure), if available
- Monitor intake and output
- Administer prescribed medications to reduce preload (e.g., furosemide, spironolactone, morphine, and nitroglycerin)

- Monitor for evidence of reduced preload (e.g., increased urine output; improvement in adventitious lung sounds; decreased BP, MAP, CVP, PCWP, CO, CI)
- Monitor for evidence of excessive medication effect (e.g., dehydration, hypotension, tachycardia, hypokalemia)
- Instruct patient on the use of medications to reduce preload
- Administer intravenous infusions (e.g., fluids, blood products) slowly to prevent a rapid increase in preload
- Restrict free water intake in patients with dilutional hyponatremia
- Avoid the use of hypotonic IV fluids
- Elevate head of bed to improve ventilation, as appropriate
- Facilitate endotracheal intubation and initiation of mechanical ventilation for patients with severe pulmonary edema, as appropriate
- Maintain prescribed mechanical ventilator settings (e.g., FiO_2, mode, volume or pressure settings, PEEP), as appropriate
- Use closed-system suction for patient with pulmonary edema on mechanical ventilation with PEEP, as appropriate
- Prepare patient for dialysis (e.g., assist with dialysis catheter insertion), as appropriate
- Maintain dialysis vascular access device
- Determine patient's weight change before and after each dialysis session

- Monitor patient's hemodynamic response during and after each dialysis session
- Determine volume of infused dialysate and returned effluent after each peritoneal dialysis exchange
- Monitor returned peritoneal effluent for indications of complications (e.g., infection, excessive bleeding, and clots)
- Reposition the patient with dependent edema frequently, as appropriate
- Monitor skin integrity in immobile patients with dependent edema
- Promote skin integrity (e.g., prevent shearing, avoid excessive moisture, and provide adequate nutrition) in immobile patients with dependent edema, as appropriate
- Instruct the patient and family on use of intake and output record, as appropriate
- Instruct patient and family on the planned interventions to treat hypervolemia
- Restrict dietary intake of sodium, as indicated
- Promote a positive body image and self-esteem if concerns are expressed as a result of excessive fluid retention

1st edition 1992; revised 2013

Background Evidence:

Heitz, U., & Horne, M. M. (2005). *Pocket guide to fluid, electrolyte, and acid-base balance* (5th ed.). Elsevier Mosby.

Leeper, B. (2006). Cardiovascular system. In M. Chulay & S. M. Burns (Eds.), *AACN essentials of critical care nursing* (pp. 215–246). McGraw-Hill.

Miller, L. R. (2006). Hemodynamic monitoring. In M. Chulay & S. M. Burns (Eds.), *AACN essentials of critical care nursing* (pp. 65–110). McGraw-Hill.

Salvador, D., Punzalan, F., & Ramos, G. (2005). Continuous infusion versus bolus injection of loop diuretics in congestive heart failure. *Cochrane Database of Systematic Reviews, 2005*(3). https://doi.org/10.1002/14651858.CD 003178.pub3

Schroeder, K. (2012). Acute renal failure. In E. T. Bope & R. D. Kellerman (Eds.), *Conn's current therapy 2012* (pp. 873–876). Elsevier Saunders.

Stark, J. (2006). The renal system. In J. G. Alspach (Ed.), *American Association of Critical Care Nurses, Core curriculum for critical care nursing* (6th ed., pp. 525–610). W. B. Saunders.

Winkel, E., & Kao, W. (2012). Heart failure. In E. T. Bope & R. D. Kellerman (Eds.), *Conn's current therapy 2012* (pp. 432–436). Elsevier Saunders.

H

Hypnosis   5920

Definition: Assisting a patient to achieve a state of attentive, focused concentration with suspension of some peripheral awareness to create changes in sensation, thoughts, or behavior

Activities:

- Obtain history of the problem to be treated by hypnosis
- Determine goals for hypnosis with patient
- Determine patient's receptivity to using hypnosis
- Correct myths and misconceptions of hypnosis
- Ensure the patient has accepted the treatment
- Evaluate the suitability of the patient by assessing his or her hypnotic suggestibility
- Determine patient's history with trance states, such as daydreaming and "highway hypnosis"
- Confirm the presence of a trusting relationship
- Prepare a quiet comfortable environment
- Take precautions to prevent interruptions
- Instruct patient on purpose for the intervention
- Instruct patient that he/she will induce the trance state and retain control
- Sit comfortably, half-facing the patient, when appropriate
- Discuss with patient the hypnotic suggestions to be used before induction
- Select an induction technique (e.g., Chevreul pendulum illusion, relaxation, imaging walking down a staircase, eye closure, arm levitation, simple muscle relaxation, visualization exercises, attention to breathing, repetition of key words/phrases, and others)
- Use patient's language as much as possible
- Give a small number of suggestions in an assertive manner
- Combine suggestions with naturally occurring events
- Convey permissive attitude to aid in trance induction
- Use a rhythmical, soothing, monotone voice during patient induction
- Pace statements with patient's respirations
- Encourage patient to take deep breaths to intensify the state of relaxation and decrease tension
- Assist patient to escape to a pleasant place, using guided imagery
- Assist the patient to identify appropriate deepening techniques (e.g., movement of a hand to the face, imagery escalation technique, fractionation, and others)
- Avoid guessing what the patient is thinking
- Assist patient to use all senses during the process
- Determine whether to use directive or nondirective imagery with the patient, as appropriate
- Facilitate quick induction through a specific cue (verbal or visual) with experience
- Instruct patient that the level of trance is not important to successful hypnosis
- Facilitate patient's coming out of the trance by counting to a prearranged number, as appropriate
- Assist patient to come out of the trance at own pace, as appropriate
- Provide positive feedback to patient after each episode
- Encourage patient to use self-induction independent of the nurse to manage problem under treatment
- Identify situations, such as painful procedures, where patient requires additional staff support for effective induction

1st edition 1992; revised 2008

Background Evidence:

Fontaine, K. L. (2005). Hypnotherapy and guided imagery. In K. L. Fountaine (Ed.), *Complementary & alternative therapies for nursing practice* (2nd ed., pp. 301–338). Prentice Hall.

Freeman, L. (Ed.). (2004). Hypnosis. In *Mosby's complementary & alternative medicine: A research-based approach* (2nd ed., pp. 237–274). Mosby.

Lynn, S. J., & Kirsch, I. (2006). *Essentials of clinical hypnosis: An evidence-based approach*. American Psychological Association.

Rankin-Box, D. (2001). Hypnosis. In D. Rankin-Box (Ed.), *The nurse's hand-book of complementary therapies* (2nd ed., pp. 208–214). Edinburgh: Bailliere Tindall.

Zahourek, R. P. (1985). *Clinical hypnosis and therapeutic suggestion in nursing.* Grune & Stratton.

Hypoglycemia Management   2130

Definition: Preventing and treating low blood glucose levels

Activities:
- Identify person at risk for hypoglycemia
- Determine ability for recognizing signs and symptoms of hypoglycemia
- Monitor blood glucose levels
- Monitor for signs and symptoms of hypoglycemia, (e.g., shakiness, tremor, sweating, nervousness, anxiety, irritability, impatience, tachycardia, palpitations, chills, clamminess, light-headedness, pallor, hunger, nausea, headache, tiredness, drowsiness, weakness, warmth, dizziness, faintness, blurred vision, nightmares, crying out in sleep, paresthesia, difficulty concentrating, difficulty speaking, incoordination, behavior change, confusion, coma, seizure)
- Administer glucagon or intravenous glucose, as indicated
- Provide simple carbohydrate if able to eat, utilizing the 15-15 rule (i.e., 15 grams of carbohydrate and check blood sugar after 15 minutes, if below 70 mg/dL, provide another 15 grams)
- Provide complex carbohydrate and protein, as indicated
- Contact emergency medical services, as necessary
- Maintain patent airway, as necessary
- Maintain IV access, as appropriate
- Protect from injury, as necessary
- Review events before hypoglycemia to determine probable cause
- Provide educational interventions on glucose awareness training
- Provide feedback regarding appropriateness of self-management of hypoglycemia
- Instruct person and significant others on signs and symptoms, risk factors, and treatment of hypoglycemia
- Instruct to have simple carbohydrate available at all times
- Instruct to obtain and carry or wear appropriate emergency identification
- Instruct significant others on use and administration of glucagon, as appropriate
- Instruct on interaction of diet, insulin or oral agents, and exercise
- Provide assistance in making self-care decisions to prevent hypoglycemia, (i.e., reducing insulin or oral agents and increasing food intake when exercising)
- Encourage self-monitoring of blood glucose levels
- Provide interdisciplinary team access and approach for consultation regarding adjustments in treatment regimen
- Collaborate with person and diabetes education team to make changes in insulin regimen, (e.g., multiple daily injections), as indicated
- Modify blood glucose goals to prevent hypoglycemia in absence of hypoglycemia symptoms
- Inform of need for routine checks of glycosylated hemoglobin (HbA1c), as prescribed
- Inform of increased risk of hypoglycemia with intensive therapy and normalization of blood glucose levels
- Instruct regarding probable changes in hypoglycemia symptoms with intensive therapy and normalization of blood glucose levels
- Use teach-back to ensure understanding

1st edition 1992; revised 2000, 2024

Background Evidence:

American Diabetes Association. (2021). *Standards of medical care in diabetes.*

American Diabetes Association. (2021). *Hypoglycemia (Low blood glucose).* https://www.diabetes.org/healthy-living/medication-treatments/blood-glucose-testing-and-control/hypoglycemia

Garg, G. K., & Vimalananda, V. (2020). Type 1 diabetes mellitus. *British Medical Journal, (BMJ) Best Practice*, 1–53.

Perry, A. G., & Potter, P. A. (2020). *Fundamentals of nursing* (10th ed.). Elsevier.

Perry, A. G., Potter, P. A., Ostendorf, W., & LaPlante, N. (2021). *Clinical nursing skills and techniques* (10th ed.). Elsevier.

Ryan, D., Burke, S. D., Lichtman, M. L., Bronich-Hall, L., Kolb, L., Rinker, J., & Yehl, K. (2020). Competencies for diabetes care and education specialists. *The Diabetes Educator*, 46(4), 384–397.

Simonson, G., Carlson, A., Martens, T., & Bergenstal, R. (2021). Type 2 diabetes mellitus in adults. *British Medical Journal, (BMJ) Best Practice*, 1–100.

Hypotension Management   4175

Definition: Preventing and treating blood pressure levels lower than normal

Activities:
- Elicit a detailed patient health history to determine hypotension risk level of patient, including medication use
- Identify possible causes of hypotension (e.g., diabetes, coronary artery disease, peripheral artery disease, heart failure, previous stroke, chronic kidney disease, proteinuria, age greater than 50 years, smokers, obesity, treatment of Parkinson's disease, treatment of epilepsy, treatment of depression; nocturnal urination)
- Measure BP to determine presence of hypotension (defined as less than 90 mm Hg systolic and or less than 60 mm Hg diastolic in the general population)
- Assure proper assessment of blood pressure (i.e., hypotensive classification is based on the average of two or more properly measured with position change, BP readings on each of two or more office visits)
- Instruct patients to keep a blood pressure diary with orthostatic blood pressure measurements taken over several days and at various different time points to increase the sensitivity for detection pending issues
- Perform an electrocardiogram, if applicable
- Perform analytical chemistry, if applicable
- Perform blood gas study, if applicable
- Perform additional diagnostic tests, as indicated

- Avoid measurement of BP for classification when contributing factors are present (e.g., recent ingestion of influential medications, allergic responses, blood loss, dehydration)
- Elicit patient's descriptive experience of hypotension (e.g., occurrences, situations, causes, time of day, food or medication intake, sleep patterns)
- Determine medication regime and influences on hypotension (e.g., diuretics, alpha blockers, beta blockers, medications for Parkinson's disease, tricyclic antidepressants)
- Address any conditions influencing hypotension, as needed
- Consider nonpharmacological treatments as first approach
- Discontinue medications that predispose to or exacerbate hypotension, as appropriate
- Educate patient on physical countermeasures to reduce gravitational blood pooling in the lower extremities (e.g., moving gradually from supine to standing positions, avoiding standing motionless, standing with legs crossed, squatting, active tensing of leg muscles)
- Encourage patient to employ approaches to improve central volume (e.g., increase salt consumption to 6 to 9 g of sodium chloride per day with 1 g sodium chloride tablets taken with each meal, if needed; increase water intake up to 2 to 3 liters per day, with rapid water ingestion [16 ounces in 3 to 4 minutes] used as a rescue measure)
- Monitor for complications (e.g., blurred vision, confusion, dizziness, syncope, pallor, cold sweating, tachycardia, dizziness, drowsiness, weakness, altered level of consciousness, seizure, shortness of breath, chest pain)
- Be alert to the need to treat worsening symptoms urgently
- Administer pharmacological agents (e.g., fludrocortisone, midodrine) and monitor effects, if applicable
- Instruct the patient and family to communicate worsening blood pressure numbers or symptoms

- Promote oral fluid intake recommended by age
- Encourage healthy eating and adequate fluid intake
- Instruct patient and family on the need to avoid tobacco, illicit drugs, and alcohol
- Instruct the patient on lifestyle modification
- Provide information and education on possible changes in lifestyle necessary to avoid future complications and control the disease process
- Evaluate as indicated vital signs, such as blood pressure, heart rate, respiratory rate, oxygen saturation, temperature, and other parameters, such as capillary blood glucose, for possible complications
- Refer to a specialist unit, as indicated

7th edition 2018

Background Evidence:

Arnold, A. C., & Shibao, C. (2013). Current concepts in orthostatic hypotension management. *Current Hypertension Reports, 15*(4), 304–312.

Ferrer-Gila, T., & Rizea, C. (2013). Orthostatic hypotension in the elderly. *Revista de Neurologia, 56*(6), 337–343. [Spanish].

Figueroa, J. J., Basford, J. R., & Low, P. A. (2010). Preventing and treating orthostatic hypotension: As easy as A, B, C. *Cleveland Clinic Journal of Medicine, 77*(5), 298–306.

Grossman, E., Voichanski, S., Grossman, C., & Leibowitz, A. (2012). The association between orthostatic hypotension and nocturnal blood pressure may explain the risk for heart failure. *Hypertension, 60*(1), e1.

Mager, D. R. (2012). Orthostatic hypotension: Pathophysiology, problems, and prevention. *Home Healthcare Nurse, 30*(9), 525–530.

Shibao, C., Grijalva, C. G., Raj, S. R., Biaggioni, I., & Griffin, M. R. (2007). Orthostatic hypotension-related hospitalizations in the United States. *The American Journal of Medicine, 120*(11), 975–980.

H

Hypothermia Induction Therapy 3790

Definition: Attaining and maintaining core body temperature below 35°C and monitoring for side effects and/or prevention of complications

Activities:
- Monitor vital signs, as appropriate
- Monitor patient's temperature, using a continuous core temperature monitoring device, as appropriate
- Place patient on a cardiac monitor
- Institute active external cooling measures (e.g., ice packs, water cooling blanket, circulating water cooling pads), as appropriate
- Institute active internal cooling measures (e.g., intravascular cooling catheters), as appropriate
- Monitor skin color and temperature
- Monitor for shivering
- Use facial or hand warming or insulative wraps to diminish shivering response, as appropriate
- Give appropriate medication to prevent or control shivering
- Monitor for and treat arrhythmias, as appropriate
- Monitor for electrolyte imbalance
- Monitor for acid-base imbalance
- Monitor intake and output
- Monitor respiratory status
- Monitor coagulation studies, including prothrombin time, activated partial thromboplastin time, and platelet counts, as indicated

- Monitor the patient closely for signs and symptoms of persistent bleeding
- Monitor white blood cell count, as appropriate
- Monitor hemodynamic status (e.g., PCWP, CO, SVR), using invasive hemodynamic monitoring, as appropriate
- Promote adequate fluid and nutritional intake

5th edition 2008

Background Evidence:

Holtzclaw, B. J. (2004). Shivering in acutely ill vulnerable populations. *AACN Clinical Issues, 15*(2), 267–279.

McIlvoy, L. H. (2005). The effect of hypothermia and hyperthermia on acute brain injury. *AACN Clinical Issues, 16*(4), 488–500.

Wright, J. E. (2005). Therapeutic hypothermia in traumatic brain injury. *Critical Care Nursing Quarterly, 28*(2), 150–161.

Zeitzer, M. B. (2005). Inducing hypothermia to decrease neurological deficit: Literature review. *Journal of Advanced Nursing, 52*(2), 189–199.

H

Hypothermia Treatment 3800

Definition: Heat loss prevention, rewarming, and surveillance of a patient whose core body temperature is abnormally low as a result of noninduced circumstances

Activities:

- Monitor patient's temperature, using most appropriate measuring device and route
- Remove patient from cold environment
- Remove patient's cold, wet clothing
- Place patient in supine position, minimizing orthostatic changes
- Minimize stimulation of the patient (i.e., handle gently and avoid excessive movement) to avoid precipitating ventricular fibrillation
- Encourage patient with uncomplicated hypothermia to consume warm, high carbohydrate liquids without alcohol or caffeine
- Share body heat, using minimal clothing to facilitate heat transfer between victim and rescuer
- Apply passive rewarming (e.g., blanket, head covering, and warm clothing)
- Apply active external rewarming (e.g., heating pad placed on truncal area before extremities, hot water bottles, forced air warmer, warmed blanket, radiant light, warmed packs, and convective air heaters)
- Avoid active external rewarming for the severely hypothermic patient
- Apply active internal rewarming or "core rewarming" (e.g., warmed IV fluids, warmed humid oxygen, cardiopulmonary bypass, hemodialysis, continuous arteriovenous rewarming, and warm lavage of body cavities)
- Monitor for complications associated with extracorporeal rewarming (e.g., acute respiratory distress syndrome, acute renal failure, and pneumonia)
- Initiate CPR for patients without spontaneous circulation, remaining aware that defibrillation attempts may be ineffective until core temperature is higher than 30° C

- Administer medications using caution (e.g., be aware of unpredictable metabolism, monitor for increased action or toxicity, and consider withholding IV medications until core temperature is higher than 30° C)
- Monitor for symptoms associated with mild hypothermia (e.g., tachypnea, dysarthria, shivering, hypertension, and diuresis), moderate hypothermia (e.g., atrial arrhythmias, hypotension, apathy, coagulopathy, and decreased reflexes), and severe hypothermia (e.g., oliguria, absent neurological reflexes, pulmonary edema, and acid-base abnormalities)
- Monitor for rewarming shock
- Monitor skin color and temperature
- Identify medical, environmental, and other factors that may precipitate hypothermia (e.g., cold water immersion, illness, traumatic injury, shock states, immobilization, weather, extremes of age, medications, alcohol intoxication, malnutrition, hypothyroidism, diabetes, and malnutrition)

1st edition 1992; revised 2013

Background Evidence:

Ireland, S., Murdoch, K., Ormrod, P., Saliba, E., Endacott, R., Fitzgerald, M., & Cameron, P. (2006). Nursing and medical staff knowledge regarding the monitoring and management of accidental or exposure hypothermia in adult major trauma patients. *International Journal of Nursing Practice*, 12(6), 308–318.

Laskowski-Jones, L. (2010). Care of patients with common environmental emergencies. In D. D. Ignatavicius & M. L. Workman (Eds.), *Medical-surgical nursing: Patient-centered collaborative care* (6th ed., pp. 141–168). Elsevier Saunders.

Smith, S. F., Duell, D. J., & Martin, B. C. (2008). *Clinical nursing skills: Basic to advanced skills* (7th ed.). Pearson: Prentice Hall.

Hypovolemia Management 4180

Definition: Expansion of intravascular fluid volume in a patient who is volume depleted

Activities:

- Weigh daily at consistent times (e.g., after voiding, before breakfast) and monitor trends
- Monitor hemodynamic status, including HR, BP, MAP, CVP, PAP, PCWP, CO, and CI, if available
- Monitor for evidence of dehydration (e.g., poor skin turgor, delayed capillary refill, weak/thready pulse, severe thirst, dry mucous membranes, and decreased urine output)
- Monitor for orthostatic hypotension and dizziness upon standing
- Monitor for sources of fluid loss (e.g., bleeding, vomiting, diarrhea, excessive perspiration, and tachypnea)
- Monitor intake and output
- Monitor vascular access device insertion site for infiltration, phlebitis, and infection, as appropriate

- Monitor for laboratory evidence of blood loss (e.g., hemoglobin, hematocrit, fecal occult blood test), if available
- Monitor for laboratory evidence of hemoconcentration (e.g., sodium, BUN, urine specific gravity), if available
- Monitor for laboratory and clinical evidence of impending acute kidney injury (e.g., increased BUN, increased creatinine, decreased GFR, myoglobinemia, and decreased urine output)
- Encourage oral fluid intake (i.e., distribute fluids over 24 hours and give fluids with meals), unless contraindicated
- Offer a beverage of choice every 1 to 2 hours when awake, unless contraindicated
- Maintain patent IV access
- Calculate fluid needs based on body surface area and size of burn, as appropriate

- Administer prescribed isotonic IV solutions (e.g., normal saline or lactated Ringer's solution) for extracellular rehydration at an appropriate flow rate, as appropriate
- Administer prescribed hypotonic IV solutions (e.g., 5% dextrose in water or 0.45% sodium chloride) for intracellular rehydration at an appropriate flow rate, as appropriate
- Administer prescribed isotonic IV fluid bolus at an appropriate flow rate to maintain hemodynamic integrity
- Administer prescribed colloid suspensions (e.g., Hespan, albumin, or Plasmanate), for replacement of intravascular volume, as appropriate
- Administer prescribed blood products to increase plasma oncotic pressure and replace blood volume, as appropriate
- Monitor for evidence of blood transfusion reaction, as appropriate
- Institute autotransfusion of blood loss, if appropriate
- Monitor for evidence of hypervolemia and pulmonary edema during IV rehydration
- Administer IV fluids at room temperature
- Use an IV pump to maintain a steady intravenous infusion flow rate
- Monitor skin integrity in immobile patients with dry skin
- Promote skin integrity (e.g., prevent shearing, avoid excessive moisture, and provide adequate nutrition) in immobile patients with dry skin, as appropriate
- Assist patient with ambulation in case of postural hypotension
- Instruct the patient to avoid rapid position changes, especially from supine to sitting or standing
- Implement modified Trendelenburg positioning (e.g., legs elevated higher than heart level with rest of body supine) when hypotensive to optimize cerebral perfusion while minimizing myocardial oxygen demand
- Monitor oral cavity for dry and/or cracked mucous membranes
- Provide oral fluids (or moistened mouth swabs) frequently to maintain oral mucous membrane integrity, unless contraindicated
- Facilitate oral cleaning (e.g., toothbrush with toothpaste, nonalcohol based mouthwash) twice daily

- Position for peripheral perfusion
- Administer prescribed vasodilators with caution (e.g., nitroglycerin, nitroprusside, and calcium channel blockers) when rewarming a postoperative patient, as appropriate
- Administer prescribed atrial natriuretic peptide (ANP) to prevent acute kidney injury, as appropriate
- Instruct the patient and/or family on the use of intake and output record, as appropriate
- Instruct the patient and/or family on measures instituted to treat the hypovolemia

1st edition 1992; revised 2013

Background Evidence:

Heitz, U., & Horne, M. M. (2005). *Pocket guide to fluid, electrolyte, and acid-base balance* (5th ed.). Elsevier Mosby.

Leeper, B. (2006). Cardiovascular system. In M. Chulay & S. M. Burns (Eds.), *AACN essentials of critical care nursing* (pp. 215–246). McGraw-Hill.

Mentes, J. C. (2008). Managing oral hydration. In E. Capezuti, D. Zwicker, M. Mezey, & T. Fulmer (Eds.), *Evidence-based geriatric nursing protocols for best practice* (3rd ed., pp. 391–402). Springer.

Miller, L. R. (2006). Hemodynamic monitoring. In M. Chulay & S. M. Burns (Eds.), *AACN essentials of critical care nursing* (pp. 65–110). McGraw-Hill.

Nigwekar, S. U., Navaneethan, S. D., Parikh, C. R., & Hix, J. K. (2009). Atrial natriuretic peptide for preventing and treating acute kidney injury. *Cochrane Database of Systematic Reviews, 2009*(4). https://doi.org/10.1002/14651858.CD006028.pub2

Smeltzer, S. C., & Bare, B. G. (2004). (10th ed.) *Brunner & Suddarth's textbook of medical surgical nursing* (Vol. 1, pp. 256–259). Lippincott Williams & Wilkins.

Stark, J. (2006). The renal system. In J. G. Alspach (Ed.), *American Association of Critical Care Nurses, Core curriculum for critical care nursing* (6th ed., pp. 525–610). W. B. Saunders.

H

Impulse Control Training 4370

Definition: Assisting the patient to mediate impulsive behavior through application of problem-solving strategies to social and interpersonal situations

Activities:

- Select a problem-solving strategy that is appropriate to the patient's developmental level and cognitive functioning
- Use a behavior modification plan to reinforce the problem-solving strategy that is being taught, as appropriate
- Assist patient to identify the problem or situation that requires thoughtful action
- Instruct patient to cue self to "stop and think" before acting impulsively
- Instruct patient to consider own thoughts and feelings before acting impulsively
- Demonstrate the steps of the problem-solving strategy in the context of situations that are meaningful to the patient
- Assist patient to identify courses of possible actions and their costs and benefits
- Assist patient to choose the most beneficial course of action
- Provide positive reinforcement (e.g., praise, rewards) for successful outcomes
- Encourage patient to self-reward for successful outcomes
- Assist patient to evaluate how unsuccessful outcomes could have been avoided by different behavioral choices
- Provide opportunities for patient to practice problem solving (e.g., role playing) within the therapeutic environment
- Encourage patient to practice impulse control strategies in social and interpersonal situations outside the therapeutic environment, followed by evaluation of outcome

2nd edition 1996; revised 2018

Background Evidence:

Fujita, K. (2011). On conceptualizing self-control as more than the effortful inhibition of impulses. *Personality and Social Psychology Review, 15*(4), 352–366.

Hofmann, W., Friese, M., & Strack, F. (2009). Impulse and self-control from a dual-systems perspective. *Perspectives on Psychological Science, 4*(20), 162–176.

Limandri, B. J., & Boyd, M. A. (2005). Personality and impulse control disorders. In M. A. Boyd (Ed.), *Psychiatric nursing: Contemporary practice* (3rd ed., pp. 420–469). Lippincott Williams & Wilkins.

Oberle, E., Schonert-Reichl, K., Lawlor, M., & Thomson, K. (2012). Mindfulness and inhibitory control in early adolescence. *The Journal of Early Adolescence, 32*(4), 565–588.

Incident Reporting 7980

Definition: Written and verbal reporting of any event in the process of patient care that is inconsistent with desired patient outcomes or routine operations of the health care facility

Activities:

- Identify events (e.g., patient falls, blood transfusion reactions, and equipment malfunction) that compromise patient safety and thereby require reporting, as defined in agency policy
- Notify physician to evaluate patient, as appropriate
- Notify nursing supervisor, as appropriate
- Document in patient record that physician was notified
- Complete incident report form(s) to include factual information, patient hospital number, medical diagnosis, and date of admission
- Document factual information about the event in the patient record, as appropriate
- Document nursing assessments and interventions after the event
- Identify and report medical device failures leading to patient injury, as appropriate
- Maintain confidentiality of incident report, according to agency policy
- Initiate Medical Device Reporting System for deaths or serious injury resulting from medical devices
- Discuss event with involved staff to determine what, if any, corrective action is necessary
- Provide feedback to all staff about lessons learned and organizational changes resulting from an incident report, as appropriate
- Promote a culture that supports the idea that voluntary event reporting is a form of passive surveillance for near misses and unsafe conditions
- Combine event reports with active surveillance methods (e.g., direct observation, chart audits) to identify and prioritize patient safety threats
- Understand that a higher workload may be related to a higher number of patient safety incidents

2nd edition 1996; revised 2018

Background Evidence:

Agency for Health Care Research and Quality. (2014). Voluntary patient safety event reporting (incident reporting). *Patient Safety Primers.* https://psnet.ahrq.gov/primers/primer/13/voluntary-patient-safety-event-reporting-incident-reporting?q=Voluntary+patient+safety+event+reporting

Besmer, M., Bressler, T., & Barrell, C. (2010). Evidence-based nursing: Using incident reports as a teaching tool. *Nursing Management, 41*(7), 16–18.

Khorsandi, M., Skouras, C., Beatson, K., & Alijani, A. (2012). Quality review of an adverse incident reporting system and root cause analysis of serious adverse surgical incidents in a teaching hospital of Scotland. *Online Patient Safety in Surgery, 6*(1). https://doi.org/10.1186/1754-9493-6-21

Nishizaki, Y., Tokuda, Y., Sato, E., Kato, K., Matsumoto, A., Takekata, M., Terai, M., Watanabe, C., Lim, Y. Y., Phde, S., & Ishikawa, R. (2010). Relationship between nursing workloads and patient safety incidents. *Journal of Multidisciplinary Healthcare, 3*, 49–54.

Incision Site Care 3440

Definition: Cleansing, monitoring, and promotion of healing in a wound that is closed with sutures, clips, or staples

Activities:

- Explain procedure using sensory preparation
- Administer analgesic medications 30 to 60 minutes prior to incision care
- Use hand hygiene and aseptic technique
- Inspect incision site for redness, swelling, signs of dehiscence, evisceration, or drainage
- Monitor healing process and signs and symptoms of infection at incision site
- Cleanse area around incision with appropriate non-cytotoxic cleansing solution and gentle friction
- Swab from clean area toward less clean area (i.e., from incision to surrounding skin; from drain insertion in circular motion spiraling outward)
- Direct any irrigation fluid to flow from least to most contaminated area
- Use swab or gauze piece only once across incision and discard
- Use sterile, cotton-tipped applicators for efficient cleansing of tight-fitting wire sutures, deep and narrow wounds, or wounds with pockets
- Cleanse area around any drain site or drainage tube last
- Maintain position of drainage tube, if indicated
- Apply incision closure strips, as appropriate
- Use reusable tape or skin barriers to avoid repeated removal of tape from sensitive skin areas
- Apply antiseptic ointment, as prescribed
- Remove sutures, staples, or clips, as indicated
- Change dressing at appropriate intervals
- Apply appropriate dressing to protect incision
- Facilitate person's viewing of incision
- Instruct on how to care for incision during bathing or showering
- Educate how to minimize stress on incision site
- Instruct how to care for incision, including signs and symptoms of infection
- Educate on reasons to notify health care provider (e.g., fever redness, swelling, wound dehiscence)
- Use teach-back to ensure understanding
- Document incision care, incision status and education provided

1st edition 1992; revised 2000, 2024

Background Evidence:

Beauchaine, D. (2021). Skin integrity and wound healing. In R. F. Craven, C. J. Hirnle, & C. J. Henshaw (Eds.), *Fundamentals of nursing: Human health and function* (8th ed.). Wolters-Kluwer.

Berman, A., Snyder, S. J., & Frandsen, G. (2018). Skin integrity and wound care. In *Kozier and Erb's Fundamentals of nursing: Concepts, process and practice* (pp. 837–857) (10th ed.). Pearson.

Boon, C. J. W. (2021). Skin integrity and wound care. In P. A. Potter, A. G. Perry, P. A. Stockert, & A. M. Hall (Eds.), *Fundamentals of nursing* (10th ed., pp. 1207–1210). Elsevier.

Perry, A. G., Potter, P. A., Ostendorf, W. R., & Laplante, N. (2022). Wound care and irrigation. In *Clinical Nursing Skills and Techniques* (10th ed.). Elsevier.

Williams, P. (2020). *Basic geriatric nursing* (7th ed.). Elsevier.

I

Infant Care 6820

Definition: Provision of developmentally-appropriate, family-centered care to the child under 1 year of age

Activities:

- Encourage consistent assignment of professional caregivers
- Monitor infant's height and weight
- Monitor intake and output
- Incorporate parent preferences for bathing, when possible
- Change diapers
- Feed infant foods that are developmentally appropriate
- Provide opportunities for nonnutritive sucking
- Keep side rails of crib up when not caring for infant
- Remove small items from crib (e.g., syringe covers and alcohol wipes)
- Monitor safety of infant's environment
- Provide developmentally appropriate safe toys and activities for infant
- Provide information to parent about child development and child rearing
- Provide visual, auditory, tactile, and kinetic stimulation during play
- Structure play and care around infant's temperament
- Talk to infant when giving care
- Encourage parent to participate in care activities (e.g., bathing, feeding, medication administration, or dressing changes)
- Instruct parent to perform special care for infant
- Reinforce parent skill in performing special care for infant
- Inform parent about infant's status
- Involve parent in decision making, providing support throughout process
- Explain rationale for treatments and procedures to parent
- Give parent the option of being present for procedure or returning upon its completion
- Apply restraints when indicated and monitor throughout use
- Comfort infant through rocking, holding, cuddling, swaddling
- Monitor infant for signs of pain, including kicking, legs drawn up, steady crying, and difficulty consoling
- Use pain management strategies (e.g., distraction, parent's involvement, positioning, swaddling, or environmental manipulation)
- Explain to parent that regression is normal during times of stress, such as illness or hospitalization
- Encourage family to visit and stay overnight in hospital
- Provide emotional and spiritual support to parent (e.g., be available to listen, assist with maintaining or creating coping strategies, or referral)
- Maintain infant's daily routine during hospitalization, when possible

- Provide quiet, uninterrupted environment during nap time and nighttime

1st edition 1992; revised 2013

Background Evidence:

Algren, C. L. (2007). Family-centered care of the child during illness and hospitalization. In M. J. Hockenberry & D. Wilson (Eds.), *Wong's nursing care of infants and children* (8th ed., pp. 1046–1082). Mosby Elsevier.

Hopia, H., Tomlinson, P. S., Paavilainen, E., & Astedt-Kurki, P. (2005). Child in hospital: Family experiences and expectations of how nurses can promote family health. *Journal of Clinical Nursing, 14*(2), 212–222.

Pillitteri, A. (2007). The family with an infant. In *Maternal and child health nursing: Care of the childbearing and childrearing family* (pp. 824–859) (5th ed.). Lippincott Williams & Wilkins.

Ward, S. L., & Hisley, S. M. (2009). Caring for the child in the hospital and in the community. In *Maternal-child nursing care: Optimizing outcomes for mothers, children, & families* (pp. 664–700). F.A. Davis.

Ward, S. L., & Hisley, S. M. (2009). Caring for the family across care settings. In *Maternal-child nursing care: Optimizing outcomes for mothers, children, & families* (pp. 701–714). F.A. Davis.

Infant Care: Eye Examination Support 6810

Definition: Reducing pain and promoting comfort during preterm infant eye examination

Activities:

- Schedule eye examination for preterm infant
- Inform parents or guardians about eye screening and examination procedures
- Ensure quiet and calm setting
- Adjust ambient light to moderate-low level
- Obtain baseline heart rate, oxygen saturation, and respiratory rate
- Apply eye drops 1 hour before examination to dilate pupils and at appropriate intervals thereafter, per manufacturer instructions and per agency protocol
- Place supine on flat surface with appropriate swaddling and arms and legs flexed
- Place small pad under head to support cervical spine and thoracic first and second vertebrae
- Offer oral glucose 10 to 15 minutes before procedure, and before body restraint
- Offer pacifier before beginning examination
- Leave pacifier in place throughout examination if suckles
- Use soft tone while talking to infant
- Ensure warm temperature of nurse hands and use only gentle touch
- Hyperextend head minimally
- Apply local anesthetic drops to eyes as indicated
- Monitor heart rate, oxygen saturation, and respiratory rate during procedure
- Ensure head stable and immobile
- Wait until ophthalmologist places eyelid retractor on left or right eye before examination
- Rate pain using appropriate pain scale for neonates or premature infants (e.g., Premature Infant Pain Profile, N-PASS, CRIES)
- Provide oxygen if oxygen saturation <85% due to maneuvers made during examination (e.g., scleral depression, traction of extraocular muscles, globe pressure)
- Stop procedure and rest infant if heart rate >200 bpm
- Maintain swaddling position throughout examination for both eyes, as indicated
- Give pacifier and maintain swaddling position until calmed down after completion of examination
- Rate pain level
- Record procedure
- Closely monitor nausea, apnea, increase in gastric residue, temporary changes in heart rate and desaturation for 24 hours after eye examination

8th edition 2024

Background Evidence:

Chuang, L., Chen, C., Huang, M., Wang, S., Ma, M., & Lin, C. (2019). A modified developmental care bundle reduces pain and stress in preterm infants undergoing examinations for retinopathy of prematurity: A randomized controlled trial. *Journal of Clinical Nursing (John Wiley & Sons, Inc.), 28*(3/4), 545–559. https://doi.org/10.1111/jocn.14645

Chuang, L., & Huang, M. (2020). The clinical application of developmental care in retinopathy of prematurity eye examinations. *Journal of Nursing, 67*(5), 82–88. https://doi.org/10.6224/JN.202010_67(5).11

Jang, E. K., Lee, H., Jo, K. S., Lee, S. M., Seo, H. J., & Huh, E. J. (2019). Comparison of the pain-relieving effects of human milk, sucrose, and distilled water during examinations for retinopathy of prematurity: A randomized controlled trial. *Child Health Nursing Research, 25*(3), 255–261. https://doi.org/10.4094/chnr.2019.25.3.255

Metreş, Ö., & Yıldız, S. (2019). Pain management with ROP position in Turkish preterm infants during eye examinations: A randomized controlled trial. *Journal of Pediatric Nursing, 49*, e81–e89. https://doi.org/10.1016/j.pedn.2019.08.013

Sloane, A. J., O'Donnell, E. A., Mackley, A. B., Reid, J. E., Greenspan, J. S., Paul, D. A., & Aghai, Z. H. (2021). Do extremely preterm infants need retinopathy of prematurity screening earlier than 31 weeks postmenstrual age? *Journal of Perinatology, 41*(2), 305–309. https://doi.org/10.1038/s41372-020-0681-6

Tan, J. B. C., Dunbar, J., Hopper, A., Wilson, C. G., & Angeles, D. M. (2019). Differential effects of the retinopathy of prematurity exam on the physiology of premature infants. *Journal of Perinatology, 39*(5), 708–716. https://doi.org/10.1038/s41372-019-0331-z

Infant Care: Newborn   6824

Definition: Provision of care to the infant during the transition from birth to extrauterine life

Activities:

- Clear secretions from oral and nasal passages
- Perform Apgar evaluation at 1 and 5 minutes after birth
- Obtain weight, length, and fronto-occipital circumference
- Monitor temperature
- Maintain adequate body temperature of newborn (i.e., dry infant immediately after birth, wrap in blanket if not to be placed in warmer or skin to skin with parent)
- Apply stockinette cap and instruct parent to keep head covered
- Monitor respiratory rate and breathing pattern
- Respond to signs of respiratory distress (e.g., tachypnea, nasal flaring, grunting, retractions, rhonchi, rales)
- Monitor heart rate and skin color
- Place skin-to-skin with parent for first 1–2 hours after birth, as appropriate
- Administer vitamin K injection, as appropriate
- Determine gestational age within 2 hours after birth (e.g., New Ballard Score)
- Compare weight with estimated gestational age
- Put to breast immediately after birth if breastfeeding preferred method of feeding
- Monitor first feeding
- Monitor suck reflex during feeding
- Hold infant during feedings, attempt to burp during and after
- Burp with head elevated
- Monitor weight, intake, and output
- Record first voiding and bowel movement
- Assist parent in giving initial bath after temperature has stabilized
- Regularly hold or touch in isolette
- Provide prophylactic eye care
- Compare maternal and newborn blood groups and types
- Swaddle to promote sleep and provide sense of security
- Position on back or hold in reclined position after feeding
- Provide information about nutritional needs, feeding techniques, and signs of infant stress during feeding
- Determine condition of cord before transfusion using umbilical vein
- Keep umbilical cord dry and exposed to air by diapering below cord
- Monitor umbilical cord for redness and drainage
- Cleanse and apply petroleum jelly dressing to circumcision
- Apply diapers loosely after circumcision
- Apply restraints when indicated and monitor appropriately throughout use
- Monitor response to circumcision and signs of bleeding
- Monitor for hypoglycemia and anomalies if mother has diabetes
- Monitor for signs of hyperbilirubinemia every 8–12 hours
- Instruct parent to recognize symptoms of hyperbilirubinemia
- Protect from sources of infection in hospital environment
- Determine readiness state before providing care
- Make eye contact and talk to newborn when giving care
- Provide quiet, soothing environment
- Respond to cues for care to facilitate development of trust
- Promote and facilitate family bonding and attachment with newborn
- Provide information and facilitate screening for metabolic disorders
- Instruct parent to recognize signs of breathing difficulty
- Instruct parent to place newborn alone and on back when sleeping, with no loose pillows or blankets
- Keep bulb syringe accessible and instruct parents on use
- Complete critical congenital heart disease screening test at 24 and 48 hours of age
- Discourage pacifier use until breastfeeding well established
- Encourage frequent diaper changes and provide education on stool transition expectation
- Ensure hearing screening conducted prior to discharge
- Conduct monitored car seat evaluation with infant, as needed
- Instruct parents on post-circumcision monitoring and care, as appropriate
- Complete discharge planning and education
- Use teach-back to ensure parental understanding

6th edition 2013; revised 2024

Background Evidence:

Garzon Maaks, D. L., Barber Starr, N., Brady, M. A., Gaylord, N. M., Driessnack, M., & Duderstadt, K. G. (2021). *Burns' pediatric primary care* (7th ed.). Elsevier.

Hockenberry, M. J., & Wilson, D. (2019). *Wong's nursing care of infants and children* (11th ed.). Elsevier.

Perry, S. E., Hockenberry, M. J., Lowdermilk, D. L., & Wilson, D. (2018). *Maternal child nursing care* (6th ed.). Elsevier.

Richardson. (2020). *Pediatric primary care: Practice guidelines for nurses* (4th ed.) Jones & Bartlett Learning.

Infant Care: Preterm   6826

Definition: Aligning caretaking practices with the preterm infant's individual developmental and physiological needs to support growth and development

Activities:

- Create a therapeutic and supportive relationship with parent
- Provide space for parent on unit and at infant's bedside
- Provide parent with accurate, factual information regarding the infant's condition, treatment, and needs
- Inform parent about developmental considerations in preterm infants
- Facilitate parent-infant bonding/attachment
- Instruct parent to recognize infant cues and states
- Demonstrate how to elicit infant's visual or auditory attention
- Assist parent in planning care that is responsive to infant cues and states
- Point out infant's self-regulatory activities (e.g., hand to mouth, sucking, use of visual or auditory stimulus)

- Provide "time out" when infant exhibits signs of stress (e.g., finger splaying, poor color, fluctuation of heart and respiratory rates)
- Instruct parent how to console infant using behavioral quieting techniques (e.g., placing hand on infant, positioning, and swaddling)
- Create individualized development plan and update regularly (e.g., Neonatal Individualized Development Care and Assessment Program [NIDCAP])
- Avoid overstimulation by stimulating one sense at a time (i.e., avoid talking while handling and looking at while feeding)
- Provide boundaries that maintain flexion of extremities while still allowing room for extension (e.g., nesting, swaddling, bunting, hammock, hat, and clothing)
- Provide supports to maintain positioning and prevent deformities (e.g., back rolls, nesting, bunting, and head donuts)
- Reposition infant frequently
- Provide midline orientation of arms to facilitate hand-to-mouth activities
- Provide water mattress and sheepskin, as appropriate
- Use smallest diaper to prevent hip abduction
- Monitor stimuli (e.g., light, noise, handling, and procedures) in infant's environment and reduce, when possible
- Decrease environmental ambient light
- Shield eyes of infant when using lights with high, foot-candles wattage
- Alter environmental lighting to provide diurnal rhythmicity
- Decrease environmental noise (i.e., turn down and respond quickly to monitor alarms and telephones and move conversation away from bedside)
- Position incubator away from sources of noise (e.g., sinks, doors, telephone, high activity, radio, and traffic pattern)
- Time infant care and feeding around sleep and wake cycle
- Gather and prepare equipment needed away from bedside
- Cluster care to promote longest possible sleep interval and energy conservation
- Position infant for sleeping in prone upright position on parent's bared chest, if appropriate
- Provide comfortable chair in quiet area for feeding
- Use slow, gentle movements when handling, feeding, and caring for infant
- Position and support throughout feeding, maintaining flexion and midline position (e.g., shoulder and truncal support, foot bracing, hand holding, use of bunting, or swaddling)
- Feed in upright position to promote tongue extension and swallowing
- Promote parent participation in feeding
- Support breastfeeding

- Monitor intake and output
- Use a pacifier during gavage feeding and between feedings for nonnutritive sucking to promote physiological stability and nutritional status
- Facilitate state transition and calming during painful, stressful-but-necessary procedures
- Establish consistent and predictable routines to promote regular sleep and wake cycles
- Provide stimulation using recorded instrumental music, mobiles, massage, rocking, and touch
- Monitor and manage oxygenation needs
- Cover eyes and genitalia with opaque shield for child receiving phototherapy
- Remove eye mask during feedings and regularly to monitor for discharge or corneal irritation
- Monitor hematocrit and administer blood transfusions, when necessary
- Inform parent about prevention measures for SIDS (Sudden Infant Death Syndrome)

6th edition 2013

Background Evidence:

Becker, P. T., Grunwald, P. C., Moorman, J., & Stuhr, S. (1991). Outcomes of developmentally supportive nursing care for very low birth weight infants. *Nursing Research, 40*(3), 150–155.

Brown, G. (2009). NICU noise and the preterm infant. *Neonatal Network, 28*(3), 165–173.

Johnston, A., Bullock, C., Graham, J., Reilly, M., Rocha, C., Hoopes, R., Jr., Van Der Meid, V., Gutierrez, S., & Abraham, M. (2006). Implementation and case-study results of potentially better practices for family-centered care: The family-centered care map. *Pediatrics, 118*(Suppl. 2), S108–S114.

Pinelli, J., & Symington, A. J. (2005). Non-nutritive sucking for promoting physiologic stability and nutrition in preterm infants. *Cochrane Database of Systematic Reviews, 2005*(4). https://doi.org/10.1002/14651858.CD001071.pub2

Symington, A. J., & Pinelli, J. (2006). Developmental care for promoting development and preventing morbidity in preterm infants. *Cochrane Database of Systematic Reviews, 2006*(2). https://doi.org/10.1002/14651858.CD001814.pub2

Wallin, L., & Eriksson, M. (2009). Newborn individual developmental care and assessment program (NIDCAP): A systematic review of the literature. *Worldviews on Evidence-Based Nursing, 6*(2), 54–69.

Ward, S. L., & Hisley, S. M. (2009). Caring for the newborn at risk. In *Maternal-child nursing care: Optimizing outcomes for mothers, children, & families* (pp. 603–637). F.A. Davis.

Infection Control   6540

Definition: Minimizing the acquisition and transmission of infectious agents

Activities:

- Follow universal precautions for all care activities
- Wash hands or use antimicrobial hand sanitizer before and after each care activity
- Promote easy access to antimicrobial hand sanitizers (i.e., hang dispenser on wall or place by doors to all care areas)
- Use PPE whenever expectation of possible exposure to infectious material

- Ensure easy access to appropriate PPE to provide care for persons with known infectious material or disease (e.g., gloves, face masks, goggles, isolation gowns)
- Promote protection of eyes, nose, and mouth
- Position persons to direct sprays and splatter away from face of caregiver
- Provide mouthpieces, pocket resuscitation masks with one-way valves, and other ventilation devices to ensure alternatives to

mouth-to-mouth resuscitation and prevent exposure of care-giver's nose and mouth to oral and respiratory fluids during resuscitation efforts

- Employ particulate respirator masks (e.g., N-95) during aero-sol-generating procedures when aerosol likely to contain certain respiratory pathogens (e.g., *M. tuberculosis*, COVID-2019, avian or pandemic influenza viruses)
- Employ safe work practices to prevent needlesticks and other sharps-related injuries (e.g., safety engineered sharps devices, appropriate disposal areas for sharps)
- Provide single person rooms when concern about transmission of infectious agent, per organization policy and ability
- Prioritize single person rooms for persons who have conditions that facilitate transmission of infectious material to other persons (e.g., draining wounds, stool incontinence, uncontained secretions, poor personal hygiene habits)
- Prioritize single person rooms for those who are at increased risk of acquisition and adverse outcomes resulting from hospital acquired infections (HAIs) (e.g., persons with immunosuppression, open wounds, indwelling catheters)
- Allocate appropriate square feet per person, as indicated by CDC guidelines (i.e., avoid overcrowding care areas)
- Isolate persons exposed to communicable disease or with diagnosis of communicable disease, per the appropriate isolation precautions (e.g., contact, airborne, droplet, bloodborne)
- Clean care area environment appropriately after each use, per agency policy
- Clean and disinfect surfaces contaminated with pathogens, including those close to person (e.g., bed rails, over bed tables) and frequently touched surfaces in care environment (e.g., door knobs, surfaces in and surrounding toilets in rooms) more frequently, compared to other surfaces (e.g., horizontal surfaces in waiting rooms)
- Use Environmental Protection Agency (EPA)-registered disinfectants that have microbiocidal activity against pathogens most likely to contaminate care environment, in accordance with manufacturer's instructions
- Clean and disinfect all contact or care items or equipment, including toys in pediatric areas and multi-use mobile devices moved in and out of rooms
- Contain, transport, and handle care equipment and instruments or devices that may be contaminated with infectious materials, per agency policy
- Remove organic material from critical and semi-critical instruments or devices, using recommended cleaning agents prior to high level disinfection and sterilization, to enable effective disinfection and sterilization processes
- Handle used textiles and fabrics with minimum agitation to avoid contamination of air, surfaces, and persons
- Post written notices indicating type of isolation for each isolated person, including visitor restrictions or activities required by anyone entering room (e.g., handwashing, PPE use, length of allowed stay, distance to maintain from person)
- Maintain isolation techniques for isolated persons, as appropriate
- Limit the number of visitors for isolated persons, as appropriate
- Post signs in public areas (e.g., entrances, cafeterias, elevators) with instructions to limit visitation if symptoms of respiratory infection, cough, or sneezing
- Provide tissues and no-touch receptacles (e.g., foot-pedal-operated lid, open, plastic-lined waste basket) for disposal of tissues
- Instruct persons on appropriate handwashing techniques and to cleanse hands on entering and leaving rooms
- Maintain basic principles of aseptic technique for preparation and administration of parenteral medications (e.g., use of sterile, single-use, disposable needle and syringe for each injection

given; prevent contamination of injection equipment and medication; use only single-dose vials)

- Use fluid infusion and administration sets (e.g., IV bags, tubing, connectors) for one person only and dispose appropriately after use
- Maintain an optimal aseptic environment during bedside insertion of central lines or any parenteral access
- Maintain an aseptic environment and aseptic handling of all IV lines and when changing all IV tubing and bottles
- Maintain a closed system when doing invasive hemodynamic monitoring
- Change peripheral IV and central line sites and dressings according to current Centers for Disease Control and Prevention guidelines
- Use appropriate wound-care technique
- Limit use of invasive devices (e.g., urinary catheters, feeding tubes) to decrease susceptibility to infection and colonization where possible
- Discontinue invasive devices (e.g., urinary catheters, IV sites) when clinically indicated, to reduce risk for infection
- Use urinary catheter care protocols and evidence-based guidelines to reduce risk of infection
- Administer antibiotic therapy or immunizing agents, as appropriate
- Maintain judicial use of antibiotics
- Instruct to take antibiotics as prescribed and until finished
- Instruct person and family about signs and symptoms of infection and when to report them to health care provider
- Instruct person and family members how to avoid infections
- Promote immunizations and vaccinations as preventative infection measures, as appropriate
- Offer immunization and vaccination opportunities to health care workers
- Provide employee health services related to infection prevention (e.g., assessment of risk, administration of recommended treatment following exposure, tuberculosis screening, influenza vaccination, respiratory protection fit testing)
- Provide and attend education annually related to control and transmission of pathogens (e.g., handwashing, use of PPE, types of isolation)
- Use teach-back to ensure understanding

1st edition 1992; revised 2000, 2024

Background Evidence:

Cochrane, J., & Jersby, M. (2019). When to wear personal protective equipment to prevent infection. *British Journal of Nursing, 28*(15), 982–984.

Hart, A. M. (2019). Preventing outpatient health care–associated infections. *Journal for Nurse Practitioners, 15*(6), 400–404.

Nielsen, C. S. R., Sanchez-Vargas, R., & Perez, A. (2019). Clostridium Difficile: Reducing infections using an evidence-based practice initiative. *Clinical Journal of Oncology Nursing, 23*(5), 482–486.

Potter, P. A., & Perry, A. G. (2021). *Fundamentals of nursing.* Elsevier.

Siegel, J.D., Rhinehart, E., Jackson, M., Chiarello, L., & The Healthcare Infection Control Practices Advisory Committee. (2019 update). 2007 Guideline for isolation precautions: Preventing transmission of infectious agents in healthcare settings. Centers for Disease Control. https://www.cdc.gov/infectioncontrol/guidelines/isolation/index.html

Spruce, L. (2020). Transmission-based precautions. *AORN Journal, 112*(5), 558–566.

Yu, S., Marshall, A. P. Li, J., & Lin, F. (2020). Interventions and strategies to prevent catheter-associated urinary tract infections with short-term indwelling urinary catheters in hospitalized patients: An integrative review. *International Journal of Nursing Practice, 26*(3), 1–17.

I

Infection Control: Intraoperative 6545

Definition: Preventing nosocomial infection in the operating room

Activities:
- Damp dust flat surfaces and lights in operating room daily
- Monitor and maintain room temperature between 20° and 24° C
- Monitor and maintain relative humidity between 20% and 60%
- Monitor and maintain laminar airflow
- Limit and control traffic into operating suite arenas
- Verify that prophylactic antibiotics have been administered, as appropriate
- Use universal precautions
- Ensure that operating personnel are wearing appropriate attire
- Use designated isolation precautions, as appropriate
- Monitor isolation techniques, as appropriate
- Verify integrity of sterile packaging and sterilization indicators
- Open sterile supplies and instruments using aseptic technique
- Scrub, gown, and glove, per agency policy
- Follow agency policy related to artificial nail enhancements and polishes for staff
- Assist with gowning and gloving of team members
- Assist with draping, ensuring protection of eyes and minimizing pressure to body parts
- Separate sterile from nonsterile supplies
- Monitor sterile field for break in sterility and correct breaks, as indicated
- Maintain integrity of catheters and intravascular lines
- Inspect skin and tissue around surgical site
- Apply drip towels to prevent pooling of antimicrobial prep solution
- Apply antimicrobial solution to surgical site, as per agency policy
- Remove drip towels
- Obtain cultures, as needed
- Contain contamination when it occurs
- Document incidences of contamination and level of break in technique
- Administer antibiotic therapy, as appropriate
- Maintain neat and orderly room to limit contamination
- Apply and secure surgical dressings
- Remove drapes and supplies to limit contamination
- Clean and sterilize instruments, as appropriate
- Coordinate cleaning and preparation of operating room after procedure

2nd edition 1996; revised 2013, 2024

Background Evidence:

Association of PeriOperative Registered Nurses. (2021). *2021 Guidelines for perioperative practice.*

Graham, L. A. (2021). Infection prevention and control. In P. A., Potter, A. G., Perry, P. A., Stockert, & A. M. Hall (Eds.), *Fundamentals of nursing* (10th ed., pp. 435–440). Elsevier.

Rothrock, J., & McEwen, D. R. (2019). *Alexander's care of the patient in surgery* (16th ed.). Elsevier.

Infection Protection 6550

Definition: Prevention and early detection of infection in a person at risk

Activities:
- Verify risk level using health history questions, including international and local travel
- Determine current level of knowledge related to acquisition and transmission of infectious agents
- Monitor aspects of preexisting conditions that increase person's infection risk (e.g., pancytopenia, immunosuppressive drugs)
- Monitor for systemic and localized signs and symptoms of infection
- Monitor vulnerability to infection (e.g., decreased ability for self-care, open wounds, recent surgery)
- Monitor absolute granulocyte count, WBC, and differential results
- Follow neutropenic precautions, as appropriate
- Limit number of visitors, if needed
- Avoid close contact between pets and immunocompromised hosts
- Screen all visitors for communicable disease
- Maintain asepsis for person at risk
- Maintain appropriate isolation techniques
- Provide appropriate skin care to edematous areas
- Inspect skin and mucous membranes for redness, extreme warmth, or drainage
- Inspect condition of any surgical incision or wound at regular intervals
- Obtain cultures as needed
- Promote sufficient rest, nutritional and fluid intake, as appropriate
- Monitor for change in energy level or malaise
- Encourage increased mobility and exercise, as appropriate
- Encourage deep breathing and coughing, as appropriate
- Administer immunizing agent, as appropriate
- Instruct to take antibiotics as prescribed
- Maintain judicial use of antibiotics
- Avoid antibiotic treatment for viral infections
- Instruct about differences between viral and bacterial infections
- Instruct about signs and symptoms of infection and when to report to health care provider
- Instruct about how to avoid infections
- Promote immunizations and vaccinations as preventative infection measures, as appropriate
- Eliminate fresh fruits, vegetables, and pepper in diets of persons with neutropenia
- Remove fresh flowers and plants from care areas, as appropriate
- Provide private room as indicated

- Ensure water safety by instituting hyperchlorination and hyper-heating, as appropriate
- Report suspected infections to infection control personnel
- Report positive cultures to infection control personnel
- Use teach-back to ensure understanding

1st edition 1992; revised 2013, 2024

Background Evidence:

Patel, P. K., Popovich, K. J., Collier, S., Lassiter, S., Mody, L., Ameling, J. M., & Meddings, J. (2019). Foundational elements of infection prevention in the STRIVE curriculum. *Annals of Internal Medicine, 171*(7), S10–S19.

Potter, P. A., & Perry, A. G. (2021). Stockert & Hall: *Fundamentals of nursing care* (10th ed.). Elsevier.

Prior, M., Delac, K., Melone, D., & Laux, L. (2020). Determining nursing education needs during a rapidly changing COVID-19 environment. *Critical Care Nursing Quarterly, 43*(4), 428–450.

Wilson, B. J., Zitella, L. J., Erb, C. H., Foster, J., Peterson, M., & Wood, S. K. (2018). Prevention of infection: A systematic review of evidence-based practice interventions for management in patients with cancer. *Clinical Journal of Oncology Nursing, 22*(2), 157–168.

Insurance Authorization 7410

Definition: Assisting the patient and provider to secure payment for health services or equipment from a third party

Activities:

- Determine whether patient's insurance company requires authorization before use of a particular service or equipment
- Understand the changes in insurance authorization as a result of the Patient Protection and Affordable Care Act of 2010
- Explain reasons for obtaining preapproval for health services or equipment
- Explain consent for release of information
- Obtain signature of patient or responsible adult on release of information form
- Obtain information and signature of patient or responsible adult on assignment of benefits form, as needed
- Provide information to third-party payer about the necessity of the health service or equipment
- Obtain or write a prescription for equipment, as appropriate
- Submit prescription for equipment to the third-party payer
- Assist with the completion of claim forms, as needed
- Facilitate communication with third-party payers, as needed
- Record evidence of preapproval (e.g., validation number) on the patient's chart, as necessary
- Inform patient or responsible adult of the status of the preapproval request
- Provide preapproval information to other departments, as necessary
- Discuss financial responsibilities of patient (e.g., out-of-pocket expenses), as appropriate
- Notify appropriate health professional if approval refused by the third-party payer
- Negotiate alternative modalities of care if approval is refused (e.g., outpatient status or change in acuity level), as appropriate
- Assist in the filing of an appeal if claim is denied, as appropriate
- Assist patient to access needed health services or equipment
- Document care provided, as required
- Collaborate with other health professionals about continued need for health services, as appropriate
- Document continued need for health services, as required
- Provide necessary information (e.g., name, Social Security number, insurance company ID number, provider) to third-party payer for billing, as needed
- Support the simplification and standardization of the preauthorization process by adopting and using standardized paper forms or Health Insurance Portability and Accountability Act (HIPAA) electronic standard transactions

2nd edition 1996; revised 2018

Background Evidence:

American Medical Association. (2011). Standardization of prior authorization process for medical services white paper. http://www.ama-assn.org/resources/doc/psa/standardization-prior-auth-whitepaper.pdf

Mathews, A. W. (2012, August 2). Remember managed care? It's quietly coming back. *Wall Street Journal.*

Rosenbaum, S. (2011). The Patient Protection and Affordable Care Act: Implications for public health policy and practice. *Public Health Reports, 126*(1), 130–135.

Intracranial Pressure (ICP) Monitoring 2590

Definition: Measurement and interpretation of patient data to regulate intracranial pressure

Activities:

- Assist with ICP monitoring device insertion
- Provide information to patient and family and significant others
- Calibrate the transducer
- Level external transducer to consistent anatomical reference point
- Prime flush system, as appropriate
- Set monitor alarms
- Record ICP pressure readings
- Monitor quality and characteristics of ICP waveform
- Monitor cerebral perfusion pressure
- Monitor neurological status
- Monitor patient's ICP and neurological response to care activities and environmental stimuli
- Monitor amount, rate, and characteristics of cerebrospinal fluid (CSF) drainage

- Maintain position of CSF collection chamber as ordered
- Monitor intake and output
- Prevent device dislodgment
- Maintain sterility of monitoring system
- Monitor pressure tubing for air bubbles, debris, or clotted blood
- Change transducer, flush system, and drainage bag, as indicated
- Change and/or reinforce insertion site dressing, as necessary
- Monitor insertion site for infection or leakage of fluid
- Obtain cerebrospinal fluid drainage samples, as appropriate
- Monitor temperature and WBC count
- Check patient for nuchal rigidity
- Administer antibiotics
- Position the patient with head and neck in a neutral position, avoiding extreme hip flexion
- Adjust head of bed to optimize cerebral perfusion
- Monitor effect of environmental stimuli on ICP
- Space nursing care to minimize ICP elevation
- Alter suctioning procedure to minimize increase in ICP with catheter introduction (e.g., give lidocaine and limit number of suction passes)
- Monitor CO_2 levels and maintain within specified parameters
- Maintain systemic arterial pressure within specified range
- Administer pharmacological agents to maintain ICP within specified range
- Notify physician for elevated ICP that does not respond to treatment protocols

1st edition 1992; revised 2008

Background Evidence:

American Association of Neuroscience Nurses. (1997). *Clinical guidelines series: Intracranial pressure monitoring.*

Arbour, R. (2004). Intracranial hypertension: Monitoring and nursing assessment. *Critical Care Nurse, 24*(5), 19–32.

Barker, E. (2002). Intracranial pressure and monitoring. In E. Barker (Ed.), *Neuroscience nursing: A spectrum of care* (2nd ed., pp. 379–408). Mosby.

Hickey, J. V. (2003). Intracranial hypertension: Theory and management of increased intracranial pressure. In J. V. Hickey (Ed.), *The clinical practice of neurological and neurosurgical nursing* (5th ed., pp. 285–318). Lippincott Williams & Wilkins.

Kirkness, C., & March, K. (2004). Intracranial pressure management. In M. K. Bader & L. R. Littlejohns (Eds.), *AANN core curriculum for neuroscience nursing* (pp. 249–267). W. B. Saunders.

Mitchell, P. H. (2001). Decreased behavioral arousal. In C. Stewart-Amidei & J. A. Kunkel (Eds.), *AANN's neuroscience nursing: Human responses to neurologic dysfunction* (2nd ed., pp. 93–118). W. B. Saunders.

Intrapartal Care   6830

Definition: Monitoring and management of stages one and two of labor

Activities:

- Determine stage of labor, risk status, and presence of ruptured membranes
- Admit to birthing area
- Obtain informed consent
- Determine childbirth preparation and goals
- Encourage family participation in labor, if consistent with personal goals
- Prepare for labor per protocol, practitioner request, and preference
- Identify emotional and psychological needs throughout labor
- Educate that length of first stage of labor varies between women
- Provide ice chips, wet washcloth, or hard candy as needed
- Encourage to empty bladder every 2 hours
- Inform of prescribed diet
- Provide supportive one-to-one care
- Assist labor coach or family in providing comfort and support
- Perform vaginal exam to determine complete cervical dilation, effacement, fetal position, and station after abdominal palpation
- Use partogram once labor established to document frequency of contractions and fetal heart rate, per protocol
- Document cervical examination per protocol
- Ensure privacy during labor process
- Ask permission to perform exams as needed
- Perform Leopold's maneuvers to determine fetal position
- Perform vaginal exams at admission and as necessary during labor, avoiding excessive manipulation
- Monitor vital signs and pain level per protocol
- Palpate contractions to determine frequency, duration, intensity, and resting tone as needed
- Perform intermittent auscultation of fetal heart rate per protocol
- Monitor fetal heart rate between contractions to establish baseline, and during and after contractions to detect decelerations or accelerations
- Apply electronic fetal monitor per protocol
- Instruct on fetal heart monitoring process and equipment
- Report abnormal fetal heart rate changes to primary practitioner
- Assist with position changes to correct abnormal fetal heart rate
- Provide clear, consistent, and evidence-based explanation about possible positions during labor
- Inform of benefits of positioning and ambulation (e.g., sitting, standing, kneeling)
- Use childbirth tools (e.g., birthing ball, peanut ball, birthing bar, hydrotherapy) to support comfortable positioning
- Educate on importance of avoiding long periods supine or in one position
- Instruct on breathing, relaxation, and visualization techniques
- Perform or assist with amniotomy per protocol
- Auscultate fetal heart rate before and after amniotomy
- Document characteristics of amniotic fluid, fetal heart rate, and contraction pattern
- Keep informed of labor progress
- Monitor coping during labor
- Instruct on pushing techniques for second stage labor
- Encourage spontaneous bearing-down efforts during the second stage
- Monitor effectiveness of pushing and length of time in second stage
- Offer warm compresses for back and suprapubic region, according to preference
- Document events of labor

• Notify primary practitioner at appropriate time to scrub for attending delivery

---

1st edition 1992; revised 1996, 2018, 2024

Background Evidence:

Cluett, E. R., Burns, E., & Cuthbert, A. (2018). Immersion in water during labor and birth. *Cochrane Database of Systematic Reviews, 5,* CD000111. https://doi.org/10.1002/14651858.CD000111.pub4

Czech, I., Fuchs, P., Fuchs, A., Lorek, M., Tobolska-Lorek, D., Drosdzol-Cop, A., & Sikora, J. (2018). Pharmacological and non-pharmacological methods of labor pain relief: Establishment of effectiveness and comparison. *International Journal of Environmental Research and Public Health, 15*(12), 2792. https://doi.org/10.3390/ijerph15122792

Lavender, T., Cuthbert, A., & Smyth, R. M. (2018). Effect of partograph use on outcomes for women in spontaneous labour at term and their babies. *Cochrane Database of Systematic Reviews, 8,* CD005461. https://doi.org/10.1002/14651858.CD005461.pub5

National Institute for Health and Care Excellence (NICE). (2019). *2019 surveillance of intrapartum care for healthy women and babies* (NICE guideline CG190). https://www.ncbi.nlm.nih.gov/books/NBK550941/

Smith, C. A., Levett, K. M., Collins, C. T., Dahlen, H. G., Ee, C. C., & Suganuma, M. (2018). Massage, reflexology and other manual methods for pain management in labour. *Cochrane Database of Systematic Reviews, 3*(3), CD009290. https://doi.org/10.1002/14651858.CD009290.pub3

World Health Organization. (2018). WHO recommendations: Intrapartum care for a positive childbirth experience.

Intrapartal Care: High-Risk Delivery   6834

Definition: Assisting with vaginal delivery of multiple or malpositioned fetuses

Activities:

• Inform patient and support person of extra procedures and personnel to anticipate during birth process
• Communicate changes in maternal or fetal status to primary practitioner, as appropriate
• Prepare appropriate equipment, including electronic fetal monitor, ultrasound, anesthesia machine, neonatal resuscitation supplies, forceps (e.g., Piper), and extra infant warmers
• Notify extra assistants to attend birth (e.g., neonatologist, neonatal intensive care nurses, anesthesiologist)
• Provide assistance for gowning and gloving obstetrical team
• Continue electronic monitoring
• Coach during second stage pushing
• Alert primary practitioner to abnormalities in maternal vital signs or fetal heart tracing(s)
• Encourage support person to assist with comfort measures
• Use universal precautions
• Perform perineal scrub
• Perform or assist with manual rotation of fetal head from occiput posterior to anterior position, as appropriate
• Record time of delivery of first twin or of breech to the level of the umbilicus
• Assist with amniotomy of additional amniotic membranes, as needed
• Continue to monitor heart rate(s) of second or third fetus
• Perform ultrasound to locate fetal position, as appropriate
• Follow fetal head with hand to promote flexion during breech delivery, as directed by primary practitioner
• Perform McRoberts maneuver, suprapubic pressure per request of physician or nurse-midwife
• Support body as primary practitioner delivers aftercoming head
• Assist with application of forceps or vacuum extractor, as needed
• Assist with administration of maternal anesthetic (e.g., intubation), as needed
• Record time of birth(s)
• Assist with neonatal resuscitation, as needed
• Document procedures (e.g., anesthesia, forceps, vacuum extraction, suprapubic pressure, McRoberts maneuver, neonatal resuscitation) used to facilitate birth
• Explain newborn characteristics related to high-risk birth (e.g., bruising and forceps marks)
• Observe closely for postpartum hemorrhage
• Assist mother to recover from anesthetic, as appropriate
• Encourage parental interaction with newborn(s) soon after delivery

---

2nd edition 1996; revised 2018

Background Evidence:

Association of Women's Health, Obstetric and Neonatal Nurses. (2013). *Basic, high-risk, and critical-care intrapartum nursing: Clinical competencies and education guide* (5th ed.).

Davidson, M., London, M., & Ladewig, P. (2016). *Old's maternal-newborn nursing and women's health across the lifespan* (10th ed.). Pearson.

Troiano, N., Harvey, C., & Chez, B. (Eds.). (2013). *High-risk and critical care obstetrics* (3rd ed.). Lippincott, Williams & Wilkins.

I

Intravenous (IV) Insertion 4190

Definition: Insertion of a cannulated needle into a peripheral vein for the purpose of administering fluids, blood, or medications

Activities:

- Verify prescription for IV therapy
- Instruct about procedure
- Maintain strict aseptic technique
- Identify allergies to any medications, iodine, or tape
- Identify if clotting problem or taking any medications that would affect clotting
- Provide emotional support, as appropriate
- Place in supine position
- Ask parents to hold and comfort child, as appropriate
- Ensure comfort in positioning
- Ask to hold still when performing venipuncture
- Remove clothing from targeted extremity
- Select appropriate vein for venipuncture, considering preference, past experience with IVs, and nondominant hand
- Consider assessment factors when examining veins for cannula insertion (e.g., age, purpose of catheter, cannula gauge, cannula material, cannula proximity to joints, condition of extremity, condition, skill of practitioner)
- Start IVs in opposite arm of arteriovenous fistulas or shunts, or conditions contraindicating cannulation (e.g., lymphedema, mastectomy, radiation therapy)
- Choose needle based on purpose and length of use (e.g., larger bore for blood administration)
- Apply heat compresses if needed for increased blood flow for vein visualization (e.g., warm dry towels)
- Apply topical analgesia as indicated per agency protocol
- Administer 1% or 2% lidocaine at insertion site based on agency protocol
- Adhere to time requirements for topical analgesia effectiveness (i.e., some topical analgesic medications require 2 hours to take effect)
- Apply tourniquet 3 to 4 inches higher than anticipated puncture site, as appropriate
- Apply enough tourniquet pressure to impede venous circulation but not arterial flow
- Instruct to hold extremity below heart to allow for maximum blood flow to selected site
- Massage arm from proximal to distal end, as appropriate
- Lightly tap puncture area after applying tourniquet, as appropriate
- Request to open and close hand several times, as appropriate
- Cleanse area with appropriate solution based on agency protocol
- Use ultrasound-guided peripheral intravenous catheter insertion for individuals with difficult intravenous access, per agency protocol

- Insert needle according to manufacturer's instructions, using only needles with sharps injury prevention features
- Determine correct placement by observing for blood in flash chamber or tubing
- Obtain blood sample from cannulated vein, if ordered
- Remove tourniquet as soon as possible
- Tape cannula securely in place
- Connect cannula to IV tubing or flush and connect to saline lock, as appropriate and per agency protocol
- Apply small transparent dressing over insertion site
- Label site dressing with date, gauge, and initials per agency protocol

1st edition 1992; revised 2013, 2024

Background Evidence:

Coventry, L. L., Jacob, A. M., Davies, H. T., Stoneman, L., Keogh, S., & Jacob, E. R. (2019). Drawing blood from peripheral intravenous cannula compared with venupuncture: A systematic review and meta-analysis. *Journal of Advanced Nursing, 75*(11), 2313–2339. https://doi.org/10.1111/jan.14078

Davis, E. M., Feinsmith, S., Amick, A. E., Sell, J., McDonald, V., Trinquero, P., Moore, A., Gappmaier, V., Colton, K., Cunningham, A., Ford, W., Feinglass, J., & Barsuk, J. H. (2021). Difficult intravenous access in the emergency department: Performance and impact of ultrasound-guided IV insertion performed by nurses. *American Journal of Emergency Medicine, 46*, 539–544. https://doi.org/10.1016/j.ajem.2020.14.013

Infusion Nursing Society. (2021). *Policies & procedures for infusion therapy: Acute care* (6th ed.).

Infusion Nursing Society. (2021). *Standards of practice* (8th ed.).

Kleidon, T., Schults, J., Rickard, C., & Ullman, A. (2021). Techniques and technologies to improve peripheral intravenous catheter insertion success and outcomes: A systematic review and meta-analysis. *Infection, Disease & Health, 26*(Sppl. 1), S10. https://doi.org/10.1016/j.idh.2021.09.035

Morata, L., & Bowers, M. (2020). Ultrasound-Guided peripheral intravenous catheter insertion: The Nurse's Manual. *Critical Care Nurse, 40*(5), 38–46. https://doi.org/10.4037/ccn2020240

Nickel, B. (2019). Peripheral intravenous access: Applying Infusion Therapy Standards of Practice to improve patient safety. *Critical Care Nurse, 39*(1), 61–71. https://doi.org/10.4037/ccn2019790

Perry, A. G., Potter, P. A., Ostendorf, W., & LaPlante, N. (2021). *Clinical nursing skills and techniques* (10th ed.). Elsevier.

Intravenous (IV) Therapy 4200

Definition: Administration and monitoring of intravenous fluids and medications

Activities:

- Check accuracy and completeness of each medication administration record (MAR) prior to administering any medications
- Follow the six rights of medication administration
- Identify using at least two identifiers (e.g., name, birth date)

- Note medical history and history of allergies
- Determine knowledge of medication and understanding of method of administration
- Perform necessary pre-medication assessments (e.g., blood pressure, pulse)

- Follow agency guidelines regarding requirements for special monitoring of person while medication administered (i.e., telemetry with heart medications)
- Use standardized concentrations and dosages of IV fluids and medications, preferably prepared and dispensed from pharmacy or commercially prepared when possible
- Instruct about procedure
- Identify if currently taking medication incompatible with medication ordered
- Review information regarding how to administer solution safely, as needed
- Calculate infusion flow rate
- Verify calculations and rates with another RN, if indicated
- Select and prepare IV infusion pump, as indicated
- Maintain strict aseptic technique with supplies that will potentially be in contact with blood stream (e.g., IV cannula, IV insertion site, IV tubing connections, IV tubing access ports, IV fluids)
- Examine solution for type, amount, expiration date, character of solution, and intact container
- Spike container with appropriate tubing
- Squeeze drip chamber once or twice
- Open tubing clamp slowly to prime tubing
- Check for IV patency before administration of IV medication
- Administer IV medications as prescribed, monitor during infusion, and monitor for results
- Trace all catheters or administration sets or add-on devices between person and fluid container before connecting or reconnecting any infusion device
- Label administration sets with infusing solution or medication both near person connection and near solution container
- Instruct person, caregivers, and unlicensed assistive personnel to obtain assistance from licensed staff whenever real or perceived need to connect or disconnect devices or infusions unless person or caregiver independently administering infusion medications (e.g., in home care setting)
- Document which solutions and medications are being infused through which device or lumen, when multiple vascular access devices (VADs) or catheter lumens are used
- Route tubing having different purposes in different directions (i.e., IV catheters routed toward head, feeding tubes routed toward feet)
- Use technology according to organizational policies and procedures (e.g., bar code, smart pump with dose-error reduction software, volume-control administration set, mini-infusion administration set), when available
- Monitor intravenous flow rate and intravenous site during infusion
- Monitor for possible complications of IV therapy (e.g., fluid overload, allergic reaction, site discomfort, infusion phlebitis, local infection)
- Monitor vital signs as indicated
- Maintain sterile, occlusive dressing for IV sites
- Perform IV site checks and care according to agency protocol
- Perform site change, tubing change and site with dressing care changes, according to agency protocol
- Follow strict drug guidelines when administering high-alert IV medications (e.g., heparin, dopamine, dobutamine, nitroglycerine, potassium, antibiotics, magnesium)
- Flush intravenous lines between administration of incompatible solutions
- Stop IV fluids and clamp IV line if IV medication found to be incompatible with IV fluids during administration (i.e., IV fluid becomes cloudy in tubing)
- Restart IV fluids with new tubing if incompatible medications in current tubing
- Record intake and output, as appropriate
- Document prescribed therapy per agency protocol
- Documentation condition of IV site prior, during, and after infusion therapy
- Maintain universal precautions when providing IV site care or therapy
- Provide person and caregiver education including infusion administration and signs and symptoms to report, including those that may occur after person leaves health care setting

1st edition 1992; revised 2004, 2024

Background Evidence:

Infusion Nursing Society. (2021). *Policies and procedures for infusion therapy: Acute care* (6th ed.).

Infusion Nursing Society. (2021). *Standards of practice* (8th ed.).

Perry, A. G., & Potter, P. A. (2020). *Fundamentals of nursing* (10th ed.). Elsevier.

Perry, A. G., Potter, P. A., Ostendorf, W., & LaPlante, N. (2021). *Clinical nursing skills and techniques* (10th ed). Elsevier.

I

Invasive Hemodynamic Monitoring   4210

Definition: Measurement and interpretation of intravascular pressure, flow, and oxygenation

Activities:

- Obtain informed consent
- Explain purpose and procedure of hemodynamic monitoring
- Assist with insertion of invasive hemodynamic lines
- Monitor blood pressure (e.g., systolic, diastolic, mean), central venous and right atrial pressure, pulmonary artery pressure (e.g., systolic, diastolic, mean), and pulmonary capillary and artery wedge pressure
- Zero and calibrate equipment every 4 to 12 hours, per policy
- Monitor hemodynamic waveforms for changes in cardiovascular function
- Compare clinical signs and symptoms with hemodynamic parameters

- Reposition to address catheter or tubing problems (e.g., tubing kinks, air bubbles, clot)
- Monitor peripheral perfusion distal to catheter insertion site every 4 hours or per protocol
- Monitor for dyspnea, fatigue, tachypnea, and orthopnea
- Refrain from inflating balloon more frequently than every 1 to 2 hours or as appropriate
- Monitor for balloon rupture (i.e., assess for resistance when inflating balloon and allow balloon to passively deflate after obtaining pulmonary capillary or artery wedge pressure)
- Prevent air emboli (i.e., remove air bubbles from tubing; if balloon rupture is suspected, refrain from attempts to reinflate balloon and clamp balloon port)

- Maintain sterility of closed-pressure system, as appropriate
- Perform sterile dressing changes and site care, per protocol
- Inspect insertion site for signs of bleeding, hematoma, pain, or infection
- Change IV solution and tubing every 24 to 72 hours, per protocol
- Monitor laboratory results
- Administer fluid or pharmacological agents to maintain hemodynamic parameters within specified range, as prescribed
- Assist with chest x-ray examination after insertion of pulmonary artery catheter
- Instruct on therapeutic use of hemodynamic monitoring catheters
- Instruct on activity restriction while catheters remain in place
- Use teach-back to ensure understanding
- Assist with removal of invasive hemodynamic lines

1st edition 1992; revised 2000, 2004, 2024

Background Evidence:

Burns, S. M., & Delgado, S. A. (2019). *AACN Essentials of Critical Care Nursing* (4th ed.). McGraw-Hill.

Knapp, R. (2020). *Hemodynamic monitoring made incredibly visual!*. Wolters Kluwer.

Laher, A. E., Watermeyer, M. J., Buchanan, S. K., Dippenaar, N., Simo, N. C. T., Motara, F., & Moolla, M. (2017). A review of hemodynamic monitoring techniques, methods and devices for the emergency physician. *American Journal of Emergency Medicine*, *35*(9), 1335–1347. https://doi.org/10.1016/j.ajem.2017.03.036

Lough, M. E., Berger, S. J., Larsen, A., & Sandoval, C. P. (2022). Cardiovascular diagnostic procedures. In L. D. Urden, K. M. Stacy, & M. E. Lough (Eds.), *Critical care nursing* (9th ed., pp. 206–297). Elsevier.

I

Journaling   4740

Definition: Promotion of writing as a means to provide opportunities to reflect upon and analyze past events, experiences, thoughts, and feelings

Activities:

- Discuss experiences with similar interventions and receptiveness to intervention
- Establish purpose and goals
- Explain various approaches to journaling and decide on a journaling technique (e.g., free flowing, topical, or intensive journaling)
- Determine a time frame to complete task
- Encourage writing without interruption at least three times a week for 20 minutes
- Ensure the environment is optimal for task completion (e.g., client is in a comfortable position, room is well lit, client has glasses)
- Minimize emotional, visual, audio, olfactory, and visceral distractions
- Maintain privacy and assure confidentiality
- Allow the person to select media and method (e.g., pen, pencil, marker, journal, computer, tape recorder, etc.)
- Gather all necessary supplies
- Instruct the person to date journal entries for future reference and reflection
- Encourage writing in the order that things occur without topic restrictions
- Encourage the describing and telling of events in terms of stories, images, and associated thoughts and feelings
- Describe experiences in terms of the five senses, as applicable
- Promote expressing deepest thoughts and feelings
- Instruct to pay no attention to punctuation, spelling, sentence structure, and/or grammar
- Determine ability to continue with intervention independently in the future
- Review journal entries at defined intervals
- Monitor achievement of the established goals

5th edition 2008

Background Evidence:

Butcher, H. K. (2004). Written expression and the potential to enhance knowing participation in change. *Visions: The Journal of Rogerian Nursing Science, 12*(1), 37–50.

Butcher, H. K., Gordon, J. K., Ko, J. W., Perkhounkova, Y., Rinner, A., Cho, J. Y., & Lutgendorf, S. (2016). Finding meaning in written emotional expression by family caregivers of persons with dementia. *The American Journal of Alzheimer's Disease and Other Dementias, 31*(8), 631–642. https://doi.org/10.1177/1533317516606113

DeSalvo, L. (1999). *Writing as a way of healing: How telling our stories transforms our lives.* Beacon Press.

Lepore, S. J., & Smyth, J. M. (2002). *The writing cure: How expressive writing promotes health and emotional well-being.* American Psychological Association.

Pennebaker, J. W. (1997). *Opening up: The healing power of expressing emotions.* Guilford.

Pennebaker, J. W. (1997). Writing about emotional experiences as a therapeutic process. *Psychological Science, 8*(3), 162–166.

Rew, L. (2005). Self-reflection: Consulting the truth within. In B. M. Dossey, L. Keegan, & C. E. Guzzetta (Eds.), *Holistic nursing: A handbook for practice* (4th ed., pp. 429–447). Jones and Bartlett.

Stone, M. (1998). Journaling with clients. *The Journal of Individual Psychology, 54*(4), 535–545.

Synder, M. (2006). Journaling. In M. Snyder & R. Lindquist (Eds.), *Complementary/alternative therapies in nursing* (5th ed., pp. 165–173). Springer.

J

Kangaroo Care 6840

Definition: Facilitation of skin-to-skin contact between parent or other caregiver and physiologically-stable preterm infant

Activities:

- Explain advantages and implications of providing skin-to-skin contact with infant
- Monitor parent factors influencing involvement in care (e.g., willingness, health, availability, and presence of support system)
- Ensure that infant's physiological status meets guidelines for participation in care
- Prepare a quiet, private, and warm environment
- Provide parent with a reclining or rocking chair
- Instruct parent to wear comfortable, open-front clothing
- Instruct parent how to transfer infant from incubator, warmer bed, or bassinet while managing equipment and tubing
- Position diaper-clad infant in prone, upright position on parent's bare chest
- Turn infant head to one side in a slightly extended position to facilitate eye contact with parent and keep airway open
- Avoid forward flexion and hyperextension of infant head
- Infant's hips and arms should be flexed
- Secure infant and parent position (i.e., tie binding cloth around infant-parent dyad, wrap parent's clothing around infant, and place blanket over dyad)
- Instruct parent how to move infant in and out of binding cloth
- Encourage parent to focus on infant rather than high technological setting and equipment
- Encourage parent to gently stroke infant in prone upright position
- Encourage parent to gently rock infant in prone upright position
- Decrease auditory stimulation of infant
- Support parent in nurturing and providing hands-on care for infant
- Instruct parent to hold infant with full, encompassing hands
- Encourage parent to identify infant's behavioral cues
- Point out infant state changes to parent
- Encourage parent to sit, stand, walk, and engage in other activities of interest while providing skin-to-skin contact
- Encourage postpartum mothers to ambulate every 90 minutes while providing skin-to-skin contact to prevent thrombolytic disease
- Instruct parent to decrease activity when infant shows signs of overstimulation, distress, or avoidance
- Encourage parent to let the infant sleep during care

- Encourage breastfeeding during care, as appropriate
- Encourage parent to provide care at least 60 minutes to avoid frequent and potentially stressful changes, if possible
- Instruct parent to gradually increase time of each skin-to-skin contact, with length eventually becoming as continuous, as possible
- Monitor parent's emotional reaction to and concerns regarding kangaroo care
- Monitor infant's physiological status (e.g., color, temperature, heart rate, and apnea)
- Instruct parent how to monitor infant's physiological status
- Support parent to continue skin-to-skin contact at home
- Discontinue care if infant becomes physiologically compromised or agitated

2nd edition 1996; revised 2013

Background Evidence:

Askin, D. F., & Wilson, D. (2007). The high-risk newborn and family. In M. J. Hockenberry & D. Wilson (Eds.), *Wong's nursing care of infants and children* (8th ed., pp. 344–421). Mosby Elsevier.

Breitbach, K. M. (2001). Kangaroo care. In M. Craft-Rosenberg & J. Denehy (Eds.), *Nursing interventions for infants, children, and families* (pp. 151–162). Sage.

Johnston, C., Filion, F., Campbell-Yeo, M., Goulet, C., Bell, L., McNaughton, K., Byron, J., Aita, M., Finley, G., & Walker, C. (2008). Kangaroo mother care diminishes pain from heel lance in very preterm neonates: A crossover trial. *BMC Pediatrics, 8*(13). https://doi.org/10.1186/1471-2431-8-13

Renfrew, M. J., Craig, D., Dyson, L., McCormick, F., Rice, S., King, S. E., Misso, K., Stenhouse, E., & Williams, A. F. (2009). Breastfeeding promotion for infants in neonatal units: A systematic review and economic analysis. *Health Technology Assessment, 13*(40), 1–146.

Smith, K. M. (2007). Sleep and kangaroo care: Clinical practice in the newborn intensive care unit where the baby sleeps. *Journal of Perinatology and Neonatal Nursing, 21*(2), 151–157.

Suman, R. P., Udani, R., & Nanavati, R. (2008). Kangaroo mother care for low-birth-weight infants: A randomized controlled trial. *Indian Pediatrics, 45*(1), 17–23.

World Health Organization Department of Reproductive Health and Research. (2003). *Kangaroo mother care: A practical guide.*

K

Labor Induction 6850

Definition: Initiation or augmentation of labor by mechanical or pharmacological methods

Activities:

- Determine medical and obstetrical indications for induction
- Review obstetrical history for pertinent information that may influence induction (e.g., gestational age, length of prior labor, placenta previa, pelvic structural deformities, prior uterine rupture, active genital herpes, umbilical cord prolapse, transverse lie, Category III fetal heart rate [FHR])
- Determine Bishop score to rate readiness of cervix for labor induction (i.e., a score of 8 or greater is more favorable for vaginal delivery)
- Monitor maternal and fetal vital signs before induction
- Perform or assist with application of mechanical or pharmacological agents at the appropriate intervals to enhance cervical readiness, as needed
- Assist with membrane stripping if greater than or equal to 39 weeks' gestation
- Monitor for side effects of procedures used to ready cervix
- Reevaluate cervical status and verify presentation before initiating further induction measures
- Perform or assist with amniotomy if cervical dilatation is adequate and vertex is well engaged
- Determine fetal heart rate by auscultation or electronic fetal monitoring postamniotomy and per protocol
- Encourage ambulation, if no contraindications are present for both mother and fetus
- Observe for onset or change in uterine activity
- Initiate IV medication (e.g., oxytocin) to stimulate uterine activity according to protocol, as needed
- Regulate uterine stimulant until birth is imminent, as needed or per protocol
- Monitor labor progress closely, being alert to signs of abnormal labor progress
- Avoid uterine tachysystole by using low dose protocol to infuse oxytocin to achieve adequate contraction frequency, duration, and relaxation
- Monitor data provided by intrauterine pressure catheter
- Observe for signs of uteroplacental insufficiency (e.g., late decelerations and Category III fetal heart rate changes) during the process of induction
- Monitor for water retention during oxytocin administration

2nd edition 1996; revised 2018

Background Evidence:

Ladewig, P., London, M., & Davidson, M. (2014). *Contemporary maternal-newborn nursing care* (8th ed.). Prentice Hall.

Mattson, S., & Smith, J. (Eds.). (2011). *Core curriculum for maternal-newborn nursing* (4th ed.). Elsevier.

Odent, M. (2013). Should we ban labor induction? *Midwifery Today, 107,* 22–23.

Wing, D. (2015). *Induction of labor. UpToDate.* http://www.uptodate.com/contents/induction-of-labor?source=search_result&search=%22Should+we+ban+labor+induction%22&selectedTitle=1%7E150

L

Labor Pain Management 6855

Definition: Alleviation or reduction of labor pain

Activities:

- Review initial level of labor pain with multidimensional scale (e.g., location, characteristics, onset, duration, frequency, intensity, severity, precipitating factors)
- Discuss initial plans for pain management during labor
- Convey it is okay if plans change
- Monitor for nonverbal cues of discomfort
- Use therapeutic communication strategies to acknowledge pain experience and convey acceptance of response to pain
- Evaluate pain measures that have been used and helped in past labor experience
- Explore and consider knowledge, beliefs, cultural influences, and values on labor pain
- Explore factors that impact pain throughout labor
- Provide information about causes of labor pain and anticipated likely discomforts from procedures
- Eliminate factors that could increase labor pain experience (e.g., fear, lack of knowledge, environmental factors, procedures, absence of family or labor coach)
- Provide continuous emotional support during labor (e.g., comfort measures, information, advocacy)
- Encourage to use whatever positions facilitate pain relief, unless not clinically indicated
- Monitor pain level during labor with multidimensional scale, as possible
- Inform about all possible non-pharmacological methods of pain management (e.g., immersion in water, massage, warm compresses, relaxation, aromatherapy, guided imagery)
- Inform about risks, benefits and efficacy of each method of pain relief
- Provide alternative methods of pain relief consistent with preferences
- Administer analgesics of choice (e.g., oral, IV, epidural)
- Monitor effects of pharmacological and non-pharmacological analgesia on person and fetus
- Assist with regional analgesia or anesthesia, as appropriate
- Monitor fetal heart rate and progression of labor during epidural analgesic effects
- Monitor satisfaction with pain management

8th edition 2024

Background Evidence:

Akköz Çevik, S., & Karaduman, S. (2020). The effect of sacral massage on labor pain and anxiety: A randomized controlled trial. *Japan Journal of Nursing Science, 17*(1), e12272.

Amiri, P., Mirghafourvand, M., Esmaeilpour, K., Kamalifard, M., & Ivanbagha, R. (2019). The effect of distraction techniques on pain and stress during labor: A randomized controlled clinical trial. *BMC Pregnancy and Childbirth, 19*(1), 534. https://doi.org/10.1186/s12884-019-2683-y

Anim-Somuah, M., Smyth, R. M., Cyna, A. M., & Cuthbert, A. (2018). Epidural versus non-epidural or no analgesia for pain management in labour. *Cochrane Database of Systematic Reviews, 5*(5).

Bohren, M. A., Hofmeyr, G. J., Sakala, C., Fukuzawa, R. K., & Cuthbert, A. (2017). Continuous support for women during childbirth. *Cochrane Database of Systematic Reviews, 7*(7), CD003766. https://doi.org/10.1002/14651858.CD003766.pub6

National Collaborating Centre for Women's and Children's Health [NICE]. (2017) Intrapartum care. Care of healthy women and their babies during childbirth - version 2 - *Clinical Guideline 190 Methods, evidence and recommendations.* https://www.nice.org.uk/guidance/cg190

Ranjbaran, M., Khorsandi, M., Matourypour, P., & Shamsi, M. (2017). Effect of massage therapy on labor pain reduction in primiparous women: A systematic review and meta-analysis of randomized controlled clinical trials in Iran. *Iranian Journal of Nursing and Midwifery Research, 22*(4), 257–261. https://doi.org/10.4103/ijnmr.IJNMR_109_16

Walker, K. F., Kibuka, M., Thornton, J. G., & Jones, N. W. (2018). Maternal position in the second stage of labour for women with epidural anaesthesia. *The Cochrane Database of Systematic Reviews, 11*(11), CD008070. https://doi.org/10.1002/14651858.CD008070.pub4

Labor Suppression 6860

Definition: Controlling uterine contractions prior to 37 weeks of gestation to prevent preterm birth

Activities:

- Review history for risk factors commonly related to preterm labor (e.g., prior patient or family history of preterm birth or abortion; multifetal gestation; uterine cervical anomalies; early cervical change; uterine irritability; infection, including periodontal disease; short interpregnancy interval; technology-induced conception; history of vaginal bleeding in first and or second trimester; positive fetal fibronectin results; extremes of pre-pregnancy body weight)
- Determine fetal age based on last menstrual period, early sonogram, fundal height measurements, date of quickening, and date of audible fetal heart tones
- Interview about onset and duration of preterm labor symptoms
- Ask about activities preceding onset of preterm labor symptoms
- Determine status of amniotic membranes
- Obtain urine and cervical cultures
- Document uterine activity using palpation as well as electronic fetal monitoring
- Obtain baseline maternal weight
- Position mother laterally to optimize placental perfusion
- Initiate oral or intravenous hydration
- Note contraindications to use of tocolytics (e.g., chorioamnionitis, preeclampsia, hemorrhage, fetal demise, or severe intrauterine growth retardation)
- Initiate oral, subcutaneous, or IV tocolytics, per physician order or protocol, if hydration does not reduce uterine activity
- Monitor maternal vital signs, fetal heart rate, and uterine activity every 15 minutes during initiation of IV tocolysis
- Monitor for side effects of tocolytic therapy, including loss of deep tendon reflexes and depressed respirations, if magnesium sulfate is administered
- Educate the patient and family about normal tocolytic side effects (e.g., tremors, headache, palpitations, anxiety, nausea, vomiting, flushing, warmth)
- Provide interventions to reduce discomforts of normal side effects (e.g., relaxation therapy, anxiety reduction, therapeutic touch)
- Educate patient and family about abnormal tocolytic side effects (e.g., chest pain, shortness of breath, tachycardia, or recurrent contractions) to report to physician

- Obtain baseline EKG, as appropriate
- Monitor intake and output
- Auscultate lungs
- Administer corticosteroid therapy, if indicated and ordered to hasten maturity of fetal lungs
- Determine patient and family knowledge of fetal development and preterm birth, as well as motivation to prolong pregnancy
- Involve patient and family in plan for home care
- Begin discharge teaching for home care, including medication regimens, activity restrictions, diet and hydration, sexual abstinence, and ways to avoid constipation
- Instruct contraction palpation techniques
- Provide written patient education material for family
- Provide referrals to assist family with child care, home maintenance, and diversional activities, as appropriate
- Discuss signs of recurrent preterm labor and reinforce the need to seek care immediately, if symptoms return and continue for 1 hour
- Provide written discharge instructions, including explicit directions for seeking medical care

2nd edition 1996; revised 2018

Background Evidence:

Chabra, S. (2014). Clearing the confusion about completed weeks of gestation. *JOGNN-Journal of Obstetric, Gynecologic, & Neonatal Nursing, 43*(3), 269.

Ladewig, P., London, M., & Davidson, M. (2014). *Contemporary maternal-newborn nursing care* (8th ed.). Prentice Hall.

Mattson, S., & Smith, J. (Eds.). (2011). *Core curriculum for maternal-newborn nursing* (4th ed.). Saunders Elsevier.

Simham, H., & Caritas, S. (2014). Inhibition of acute preterm labor. In V. A. Barss (Ed.), *UpToDate.* http://www.uptodate.com/contents/inhibition-of-acute-preterm-labor?source=search_result&search=Inhibition+of+acute+preterm+labor&selectedTitle=1%7E150

Laboratory Data Interpretation   7690

Definition: Critical analysis of patient laboratory data in order to assist with clinical decision-making

Activities:
- Be familiar with accepted abbreviations for particular institution
- Use the reference ranges from the laboratory that is performing the particular test(s)
- Recognize physiological factors that can affect laboratory values, including race, gender, age, pregnancy, menstrual cycle, diet (especially hydration), time of day, activity level, and stress
- Recognize the effect of drugs on laboratory values, including prescription drugs, as well as over-the-counter medications
- Note time and site of specimen collection, as applicable
- Use peak drug levels when testing for toxicity
- Recognize that trough drug levels are useful for demonstrating satisfactory therapeutic level
- Consider influences of pharmacokinetics (e.g., half-life, peak, protein binding, and excretion) when evaluating toxic and therapeutic levels of drugs
- Consider that multiple test abnormalities are more likely to be significant than single test abnormalities
- Compare test results with other related laboratory and diagnostic tests
- Compare results with previous values obtained when the patient was not ill (if available) to determine baseline values
- Monitor sequential test results for trends or gross changes
- Consult appropriate references for clinical implication of unfamiliar tests
- Recognize that incorrect test results most often result from clerical errors
- Perform confirmation of grossly abnormal test results with close attention to patient and specimen identification, condition of specimen, and prompt delivery to the laboratory
- Report results of laboratory tests to patient, as appropriate
- Send split samples to the laboratory for verification of results, if appropriate
- Report sudden changes in laboratory values to physician immediately
- Report critical values (as determined by institution) to physician immediately
- Analyze whether results obtained are consistent with patient behavior and clinical status

2nd edition 1996; revised 2018

Background Evidence:
Amarillo Medical Specialists. (2010). *How to interpret and understand your blood test results.* http://www.amarillomed.com/howto

Chernecky, C. C., & Berger, B. J. (2013). *Laboratory tests and diagnostic procedures* (6th ed.). Elsevier Saunders.

Pagana, K. D., & Pagana, T. J. (2014). *Mosby's manual of diagnostic and laboratory tests* (5th ed.). Elsevier Mosby.

Xiong Lian, J. (2010). Interpreting and using blood gas analysis. *Nursing 2010 Critical Care, 5*(3), 26–36.

L

Lactation Counseling   5244

Definition: Assisting in the establishment and maintenance of successful breastfeeding

Activities:
- Provide information about psychological and physiological benefits of breastfeeding
- Determine mother's desire and motivation to breastfeed as well as perception of breastfeeding
- Correct misconceptions, misinformation, and inaccuracies about breastfeeding
- Encourage mother's significant other, family, or friends to provide support (i.e., offer praise, encouragement, and reassurance, perform household tasks, and ensure that mother is receiving adequate rest and nutrition)
- Provide educational material, as needed
- Encourage attendance to breastfeeding classes and support groups
- Provide mother the opportunity to breastfeed after birth, when possible
- Instruct on infant's feeding cues (e.g., rooting, sucking, and quiet alertness)
- Assist in ensuring proper infant attachment to breast (i.e., monitor proper infant alignment, areolar grasp and compression, and audible swallowing)
- Instruct on various feeding positions (e.g., cross-cradle, football hold, and side-lying)
- Instruct mother on signs of milk transfer (e.g., milk leakage, audible swallowing, and "let down" sensations)
- Discuss ways to facilitate milk transfer (e.g., relaxation techniques, breast massage, and a quiet environment)
- Inform about the difference between nutritive and nonnutritive sucking
- Monitor infant's ability to suck
- Demonstrate suck training (i.e., use a clean finger to stimulate suck reflex and latch on), if necessary
- Instruct mother to allow infant to finish first breast before offering second breast
- Instruct on how to break suction of nursing infant, if necessary
- Instruct mother on nipple care
- Monitor for nipple pain and impaired skin integrity of nipples
- Discuss techniques to avoid or minimize engorgement and associated discomfort (e.g., frequent feedings, breast massage, warm compresses, milk expression, ice packs applied after feeding or pumping, and anti-inflammatory medications)
- Instruct on signs, symptoms, and management strategies for plugged ducts, mastitis, and candidiasis infection
- Discuss needs for adequate rest, hydration, and well-balanced diet
- Assist in determining need for supplemental feedings, pacifiers, and nipple shields
- Encourage mother to wear a well-fitting, supportive bra
- Instruct on record keeping of nursing and pumping sessions, if indicated

- Instruct about infant stool and urination patterns
- Discuss frequency of normal feeding patterns, including cluster feedings and growth spurts
- Encourage continued lactation upon return to work or school
- Discuss options for milk expression, including nonelectrical pumping (e.g., hand and manual) and electrical pumping (e.g., single and double; hospital-grade pump for mother of preterm infant)
- Instruct on appropriate handling of expressed milk (e.g., collection, storage, thawing, preparation, fortification, and warming)
- Instruct patient to contact lactation consultant to assist in determining status of milk supply (i.e., whether insufficiency is perceived or actual)
- Discuss strategies aimed at optimizing milk supply (e.g., breast massage, frequent milk expression, complete emptying of breasts, kangaroo care, and medications)
- Provide instruction and support in accordance with health care institution's policy on lactation for the mother of preterm infant (i.e., instruct on frequency of pumping, when to expect milk supply to increase, normal feeding patterns based on gestational age, and weaning from pump when infant is able to nurse well)
- Instruct on signs and symptoms warranting reporting to a health care practitioner or lactation consultant
- Provide discharge instructions and arrange for follow-up care tailored to patient's specific needs (e.g., mother of healthy term infant, multiples, preterm infant, or ill infant)
- Refer to a lactation consultant
- Assist with re-lactation, if needed
- Discuss options for weaning

- Instruct mother to consult her health care practitioner before taking any medications when breastfeeding, including over-the-counter medications and oral contraceptives
- Discuss methods of contraception
- Encourage employers to provide opportunities for lactating mothers to express and store breast milk during the workday

2nd edition 1996; revised 2000, 2013

Background Evidence:

Dyson, L., McCormick, F. M., & Renfrew, M. J. (2005). Interventions for promoting the initiation of breastfeeding. *Cochrane Database of Systematic Reviews, 2005*(2). https://doi.org/10.1002/14651858.CD001688.pub2

Hill, P. D. (2001). Lactation counseling. In M. Craft-Rosenberg & J. Denehy (Eds.), *Nursing interventions for infants, children, and families* (pp. 61–76). Sage.

Kramer, M. S., & Kakuma, R. (2002). *The optimal duration of exclusive breastfeeding: A systematic review*. Geneva, Switzerland: World Health Organization.

Lang, S. (2002). *Breastfeeding special care babies* (2nd ed.). London: Bailliere Tindall.

Riordan, J. (2005). *Breastfeeding and human lactation* (3rd ed.). Jones & Bartlett.

Walker, M. (2006). *Breastfeeding management for the clinician: Using the evidence*. Jones & Bartlett.

Ward, S. L., & Hisley, S. M. (2009). Caring for the postpartal woman and her family. In *Maternal-child nursing care: Optimizing outcomes for mothers, children, & families* (pp. 469–509). F.A. Davis.

L

Lactation Suppression   6870

Definition: Facilitating the cessation of milk production while minimizing painful engorgement

Activities:

- Discuss options for milk expression (e.g., hand, manual, and electrical pumping)
- Instruct patient to express enough milk via hand, manual, or electrical pumping to reduce breast pressure but not enough to empty breast
- Assist patient in securing a good quality breast pump for use
- Assist patient in determining schedule (e.g., frequency and duration) for milk expression based on individual factors (e.g., length of time after giving birth, frequency of emptying breasts, and amount of milk currently being produced)
- Monitor breast engorgement and associated discomfort or pain
- Instruct patient on measures to reduce discomfort or pain (i.e., ice packs or cold cabbage leaves applied to breasts; analgesics)
- Administer lactation suppression drug, if appropriate
- Encourage patient to wear supportive, well-fitting bra continuously until lactation is suppressed
- Provide anticipatory guidance on physiological changes (i.e., uterine cramping and presence of scant milk post-lactation suppression)

- Discuss feelings, concerns, or issues patient may have pertaining to lactation cessation

1st edition 1992; revised 2013

Background Evidence:

Moore, D. B., & Catlin, A. (2003). Pediatric ethics, issues, & commentary. Lactation suppression: Forgotten aspect of care for the mother of a dying child. *Pediatric Nursing, 29*(5), 383–384.

Oladapo, O. T., & Fawole, B. (2009). Treatments for suppression of lactation. *Cochrane Database of Systematic Reviews*, CD005937. https://doi.org/10.1002/14651858.CD005937pub2

Pillitteri, A. (2007). Nutritional needs of a newborn. In *Maternal and child health nursing: Care of the childbearing and childrearing family* (pp. 722–746) (5th ed.). Lippincott Williams & Wilkins.

Riordan, J. (2005). *Breastfeeding and human lactation* (3rd ed.). Jones and Bartlett.

Walker, M. (2006). *Breastfeeding management for the clinician: Using the evidence*. Jones & Bartlett.

Laser Precautions   6560

Definition: Limiting the risk of laser-related injury to the patient and others

Activities:

- Assure all personnel working in a laser environment have knowledge of established laser safety, including review of safety information supplied by the laser manufacturer
- Assure all personnel operating laser equipment have proper training
- Determine the nominal hazard zone (i.e., the space in which the level of direct, reflected, or scattered radiation used during normal laser operation exceeds the applicable maximum permissible exposure)
- Place clearly marked laser signs at all entrances to laser treatment areas when lasers are in use
- Assure that all doors and windows in the nominal hazard zone remain closed
- Assure that windows, including door windows, are covered with a barrier that blocks transmission of a beam to the type of laser being used, as appropriate
- Implement procedures to prevent accidental activation or misdirection of laser beams
- Restrict access to laser keys to authorized personnel
- Place lasers in standby mode when not in active use
- Place laser foot switch in a position convenient to the operator, with the activation mechanism identified
- Remove other pedals from the area
- Assure laser user is the only one to activate the device with the foot pedal
- Assure that laser assistant does not have competing responsibilities that would require leaving the laser unattended during active use
- Provide for ease of access to the emergency shut off switch to disable the laser in case of a component breakdown or untoward event
- Minimize reflective surfaces during laser surgery
- Provide appropriate laser, fibers, filters, lenses, and attachments, as appropriate
- Assure that persons in the nominal hazard zone wear protective eyewear or use filters of specific wavelength and optical density for the laser in use
- Assure that correct laser wavelength and optical density eye protection is available at the entrance to a room where a laser is in use
- Assure that patient's eyes and eyelids are protected from the laser beam
- Verify that instruments and supplies are laser safe
- Verify that ointments and solutions are nonflammable
- Set up and connect plume evacuator, as appropriate
- Remove surgical smoke by use of a smoke evacuation system in both open and minimally invasive procedures to prevent occupational exposure to laser-generated airborne contaminants
- Consider used smoke evacuator filters, tubing, and wands potentially infectious waste and handle using standard precautions; dispose of as biohazardous waste
- Assure that personnel wear respiratory protection (e.g., fit-tested surgical N95 filtering face piece respirator, high-filtration surgical mask) during procedures that generate surgical smoke
- Check fire-extinguishing supplies and equipment
- Assure that personnel are prepared to extinguish fires using the appropriate extinguisher per laser type based on manufacturer's suggestions
- Set up laser, as per protocol
- Inspect electrical cords
- Inspect laser fibers for breaks
- Activate area entryway control system, as appropriate
- Test fire laser
- Instruct patient about importance of not moving during laser use, as appropriate
- Immobilize patient's body part, as appropriate
- Protect tissue around laser site with moistened towels or sponges
- Protect exposed tissues around surgical site with saline-saturated materials when lasers with a thermal effect are being used
- Provide a rectal pack, as appropriate
- Adjust laser settings as per physician or agency protocol
- Monitor patient for potential injury
- Monitor environment for possible fire, adhering to local, state and federal regulations pertaining to laser use
- Monitor environment for flammable substance or breaks in precautions, assuring that laser surgery is not performed in an oxygen-rich environment
- Assure that laser-resistant endotracheal tubes are used to minimize the potential for fire during laser procedures involving the patient's airway or digestive tract
- Return laser key to designated secure location
- Sterilize laser lenses, as appropriate
- Record information, as per protocol
- Use a laser safety checklist
- Provide a laser log as an adjunct to the perioperative documentation, as appropriate
- Document service and maintenance activities

2nd edition 1996; revised 2018

Background Evidence:

Association of Operating Room Nurses. (2014). *Perioperative standards and recommended practices.*

Castelluccio, D. (2012). Implementing AORN recommended practices for laser safety. *AORN Journal, 95*(5), 612–627.

Simon, M. (2011). Laser safety: Practical measures and latest legislative requirements. *Journal of Perioperative Practice, 21*(9), 299–303.

Smeltzer, S. C., & Bare, B. G. (2004). Intraoperative nursing management (10th ed.) *Brunner & Suddarth's textbook of medical surgical nursing* (Vol. 1, pp. 417–435). Lippincott Williams & Wilkins.

L

Latex Precautions 6570

Definition: Reducing the risk of a systemic reaction to latex

Activities:
- Determine if person has latex allergy
- Determine if history of neural tube defect (e.g., spina bifida) or congenital urological condition (e.g., exstrophy of the bladder)
- Determine allergies to foods such as bananas, kiwi, avocado, mango, and chestnuts
- Determine type of reaction to latex or other allergies in the past
- Determine history of systemic reactions to natural rubber latex (e.g., facial or scleral edema, tearing eyes, urticaria, rhinitis, wheezing)
- Refer to allergist for allergy testing, as appropriate
- Record allergy or risk in medical record
- Place allergy band on person
- Post sign indicating latex precautions
- Survey environment and remove latex products
- Use non-latex substitutes in environment wherever possible (i.e., avoid balloons, rubber bands, review bandage packages for content, ensure emergency kits in schools have only latex free products)
- Monitor for signs and symptoms of systemic reaction
- Report information to health care provider, pharmacist, and other care providers, as indicated
- Administer medications, as appropriate
- Instruct about risk factors for developing latex allergy
- Instruct about signs and symptoms of reaction
- Instruct about latex content in household products and substitution with nonlatex products, as appropriate
- Provide written list of non-latex substitutes for household products
- Instruct to wear health care alert tag
- Instruct person and family about emergency treatment (e.g., epinephrine), as appropriate
- Instruct visitors about latex-free environment (e.g., latex balloons)
- Ensure yearly education for staff related to latex allergic reactions and treatments
- Use teach-back to ensure understanding

2nd edition 1996; revised 2004, 2024

Background Evidence:

Berman, A., Snyder, S. J., & Frandsen, G. (2018). Asepsis. In *Kozier and Erb's Fundamentals of nursing: Concepts, process and practice* (pp. 621–622) (10th ed.). Pearson.

Leppert, K. (2021). Perioperative nursing. In R. F., Craven, C. J., Hirnle, & C. J. Henshaw (Eds.), *Fundamentals of nursing: Human health and function* (8th ed.). Wolters-Kluwer.

Liberatore, K. (2019). Protecting patients with latex allergies. *AJN, American Journal of Nursing, 119*(1), 60–63. https://doi.org/10.1097/01. NAJ.0000552616.96652.72

Potter, P. A., Perry, A. G., Stockert, P. A., & Hall, A. M. (2021). *Fundamentals of Nursing* (10th ed.). Elsevier.

Laughter Yoga 5930

Definition: Use of prolonged voluntary laughter assisted by chants and exercises such as clapping, meditation, body movements, and stretching

Activities:
- Evaluate readiness and willingness of individual or group
- Identify mutual goals and desired specific change in behavior or physiology with individual (e.g., stress reduction, increased sense of well-being, decreased pain, better sleep quality)
- Provide calm, comfortable, and private environment to ensure personal comfort
- Determine frequency and duration of sessions (i.e., usually 25–30 minutes)
- Obtain consent, if indicated
- Begin with 10 minutes warm-up exercises (e.g., deep belly breathing, body stretching, gentle neck and shoulder stretches, smiling to loosen up face muscles)
- Vary warmup with additional stretches, sounds, and movements (e.g., lion roar with belly laugh, clapping hands rhythmically with chanted words, deep breathing using abdomen to fill lungs)
- Follow warmup with 15 minutes of physical activity (i.e., use left hand to tap five times from shoulder to wrist on right side and repeat for left side; next tap five times down both legs) while chanting repetitively
- Ensure repeated chanting with physical activity, and progressively increase tapping and chanting
- Increase activity slowly to include playful exercises (e.g., singing a nonsense song and laughing after each verse, dancing around room while laughing, miming pretend scenario and laughing throughout or at end)
- Encourage individual to use deep breathing exercises throughout session
- Incorporate various exuberant and amusing laughs with movements
- Demonstrate movements and laughter if needed to facilitate understanding
- Encourage happy feelings and upbeat mood using cheerful activities (i.e., make wishes and rejoice as if wishes had come true)
- Stop session immediately if anyone uncomfortable or having pain

- Use body relaxation, smiling, and deep breathing in final 5 minutes
- Monitor physical, social, mental, emotional, spiritual responses

8th edition 2024

Background Evidence:

Bressington, D., Yu, C., Wong, W., Ng, T. C., & Chien, W. T. (2018). The effects of group-based laughter yoga interventions on mental health in adults: A systematic review. *Journal of Psychiatric Mental Health Nursing, 25*(8), 517–527. https://doi.org/10.1111/jpm.12491

Kuru Alici, N., & Arikan Dönmez, A. (2020). A systematic review of the effect of laughter yoga on physical function and psychosocial outcomes in older adults. *Complementary Therapeutic Clinical Practices, 41*, 101252. https://doi.org/10.1016/j.ctcp.2020.101252

Memarian, A., Sanatkaran, A., & Bahari, S. M. (2017). The effect of laughter yoga exercises on anxiety and sleep quality in patients suffering from Parkinson's disease. *Biomedical Research and Therapy, 4*(7), 1463–1479. https://doi.org/10.15419/bmrat.v4i07.200

Rezaei, S., Mahfeli, M., Mousavi, S. V., & Poorabolghasem Hosseini, S. (2019). The effect of laughter yoga on the quality of life of elderly nursing home residents. *Caspian Journal of Neurological Science, 5*(1), 7–15. http://cjns.gums.ac.ir/article-1-254-en.html

Shattla, S. I., Mabrouk, S. M., & Abed, G. A. (2019). Effectiveness of laughter yoga therapy on job burnout syndromes among psychiatric nurses. *International Journal of Nursing, 6*(1), 33–47.

Tanaka, A., Tokuda, N., & Ichihara, K. (2018). Psychological and physiological effects of laughter yoga sessions in Japan: A pilot study. *Nursing in Health Sciences, 20*(3), 304–312. https://doi.org/10.1111/nhs.12562

van der Wal, N., & Kok, R. N. (2019). Laughter-inducing therapies: Systematic review and meta-analysis. *Social Science & Medicine, 232*, 473–488. https://doi.org/10.1016/j.socscimed.2019.02.018

Learning Facilitation 5520

Definition: Enhancing willingness and ability to receive, process, and comprehend information

Activities:

- Determine willingness and ability to receive, process, and comprehend information
- Provide environment conducive to learning and void of distractions
- Meet basic physiological needs (e.g., hunger, thirst, warmth, pain, fatigue)
- Encourage active participation
- Enlist participation of family and others, as appropriate
- Establish mutual, realistic learning goals and objectives
- Tailor content to cognitive, psychomotor, and emotional abilities
- Provide information appropriate to developmental level
- Arrange information in logical sequence
- Adapt information to comply with lifestyle, routines, and beliefs
- Use multiple teaching modalities, as appropriate
- Provide instructional pamphlets, videos, and online resources, as appropriate
- Ensure that educational material current
- Use plain language, short words and sentences, and avoid medical jargon
- Relate new content to previous knowledge, as appropriate
- Encourage sharing of valid experiences throughout learning experience
- Use self-paced instruction, when possible
- Encourage free expression of different opinions and ideas
- Repeat important information
- Provide verbal prompts and reminders, as appropriate
- Ensure that consistent information provided by interprofessional team
- Provide opportunities for practice, as appropriate
- Provide frequent feedback about learning progress
- Correct information misinterpretations, as appropriate
- Provide time for questions and concerns
- Answer questions in clear, concise manner
- Refer to appropriate resources including support groups
- Use teach-back to ensure understanding

1st edition 1992; revised 2013, 2024

Background Evidence:

Cutilli, C. C. (2021). Excellence in patient education evidence-based education that "Sticks" and improves patient outcomes. *Nursing Clinics of North America, 56*, 401–412. https://doi.org/10.1016/j.cnur.2021.04.006

Guthrie, K. L. (2020). *Transforming learning: Instructional and assessment strategies for. leadership education.* Information Age Publishing.

Kennedy, M. B., & Parish, A. l. (2021). Educational theory and cognitive science. *practical principles to improve patient education. Nursing Clinics of North America, 56*, 401–412. https://doi.org/10.1016/j.cnur.2021.04.006

Goldman, J., Smeraglio, A., Lo, L., Kuper, A., & Wong, B. M. (2021). Theory in quality improvement and patient safety education: A scoping review. *Perspectives in Medical Education, 10*, 319–326. https://doi.org/10.1007/s40037-021-00686-5

L

Leech Therapy 3460

Definition: Application of medicinal leeches to improve venous blood flow

Activities:

- Reassure that leech therapy accepted health care treatment
- Obtain informed consent
- Obtain complete blood cell count and other laboratory tests, per agency protocol
- Administer prophylactic antibiotic, as prescribed
- Cleanse treatment site with soap and water, and rinse
- Direct head of leech toward treatment site and allow to attach
- Use petrolatum or transparent adhesive dressing to cover treatment site, as prescribed

- Surround site with towels or gauze to prevent leech from migrating
- Place drop of blood on treatment site if slow to attach
- Keep in place for 30–90 minutes or as prescribed
- Dispose in biohazardous waste according to agency policy
- Monitor for adverse reactions (e.g., excessive bleeding, hypersensitivity reactions, infection)
- Instruct not to touch or remove leeches once applied
- Remove leeches that do not drop off by gently stroking with alcohol pad
- Refrigerate unused leeches in container filled with salt solution (using spring or distilled water) covered with netting
- Handle leeches carefully after feeding to prevent regurgitation of gut contents
- Place leeches in small container of alcohol for incineration
- Cleanse treated area every 1 to 2 hours with half-and-half solution of hydrogen peroxide and sterile water to prevent bloody drainage from hardening and constricting blood flow

- Monitor hemoglobin and hematocrit at least daily, as appropriate
- Document response to treatment

2nd edition 1996; revised 2004, 2024

Background Evidence:

del Rosario, C., & Barkley, J. T. (2017). Postoperative graft and flap care: What clinical nurses need to know. *MEDSURG Nursing, 26*(3), 180–192.

Labarite, A., & Parsh, B. (2020). How to manage leech therapy. *Nursing, 50*(11), 11–12. https://doi.org/10.1097/01.NURSE.0000718916.16465.aa

Spiers, E. (2018). Managing vascular compromise of hand and digit replantation following traumatic amputation. *British Journal of Nursing, 27*(20), S50–S56. https://doi.org/10.12968/bjon.2018.27.Sup20.S50

Şenel, E., Taylan Özkan, A., & Mumcuoglu, K. Y. (2020). Scientometric analysis of medicinal leech therapy. *Journal of Ayurveda and Integrative Medicine, 11*(4), 534–538. https://doi.org/10.1016/j.jaim.2018.11.006

Life Skills Enhancement 5326

Definition: Developing an individual's ability to independently and effectively deal with the demands and challenges of everyday life

Activities:

- Establish rapport by using empathy, warmth, spontaneity, organization, patience, and persistence
- Determine the life skill learning needs of the patient, family, group, or community
- Appraise the patient's educational level
- Determine level of knowledge of the life skill
- Appraise the patient's current level of skill and understanding of the content
- Appraise the patient's learning style
- Mutually agree upon goals for the life skills program
- Determine number of sessions and length of time of the program
- Enhance motivation by setting achievable incremental goals
- Appraise the patient's cognitive, psychomotor, and affective abilities and disabilities
- Determine the patient's ability to learn specific information (i.e., consider the patient's developmental level, physiological status, orientation, pain, fatigue, unfulfilled basic needs, emotional state, and adaptation to illness)
- Determine the patient's motivation to learn specific information (i.e., consider the patient's health beliefs, past noncompliance, bad experiences with health care or learning, and conflicting goals)
- Select appropriate teaching methods and strategies
- Select appropriate educational materials
- Tailor the content to the patient's cognitive, psychomotor, and affective abilities and disabilities
- Break more complex skills into their stepwise components to enable incremental progress
- Adjust instruction to facilitate learning, as appropriate
- Provide an environment conducive to learning
- Use role-playing of appropriate behaviors with scenarios that simulate real life interpersonal interactions
- Provide positive feedback contingent on improvements in the patient's improved learning skill
- Use assignments to practice and enhance the performance of new skills in real life situations

- Instruct on strategies designed to enhance communication skills, if needed
- Provide assertiveness training, if needed
- Use strategies to enhance the patient's self awareness
- Provide appropriate social skills training, if needed
- Assist the patient to solve problems in a constructive manner
- Instruct patient how to manage conflict, if needed
- Instruct patient in setting priorities and decision making
- Assist patient in values clarification
- Provide instruction on time management, if needed
- Provide instruction on diet, nutrition, and food preparation, if needed
- Instruct patient in the use of stress management techniques, as appropriate
- Instruct patient on how to manage his or her illness symptoms, if appropriate
- Instruct patient on medication management, if appropriate
- Instruct the patient on workplace fundamentals (e.g., improving job performance, leaning about specific workplace and performance expectations, making friends and appropriate socializing)
- Identify and arrange for participation in leisure activities
- Provide assistance in managing finances and creating a budget, if indicated
- Include the family or significant others, as appropriate

6th edition 2013

Background Evidence:

Bartels, S., Forester, B., Mueser, K., Miles, K., Dums, A., Pratt, & Perkins, L. (2004). Enhanced skills training and health care management for older persons with severe mental illness. *Community Mental Health Journal, 40*(1), 75–90.

Bellack, A. S., Mueser, K. T., Gingerich, S., & Agresta, J. (2004). *Social skills training for schizophrenia: A step-by-step guide* (2nd ed.). Guilford Press.

Grawe, R. W., Hagen, R., Espeland, B., & Mueser, K. T. (2007). The better life program: Effects of group skills training for persons with severe mental illness and substance abuse disorders. *Journal of Mental Health*, *16*(5), 625–634.

Liberman, R. P. (2007). Dissemination and adoption of social skills training: Social validation of an evidence-based treatment for the mentally disabled. *Journal of Mental Health*, *16*(5), 595–623.

Liberman, R. P., Glynn, S. M., Blair, K. E., Ross, D., & Marder, S. R. (2002). In vivo amplified skills training: Promoting generalization of independent living skills for clients with schizophrenia. *Psychiatry*, *65*(2), 137–155.

World Health Organization. (1999). *Partners in life skills education*: Conclusions from a United Nations inter-agency meeting.

Limit Setting 4380

Definition: Establishing the parameters of desirable and acceptable patient behavior

Activities:

- Use a consistent, matter-of-fact, nonjudgmental approach
- State limit or identify (with patient input, when appropriate) undesirable patient behavior
- Communicate the limit in positive terms (e.g., "keep your clothes on," rather than "that behavior is inappropriate")
- Discuss concerns with patient about behavior
- Establish consequences (with patient input, when appropriate) for occurrence or nonoccurrence of desired behaviors
- Discuss with patient what is desirable behavior in a given situation or setting, when appropriate
- Establish reasonable expectations for patient behavior based on the situation and the patient
- Avoid arguing or bargaining about the consequences and established behavioral expectations with the patient
- Communicate the established consequences and behavioral expectations to the patient in a language that is easily understood and nonpunitive
- Communicate the established consequences and behavioral expectations with the treatment team for consistency and continuity in care
- Assist patient to show the desired behaviors, when necessary and appropriate

- Monitor patient for occurrence or nonoccurrence of the desired behaviors
- Initiate the established consequences for the occurrence or nonoccurrence of the desired behaviors
- Modify consequences and behavioral expectations, as needed, to accommodate reasonable changes in the patient's situation
- Decrease limit setting as patient behavior approximates the desired behaviors

1st edition 1992; revised 2008

Background Evidence:

Deering, C. (2006). Therapeutic relationships and communication. In W. Mohr (Ed.), *Psychiatric mental health nursing* (6th ed., pp. 55–78). Lippincott Williams & Wilkins.

Lowe, T., Wellman, N., & Taylor, R. (2003). Limit-setting and decision-making in the management of aggression. *Journal of Advanced Nursing*, *41*(2), 154–161.

Rickelman, B. L. (2006). The client who displays angry, aggressive, or violent behavior. In W. Mohr (Ed.), *Psychiatric mental health nursing* (6th ed., pp. 659–686). Lippincott Williams & Wilkins.

Videbeck, S. L. (2006). *Psychiatric mental health nursing* (3rd ed.). Lippincott Williams & Wilkins.

Listening Visits 5328

Definition: Empathic listening to genuinely understand an individual's situation and work collaboratively over a number of home visits to identify and generate solutions to reduce depressive symptoms

Activities:

- Screen for depression to establish baseline
- Establish the purpose and proposed number of visits
- Establish an agreeable place and time for the visits
- Display interest in the patient
- Maintain patient confidentiality and privacy
- Use personal strengths to establish relationship with patient
- Use open-ended questions to encourage expression of thoughts, feelings, and concerns
- Use silence to encourage the expression of thoughts, feelings, and concerns
- Avoid barriers to active listening (i.e., minimizing feelings, offering easy solutions, interrupting, talking about self, and premature closure)
- Focus completely on the interaction by suppressing prejudice, bias, assumptions, preoccupying personal concerns, and other distractions
- Use nonverbal behavior to facilitate communication (i.e., be aware of physical stance conveying nonverbal messages)

- Listen for the unexpressed message and feeling, as well as content, of the conversation
- Explore patient's behavior, feelings, and cognition about a situation
- Assist patient to name feelings and emotion, associated with situation
- Clarify the message through the use of questions and feedback
- Identify the predominant themes
- Assist patient to generate a comprehensive list of current problems
- Assist patient to identify most important problem
- Assist patient to generate a list of solutions
- Assist patient to evaluate the disadvantages and advantages of the list generated
- Encourage patient to select desired solutions
- Assist patient to develop a plan to carry out the solution
- Explore progress toward resolution of the problem at subsequent visit

L

- Evaluate depression symptoms at appropriate intervals
- Refer patient to other health care providers, as necessary

6th edition 2013

Background Evidence:

Cooper, P. J., Murray, L., Wilson, A., & Romaniuk, H. (2003). Controlled trial of the short- and long-term effect of psychological treatment of post-partum depression. Impact on maternal mood. *British Journal of Psychiatry*, *182*(5), 412–419.

Holden, J. M., Sagovsky, R., & Cox, J. L. (1989). Counselling in a general practice setting: Controlled study of health visitor intervention in treatment of postnatal depression. *British Medical Journal*, *298*(6668), 223–226.

Morrell, C. J., Slade, P., Warner, R., Paley, G., Dixon, S., Walters, S. J., Brugha, T., Barkham, M., Parry, G., & Nicholl, J. (2009). Clinical effectiveness of health visitor training in psychologically informed approaches for depression in postnatal women: Pragmatic cluster randomised trial in primary care. *British Medical Journal*, *338*, a3045. https://doi.org/10.1136/bmj.a3045

Segre, L. S. (2011). Postpartum depression. In M. C. Rosenberg & S. R. Pehler (Eds.), *Encyclopedia of family health* (pp. 833–835). Sage.

Wickberg, B., & Hwang, C. P. (1996). Counselling of postnatal depression: A controlled study on a population based Swedish sample. *Journal of Affective Disorders*, *39*(3), 209–216.

Lower Extremity Monitoring 3480

Definition: Collection, analysis, and use of person data to categorize risk and prevent injury to the lower extremities

Activities:

- Review history of lower extremity injuries and recent changes
- Determine current mobility and perception of mobility status (i.e., walks without assistance, walks with assistance of device, does not walk, uses wheelchair)
- Determine evidence of poor hygiene, edema, presence of toenail changes (e.g., thickening, fungal infection, improper trimming, nail care)
- Determine color, temperature, hydration, hair growth, texture, deformities, and skin condition
- Monitor muscle strength and joint mobility in ankle and foot
- Determine evidence of lower extremity pressure areas (i.e., presence of localized redness, increased temperatures, blisters, corns, or callus formation)
- Inquire about paresthesia (e.g., numbness, tingling, burning)
- Monitor lower extremity pulses
- Determine ankle brachial index, as prescribed
- Determine presence of intermittent claudication, rest pain, or night pain
- Determine capillary refill time
- Monitor level of protective sensation using approved tests of sensory loss (e.g., Semmes-Weinstein nylon monofilament)
- Determine vibration perception threshold
- Determine proprioceptive responses
- Elicit deep tendon reflexes (i.e., ankle and knee), as indicated
- Monitor gait and weight distribution on feet (e.g., observe walking, determine wear pattern on shoes)
- Monitor appropriateness and condition of shoes and socks
- Perform ongoing surveillance of lower extremities to determine need for referral at least four times per year or as prescribed
- Determine specialty foot care services required
- Consult with health care provider regarding recommendation for further evaluation and therapy (e.g., x-ray), as needed
- Provide with information about recommended specialty foot care services
- Determine preference for referral to health professional or agency, as appropriate
- Provide assistance in obtaining necessary financial resources, as appropriate
- Instruct on lower extremity care needs
- Use teach-back to ensure understanding

4th edition 2004; revised 2024

Background Evidence:

Aziz, M. G. (2021). Hygiene and self-care. In R. F., Craven, C. J., Hirnle, & C. J. Henshaw (Eds.), *Fundamentals of nursing: Human health and function* (8th ed.). Wolters-Kluwer.

Berman, A., Snyder, S. J., & Frandsen, G. (2018). Hygiene. In *Kozier and Erb's Fundamentals of nursing: Concepts, process and practice* (pp. 684–688) (10th ed.). Pearson.

Perry, A. G., Potter, P. A., Ostendorf, W. R., & Laplante, N. (2022). Personal hygiene and bedmaking. In *Clinical Nursing Skills and Techniques* (10th ed.). Elsevier.

Porter-O'Grady, T. (2021). Wound and foot care nursing on the streets of the city: A view from here. *Journal of Wound, Ostomy & Continence Nursing*, *48*(1), 69–74.

Potter, P. A., Perry, A. G., Stockert, P. A., & Hall, A. M. (2021). *Fundamentals of Nursing* (10th ed.). Elsevier.

Trelease, J., & Simmons, J. (2021). Getting ready for foot care certification: Intervention and treatment for dermatological conditions affecting the feet and lower extremities. *Journal of Wound, Ostomy & Continence Nursing*, *48*(3), 262–264.

Williams, P. (2020). *Basic geriatric nursing* (7th ed.). Elsevier.

L

Malignant Hyperthermia Precautions 3840

Definition: Prevention or reduction of hypermetabolic response to pharmacological agents used during surgery

Activities:

- Ask patient about personal or family history of malignant hyperthermia, unexpected deaths from anesthetic, muscle disorder, or unexplained postoperative fever
- Refer patient with family history of malignant hyperthermia for further testing to determine risk (e.g., muscle contracture test, molecular genetic test)
- Notify surgical team of patient history or risk status
- Maintain emergency equipment for malignant hyperthermia, per protocol
- Review malignant hyperthermia emergency care with staff, per protocol
- Monitor vital signs, including core body temperature
- Provide anesthesia machine free of precipitating anesthetic agents for patient at-risk for malignant hyperthermia or discontinue use of anesthesia machine for patient experiencing malignant hyperthermia
- Place cooling water mattress under patient at-risk for malignant hyperthermia at start of procedure
- Use non-triggering anesthetic agents for patient at-risk for or experiencing malignant hyperthermia (e.g., opioids, benzodiazepines, local anesthetics, nitrous oxide, and barbiturates)
- Avoid or discontinue use of triggering agents (e.g., succinylcholine used alone or in conjunction with volatile inhalation agents such as halothane, enflurane, isoflurane, sevoflurane, or desflurane)
- Monitor for signs of malignant hyperthermia (e.g., hypercarbia, hyperthermia, tachycardia, tachypnea, metabolic acidosis, arrhythmias, cyanosis, mottled skin, muscle rigidity, profuse sweating, and unstable blood pressure)
- Discontinue procedure, if possible
- Provide emergency management supplies
- Obtain blood and urine samples
- Monitor for abnormalities in laboratory values (e.g., increased end-tidal carbon dioxide level with decreased oxygen saturation, increased serum calcium, increased potassium, unexplained metabolic acidosis, hematuria, and myoglobinuria)
- Monitor electrocardiography results
- Intubate or assist with intubation if endotracheal tube is not already in place
- Hyperventilate with 100% oxygen using highest flow rate possible
- Prepare and administer medications (e.g., dantrolene sodium, sodium bicarbonate, insulin, antidysrhythmic agents other than calcium channel blockers, and osmotic or loop diuretics)
- Administer iced saline
- Apply cooling blanket or commercial cooling device over torso
- Rub or wrap extremities with cold, wet, or iced towels
- Lavage stomach, bladder, rectum, and open body cavities with sterile, iced, normal saline
- Insert nasogastric tube, rectal tube, and urinary catheter, as necessary
- Monitor urine output
- Administer sufficient IV fluids to maintain urine output
- Initiate second IV line
- Assist with arterial and central venous pressure line insertion
- Avoid use of drugs, including calcium chloride or gluconate, cardiac glycosides, adrenergics, atropine, and lactated ringer solutions
- Decrease environmental stimuli
- Observe for signs of late complications (e.g., consumption coagulopathy, renal failure, hypothermia, pulmonary edema, hyperkalemia, neurological sequelae, muscle necrosis, and reoccurrence of symptoms after treatment of initial episode)
- Provide patient and family education (i.e., discuss needed precautions for future anesthetic administration, discuss methods for determining malignant hyperthermia risk)
- Refer patient and family to Malignant Hyperthermia Association of the United States
- Refer for genetic counseling
- Report incident to the North American Malignant Hyperthermia Registry and the Medic Alert Hotline

2nd edition 1996; revised 2013

Background Evidence:

Chard, R. (2010). Care of intraoperative patients. In D. D. Ignatavicius & M. L. Workman (Eds.), *Medical-surgical nursing: Patient-centered collaborative care* (6th ed., pp. 264–284). Saunders Elsevier.

Hernandez, J. F., Secrest, J. A., Hill, L., & McClarty, S. J. (2009). Scientific advances in the genetic understanding and diagnosis of malignant hyperthermia. *Journal of PeriAnesthesia Nursing, 24*(1), 19–34.

Hommertzheim, R., & Steinke, E. E. (2006). Malignant hyperthermia: The perioperative nurse's role. *AORN Journal, 83*(1), 149–164.

Kaplow, R. (2010). Care of postanesthesia patients. *Critical Care Nursing, 30*(1), 60–62.

Nagelhout, J. J., & Plaus, K. L. (2010). *Handbook of nurse anesthesia* (4th ed.). Saunders Elsevier.

M

Massage 1480

Definition: Stimulation of the skin and underlying tissues with varying degrees of hand pressure to decrease pain, produce relaxation, and/or improve circulation

Activities:

- Screen for contraindications such as decreased platelets, decreased skin integrity, deep vein thrombosis, areas with open lesions, redness or inflammation, tumors, and hypersensitivity to touch
- Assess the client's willingness to have a massage
- Establish a period of time for massage that achieves the desired response
- Select the area or areas of the body to be massaged
- Wash hands with warm water
- Prepare a warm, comfortable, private environment without distractions

- Place in a comfortable position that facilitates massage
- Drape to expose only area to be massaged, as needed
- Drape unexposed areas with blankets, sheets, or bath towels, as needed
- Use lotion, oil, or dry powder to reduce friction (no lotion or oils on head or scalp), assessing for any sensitivity or contraindications
- Warm lotion or oil in palm of hands or by running bottle under warm water for several minutes
- Massage using continuous, even, long strokes; kneading; or vibration with palms, fingers, and thumbs
- Adapt massage area, technique, and pressure to patient's perception of comfort and purpose of massage
- Massage the hands or feet, if other areas are inconvenient, or if more comfortable for the patient
- Encourage patient to deep breathe and relax during massage
- Encourage patient to advise of any part of the massage that is uncomfortable
- Instruct patient at completion of massage to rest until ready and then to move slowly
- Use massage alone or in conjunction with other measures, as appropriate
- Evaluate and document response to massage

1st edition 1992; revised 2008

Background Evidence:

Altman, G. B. (2004). *Delmar's fundamental and advanced nursing skills* (2nd ed.). Delmar Learning.

Coe, A. B., & Anthony, M. L. (2005). Understanding bodywork for the patient with cancer. *Clinical Journal of Oncology Nursing, 9*(6), 733–739.

Fontaine, K. L. (2005). *Complementary and alternative therapies for nursing practice* (2nd ed.). Pearson Prentice Hall.

Smith, M. C., Kemp, J., Hemphill, L., & Vojir, C. P. (2002). Outcomes of therapeutic massage for hospitalized cancer patients. *Journal of Nursing Scholarship, 34*(3), 257–262.

Smith, S. F., Duell, D. J., & Martin, B. C. (2004). *Clinical nursing skills: Basic to advanced skills* (6th ed.). Prentice Hall.

Snyder, M., & Tseng, Y. (2002). Massage. In M. Snyder & R. Lindquist (Eds.), *Complementary/alternative therapies in nursing* (4th ed., pp. 223–233). Springer.

Wang, H. L., & Keck, J. F. (2004). Foot and hand massage as an intervention for postoperative pain. *Pain Management Nursing, 5*(2), 59–65.

Mechanical Ventilation Management: Invasive   3300

Definition: Assisting the patient receiving artificial breathing support through a device inserted into the trachea

Activities:

- Monitor for conditions indicating a need for ventilation support (e.g., respiratory muscle fatigue, neurological dysfunction secondary to trauma, anesthesia, drug overdose, refractory respiratory acidosis)
- Monitor for impending respiratory failure
- Consult with other health care personnel in selection of a ventilator mode (initial mode usually volume control with breath rate, FiO_2 level and targeted tidal volume specified)
- Obtain baseline total body assessment of patient initially and with each change of caregiver
- Initiate setup and application of the ventilator
- Ensure that ventilator alarms are on
- Instruct the patient and family about the rationale and expected sensations associated with use of mechanical ventilators
- Routinely monitor ventilator settings, including temperature and humidification of inspired air
- Check all ventilator connections regularly
- Monitor for decrease in exhaled volume and increase in inspiratory pressure
- Administer muscle paralyzing agents, sedatives, and narcotic analgesics, as appropriate
- Monitor for activities that increase oxygen consumption (e.g., fever, shivering, seizures, pain, or basic nursing activities) that may supersede ventilator support settings and cause oxygen desaturation
- Monitor for factors that increase patient/ventilator work of breathing (e.g., morbid obesity, pregnancy, massive ascites, lowered head of bed, biting of ET, condensation in ventilator tubes, clogged filters)
- Monitor for symptoms that indicate increased work of breathing (e.g., increased heart or respiratory rate, increased blood pressure, diaphoresis, changes in mental status)
- Monitor the effectiveness of mechanical ventilation on patient's physiological and psychological status
- Initiate relaxation techniques, as appropriate
- Provide care to alleviate patient distress (e.g., positioning, tracheobronchial toileting, bronchodilator therapy, sedation and/or analgesia, frequent equipment checks)
- Provide patient with a means for communication (e.g., paper and pencil, alphabet board)
- Empty condensed water from water traps
- Ensure change of ventilator circuits every 24 hours
- Use aseptic technique in all suctioning procedures and as appropriate
- Monitor ventilator pressure readings, patient/ventilator synchronicity, and patient breath sounds
- Perform suctioning based on presence of adventitious breath sounds and/or increased inspiratory pressure
- Monitor pulmonary secretions for amount, color, and consistency and regularly document findings
- Stop NG feedings during suctioning and 30 to 60 minutes before chest physiotherapy
- Silence ventilator alarms during suctioning to decrease frequency of false alarms
- Monitor patient's progress on current ventilator settings and make appropriate changes, as ordered
- Monitor for adverse effects of mechanical ventilation (e.g., tracheal deviation, infection, barotrauma, volutrauma, reduced cardiac output, gastric distension, subcutaneous emphysema)
- Monitor for mucosal damage to oral, nasal, tracheal, or laryngeal tissue from pressure from artificial airways, high cuff pressures, or unplanned extubations
- Use commercial tube holders rather than tape or strings to fixate artificial airways to prevent unplanned extubations

- Position to facilitate ventilation/perfusion matching ("good lung down"), as appropriate
- Collaborate with physician to use pressure support or PEEP to minimize alveolar hypoventilation, as appropriate
- Collaborate routinely with physician and respiratory therapist to coordinate care and assist patient to tolerate therapy
- Perform chest physiotherapy, as appropriate
- Promote adequate fluid and nutritional intake
- Promote routine assessments for weaning criteria (e.g., hemodynamic, cerebral, metabolic stability, resolution of condition prompting intubation, ability to maintain patent airway, ability to initiate respiratory effort)
- Provide routine oral care with soft moist swabs, antiseptic agent, and gentle suctioning
- Monitor effects of ventilator changes on oxygenation: ABG, SaO_2, SvO_2, end-tidal CO_2, Qsp/Qt, A-aDO_2, patient's subjective response
- Monitor degree of shunt, vital capacity, Vd/Vt, MVV, inspiratory force, and FEV1 for readiness to wean from mechanical ventilation based on agency protocol
- Document all changes to ventilator settings with rationale for changes
- Document all patient responses to ventilator and ventilator changes (e.g., chest movement observation/auscultation, changes in x-ray, changes in ABGs)
- Monitor for post-extubation complications (e.g., stridor, glottic swelling, laryngospasm, tracheal stenosis)

- Ensure emergency equipment at bedside at all times (e.g., manual resuscitation bag connected to oxygen, masks, suction equipment/supplies), including preparations for power failures

1st edition 1992; revised 2000, 2008

Background Evidence:

American Association of Critical-Care Nurses. (2006). In J. G. Alspach (Ed.), *Core curriculum for critical care nursing* (6th ed.). Saunders Elsevier.

American Heart Association. (2005). 2005 American Heart Association guidelines for cardiopulmonary resuscitation and emergency cardiovascular care. *Circulation, 112*(24 Suppl.), IV-1–IV-211.

Fenstermacher, D., & Hong, D. (2004). Mechanical ventilation: What have we learned? *Critical Care Nursing Quarterly, 27*(3), 258–294.

Knipper, J. S., & Alpen, M. A. (1992). Ventilatory support. In G. M. Bulechek & J. C. McCloskey (Eds.), *Nursing interventions: Essential nursing treatments* (2nd ed., pp. 531–543). W.B. Saunders.

Manno, M. S. (2005). Managing mechanical ventilation. *Nursing, 2005, 35*(12), 36–42.

Smeltzer, S. C., & Bare, B. G. (2004). (10th ed.) *Brunner & Suddarth's textbook of medical-surgical nursing* (Vol. 1). Lippincott Williams and Wilkins.

Urden, L. D., Stacy, K. M., & Lough, M. E. (2006). *Thelan's critical care nursing: Diagnosis and management* (5th ed.). Mosby Elsevier.

Wiegand, D., & Carlson, K. (Eds.). (2005). *AACN procedure manual for critical care* (5th ed.). Elsevier Saunders.

Mechanical Ventilation Management: Noninvasive   3302

M

Definition: Assisting a patient receiving artificial breathing support that does not necessitate a device inserted into the trachea

Activities:

- Monitor for conditions indicating appropriateness of noninvasive ventilation support (e.g., acute exacerbations of COPD, asthma, noncardiogenic and cardiogenic pulmonary edema, acute respiratory failure due to community acquired pneumonia, obesity hypoventilation syndrome, obstructive sleep apnea)
- Monitor for contraindications to noninvasive ventilation support (e.g., hemodynamic instability, cardiovascular or respiratory arrest, unstable angina, acute myocardial infarction, refractory hypoxemia, severe respiratory acidosis, decreased level of consciousness, problems with securing/placing noninvasive equipment, facial trauma, inability to cooperate, morbidly obese, thick secretions, or bleeding)
- Consult with other health care personnel in selection of a noninvasive ventilator type (e.g., pressure limited [bilevel positive airway pressure], volume-cycled flow-limited, or CPAP)
- Consult with other health care personnel and patient in selection of noninvasive device (e.g., nasal or face mask, nasal plugs, nasal pillow, helmet, oral mouthpiece)
- Obtain baseline total body assessment of patient initially and with each change of caregiver
- Instruct the patient and family about the rationale and expected sensations associated with use of noninvasive mechanical ventilators and devices
- Place patient in semi-Fowler position
- Apply noninvasive device, assuring adequate fit and avoidance of large air leaks (take particular care with edentulous or bearded patients)

- Apply facial protection to avoid pressure damage to skin, as needed
- Initiate setup and application of the ventilator
- Observe patient continuously in first hour after application to assess tolerance
- Ensure that ventilator alarms are on
- Routinely monitor ventilator settings, including temperature and humidification of inspired air
- Check all ventilator connections regularly
- Monitor for decrease in exhaled volume and increase in inspiratory pressure
- Monitor for activities that increase oxygen consumption (e.g., fever, shivering, seizures, pain, or basic nursing activities) that may supersede ventilator support settings and cause oxygen desaturation
- Monitor for symptoms that indicate increased work of breathing (e.g., increased heart or respiratory rate, increased blood pressure, diaphoresis, changes in mental status)
- Monitor the effectiveness of mechanical ventilation on patient's physiological and psychological status
- Initiate relaxation techniques, as appropriate
- Ensure periods of rest daily (e.g., 15 to 30 minutes every 4 to 6 hours)
- Provide care to alleviate patient distress (e.g., positioning; treat side effects such as rhinitis, dry throat, or epistaxis; give sedation and/or analgesia; frequent equipment checks; cleansing or change of noninvasive device)
- Provide patient with a means for communication (e.g., paper and pencil, alphabet board)

- Empty condensed water from water traps
- Ensure change of ventilator circuits every 24 hours
- Use aseptic technique, as appropriate
- Monitor patient and ventilator synchronicity and patient breath sounds
- Monitor patient's progress on current ventilator settings and make appropriate changes, as ordered
- Monitor for adverse effects (e.g., eye irritation, skin breakdown, occluded airway from jaw displacement with mask, dyspnea, anxiety, claustrophobia, gastric distension)
- Monitor for mucosal damage to oral, nasal, tracheal, or laryngeal tissue
- Monitor pulmonary secretions for amount, color, and consistency and regularly document findings
- Collaborate routinely with physician and respiratory therapist to coordinate care and assist patient to tolerate therapy
- Perform chest physiotherapy, as appropriate
- Promote adequate fluid and nutritional intake
- Promote routine assessments for weaning criteria (e.g., resolution of condition prompting ventilation, ability to maintain adequate respiratory effort)
- Provide routine oral care with soft moist swabs, antiseptic agent, and gentle suctioning
- Document all changes to ventilator settings with rationale for changes
- Document all patient responses to ventilator and ventilator changes (e.g., chest movement observation/auscultation, changes in x-ray, changes in ABGs)

- Ensure emergency equipment at bedside at all times (e.g., manual resuscitation bag connected to oxygen, masks, suction equipment/supplies) including preparations for power failures

5th edition 2008

Background Evidence:

American Association of Critical-Care Nurses. (2006). In J. G. Alspach (Ed.), *Core curriculum for critical care nursing* (6th ed.). Saunders Elsevier.

American Heart Association. (2005). 2005 American Heart Association guidelines for cardiopulmonary resuscitation and emergency cardiovascular care. *Circulation, 112*(24 Suppl.), IV-1–IV-211.

Fenstermacher, D., & Hong, D. (2004). Mechanical ventilation: What have we learned? *Critical Care Nursing Quarterly, 27*(3), 258–294.

Knipper, J. S., & Alpen, M. A. (1992). Ventilatory support. In G. M. Bulechek & J. C. McCloskey (Eds.), *Nursing interventions: Essential nursing treatments* (2nd ed., pp. 531–543). W.B. Saunders.

Manno, M. S. (2005). Managing mechanical ventilation. *Nursing 2005, 35*(12), 36–42.

Smeltzer, S. C., & Bare, B. G. (2004). *Brunner & Suddarth's textbook of medical-surgical nursing* (10th ed.). Lippincott Williams and Wilkins.

Stoltzfus, S. (2006). The role of noninvasive mechanical ventilation: CPAP and BiPAP in the treatment of congestive heart failure. *Dimensions of Critical Care Nursing, 25*(2), 66–70.

Urden, L. D., Stacy, K. M., & Lough, M. E. (2006). *Thelan's critical care nursing: Diagnosis and management* (5th ed.). Mosby Elsevier.

Wiegand, D., & Carlson, K. (Eds.). (2005). *AACN procedure manual for critical care* (5th ed.). Elsevier Saunders.

M

Mechanical Ventilation Management: Pneumonia Prevention   3304

Definition: Care of a patient at risk for developing ventilator-associated pneumonia

Activities:

- Wash hands before and after patient care activity, particularly after emptying fluids from ventilator circuitry
- Wear gloves and protective equipment and clothing for oral care and change gloves to prevent cross-contamination during oral care
- Monitor oral cavity, lips, tongue, buccal mucosa, and condition of teeth
- Monitor oral cavity for dental plaque, inflammation, bleeding, candidiasis, purulent matter, calculus, and staining
- Brush teeth and tongue with toothpaste or an antiseptic oral rinse using circular motion with a soft toothbrush or suction toothbrush
- Rinse toothbrush after each use and change at regular intervals
- Brush gingiva gently if patient is edentulous
- Assist with the application of a debriding agent or mouth wash to gingiva, teeth, and tongue with swab, according to agency protocol
- Use water rinses instead of a debriding agent with patients who have mucositis or altered oral mucosa
- Assist with swabbing perpendicular to gum line, applying gentle pressure to help facilitate the removal of debris and mucus
- Consider providone-iodine oral antiseptic in patients with severe head injury
- Consult dentistry, if needed
- Apply oral moisturizer to oral mucosa and lips, as needed
- Facilitate use of yankauer or soft suction for oral care, as needed

- Facilitate subglottic suctioning before repositioning patient supine (bed, chair, road trip), repositioning endotracheal tube (ET), and deflating the ET cuff
- Suction the trachea, then oral cavity, and then nasal pharynx to remove secretions above the endotracheal tube cuff to decrease the risk of aspiration
- Rinse yankauer and inline, deep suction lines after each use and change every day
- Consider use of continuous subglottic suctioning and drainage with specifically designed endotracheal tube in patients who have mechanical ventilation longer than 72 hours
- Keep head of bed elevated to 30 to 45 degrees unless contraindicated (i.e., hemodynamic instability), particularly during enteral tube feedings
- Turn patient frequently (at least every 2 hours)
- Facilitate daily interruptions of sedation, in consultation with the physician team
- Consider using a cuffed endotracheal tube with inline or subglottic suctioning
- Maintain an endotracheal cuff pressure of at least 20 cm
- Monitor the depth of the endotracheal tube
- Consider use of oral intubation over nasal intubation
- Keep endotracheal tube tapes clean and dry
- Monitor the effectiveness of mechanical ventilation on patient's physiological and psychosocial status
- Check all ventilator connections regularly
- Monitor daily for evidence of readiness for extubation

- Monitor patient for signs and symptoms of respiratory infection (e.g., restlessness, coughing, fever, increased heart rate, change in secretions, leukocytosis, infiltrates in chest x-ray)
- Monitor and document oxygen saturation
- Avoid histamine receptor blocking agents and proton pump inhibitors unless patient is at high risk for developing a stress ulcer
- Instruct patient and family about oral care routine

6th edition 2013

Background Evidence:

Cason, C. L., Tyner, T., Saunders, S., & Broome, L. (2007). Nurses' implementation of guidelines for ventilator-associated pneumonia from the Centers for Disease Control and Prevention. *American Journal of Critical Care, 16*(1), 28–36.

Chan, E. Y., Ruest, A., Meade, M., & Cook, D. J. (2007). Oral decontamination for prevention of pneumonia in mechanically ventilated adults: Systematic review and meta-analysis. *British Medical Journal, 334*(7599), 889.

Efraiti, S., Deutsch, I., Antonelli, M., Hockey, P., Rozenblum, R., & Gurman, G. M. (2010). Ventilator-associated pneumonia: Current status and future recommendations. *Journal of Clinical Monitoring and Computing, 24*(2), 161–168.

Munro, C. L., Grap, M. J., Jablonski, R., & Boyle, A. (2006). Oral health measurement in nursing research: State of the science. *Biological Research for Nursing, 8*(1), 35–42.

Muscadere, J., Dodek, P., Keenan, S., Fowler, R., Cook, D., & Heyland, D. (2008). Comprehensive evidence-based clinical practice guidelines for ventilator-associated pneumonia: Prevention. *Journal of Critical Care, 23*(1), 126–137.

Pineda, L. A., Saliba, R. G., & El Solh, A. A. (2006). Effect of oral decontamination with chlorhexidine on the incidence of nosocomial pneumonia: A meta-analysis. *Critical Care, 10*(1), R35.

Tablan, O., Anderson, L., Besser, R., Bridges, C., & Hajjeh, R. (2003). *Guidelines for preventing health-care-associated pneumonia*. Atlanta, GA: Centers for Disease Control and Prevention.

Tolentino-Delosreyes, A., Ruppert, S., & Shiao, S. (2007). Evidence-based practice: Use of the ventilator bundle to prevent ventilator-associated pneumonia. *American Journal of Critical Care, 16*(1), 20–27.

Mechanical Ventilatory Weaning   3310

Definition: Assisting the patient to breathe without the aid of a mechanical ventilator

Activities:

- Determine patient readiness for weaning (hemodynamically stable, condition requiring ventilation resolved, current condition optimal for weaning)
- Monitor predictors of ability to tolerate weaning based on agency protocol (e.g., degree of shunt, vital capacity, Vd/Vt, MVV, inspiratory force, FEV_1, negative inspiratory pressure)
- Monitor to assure patient is free of significant infection before weaning
- Monitor for optimal fluid and electrolyte status
- Collaborate with other health team members to optimize patient's nutritional status, assuring that 50% of the diet's nonprotein caloric source is fat rather than carbohydrate
- Position patient for best use of ventilatory muscles and to optimize diaphragmatic descent
- Suction the airway, as needed
- Administer chest physiotherapy, as appropriate
- Consult with other health care personnel in selecting a method for weaning
- Initiate weaning with trial periods (30 to 120 minutes of ventilator-assisted spontaneous breathing)
- Alternate periods of weaning trials with sufficient periods of rest and sleep
- Avoid delaying return of patient with fatigued respiratory muscles to mechanical ventilation
- Set a schedule to coordinate other patient care activities with weaning trials
- Promote the best use of the patient's energy by initiating weaning trials after the patient is well rested
- Monitor for signs of respiratory muscle fatigue (e.g., abrupt rise in $PaCO_2$; rapid, shallow ventilation; paradoxical abdominal wall motion), hypoxemia, and tissue hypoxia when weaning is in process
- Administer medications that promote airway patency and gas exchange
- Set discrete, attainable goals with the patient for weaning
- Use relaxation techniques, as appropriate
- Coach the patient during difficult weaning trials
- Assist the patient to distinguish spontaneous breaths from mechanically delivered breaths
- Minimize excessive work of breathing that is nontherapeutic by eliminating extra dead space, adding pressure support, administering bronchodilators, and maintaining airway patency, as appropriate
- Avoid pharmacological sedation during weaning trials, as appropriate
- Provide some means of patient control during weaning
- Stay with the patient and provide support during initial weaning attempts
- Instruct patient about ventilator setting changes that increase the work of breathing, as appropriate
- Provide the patient with positive reinforcement and frequent progress reports
- Consider using alternate methods of weaning as determined by patient's response to the current method
- Instruct the patient and family about what to expect during various stages of weaning
- Prepare discharge arrangements through multidisciplinary involvement with patient and family

1st edition 1992; revised 1996, 2008

Background Evidence:

American Association of Critical-Care Nurses. (2006). In J. G. Alspach (Ed.), *Core curriculum for critical care nursing* (6th ed.). Saunders Elsevier.

A Collective Task Force Facilitated by the American College of Chest Physicians, the American Association of Respiratory Care and the American College of Critical Care Medicine. (2002). Evidence-based guidelines for weaning and discontinuing ventilatory support. *Respiratory Care, 47*(1), 69–90.

Fenstermacher, D., & Hong, D. (2004). Mechanical ventilation: What have we learned? *Critical Care Nursing Quarterly, 27*(3), 258–294.

Manno, M. S. (2005). Managing mechanical ventilation. *Nursing 2005, 35*(12), 36–42.

M

Phelan, B. A., Cooper, D. A., & Sangkachand, P. (2002). Prolonged mechanical ventilation and tracheostomy in the elderly. *AACN Clinical Issue, 13*(1), 84–93.

Smeltzer, S. C., & Bare, B. G. (2004). *Brunner & Suddarth's textbook of medical-surgical nursing* (10th ed.). Lippincott Williams and Wilkins.

Urden, L. D., Stacy, K. M., & Lough, M. E. (2006). *Thelan's critical care nursing: Diagnosis and management* (5th ed.). Mosby Elsevier.

Wiegand, D., & Carlson, K. (Eds.). (2005). *AACN procedure manual for critical care* (5th ed.). Elsevier Saunders.

Medication Administration 2300

Definition: Preparing, administering, and evaluating the effectiveness of prescription and nonprescription medication

Activities:

- Follow agency policies and procedures for accurate and safe administration of medications
- Promote environment that maximizes safe and efficient administration of medications
- Familiarize self with condition of person receiving medications, and indications and information related to medication (e.g., dosage ranges, expected therapeutic effects, possible adverse reactions, interactions with other medications)
- Instruct on each medication's purpose, and answer questions appropriately
- Follow six rights of medication administration (e.g., right person, right medication, right dose, right route, right time, right documentation)
- Identify using at least two identifiers (e.g., name, birthdate)
- Prepare medications for only one person at a time
- Prepare medications using appropriate equipment and techniques for medication administration modality
- Ensure medication prescriptive orders contain person name, medication name, amount and frequency of dose, route of administration, reason for medication, and appropriate signature for authorization
- Clarify medication prescriptive orders that are missing any required information, prior to administration
- Verify changes in medication form before administering (e.g., crushed enteric tablets, oral liquids in intravenous syringe, unusual packaging)
- Decline to administer medications that may jeopardize person safety
- Look only at one person's medication administration record (MAR), computer printouts or computer medication administration screen at a time
- Use medication distribution system as required by institution policies and procedures (e.g., unit dose, automated medication-dispensing system)
- Avoid administering any medication not properly labeled, with broken medication seals, or expired
- Dispose of unused or expired medications according to agency guidelines
- Calculate medication dose as necessary
- Double check all calculations
- Avoid interruptions when preparing, verifying, or administering medications
- Prescribe or recommend medications, as appropriate, according to prescriptive authority
- Administer medications according to prescriptive authority, protocol, policy, and procedure
- Use health provider prescriptions, agency policies, and procedures to guide appropriate method of medication administration (i.e., scan patient ID bracelet and scan medication bar-code)
- Note allergies before delivery of medication and hold medications, as appropriate

- Monitor for possible medication allergies, interactions, and contraindications, including over-the-counter medications and herbal remedies
- Verify with person or caregivers of each medication type, reason for administration, expected actions, and adverse effects before administering, as persons often able to identify inappropriate medications
- Answer all questions before administering medications to ensure knowledge of medication regime
- Check record for previous medication count when preparing controlled substance medications, and ensure current count and available supply match
- Sign out controlled substances according to agency protocol
- Report any discrepancies in controlled substance counts immediately
- Ensure that hypnotics, narcotics, and antibiotics are either discontinued or reordered on their renewal date
- Do not leave medications unattended
- Ensure person takes all medications
- Document medications only after given and observed
- Stay with person until all medications ingested
- Give time-critical medications at exact time ordered (i.e., no later than 30 minutes before or after time ordered)
- Perform necessary pre-medication assessments (e.g., blood pressure, pulse)
- Monitor vital signs and laboratory values before and after medication administration, as appropriate
- Assist person in taking medication, as needed
- Give medication using appropriate technique and route
- Use aseptic technique for all parenteral medication administration
- Instruct person and family about expected actions and adverse effects of medication
- Validate and document understanding of expected actions and adverse effects of medication
- Monitor to determine need for PRN medications, as appropriate
- Monitor for therapeutic effect of all medications
- Monitor for adverse effects, toxicity, and interactions of administered medications
- Document medication administration and person responsiveness (i.e., include medication generic name, dose, time, route, reason for administration, and effect achieved), according to agency protocol
- Use teach-back to ensure understanding

1st edition 1992; revised 2013, 2024

Background Evidence:

Berman, A., Snyder, S. J., & Frandsen, G. (2018). Medications. In *Kozier and Erb's fundamentals of nursing: Concepts, process and practice* (pp. 750–829) (10th ed.). Pearson.

Boyer, M. J. (2020). *Math for nurses* (10th ed.). Wolters-Kluwer.

Kirby, N. (2021). Medication administration. In R. F. Craven, C. J. Hirnle, & C. J. Henshaw (Eds.), *Fundamentals of nursing: Human health and function* (8th ed., pp. 410–471). Wolters-Kluwer.

Potter, P. A., Ostendorf, W. R., & LaPlante, N. (2018). Nonparenteral medications. In *Clinical nursing skills and techniques* (pp. 523–579) (9th ed.). Mosby.

Potter, P. A., Ostendorf, W. R., & LaPlante, N. (2018). Parenteral medications. In *Clinical nursing skills and techniques* (pp. 580–628) (9th ed.). Mosby.

Potter, P. A., Ostendorf, W. R., & LaPlante, N. (2018). Safe medication preparation. In *Clinical nursing skills and techniques* (pp. 501–522) (9th ed.). Mosby.

Sanoski, C. A., & Vallerand, A. H. (2021). *Davis's drug guide for nurses* (17th ed.). F.A. Davis.

Williams, P. A. (2020). Medications and older adults. In *Basic geriatric nursing* (pp. 132–149) (7th ed.). Elsevier.

Medication Administration: Continuous Subcutaneous Infusion   2321

Definition: Preparing and providing medications as a continuous infusion via the subcutaneous route

Activities:

- Follow agency policies and procedures for accurate and safe administration of medications
- Promote environment that maximizes safe and efficient administration of medications
- Familiarize self with condition of person receiving medications, and indications and information related to medication (e.g., dosage ranges, expected therapeutic effects, possible adverse reactions, interactions with other medications)
- Check accuracy and completeness of each medication administration record (MAR) prior to giving any medications
- Review health history and history of allergies
- Determine person's knowledge of medication and understanding of method of administration
- Instruct on medication purpose and answer questions appropriately
- Follow six rights of medication administration (e.g., right person, right medication, right dose, right route, right time, right documentation)
- Identify using at least two identifiers (e.g., name, birthdate)
- Perform necessary pre-medication evaluations (e.g., blood pressure, pulse, blood sugar assessment, pain level)
- Obtain and program medication administration pump
- Ensure medication administration pump has safety features (e.g., lockout intervals, warning alarms)
- Verify prefilled medication container with MAR and one other licensed staff
- Obtain small winged IV catheter with attached tubing
- Use needle with shortest length and smallest gauge necessary to establish and maintain infusion
- Prime needle and pump tubing using aseptic technique
- Position person supine, drape and provide privacy
- Select appropriate injection site free from irritation, bony prominences and waistline (i.e., most common sites are under subclavian and abdomen)
- Select injection site considering medication (i.e., pain medications best delivery in upper chest, insulin absorbed most consistently in abdomen)
- Select injection site where pump tubing not disturbed
- Clean injection site twice (i.e., alcohol followed by antiseptic) and allow both to dry
- Gently pinch or lift up skin
- Insert needle at 45-to-90-degree angle, release skinfold and secure wings of needle
- Place occlusive, transparent dressing over insertion site
- Instruct to alert staff if site becomes painful, red, swollen, or leaks
- Monitor for any allergic reactions
- Rotate sites as needed for complications
- Remove needle and place new needle in different site if complains of localized pain or burning at site, or site appears red, swollen, or leaking
- Stop infusion immediately if signs of allergic reactions and follow agency guidelines for appropriate response to allergic reaction
- Instruct on need for medication alert bracelet
- Monitor for expected and unexpected medication effects
- Document medication administration and responsiveness according to agency guidelines

8th edition 2024

Background Evidence:

Alvarenga, C. S., La Banca, R. O., Neris, R. R., de Cássia Sparapani, V., Fuentealba-Torres, M., Cartagena-Ramos, D., Leal, C. L., Esper, M. V., & Nascimento, L. C. (2022). Use of continuous subcutaneous insulin infusion in children and adolescents with type 1 diabetes mellitus: A systematic mapping review. *BMC Endocrine Disorders, 22*(1), 1–15. https://doi.org/10.1186/s12902-022-00950-7

Berman, A., Snyder, S. J., & Frandsen, G. (2018). Medications. In *Kozier and Erb's fundamentals of nursing: Concepts, process and practice* (pp. 794–797) (10th ed.) Pearson.

Cicero, T. (2021). Intravenous therapy. In R. F. Craven, C. J. Hirnle, & C. J. Henshaw (Eds.), *Fundamentals of nursing: Human health and function* (8th ed., pp. 472–541). Wolters-Kluwer.

Kirby, N. (2021). Medication administration. In R. F. Craven, C. J. Hirnle, & C. J. Henshaw (Eds.), *Fundamentals of nursing: Human health and function* (8th ed., pp. 410–471). Wolters-Kluwer.

McGaugh, S. M., Zaharieva, D. P., Pooni, R., D'Souza, N. C., Vienneau, T., Ly, T. T., & Riddell, M. C. (2021). Carbohydrate requirements for prolonged, fasted exercise with and without basal rate reductions in adults with type 1 diabetes on continuous subcutaneous insulin infusion. *Diabetes Care, 44*(2), 610–613. https://doi.org/10.2337/dc20-1554

Potter, P. A., Ostendorf, W. R., & LaPlante, N. (2018). Administering continuous subcutaneous medications. In *Clinical nursing skills and techniques* (pp. 620–628) (9th ed.). Mosby.

Sanoski, C. A., & Vallerand, A. H. (2021). *Davis's drug guide for nurses* (17th ed.). F.A. Davis.

M

Medication Administration: Ear   2308

Definition: Preparing and instilling otic medications

Activities:

- Follow agency policies and procedures for accurate and safe administration of medications
- Promote environment that maximizes safe and efficient administration of medications
- Familiarize self with condition of person receiving medications, and indications and information related to medication (e.g., dosage ranges, expected therapeutic effects, possible adverse reactions, interactions with other medications)
- Check accuracy and completeness of each medication administration record (MAR) prior to giving any medications
- Review health history and history of allergies
- Determine person's knowledge of medication and understanding of method of administration
- Instruct on medication purpose and answer questions appropriately
- Follow six rights of medication administration (e.g., right person, right medication, right dose, right route, right time, right documentation)
- Identify using at least two identifiers (e.g., name, birthdate)
- Perform necessary pre-medication evaluations (e.g., blood pressure, pulse, blood sugar assessment, pain level)
- Position in side-lying position with ear to be treated facing up or have sit in chair
- Cleanse pinna and meatus of ear canal with cotton tipped applicators
- Warm medication prior to instilling (i.e., place in warm water for short time, hold tightly in hand)
- Straighten ear canal by pulling auricle down and back for child or upward and outward for adult
- Instill medication holding dropper above ear canal and placing drops on side of auditory canal to allow drops to flow in (i.e.,

avoid instilling drops into auricular opening as causes increased discomfort)
- Use flexible rubber tip where possible to avoid injury due to sudden motion
- Instruct to remain in side-lying position 5 to 10 minutes
- Apply gentle pressure or massage to tragus of ear with finger
- Place cotton ball or wick in outer ear to keep medication in ear canal, as indicated
- Remove cotton ball after 15 minutes
- Wait 5 to 10 minutes to instill drops in other ear, as prescribed
- Instruct related to self-administration technique, as appropriate
- Document medication administration and responsiveness according to agency protocol
- Use teach-back to ensure understanding

3rd edition 2000; revised 2004, 2024

Background Evidence:

Berman, A., Snyder, S. J., & Frandsen, G. (2018). Medications. In *Kozier and Erb's Fundamentals of nursing: Concepts, process and practice* (pp. 815–817) (10th ed.). Pearson.

Boyer, M. J. (2020). *Math for nurses* (10th ed.). Wolters-Kluwer.

Kirby, N. (2021). Medication administration. In R. F. Craven, C. J. Hirnle, & C. J. Henshaw (Eds.), *Fundamentals of nursing: Human health and function* (8th ed., pp. 410–471). Wolters-Kluwer.

Potter, P. A., Ostendorf, W. R., & LaPlante, N. (2018). Administering ear medications. In *Clinical nursing skills and techniques* (pp. 547–550) (9th ed.). Mosby.

Sanoski, C. A., & Vallerand, A. H. (2021). *Davis's drug guide for nurses* (17th ed.). F.A. Davis.

M

Medication Administration: Enteral   2301

Definition: Delivering medications through a tube inserted into the gastrointestinal system

Activities:

- Follow agency policies and procedures for accurate and safe administration of medications
- Promote environment that maximizes safe and efficient administration of medications
- Familiarize self with condition of person receiving medications, and indications and information related to medication (e.g., dosage ranges, expected therapeutic effects, possible adverse reactions, interactions with other medications)
- Check accuracy and completeness of each medication administration record (MAR) prior to giving any medications
- Review health history and history of allergies
- Determine person's knowledge of medication and understanding of method of administration
- Instruct on medication purpose and answer questions appropriately
- Follow six rights of medication administration (e.g., right person, right medication, right dose, right route, right time, right documentation)

- Identify using at least two identifiers (e.g., name, birthdate)
- Perform necessary pre-medication evaluations (e.g., blood pressure, pulse, blood sugar assessment, pain level)
- Determine any contraindications to receiving oral medication via tube (e.g., bowel inflammation, reduced peristalsis, recent gastrointestinal surgery, attached to gastric suction)
- Ensure correct tubes selected for medications
- Ensure medication compatibility with enteral tube feeding solution, if indicated
- Schedule medication to be in accord with formula feeding times, if indicated
- Obtain liquid dosage form of medication if available
- Consult with pharmacist before deciding to alter form of any medication, as needed
- Avoid crushing sublingual, sustained-release, chewable, long-acting, or enteric-coated medications
- Contact health care provider for substitute medication if formulation alternatives are unavailable for medications that cannot be altered

- Prepare medication (e.g., crush, mix with fluids, open capsules, pierce gel capsule with sterile needle or dissolve) as noted in pharmacological instructions
- Adjust water amount if needed for fluid restrictions
- Stop enteral tube feeding and flush tube with 15 mL water prior to administering medication
- Administer medications individually to avoid clogging enteral tube
- Ensure medications are dissolved before administering
- Inform of expected actions and possible adverse effects of each medication
- Use correct syringe for enteral tube medication administration
- Check placement of tube by aspirating gastrointestinal contents, checking pH level and color of 5 to 10 mL of aspirate (i.e., gastric content pH < or = 5.5, color greenish to tan or off white; pulmonary content pH >6, color clear to light yellow with mucus), or obtaining x-ray film, as per agency guidelines
- Place in high Fowler's position during medication administration if not contraindicated
- Aspirate stomach contents, return aspirate by flushing with 30 mL of air or appropriate amount for age, and flush tube with 30 mL of water, as appropriate
- Determine gastric residual volume and hold medications if greater that 200 mL
- Recheck gastric residual volume in 30 to 60 minutes if holding medications for excessive residual volume, assuring feedings also held
- Contact health care provider if medications held for excessive gastric residual volume after second check
- Remove plunger from syringe and connect to pinched or kinked tube
- Flush tube with 15 to 30 mL of water after releasing pinched or kinked tube
- Raise or lower barrel of syringe to adjust flow as needed
- Pinch or clamp tube before all water instilled to avoid excess air entering stomach
- Pour medication into syringe and release pinched tube
- Administer medication by allowing medication to flow freely from barrel of syringe, using plunger only as needed to facilitate flow
- Flush tube with 15 to 30 mL of warm water, or appropriate amount for age, after each medication administration
- Follow last dose of medication with 30 to 60 mL of water or appropriate amount for age
- Record total amount of fluid flushes on I & O record
- Resume tube feedings as prescribed

- Hold feeding solution for additional 30 to 60 minutes if medications not compatible with feeding solution
- Disconnect suction and keep tube clamped for 20 to 30 minutes to enhance adsorption if medications given through tube used for decompression
- Rinse and replace syringe to storage area at bedside
- Keep head of bed elevated a minimum of 30 degrees for 1 hour after medication administration
- Monitor for therapeutic effects, adverse effect, drug toxicity, and drug interactions
- Document medication administration and responsiveness according to agency guidelines

1st edition 1992; revised 1996, 2004, 2024

Background Evidence:

Alsaeed, D., Furniss, D., Blandford, A., Smith, F., & Orlu, M. (2018). Carers' experiences of home enteral feeding: A survey exploring medicines administration challenges and strategies. *Journal of Clinical Pharmacy & Therapeutics, 43*(3), 359–365. https://doi.org/10.1111/jcpt.12664

Berman, A., Snyder, S. J., & Frandsen, G. (2018). Medications. In *Kozier and Erb's Fundamentals of nursing: Concepts, process and practice* (pp. 780–781) (10th ed.). Pearson.

Kirby, N. (2021). Medication administration. In R. F. Craven, C. J. Hirnle, & C. J. Henshaw (Eds.), *Fundamentals of nursing: Human health and function* (8th ed., pp. 410–471). Wolters-Kluwer.

Li, T., Eisenhart, A., & Costello, J. (2017). Development of a medication review service for patients with enteral tubes in a community teaching hospital. *American Journal of Health-System Pharmacy, 74*, S47–S51. https://doi.org/10.2146/ajhp160519

Portela Beserra, M. P., Gonçalves de Oliveira, C. L. C., Portela, M. P., de Oliveira Lopes, M. V., de França Fonteles, M. M., Beserra, M. P. P., De Oliveira, C. L. C. G., Lopes, M. V., de, O., Fonteles, M. M., & de, F. (2017). Drugs via enteral feeding tubes in inpatients: dispersion analysis and safe use of dispensers. *Nutricion Hospitalaria, 34*(2), 257–263. https://doi.org/10.20960/nh.486

Potter, P. A., Ostendorf, W. R., & LaPlante, N. (2018). Administering medications through a feeding tube. In *Clinical nursing skills and techniques* (pp. 530–536) (9th ed.). Mosby.

Sanoski, C. A., & Vallerand, A. H. (2021). *Davis's drug guide for nurses* (17th ed.). F.A. Davis.

Smith, S. F., Duell, D. J., Martin, B. C., Aebersold, M. L., & Gonzalez, L. (2017). Administering medications per enteral (NG or NI) feeding tube. In *Clinical nursing skills: Basic to advanced skills* (pp. 585–586) (9th ed.). Pearson.

M

Medication Administration: Eye   2310

Definition: Preparing and instilling ophthalmic medications

Activities:

- Follow agency policies and procedures for accurate and safe administration of medications
- Promote environment that maximizes safe and efficient administration of medications
- Familiarize self with condition of person receiving medications, and indications and information related to medication (e.g., dosage ranges, expected therapeutic effects, possible adverse reactions, interactions with other medications)
- Check accuracy and completeness of each medication administration record (MAR) prior to giving any medications

- Review health history and history of allergies
- Determine person's knowledge of medication and understanding of method of administration
- Instruct on medication purpose and answer questions appropriately
- Follow six rights of medication administration (e.g., right person, right medication, right dose, right route, right time, right documentation)
- Identify using at least two identifiers (e.g., name, birthdate)
- Perform necessary pre-medication evaluations (e.g., blood pressure, pulse, blood sugar assessment, pain level)

- Position supine or sitting in chair with neck slightly hyperextended and eyes looking up
- Provide with tissues to blot medication or tears as indicated
- Cleanse eyelid and eyelashes of any drainage, ensuring that each area of cleansing surface used only once and moving from inner toward outer canthus
- Place finger or thumb on lower bony orbit and gently pull lower lid down
- Place other hand on forehead holding medication container in this hand
- Instill medication onto conjunctival sac using aseptic technique
- Avoid touching eyelids, lashes, or eyeball with either hand or with medication applicator
- Avoid dropping solution directly onto cornea as this causes increased discomfort
- Release lower lid and instruct to close eye
- Repeat medication administration if blinks or closes eye, causing medication to land on outer lid margins
- Apply gentle pressure to nasolacrimal duct if medication has systemic effects
- Avoid pressure directly against eyeball
- Instruct to close eye gently to help distribute medication
- Apply eye patch if indicated
- Tape eye patch securely, avoiding pressure to eye
- Monitor for local, systemic, and adverse effects of medication
- Explain that some medications may cause blurred vision

- Advise that wearing sunglasses decreases photophobia effect of dilation medications
- Instruct not to drive or perform activities that require acute vision if receiving medications that affect vision (i.e., medications that dilate pupil or paralyze ciliary muscles)
- Instruct related to self-administration technique, as appropriate
- Document medication administration and responsiveness according to agency protocol
- Use teach-back to ensure understanding

3rd edition 2000; revised 2024

Background Evidence:

Berman, A., Snyder, S. J., & Frandsen, G. (2018). Medications. In *Kozier and Erb's Fundamentals of nursing: Concepts, process and practice* (pp. 813–815) (10th ed.). Pearson.

Kirby, N. (2021). Medication administration. In R. F. Craven, C. J. Hirnle, & C. J. Henshaw (Eds.), *Fundamentals of nursing: Human health and function* (8th ed., pp. 410–471). Wolters-Kluwer.

Potter, P. A., Ostendorf, W. R., & LaPlante, N. (2018). Administering ophthalmic medications. In *Clinical nursing skills and techniques* (pp. 541–547) (9th ed.). Mosby.

Sanoski, C. A., & Vallerand, A. H. (2021). *Davis's drug guide for nurses* (17th ed.). F.A. Davis.

Medication Administration: Inhalation   2311

M

Definition: Preparing and administering inhaled medications

Activities:

- Follow agency policies and procedures for accurate and safe administration of medications
- Promote environment that maximizes safe and efficient administration of medications
- Familiarize self with condition of person receiving medications, and indications and information related to medication (e.g., dosage ranges, expected therapeutic effects, possible adverse reactions, interactions with other medications)
- Check accuracy and completeness of each medication administration record (MAR) prior to giving any medications
- Review health history and history of allergies
- Determine person's knowledge of medication and understanding of method of administration
- Instruct on medication purpose and answer questions appropriately
- Follow six rights of medication administration (e.g., right person, right medication, right dose, right route, right time, right documentation)
- Identify using at least two identifiers (e.g., name, birthdate)
- Perform necessary pre-medication evaluations (e.g., blood pressure, pulse, blood sugar assessment, pain level)
- Determine ability to manipulate and administer medication
- Assist to use inhaler as prescribed
- Have demonstrate how to use device if previously instructed
- Correct techniques as needed for current device and medication
- Instruct on use of aero-chamber or spacer with inhaler, as appropriate
- Instruct on use of breath-activated metered dose-inhalers, as appropriate
- Shake inhaler, remove inhaler cap and hold inhaler upside down to administer medication

- Assist to position inhaler in mouth or nose, tilt head back slightly and exhale completely
- Instruct to press down on inhaler to release medication while inhaling slowly
- Have person take slow, deep breaths, with brief end-inspiratory pause, and passive exhalation when using nebulizer
- Have person hold breath for 10 seconds, as appropriate
- Have person exhale slowly through nose or pursed lips
- Instruct to repeat inhalations as ordered, per inhalation medication instructions
- Instruct to wait between inhalations if two metered-dose inhalers are prescribed, per agency protocol
- Instruct in removing medication canister and cleaning inhaler in warm water
- Instruct in determining if inhaler actually releasing spray
- Instruct in determining when inhaler empty
- Instruct on use of nebulizer as needed (e.g., breathing through mouth or nose during use, medications and dosage, use and cleaning of nebulizer and equipment)
- Monitor respirations and auscultate lungs, as appropriate
- Monitor for effects of medication and instruct person and caregivers on desired effects and possible side effects of medication
- Instruct and monitor self-administration technique, as appropriate
- Document medication administration and responsiveness according to agency protocol
- Use teach-back to ensure understanding

3rd edition 2000; revised 2004, 2024

Background Evidence:

Berman, A., Snyder, S. J., & Frandsen, G. (2018). Medications. In *Kozier and Erb's Fundamentals of nursing: Concepts, process and practice* (pp. 821–823) (10th ed.). Pearson.

Garzon Maaks, D. L., Barber Starr, N., Brady, M. A., Gaylord, N. M., Driessnack, M., & Duderstadt, K. (2021). *Burns' pediatric primary care* (7th ed.). Elsevier.

Kirby, N. (2021). Medication administration. In R. F. Craven, C. J. Hirnle, & C. J. Henshaw (Eds.), *Fundamentals of nursing: Human health and function* (8th ed., pp. 410–471). Wolters-Kluwer.

Potter, P. A., Ostendorf, W. R., & LaPlante, N. (2018). Using metered-dose inhalers, using dry powder inhaled medications, using small-volume nebulizers. In *Clinical nursing skills and techniques* (pp. 554–565) (9th ed.). Mosby.

Richardson, B. (2020). *Pediatric primary care: Practice guidelines for nurses* (4th ed). Jones & Bartlett Learning.

Sanoski, C. A., & Vallerand, A. H. (2021). *Davis's drug guide for nurses* (17th ed.). F.A. Davis.

Medication Administration: Interpleural   2302

Definition: Administration of medication through a catheter for diffusion within the pleural cavity

Activities:

- Follow agency policies and procedures for accurate and safe administration of medications
- Promote environment that maximizes safe and efficient administration of medications
- Familiarize self with condition of person receiving medications, and indications and information related to medication (e.g., dosage ranges, expected therapeutic effects, possible adverse reactions, interactions with other medications)
- Check accuracy and completeness of each medication administration record (MAR) prior to giving any medications
- Review health history and history of allergies
- Determine person's knowledge of medication and understanding of method of administration
- Instruct on medication purpose and answer questions appropriately
- Follow six rights of medication administration (e.g., right person, right medication, right dose, right route, right time, right documentation)
- Identify using at least two identifiers (e.g., name, birthdate)
- Perform necessary pre-medication evaluations (e.g., blood pressure, pulse, blood sugar assessment, pain level)
- Follow agency policies and protocols for management and monitoring of interpleural catheters
- Determine comfort level
- Instruct about purpose, benefits, and rationale for use of interpleural catheter and medication
- Monitor vital signs
- Maintain aseptic technique
- Affirm correct catheter placement with chest x-ray examination, as appropriate
- Monitor pain before and after catheter insertion, as appropriate
- Conduct time-out immediately before starting procedure to perform final assessment that correct person, site, positioning, and procedure are identified and all relevant information and necessary equipment are available
- Aspirate interpleural catheter fluid before all injections of medication
- Check for absence of blood return before medication administration
- Observe aspirate for color and amount of return
- Withhold medication if more than 2 cc of fluid returns when checking interpleural catheter
- Prepare all medications aseptically
- Administer medication for pain relief through interpleural catheter intermittently or by continuous drip
- Position to avoid pressure on interpleural catheter

- Use monitoring modalities to interpret physiological responses and initiate nursing interventions to ensure optimal care
- Monitor for shortness of breath or unequal or abnormal breath sounds
- Note any leakage that may occur from interpleural catheter
- Observe for pain relief, side effects, or adverse reactions from medication administered
- Connect catheter to medication administration pump, as appropriate
- Document medication administration following established agency policies
- Provide for total care needs while receiving analgesia, as needed
- Anticipate potential complications of analgesia technique in relation to device and medications being used
- Recognize emergency situations and institute treatment in compliance with established agency policies, procedures, and guidelines
- Encourage early ambulation with use of interpleural catheter, as appropriate
- Change dressing, as appropriate
- Observe for signs and symptoms of infection at interpleural catheter insertion site
- Remove interpleural catheter as ordered and per agency policy
- Use teach-back to ensure understanding

1st edition 1992; revised 2013, 2024

Background Evidence:

Banka, R., Ellayeh, M., & Rahman, N. (2021). Pleurodesis. In *Reference Module in Biomedical Sciences*. Elsevier. https://doi.org/10.1016/B978-0-08-102723-3.00143-8

Cheng, G. S., & Ilfeld, B. M. (2018). An evidence-based review of the efficacy of perioperative analgesic techniques for breast cancer-related surgery. *Pain Medicine, 18*(7), 1344–1365.

Dhanjal, S., & Shannon, C. (2020). Interpleural analgesia. In *StatPearls*. StatPearls Publishing. https://www.ncbi.nlm.nih.gov/books/NBK526020/

Koshini, S. (2020). *A comparative randomized study of thoracic paravertebral block versus inter pleural block for post operative analgesia after modified radical mastectomy, cholecystectomy and nephrectomy surgeries.* Chengalpattu: Doctoral dissertation, Chengalpattu Medical College and Hospital.

Rajaretnam, N., Smith, N., Massey, L., Rockett, M., & Aroori, S. (2020). Is epidural analgesia still the gold standard analgesic technique for pancreaticoduodenectomy? *HPB, 22*, S306.

Spasova, A. (2021). *Interpleural analgesia in the treatment of pain syndromes: Methodology and clinical application.* Sciencia Scripts.

M

Medication Administration: Intradermal   2312

Definition: Preparing and providing medications via the intradermal route

Activities:
- Follow agency policies and procedures for accurate and safe administration of medications
- Promote environment that maximizes safe and efficient administration of medications
- Familiarize self with condition of person receiving medications, and indications and information related to medication (e.g., dosage ranges, expected therapeutic effects, possible adverse reactions, interactions with other medications)
- Check accuracy and completeness of each medication administration record (MAR) prior to giving any medications
- Review health history and history of allergies
- Determine person's knowledge of medication and understanding of method of administration
- Instruct on medication purpose and answer questions appropriately
- Follow six rights of medication administration (e.g., right person, right medication, right dose, right route, right time, right documentation)
- Identify using at least two identifiers (e.g., name, birthdate)
- Perform necessary pre-medication evaluations (e.g., blood pressure, pulse, blood sugar assessment, pain level)
- Determine understanding of purpose of skin testing
- Select correct needle and syringe based on type of injection
- Prepare dose correctly from ampule or vial following manufacturer's directions
- Select appropriate injection site and inspect skin to avoid areas with bruises, inflammation, edema, lesions, or discoloration
- Insert needle at a 5-to-15-degree angle
- Inject medication slowly, watching for small bleb on skin surface
- Inject only small amounts of medication (e.g., 0.01–0.1 mL)
- Watch carefully for bleeding at site after needle withdrawal, or lack of bleb appearance, which invalidates test results as medication entering SQ tissue
- Monitor for allergic reaction
- Mark injection site and read site at appropriate interval after injection (e.g., 48–72 hours)
- Monitor for expected effects of specific allergen or medication
- Document area of injection and appearance of skin at injection site
- Document appearance of injection site after appropriate interval
- Use teach-back to ensure understanding

3rd edition 2000; revised 2024

Background Evidence:
Berman, A., Snyder, S. J., & Frandsen, G. (2018). Medications. In *Kozier and Erb's Fundamentals of nursing: Concepts, process and practice* (pp. 792–793) (10th ed.). Pearson.

Kirby, N. (2021). Medication administration. In R. F. Craven, C. J. Hirnle, & C. J. Henshaw (Eds.), *Fundamentals of nursing: Human health and function* (8th ed., pp. 410–471). Wolters-Kluwer.

Potter, P. A., Ostendorf, W. R., & LaPlante, N. (2018). *Clinical nursing skills and techniques* (pp. 589–593) (9th ed.). Administering intramuscular injections. Mosby.

Sanoski, C. A., & Vallerand, A. H. (2021). *Davis's drug guide for nurses* (17th ed.). F.A. Davis.

Medication Administration: Intramuscular (IM)   2313

Definition: Preparing and providing medications via the intramuscular route

Activities:
- Follow agency policies and procedures for accurate and safe administration of medications
- Promote environment that maximizes safe and efficient administration of medications
- Familiarize self with condition of person receiving medications, and indications and information related to medication (e.g., dosage ranges, expected therapeutic effects, possible adverse reactions, interactions with other medications)
- Check accuracy and completeness of each medication administration record (MAR) prior to giving any medications
- Review health history and history of allergies
- Determine person's knowledge of medication and understanding of method of administration
- Instruct on medication purpose and answer questions appropriately
- Follow six rights of medication administration (e.g., right person, right medication, right dose, right route, right time, right documentation)
- Identify using at least two identifiers (e.g., name, birthdate)
- Perform necessary pre-medication evaluations (e.g., blood pressure, pulse, blood sugar assessment, pain level)
- Consider indications and contraindications for intramuscular injection
- Select correct needle and syringe based on person and medication information (e.g., viscosity of medication, amount of medication, injection site, person weight, amount of adipose tissue)
- Investigate alternative routes when unable to select longer and heavier gauge needle for obese persons where amount of fat interferes with ability to reach muscle tissue
- Avoid emaciated or atrophied muscles for injection
- Discard mixed medications that are not properly labeled
- Prepare dose correctly from ampule, vial, or prefilled syringe per manufacturer's directions
- Select appropriate injection site (e.g., ventrogluteal, vastus lateralis, deltoid)
- Rotate injection sites to decrease risk for hypertrophy when giving regularly scheduled injections
- Palpate site for edema, masses, or tenderness to avoid areas of scarring, bruising, abrasion, or infection
- Position nondominant hand at proper anatomical landmark, spread skin tightly
- Administer injection using aseptic technique and proper protocol

M

- Inject needle quickly at a 90-degree angle
- Follow agency policy related to aspiration before injection as no longer recommended due to increased discomfort with aspiration
- Use aspiration if indicated
- Inject medication slowly if no blood aspirated
- Wait 10 seconds after injecting medication, then smoothly withdraw needle and release skin
- Apply gentle pressure at injection site and avoid massaging site
- Monitor for acute pain at injection site
- Avoid injecting large volumes of medication (i.e., maximum dosages are 4–5 mL for adults, 2 mL for children, older adults and thin persons, 1 mL for small children and older infants, 0.5 mL for smaller infants)
- Use Z-track method (i.e., pull overlying skin and SQ tissue approximately 2.5–3.5 cm [1–1.5 inches] laterally to side with ulnar side of non-dominant hand, hold skin in place until injection complete then release skin) as indicated
- Monitor for sensory or motor alteration at or distal to injection site

- Monitor for expected and unexpected medication effects
- Document medication administration and responsiveness according to agency protocol

3rd edition 2000; revised 2004, 2024

Background Evidence:

Berman, A., Snyder, S. J., & Frandsen, G. (2018). Medications. In *Kozier and Erb's Fundamentals of nursing: Concepts, process and practice* (pp. 801–802) (10th ed.). Pearson.

Kirby, N. (2021). Medication administration. In R. F. Craven, C. J. Hirnle, & C. J. Henshaw (Eds.), *Fundamentals of nursing: Human health and function* (8th ed., pp. 410–471). Wolters-Kluwer.

Potter, P. A., Ostendorf, W. R., & LaPlante, N. (2018). Administering intramuscular injections. In *Clinical nursing skills and techniques* (pp. 600–607) (9th ed.). Mosby.

Sanoski, C. A., & Vallerand, A. H. (2021). *Davis's drug guide for nurses* (17th ed.). F.A. Davis.

Medication Administration: Intraocular Disk   2322

Definition: Preparing and inserting intraocular disk medications

Activities:

- Follow agency policies and procedures for accurate and safe administration of medications
- Promote environment that maximizes safe and efficient administration of medications
- Familiarize self with condition of person receiving medications, and indications and information related to medication (e.g., dosage ranges, expected therapeutic effects, possible adverse reactions, interactions with other medications)
- Check accuracy and completeness of each medication administration record (MAR) prior to giving any medications
- Review health history and history of allergies
- Determine person's knowledge of medication and understanding of method of administration
- Instruct on medication purpose and answer questions appropriately
- Follow six rights of medication administration (e.g., right person, right medication, right dose, right route, right time, right documentation)
- Identify using at least two identifiers (e.g., name, birthdate)
- Perform necessary pre-medication evaluations (e.g., blood pressure, pulse, blood sugar assessment, pain level)
- Position supine or sitting in chair with neck slightly hyperextended and eyes looking up
- Provide with tissues to blot medication or tears as indicated
- Cleanse eyelid and eyelashes of any drainage, assuring that each area of cleansing surface used only once, moving from inner toward outer canthus
- Gently press fingertip against disk to assure adherence to finger
- Moisten fingertip as needed with sterile saline if disk not adhering
- Position convex side of disk on fingertip

- Pull lower eyelid down and away from eye
- Ask to look up
- Place disk in conjunctival sac so floats on sclera between iris and lower eyelid
- Pull lower eyelid out and over disk, ensuring disk covered by lower eyelid and no longer visible
- Ensure disk not placed on cornea or under upper eye lid
- Remove after prescribed time period unless disk to be dissolved in eye
- Remove by gently pulling lower lid down
- Pinch disk between thumb and forefinger to remove
- Monitor for local, systemic, and adverse effects of medication
- Instruct related to self-administration technique, as appropriate
- Document medication administration and responsiveness according to agency protocol
- Use teach-back to ensure understanding

8th edition 2024

Background Evidence:

Berman, A., Snyder, S. J., & Frandsen, G. (2018). Medications. In *Kozier and Erb's Fundamentals of nursing: Concepts, process and practice* (pp. 813–815) (10th ed.). Pearson.

Kirby, N. (2021). Medication administration. In R. F. Craven, C. J. Hirnle, & C. J. Henshaw (Eds.), *Fundamentals of nursing: Human health and function* (8th ed., pp. 410–471). Wolters-Kluwer.

Potter, P. A., Ostendorf, W. R., & LaPlante, N. (2018). Administering ophthalmic medications. In *Clinical nursing skills and techniques* (pp. 541–547) (9th ed.). Mosby.

Sanoski, C. A., & Vallerand, A. H. (2021). *Davis's drug guide for nurses* (17th ed.). F.A. Davis.

M

Medication Administration: Intraosseous 2303

Definition: Insertion of a needle through the bone cortex into the medullary cavity for the purpose of short-term, emergency administration of fluid, blood, or medication

Activities:

- Follow agency policies and procedures for accurate and safe administration of medications
- Promote environment that maximizes safe and efficient administration of medications
- Familiarize self with condition of person receiving medications, and indications and information related to medication (e.g., dosage ranges, expected therapeutic effects, possible adverse reactions, interactions with other medications)
- Check accuracy and completeness of each medication administration record (MAR) prior to giving any medications
- Review health history and history of allergies
- Determine person's knowledge of medication and understanding of method of administration
- Instruct on medication purpose and answer questions appropriately
- Follow six rights of medication administration (e.g., right person, right medication, right dose, right route, right time, right documentation)
- Identify using at least two identifiers (e.g., name, birthdate)
- Perform necessary pre-medication evaluations (e.g., blood pressure, pulse, blood sugar assessment, pain level)
- Administer medications within scope of practice and agency guidelines
- Determine appropriateness of person for therapy, establishing responsiveness and emergent need
- Restrict intraosseous access in contraindicated situations (e.g., compartment syndrome in target extremity, previously used intraosseous site or recent failed intraosseous attempt, fractures at or above site, previous orthopedic surgery or hardware, presence of infection or severe burns near insertion site, local vascular compromise)
- Avoid use of intraosseous access in presence of bone diseases (e.g., osteogenesis imperfecta, osteopetrosis, osteoporosis)
- Use appropriate intraosseous device for age and condition, preferably safety-engineered intraosseous device
- Select appropriate intraosseous site based on clinical situation and in accordance with manufacturers' directions for device use
- Consider sites most commonly used in both adults and children (e.g., proximal and distal tibia, proximal humerus, distal femur for children, sternum in adults)
- Ensure proper landmarks identified prior to insertion, when clinically possible, to avoid complications related to improper placement
- Ensure correct needle size with drill or driver for intraosseous device, matching with body mass index
- Choose appropriate size needle with stylet for non-drill or driver devices
- Consider use of subcutaneous lidocaine as local anesthetic prior to insertion at intended site
- Immobilize extremity and perform skin antisepsis using an appropriate solution (e.g., alcohol-based chlorhexidine, povidone-iodine, 70% alcohol) based on agency policies and procedures
- Administer 1% lidocaine at insertion point, as appropriate
- Insert needle with stylet at 60-to-90-degree angle directed inferiorly
- Remove inner stylet, as necessary

- Confirm correct placement of intraosseous device using correct needle position, sensation of loss of resistance upon bone penetration, and absence of any signs of infiltration upon flushing with 5 to 10 mL (adult) or 2 to 5 mL (pediatric) preservative-free 0.9% sodium chloride
- Aspirate blood or bone marrow to confirm placement where possible, although not an indication of improper placement if other indications of placement confirmation are present
- Consider use of color Doppler ultrasound to confirm initial placement and confirm position after person movement
- Flush needle with solution according to agency protocol
- Secure needle in place with tape and apply appropriate sterile dressing according to agency protocol
- Connect tubing to needle and allow fluids to run by gravity or under pressure, as required by flow rate
- Anchor IV lines to extremity
- Ensure compatibility of medications and fluids in infusion
- Determine flow rate and adjust accordingly
- Monitor for signs and symptoms of extravasation of fluids or medications, infection, or fat embolism
- Reduce risk for infiltration or extravasation by avoiding multiple attempts at intraosseous access at same site, ensuring proper needle placement, securing intraosseous device, rechecking intraosseous placement with transport or repositioning of person, and before infusing highly irritating solutions or known vesicants and large-volume infusions
- Ensure ongoing and frequent assessment of intraosseous site and extremity, including palpation and calf circumference for tibial placement
- Limit infusion time to less than 24 hours, not to exceed 48 hours total
- Promptly remove intraosseous device within 24 hours, when therapy complete, or if signs of dysfunction occur
- Follow manufacturers' directions for use and removal of intraosseous device to reduce risk of complications
- Document site, needle type and size, type of fluid and medication, flow rate, and response as per agency protocol
- Report response to therapy according to agency protocol
- Establish IV access and discontinue intraosseous line after condition stabilizes
- Improve appropriate use of intraosseous route through education and competency programs
- Include initial and ongoing validation of safe insertion knowledge and skills through demonstration, demonstration of appropriate device management, and ability to recognize complications related to intraosseous access in all competency programs

2nd edition 1996; revised 2004, 2024

Background Evidence:

Infusion Nurses Society. (2021). Infusion therapy standards of practice, 8th edition. *Journal of Infusion Nursing, 39*(1S), 1–179.

Kirby, N. (2021). Medication administration. In R. F. Craven, C. J. Hirnle, & C. J. Henshaw (Eds.), *Fundamentals of nursing: Human health and function* (8th ed., pp. 410–471). Wolters-Kluwer.

Konopka, E., Webb, K., Reserva, J., Moy, L., Ton-That, H., Speiser, J., & Tung, R. (2021). Cutaneous complications associated with intraosseous access placement. *Cutis, 107*(6), E31–E33. https://doi.org/10.12788/cutis.0303

Nguyen, L., Suarez, S., Daniels, J., Sanchez, C., Landry, K., & Redfield, C. (2019). Effect of intravenous versus intraosseous access in prehospital cardiac arrest. *Air Medical Journal, 38*(3), 147–149. https://doi.org/10.1016/j.amj.2019.02.005

Potter, P. A., Ostendorf, W. R., & LaPlante, N. (2018). Safe medication preparation. In *Clinical nursing skills and techniques* (pp. 501–522) (9th ed.). Mosby.

Sanoski, C. A., & Vallerand, A. H. (2021). *Davis's drug guide for nurses* (17th ed.). F.A. Davis.

Santos, A. P., Conkin, R., & Dowd, K. (2017). Needle break: Complication and management of intraosseous vascular access. *American Surgeon, 83*(1), e18–e20. https://doi.org/10.1177/000313481708300112

Medication Administration: Intraspinal   2319

Definition: Administration and monitoring of medication via an established epidural or intrathecal route

Activities:

- Follow agency policies and procedures for accurate and safe administration of medications
- Promote environment that maximizes safe and efficient administration of medications
- Familiarize self with condition of person receiving medications, and indications and information related to medication (e.g., dosage ranges, expected therapeutic effects, possible adverse reactions, interactions with other medications)
- Check accuracy and completeness of each medication administration record (MAR) prior to giving any medications
- Review health history and history of allergies
- Determine person's knowledge of medication and understanding of method of administration
- Instruct on medication purpose and answer questions appropriately
- Follow six rights of medication administration (e.g., right person, right medication, right dose, right route, right time, right documentation)
- Identify using at least two identifiers (e.g., name, birthdate)
- Perform necessary pre-medication evaluations (e.g., blood pressure, pulse, blood sugar assessment, pain level)
- Administer medications within scope of practice and agency guidelines
- Maintain aseptic technique
- Ensure intraspinal access devices and administration sets are identified and labeled as specialized infusion administration system and differentiated from other infusion administration and access systems
- Use only medications that are free of preservatives
- Filter intraspinal infusion solutions using 0.2-micron, surfactant-free, particulate-retentive, and air-eliminating filter
- Use different delivery devices, systems, and connectors for medications to be administered via intraspinal and other parenteral routes
- Prepare and store intrathecal medications separately, and clearly label "For Intrathecal Use"
- Perform independent double check with another qualified health care provider prior to administration of medication, or when syringe or medication container, rate, or concentration changed
- Verify safety of medication for intraventricular or intrathecal route and verify medication mixture with preservative-free 0.9% sodium chloride or other appropriate solution
- Wear mask during all intraspinal medication injections to reduce risk of droplet transmission of oropharyngeal flora
- Monitor vital signs, comfort level, neurological status, mobility, and motor and sensory functions
- Confirm placement of intraspinal access device before any infusion or medication administration
- Aspirate epidural access devices prior to medication administration to ascertain absence of spinal fluid and blood
- Notify health care provider if greater than 0.5 mL of serous fluid is aspirated and do not administer medication as indicative of catheter migration into intrathecal space
- Aspirate intrathecal and ventricular access devices prior to medication administration to ascertain presence of spinal fluid and absence of blood
- Aseptically prepare preservative-free medication through filter needle
- Inject medication slowly per health care provider order and according to agency protocol
- Use only aqueous chlorhexidine solution or povidone iodine solution for device access or site care
- Allow any skin antiseptic agent to fully dry as all antiseptic agents have neurotoxic potential
- Monitor epidural or intrathecal catheter insertion site for signs of infection
- Apply and maintain clean, dry, and intact sterile dressing over insertion site
- Secure access site with securement product or tape tension loop of tubing to body to reduce risk of accidental dislodgement
- Perform site care and dressing changes over tunneled and accessed implanted epidural device in accordance with agency policy
- Use transparent semipermeable dressing to allow for site visualization, and chlorhexidine-impregnated dressings for epidural access device when possible
- Monitor dressing on epidural or intrathecal catheter insertion site for presence of clear drainage
- Notify health care provider if epidural or intrathecal dressing is wet
- Secure catheter to skin and tape all tubing connections, as appropriate
- Mark tubing as either intrathecal or epidural, as appropriate
- Trace all catheters, administration sets or add-on devices between person and container before connecting or reconnecting any infusion device, at each care transition to new setting or service, and as part of handoff process
- Check infusion pump for proper calibration and operation per agency protocol
- Use electronic infusion pump with anti–free-flow protection to administer continuous infusions
- Use administration set without any injection ports to reduce risk of inadvertent intraspinal access
- Monitor infusion set up, flow rate, and solution at regular intervals
- Monitor for central nervous system infection (e.g., fever, change in level of consciousness, nausea, vomiting)

M

- Determine current anticoagulation therapy prior to insertion or removal of intraspinal lines
- Withhold anticoagulants before intraspinal insertion and before removal due to risk for epidural hematoma and paralysis
- Maintain peripheral IV access for at least 24 hours after insertion due to potential need for naloxone administration in event of respiratory depression
- Monitor after initiating or restarting an intraspinal infusion for at least first 24 hours, in time frames of every 1 to 2 hours until stable, then every 4 hours, or with each home visit
- Instruct related to principles of intraspinal access device placement and what to expect during insertion procedure
- Instruct related to importance of reporting alcohol use and all medications used, including prescription, over-the-counter, and complementary medications
- Instruct related to signs and symptoms to report, including changes in pain perception, new or worsening side effects, and fever
- Instruct related to clinical signs of overdose, including dizziness, sedation, euphoria, anxiety, seizures, and respiratory depression
- Instruct persons with implanted infusion pump systems not to bend or twist at waist for 6 weeks and use overall caution with active repetitive bending or twisting of spine as may increase risk for catheter damage or dislodgement
- Document medication administration and response according to agency guidelines
- Use teach-back to ensure understanding

4th edition 2004; revised 2024

Background Evidence:

Hess, S. R., Lahaye, L. A., Waligora, A. C., Sima, A. P., Jiranek, W. A., & Golladay, G. J. (2019). Safety and side-effect profile of intrathecal morphine in a diverse patient population undergoing total knee and hip arthroplasty. *European Journal of Orthopaedic Surgery & Traumatology, 29*(1), 125–129. https://doi.org/10.1007/s00590-018-2293-9

Infusion Nurses Society. (2021). Infusion therapy standards of practice, 8th edition. *Journal of Intravenous Nursing, 39*(1S), 1–179.

Kirby, N. (2021). Medication administration. In R. F. Craven, C. J. Hirnle, & C. J. Henshaw (Eds.), *Fundamentals of nursing: Human health and function* (8th ed., pp. 410–471). Wolters-Kluwer.

Pittelkow, T. P., Bendel, M. A., Strand, J. J., & Moeschler, S. M. (2019). Curing opioid toxicity with intrathecal targeted drug delivery. *Case Reports in Medicine, 2019.* https://doi.org/10.1155/2019/3428576

Potter, P. A., Ostendorf, W. R., & LaPlante, N. (2018). Parenteral medications. In *Clinical nursing skills and techniques* (pp. 580–628) (9th ed.). Mosby.

Potter, P. A., Ostendorf, W. R., & LaPlante, N. (2018). Safe medication preparation. In *Clinical nursing skills and techniques* (pp. 501–522) (9th ed.). Mosby.

Sanoski, C. A., & Vallerand, A. H. (2021). *Davis's drug guide for nurses* (17th ed.). F.A. Davis.

Scanlon, M. M., Gazelka, H. M., Moeschler, S. M., Hoelzer, B. C., Hooten, W. M., Bendel, M. A., & Lamer, T. J. (2017). Surgical site infections in cancer patients with intrathecal drug delivery devices. *Pain Medicine, 18*(3), 520–525. https://doi.org/10.1093/pm/pnw203

Vice-O'Con, K. (2018). Pharmacologic methods for preventing pruritus in patients receiving intrathecal opioids for cesarean delivery. *AANA Journal, 86*(1), 59–66.

M

Medication Administration: Intravenous (IV)   2314

Definition: Preparing and infusing medications via the intravenous route

Activities:

- Follow agency policies and procedures for accurate and safe administration of medications
- Promote environment that maximizes safe and efficient administration of medications
- Familiarize self with condition of person receiving medications, and indications and information related to medication (e.g., dosage ranges, expected therapeutic effects, possible adverse reactions, interactions with other medications)
- Check accuracy and completeness of each medication administration record (MAR) prior to giving any medications
- Review health history and history of allergies
- Determine person's knowledge of medication and understanding of method of administration
- Instruct on medication purpose and answer questions appropriately
- Follow six rights of medication administration (e.g., right person, right medication, right dose, right route, right time, right documentation)
- Identify using at least two identifiers (e.g., name, birthdate)
- Perform necessary pre-medication evaluations (e.g., blood pressure, pulse, blood sugar assessment, pain level)
- Confirm agency guidelines regarding requirements for special monitoring while medication administered (i.e., telemetry with heart medications)
- Use standardized concentrations and dosages of IV medications, preferably prepared and dispensed from pharmacy or commercially prepared when possible
- Avoid preparing high-alert IV medications (e.g., chemotherapy, heparin, dopamine, dobutamine, nitroglycerin, potassium, antibiotics, magnesium) on care unit
- Use only standardized infusion concentrations of high-alert IV medications
- Perform independent double check by two licensed staff for high-alert medications, according to agency guidelines
- Check for IV medication incompatibilities
- Avoid mixing incompatible medications in same IV line or solution
- Initiate additional IV site if required to administer incompatible medications, or if current IV line contains medication that cannot be interrupted or stopped temporarily
- Limit use of add-on infusion devices (e.g., extension sets) to single IV line to reduce risk of contamination or accidental disconnection
- Use technology according to agency policies and procedures (e.g., bar code, smart pump with dose-error reduction software, volume-control administration set, mini-infusion administration set), when available
- Label all medications prepared in syringes
- Discard and do not use any medication syringes that are unlabeled unless medication prepared at bedside and immediately administered without break in process
- Note expiration date of medications and solutions
- Set up proper equipment for medication administration

- Prepare appropriate concentration of IV medication from ampule or vial
- Do not dilute IV push medications unless recommended by manufacturer, agency policy, or reference literature
- Verify placement and patency of IV catheter within vein
- Maintain sterility of IV system
- Perform disinfection of connection surfaces (e.g., needleless connectors, injection ports) before medication administration, flushing, and locking procedures
- Administer IV medication at rate recommended by manufacturer, agency policy, or reference literature
- Select injection port of IV tubing closest to person, occlude IV line above port, and aspirate for blood return before injecting intravenous bolus into existing line
- Observe area above IV catheter insertion point for puffiness or swelling during administration and for 48 hours after IV push
- Discontinue medication administration if puffiness or swelling occurs and remove IV catheter as infiltrated
- Flush intravenous lock with appropriate solution before and after medication administration as per agency protocol
- Connect infusion tubing for IV piggyback medications to medication bag and fill tubing by opening regulator flow clamp
- Hang piggyback medication bag above level of primary fluid bag and connect to appropriate connector of primary infusion line
- Regulate flow with slide clamp or with IV pump infusion rate
- Ensure primary infusion automatically begins after piggyback solution is empty
- Observe closely for adverse reactions during administration and several minutes thereafter
- Stop delivering medication immediately if adverse reaction noted
- Follow agency guidelines for appropriate response to allergic reaction (e.g., administration of antihistamine)
- Stop delivering medication immediately if IV site shows symptoms of infiltration or phlebitis
- Determine how much damage IV medication can produce in subcutaneous tissue
- Follow agency guidelines for IV extravasation care
- Stop IV fluids and clamp IV line if IV medication found to be incompatible with IV fluids during administration (i.e., IV fluid becomes cloudy in tubing)
- Restart IV fluids with new tubing if incompatible medications in current tubing
- Cleanse injection port to IV fluid container with antiseptic or alcohol swabs prior to adding medication to IV fluid container
- Mix solution gently by rotating bag or bottle if adding medication to IV fluid container
- Determine that current IV solution is sufficient for adding medication, when adding to an existing infusion
- Complete medication additive label and apply to IV fluid container, as appropriate

- Trace all catheters or administration sets or add-on devices between person and fluid container before connecting or reconnecting any infusion device
- Label administration sets with infusing solution or medication both near person connection and near solution container
- Instruct person, caregivers, and unlicensed assistive personnel to obtain assistance from licensed staff whenever real or perceived need to connect or disconnect devices or infusions unless person or caregiver independently administering infusion medications (e.g., in home care setting)
- Document which solutions and medications are being infused through which device or lumen, when multiple vascular access devices (VADs) or catheter lumens are used
- Route tubing having different purposes in different directions (i.e., IV catheters routed toward head, feeding tubes routed toward feet)
- Dispose of needles, syringes, and equipment according to agency practice
- Maintain IV access, as appropriate
- Follow agency practice related to recommended changes for IV site, IV tubing, and IV fluids
- Monitor to determine response to medication
- Monitor IV setup, flow rate, and solution at regular intervals per agency protocol
- Monitor for infiltration and phlebitis at infusion site
- Provide person and caregiver education including infusion administration and signs and symptoms to report, including those that may occur after person leaves health care setting
- Document medication administration and person responsiveness according to agency protocol
- Use teach-back to ensure understanding

3rd edition 2000; revised 2004, 2024

M

Background Evidence:

Berman, A., Snyder, S. J., & Frandsen, G. (2018). Medications. In *Kozier and Erb's Fundamentals of nursing: Concepts, process and practice* (pp. 803–811) (10th ed.). Pearson.

Cicero, T. (2021). Intravenous therapy. In R. F. Craven, C. J. Hirnle, & C. J. Henshaw (Eds.), *Fundamentals of nursing: Human health and function* (8th ed., pp. 472–541). Wolters-Kluwer.

Gorski, L. A. (2017). The 2016 Infusion Therapy Standards of Practice. *Home Healthcare Now*, 35(1), 10–18. https://doi.org/10.1097/NHH.0000 000000000481

Infusion Nursing Society. (2021). *Policies and procedures for infusion therapy: Acute care* (6tj ed.).

Infusion Nursing Society. (2021). *Standards of practice* (8th ed.).

Potter, P. A., Ostendorf, W. R., & LaPlante, N. (2018). Parenteral medications. In *Clinical nursing skills and techniques* (pp. 607–619) (9th ed.). Mosby.

Sanoski, C. A., & Vallerand, A. H. (2021). *Davis's drug guide for nurses* (17th ed.). F.A. Davis.

Medication Administration: Nasal   2320

Definition: Preparing and providing medications via nasal passages

Activities:

- Follow agency policies and procedures for accurate and safe administration of medications
- Promote environment that maximizes safe and efficient administration of medications

- Familiarize self with condition of person receiving medications, and indications and information related to medication (e.g., dosage ranges, expected therapeutic effects, possible adverse reactions, interactions with other medications)

- Check accuracy and completeness of each medication administration record (MAR) prior to giving any medications
- Review health history and history of allergies
- Determine person's knowledge of medication and understanding of method of administration
- Instruct on medication purpose and answer questions appropriately
- Follow six rights of medication administration (e.g., right person, right medication, right dose, right route, right time, right documentation)
- Identify using at least two identifiers (e.g., name, birthdate)
- Perform necessary pre-medication evaluations (e.g., blood pressure, pulse, blood sugar assessment, pain level)
- Instruct to blow nose gently before administration of nasal medication unless contraindicated
- Assist to supine position and place head appropriately, depending on which sinuses are to be medicated when administering nose drops
- Place in supine position with head over edge of bed or with pillow under shoulders to tip head backward, when instilling medication into sinus areas
- Turn head to side of sinus area to be treated, when instilling drops into maxillary or frontal sinuses
- Have person remain supine with head tipped backward for ethmoid or sphenoid sinuses
- Instruct to breathe through mouth during administration when administering nose drops
- Hold dropper 1 cm above nares and instill prescribed number of drops
- Instruct to remain supine for 5 minutes after administering nose drops
- Instruct to remain upright and to not tilt head backward when administering nasal spray
- Insert nozzle into nostril and squeeze bottle quickly and firmly when administering nasal spray
- Aim spray applicator top toward the midline of nose

- Administer spray during inhalation
- Instruct not to blow nose for several minutes after administration
- Keep children in upright position during administration to avoid swallowing of excess spray
- Instruct on medication insertion via nasal packing or tampon (e.g., leave in place for prescribed time, do not blow nose, medication intended effects)
- Instruct to avoid using decongestant nasal sprays too frequently or for several days, as rebound nasal congestion can occur
- Instruct to alternate nares if using irritating medications regularly (e.g., calcitonin)
- Instruct that each family member should have different dropper or spray applicator
- Instruct to use OTC nasal sprays or nose drops for one illness only and then discard
- Monitor to determine response to medication
- Document medication administration and response according to agency protocol
- Use teach-back to ensure understanding

4th edition 2004; revised 2024

Background Evidence:

Berman, A., Snyder, S. J., & Frandsen, G. (2018). Medications. In *Kozier and Erb's Fundamentals of nursing: Concepts, process and practice* (pp. 817–818) (10th ed.). Pearson.

Kirby, N. (2021). Medication administration. In R. F. Craven, C. J. Hirnle, & C. J. Henshaw (Eds.), *Fundamentals of nursing: Human health and function* (8th ed., pp. 410–471). Wolters-Kluwer.

Potter, P. A., Ostendorf, W. R., & LaPlante, N. (2018). Administering nasal instillations. *In Clinical nursing skills and techniques* (pp. 550–554) (9th ed.). Mosby.

Sanoski, C. A., & Vallerand, A. H. (2021). *Davis's drug guide for nurses* (17th ed.). F.A. Davis.

Medication Administration: Oral   2304

Definition: Preparing and providing medications by mouth

Activities:

- Follow agency policies and procedures for accurate and safe administration of medications
- Promote environment that maximizes safe and efficient administration of medications
- Familiarize self with condition of person receiving medications, and indications and information related to medication (e.g., dosage ranges, expected therapeutic effects, possible adverse reactions, interactions with other medications)
- Check accuracy and completeness of each medication administration record (MAR) prior to giving any medications
- Review health history and history of allergies
- Determine person's knowledge of medication and understanding of method of administration
- Instruct on medication purpose and answer questions appropriately
- Follow six rights of medication administration (e.g., right person, right medication, right dose, right route, right time, right documentation)
- Identify using at least two identifiers (e.g., name, birthdate)
- Perform necessary pre-medication evaluations (e.g., blood pressure, pulse, blood sugar assessment, pain level)

- Prepare medications for one person at a time
- Look only at one MAR, computer printout, or computer medication administration screen at a time
- Determine preference for fluids and determine if medications can be given with these fluids, maintaining fluid restrictions if ordered
- Determine any contraindications to receiving oral medication (e.g., difficulty swallowing, nausea or vomiting, bowel inflammation, reduced peristalsis, recent gastrointestinal surgery, attached to gastric suction, NPO, decreased level of consciousness)
- Give time-critical medications at exact time ordered (i.e., no later than 30 minutes before or after time ordered)
- Place in sitting or Fowler's position prior to administering medications
- Keep in same position for 30 minutes after medications given
- Use side lying position if unable to sit
- Assist with taking medications by holding cup, placing single pill in mouth at one time
- Do not rush or force medication administration
- Evaluate swallowing ability and risk for aspiration using dysphagia screening tool prior to drug administration, as indicated

- Check for possible drug interactions and contraindications
- Note expiration date on medication container or wrapper and discard medications that are expired
- Give medications on empty stomach, with food, or 2 to 3 hours after eating, as indicated by type of medication
- Avoid handling or preparing medications unless gloved
- Mix offensive-tasting medications with food or fluids, as appropriate
- Mix medication with flavored syrup from pharmacy, as appropriate
- Crush medication and mix with small amount of soft food (e.g., applesauce, pudding), as required by condition or age
- Do not crush or split enteric coated medications as medication may be released too early, become inactivated or fail to reach intended site of action
- Caution against chewing or swallowing lozenges
- Add tablet or powder to glass of water at bedside for effervescent medications and administer immediately after dissolving
- Inform of expected actions and possible adverse effects of medications
- Instruct of proper administration of sublingual medication
- Place sublingual medications under tongue and instruct not to swallow but to allow to dissolve slowly
- Place buccal medication in mouth against mucous membranes of cheek until dissolves
- Instruct not to eat or drink until sublingual or buccal medication completely dissolved
- Ensure takes all medications
- Do not leave medications unattended
- Document medications only after given and observed
- Stay with person until all medications ingested
- Monitor for possible aspiration, as appropriate

- Perform mouth checks after delivery of medications, as appropriate
- Return to position of comfort 30 minutes after medication administration
- Use automated, computer-controlled drug dispensing or unit-dose medication carts as per agency policy
- Instruct person or family member on how to administer medication
- Monitor for therapeutic effects, adverse effect, drug toxicity, and drug interactions
- Document medications administered and responsiveness according to agency protocol
- Use teach-back to ensure understanding

1st edition 1992; revised 2000, 2004, 2024

Background Evidence:

Berman, A., Snyder, S. J., & Frandsen, G. (2018). Medications. In *Kozier and Erb's fundamentals of nursing: Concepts, process and practice* (pp. 792–793) (10th ed.). Pearson.

Boyer, M. J. (2020). *Math for nurses* (10th ed.). Wolters-Kluwer.

Kirby, N. (2021). Medication administration. In R. F. Craven, C. J. Hirnle, & C. J. Henshaw (Eds.), *Fundamentals of nursing: Human health and function* (8th ed., pp. 410–471). Wolters-Kluwer.

Potter, P. A., Ostendorf, W. R., & LaPlante, N. (2018). Administering intramuscular injections. In *Clinical nursing skills and techniques* (pp. 589–593) (9th ed.). Mosby.

Sanoski, C. A., & Vallerand, A. H. (2021). *Davis's drug guide for nurses* (17th ed.). F.A. Davis.

Medication Administration: Rectal   2315

M

Definition: Preparing and inserting rectal suppositories, pills, capsules, or tablets

Activities:

- Follow agency policies and procedures for accurate and safe administration of medications
- Promote environment that maximizes safe and efficient administration of medications
- Familiarize self with condition of person receiving medications, and indications and information related to medication (e.g., dosage ranges, expected therapeutic effects, possible adverse reactions, interactions with other medications)
- Check accuracy and completeness of each medication administration record (MAR) prior to giving any medications
- Review health history and history of allergies
- Determine person's knowledge of medication and understanding of method of administration
- Instruct on medication purpose and answer questions appropriately
- Follow six rights of medication administration (e.g., right person, right medication, right dose, right route, right time, right documentation)
- Identify using at least two identifiers (e.g., name, birthdate)
- Perform necessary pre-medication evaluations (e.g., blood pressure, pulse, blood sugar assessment, pain level)
- Review medical record for history of rectal surgery, bleeding, or contraindications to rectal medication
- Determine if any presenting signs and symptoms of gastrointestinal alterations (e.g., constipation, diarrhea)
- Determine ability to retain medication
- Assist to side-lying (left lateral) position with upper leg flexed upward

- Maintain privacy where possible, draping with bedclothes or towels, allowing exposure of buttocks
- Lubricate gloved index finger of dominant hand and rounded end of suppository
- Lubricate pill, capsule, or tablet in similar manner as suppository, as indicated
- Instruct to take slow deep breaths through mouth and to relax anal sphincter
- Retract buttocks
- Insert suppository, pill, tablet, or capsule gently through anus, past internal anal sphincter, and against rectal wall (i.e., 4 inches or 10 cm for adults, 2 inches or 5 cm for children)
- Avoid embedding medications in feces
- Press buttocks together for a few minutes
- Instruct to remain flat or on side for 5 minutes
- Instruct to retain medication according to manufacturer instructions
- Place in supine position to insert medication through colostomy
- Use lubricant and same technique as insertion via anal area, for colostomy suppository or medications
- Monitor for effects of medication
- Instruct related to self-administration technique as appropriate
- Ensure person aware to remove foil wrapper before administering suppositories
- Ensure person same effect obtained from rectal administration of medications as with oral
- Ensure ability to manipulate medications or applicator if self-administering

- Document medication administration and responsiveness according to agency protocol
- Use teach-back to ensure understanding

3rd edition 2000; revised 2004, 2024

Background Evidence:

Berman, A., Snyder, S. J., & Frandsen, G. (2018). Medications. In *Kozier and Erb's Fundamentals of nursing: Concepts, process and practice* (pp. 820–821) (10th ed.). Pearson.

Hua, S. (2019). Physiological and pharmaceutical considerations for rectal drug formulations. *Frontiers in Pharmacology, 10,* 1196. https://doi.org/10.3389/fphar.2019.01196

Kirby, N. (2021). Medication administration. In R. F. Craven, C. J. Hirnle, & C. J. Henshaw (Eds.), *Fundamentals of nursing: Human health and function* (8th ed., pp. 410–471). Wolters-Kluwer.

Lam, S. H. F., Li, D. R., Hong, C. E., & Vilke, G. M. (2018). Systematic review: Rectal administration of medications for pediatric procedural sedation. *Journal of Emergency Medicine, 55*(1), 51–63. https://doi.org/10.1016/j.jemermed.2018.04.025

Lindauer, A., Sexson, K., & Harvath, T. A. (2017). Teaching caregivers to administer eye drops, transdermal patches, and suppositories. *AJN American Journal of Nursing, 117*(1), 54–59. https://doi.org/10.1097/01.NAJ.0000511568.58187.36

Potter, P. A., Ostendorf, W. R., & LaPlante, N. (2018). Administering rectal suppositories. In *Clinical nursing skills and techniques* (pp. 569–580) (9th ed.). Mosby.

Sanoski, C. A., & Vallerand, A. H. (2021). *Davis's drug guide for nurses* (17th ed.). F.A. Davis.

Selge, C., Bausewein, C., & Remi, C. (2018). Rectal administration of baclofen at the end of life. *Journal of Pain & Symptom Management, 56*(5), e1–e3. https://doi.org/10.1016/j.jpainsymman.2018.07.023

Medication Administration: Skin   2316

Definition: Preparing and applying medications to the epidermis

Activities:

- Follow agency policies and procedures for accurate and safe administration of medications
- Promote environment that maximizes safe and efficient administration of medications
- Familiarize self with condition of person receiving medications, and indications and information related to medication (e.g., dosage ranges, expected therapeutic effects, possible adverse reactions, interactions with other medications)
- Check accuracy and completeness of each medication administration record (MAR) prior to giving any medications
- Review health history and history of allergies
- Determine person's knowledge of medication and understanding of method of administration
- Instruct on medication purpose and answer questions appropriately
- Follow six rights of medication administration (e.g., right person, right medication, right dose, right route, right time, right documentation)
- Identify using at least two identifiers (e.g., name, birthdate)
- Perform necessary pre-medication evaluations (e.g., blood pressure, pulse, blood sugar assessment, pain level)
- Determine skin condition over area where medication will be applied
- Cleanse area if needed as skin encrustations and dead tissue block contact of medication with affected tissue
- Remove previous dose of medication and cleanse skin
- Avoid applying new medication over previously applied medication as decreases therapeutic benefit
- Expose affected areas only, keeping unaffected areas covered as indicated
- Measure correct amount of topically applied systemic medications, using standardized measurement devices
- Apply topical agent to thickness as prescribed
- Apply topical agent while skin still damp, if skin excessively dry
- Apply transdermal patches and topical medications to areas of skin without hair, as appropriate
- Instruct that transdermal patch cannot be cut as changes in patch size changes dosage
- Instruct to notify health care provider to change order if new strength of medication needed
- Soften medication as needed by rubbing briskly between gloved hands
- Spread medication evenly over skin, as appropriate
- Use long, even strokes when applying medication, following direction of hair growth
- Rotate application sites of topical systemic medications
- Instruct that skin may feel oily after application
- Write date, time, and initials on antianginal applications that use dose application papers
- Shake aerosol containers vigorously prior to application
- Use recommended distance for holding sprayer to apply medication
- Instruct to turn face away or briefly cover face with towel, as indicated
- Shake suspension-based medications as indicated per directions
- Apply suspension-based medications to gauze dressing or pad and apply stroking in direction of hair growth
- Apply powder medications when skin surface thoroughly dry
- Cover face appropriately if near to application area
- Dust skin lightly with power and cover with dressing as indicated
- Monitor for local, systemic, and adverse effects of medication
- Instruct related to self-administration techniques, as appropriate
- Document medication administration and responsiveness according to agency protocol
- Use teach-back to ensure understanding

3rd edition 2000; revised 2024

Background Evidence:

Berman, A., Snyder, S. J., & Frandsen, G. (2018). Medications. In *Kozier and Erb's Fundamentals of nursing: Concepts, process and practice* (pp. 759–813) (10th ed.). Pearson.

Kirby, N. (2021). Medication administration. In R. F. Craven, C. J. Hirnle, & C. J. Henshaw (Eds.), *Fundamentals of nursing: Human health and function* (8th ed., pp. 410–471). Wolters-Kluwer.

Potter, P. A., Ostendorf, W. R., & LaPlante, N. (2018). Administering topical medications to the skin. In *Clinical nursing skills and techniques* (pp. 536–541) (9th ed.). Mosby.

Sanoski, C. A., & Vallerand, A. H. (2021). *Davis's drug guide for nurses* (17th ed.). F.A. Davis.

Medication Administration: Subcutaneous   2317

Definition: Preparing and providing medications via the subcutaneous route

Activities:

- Follow agency policies and procedures for accurate and safe administration of medications
- Promote environment that maximizes safe and efficient administration of medications
- Familiarize self with condition of person receiving medications, and indications and information related to medication (e.g., dosage ranges, expected therapeutic effects, possible adverse reactions, interactions with other medications)
- Check accuracy and completeness of each medication administration record (MAR) prior to giving any medications
- Review health history and history of allergies
- Determine person's knowledge of medication and understanding of method of administration
- Instruct on medication purpose and answer questions appropriately
- Follow six rights of medication administration (e.g., right person, right medication, right dose, right route, right time, right documentation)
- Identify using at least two identifiers (e.g., name, birthdate)
- Perform necessary pre-medication evaluations (e.g., blood pressure, pulse, blood sugar assessment, pain level)
- Consider indications and contraindications for subcutaneous injection
- Select correct needle and syringe based on person and medication information
- Prepare dose correctly from ampule or vial, per manufacturer's directions
- Select appropriate injection site (e.g., outer aspects of upper arms, abdomen, anterior thighs)
- Rotate insulin injection sites systematically within one anatomical region
- Use shorter needles for insulin in persons with BMI of 25 or less
- Have self-administer insulin whenever possible
- Store vials of insulin in refrigerator, not freezer
- Keep vials currently being used at room temperature
- Do not inject cold insulin
- Palpate injection site for edema, masses, or tenderness and avoid those areas
- Avoid areas of scarring, bruising, abrasion, or infection
- Use abdominal sites when administering heparin subcutaneously, keeping at least 5 cm (2 inches) away from umbilicus
- Ensure not taking herbal medications that interact with heparin (e.g., garlic, ginger, ginkgo, horse chestnut, feverfew)
- Do not expel air from prefilled low-molecular-weight syringes unless dosage must be changed

- Do not aspirate when giving heparin injections
- Administer injection using aseptic technique
- Inject needle quickly at a 45-to-90-degree angle, depending on size of person
- Limit medication to small volume depending on person (i.e., 0.5–1.5 mL adults, up to 0.5 mL in children) and water-soluble medications
- Select needle-less system or needle based on needs
- Use abdominal sites for thin persons
- Ensure medication reaches SQ tissue by inserting at 90-degree angle if can grasp 5 cm (2 inches) of tissue; insert at 45-degree angle if can only grasp 2.5 cm (1 inch)
- Apply gentle pressure to site and avoid massaging site
- Monitor for expected and unexpected medication effects
- Instruct person and family regarding injection technique for regular hypodermic needles and medication, as well as with injection pens
- Ensure learns techniques of self-administration when regular injections required
- Use return demonstrations of injection techniques to validate learning
- Instruct person and family to observe injection sites for complications and immediately report complications to health care provider
- Ensure priming of injection pen before administration of medication
- Document medication administration and responsiveness according to agency protocol
- Use teach-back to ensure understanding

3rd edition 2000; revised 2004, 2024

Background Evidence:

Berman, A., Snyder, S. J., & Frandsen, G. (2018). Medications. In *Kozier and Erb's fundamentals of nursing: Concepts, process and practice* (pp. 794–797) (10th ed.). Pearson.

Kirby, N. (2021). Medication administration. In R. F. Craven, C. J. Hirnle, & C. J. Henshaw (Eds.), *Fundamentals of nursing: Human health and function* (8th ed., pp. 410–471). Wolters-Kluwer.

Potter, P. A., Ostendorf, W. R., & LaPlante, N. (2018). Administering intramuscular injections. In *Clinical nursing skills and techniques* (pp. 593–600) (9th ed.). Mosby.

Sanoski, C. A., & Vallerand, A. H. (2021). *Davis's drug guide for nurses* (17th ed.). F.A. Davis.

M

Medication Administration: Vaginal   2318

Definition: Preparing and inserting vaginal medications

Activities:

- Follow agency policies and procedures for accurate and safe administration of medications
- Promote environment that maximizes safe and efficient administration of medications
- Familiarize self with condition of person receiving medications, and indications and information related to medication (e.g.,

    dosage ranges, expected therapeutic effects, possible adverse reactions, interactions with other medications)
- Check accuracy and completeness of each medication administration record (MAR) prior to giving any medications
- Review health history and history of allergies
- Determine person's knowledge of medication and understanding of method of administration

- Instruct on medication purpose and answer questions appropriately
- Follow six rights of medication administration (e.g., right person, right medication, right dose, right route, right time, right documentation)
- Identify using at least two identifiers (e.g., name, birthdate)
- Perform necessary pre-medication evaluations (e.g., blood pressure, pulse, blood sugar assessment, pain level)
- Have void before administration
- Assure privacy with draped abdomen or lower extremities, as indicated
- Assure adequate lighting using room light or portable gooseneck lamp, as indicated
- Apply water-soluble lubricant to rounded end of suppository or tablet
- Lubricate gloved index finger of dominant hand
- Gently separate folds of labia in front to back direction
- Insert rounded end of suppository, tablet, or capsule along posterior wall of vaginal canal 3 to 4 inches (7–10 cm) or insert applicator approximately 2 to 3 inches (5–7 cm)
- Withdraw finger and cleanse area of excess lubricant
- Use same positioning and techniques for jelly, cream or foam applications, filling applicator using medication directions
- Insert applicator 2 to 3 inches (5–7.5 cm) and push applicator plunger to deposit medication
- Instruct to remain on back for at least 10 minutes
- Use same positioning for vaginal douche or irrigation, adding bedpan and absorbent pad underneath
- Assure douche or irrigation at body temperature
- Prime tubing or nozzle of container
- Separate labial folds and insert nozzle, directing toward sacrum following vaginal floor
- Raise container 12 to 20 inches (30–50 cm) above level of vagina
- Allow solution to flow while rotating nozzle
- Administer entire solution
- Withdraw nozzle and assist to sitting position, remaining on bedpan for a few minutes
- Clean and dry perineum as indicated after medication administration
- Offer perineal pad as indicated
- Cleanse all equipment including applicator, after each use
- Maintain good perineal hygiene
- Monitor for effects of medication
- Instruct self-administration technique, as appropriate
- Instruct to take all of medications as prescribed, to ensure effectiveness of treatment
- Instruct to abstain from sexual intercourse as indicated by medication
- Instruct to continue taking medications during menstruation
- Instruct to avoid excessive use of vaginal medications, as leads to irritation of vaginal mucosa
- Document medication administration and responsiveness according to agency protocol
- Use teach-back to ensure understanding

3rd edition 2000; revised 2004, 2024

Background Evidence:

Berman, A., Snyder, S. J., & Frandsen, G. (2018). Medications. In *Kozier and Erb's Fundamentals of nursing: Concepts, process and practice* (pp. 818–820) (10th ed.). Pearson.

Kirby, N. (2021). Medication administration. In R. F. Craven, C. J. Hirnle, & C. J. Henshaw (Eds.), *Fundamentals of nursing: Human health and function* (8th ed., pp. 410–471). Wolters-Kluwer.

Potter, P. A., Ostendorf, W. R., & LaPlante, N. (2018). Administering vaginal instillations. In *Clinical nursing skills and techniques* (pp. 565–569) (9th ed.). Mosby.

Sanoski, C. A., & Vallerand, A. H. (2021). *Davis's drug guide for nurses* (17th ed.). F.A. Davis.

M

Medication Administration: Ventricular Reservoir   2307

Definition: Administration and monitoring of medication through an indwelling catheter into the lateral ventricle of the brain

Activities:

- Follow agency policies and procedures for accurate and safe administration of medications
- Promote environment that maximizes safe and efficient administration of medications
- Familiarize self with condition of person receiving medications, and indications and information related to medication (e.g., dosage ranges, expected therapeutic effects, possible adverse reactions, interactions with other medications)
- Check accuracy and completeness of each medication administration record (MAR) prior to giving any medications
- Review health history and history of allergies
- Determine person's knowledge of medication and understanding of method of administration
- Instruct on medication purpose and answer questions appropriately
- Follow six rights of medication administration (e.g., right person, right medication, right dose, right route, right time, right documentation)
- Identify using at least two identifiers (e.g., name, birthdate)
- Perform necessary pre-medication evaluations (e.g., blood pressure, pulse, blood sugar assessment, pain level)
- Determine comfort level
- Monitor neurological status and vital signs
- Remove hair over reservoir as per agency protocol
- Maintain aseptic technique, including wearing of masks to avoid droplet transmission of oropharyngeal flora
- Prepare scalp with antiseptic scrub, using aqueous chlorhexidine solution or povidone iodine solution and allowing to dry completely before access
- Fill reservoir with cerebral spinal fluid by applying pressure gently with index finger
- Pierce reservoir with smaller or thinner needle, in oblique fashion and then aspirate while noting color and opacity of cerebral spinal fluid
- Collect cerebral spinal fluid specimen, as appropriate per order or agency protocol
- Evaluate cerebral spinal fluid for blood or cloudy returns before injection of medication
- Prepare and store intrathecal medications separately and clearly labeled "For Intrathecal Use"
- Perform independent double check with another qualified licensed health care provider prior to medication administration and when syringe or medication container, rate, or concentration changed

- Verify safety of intraventricular route and its mixture with preservative-free 0.9% sodium chloride or solutions for chemotherapies (e.g., methotrexate sodium, cytarabine)
- Inject medication slowly per health care provider order and according to agency protocol, using appropriate size needles with filters
- Use only medications without preservatives for ventricular reservoirs
- Apply pressure with index finger to reservoir to ensure mixing of medication with cerebral spinal fluid
- Ensure availability of naloxone to treat inadvertent overdoses
- Ensure reservoir never allowed to be empty
- Ensure strict attention to needle placement to avoid accidental injection into surrounding tissue
- Consider use of ultrasound to access pump septum, if indicated
- Apply dressing to site, as appropriate
- Observe site for signs of bleeding and CSF leakage
- Monitor for 2 hours in supine position for any neurological deterioration
- Maintain peripheral IV access for at least 24 hours due to potential need for naloxone administration for respiratory depression
- Monitor for central nervous system infection (e.g., fever, change in level of consciousness, nausea, vomiting)
- Document medication administration and response according to agency protocol

Background Evidence:

Berman, A., Snyder, S. J., & Frandsen, G. (2018). *Kozier and Erb's fundamentals of nursing: Concepts, process and practice* (pp. 750–829) (10th ed.). Pearson.

Infusion Nurses Society. (2021). Infusion therapy standards of practice 8th edition. *Journal of Intravenous Nursing, 39*(1S), 1–179.

Jeston, S. (2020). *Ventricular reservoir management in neonates.* The Royal Children's Hospital in Melbourne. https://www.rch.org.au/rchcpg/hospital_clinical_guideline_index/Ventricular_reservoir_management_in_Neonates/

Kirby, N. (2021). Medication administration. In R. F. Craven, C. J. Hirnle, & C. J. Henshaw (Eds.), *Fundamentals of nursing: Human health and function* (8th ed., pp. 410–471). Wolters-Kluwer.

Potter, P. A., Ostendorf, W. R., & LaPlante, N. (2018). Parenteral medications. In *Clinical nursing skills and techniques* (pp. 580–628) (9th ed.). Mosby.

Potter, P. A., Ostendorf, W. R., & LaPlante, N. (2018). Safe medication preparation: *Clinical nursing skills and techniques* (pp. 501–522) (9th ed.). Mosby.

Sanoski, C. A., & Vallerand, A. H. (2021). *Davis's drug guide for nurses* (17th ed.). F.A. Davis.

Zubair, A., & De Jesus, O. (2021). Ommaya Reservoir. In *StatPearls*. StatPearls Publishing. https://www.ncbi.nlm.nih.gov/books/NBK559011/

2nd edition 1996; revised 2000, 2004, 2024

Medication Deprescribing

2370

M

Definition: Intentional tapering, discontinuing, or withdrawing drugs to manage polypharmacy or reduce risk of adverse side effects

Activities:

- Determine goals of medication therapy
- Obtain complete medication history (i.e., examining medication vials or list, communicating with health care providers and pharmacy)
- Verify medication history with person and family
- Reconcile medication list for duplicate prescriptions
- Document current drug name, dosage, frequency, and route on medication list
- Determine if prescribed medication still indicated and clinically appropriate
- Consult with other health care professionals to minimize number and frequency of medications needed for therapeutic effect
- Evaluate risks and benefits of tapering or discontinuing any medication on list
- Consult published guidelines on appropriateness of medication use (i.e., Beers Criteria for potentially inappropriate medication use in older adults)
- Prioritize medications to discontinue based on clinical guidelines
- Follow published evidence-based recommendations to guide medication discontinuation or tapering
- Share decision-making with other health care providers, person, and family
- Provide written instructions for medication discontinuation or taper schedule for person and family, as appropriate
- Monitor for potential adverse events from medication discontinuation
- Evaluate need for restarting therapy

8th edition 2024

Background Evidence:

Chou, J., Tong, M., & Brandt, N. (2019). Combating polypharmacy through deprescribing potentially inappropriate medications. *Journal of Gerontological Nursing, 45*(1), 9–15.

Farrell, B., Richardson, L., Raman-Wilms, L., de Launay, D., Alsabbagh, M. W., & Conklin, J. (2018). Self-efficacy for deprescribing: A survey for health care professionals using evidence-based deprescribing guidelines. *Research in Social & Administrative Pharmacy: RSAP, 14*(1), 18–25. https://doi.org/10.1016/j.sapharm.2017.01.003

Murdoch, V. (2020). Inappropriate use of diuretics and antibiotics for wet or 'leaky' legs. *Journal of Community Nursing, 34*(4), 58–62.

Nierop-van Baalen, C., Grypdonck, M., Hecke, A., & Verhaeghe, S. (2020). Associated factors of hope in cancer patients during treatment: A systematic literature review. *Journal of Advanced Nursing, 76*(7), 1520–1537.

Sun, W., Tahsin, F., Lam, A., & Pizzaccalla, A. (2019). Raising awareness about the critical importance of the nursing role in deprescribing medication for older adults. *The Journal of the Gerontological Nursing Association, 40*(4), 17–22.

Tjia, J., DeSanto-Madeya, S., Mazor, K., Han, P., Nguyen, B., Curran, T., Gallagher, J., & Clayton, M. (2019). Nurses' perspectives on family caregiver medication management support and deprescribing. *Journal of Hospice & Palliative Nursing, 21*(4), 312–318.

Medication Management 2380

Definition: Facilitation of safe and effective use of medications

Activities:

- Use standardized tool to elicit all medication information, including prescribed medications, non-prescription medications, and dietary and herbal supplements
- Determine medications needed and administer according to prescriptive authority or protocol
- Identify types and amounts of non-prescription medications used
- Provide information about use of non-prescription medications and how may influence existing condition
- Determine if using culturally based home health remedies and possible effects on use of non-prescription and prescribed medications
- Monitor effectiveness of medication administration modality
- Monitor therapeutic effect of medication
- Monitor for signs and symptoms of medication toxicity or adverse effects
- Monitor serum blood levels (e.g., electrolytes, prothrombin, medications), as appropriate
- Monitor for nontherapeutic medication interactions
- Review periodically with person and family types and amounts of medications taken
- Discuss financial concerns related to medication regimen and ability to obtain needed medications
- Determine ability to self-medicate or need for medication administration assistance
- Discard old, discontinued, or contraindicated medications
- Facilitate changes in medication with health care provider, as appropriate
- Monitor for response to changes in medication regimen
- Determine knowledge about medication regimen
- Determine factors that preclude person from taking medications as prescribed
- Develop strategies to enhance concordance with prescribed medication regimen (i.e., manage side effects of medications, use lower cost generic versions when appropriate, use medication delivery services)
- Investigate possible financial resources for acquisition of prescribed medications, as appropriate
- Determine effect of medication use on lifestyle
- Provide alternatives for timing and modality of self-administered medications to minimize undesired lifestyle effects
- Assist in making necessary lifestyle adjustments associated with medications, as appropriate
- Consult with other health care professionals to minimize number and frequency of medications needed for therapeutic effect
- Communicate clearly with other health care professionals to incorporate person's priorities and preferences
- Obtain health care provider order for self-medication, as appropriate
- Instruct in method of medications administration, as appropriate
- Instruct in expected action and side effects of medication
- Instruct when to seek medical attention
- Provide written and visual information to enhance self-administration of medications, as appropriate
- Establish protocol for storage, restocking, and monitoring of medications left at bedside for self-medication purposes
- Review strategies for managing medication regimen
- Provide list of resources to contact for further information about medication regimen
- Contact post discharge, as appropriate, to answer questions and discuss concerns associated with medication regime
- Encourage to have screening tests to determine medication effects, as needed
- Use teach-back to ensure understanding

1st edition 1992; revised 1996, 2000, 2004, 2024

Background Evidence:

Berman, A., Snyder, S. J., & Frandsen, G. (2018). *Kozier and Erb's Fundamentals of nursing: Concepts, process and practice* (pp. 750–829) (10th ed.). Pearson.

Kirby, N. (2021). Medication administration. In R. F. Craven, C. J. Hirnle, & C. J. Henshaw (Eds.), *Fundamentals of nursing: Human health and function* (8th ed., pp. 410–471). Wolters-Kluwer.

Potter, P. A., Ostendorf, W. R., & LaPlante, N. (2018). Safe medication preparation. In *Clinical nursing skills and techniques* (pp. 501–522) (9th ed.). Mosby.

Sanoski, C. A., & Vallerand, A. H. (2021). *Davis's drug guide for nurses* (17th ed.). F.A. Davis.

Tomlinson, J., Cheong, V., Fylan, B., Silcock, J., Smith, H., Karban, K., & Blenkinsopp, A. (2020). Successful care transitions for older people: A systematic review and meta-analysis of the effects of interventions that support medication continuity. *Age and Ageing, 49*(4), 558–569. https://doi.org/10.1093/ageing/afaa002

Williams, P. (2020). Medications and older adults. In *Basic geriatric nursing* (pp. 132–149) (7th ed.). Elsevier.

Medication Management: Medical Cannabis 2385

Definition: Preparing, administering, or evaluating the effectiveness of medical marijuana

Activities:

- Determine current stage of legalization of medical and recreational cannabis use in state of practice
- Determine principles of local medical marijuana dispensaries (e.g., how persons qualify, who can obtain cannabis from dispensary)
- Provide certification for qualifying conditions (e.g., cachexia, chemotherapy induced nausea and vomiting, chronic pain, neuropathies)
- Instruct on medications to be given, and answer questions appropriately
- Follow six rights of medication administration (e.g., right person, right medication, right dose, right route, right time, right documentation)
- Document dosages and responses in record

- Monitor for undesirable side effects or toxicities of cannabis (e.g., hallucinations, dry eye, paranoia, decreased blood pressure, impaired attention or memory)
- Instruct to titrate own dose using principle of "start low, go slow" and monitoring efficacy and adverse effects
- Instruct to regularly track dose, symptoms, relief, and adverse effects in journal
- Instruct to store safely, in locked area and out of reach of children, and dispose of properly (i.e., collection receptacle located in pharmacy)
- Communicate findings of clinical encounter with other health care providers
- Administer cannabis only in medical marijuana approved programs as registered caregiver
- Administer FDA-approved synthetic THC drugs (e.g., dronabinol, nabilone) as per facility formulary and policy
- Use teach-back to ensure understanding

8th edition, 2024

Background Evidence:

Campbell, C. T., Phillips, M. S., & Manasco, K. (2017). Cannabinoids in pediatrics. *The Journal of Pediatric Pharmacology and Therapeutics, 22*(3), 176–185.

National Academies of Sciences, Engineering, and Medicine. (2017). *The health effects of cannabis and cannabinoids: The current state of evidence and recommendations for research.* National Academies Press.

National Conference of State Legislatures (NCSL). (2017). *State Medical Marijuana Laws.* http://www.ncsl.org/research/health/state-medical-marijuana-laws.aspx

Russell, K. A. (2019). Caring for patients using medical marijuana. *Journal of Nursing Regulation, 10*(3), 47–59.

Russell, K. A., & Duderstadt, K. G. (2019). Medical marijuana guidelines for practice: Health policy implications. *Journal of Pediatric Healthcare, 33*(6), 722–726.

The National Council of State Boards of Nursing (NCSBN) Medical Marijuana Guidelines Committee. (2018). The NCSBN national nursing guidelines for medical marijuana. *Journal of Nursing Regulation, 9*(2. Suppl.), S5. https://doi.org/10.1016/S2155-8256(18)30082-6

Medication Management: Wearable Infusion Device   2398

Definition: Facilitating self-administration of continuous or intermittent medication infusion via a delivery device

Activities:

- Determine understanding of medication and method of administration
- Determine ability to control infusion
- Obtain consent or agreement for self-management
- Collaborate with treatment team to ensure accurate communication of infusion plan
- Determine type of pump and necessary steps for programming and use (e.g., continuous or intermittent, basal dose rate adjustment, continuous closed loop glucose monitoring, hybrid closed loop monitoring)
- Develop medication self-administration plan of care
- Ensure care measures in place for emergent episodes of health (e.g., hypoglycemia, hyperglycemia)
- Instruct person, family, and caregivers on plan of care, including blood level monitoring, dose adjustments (e.g., basal, continuous, bolus), and requirements for safe medication administration
- Review needed medication adjustments with activity changes
- Review diet changes required with medication administration
- Instruct person, family, and care providers related to delivery device operations
- Ensure person, family, and care providers have competency with delivery device operations
- Identify pump issues with untoward health episodes (e.g., kinked tubes, leaking catheter set, dislodgement of cannula, hematoma at insertion sites, incorrect programming, low battery, empty medication cartridge)
- Ensure criteria for emergency management of device including possible discontinuation of medication infusion
- Develop plan for labeling and storage of device when temporary cessation or discontinuation occurs
- Monitor psychological status, self-care behavior, education, and training before and during use of device
- Ensure basic physiologic monitoring maintained (e.g., respiratory patterns, blood sugar values, insulin infusion rate, diet, exercise), as indicated by type of medication administered
- Examine insertion site regularly for redness, pain, signs of infection or signs of lipodystrophy, assuring rotation of site as indicated
- Ensure site rotated every 2 to 3 days
- Assist with adjustments to pump infusion as indicated
- Assist with adjustments to pump location as indicated (i.e., removal for activities such as bathing, swimming, contact sports)
- Provide ongoing motivation, education and support as indicated, particularly to school age children and adolescents
- Ensure access to device manufacturer and contact information
- Instruct in accessing device data (e.g., dose, infusion time, blood values)
- Obtain supplies related to brand of pump (e.g., tubing, needles, arm band, batteries)
- Perform pump maintenance in required time frame
- Ensure monitoring requirements and best practice assessments consistent with institutional policies
- Ensure documentation includes device used, medication administered, method of device management, and monitoring requirements per institutional documentation policies
- Provide nurse contact information for post-discharge issues
- Instruct to carry identification of device information
- Use teach-back to ensure understanding

8th edition 2024

Background Evidence:

Bostelman, C. (2019). 5-Fluorouracil infiltrations and ambulatory pumps: Education, prevention, and management considerations. *Clinical Journal of Oncology Nursing, 23*(5), 537–539. https://doi.org/10.1188/19.CJON.537-539

Cinar, A. (2019). Automated insulin delivery algorithms. *Diabetes Spectrum, 32*(3), 209–214. https://doi.org/10.2337/ds18-0100

Collard, S. S., Regmi, P. R., Hood, K. K., Laffel, L., Weissberg, B. J., Naranjo, D., & Barnard, K. K. (2020). Exercising with an automated insulin delivery system: Qualitative insight into the hopes and expectations of people with

M

type 1 diabetes. *Practical Diabetes*, *37*(1), 19–23. https://doi.org/10.1002/pdi.2255

Grissinger, M. (2018). Ambulatory pump safety: Managing home infusion patients admitted to the emergency department and hospital. *Pharmacy & Therapeutics*, *43*(8), 450–45.

Heile, M., Hollstegge, B., Broxterman, L., Cai, A., & Close, K. (2020). Automated insulin delivery: Easy enough to use in primary care?. *Clinical Diabetes*, 474–485. https://doi.org/10.2337/cd20-0050

Latham, J. (2019). The artificial pancreas: What school nurses need to know. *NASN School Nurse*, *34*(2), 86–89. https://doi.org/10.1177/1942602X18804491

Paparella, S. F. (2018). Ambulatory infusion pumps: Coming to an Emergency Department near you. *Journal of Emergency Nursing*, *44*(5), 517–519.

Ramkissoon, C., Herrero, P., Bondia, J., & Vehi, J. (2018). Unannounced meals in the artificial pancreas: Detection using continuous glucose monitoring. *Sensors*, *18*(3), E884. https://doi.org/10.3390/s18030884

Turksoy, K., Frantz, N., Quinn, L., Dumin, M., Kilkus, J., Hibner, B., Cinar, A., & Littlejohn, E. (2017). Automated insulin delivery: The light at the end of the tunnel. *Journal of Pediatrics*, *186*, 17–28. https://doi.org/10.1016/j.jpeds.2017.0055

Medication Prescribing 2390

Definition: Prescribing medication for health promotion

Activities:

- Evaluate signs and symptoms of current health problem
- Determine past health history and medication use
- Review current medications and indications for each medication's use
- Identify known allergies and reactions
- Determine ability to administer medication
- Identify medications indicated for current problems
- Compare new medications with current medications to ensure compatibility, potentially inappropriate medications, drug-drug interactions, and drug-disease interactions in persons with comorbidities
- Prescribe medications according to prescriptive authority and protocol
- Write prescription, using name of medication and including dose and directions for administration
- Spell out problematic abbreviations that are easily misunderstood (e.g., micrograms, milligrams, units)
- Verify that decimal points used in dosages are clearly seen by using leading zeros (e.g., 0.2 vs. .2)
- Avoid use of trailing zeros (e.g., 2 vs. 2.0)
- Use electronic prescribing methods, as available
- Use standardized abbreviations, acronyms, and symbols
- Verify that all medication orders are written accurately, completely, and with necessary discrimination for intended use
- Follow recommendations for starting doses of medication (e.g., milligrams per kilogram body weight, body surface area, lowest effective dose)
- Use appropriate laboratory monitoring of medication effects, as indicated
- Consult with pharmacist, as appropriate
- Seek regular input from pharmacist to reduce inappropriate prescribing
- Consult reliable references as necessary
- Simplify medication regimen by using once-daily dosing and generic drugs where possible
- Initiate medications one at a time at lowest dose possible
- Identify risks and benefits of any new medication prior to prescribing
- Regularly review medication list to reduce inappropriate prescribing and polypharmacy
- Instruct about method of drug administration, as appropriate
- Instruct about rationale for use, expected action and side effects of medication
- Consider potential adverse drug event as cause of any new symptom
- Avoid "prescribing cascade" in which medications are started to treat adverse drug event
- Provide alternatives for timing and modality of self-administered medications to minimize lifestyle effects
- Instruct about how to fill prescription as necessary
- Encourage to use one pharmacy and inform pharmacist of any medication changes to decrease risk of error
- Instruct about when to seek additional assistance
- Verify compliance with medication regime routinely
- Monitor for therapeutic and adverse effects of medication, as appropriate
- Revisit medication efficacy and continued use as needed for each medication
- Discontinue medications with reported intolerable side effects, lack of therapeutic effects, or lack of compliance with regime
- Maintain knowledge of medications used in practice, including indications for use, precautions, adverse effects, toxic effects, and dosing information, as required by prescriptive authority rules and regulations
- Use teach-back to ensure understanding

2nd edition 1996; revised 2004, 2024

Background Evidence:

Anderson, R., & Ferguson, R. (2020). A nurse practitioner–led medication reconciliation process to reduce hospital readmissions from a skilled nursing facility. *Journal of the American Association of Nurse Practitioners*, *32*(2), 160–167.

Fong, J., Buckley, T., Cashin, A., & Pont, L. (2017). Nurse practitioner prescribing in Australia: A comprehensive literature review. *Australian Critical Care*, *30*(5), 252–259. https://doi.org/10.1016/j.aucc.2016.11.003

Fong, J., Cashin, A., & Buckley, T. (2020). Models of prescribing, scope of practice, and medicines prescribed, a survey of nurse practitioners. *Journal of Advanced Nursing (John Wiley & Sons, Inc.)*, *76*(9), 2311–2322. https://doi.org/10.1111/jan.14444

Granara, B., & Laurent, J. (2017). Provider attitudes and practice patterns of obesity management with pharmacotherapy. *Journal of the American Association of Nurse Practitioners*, *29*(9), 543–550.

Hanson, C. M., & Cahill, M. (2019). Understanding regulatory, legal and credentialing requirements. In *Hamric and Hanson's Advanced Practice Nursing: An Integrative approach* (pp. 572–575) (6th ed.). Elsevier.

Kulsick, C., Votta, J., Wright, W. L., White, P., & Strowman, S. (2021). Enhancing medication adherence in older adults at two nurse practitioner–owned clinics. *Journal of the American Association of Nurse Practitioners*, *33*(7), 553–562. https://doi.org/10.1097/JXX.0000000000000414

Nissen, L. (2018). Prescribing in the future. *Lamp*, *75*(10), 24–25.

Stitzlein Davies, P. (2017). Opioids for pain management in older adults: Strategies for safe prescribing. *Nurse Practitioner*, *42*(2), 20–29. https://doi.org/10.1097/01.NPR.0000511772.62176.10

M

Medication Reconciliation   2395

Definition: Creating an accurate list of all medications a person is taking

Activities:

- Reconcile medications at all transition points including admission, transfer, and discharge
- Reconcile medications with changes in condition or with medication changes
- Use standardized tool to elicit all medication information, including prescribed medications, over-the-counter medications, and dietary and herbal supplements
- Eliminate distractions and go slowly when reconciling medications
- Collect list of medications when admitted to health care institution, seen in outpatient setting, or transferred between units or institutions
- Obtain complete medication history by examining medication vials or list, verifying with person and family, and communicating with health care providers and pharmacy, as needed
- Document drug name, dosage, frequency, and route on medication list
- Determine when medications were last taken
- Compare medication list to indications and medical history to ensure complete and accurate list
- Compare medications currently taking or should be taking, with newly ordered medications, to address duplication, omissions, interactions, and need to continue current medications
- Compare initial home medication list, current medication orders, and discharge medication orders to ensure medications appropriately continued, resumed, or discontinued upon discharge
- Communicate discrepancies to ordering practitioners as needed
- Provide with written information about medications to take upon discharge, for each medication
- Explain importance of managing medication information upon discharge
- Instruct to maintain updated medication list and reconcile with health care provider at each appointment or hospital admission
- Instruct to obtain all medications through one pharmacy to decrease risk of error
- Instruct to take active role in medication management
- Use teach-back to ensure understanding

5th edition 2008; revised 2024

Background Evidence:

Berman, A., Snyder, S. J., & Frandsen, G. (2018). *Kozier and Erb's Fundamentals of nursing: Concepts, process and practice* (pp. 750–829) (10th ed.). Pearson.

Fredericks, T. (2018). Medication reconciliation. *MEDSURG Nursing, 27*(5), 329–330.

Guisado-Gil, A. B., Mejías-Trueba, M., Alfaro-Lara, E. R., Sánchez-Hidalgo, M., Ramírez-Duque, N., & Santos-Rubio, M. D. (2020). Impact of medication reconciliation on health outcomes: An overview of systematic reviews. *Research in Social & Administrative Pharmacy, 16*(8), 995–1002. https://doi.org/10.1016/j.sapharm.2019.10.011

Institute for Healthcare Improvement. (2018). Reconcile medications at all transition points. http://www.ihi.org/resources/Pages/Changes/Reconcile MedicationsatAllTransitionPoints.aspx

Marien, S., Krug, B., & Spinewine, A. (2017). Electronic tools to support medication reconciliation: A systematic review. *Journal of the American Medical Informatics Association, 24*(1), 227–240. https://doi.org/10.1093/jamia/ocw068

Ostendorf, W. R. (2021). Medication administration. In P. A. Potter, A. G. Perry, P. A. Stockert, & A. Hall (Eds.), *Fundamentals of nursing* (10th ed., pp. 606–607). Elsevier.

Potter, P. A., Ostendorf, W. R., & LaPlante, N. (2018).). Safe medication preparation. *In Clinical nursing skills and techniques* (pp. 501–522) (9th ed.). Mosby.

Romanoski, M. (2018). Improving practice—Reconciliation of medications. *Geriatric Nursing, 39*(6), 723–724. https://doi.org/10.1016/j.gerinurse.2018.10.010

Sanoski, C. A., & Vallerand, A. H. (2021). *Davis's drug guide for nurses* (17th ed.). F.A. Davis.

The Joint Commission. (2018). Ambulatory health care national patient safety goals. https://www.jointcommission.org/assets/1/6/2018_AHC_NPSG_goals_final.pdf

Tong, M., Hye Young Oh, Thomas, J., Patel, S., Hardesty, J. L., & Brandt, N. J. (2017). Nursing home medication reconciliation. *Journal of Gerontological Nursing, 43*(4), 9–14. https://doi.org/10.3928/00989134-20170313-04

M

Meditation Facilitation   5960

Definition: Facilitating a relaxed internal state of expanded awareness in the present moment by concentrating focus on a sound, object, visual image, the breath, or movement

Activities:

- Discuss the patient's previous experience with meditation
- Discuss the patient's desire to learn meditation
- Explain that during meditation one is calm, yet alert
- Provide quiet time, free of interruptions
- Select a calm and peaceful environment
- Suggest the patient wear comfortable clothing
- Decide how long the meditation session will be
- Instruct patient to sit in a comfortable position with the back straight and hands resting in the lap, if possible
- Inform the patient that the eyes can be closed or open, gently glancing down about three feet in front
- Help the patient choose an object to focus the attention on such as a breath, a word, or the body as a whole
- Instruct the patient to focus attention on the chosen object, and when the mind wanders off in thought, to let go of the thought and gently bring attention back to the chosen object
- Instruct the patient to just sit free of thought if the object of awareness becomes subtler or fades away

- Instruct to return attention to the chosen object whenever thoughts arise in the mind rather than engaging in thinking or daydreaming
- Encourage patient to meditate for about 10 minutes each day, eventually increasing the time as desired to about 25 minutes or twice a day
- Suggest meditation groups in which the patient can receive support and further instruction in meditation

1st edition 1992; revised 2000, 2018

Background Evidence:

Austin, J. H. (2011). *Meditating selflessly: Practical neural Zen.* Massachusetts Institute of Technology Press.

Kabat-Zinn, J. (2012). *Mindfulness for beginners: Reclaiming the present moment and your life.* Sounds-True.

Lutz, A., Slagter, H., Dunne, J., & Davidson, R. (2008). Attention regulation and monitoring in meditation. *Trends in Cognitive Sciences, 12*(4), 163–169.

Watson, J. (2008). *Nursing: Philosophy and science of caring (revised).* University Press of Colorado.

Memory Training 4760

Definition: Facilitation of memory

Activities:

- Discuss any memory problems experienced
- Stimulate memory by repeating last expressed thought, as appropriate
- Reminisce about past experiences, as appropriate
- Mutually develop memory training plan (e.g., type of memory training techniques, frequency, length of sessions, length of program)
- Implement memory techniques (e.g., visual imagery, mnemonic devices, memory games, memory cues, association techniques, making lists)
- Provide and assist with use of memory training apps, websites, or computer programs
- Assist in associate-learning tasks (i.e., practice learning and recalling verbal and pictorial information presented)
- Provide for orientation training (e.g., rehearsing personal information, dates), as appropriate
- Provide opportunity for concentration (i.e., matching pairs of cards), as appropriate
- Provide opportunity to use memory for recent events (i.e., question about recent outing)
- Provide for picture recognition memory, as appropriate
- Structure teaching methods according to person's organization of information
- Refer for neurological testing as appropriate
- Refer for occupational and activity therapy as appropriate
- Encourage to participate in group memory training programs, as appropriate
- Monitor behavior during training
- Identify and correct errors in orientation, as appropriate
- Monitor changes in memory with training

1st edition 1992; revised 2004, 2024

Background Evidence:

Dentz, A., Guay, M. C., Parent, V., & Romo, L. (2020). Working memory training for adults with ADHD. *Journal of Attention Disorders, 24*(6), 918–927.

McDougall, G. J., McDonough, I. M., & LaRocca, M. (2019). Memory training for adults with probable mild cognitive impairment: A pilot study. *Aging & Mental Health, 23*(10), 1433–1441.

Pang, S. H., Lim, S. F., & Siah, C. J. (2021). Online memory training intervention for early-stage dementia: A systematic review and meta-analysis. *Journal of Advanced Nursing, 77*(3), 1141–1154.

Sala, G., & Gobet, F. (2020). Working memory training in typically developing children: A multilevel meta-analysis. *Psychonomic Bulletin & Review, 27*(3), 423–434.

Yang, H. -L., Chan, P. -T., Chang, P. -C., Chiu, H. -L., Sheen Hsiao, S. -T., Chu, H., & Chou, K. -R. (2018). Memory-focused interventions for people with cognitive disorders: A systematic review and meta-analysis of randomized controlled studies. *International Journal of Nursing Studies, 78*, 44–51. https://doi.org/10.1016/j.ijnurstu.2017.08.005

Milieu Therapy 4390

Definition: Use of people, resources, and events in the patient's immediate environment to promote optimal psychosocial functioning

Activities:

- Determine factors in environment that contribute to patient's behavior
- Regulate environmental factors to maximize adaptive behavior and minimize maladaptive behavior
- Consider needs of others in addition to needs of particular individual
- Provide self-care resources for use by patient
- Enhance the normality of the environment through use of clocks, calendars, railings, furniture, etc.
- Facilitate open communication among patient, nurses, and other staff
- Build a therapeutic rapport with individuals conveying genuine regard, respect, care, and compassion
- Model effective interpersonal, distress tolerance, and emotion regulation skills
- Be neither too rigid nor too flexible with rules
- Define clear and consistent rules and policies for patients, family members, and staff
- Notice and reinforce new, adaptive behaviors
- Provide descriptions of problematic behavior in objective, nonjudgmental, nonpejorative terms, avoiding stigmatizing labels
- Include patient in decisions about own care

M

- Define treatment goals collaboratively with the patient, linking privileges to goal progress and achievement, when appropriate
- Communicate individual patient treatment goals with all staff members
- Provide one-on-one nursing care, as appropriate
- Check on the patient regularly
- Support formal and informal group activities to promote sharing, cooperation, compromise, and leadership
- Provide time and space for rehearsal of new behaviors in order to build mastery and adapt to future environments
- Examine own attitudes toward issues of patients' rights, self-determination, social control, and deviancy
- Use empathy when interpreting the behaviors of patients and colleagues
- Ensure staff presence and supervision
- Minimize restrictions that diminish privacy or self-control, when appropriate
- Encourage use of personal property
- Minimize as much as possible the use of locked doors, medications, and strict regulations of activity or property
- Provide a telephone in a private space, when appropriate
- Encouraging appropriate patient-to-patient interactions
- Provide attractively furnished areas for private conversations with other patients, family, and friends
- Provide books, magazines, and arts and crafts materials in accordance with patient's recreational, cultural, and educational background and needs
- Monitor individual behavior that may be disruptive or detrimental to overall well-being of others
- Respond to disruptive or detrimental behavior safely, utilizing least restrictive measures

- Prevent use of physical, mechanical, and chemical restraint, when possible
- Limit the number of unmedicated psychotic patients at any time through controlled admissions and varying lengths of medication-free trials, as appropriate

1st edition 1992; revised 1996, 2018

Background Evidence:

Bak, J., Brandt-Christensen, M., Sestoft, D. M., & Zoffman, V. (2012). Mechanical restraint—Which interventions prevent episodes of mechanical restraint?—A systematic review. *Perspectives in Psychiatric Care*, 48(2), 83–94.

Mahoney, J., Palyo, N., Napier, G., & Giordano, J. (2009). The therapeutic milieu reconceptualized for the 21st century. *Archives of Psychiatric Nursing*, 23(6), 423–429.

Oeye, C., Bjelland, A., Skorpen, A., & Anderssen, N. (2009). Raising adults as children? A report on milieu therapy in a psychiatric ward in Norway. *Issues in Mental Health Nursing*, 30(3), 151–158.

Sadock, B. J., & Sadock, V. A. (2007). *Kaplan & Sadock's synopsis of psychiatry: Behavioral sciences/clinical psychiatry* (pp. 970–971) (10th ed.). Wolters Kluwer Health/Lippincott Williams & Wilkins.

Swenson, C. R., Witterholt, S., & Bohus, M. (2007). Dialectical behavior therapy on inpatient units. In L. A. Dimeff & K. Koerner (Eds.), *Dialectical behavior therapy in clinical practice: Applications across disorders and settings* (pp. 69–111). The Guilford Press.

Thibeault, C., Trudeau, K., d'Entremont, M., & Brown, T. (2010). Understanding the milieu experiences of patients on an acute inpatient psychiatric unit. *Archives of Psychiatric Nursing*, 24(4), 216–226.

M

Mood Management   5330

Definition: Providing for safety, stabilization, recovery, and maintenance for a person experiencing depression or elevated mood

Activities:

- Review initial assessment of mood (e.g., signs, symptoms, personal history)
- Evaluate for changes in mood on regular basis as treatment progresses
- Administer self-report questionnaires (e.g., PHQ-9, Hamilton Depression Scale, Geriatric Depression Scale, Beck Depression Inventory, Social Functioning Questionnaire, other depression and functional status scales), as appropriate
- Determine whether safety risk to self or others
- Consider hospitalization if severity of mood disorder poses safety risk, person unable to meet self-care needs, or lacks sufficient social support
- Initiate necessary precautions to safeguard those at risk for physical harm (e.g., suicide, self-harm, elopement, violence)
- Provide or refer for substance abuse treatment, when contributing factor to mood disorder
- Adjust or discontinue medications contributing to mood disorders, per appropriately licensed practitioner
- Refer for evaluation or treatment for underlying medical illness that may be contributing to dysfunctional mood (e.g., thyroid disorders)
- Monitor self-care ability (e.g., grooming, hygiene, food and fluid intake, elimination)
- Assist with self-care, as needed

- Monitor physical status (e.g., body weight, hydration)
- Monitor and regulate level of activity and stimulation in environment in accord with needs
- Assist to maintain normal cycle of sleep and wakefulness (e.g., scheduled rest times, relaxation techniques, sedating medications, limit caffeine)
- Assist to assume increasing responsibility for self-care
- Provide opportunity for physical activity (e.g., walking, riding exercise bike)
- Monitor cognitive functioning (e.g., concentration, attention, memory, ability to process information, decision-making ability)
- Use simple, concrete, here-and-now language during interactions if cognitively compromised
- Use memory aides and visual cues to assist if cognitively compromised
- Limit decision-making opportunities if cognitively compromised
- Provide instruction on use of decision-making skills, as needed
- Encourage to engage in increasingly more complex decision-making
- Encourage to take active role in treatment and rehabilitation, as appropriate
- Provide or refer for psychotherapy (e.g., cognitive behavioral, interpersonal, marital, family, group), when appropriate

- Interact at regular intervals to convey caring and provide opportunity to talk about feelings
- Help to consciously self-monitor mood (e.g., 1–10 rating scale, journaling)
- Help identify thoughts and feelings underlying dysfunctional mood
- Limit amount of time allowed to express negative feelings or accounts of past failures
- Assist to ventilate feelings in appropriate manner (e.g., punching bag, art therapy, vigorous physical activity)
- Help identify precipitants of dysfunctional mood (e.g., chemical imbalances, situational stressors, grief and loss, physical problems)
- Help identify aspects of precipitants that can or cannot be changed
- Assist in identification of available resources, personal strengths, and abilities to use in modifying precipitants of dysfunctional mood
- Provide instruction on new coping and problem-solving skills
- Encourage to engage in social interactions and activities with others
- Provide social skills and assertiveness training as needed
- Provide feedback regarding appropriateness of social behaviors
- Use limit setting and behavioral management strategies to assist in refraining from intrusive and disruptive behavior
- Use restrictive interventions only if necessary (e.g., area restriction, seclusion, physical restraint, chemical restraint), to manage unsafe or inappropriate behavior not responsive to less restrictive behavior management interventions
- Manage and treat hallucinations or delusions that may accompany mood disorder
- Prescribe, adjust, and discontinue medications used to treat dysfunctional mood, per appropriately licensed practitioner
- Administer mood-stabilizing medications (e.g., antidepressants, lithium, anticonvulsants, antipsychotics, anxiolytics, hormones, vitamins)
- Monitor for medication side effects
- Treat medication side effects or adverse drug reactions
- Monitor serum blood levels of medications (e.g., tricyclic antidepressants, lithium, anticonvulsants), as appropriate
- Promote medication concordance

- Assist with provision of electroconvulsive therapy (ECT) treatments when indicated
- Monitor physiological and mental status immediately after ECT
- Assist with provision of phototherapy to elevate mood
- Explain ECT or phototherapy procedures
- Monitor response to ECT or phototherapy
- Provide medication teaching
- Provide illness teaching if dysfunctional mood is illness based (e.g., depression, mania, premenstrual syndrome)
- Provide guidance about development and maintenance of support systems (e.g., family, friends, spiritual resources, support groups, counseling)
- Assist to anticipate and cope with life changes (e.g., new job, leave of absence from work, new peer group)
- Provide follow-up at appropriate intervals, as needed
- Use teach-back to ensure understanding

2nd edition 1996; revised 2000; 2024

Background Evidence:

Bingham, K. S., Flint, A. J., & Mulsant, B. H. (2019). Management of late-life depression in the context of cognitive impairment: A review of the recent literature. *Current Psychiatry Reports, 21*(8), 74.

Butcher, H. K., & Ingram, T. (2018). Secondary suicide prevention in later life. *Journal of Gerontological Nursing, 44*(11), 20–32.

Butcher, H. (2017). Reactive depression. In M. Maas, J. Specht, P. Mobily, D. Schoenfelder, & A. Stineman (Eds.). *Care of older persons for optimum quality of life: Nursing diagnoses, outcomes, and interventions* (Vol. 3). Iowa City, Iowa: University of Iowa College of Nursing Barbara and Richard Csomay Center for Gerontological Excellence.

D'Anci, K. E., Uhl, S., Giradi, G., & Martin, C. (2019). Treatments for the prevention and management of suicide: A systematic review. *Annals of Internal Medicine, 171*(5), 334–342.

Edwards, G., Nuckols, T., Herrera, N., Danovitch, I., & Iskak, W. W. (2019). Improving depression management in patients with medical illness using collaborative care: Linking treatment from the inpatient to the outpatient setting. *Innovations in Clinical Neuroscience, 16*(11/12), 19–24.

Malhi, G. S., & Mann, J. J. (2018). Depression. *Lancet, 392*(10161), 2299–2312.

Oquendo, M. A. (2019). Developing effective strategies for the management of depression and suicidal thoughts. *Revista brasileira de psiquiatria, 41*(5), 375.

Motivational Interviewing 4395

Definition: Use of a collaborative person-centered conversational approach for strengthening motivation and commitment to change

Activities:

- Establish partnership based on trust and respect
- Display interest in person
- Demonstrate unconditional acceptance
- Convey absolute worth and compassion
- Encourage expression of thought and feelings
- Mutually establish purpose and goals for conversation
- Ask what change they would like to make
- Ask why they want to make change
- Elicit perspective about concerns, issues, or problems
- Use reflective listening (e.g., mirror what person saying by repeating what was expressed)
- Guide in connecting feelings to thoughts
- Strive for mutual understanding of experience
- Affirm efforts and strengths

- Offer information designed to provide deeper understanding of concerns, with permission
- Assist in defining needed change
- Assist in developing own solutions (i.e., ask how to go about making change to have succuss)
- Focus on resolving ambivalence about making desired changes
- Ask to identify at least three reasons for making change
- Collaboratively explore motivation and commitment to making change (i.e., ask how important it is to make change)
- Recognize that true power for change rests within person
- Help identify achievements already made toward making desired changes
- Assist to identify barriers limiting change
- Mutually explore strategies to overcome barriers limiting change

- Evoke plan for change while reinforcing positive motivations for change
- Conclude with summary of conversation and plan for change

8th edition 2024

Background Evidence:

Frost, H., Campbell, P., Maxwell, M., O'Carroll, R. E., Dombrowski, R. U., Williams, B., Cheyne, H., Coles, E., & Pollock, A. (2018). Effectiveness of motivational interviewing on adult behavior change in health and social care settings: A systematic review of reviews. *PLoS ONE, 13*(10), e0204890. https://doi.org/10.1371/journal.pone.0204890

Miller, W. R., & Rollnick, S. (2013). *Motivational interviewing: Helping people change* (3rd ed.). Guilford.

Palacio, A., Garay, D., Langer, B., Taylor, J., Wood, B., & Tamariz, L. (2016). Motivational interviewing improves medication adherence: A systematic review and meta-analysis. *Journal of General Internal Medicine*, (8), 929–940. https://doi.org/10.1007/s11606-016-3685-3

Seigart, D., Veltman, M., Willhaus, J., & Letterle, C. (2018). Implementation of motivational interviewing training in an undergraduate nursing curriculum: Identifying adolescents at risk for substance use. *International Journal of Research in Public Health, 15*(8), 1623. https://doi.org/10.3390/ijerph15081623

Stallings, D. T., & Schneider, J. K. (2018). Motivational interviewing and fat consumption in older adults: A meta-analysis. *Journal of Gerontological Nursing, 44*(11), 33–43. https://doi.org/10.3928/00989134-20180817-01

Vallabhan, M. K., Jimenez, E. Y., Nash, J. L., Gonzales-Pacheco, D., Coakley, K. E., Noe, S. R., DeBlieck, C. J., Summers, L. C., Feldstein-Ewing, S. W., & Kong, A. S. (2018). Motivational interviewing to treat adolescents with obesity: A meta-analysis. *Pediatrics, 142*(5), e20180733. https://doi.org/10.1542/peds.2018-0733

Widder, R. (2017). Learning to use motivational interviewing effectively: Modules. *Journal Continuing Education in Nursing, 48*(7), 312–319. https://doi.org/10.3928/00220124-20170616-08

Multidisciplinary Care Conference   8020

Definition: Planning and evaluating patient care with health professionals from other disciplines

Activities:

- Designate a leader who plans and schedules regular and as needed patient care conferences involving the core health care professionals
- Arrange for the health care team members to meet face to face or by videoconference
- Facilitate communication and collaboration among multidisciplinary team members to enassure effective and focused discussions that enable the team members to problem solve and efficiently provide for patient's needs
- Summarize health status data pertinent to planning patient care
- Identify current nursing diagnoses
- Establish mutually agreeable goals
- Involve patient's family members in planning care, as appropriate
- Describe nursing interventions being implemented
- Use the appropriate clinical protocols and evidence-based practice guidelines in planning treatment and care options
- Clarify responsibilities related to implementation of patient's plan of care
- Seek input from all multidisciplinary team members involved in the planning conference
- Describe patient and family responses to nursing interventions
- Seek input about effectiveness of nursing interventions

- Provide data to facilitate evaluation of patient's plan of care
- Discuss progress toward desired patient outcomes
- Recommend changes in treatment plan, as necessary
- Revise the patient's critical pathway or plan of care, as necessary
- Review discharge plans
- Discuss referrals, as appropriate
- Document treatment plans in the interdisciplinary progress notes

2nd edition 1996; revised 2018

Background Evidence:

Berman, A., & Snyder, S. (2012). *Kozier & Erb's fundamentals of nursing: Concepts, process, and practice* (9th ed.). Pearson Education.

Bodenheimer, T. (2008). Coordinating care—a perilous journey through the health care system. *New England Journal of Medicine, 358*(10), 1064–1071.

Ministry of Health. (2012). *Guidance for implementing high-quality multidisciplinary meetings: Achieving best practice cancer care.* Wellington, New Zealand.

Van Houdt, S., De Lepeleire, J., Driessche, K., Thijs, G., & Buntinx, F. (2011). Multidisciplinary team meetings about a patient in primary care: An explorative study. *Journal of Primary Care & Community Health, 2*(2), 72–76.

Music Therapy   4400

Definition: Using music to help achieve a specific change in behavior, feeling, or physiology

Activities:

- Define specific desired change in behavior and physiology (e.g., relaxation, stimulation, concentration, pain reduction)
- Identify musical preferences
- Inform of purpose of music experience
- Choose music selections representative of preferences
- Assist in assuming comfortable position

- Limit extraneous stimuli (e.g., lights, sounds, visitors, telephone calls) during listening experience
- Make music equipment available to individual
- Ensure equipment in good working order
- Provide listening device, as indicated
- Ensure that volume adequate
- Avoid turning music on and leaving on for long periods

M

- Facilitate active participation (e.g., playing instrument, singing) if desired and feasible in setting
- Monitor vital signs, if indicated
- Monitor sleep quality, duration, and response

1st edition 1992; revised 2000, 2004, 2024

Background Evidence:

Cheng, J., Zhang, H., Bao, H., & Hong, H. (2021). Music-based interventions for pain relief in patients undergoing hemodialysis: A PRISMA-compliant systematic review and meta-analysis. *Medicine, 100*(2), e24102. https://doi.org/10.1097/MD.0000000000024102

Govindan, R., Kommu, J., & Bhaskarapillai, B. (2020). The effectiveness of nurses implemented music add-on therapy in children with behavioral problems. *Indian Journal of Psychological Medicine, 42*(3), 274–280. https://doi.org/10.4103/IJPSYM.IJPSYM_240_19

Jing Huang, Xiaohui Yuan, Nan Zhang, Hui Qiu, & Xiangdong Chen. (2021). Music therapy in adults with COPD. *Respiratory Care, 66*(3), 501–509. https://doi.org/10.4187/respcare.07489

Tang, Q., Huang, Z., Zhou, H., & Ye, P. (2020). Effects of music therapy on depression: A meta-analysis of randomized controlled trials. *PLoS ONE, 15*(11), e0240862. https://doi.org/10.1371/journal.pone.0240862

Wurjatmiko, A. T. (2019). The effects of music therapy intervention on the pain and anxiety levels of cancer patient: A systematic review. *International Journal of Nursing Education, 11*(4), 14–18. https://doi.org/10.5958/0974-9357.2019.00079.5

Mutual Goal Setting 4410

Definition: Collaborating with patient to identify and prioritize care goals, then developing a plan for achieving those goals

Activities:

- Encourage the identification of specific life values
- Assist patient and significant other to develop realistic expectations of themselves in performance of their roles
- Determine patient's recognition of own problem
- Encourage the patient to identify own strengths and abilities
- Assist the patient in identifying realistic, attainable goals
- Construct and use goal attainment scaling, as appropriate
- Identify with patient the goals of care
- State goals in positive terms
- Assist the patient in breaking down complex goals into small, manageable steps
- Recognize the patient's value and belief system when establishing goals
- Encourage the patient to state goals clearly, avoiding the use of alternatives
- Avoid imposing personal values on patient during goal setting
- Explain to the patient that only one behavior should be modified at a time
- Assist the patient in prioritizing (weighting) identified goals
- Clarify with the patient the roles of the health care provider and the patient, respectively
- Explore with the patient ways to best achieve the goals
- Assist the patient in examining available resources to meet the goals
- Assist the patient in developing a plan to meet the goals
- Assist the patient in setting realistic time limits
- Assist the patient in prioritizing activities used for goal achievement
- Appraise the patient's current level of functioning with regard to each goal
- Facilitate the patient in identification of individualized, expected outcomes for each goal
- Assist the patient in identifying a specific measurement indicator (e.g., behavior, social event) for each goal
- Prepare behavioral outcomes for use in goal attainment scaling
- Help the patient focus on expected rather than desired outcomes
- Encourage the acceptance of partial goal satisfaction
- Develop a scale of upper and lower levels related to expected outcomes for each goal
- Identify scale levels that are defined by behavioral or social events for each goal
- Assist the patient in specifying the period of time in which each indicator will be measured
- Explore with the patient the methods of measuring progress toward goals
- Coordinate with the patient periodic review dates for assessment of progress toward goals
- Review the scale (as developed with the patient) during review dates for assessment of progress
- Calculate a goal attainment score
- Reevaluate goals and plan, as appropriate

1st edition 1992; revised 2000

Background Evidence:

Boyd, M. A. (2005). Psychiatric-mental health nursing interventions. In M. A. Boyd (Ed.), *Psychiatric nursing: Contemporary practice* (3rd ed., pp. 218–232). Lippincott Williams & Wilkins.

Hefferin, E. A. (1979). Health goal setting: Patient-nurse collaboration at Veterans Administration facilities. *Military Medicine, 144*(12), 814–822.

Horsley, J. A., Crane, J., Haller, K. B., & Reynolds, M. A. (1982). Mutual goal setting in patient care. *CURN Project.* Grune & Stratton.

Simons, M. R. (1992). Interventions related to compliance. *Nursing Clinics of North America, 27*(2), 477–494.

Stanley, B. (1984). Evaluation of treatment goals: The use of goal attainment scaling. *Journal of Advanced Nursing, 9*(4), 351–356.

Webster, J. (2002). Client-centered goal planning. *Nursing Times, 98*(6), 36–37.

Nail Care 1680

Definition: Promotion of clean, neat, attractive nails and prevention of skin lesions related to improper care of nails

Activities:

- Monitor or assist with cleaning and trimming of nails according to self-care ability
- Instruct to keep nails clean and dry
- Cut nails straight across with sharp nail scissors or clippers but round slightly at tips for maximum strength when trimming, and reduced occurrence of ingrown toenails
- Keep nails shaped and free of snags by filing with emery board
- File nail in same direction with emery board, as filing back and forth weakens nail
- Leave cuticles alone as they protect nail roots from infection (i.e., avoid cutting cuticles or pushing them back)
- Instruct not to bite fingernails or remove cuticle, as can damage nail
- Instruct not to use nails for tools, to avoid chips and cracks
- Trim toenails less frequently than fingernails as toenails grow more slowly
- Trim toenails regularly when soft after taking baths to minimize risk of trauma and injury
- Soak feet in warm salt water for 5 to 10 minutes when toenails thick and difficult to cut
- Avoid "digging out" ingrown toenails, especially if infected and sore
- Recommend specialist for ingrown toenail care
- Instruct to wear shoes that fit properly and to alternate shoes worn each day
- Instruct to wear flip flops at pools and in public showers to reduce risk of fungal infections
- Use proper tools (e.g., nail clipper or nail scissors for fingernails, toenail clipper for toenails) and disinfect tools monthly
- Monitor nails for changes in color, texture, or shape
- Consult specialist for unusual nail changes to determine if signs of disease or infection (e.g., dark streaks, redness and swelling, clubbing, thick and overgrown)
- Remove nail polish before surgery, as appropriate
- Assist to apply nail polish if desired
- Educate on all aspects of nail care
- Reinforce information provided by other health professionals, as appropriate
- Provide written nail care guidelines
- Document instruction as indicated
- Use teach-back to ensure understanding

1st edition 1992; revised 2004, 2024

Background Evidence:

Akbayrak, A., Kasap, T., Takçı, Z., & Seçkin, H. Y. (2021). Frequency of nail abnormalities in children and adolescents admitted to a dermatology outpatient clinic. *Journal of Pediatric Research, 8*(1), 69–74.

Aziz, M. G. (2021). Hygiene and self-care. In R. F. Craven, C. J. Hirnle, & C. J. Henshaw (Eds.), *Fundamentals of nursing: Human health and function* (8th ed.). Wolters-Kluwer.

Berman, A., Snyder, S. J., & Frandsen, G. (2018). Hygiene. In *Kozier and Erb's Fundamentals of nursing: Concepts, process and practice* (pp. 688–689) (10th ed.). Pearson.

Chapman, S. (2017). Foot care for people with diabetes: Prevention of complications and treatment. *British Journal of Community Nursing, 22*(5), 226–229.

Perry, A. G., Potter, P. A., Ostendorf, W. R., & Laplante, N. (2022). Personal hygiene and bedmaking. In *Clinical Nursing Skills and Techniques* (10th ed.). Elsevier.

Porter-O'Grady, T. (2021). Wound and foot care nursing on the streets of the city: A view from here. *Journal of Wound, Ostomy & Continence Nursing, 48*(1), 69–74.

Potter, P. A., Perry, A. G., Stockert, P. A., & Hall, A. M. (2021). *Fundamentals of nursing* (10th ed.). Elsevier.

Williams, P. (2020). *Basic geriatric nursing* (7th ed.). Elsevier.

N

Nasal Irrigation 3316

Definition: Enhancing nasal mucosa functioning using saline lavage

Activities:

- Consider contraindications before procedure (e.g., patients with facial trauma not fully healed and patients with neurological or musculoskeletal problems that increase aspiration risk)
- Prepare irrigating solution using premade packets or household ingredients
- Mix 1 teaspoon salt and ½ teaspoon baking soda with 1 pint lukewarm, potable water, adjusting salinity and temperature of solution according to institutional guidelines or patient preference, if necessary
- Use salt that does not contain iodine, anticaking agents, or preservatives to avoid irritation to the nasal mucosa (i.e., use kosher, canning, or pickling salt)
- Draw up solution using low positive pressure device (e.g., bulb syringe or spray bottle) or gravity-based pressure device (e.g., Neti Pot or other commercial nasal saline rinse product)
- Position patient over sink or basin with head tilted downward and rotated so that one nostril is higher than the other
- Gently insert applicator tip or spout into upper most nostril until a comfortable seal is formed, avoiding pressing tip or spout into the septum
- Instill approximately half of prepared solution into nostril
- Instruct patient to breathe normally through mouth
- Monitor evacuation of fluid return from lower nostril (e.g., amount, color, consistency)
- Repeat procedure in other nostril
- Adjust head position, to avoid the draining of solution into back of throat or ears, as needed
- Encourage patient to blow nose gently
- Irrigate nasal passages 1 to 3 times per day or as prescribed
- Cleanse irrigating device after each use
- Prepare fresh solution daily

- Discontinue if patient experiences pain, nosebleeds, or other problems
- Instruct patient on techniques for self-irrigation
- Administer nasal medication, if necessary
- Provide referral to health care provider

6th edition 2013

Background Evidence:

Azar, A. E., & Muller, B. A. (2006). A practical evidence-based approach to rhinosinusitis. *The Journal of Respiratory Disease, 27*(9), 372–379.

Harvey, R., Hannan, S. A., Badia, L., & Scadding, G. (2007). Nasal saline irrigations for the symptoms of chronic rhinosinusitis. *Cochrane Database*

of Systematic Reviews, (3). https://doi.org/10.1002/14651858.CD006394.pub2

Kassel, J. C., King, D., & Spurling, G. K. P. (2010). Saline nasal irrigation for acute upper respiratory tract infections. *Cochrane Database of Systematic Reviews, 2010*(3). https://doi.org/10.1002/14651858.CD006821.pub2

Moyad, M. A. (2009). Conventional and alternative medical advice for cold and flu prevention: What should be recommended and what should be avoided? *Urologic Nursing, 29*(6), 455–458.

Rabago, D., & Zgierska, A. (2009). Saline nasal irrigation for upper respiratory conditions. *American Family Physician, 80*(10), 1117–1119, 1121–1122.

Steele, R. W. (2005). Chronic sinusitis in children. *Clinical Pediatrics, 44*(6), 465–471.

Nasogastric Intubation 1080

Definition: Insertion of a tube through the naris into the gastrointestinal tract

Activities:

- Verify that the patient has no contraindications for nasal placement (e.g., basilar skull fracture; facial, nasal, or sinus trauma; esophageal varices or stricture; or clotting abnormalities)
- Select type and size of tube to insert (i.e., small bore tubes are used for feeding and administering medications whereas large bore tube are used for gastric drainage; some have electromagnetic guidance systems)
- Explain to the patient and family the rationale for using a nasogastric tube
- Place patient in a supine position with head of bed elevated at least 30 degrees, unless contraindicated
- Determine the length of tube to be inserted into stomach by measuring the tube from the tip of the nose to the tip of the earlobe and to the bottom of the xiphoid process
- Add additional length if the tube is to pass through the pyloric sphincter
- Provide the patient with a glass of water to swallow during insertion, as appropriate
- Lubricate the distal end of the tube with water or water-soluble jelly
- Insert the tube into the naris and advance along the base of the nostril to the posterior pharynx
- Instruct patient to swallow and advance the tube to the predetermined marking
- Position the patient on right side to facilitate movement of the tube into the duodenum, as appropriate
- Administer medication to increase peristalsis, as appropriate

- Apply skin preparation to the nose and securing surface of the face
- Tape the tube securely to the nose so that the tube does not press against the skin of the naris
- Record the tube depth
- Label the tube with the date and time of placement
- Obtain radiograph to confirm placement of the tube in the gastrointestinal tract

1st edition 1992; revised 1996, 2018

Background Evidence:

Baskin, W. N. (2006). Acute complications associated with bedside placement of feeding tubes. *Nutrition in Clinical Practice, 21*(1), 40–55.

Durai, R., Venkatraman, R., & Ng, P. (2009). Nasogastric tubes: Insertion technique and confirming the correct position. *Nursing Times, 105*(16), 12–13.

Ecklund, M. (2011). Small-bore feeding tube insertion and care. In D. Wiegand (Ed.), *AACN procedure manual for critical care* (6th ed., pp. 1206–1210). Elsevier Saunders.

Klingman, L. (2013). Bowel elimination. In P. Potter, A. Perry, P. Stockert, & A. Hall (Eds.), *Fundamentals of nursing* (8th ed., pp. 1087–1126). Elsevier Mosby.

Roberts, S., Echeverria, P., & Gabriel, S. (2007). Devices and techniques for bedside enteral feeding tube placement. *Nutrition in Clinical Practice, 22*(4), 412–420.

Nausea Management 1450

Definition: Prevention and alleviation of nausea

Activities:

- Determine branch of emetic pathway involved (e.g., vestibular system, chemoreceptor trigger zone)
- Ascertain severity and intensity of symptoms using an assessment tool or scale (e.g., Self-Care Journal, Visual Analog Scales, Duke Descriptive Scales, Rhodes Index of Nausea and Vomiting, NOC Nausea & Vomiting Control)

- Evaluate precipitating and relieving factors (e.g., movement, food, fluids, hunger, aromas), and characteristics (e.g., duration, frequency)
- Observe for nonverbal cues of discomfort, especially for infants, children, and those unable to communicate effectively, such as individuals with Alzheimer's disease
- Evaluate past experiences with nausea (e.g., pregnancy, car sickness, medication, anesthesia)

- Obtain complete pretreatment history
- Obtain dietary history containing likes, dislikes, and cultural food preferences
- Provide effective antiemetic drugs to prevent nausea when possible (i.e., avoid nausea related to pregnancy)
- Administer medication via appropriate routes considering condition and needs (e.g., intravascular, oral, rectal, intramuscular)
- Administer medication considering two or more antiemetics may be required to achieve adequate symptom control, depending upon cause
- Prescribe medication specific to nausea etiology (i.e., antiemetics vary in their mechanisms of action, are dependent upon cause and receptor)
- Control environmental factors that may evoke nausea (e.g., aversive smells, sound, unpleasant visual stimulation)
- Reduce or eliminate personal factors that precipitate or increase nausea (e.g., anxiety, fear, fatigue, lack of knowledge)
- Identify strategies that have been successful in relieving nausea
- Employ multimodal approach that incorporates both pharmacological and non-pharmacological management methods
- Collaborate with person when selecting nausea control strategy
- Consider cultural influence on nausea response when implementing interventions
- Encourage to be persistent with health providers in obtaining pharmacological and non-pharmacological relief
- Instruct on use of non-pharmacological techniques (e.g., biofeedback, hypnosis, relaxation, guided imagery, music therapy, distraction, acupressure) to manage nausea
- Encourage use of non-pharmacological techniques before, during, and after treatments; before nausea occurs or increases; and along with other nausea control measures
- Inform other health care professionals and family members of any non-pharmacological strategies being used
- Promote adequate rest and sleep to facilitate nausea relief
- Use frequent oral hygiene to promote comfort unless stimulates nausea
- Encourage eating small amounts of food that are appealing, if not contraindicated
- Instruct in high carbohydrate and low-fat food, as appropriate
- Give cold, clear liquid, and odorless, colorless food, as appropriate
- Monitor recorded intake for nutritional content and calories
- Evaluate effect of nausea experience on quality of life (e.g., appetite, activity, job performance, role responsibility, sleep)
- Provide information about nausea (e.g., causes, duration)
- Provide emotional support
- Encourage to learn strategies for managing own nausea
- Provide anti-nausea measures preventively if indicated
- Monitor effects of nausea management
- Use teach-back to ensure understanding

3rd edition 2000; revised 2024

Background Evidence:

Dilek, B., & Necmiye, C. (2020). Usage of aromatherapy in symptom management in cancer patients: A systematic review. *International Journal of Caring Sciences, 13*(1), 537–546.

Ford, C., & Park, L. (2020). Assessing and managing nausea and vomiting in adults. *British Journal of Nursing, 29*(11), 602–605.

Momami, T., & Berry, D. (2017). Integrative therapeutic approaches for the management and control of nausea in children undergoing cancer treatment: A systematic review of literature. *Journal of Pediatric Oncology Nursing, 34*(3), 173–184.

Moorhead, S., Swanson, E., Johnson, M., & Maas, M. L. (2018). *Nursing Outcomes Classification (NOC): Measurement of Health Outcomes.* Elsevier.

Walsh, D., Davis, M., Ripamonti, C., Bruera, E., Davies, A., & Molassiotis, A. (2017). 2016 Updated MASCC/ESMO consensus recommendations: Management of nausea and vomiting in advanced cancer. (Systematic Review). *Supportive Care in Cancer, 25*, 333–340.

Zorba, P., & Ozdemir, L. (2018). The preliminary effects of massage and inhalation aromatherapy on chemotherapy-induced acute nausea and vomiting: A quasi-randomized controlled pilot trial. *Cancer Nursing, 41*(5), 359–366.

Neurologic Monitoring — 2620

Definition: Collection and analysis of patient data to prevent or minimize neurologic complications

Activities:

- Monitor level of consciousness
- Monitor level of orientation
- Monitor trend of Glasgow Coma Scale
- Monitor recent memory, attention span, past memory, mood, affect, and behaviors
- Monitor sense of smell
- Monitor for visual disturbance (e.g., diplopia, nystagmus, visual-field cuts, blurred vision, visual acuity)
- Monitor pupillary size, shape, symmetry, and reactivity
- Monitor EOMs and gaze characteristics
- Monitor for tracking response
- Monitor corneal reflex
- Monitor facial symmetry
- Monitor cough and gag reflex
- Monitor tongue protrusion
- Monitor muscle tone, motor movement, gait, and proprioception, comparing both sides of body simultaneously
- Monitor for pronator drift, comparing both sides of body simultaneously
- Monitor grip strength, comparing both sides of body simultaneously
- Monitor for tremor, comparing both sides of body simultaneously
- Monitor vital signs (e.g., temperature, blood pressure, pulse, respirations)
- Monitor respiratory status (e.g., ABG levels, pulse oximetry, depth, pattern, rate, effort)
- Monitor invasive hemodynamic parameters, as appropriate
- Monitor ICP and CPP
- Note complaint of headache
- Monitor speech characteristics (e.g., fluency, presence of aphasias, or word-finding difficulty)
- Monitor response to stimuli (e.g., verbal, tactile, noxious)
- Monitor sharp and dull or hot and cold discrimination
- Monitor for numbness and tingling
- Monitor sweating patterns
- Monitor Babinski response
- Monitor for Cushing response (i.e., rising systolic pressure with widening pulse and bradycardia)

- Monitor craniotomy or laminectomy dressing for drainage
- Monitor response to medications
- Consult with co-workers to confirm data, as appropriate
- Identify emerging patterns in data
- Increase frequency of neurological monitoring, as appropriate
- Avoid activities that increase intracranial pressure
- Space required nursing activities that increase intracranial pressure
- Notify physician of change in patient condition
- Institute emergency protocols, as needed
- Institute agency protocol for specific neurological condition (e.g., stroke, tumor, aneurism, trauma), as needed

1st edition 1992; revised 1996, 2018

Background Evidence:

American Association of Critical Care Nurses. (2006). In J. G. Alspach (Ed.), *Core curriculum for critical care nursing* (6th ed.). W.B. Saunders.

Barker, E. (2008). *Neuroscience nursing: A spectrum of care* (3rd ed.). Mosby Elsevier.

Crimlisk, J. T., & Grande, M. M. (2004). Neurologic assessment skills for the acute medical surgical nurse. *Orthopaedic Nursing, 23*(1), 3–11.

Rank, W. (2010). Simplifying neuro assessment. *Nursing made incredibly easy, 8*(2), 15–19.

Timby, B. K., & Smith, N. E. (2007). Introduction to the nervous system. In *Introductory medical-surgical nursing* (pp. 653–665) (9th ed.). Lippincott Williams & Wilkins.

Woodward, S., & Mestecky, A. (Eds.). (2011). *Neuroscience nursing: Evidence-based practice.* Wiley-Blackwell.

Neutropenic Precautions 6580

Definition: Minimizing or eliminating the acquisition and transmission of infectious agents in immunocompromised persons

Activities:

- Verify health history, including preexisting conditions, medications and treatments, to determine risk level
- Determine baseline status of immune system via bloodwork and physical examination
- Institute protective isolation precautions as indicated
- Provide private room as indicated, or ensure appropriate square feet per person as required by CDC guidelines, when unable to provide private room
- Place notice on door indicating requirements for anyone entering room (e.g., hand washing, PPE)
- Restrict microorganisms in environment where possible, using positive pressure isolation room (i.e., clean air pumped into room continuously creating air pressure such that microbes unable to enter)
- Use isolation rooms with high-efficiency particulate air (HEPA) filter systems where possible
- Ensure all equipment and furniture in room disinfected
- Use disposable and dedicated equipment where possible
- Leave reusable equipment in room and disinfect after each use (e.g., thermometers, blood pressure machines, ECG machines, IV poles)
- Ensure team members adhere to strict aseptic technique at all times
- Require hand washing with soap and water or antimicrobial solutions prior to entering, as indicated
- Require all persons entering room to wear proper PPE, as indicated
- Restrict or deny visits with children or those with colds, flu or other illnesses, as indicated
- Minimize room traffic by allowing only necessary personnel to enter and exit
- Ensure door remains shut at all times
- Monitor body temperature, laboratory work, and vital signs closely to ensure awareness of immunocompromised status at all times
- Obtain fever workup for temperature of 38.3° C (101° F) once, or 38.0° C (100.4° F) two times, 4 hours apart (e.g., blood cultures, urine cultures, open wound cultures)

- Ensure empiric antimicrobial therapy started within 2 hours of fever workup
- Ensure person follows neutropenic diet (i.e., well-cooked foods; no foods that might have bacteria, such as unwashed fruit)
- Provide bottled or filtered water for fluid intake, as tolerated
- Avoid using tap water for fluid intake
- Avoid scratching, cutting, or nicking person's skin
- Avoid permanent or semipermanent venous access devices when functionally or quantitatively neutropenic
- Change IV tubing per organization protocol unless blood, lipids, or parenteral nutrition are infused through IV lines, then change IV tubing daily
- Avoid rectal medical procedures (e.g., enemas, suppositories)
- Ensure performs frequent oral care including toothbrushing and gentle flossing as tolerated
- Ensure uses antimicrobial mouth rinses when poor oral hygiene or gingivitis present
- Ensure wears mask whenever necessary to leave room (e.g., x-ray, CT scan, surgical procedure)
- Restrict flowers, potted plants, floral arrangements with water in vases, and dried flower arrangements
- Ensure that regular cleaning of room, including damp dusting, performed
- Monitor emotional status for heightened anxiety and fearful episodes related to isolation
- Provide support as indicated for emotional needs
- Clean environment appropriately after discharge
- Determine current level of knowledge related to acquisition and transmission of infectious agents
- Determine current infection control practices and tailor instruction to learning needs
- Instruct about preexisting conditions that increase infection risk
- Instruct on condition and need for isolation, and how to follow precautions
- Instruct on conducting isolation precautions at home if needed after discharge
- Instruct to stay as clean as possible

- Instruct to wash hands often, including before and after eating or using bathroom
- Inform to shower daily, being sure to clean sweaty areas like feet, armpits, and groin
- Encourage to ask others to wash hands often, particularly visiting friends and family
- Educate to avoid intercourse, but if having sex, always use water-soluble lubricant
- Instruct to avoid anyone who is ill, even if just mild cold
- Instruct to avoid recently vaccinated persons, child or adult
- Inform to stay away from large crowds, including public transportation, restaurants, and stores
- Educate to avoid animals completely if possible and especially avoid touching animal waste
- Instruct to take measures to prevent constipation as straining from constipation can irritate rectal area (i.e., eat enough fiber and drink five to six glasses of water daily)
- Inform to avoid live plants when possible
- Instruct to use gloves when outside in garden or lawn area
- Inform to avoid tampons and use pads to decrease risk for toxic shock syndrome
- Educate to practice good oral care (i.e., brush teeth after eating and before bed, using soft toothbrush and brushing gently)
- Instruct to always wear sunscreen with high sun protection factor
- Educate to keep IV lines clean (i.e., ensure IV always dry and clean and without redness or pain every day)
- Instruct to avoid cuts and injuries such as scratches (i.e., avoid sharp objects, be sure to wear gloves while cleaning)
- Instruct to delay or avoid dental work or vaccines, unless have health care provider approval
- Instruct to practice kitchen hygiene when preparing meals (e.g., wash hands before and after preparing food and eating; use clean utensils, glasses, plates and wash after each use; wash fresh fruits and vegetables well)
- Educate to avoid uncooked and raw foods (e.g., raw or unwashed fruits and vegetables; raw or undercooked meat, including beef, pork, chicken, fish; uncooked grains, raw nuts, honey)
- Instruct to cook meat until safe internal temperature, using food thermometer to check
- Educate to avoid cross-contamination when preparing foods, keeping raw meat away from cooked foods

- Instruct not to share food or drinks with other people, and avoid self-serve stations like bulk food bins, buffets, and salad bars
- Inform to seek health care attention immediately if any signs or symptoms of infection as infections that occur during neutropenia are life-threatening and require emergency care
- Educate to check temperature twice daily,
- Instruct on signs and symptoms of infection (e.g., fever, chills or sweats, persistent cough, sore throat, difficulty breathing, any new pain, vomiting, diarrhea, bloody urine, skin rash, redness or swelling at IV site)
- Inform to attend all follow-up appointments and see health care provider if exposure to infected persons
- Use teach-back to ensure understanding

8th edition 2024

Background Evidence:

Alsharawneh, A. (2021). Effect of under-triage on the outcomes of cancer patients with febrile neutropenia, sepsis, and septic shock. *Clinical Nursing Research, 30*(8), 1127–1134. https://doi.org/10.1177/1054773821999688

Blackburn, L. B., Bender, S., & Brown, S. (2019). Acute leukemia: diagnosis and treatment. *Seminars in Oncology Nursing, 35*(6), 150950. https://doi.org/10.1016/j.soncn.2019.150950

Beaudry, J., & Scotto DiMaso, K. (2020). Central line care: Reducing central line–associated bloodstream infections on a hematologic malignancy and stem cell transplant unit. *Clinical Journal of Oncology Nursing, 24*(2), 148–152. https://doi.org/10.1188/20.CJON.148-152

Carrico, R. M., Garrett, H., Balcom, D., & Burton-Glowicz, J. (2019). Infection prevention and control core practices: A roadmap for nursing practice. *The Nurse Practitioner, 44*(3), 50–55.

Centers for Disease Control and Prevention. (2017). *Core infection prevention and control practices for safe healthcare delivery in all settings: Recommendations of the Healthcare Infection Control Practices Advisory Committee.* www.cdc.gov/hicpac/pdf/core-practices.pdf

Patel, P. K., Popovich, K. J., Collier, S., Lassiter, S., Mody, L., Ameling, J. M., & Meddings, J. (2019). Foundational elements of infection prevention in the STRIVE curriculum. *Annals of Internal Medicine, 171*(7), S10–S19.

Tavakoli, A., & Carannante, A. (2021). Nursing care of oncology patients with sepsis. *Seminars in Oncology Nursing, 37*(2), 151130. https://doi.org/10.1016/j.soncn.2021.151130

N

Nonnutritive Sucking   6900

Definition: Provision of sucking opportunities for the infant

Activities:
- Select smooth pacifier or pacifier substitute that meets standards to prevent airway obstruction
- Use clean pacifier (e.g., sterilize daily, used with only one infant, no contact with contaminated areas)
- Place largest soft pacifier infant can tolerate on top of infant's tongue
- Position infant to allow tongue to drop to floor of mouth
- Position thumb and index finger under infant's mandible to support sucking reflex, if needed
- Move infant's tongue rhythmically with pacifier if needed to encourage sucking
- Rub infant's cheek gently to stimulate suck reflex

- Provide pacifier or gloved finger to encourage sucking during tube feeding and for 5 minutes after tube feeding
- Provide pacifier or gloved finger to encourage sucking at least every 4 hours for infants receiving long-term hyperalimentation
- Use pacifier or gloved finger after feedings if infant demonstrates continual need to suck
- Rock and hold baby while sucking on pacifier or gloved finger when possible
- Play soft, appropriate music
- Position to prevent loss of pacifier
- Inform parents on importance of meeting sucking needs
- Encourage breastfeeding mother to allow nonnutritive sucking at breast after feeding complete

- Inform of alternatives to nipple sucking (e.g., thumb, finger, pacifier)
- Instruct on use of nonnutritive sucking
- Use teach-back to ensure understanding

1st edition 1992; revised 2000, 2024

Background Evidence:

Bakker, L., Jackson, B., & Miles, A. (2021). Oral-feeding guidelines for preterm neonates in the NICU: A scoping review. *Journal of Perinatology, 41*(1), 140–149. https://doi.org/10.1038/s41372-020-00887-6

Grassi, A., Sgherri, G., Chorna, O., Marchi, V., Gagliardi, L., Cecchi, F., Laschi, C., & Guzzetta, A. (2019). Early intervention to improve sucking in preterm newborns: A systematic review of quantitative studies. *Advances in Neonatal Care, 19*(2), 97–109. https://doi.org/10.1097/ANC.0000000000000543

Hockenberry, M. J., Rodgers, C. C., & Wilson, D. (2022). *Wong's essentials of pediatric nursing.* Elsevier.

John, H. B., Suraj, C., Padankatti, S. M., Sebastian, T., & Rajapandian, E. (2019). Nonnutritive sucking at the mother's breast facilitates oral feeding skills in premature infants: A pilot study. *Advances in Neonatal Care, 19*(2), 110–117. https://doi.org/10.1097/ANC.0000000000000545

Matson, S., & Smith, J. E. (2016). *Core curriculum for maternal-newborn nursing.* Elsevier.

Ostadi, M., Jokar, F., Armanian, A. M., Namnabati, M., Kazemi, Y., & Poorjavad, M. (2021). The effects of swallowing exercise and non-nutritive sucking exercise on oral feeding readiness in preterm infants: A randomized controlled trial. *International Journal of Pediatric Otorhinolaryngology, 142*, 110602. https://doi.org/10.1016/j.ijporl.2020.110602

Ziegler, A., Maron, J. L., Barlow, S. M., & Davis, J. M. (2020). Effect of pacifier design on nonnutritive suck maturation and weight gain in preterm infants: A pilot study. *Current Therapies in Research Clinical Experience, 93*, 100617. https://doi.org/10.1016/j.curtheres.2020.100617

Normalization Promotion   7200

Definition: Assisting parents and other family members of children with chronic illnesses or disabilities in providing normal life experiences for their children and families

Activities:

- Assist the family in accepting the child's condition
- Promote development of membership of child into family system without letting child become central focus of family
- Assist family to view the child as a child first, rather than as a chronically ill or disabled individual
- Provide opportunities for child to have normal childhood experiences
- Encourage interaction with healthy peers
- Deemphasize uniqueness of child's condition
- Encourage parents to make child appear as normal as possible
- Assist family in avoiding potentially embarrassing situations with child
- Encourage the family to modify preconceived developmental expectations by focusing more on smaller unexpected achievements
- Assist family in making changes in home environment that decrease reminders of child's special needs
- Determine accessibility of activity and child's ability to participate in activity
- Identify adaptations needed to accommodate child's limitations, so child can participate in normal activities
- Communicate information about child's condition to those who need this information to provide safe supervision or appropriate educational opportunities for child
- Assist family in altering prescribed therapeutic regime to fit normal schedule, when appropriate
- Assist family in advocating for child in school system to ensure access to appropriate education programs
- Encourage child to participate in school and community activities appropriate for developmental and ability level
- Encourage parents to have same parenting expectations and techniques for all children in family
- Encourage parents to spend time with all children in family
- Involve siblings in care and activities of child, as appropriate
- Determine need for respite care for parents or other care providers
- Identify resources for respite care in community
- Encourage parents to take time to care for their personal needs
- Provide information to family about child's condition, treatment, and associated support groups for families
- Encourage parents to balance involvement in special programs for child's special needs and normal family and community activities
- Encourage family to maintain usual social network and support system
- Encourage family to maintain usual family habits, rituals, and routines

2nd edition 1996; revised 2018

Background Evidence:

Deatrick, J., Knafl, K., & Murphy-Moore, C. (1999). Clarifying the concept of normalization. *Image: The Journal of Nursing Scholarship, 31*(3), 209–214.

Knafl, K., Deatrick, J., & Gallo, A. (2008). The interplay of concepts, data, and methods in the development of the family management style framework. *Journal of Family Nursing, 14*(4), 412–428.

Peck, B., & Lillibridge, J. (2005). Normalization behaviours of rural fathers living with chronically-ill children: An Australian experience. *Journal of Child Health Care, 9*(1), 31–45.

Protudjer, J., Kozyrskyj, A., Becker, A., & Marchessault, G. (2009). Normalization strategies of children with asthma. *Qualitative Health Research, 19*(1), 94–104.

Rehm, R., & Bradley, J. (2005). Normalization in families raising a child who is medically fragile/technology dependent and developmentally delayed. *Qualitative Health Research, 15*(6), 807–820.

Rehm, R., & Franck, L. (2000). Long-term goals and normalization strategies of children and families affected by HIV/AIDS. *Advances in Nursing Science, 23*(1), 69–82.

Seligman, M., & Darling, R. (2007). *Ordinary families, special children: A systems approach to childhood disability* (3rd ed.). Guilford Press.

N

Nutrition Management 1100

Definition: Providing and promoting a balanced intake of nutrients

Activities:

- Determine patient's nutritional status and ability to meet nutritional needs
- Identify patient's food allergies or intolerances
- Determine patient's food preferences
- Instruct patient about nutritional needs (i.e., discuss dietary guidelines and food pyramids)
- Assist patient in determining guidelines or food pyramids (e.g., Vegetarian Food Pyramid, Food Guide Pyramid, and Food Pyramid for Seniors over 70) most suited in meeting nutritional needs and preferences
- Determine number of calories and type of nutrients needed to meet nutrition requirements
- Provide food selection, offering guidance toward healthier choices, if necessary
- Adjust diet (i.e., provide high protein foods, suggest using herbs and spices as an alternative to salt, provide sugar substitute, increase or decrease calories, increase or decrease vitamins, minerals, or supplements), as necessary
- Provide optimal environment for meal consumption (e.g., clean, well-ventilated, relaxed, and free from strong odors)
- Perform or assist patient with oral care before eating
- Ensure patient uses well-fitting dentures, if appropriate
- Administer medications before eating (e.g., pain relief, antiemetics), if needed
- Encourage patient to sit in upright position in chair, if possible
- Ensure food is served in attractive manner and at temperature most suited for optimal consumption
- Encourage family to bring patient's favorite foods while in hospital or care facility, as appropriate
- Assist patient with opening packages, cutting food, and eating, if needed
- Instruct patient on necessary diet modifications (e.g., NPO, clear liquid, full liquid, soft, or diet as tolerated), as necessary
- Instruct patient on diet requirements for disease state (i.e., for patients with renal disease, restrict sodium, potassium, protein, and fluids)
- Instruct patient on specific dietary needs based on development or age (e.g., increased calcium, protein, fluid, and calories for lactating women; increased fiber intake to prevent constipation among older adults)
- Offer nutrient-dense snacks
- Ensure that diet includes foods high in fiber content to prevent constipation
- Monitor calorie and dietary intake
- Monitor trends in weight loss and gain
- Instruct patient to monitor calorie and dietary intake (e.g., food diary)
- Encourage safe food preparation and preservation techniques
- Assist patient in accessing community nutritional programs (e.g., Women, Infants, and Children, food stamps, and home-delivered meals)
- Provide referral

1st edition 1992; revised 2013

Background Evidence:

Craven, R. F., & Hirnle, C. J. (2009). *Nutrition. In Fundamentals of nursing: Human health and function* (pp. 947–988) (6th ed.). Lippincott Williams & Wilkins.

Ignatavicius, D. D. (2010). Care of patients with malnutrition and obesity. In D. D. Ignatavicius & M. L. Workman (Eds.), *Medical-surgical nursing: Patient-centered collaborative care* (6th ed., pp. 1386–1410). Saunders Elsevier.

Kaiser, L., Allen, L. H., & American Dietetic Association. (2008). Position of the American Dietetic Association: Nutrition and lifestyle for a healthy pregnancy outcome. *Journal of the American Dietetic Association, 108*(3), 553–561.

U.S. Department of Agriculture and U.S. Department of Health and Human Services. (2010). *Dietary guidelines for Americans, 2010* (7th ed.). Government Printing Office.

N

Nutrition Therapy 1120

Definition: Administration of food and fluids to support metabolic processes of a person with a chronic condition

Activities:

- Review information on nutritional status
- Identify nutritional risks
- Measure weight and height, and length as indicated for pediatric persons
- Measure head circumference for children less than 36 months
- Screen fluid intake for dehydration
- Start nutritional support as soon as possible, as appropriate
- Monitor food and fluid ingested and calculate daily caloric intake, as appropriate
- Monitor appropriateness of prescribed diet to meet daily nutritional needs, as appropriate
- Eliminate potential causes of malnutrition and dehydration, as soon as possible
- Evaluate need for intravenous fluids
- Initiate prescribed number of calories and type of nutrients needed to meet requirements, as appropriate
- Determine food preferences
- Consider cultural and religious preferences
- Consider nutrition therapy for persons who have limited food and fluid intake
- Offer nutritional supplements, as appropriate
- Evaluate concordance with nutritional supplement consumption routinely
- Encourage to select semisoft food if lack of saliva hinders swallowing
- Ensure that diet includes foods high in fiber content to prevent constipation, as appropriate
- Offer mealtime assistance to support adequate dietary intake, as appropriate

- Determine need for enteral tube or parenteral feedings
- Manage enteral feeding or parenteral nutrition, as needed
- Evaluate benefits and potential risks of enteral nutrition routinely
- Discontinue use of tube feedings as oral intake tolerated
- Administer hyperalimentation fluids, as appropriate
- Encourage bringing home-cooked food to institution, as appropriate
- Offer herbs and spices as alternative to salt
- Structure environment to create pleasant and relaxing atmosphere
- Encourage to share mealtimes with others, as appropriate
- Present food in attractive, pleasing manner, giving consideration to color, texture, and variety
- Modify consistency of foods, such as soft foods that require little chewing, as necessary
- Encourage adequate dental and mouth care
- Assist to sitting position before eating or feeding
- Measure blood glucose initially after artificial nutrition initiation and at least every 4 hours, for first 2 days, as appropriate
- Monitor laboratory values such as electrolytes, as appropriate
- Instruct about nutritional information and prescribed diet
- Refer for diet teaching and planning, as needed
- Provide written examples of prescribed diet
- Check medications and alter where possible to minimize adverse effects
- Offer nutritional counseling through individual sessions, group sessions, telephone contacts, and written advice, as appropriate
- Encourage physical activity to maintain or improve muscle mass and function
- Use teach-back to ensure understanding

1st edition 1992; revised 2004, 2024

Background Evidence:

Dudek, S. G. (2021). *Nutrition essentials for nursing practice* (8th ed.). Wolters Kluwer.

Koontalay, A., Sangsaikaew, A., & Khamrassame, A. (2020). Effect of a clinical nursing practice guideline of enteral nutrition care on the duration of mechanical ventilator for critically ill patients. *Asian Nursing Research*, *14*(1), 17–23. https://doi.org/10.1016/j.anr.2019.12.001

Mehta, N. M., Skillman, H. E., Irving, S. Y., Coss-Bu, J. A., Vermilyea, S., Farrington, E. A., McKeever, L., Hall, A. M., Goday, P. S., & Braunschweig, C. (2017). Guidelines for the provision and assessment of nutrition support therapy in the pediatric critically ill patient: Society of Critical Care Medicine and American Society for Parenteral and Enteral Nutrition. *JPEN. Journal of Parenteral and Enteral Nutrition, 41*(5), 706–742. https://doi.org/10.1177/0148607117711387

Singer, P., Blaser, A. R., Berger, M. M., Alhazzani, W., Calder, P. C., Casaer, M. P., Hiesmayr, M., Mayer, K., Montejo, J. C., Pichard, C., Preiser, J. C., van Zanten, A., Oczkowski, S., Szczeklik, W., & Bischoff, S. C. (2019). ESPEN guideline on clinical nutrition in the intensive care unit. *Clinical Nutrition (Edinburgh, Scotland), 38*(1), 48–79. https://doi.org/10.1016/j.clnu.2018.08.037

Tume, L. N., Valla, F. V., Joosten, K., Jotterand Chaparro, C., Latten, L., Marino, L. V., Macleod, I., Moullet, C., Pathan, N., Rooze, S., van Rosmalen, J., & Verbruggen, S. (2020). Nutritional support for children during critical illness: European Society of Pediatric and Neonatal Intensive Care (ESPNIC) metabolism, endocrine and nutrition section position statement and clinical recommendations. *Intensive Care Medicine, 46*(3), 411–425. https://doi.org/10.1007/s00134-019-05922-5

Volkert, D., Beck, A. M., Cederholm, T., Cruz-Jentoft, A., Goisser, S., Hooper, L., Kiesswetter, E., Maggio, M., Raynaud-Simon, A., Sieber, C. C., Sobotka, L., van Asselt, D., Wirth, R., & Bischoff, S. C. (2019). ESPEN Guideline on Clinical Nutrition and Hydration in Geriatrics. *Clinical Nutrition (Edinburgh, Scotland), 38*(1), 10–47. https://doi.org/10.1016/j.clnu.2018.05.024

N

Nutritional Counseling   5246

Definition: Use of an interactive helping process focusing on the need for diet modification

Activities:

- Establish a therapeutic relationship based on trust and respect
- Establish the length of the counseling relationship
- Determine patient's food intake and eating habits
- Facilitate identification of eating behaviors to be changed
- Establish realistic short-term and long-term goals for change in the nutritional status
- Use accepted nutritional standards to assist client in evaluating adequacy of dietary intake
- Provide information about the health need for diet modification (e.g., weight loss, weight gain, sodium restriction, cholesterol reduction, fluid restriction), as necessary
- Post attractive food guide material in the patient's room
- Help patient to consider factors of age, stage of growth and development, past eating experiences, injury, disease, culture, and finances in planning ways to meet nutritional requirements
- Discuss patient's knowledge of the basic four food groups, as well as perceptions of the needed diet modification
- Discuss nutritional requirements and patient's perceptions of prescribed or recommended diet
- Discuss patient's food likes and dislikes
- Assist patient to record what is usually eaten in a 24-hour period
- Review with patient measurements of fluid intake and output, hemoglobin values, blood pressure readings, or weight gains and losses, as appropriate
- Discuss food buying habits and budget constraints
- Discuss the meaning of food to patient
- Determine attitudes and beliefs of significant others about food, eating, and the patient's needed nutritional change
- Evaluate progress of dietary modification goals at regular intervals
- Assist patient in stating feelings and concerns about achievement of goals
- Praise efforts to achieve goals
- Encourage use of the Internet to access useful information on diet, recipes, and lifestyle modification, as appropriate
- Provide referral to or consultation with other members of the health care team, as appropriate

1st edition 1992; revised 1996, 2018

Background Evidence:

Dudek, S. G. (2014). *Nutrition essentials for nursing practice* (7th ed.). Lippincott Williams & Wilkins.

Franklin, B.A. (2010). *Counseling patients to favorably modify dietary and physical activity practices: The challenge of change.* http://pt.wkhealth.com/pt/re/chf/addcontent.14354749.htm;jsessionid=X8QJKPvRb9psL40CM0G1KyrRB2xqVKpLpyp1vvQG5fv3Gd40nwHB!-1552860756!181195628!8091!-1

Wardlaw, G., & Smith, A. (2012). *Contemporary nutrition* (9th ed.). McGraw-Hill.

Nutritional Monitoring 1160

Definition: Collection and analysis of patient data pertaining to nutrient intake

Activities:
- Weigh patient
- Monitor growth and development
- Obtain anthropometric measurements of body composition (e.g., body mass index, waist measurement, and skinfold measures)
- Monitor trends in weight loss and gain (i.e., in pediatric patients, plot height and weight on standardized growth chart)
- Identify recent changes in body weight
- Determine appropriate amount of weight gain during antepartum period
- Monitor skin turgor and mobility
- Identify abnormalities in skin (e.g., excessive bruising, poor wound healing, and bleeding)
- Identify abnormalities in hair (e.g., dry, thin, course, and breaks easily)
- Monitor for nausea and vomiting
- Identify abnormalities in bowel elimination (e.g., diarrhea, blood, mucus, and irregular or painful elimination)
- Monitor caloric and dietary intake
- Identify recent changes in appetite and activity
- Monitor type and amount of usual exercise
- Discuss role of social and emotional aspects of food consumption
- Determine meal patterns (e.g., food likes and dislikes, overconsumption of fast food, missed meals, hurried eating, parent-child interaction during feeding, frequency and length of infant feedings)
- Monitor for pale, reddened, and dry conjunctival tissue
- Identify abnormalities in nails (e.g., spoon-shaped, cracked, split, broken, brittle, and ridged nails)
- Perform swallowing evaluation (e.g., motor function of facial, oral, and tongue muscles, swallowing reflex, and gag reflex)
- Identify abnormalities in oral cavity (e.g., inflammation; spongy, receding, or bleeding gums; dry, cracked lips; sores; scarlet, raw tongue; and hyperemic and hypertrophic papillae)
- Monitor mental state (e.g., confusion, depression, and anxiety)
- Identify abnormalities in musculoskeletal system (e.g., muscle wasting, painful joints, bone fractures, poor posture)
- Conduct laboratory testing, monitoring results (e.g., cholesterol, serum albumin, transferrin, prealbumin, 24-hour urinary nitrogen, blood urea nitrogen, creatinine, hemoglobin, hematocrit, cellular immunity, total lymphocyte count, and electrolyte levels)
- Determine energy recommendation (e.g., Recommended Dietary Allowance) based on patient factors (e.g., age, weight, height, gender, and physical activity level)
- Determine factors affecting nutritional intake (e.g., knowledge, availability, and accessibility of quality food products in all food categories; religious and cultural influences; gender; ability to prepare food; social isolation; hospitalization; inadequate chewing; impaired swallowing; periodontal disease; poor-fitting dentures; decreased taste sensitivity; use of drugs or medications; and disease or postsurgical states)
- Review other sources of data pertaining to nutritional status (e.g., patient food diary and written logs)
- Initiate treatment or provide referral, as appropriate

1st edition 1992; revised 2013

Background Evidence:

Craven, R. F., & Hirnle, C. J. (2009). Nutrition. In *Fundamentals of nursing: Human health and function* (pp. 947–988) (6th ed.). Lippincott Williams & Wilkins.

Dudek, S. G. (2007). *Nutrition essentials for nursing practice* (5th rev. ed.). Lippincott Williams & Wilkins.

Roman-Vinas, B., Serra-Majem, L., Ribas-Barba, L., Ngo, J., Garcia-Alvarez, A., Wijnhoven, T., Tabacchi, G., Branca, F., de Vries, J., & de Groot, L. C. P. G. M. (2009). Overview of methods used to evaluate the adequacy of nutrient intakes for individuals and populations. *British Journal of Nutrition, 101*(Suppl. 2), S6–S11.

Smith, S. F., Duell, D. J., & Martin, B. C. (2008). *Clinical nursing skills: Basic to advanced skills* (pp. 208–248) (7th ed.). Pearson Prentice Hall.

N

Oral Health Maintenance 1710

Definition: Maintenance and promotion of oral hygiene and dental health for the person at risk for developing oral or dental lesions

Activities:

- Establish mouth care routine, including regular oral inspections with oral health measurement tools
- Apply lubricant to moisten lips and oral mucosa as needed
- Monitor teeth for color, shine, and presence of debris
- Encourage and assist to rinse mouth if able
- Facilitate toothbrushing and flossing at regular intervals (e.g., after meals, bedtime)
- Encourage parents to have children begin regular toothbrushing and flossing at preschool age
- Recommend use of soft-bristled toothbrush
- Instruct to brush teeth, gums, and tongue
- Instruct on proper toothbrushing technique required for oral hygiene (e.g., Sulcular, Bass, Stillman Charter)
- Instruct and assist to perform oral hygiene after eating and as often as needed
- Perform oral hygiene including toothbrushing and flossing if person unable, twice daily minimally
- Combine toothbrushing with oral antiseptics for at-risk persons
- Inspect mouth as needed to ensure teeth are clean
- Rinse mouth vigorously with water if unable to do brushing or flossing
- Monitor for signs and symptoms of glossitis and stomatitis, or bacterial colonization
- Consult provider or dentist about readjustment of wires and appliances and alternative methods of oral care if irritation of oral mucous membranes occurs from these devices
- Consult provider if oral dryness, irritation, and discomfort persist, or if bacterial or yeast colonization noted
- Recommend healthy diet with coarse, fibrous foods (e.g., fruits, vegetables) and adequate water intake with fluoridated water
- Schedule topical applications of fluoride if fluoridated water unavailable
- Monitor for therapeutic effects of topical anesthetics, oral protective pastes, and topical or systemic analgesics, as appropriate
- Identify any risk for development of stomatitis secondary to drug therapy
- Arrange for dental checkups as needed (e.g., every 6 months)
- Determine type of artificial teeth (e.g., lower plate, upper plate, bridge, full set)
- Ensure artificial teeth are to be removed for cleansing (e.g., fixed bridge)
- Ensure artificial teeth are well-fitted and do not cause undue discomfort
- Determine current routine for cleaning (e.g., daily, after meals, soaking, brushing)
- Use toothpaste or soaking materials appropriate for teeth (e.g., dentifrice, effervescent tablets) and cleaning compounds as indicated for plates
- Follow manufacturer directions related to how long or how frequently dentures to be soaked, and how to store dentures overnight
- Notify dentist if loose or ill-fitting dentures
- Encourage denture wearers to brush gums and tongue and rinse oral cavity daily
- Instruct on care and application of dentures
- Discourage smoking, tobacco chewing, and excessive intake of foods and drinks high in sugar between meals
- Instruct to chew sugarless gum to increase saliva and cleanse teeth between meals if indicated
- Use teach-back to ensure understanding

1st edition 1992; revised 2004, 2024

Background Evidence:

Berman, A., Snyder, S. J., & Frandsen, G. (2018). Hygiene. In *Kozier and Erb's fundamentals of nursing: Concepts, process and practice* (pp. 669–685) (10th ed.). Pearson.

Craven, R. F., Hirnle, C. J., & Henshaw, C. J. (2021). Self-care and hygiene. In *Fundamentals of nursing: Human health and function* (8th ed.). Wolters-Kluwer.

Hockenberry, M. J., Rodgers, C. C., & Wilson, D. (2022). *Wong's essentials of pediatric nursing* (11th ed.). Elsevier.

Lim, C., Lee, H., & Park, G. (2021). Effects of oral care interventions on oral health and oral health-related quality of life among denture-wearing older adults. *Korean Journal of Adult Nursing, 33*(1), 76–86.

Perry, A. G., Potter, P. A., Ostendorf, W. R., & LaPlante, N. (2021). *Clinical nursing skills and technique* (10th ed.). Mosby.

Potter, P. A., Perry, A. G., Stockert, P. A., & Hall, A. M. (2021). *Fundamentals of Nursing* (10th ed.). Elsevier.

Williams, P. (2020). *Basic geriatric nursing* (7th ed). Elsevier.

Winning, L., Lundy, F. T., Blackwood, B., McAuley, D. F., & Karim, I. E. (2021). Oral health care for the critically ill: A narrative review. *Critical Care, 25*, 1–8. https://doi.org/10.1186/s13054-021-03765-5

Oral Health Promotion 1720

Definition: Promotion of oral hygiene and dental care for a person with normal oral and dental health

Activities:

- Monitor condition of mouth (e.g., lips, tongue, mucous membranes, teeth, gums, dental appliances and their fit)
- Provide regular oral health screening and risk assessment
- Determine usual dental hygiene routine, identifying areas to be addressed, if necessary
- Instruct on frequency and quality of proper oral health care (e.g., flossing, brushing, and rinsing; adequate nutrition; use of fluoride-containing water, supplement, or other preventive product; other considerations based on developmental level and self-care ability)
- Assist in brushing teeth, gums, and tongue, rinsing, and flossing as needed
- Assist with dentures in oral care as needed (i.e., remove, cleanse, reinsert dentures; brush gums, remaining teeth, and tongue; massage gums with brush or fingers)

O

- Provide oral care using appropriate precautions (i.e., turn head to side or place in side-lying position, when possible, insert bite block or padded tongue blade, avoid putting fingers in mouth, use small amounts of liquid, use bulb syringe or other suction devices)
- Cleanse infant's mouth using dry gauze or washcloth
- Apply lubricant to moisten lips and oral mucosa as needed
- Assist in identifying and obtaining oral care products most suited to meet needs (e.g., toothbrush with easy-to-grasp handle, powered toothbrush, dental floss holder, immersion cleanser for dentures, athletic mouthguard)
- Instruct on role of sugar in development of caries (i.e., encourage to limit natural sugar intake; suggest use of artificial sweeteners in diet, particularly xylitol; and instruct parent on appropriate use of bottles and sippy cups and their contents)
- Discourage smoking and tobacco chewing (i.e., instruct on effects of tobacco use, implement tobacco-use prevention measures, and provide tobacco-cessation assistance)
- Discuss importance of regular dental checkups, including timing of child's first visit to dental health professional
- Provide community-level services (i.e., assist in meeting needs for transportation and translational services, use health fairs and cultural events as opportunities for education, and develop public service announcements)

- Provide referral as needed
- Use teach-back to ensure understanding

1st edition 1992; revised 2013, 2024

Background Evidence:

Berman, A., Snyder, S. J., & Frandsen, G. (2018). Hygiene. In *Kozier and Erb's fundamentals of nursing: Concepts, process and practice* (pp. 669–685) (10th ed.). Pearson.

Craven, R. F., Hirnle, C. J., & Henshaw, C. J. (2021). Self-care and hygiene. In *Fundamentals of nursing: Human health and function* (8th ed.). Wolters-Kluwer.

Hockenberry, M. J., Rodgers, C. C., & Wilson, D. (2022). *Wong's essentials of pediatric nursing* (11th ed.). Elsevier.

Perry, A. G., Potter, P. A., Ostendorf, W. R., & LaPlante, N. (2021). *Clinical nursing skills and technique* (10th ed.). Mosby.

Potter, P. A., Perry, A. G., Stockert, P. A., & Hall, A. M. (2021). *Fundamentals of Nursing* (10th ed.). Elsevier.

Williams, P. (2020). *Basic geriatric nursing* (7th ed). Elsevier.

Winning, L., Lundy, F. T., Blackwood, B., McAuley, D. F., & Karim, I. E. (2021). Oral health care for the critically ill: A narrative review. *Critical Care, 25*, 1–8. https://doi.org/10.1186/s13054-021-03765-5

Oral Health Restoration 1730

Definition: Promotion of healing for a person who has an oral mucosa or dental lesion

Activities:

- Monitor condition of mouth (e.g., lips, tongue, mucous membranes, teeth, gums, dental appliances and their fit), including character of abnormalities (e.g., size, color, location of internal or external lesions or inflammation, signs of infection)
- Monitor changes in taste, swallowing, quality of voice, and comfort
- Obtain order from health care provider to perform routine oral hygiene, if applicable
- Encourage maintenance of identified oral health schedule
- Instruct to use soft-bristled toothbrush or disposable mouth sponge
- Instruct on appropriate selection of floss use and type (i.e., avoid use if at-risk for bleeding; use waxed floss to prevent tissue trauma)
- Administer mouth rinse (e.g., anesthetic, effervescent, saline, coating, antifungal or antibacterial solution)
- Administer medication (e.g., analgesics, anesthetics, antimicrobials, anti-inflammatory agents), if needed
- Remove dentures, encouraging to use only for meals
- Apply lubricant to moisten lips and oral mucosa as needed
- Discourage smoking, tobacco chewing, vaping or alcohol consumption
- Instruct on frequency and quality of proper oral health care
- Instruct to avoid oral hygiene products containing glycerin, alcohol, or other drying agents
- Instruct to keep toothbrushes and other oral equipment clean
- Discuss importance of adequate nutritional intake (i.e., address malnutrition caused by deficiencies in folate, zinc, iron, and complex B vitamins; encourage consumption of high-protein, high vitamin C-containing foods)

- Avoid spicy, salty, acidic, dry, rough, or hard foods
- Avoid foods causing allergenic response (e.g., coffee, cheese, nuts, citrus fruits, gluten, potatoes) if applicable
- Encourage to increase water intake
- Instruct to avoid hot foods and liquids
- Instruct on signs and symptoms of stomatitis, including when to report to health care provider
- Provide referral as indicated
- Use teach-back to ensure understanding

1st edition 1992; revised 2013, 2024

Background Evidence:

Cromar, K. C., & Rebar, C. R. (2021). Care of patients with oral cavity problems. In D. D. Ignatavicius, M. L. Workman, C. R. Rebar, & N. M. Heimgartner (Eds.), *Medical-surgical nursing: Concepts for interprofessional collaborative care* (10th ed.). Elsevier.

Hazara, R. (2020). Oral health in older adults. *British Journal of Community Nursing, 25*(8), 396–401. https://doi.org/10.12968/bjcn.2020.25.8.396

Jenson, H. (2018). Improving oral care in hospitalized non-ventilated patients: Standardizing products and protocol. *MEDSURG Nursing, 27*(1), 38–45.

Martin, K., Johnston, L., & Archer, N. (2020). Oral conditions in the community patient: part 2—systemic complications of poor oral health. *British Journal of Community Nursing, 25*(11), 532–536. https://doi.org/10.12968/bjcn.2020.25.11.532

Pai, R. R., Ongole, R., & Banerjee, S. (2019). Oral care in cancer nursing: Practice and barriers. *Indian Journal of Dental Research, 30*(2), 226–230. https://doi.org/10.4103/ijdr.IJDR_343_17

O

Order Transcription 8060

Definition: Transferring information from order sheets to the nursing patient care planning and documentation system

Activities:
- Ensure that order sheet is labeled with accurate patient identification
- Ensure that order sheet is in correct patient chart
- Ensure that orders are written or cosigned by a licensed health care provider with clinical privileges
- Repeat verbal order back to the physician to ensure accuracy
- Avoid taking verbal orders by or through other providers
- Ensure that verbal orders are documented per agency policy before noting
- Assist a physician who lacks computer skills with computerized order entry using the physician's log-in name and confirmation that the order is correct
- Clarify confusing or illegible orders
- Clarify unclear abbreviations in orders
- Evaluate appropriateness of orders and ensure that all needed information is provided
- Consult with a pharmacist whenever you have doubts about an unfamiliar drug or dose that is prescribed
- Document any disagreement with a physician's order after discussion of the order with the physician and a supervisor
- Sign name, title, date, and time to each order noted
- Transfer order to appropriate electronic document, worksheet, medication form, laboratory slip, care plan, or Kardex
- Schedule appointments, as appropriate
- Note start and stop dates on medications, per agency policy
- Note patient allergies when transcribing medication orders
- Inform team members to initiate treatment
- Participate in the development and improvement of a computerized order entry system for physicians and other providers who write orders

2nd edition 1996; revised 2018

Background Evidence:
Buppert, C. (2012). Who can enter computerized orders for physicians? *Medscape.* http://www.medscape.com/viewarticle/764357

Kazemi, A., Fors, U., Tofighi, S., Tessma, M., & Ellenius, J. (2010). Physician order entry or nurse order entry? Comparison of two implementation strategies for a computerized order entry system aimed at reducing dosing medication errors. *Journal of Medical Internet Research, 12*(1), e5.

Potter, P., Perry, A., Stockert, P., & Hall, A. (Eds.). (2013). *Fundamentals of nursing* (8th ed.). Elsevier Mosby.

Radley, D., Wasserman, M., Olsho, L., Shoemaker, S., Spranca, M., & Bradshaw, B. (2013). Reduction in medication errors in hospitals due to adoption of computerized provider order entry systems. *JAMIA: Journal of the American Medical Informatics Association, 20*(3), 470–476.

Organ Procurement 6260

Definition: Care of the donor and family to ensure timely retrieval of vital organs and tissue for transplant

Activities:
- Review regulatory requirements and institutional policy and procedures for organ donation (i.e., in the United States, Center for Medicare and Medicaid Services and the Joint Commission mandate that every patient for whom death is imminent must be referred to the local Organ Procurement Organization [OPO] responsible for approaching the patient and family for possible organ donation)
- Participate in health care team discussions concerning the patient's condition, prognosis, and plan of care so all can speak with uniformity
- Verify that the OPO coordinator has been alerted if the patient has a life-threatening illness or injury
- Monitor vital signs and fluid status
- Obtain laboratory samples as prescribed (e.g., CBC, electrolyte levels, liver and renal function tests, hepatitis and HIV testing)
- Assist with the determination of brain death, as appropriate
- Ensure that brain death criteria have been met and documented
- Realize that the OPO coordinator will make the request for donation and prescribe the appropriate testing for donation
- Provide a private space where the OPO coordinator can approach the family to discuss organ donation
- Obtain blood samples for blood and tissue typing as directed by the OPO coordinator
- Administer IV fluids and vasoactive medications as prescribed
- Prepare the family for what to expect during withdrawal of life-support therapy, as appropriate
- Support the family through the end-of-life process
- Assist with transfer of the patient to the operating room as directed by the OPO coordinator
- Provide a mechanism for the family to obtain information about the organ recovery procedures
- Offer family postmortem viewing of the body, when possible
- Allow family time for grieving
- Understand that ethical dilemmas may arise related to organ allocation, transplant candidacy, and available technologies
- Help patients and families access quality health care information about organ donation and transplant
- Conduct community education programs about organ donation and transplant

2nd edition 1996; revised 2018

Background Evidence:
International Transplant Nurses Society. (2016). *Transplant nursing: Scope and standards of practice* (2nd ed.).

Mercer, L. (2013). Improving the rates of organ donation for transplantation. *Nursing Standard, 27*(26), 35–40.

Nierste, D. (2013). Issues in organ procurement, allocation, and transplantation. *Journal of Christian Nursing, 30*(2), 80–87.

Paramesh, A. S. (2013). What's new in the transplant OR? *AORN Journal, 97*(4), 435–447.

Wiegand, D. (Ed.). (2011). *AACN procedure manual for critical care* (6th ed., pp. 1224–1235). Saunders Elsevier.

Ostomy Care 0480

Definition: Maintenance of elimination through a stoma and care of surrounding tissue

Activities:

- Determine type of ostomy (e.g., bowel, bladder, continent, incontinent)
- Determine current level of knowledge related to ostomies, ostomy equipment, and required cares
- Determine comfort level and usual patterns with care of ostomy
- Explain procedure and establish level of participation
- Provide for privacy
- Assist to comfortable position either sitting or lying on bed, or sitting or standing in bathroom
- Empty pouch of ostomy bag and remove ostomy skin barrier
- Do not throw away reusable ostomy bag clamp
- Note consistency, color, and amount of stool or urine, including odor to urine, if any
- Clean and dry peristomal skin and stoma
- Note stoma appearance including size, (e.g., protruding, retracted)
- Note peristomal skin condition including signs of irritation
- Use gauze to cover stoma while cleansing and preparing peristomal skin
- Prepare peristomal area according to ostomy bag design (i.e., cut wafer to fit or ensure pre-designed wafer is correct size and shape, ensure skin clean and dry)
- Attach ostomy bag following directions on wafer or pre-fit bag
- Close ostomy bag per design directions
- Cover stoma with dressing or bandage if not using ostomy bag
- Instruct to empty continent urinary diversion devices (e.g., Indiana pouch) when feel sensation of fullness or at regular intervals (e.g., every 4–6 hours) using urinary catheterization equipment
- Instruct to empty ostomy bag and urinary diversion bags when one third to one half full of urine, stool, or gas
- Instruct to empty pouch moving feces down pouch sides with fingers and wipe end of pouch with tissue or premoistened towelette
- Irrigate ostomy using cone on enema catheter tip, in amounts of 300 to 500 mL, as indicated
- Instruct on ability to establish regular evacuation pattern with routine irrigation, if indicated
- Instruct on use of ostomy equipment and care
- Assist in obtaining needed equipment
- Monitor for incision and stoma healing
- Monitor for postop complications (e.g., intestinal obstruction, paralytic ileus, anastomotic leaks, mucocutaneous separation)
- Monitor stoma and surrounding tissue healing and adaptation to ostomy equipment
- Instruct when to change ostomy bag to new bag, as appropriate
- Assist in providing self-care
- Encourage to express feelings and concerns about changes in body image
- Explain what ostomy care will mean to day-to-day routine
- Assist to plan time for care routine
- Instruct how to monitor for complications (e.g., mechanical breakdown, chemical breakdown, rash, leaks, dehydration, infection)
- Instruct on mechanisms to reduce odor
- Monitor elimination patterns
- Assist to identify factors that affect elimination pattern
- Instruct in appropriate diet and expected changes in elimination function
- Provide support and assistance as develops skill in caring for stoma and surrounding tissue
- Instruct to chew foods thoroughly, avoid foods that caused digestive upset in past, add new foods one at a time, and drink plenty of fluids
- Instruct in Kegel exercises if has ileoanal reservoir
- Discuss concerns about sexual functioning, as appropriate
- Encourage visitation by persons from support group who have same condition
- Express confidence that can resume normal life with ostomy
- Encourage participation in ostomy support groups after discharge
- Notify wound ostomy nurse for follow-up and continued instruction, as appropriate
- Use teach-back to ensure understanding

1st edition 1992; revised 2000, 2004, 2024

Background Evidence:

Beauchaine, D. (2018). Urinary elimination. In R. F. Craven, C. J. Hirnle, & C. J. Henshaw (Eds.), *Fundamentals of nursing: Human health and function* (8th ed., pp. pp.1096–1114). Wolters-Kluwer.

Berman, A., Snyder, S. J., & Frandsen, G. (2018). Fecal elimination. In *Kozier and Erb's fundamentals of nursing: Concepts, process and practice* (pp. 1232–1237) (10th ed). Pearson.

Berman, A., Snyder, S. J., & Frandsen, G. (2018). Urinary elimination. In *Kozier and Erb's fundamentals of nursing: Concepts, process and practice* (pp. 1202–1204) (10th ed.). Pearson.

Berti-Hearn, L., & Elliott, B. (2018). A resource guide to improve nursing care and transition to self-care for patients with ostomies. *Home Healthcare Now, 36*(1), 43–49. https://doi.org/10.1097/NHH.0000000000000643

Potter, P. A., Ostendorf, W. R., & LaPlante, N. (2018). *Clinical nursing skills and techniques* (pp. 830–860) (9th ed.). Ostomy care. Mosby.

Stelton, S. (2019). CE: Stoma and peristomal skin care: A clinical review. *AJN, American Journal of Nursing, 119*(6), 38–45. https://doi.org/10.1097/01.NAJ.0000559781.86311.64

Westvang, N. (2018). Bowel elimination. In R. F. Craven, C. J. Hirnle, & C. J. Henshaw (Eds.), *Fundamentals of nursing: Human health and function* (8th ed., pp. 1152–1304). Wolters-Kluwer.

O

Oxygen Therapy 3320

Definition: Administration of oxygen and monitoring of its effectiveness

Activities:

- Verify order for oxygen therapy before administering, as indicated
- Instruct on oxygen therapy, role in delivery, and need to avoid smoking
- Ensure pulse oximetry available to monitor response to therapy, as indicated
- Document baseline observations including saturations, respiratory rate, blood pressure, and pulse
- Maintain airway patency
- Monitor respiratory effort, skin color, and level of consciousness
- Clear oral, nasal, and tracheal secretions to optimize airway patency
- Position for optimum breathing efficiency (e.g., high or semi-fowlers)
- Insert flow meter into outlet and attach appropriate oxygen tubing and delivery device (e.g., mask, nasal cannula, ET tube)
- Adjust method of delivery to accommodate age (e.g., oxygen tent or isolette for small children and neonates)
- Attach humidifying unit to the flow meter, as indicated (i.e., oxygen must be humidified to avoid mucosal drying when delivery bypasses oral cavity or when delivered at levels higher than 6 L/min)
- Ensure flow meter at appropriate dose
- Place appropriate signage around room or at home
- Monitor oxygen liter flow
- Monitor position of oxygen delivery device
- Plan nursing care so tent or isolette is entered as little as possible to prevent oxygen levels from dropping
- Provide children with favorite toy or blanket when fearful of tent
- Instruct about importance of leaving oxygen delivery device on (i.e., oxygen will ease dyspnea or discomfort)
- Encourage to breathe through nose if using nasal cannula
- Instruct concerning safety precautions associated with oxygen use
- Check oxygen delivery device routinely to ensure that prescribed concentration delivered (i.e., tubing not kinked, mask or cannula in wrong position)
- Monitor effectiveness of oxygen therapy (e.g., pulse oximetry, ABGs)
- Ensure replacement of oxygen mask or cannula whenever device removed
- Monitor ability to tolerate removal of oxygen when eating
- Change oxygen delivery device from mask to nasal cannula during meals, as tolerated
- Observe for signs of oxygen-induced hypoventilation (e.g., anxiety, decreased level of consciousness, inability to concentrate, fatigue, dizziness, cardiac dysrhythmias, pallor, cyanosis, dyspnea)
- Monitor for signs of oxygen toxicity and absorption atelectasis

- Monitor oxygen equipment to ensure not interfering with attempts to breathe
- Monitor anxiety related to need for oxygen therapy
- Monitor for skin breakdown from friction of oxygen device
- Provide for oxygen during transport
- Instruct to obtain supplementary oxygen prescription before air travel or trips to high altitude, as appropriate
- Consult with other health care professionals regarding use of supplemental oxygen during activity or sleep
- Instruct about use of oxygen at home (e.g., how to use equipment, when to have oxygen refilled, no smoking)
- Encourage to use oxygen vendor whose services include trained personnel to instruct in use and maintenance of equipment, 24-hour emergency service, and monthly follow-up visits for equipment maintenance and instruction
- Arrange for use of oxygen devices that facilitate mobility and instruct accordingly
- Convert to alternate oxygen delivery device to promote comfort, as appropriate
- Encourage to share fears and concerns about oxygen therapy
- Refer to local support group that uses home oxygen, as indicated
- Use teach-back to ensure understanding

1st edition 1992; revised 2000, 2024

Background Evidence:

Atkinson, D. (2017). Ambulatory and short- burst oxygen for interstitial lung disease. *Nursing Standard, 32*(14), 41–42. https://doi.org/10.7748/ns.2017.e11008

Craven, R. F., Hirnle, C. J., & Henshaw, C. J. (2021). Oxygen therapy. In *Fundamentals of nursing: Human health and function* (pp. 925–927) (9th ed.). Wolters-Kluwer.

Duan, L., Xie, C., & Zhao, N. (2022). Effect of high-flow nasal cannula oxygen therapy in patients with chronic obstructive pulmonary disease: A meta-analysis. *Journal of Clinical Nursing, 31*(1/2), 87–98. https://doi.org/10.1111/jocn.15957

Ford, C., & Robertson, M. (2021). Oxygen therapy in a hospital setting. *British Journal of Nursing, 30*(2), 96–100. https://doi.org/10.12968/bjon.2021.30.2.96

Karabey, T., & Aybek, S. D. (2021). Oxidative stress, COVID-19 and nursing care. *International Journal of Caring Sciences, 14*(3), 1763–1770.

Perry, A. G., Potter, P. A., Ostendorf, W. R., & LaPlante, N. (2021). *Clinical nursing skills and techniques* (10th ed.). Mosby.

Pruitt, B. (2021). High-flow oxygen therapy and BiPAP: Two complementary strategies to fight respiratory failure. *RT: The Journal for Respiratory Care Practitioners, 34*(3), 26–29.

Pruitt, B. (2021). Pediatric oxygen therapy and humidification. *RT: The Journal for Respiratory Care Practitioners, 34*(6), 8–11.

Siela, D., & Kidd, M. (2017). Oxygen requirements for acutely and critically ill patients. *Critical Care Nurse, 37*(4), 58–70.

O

Pacemaker Management: Permanent   4091

Definition: Care of the patient receiving permanent support of cardiac pumping through the insertion and use of a pacemaker

Activities:

- Provide information to patient and family related to pacemaker implantation (e.g., indications, functions, universal programming codes, potential complications)
- Provide concrete, objective information related to the effects of pacemaker therapy to reduce patient uncertainty, fear, and anxiety about treatment-related symptoms
- Document pertinent data in patient permanent record for initial insertion of pacemaker (e.g., manufacturer, model number, serial number, implant date, mode of operation, programmed parameters, upper and lower rate limits for rate-responsive devices, type of lead fixation, unipolar or bipolar lead system, capability for pacing and/or shock delivery, delivery system for shocks)
- Assure confirmation of pacemaker placement post-implantation in initial insertion with baseline chest x-ray
- Monitor for signs of improved cardiac output at specified intervals after initiation of pacing (e.g., improved urine output, warm and dry skin, freedom from chest pain, stable vital signs, absence of JVD and crackles, improved level of consciousness), per facility protocol
- Palpate peripheral pulses at specified intervals per facility protocol to ensure adequate perfusion with paced beats
- Monitor for potential complications associated with pacemaker insertion (e.g., pneumothorax, hemothorax, myocardial perforation, cardiac tamponade, hematoma, PVCs, infections, hiccups, muscle twitches)
- Monitor for failure to pace and determine cause (e.g., lead dislodgement, fracture, or migration), as appropriate
- Monitor for failure to capture and determine cause (e.g., lead dislodgement or malposition, pacing at voltage lower than capture threshold, faulty connections, lead fracture, ventricular perforation), as appropriate
- Monitor for failure to sense and determine cause (e.g., sensitivity set too high, malposition of catheter lead, lead fracture, lead insulation break), as appropriate
- Obtain chest x-ray immediately in the event of suspected lead fracture, patch crinkling, lead dislodgement, or lead migration
- Monitor for symptoms of arrhythmias, ischemia, or heart failure (e.g., dizziness, syncope, palpitations, chest pain, shortness of breath), particularly with each outpatient contact
- Monitor for pacemaker problems that have occurred between scheduled checkup visits
- Monitor for arm swelling or increased warmth on side ipsilateral to implanted endovascular leads
- Monitor for redness or swelling at the device site
- Perform a comprehensive appraisal of peripheral circulation (i.e., check peripheral pulses, edema, capillary refill, skin temperature, and diaphoresis) in any initial assessment of pacemaker patients and before initiating corrective actions
- Determine type and mode of pacemaker, including universal pacemaker code information for the five positions, before initiating corrective actions
- Gather additional data if possible, from patient's permanent record (e.g., date of implantation, frequency of use, programming changes and parameters) before initiating corrective actions
- Ensure ongoing monitoring of bedside ECG by qualified individuals
- Note frequency and duration of dysrhythmias
- Monitor hemodynamic response to dysrhythmias
- Facilitate acquisition of a 12-lead ECG, as appropriate
- Monitor sensorium and cognitive abilities
- Monitor blood pressure at specified intervals and with changes in patient condition
- Monitor heart rate and rhythm at specified intervals and with changes in patient condition
- Monitor drug and electrolyte levels for patients receiving concurrent antiarrhythmic medications
- Monitor for metabolic conditions with adverse effects on pacemakers (acid-base disturbances, myocardial ischemia, hyperkalemia, severe hyperglycemia [greater than 600 mg/dL], renal failure, hypothyroidism)
- Instruct patient regarding the potential hazards for electromagnetic interference from outside sources (i.e., keep at least 6 inches away from sources of interference, do not leave cell phones in the "on" mode in a shirt pocket over the pacemaker)
- Instruct patient regarding the sources of highest electromagnetic interference (e.g., arc welding equipment, electronic muscle stimulators, radio transmitters, concert speakers, large motor-generator systems, electric drills, handheld metal detectors, magnetic resonance imaging, radiation treatments)
- Instruct patient to check manufacturer warnings when in doubt about household appliances
- Instruct patient regarding the potential hazards from environmental interactions (e.g., inappropriate pacing or rhythm sensing, shortened generator life, cardiac arrhythmias, cardiac arrest)
- Instruct patient regarding the potential hazards from metabolic disruptions (e.g., potential to increase pacer or capture thresholds)
- Instruct patient on the need for regular checkups with primary cardiologist
- Instruct patient to consult primary cardiologist for all changes in medications
- Instruct patient with new pacemaker to refrain from operating motor vehicles until permitted, per primary cardiologist (usually 3 months minimally)
- Instruct patient in the need for regular monitoring of pacemaker sensing and capture thresholds
- Instruct patient in the need for regular interrogation of pacemaker by cardiologist for evidence of electromagnetic interference
- Instruct patient in the need to obtain chest x-ray at least annually for continued pacemaker placement confirmation
- Instruct patient of the signs and symptoms of dysfunctional pacemaker (e.g., bradycardia less than 30 beats per minute, dizziness, weakness, fatigue, chest discomfort, angina, shortness of breath, orthopnea, pedal edema, paroxysmal nocturnal dyspnea, dyspnea on exertion, hypotension, near-syncope, frank syncope, cardiac arrest)
- Instruct patient to carry manufacturer identification card at all times

P

- Instruct patient to wear a medical alert bracelet or necklace that identifies patient as a pacemaker patient
- Instruct patient on the special considerations at government security gates or the airport (e.g., always inform security guard of implantable pacemaker, walk through security gates, DO NOT allow handheld metal detectors near the device site, always walk quickly through metal detection devices or ask to be searched by hand, do not lean on or stand near detection devices for long periods)
- Instruct patient that handheld metal detectors contain magnets that can reset the pacemaker and cause malfunction
- Instruct patient's family that no harm comes to a person touching a patient who is receiving a pacemaker discharge

5th edition 2008

Background Evidence:

American Association of Critical-Care Nurses. (2006). In J. G. Alspach (Ed.), *Core curriculum for critical care nursing* (6th ed.). Saunders Elsevier.

Geiter, H. B., Jr. (2004). Getting back to basics with permanent pacemakers, Part 1. *Nursing 2004, 34*(10), 32cc1–32cc4.

Geiter, H. B., Jr. (2004). Getting back to basics with permanent pacemakers, Part 2. *Nursing 2004, 34*(11), 32cc1–32cc2.

Hogle, W. P. (2001). Pacing the standard of nursing practice in radiation oncology. *Clinical Journal of Oncology Nursing, 5*(6), 253–256, 267–268.

Mattingly, E. (2004). Arrhythmia management devices and electromagnetic interference. *AANA Journal, 73*(2), 129–136.

Smeltzer, S. C., & Bare, B. G. (2004). *Brunner & Suddarth's textbook of medical-surgical nursing* (10th ed.). Lippincott, Williams and Wilkins.

Yeo, T. P., & Berg, N. C. (2005). Counseling patients with implanted cardiac devices. *The Nurse Practitioner, 29*(12), 58–65.

Pacemaker Management: Temporary   4092

Definition: Temporary support of cardiac pumping through the insertion and use of a temporary pacemaker

Activities:

- Determine indications for temporary pacing and duration of intended pacing support
- Determine intended mechanics of pacing (e.g., internal or external, unipolar or bipolar, transthoracic, epicardial, or central venous catheter), including appropriateness of type of pulse generator selected
- Perform a comprehensive appraisal of peripheral circulation (i.e., check peripheral pulses, edema, capillary refill), skin temperature, and diaphoresis
- Ensure ongoing monitoring of bedside ECG by qualified individuals
- Note frequency and duration of dysrhythmias
- Monitor hemodynamic response to dysrhythmias
- Facilitate acquisition of a 12-lead ECG, as appropriate
- Monitor sensorium and cognitive abilities
- Monitor blood pressure at specified intervals and with changes in patient condition
- Monitor heart rate and rhythm at specified intervals and with changes in patient condition
- Instruct patient regarding the chosen pacemaker (e.g., purpose, indications, mechanics, duration)
- Ensure externally paced patients are aware of possibility of discomfort and availability of sedation for comfort and/or relaxation
- Obtain informed consent for insertion of the selected temporary pacemaker
- Prepare skin on chest and back by washing with soap and water and trim body hair with scissors, not razor, as necessary
- Prepare the chosen pacemaker for use, per facility protocol (i.e., ensure battery is fresh, identify atrial and ventricular wire sets, identify positive and negative leads for each pair of wires, identification labels, as indicated/preferred)
- Assist with insertion or placement of selected device, as appropriate
- Apply external transcutaneous pacemaker electrodes to clean, dry skin on the left anterior chest and to the posterior chest, as appropriate
- Provide sedation and analgesia for patients with external transcutaneous pacemaker, as indicated
- Set rate according to patient need as directed by physician (general guidelines: 90 to 110 beats per minute surgical patients, 70 to 90 beats per minute medical patients, 80 beats per minute cardiac arrest patients)
- Set the milliamperage according to patient (general adult guidelines: nonurgent 10 mA; emergent 15 to 20 mA); increase mA until capture is present
- Monitor patient response to mA setting at regular intervals in anticipation of fluctuations resulting from endothelial sheath formation around electrode tips
- Set the sensitivity (general adult guidelines: 2 to 5 millivolt, if failure to sense occurs, turn millivolt DOWN; if sensing beats not actually present, turn millivolt UP)
- Initiate pacing by slowly increasing mA level delivered until consistent capture (capture threshold) occurs (general guidelines of mA output at 1.5 to 3 times higher than threshold, and minimally 15 to 20 mA in emergent conditions)
- Obtain chest x-ray examination after insertion of invasive temporary pacemaker
- Monitor for presence of paced rhythm or resolution of initiating dysrhythmia
- Monitor for signs of improved cardiac output at specified intervals after initiation of pacing (e.g., improved urine output, warm and dry skin, freedom from chest pain, stable vital signs, absence of JVD and crackles, improved level of consciousness), per facility protocol
- Palpate peripheral pulses at specified intervals per facility protocol to ensure adequate perfusion with paced beats
- Inspect skin frequently to prevent potential burns for patients with external transcutaneous pacemaker
- Monitor for potential complications associated with pacemaker insertion (e.g., pneumothorax, hemothorax, myocardial perforation, cardiac tamponade, hematoma, PVCs, infections, hiccups, muscle twitches)
- Observe for changes in cardiac or hemodynamic status that indicate a need for modifications in pacemaker status
- Monitor for failure to pace and determine cause (e.g., battery failure, lead dislodgement, wire fracture, disconnected wire or cable), as appropriate
- Monitor for failure to capture and determine cause (e.g., lead dislodgement or malposition, battery failure, pacing at voltage lower than capture threshold, faulty connections, lead fracture, ventricular perforation), as appropriate

P

- Monitor for failure to sense and determine cause (e.g., sensitivity set too high, battery failure, malposition of catheter lead, lead fracture, pulse generator failure, lead insulation break), as appropriate
- Monitor for conditions that potentially influence capture and sensing (e.g., fluid status changes, pericardial effusion, electrolyte or metabolic abnormalities, certain medications, tissue inflammation, tissue fibrosis, tissue necrosis)
- Perform capture and sensitivity threshold testing every 24 to 48 hours with newly inserted pacers to determine best generator settings (contraindicated in patients paced 90% or more of the time)
- Perform threshold testing separately for atrial and ventricular chambers
- Provide appropriate incisional care for pacemakers with insertion sites (e.g., dressing change, antimicrobial and sterile occlusive dressing per facility protocol)
- Ensure that all equipment is grounded, in good working order, and carefully located (e.g., in a location from which it will not be dropped on the floor)
- Ensure that wires are of a length to deter inadvertent dislodging of electrodes
- Wear gloves when adjusting electrodes
- Insulate electrode wires when not in use (e.g., cover unused thoracic wires with the fingertip of a disposable glove)

- Instruct patient and family member(s) regarding symptoms to report (e.g., dizziness, fainting, prolonged weakness, nausea, palpitations, chest pain, difficulty breathing, discomfort at insertion or external electrode site, electrical shocks)
- Teach patient and family member(s) precautions and restrictions required when temporary pacemaker is in place (e.g., limitation of movement, avoid handling the pacemaker)

4th edition 2004; revised 2008

Background Evidence:

American Association of Critical-Care Nurses. (2006). In J. G. Alspach (Ed.), *Core curriculum for critical care nursing* (6th ed.). Saunders Elsevier.

Overbay, D., & Criddle, L. (2004). Mastering temporary invasive cardiac pacing. *Critical Care Nurse, 24*(3), 25–32.

Smeltzer, S. C., & Bare, B. G. (2004). *Brunner & Suddarth's textbook of medical-surgical nursing* (10th ed.). Lippincott Williams and Wilkins.

Wiegand, D., & Carlson, K. (Eds.). (2005). *AACN procedure manual for critical care* (5th ed.). Elsevier Saunders.

Yeo, T. P., & Berg, N. C. (2005). Counseling patients with implanted cardiac devices. *The Nurse Practitioner, 29*(12), 58–65.

Pain Management: Acute   1410

Definition: Alleviation or reduction of pain to a level that is acceptable to the patient in the immediate healing period following tissue damage from an identifiable cause such as trauma, surgery, or injury

Activities:

- Perform a comprehensive assessment of pain to include location, onset, duration, frequency, and intensity of pain, as well as alleviating and precipitating factors
- Identify pain intensity during movements such as required recovery activities (e.g., coughing and deep breathing, ambulation, transfers to chair)
- Explore patient's knowledge and beliefs about pain, including cultural influences
- Monitor pain using a valid and reliable rating tool appropriate for age and ability to communicate
- Observe for nonverbal cues of discomfort, especially in those unable to communicate effectively
- Question patient regarding the level of pain that allows a state of comfort and appropriate function and attempt to keep pain at or lower than identified level
- Ensure that the patient receives prompt analgesic care before the pain becomes severe or before pain-inducing activities
- Administer analgesics around-the-clock the first 24 to 48 hours after surgery, trauma, or injury except if sedation or respiratory status indicates otherwise
- Monitor sedation and respiratory status before administering opioids and at regular intervals when opioids are administered
- Follow agency protocols in selecting analgesic and dosage
- Use combination analgesics (e.g., opioids plus nonopioids), if pain level is severe
- Select and implement intervention options tailored to the patient's risks benefits and preferences (e.g., pharmacological, non-pharmacological, interpersonal) to facilitate pain relief, as appropriate
- Avoid use of analgesics that may have adverse effects in older adults

- Administer analgesics using the least invasive route available, avoiding the intramuscular route
- Provide PCA and intraspinal routes of administration, when appropriate
- Incorporate non-pharmacological interventions to the pain etiology and patient preference, as appropriate
- Modify pain control measures on the basis of the patient's response to treatment
- Prevent or manage medication side effects
- Notify physician if pain control measures are unsuccessful
- Provide accurate information to the family about the patient's pain experience

7th edition 2018

Background Evidence:

American Geriatrics Society 2012 Beers Criteria Update Expert Panel. (2012). American Geriatrics Society updated Beers criteria for potentially inappropriate medication use in older adults. *Journal of the American Geriatrics Society, 60*(4), 616–631.

American Society for Pain Management Nursing. (2010). In B. St Marie (Ed.), *Core curriculum for pain management nursing* (2nd ed.). Kendall Hunt.

Cason, L. (2013). Pain management. In P. Potter, A. Perry, P. Stockert, & A. Hall (Eds.), *Fundamentals of nursing* (8th ed., pp. 962–995). Elsevier Mosby.

D'Arcy, Y. (2011). *Compact clinical guide to chronic pain management: An evidence-based approach for nurses.* Springer.

Pasero, C., & McCaffery, M. (2011). *Pain assessment and pharmacological management.* Mosby Elsevier.

P

Pain Management: Chronic 1415

Definition: Alleviation or reduction of persistent pain that continues beyond the normal healing period, assumed to be three months, to a level that is acceptable to the patient

Activities:

- Perform a comprehensive assessment of pain to include location, onset, duration, frequency, and intensity of pain, as well as alleviating and precipitating factors
- Use a valid and reliable chronic pain assessment tool (e.g., Brief Pain Inventory-Short Form, McGill Pain Questionnaire-Short Form, Fibromyalgia Impact Questionnaire)
- Explore patient's knowledge and beliefs about pain, including cultural influences
- Determine the effect of the pain experience on quality of life (e.g., sleep, appetite, activity, cognition, mood, relationships, job performance, and role responsibilities)
- Evaluate with patient the effectiveness of past pain control measures
- Control environmental factors that may influence the patient's pain experience
- Question the patient regarding pain at frequent intervals, often at the same time as checking vital signs or at every office visit
- Question patient regarding the level of pain that allows a state of comfort and appropriate function and attempt to keep pain at or lower than identified level
- Ensure that the patient receives prompt analgesic care before the pain become severe or before pain-inducing activities
- Select and implement intervention options tailored to the patient's risks benefits and preferences (e.g., pharmacological, non-pharmacological, interpersonal) to facilitate pain relief, as appropriate
- Instruct patient and family about principles of pain management
- Encourage patient to monitor own pain and to use self-management approaches
- Encourage appropriate use of non-pharmacological techniques (e.g., biofeedback, TENS, hypnosis, relaxation, guided imagery, music therapy, distraction, play therapy, activity therapy, acupressure, heat and cold application, and massage) and pharmacological options as pain control measures
- Avoid use of analgesics that may have adverse effects in older adults
- Collaborate with patient, family, and other health professionals to select and implement pain control measures
- Prevent or manage medication side effects
- Evaluate the effectiveness of pain control measures through ongoing monitoring of the pain experience
- Watch for signs of depression (e.g., sleeplessness, not eating, flat affect statements of depression, or suicidal ideation)
- Watch for signs of anxiety or fear (e.g., irritability, tension, worry, fear of movement)
- Modify pain control measures on the basis of the patient's response to treatment
- Incorporate the family in the pain relief modality, when possible
- Utilize a multidisciplinary approach to pain management, when appropriate
- Consider referrals for patient and family to support groups and other resources, as appropriate
- Evaluate patient satisfaction with pain management at specified intervals

7th edition 2018

Background Evidence:

American Geriatrics Society 2012 Beers Criteria Update Expert Panel. (2012). American Geriatrics Society updated Beers criteria for potentially inappropriate medication use in older adults. *Journal of the American Geriatrics Society, 60*(4), 616–631.

American Society for Pain Management Nursing. (2010). In B. St Marie (Ed.), *Core curriculum for pain management nursing* (2nd ed.). Kendall Hunt.

American Society of Anesthesiologists Task Force on Chronic Pain Management, & American Society of Regional Anesthesia and Pain Medicine. (2010). Practice guidelines for chronic pain management. *Anesthesiology, 112*(4), 810–833.

Cason, L. (2013). Pain management. In P. Potter, A. Perry, P. Stockert, & A. Hall (Eds.), *Fundamentals of nursing* (8th ed., pp. 962–995). Elsevier Mosby.

D'Arcy, Y. (2011). *Compact clinical guide to chronic pain management: An evidence-based approach for nurses.* Springer.

Pasero, C., & McCaffery, M. (2011). *Pain assessment and pharmacological management.* Mosby Elsevier.

Pandemic Precautions 6592

Definition: Promotion of strategies to safeguard persons from spread of an infectious disease

Activities:

- Provide scientific and factually based information on pandemic precautions
- Avoid stigmatization and marginalization during discussions regarding pandemic precautions
- Identify reasons for resistance to pandemic precautions, as needed
- Discuss high-risk areas that may increase likelihood for contracting pandemic-related disease (e.g., industrial or food processing facilities, correctional facilities, healthcare facilities, service industries)
- Determine living arrangements to identify congregate setting, multigenerational home, or homelessness status, which may contribute to disease spread
- Identify specific behaviors that would influence increased likelihood of contracting pandemic-related disease
- Educate on common symptoms associated with pandemic-related disease
- Identify ways to monitor health daily
- Encourage frequent handwashing of at least 20 seconds with soap and water after being in public spaces, touching face, or contact with high-touch surfaces

- Educate to use hand sanitizer with at least 60% alcohol if hands are not visibly soiled and soap and water are not available
- Identify measures for decontaminating high touch surfaces at home and workplace
- Demonstrate proper mechanics for covering coughs and sneezes
- Educate on scientific rationale and proper technique for wearing face masks
- Educate on use of vaccinations, based on availability, to help reduce transmission of pandemic-related disease
- Instruct to maintain physical distance from others as close contact with individuals in pre-symptomatic or asymptomatic phase may lead to infection
- Discuss benefits of stay-at-home orders and state-based mandates for masking on reducing transmission of pandemic-related disease
- Discuss impact of poorly ventilated spaces and crowded areas on spread of disease during pandemics
- Educate persons and family members on appropriate self-isolation and quarantine procedures if someone in person's home diagnosed with pandemic-related disease
- Identify potential contacts with persons that were diagnosed with pandemic-related disease, including prior to diagnosis, as needed
- Identify local, state, regional, and national resources available to provide supplies and resources to persons

8th edition 2024

Background Evidence:

Centers for Disease Control and Prevention. (2020). *Coronavirus disease 2019 (COVID-19): How to protect yourself.* https://www.cdc.gov/coronavirus/2019-ncov/prevent-getting-sick/prevention.html

Centers for Disease Control and Prevention. (2020). *Social distancing. Centers for Disease Control and Prevention website.* https://www.cdc.gov/coronavirus/2019-ncov/prevent-getting-sick/social-distancing.html

Lynteris, C., & Poleykett, B. (2018). The anthropology of epidemic control: Technologies and Materialities. *Medical Anthropology, 37*(6), 433–441. https://doi.org/10.1080/01459740.2018.1484740

Maragakis, L. L. (2020). *Coronavirus, social and physical distancing and self-quarantine.* John Hopkins Website, Health. https://www.hopkinsmedicine.org/health/conditions-and-diseases/coronavirus/coronavirus-social-distancing-and-self-quarantine

Mukherji, A., Gupta, T., & Agarwal, J. P. (2020). Time, distance, shielding and ALARA; drawing similarities between measures for radiation protection and Coronavirus disease pandemic response. *Indian Journal of Cancer, 57*(2), 221–223.

Nicola, M., O'Neill, N., Sohrabi, C., Khan, M., Agha, M., & Agha, R. (2020). Evidence based management guideline for the COVID-19 pandemic. *International Journal of Surgery, 77*, 206–216.

Purba, A. K. (2020). How should the role of the nurse change in response to Covid-19? *Nursing Times, 116*(6), 25–28.

Wee, L., Sim, X., Conceicao, E., Aung, M., Tan, K., Ko, K., Wong, H., Wijaya, L., Tan, B., Venkatachalam, I., & Ling, M. (2020). Containing COVID-19 outside the isolation ward: The impact of an infection control bundle on environmental contamination and transmission in a cohorted general ward. *American Journal of Infection Control, 48*(9), 1056–1061.

Parent Education: Adolescent   5562

Definition: Assisting parents to understand and help their adolescent children

Activities:

- Ask parents to describe the characteristics of their adolescent child
- Discuss parent-child relationship during earlier, school-aged years
- Understand the relationship between the parent's behavior and child's age-appropriate goals
- Identify personal factors that effect on the success of the educational program (e.g., cultural values, presence of any negative experiences with social service providers, language barriers, time commitment, scheduling issues, travel, and general lack of interest)
- Identify the presence of family stressors (e.g., parental depression, drug addiction, alcoholism, low literacy, limited education, domestic violence, marital conflict, blending of families after divorce, and excessive punishment of children)
- Discuss disciplining of parents, themselves, when they were adolescents
- Instruct parent on normal physiological, emotional, and cognitive characteristics of adolescents
- Identify developmental tasks or goals of the adolescent period of life
- Identify defense mechanisms used most commonly by adolescents, such as denial and intellectualization
- Address the effects of adolescent cognitive development on information processing
- Address the effects of adolescent cognitive development on decision making
- Have parents describe methods of discipline used before adolescent years and their feelings of success with these measures
- Provide online resources, books, and literature designed to teach parents about teen parenting
- Describe the importance of power and control issues for both parents and adolescents during adolescent years
- Instruct parents about essential communication skills that will increase their ability to empathize with their adolescent and assist their adolescent to problem solve
- Instruct parents about methods of communicating their love to adolescents
- Explore parallels between school-aged dependency on parents and adolescent dependency on peer group
- Reinforce normalcy of adolescent vacillation between desire for independence and regression to dependence
- Discuss effects of adolescent separation from parents on spousal relationships
- Share strategies for managing adolescent's perception of parental rejection
- Facilitate expression of parental feelings
- Assist parents to identify reasons for their responses to adolescents
- Identify avenues to assist adolescent to manage anger
- Instruct parents how to use conflict for mutual understanding and family growth
- Role play strategies for managing family conflict
- Discuss with parents issues over which they will accept compromise and issues over which they cannot compromise
- Discuss necessity and legitimacy of limit setting for adolescents
- Address strategies for limit setting for adolescents
- Instruct parents to use reality and consequences to manage adolescent behavior

P

• Refer parents to support group or parenting classes, as appropriate

---

1st edition 1992; revised 2013

Background Evidence:

American Academy of Child and Adolescent Psychiatry. (1999). In D. Pruitt (Ed.), *Your adolescent: Emotional, behavioral, and cognitive development from early adolescence through the teen years.* Harper Collins.

Cline, F., & Fay, J. (2006). *Parenting teens with love and logic: Preparing adolescents for responsible adulthood (updated and expanded ed.).* Piñon Press.

Dinkmeyer, D., Sr., McKay, G. D., McKay, J. L., & Dinkmeyer, D., Jr. (2007). *Parenting teenagers: Systematic training for effective parenting of teens.* STEP.

Pillitteri, A. (2007). The family with an adolescent. In *Maternal and child health nursing: Care of the childbearing and childrearing family* (pp. 941–974) (5th ed.). Lippincott Williams & Wilkins.

Parent Education: Childrearing Family 5566

Definition: Assisting parents to understand and promote the physical, psychological, and social growth and development of their toddler, preschool, or school-aged child

Activities:

• Ask parent to describe the behaviors of the child
• Understand the relationship between the parent's behavior and child's age-appropriate goals
• Design an education program that builds on the family's strengths
• Involve parents in the design and content of the education program
• Identify personal factors that effect on the success of the education program (e.g., cultural values, presence of any negative experiences with social service providers, language barriers, time commitment, scheduling issues, travel, and general lack of interest)
• Identify the presence of family stressors (e.g., parental depression, drug addiction, alcoholism, low literacy, limited education, domestic violence, marital conflict, blending of families after divorce, and excessive punishment of children)
• Identify appropriate developmental tasks or goals for the child
• Identify defense mechanisms used most by age group
• Facilitate parents' discussion of methods of discipline available, selection, and results obtained
• Instruct parent on normal physiological, emotional, and behavioral characteristics of child
• Provide online resources, books, and literature designed to teach parents about parenting
• Provide parents with readings and other materials that will be helpful in performing parenting role
• Instruct parents on the importance of a balanced diet, three meals a day, and nutritious snacks
• Review nutritional requirements for specific age groups
• Review dental hygiene facts with parents
• Review grooming facts with parents
• Review safety issues with parents (e.g., children meeting strangers, water safety, bicycle safety)
• Discuss avenues parents can use to assist children in managing anger
• Discuss approaches parents can use to assist children to express feelings positively
• Help parents identify evaluation criteria for day care and school settings
• Inform parents of community resources
• Identify and instruct parents on how to use a variety of strategies in managing child's behavior
• Encourage parents to try different childrearing strategies, as appropriate
• Encourage parents to observe other parents interacting with children
• Role play childrearing techniques and communication skills
• Refer parents to support group or parenting classes, as appropriate

---

1st edition 1992; revised 2013

Background Evidence:

American Academy of Child, & Adolescent Psychiatry. (1998). In D. Pruitt (Ed.), *Your child: Emotional, behavioral, and cognitive development from birth to preadolescence.* HarperCollins.

Hockenberry, M. J., Wilson, D., & Winkelstein, M. (Eds.). (2005). *Wong's essentials of pediatric nursing* (7th ed.). Elsevier Mosby.

Licence, K. (2004). Promoting and protecting the health of children and young people. *Child: Care, Health, and Development, 30*(6), 623–635.

Riesch, S. K., Anderson, L. S., & Krueger, H. A. (2006). Parent–child communication processes: Preventing children's health-risk behavior. *Journal for Specialists in Pediatric Nursing, 11*(1), 41–56.

Schor, E. (1999). *Caring for your school age child: Ages 5 to 12.* Bantam.

Shelov, S., & Altman, T. R. (2009). *Caring for your baby and young child: Birth to age 5* (5th ed.). Bantam.

Shonkoff, J.P., & Phillips. D.A. (Eds.). (2000). *From neurons to neighborhoods: The science of early childhood development.*

Parent Education: Infant 5568

Definition: Instruction on nurturing and physical care needed during the first year of life

Activities:

• Determine knowledge and readiness and ability to learn about infant care
• Monitor learning needs of family
• Provide anticipatory guidance about developmental changes
• Assist in articulating ways to integrate infant into family system
• Instruct on skills to care for infant
• Encourage to practice exclusive breastfeeding until 6 months of age
• Provide anticipatory guidance about signs of breastfeeding problems
• Instruct on formula preparation and selection
• Provide information about risks and necessity of using pacifiers

- Provide guidance about introduction of solid foods after 6 months of age
- Provide guidance about risks of infant obesity
- Instruct on appropriate fluoride supplementation
- Give information about developing dentition and oral hygiene
- Discuss alternatives to bedtime bottle to prevent bottle caries
- Provide anticipatory guidance about changing elimination patterns
- Instruct on how to treat and prevent diaper rash
- Provide anticipatory guidance about changing sleep patterns
- Instruct about infant sleeping positions
- Demonstrate ways to stimulate infant's development
- Encourage to hold, cuddle, massage, and touch infant
- Encourage to talk and read to infant
- Encourage to provide pleasurable auditory and visual stimulation
- Encourage to play with infant
- Give examples of safe toys or available items in home that can be used as toys
- Encourage to attend parenting classes
- Provide written materials appropriate to identified knowledge needs
- Reinforce ability to apply teaching to childcare skills
- Provide support when learning infant caretaking skills
- Assist in interpreting infant cues, nonverbal cues, crying, and vocalizations
- Provide information on newborn behavioral characteristics
- Demonstrate reflexes and explain their significance to infant care
- Discuss infant's capabilities for interaction
- Assist to identify behavioral characteristics of infant
- Explain and demonstrate infant clinical condition
- Demonstrate quieting techniques
- Monitor skill in recognizing infant's physiological needs
- Reinforce caregiver role behaviors
- Reinforce skills parent does well in caring for infant to promote confidence
- Provide information about making home environment safe for infant
- Provide information about safety needs of infant when in motor vehicle
- Instruct on how to reach health professionals

- Place follow-up call 1 to 2 weeks after encounter
- Provide information about community resources
- Provide information about importance of having infant vaccinated
- Provide guidance about infant exposure to electronic devices
- Encourage participation in routine consultations to monitor infant growth and development
- Use teach-back to ensure understanding

3rd edition 2000; revised 2024

Background Evidence:

Hockenberry, M. J., Rodgers, C. C., & Wilson, D. (2022). *Wong's essentials of pediatric nursing* (11th ed.). Elsevier.

Kaufman, J., Ryan, R., Walsh, L., Horey, D., Leask, J., Robinson, P., & Hill, S. (2018). Face-to-face interventions for informing or educating parents about early childhood vaccination. *The Cochrane Database of Systematic Reviews*, 5(5), CD010038. https://doi.org/10.1002/14651858.CD010038.pub3

Mahesh, P., Gunathunga, M. W., Arnold, S. M., Jayasinghe, C., Pathirana, S., Makarim, M. F., Manawadu, P. M., & Senanayake, S. J. (2018). Effectiveness of targeting fathers for breastfeeding promotion: Systematic review and meta-analysis. *British Medical Community Public Health*, 18(1), 1140. https://doi.org/10.1186/s12889-018-6037-x

Matson, S., & Smith, J. E. (2016). *Core curriculum for maternal-newborn nursing*. Elsevier.

Matvienko-Sikar, K., Griffin, C., McGrath, N., Toomey, E., Byrne, M., Kelly, C., Heary, C., Devane, D., & Kearney, P. M. (2019). Developing a core outcome set for childhood obesity prevention: A systematic review. *Maternal & Child Nutrition*, 15(1), e12680. https://doi.org/10.1111/mcn.12680

Rayce, S. B., Rasmussen, I. S., Klest, S. K., Patras, J., & Pontoppidan, M. (2017). Effects of parenting interventions for at-risk parents with infants: A systematic review and meta-analyses. *British Medical Journal Open*, 7(12), e015707. https://doi.org/10.1136/bmjopen-2016-015707

Wan, M. W., Fitch-Bunce, C., Heron, K., & Lester, E. (2021). Infant screen media usage and social-emotional functioning. *Infant Behavior & Development*, 62, 101509. https://doi.org/10.1016/j.infbeh.2020.101509

P

Parenting Promotion   8300

Definition: Providing parenting information, support, and coordination of comprehensive services to high-risk families

Activities:

- Examine structure of family environment (i.e., adequate provision of inputs, safe space for child and family)
- Identify and enroll high-risk families in follow-up program
- Encourage mothers to receive early and regular prenatal care
- Visit mothers in hospital before discharge to begin establishing trusting relationship and schedule follow-up visit
- Make home visits as indicated by level of risk
- Assist parents with realistic expectations appropriate to developmental and ability level of child
- Assist parents with role transition and expectations of parenthood
- Refer to male home visitors to work with fathers, as appropriate
- Provide information according to family knowledge level
- Provide pamphlets, books, and other materials to develop parenting skills
- Discuss age-appropriate behavior management strategies
- Assist parents to identify unique temperament of infant
- Instruct parents to respond to behavior cues exhibited by their infant

- Model and encourage parental interaction with children
- Refer to parent support groups, as appropriate
- Assist parents in developing, maintaining, and using social support systems
- Listen to parents' problems and concerns non-judgmentally
- Provide positive feedback and structured successes at parenting skills to foster self-esteem
- Assist parents to develop social skills
- Instruct on and model coping skills
- Enhance problem-solving skills through role modeling, practice, and reinforcement
- Provide toys through toy lending library
- Monitor child health status, well-child checks, and immunization status
- Monitor parental health status and health maintenance activities
- Arrange transportation to well-child visits or other services as necessary
- Refer to community resources, as appropriate
- Coordinate community agencies working with family
- Provide linkage to job training or employment as needed

- Inform parents where to receive family planning services
- Monitor consistent and correct use of contraceptives, as appropriate
- Assist in arranging daycare as needed
- Refer for respite care, as appropriate
- Refer to domestic violence center as needed
- Refer for substance abuse treatment as needed
- Collect and record data as indicated for follow-up and program evaluation

3rd edition 2000; revised 2024

Background Evidence:

Beatson, R., Molloy, C., Perini, N., Harrop, C., & Goldfeld, S. (2021). Systematic review: An exploration of core componentry characterizing effective sustained nurse home visiting programs. *Journal of Advanced Nursing, 77*(6), 2581–2594. https://doi.org/10.1111/jan.14755

Molloy, C., Beatson, R., Harrop, C., Perini, N., & Goldfeld, S. (2021). Systematic review: Effects of sustained nurse home visiting programs for disadvantaged mothers and children. *Journal of Advanced Nursing, 77*(1), 147–161. https://doi.org/10.1111/jan.14576

Moon, D. J., Lauer, S. J., & Unell, B. (2021). Behavior Checker® staff training for positive parenting in primary care: changes in the knowledge, attitudes, and confidence. *Journal of Child & Family Studies, 30*(4), 932–940. https://doi.org/10.1007/s10826-021-01917-3

Ruiz, C. M., Drummond, J. D., Beeman, I., & Lach, L. M. (2017). Parenting for the promotion of adolescent mental health: A scoping review of programmes targeting ethnoculturally diverse families. *Health & Social Care in the Community, 25*(2), 743–757. https://doi.org/10.1111/hsc.12364

Tully, L. A., Piotrowska, P. J., Collins, D. A. J., Mairet, K. S., Black, N., Kimonis, E. R., Hawes, D. J., Moul, C., Lenroot, R. K., Frick, P. J., Anderson, V., & Dadds, M. R. (2017). Optimising child outcomes from parenting interventions: fathers' experiences, preferences and barriers to participation. *BMC Public Health, 17*, 1–14. https://doi.org/10.1186/s12889-017-4426-1

Williams, M. E., Hoare, Z., Owen, D. A., & Hutchings, J. (2020). Feasibility study of the enhancing parenting skills programme. *Journal of Child & Family Studies, 29*(3), 686–698. https://doi.org/10.1007/s10826-019-01581-8

Pass Facilitation 7440

Definition: Arranging a leave for a patient from a health care facility

Activities:

- Obtain physician order for pass, as appropriate
- Establish objectives for the pass
- Provide information about restrictions and length of time for pass
- Provide information needed for emergency use on pass
- Provide information on Medicare coverage for leave or "bed-hold" fee, as appropriate
- Determine who is responsible for patient, as appropriate
- Discuss pass with responsible person describing nursing care and self-care, as needed
- Obtain medications to be taken on pass and instruct responsible person
- Provide assistive devices and equipment, as appropriate
- Offer suggestions for appropriate pass activities, as needed
- Help pack personal belongings for pass, as needed
- Provide time for patient, family, and friends to ask questions and express concerns
- Instruct appropriate person on the information that is needed about medication, food, alcohol intake, and activities when on pass
- Provide written instructions, as needed
- Obtain signature of patient or responsible person on "sign-out" form
- Document on sign-out form the date and time of departure; name, strength, dose, and quantity of medications provided; directions given; and other pertinent actions
- Evaluate whether objectives for pass were met on return
- Verify that medications were taken as instructed on return

2nd edition 1996; revised 2018

Background Evidence:

Alper, E., O'Malley, T. A., & Greenwald, J. (2013). *Hospital discharge.* UpToDate. http://www.uptodate.com/contents/hospital-discharge

BC Children's Hospital. (2011). *Leave of absence—Patient (day/overnight pass).* http://bccwhcms.medworxx.com/Site_Published/bcc/document_render. aspx?documentRender.IdType=30&documentRender.GenericField= 1&documentRender.Id=3827

BC Children's Hospital. (2013). *Dispensing medication to patients granted temporary leave of absence from hospital ("pass meds").* http://bccwhcms. medworxx.com/Site_Published/bcc/document_render.aspx? documentRender.IdType=30&documentRender.GenericField=1& documentRender.Id=7855

Patient-Controlled Analgesia (PCA) Assistance 2400

Definition: Facilitating patient control of analgesic administration and regulation

Activities:

- Collaborate with physicians, patient, and family members in selecting the type of narcotic to be used
- Recommend administration of aspirin and nonsteroidal anti-inflammatory drugs in conjunction with narcotics, as appropriate
- Recommend discontinuation of opioid administration by other routes
- Avoid use of meperidine hydrochloride (Demerol)
- Ensure that patient is not allergic to analgesic to be administered
- Instruct patient and family to monitor pain intensity, quality, and duration
- Instruct patient and family to monitor respiratory rate and blood pressure
- Establish nasogastric, venous, subcutaneous, or spinal access, as appropriate
- Validate that the patient can use a PCA device (i.e., is able to communicate, comprehend explanations, and follow directions)
- Collaborate with patient and family to select appropriate type of patient-controlled infusion device

- Instruct patient and family members how to use the PCA device
- Assist patient and family to calculate appropriate concentration of drug to fluid, considering the amount of fluid delivered per hour via the PCA device
- Assist patient or family member to administer an appropriate bolus loading dose of analgesic
- Instruct the patient and family to set an appropriate basal infusion rate on the PCA device
- Assist the patient and family to set the appropriate lockout interval on the PCA device
- Assist the patient and family in setting appropriate demand doses on the PCA device
- Consult with patient, family members, and physician to adjust lockout interval, basal rate, and demand dosage, according to patient responsiveness
- Instruct patient how to titrate doses up or down, depending on respiratory rate, pain intensity, and pain quality
- Instruct patient and family members about the action and side effects of pain-relieving agents
- Document patient's pain, amount and frequency of drug dosing, and response to pain treatment in a pain flow sheet
- Monitor closely for respiratory depression in at-risk patients (e.g., older than 70 years; history of sleep apnea; concurrent use of PCA with a central nervous system depressant; obesity; upper abdominal or thoracic surgery and PCA bolus of greater than 1 mg; history of renal, hepatic, pulmonary, or cardiac impairment)
- Recommend a bowel regimen to avoid constipation
- Consult with clinical pain experts for a patient who is having difficulty achieving pain control

1st edition 1992; revised 2013

Background Evidence:

Berman, A., Snyder, S., Kozier, B., & Erb, G. (2008). Pain management. In *Kozier & Erb's fundamentals of nursing: Concepts, processes, and practice* (pp. 1187–1230) (8th ed.). Prentice Hall.

Chumbley, G., & Mountford, L. (2010). Patient-controlled analgesia infusion pumps for adults. *Nursing Standard, 25*(8), 35–40.

Craft, J. (2010). Patient-controlled analgesia: Is it worth the painful prescribing process? *Baylor University Medical Center Proceedings, 23*(4), 434–438.

Franson, H. (2010). Postoperative patient-controlled analgesia in the pediatric population: A literature review. *AANA Journal, 78*(5), 374–378.

Patient Identification   6574

Definition: Positive verification of a patient's identity

Activities:
- Explain to the patient the importance of proper identification throughout the health encounter
- Ask the patient his/her first name, last name, and date of birth
- Verify that the information provided by the patient is the same as the information in the identification device (e.g., wristbands, bed tag, fingerprint recognition software, palm vein scanner), and medical record
- Select the most appropriate location(s) for placing the identification device(s)
- Ensure that identification devices are put in appropriate locations
- Have on hand a number of replacement bands and an easy process for a new bracelet to be stamped and applied should a wristband be removed
- Standardize the format of the wristbands across the health care institution
- Compare the information provided by the patient with the information in the identification device before every administration of care (e.g., administering medications, performing invasive procedures, conducting diagnostic tests, transferring patient)
- Use at least two patient identifiers when laboratory samples are obtained or when medications or blood products are administered
- Conduct verification of patient at multiple points in time when procedure is complex and involves several stages
- Use identification by family member or good friend when patient cannot provide information
- Institute a "stop-the-line" policy if a misidentification error is suspected (i.e., do not carry out the intended action until positive identification is made)
- Educate the patient about the risks related to an incorrect identification
- Compare the information provided by a family member with the information in the identification device to confirm a patient's death
- Ensure a best practice for patient identification by instituting a clearly written, easy to understand, agency policy

6th edition, 2013

Background Evidence:

Association of periOperative Registered Nurses. (2006). Best practices for preventing wrong site, wrong person, and wrong procedure errors in perioperative settings. *AORN Journal, 84*(Suppl. 1), S13–S29.

Beyea, S. C. (2003). Patient identification: A crucial aspect on patient safety. *AORN Journal, 78*(3), 478–481.

Bittle, M. J., Charache, P., & Wassilchalk, D. M. (2007). Registration-associated patient misidentification in an academic medical centre: Causes and corrections. *Joint Commission Journal on Quality and Patient Safety, 33*(1), 25–33.

Clarke, J. R., Johnson, J., & Finley, E. (2007). Getting surgery right. *Annals of Surgery, 246*(3), 395–403.

Edwards, P. (2008). Ensuring correct site surgery. *Journal of Perioperative Practice, 18*(4), 168–171.

Gray, J. E., Suresh, G., Ursprung, R., Edwards, W. H., Nickerson, J., Shiono, P. H., Plsek, P., Goldmann, D. A., & Horbar, J. (2006). Patient misidentification in the neonatal intensive care unit: Quantification of risk. *Pediatrics, 117*(1), e43–e47.

Hain, P., Joers, B., Rush, M., Slayton, J., Throop, P., Hoagg, S., Allen, L., Grantham, J., & Deshpande, J. (2010). An intervention to decrease patient identification band errors in a children's hospital. *Quality Safety in Health Care, 19*(3), 244–247.

High Tech Patient ID, Information technologists design system to recognize palm vein patterns. (2007) *Science Daily.* http://www.sciencedaily.com/videos/2007/1009-high_tech_patient_id.htm

P

Patient Rights Protection   7460

Definition: Provision of respect, privacy, confidentiality, informed consent, and treatment without discrimination, coercion, or abuse

Activities:

- Provide with written statement of rights as recipient of care, in preferred language (e.g., American Hospital Association Patient Bill of Rights)
- Provide interpreter if unable to understand written or verbal explanations of rights
- Provide environment conducive for private conversations
- Protect privacy during all care activities
- Determine whether wishes about health care are known (e.g., living will, durable power of attorney for health care)
- Determine who is legally empowered to give consent for treatment or research
- Work with health care providers to honor wishes
- Refrain from forcing treatment
- Ensure cultural and religious preferences are respected
- Know legal status of living wills in current state
- Honor wishes expressed in living will or durable power of attorney for health care, and "Do Not Resuscitate" orders
- Document in health care record mental competency to make decisions, as appropriate
- Provide appropriate pain management for acute, chronic, and terminal conditions
- Intervene in situations involving unsafe or inadequate care
- Be aware of mandatory reporting requirements in the state
- Maintain privacy and confidentiality of health information
- Document issues related to person's rights, per agency policy

Background Evidence:

Abbasinia, M., Ahmadi, F., & Kazemnejad, A. (2020). Patient advocacy in nursing: A concept analysis. *Nursing Ethics, 27*(1), 141–151. https://doi.org/10.1177/0969733019832950

Berman, A., Snyder, S. J., & Frandsen, G. (2018). *Kozier and Erb's fundamentals of nursing: Concepts, process and practice* (10th ed.). Pearson.

Craven, R. F., Hirnle, C. J., & Henshaw, C. J. (2021). *Fundamentals of nursing: Human health and function* (8th ed.). Wolters-Kluwer.

Khademi, M., Mohammadi, E., & Vanaki, Z. (2019). On the violation of hospitalized patients' rights: A qualitative study. *Nursing Ethics, 26*(2), 576–586. https://doi.org/10.1177/0969733017709334

Potter, P. A., Perry, A. G., Stockert, P. A., & Hall, A. M. (2021). *Fundamentals of nursing* (10th ed.). Elsevier.

Tønnessen, S., Scott, A., & Nortvedt, P. (2020). Safe and competent nursing care: An argument for a minimum standard? *Nursing Ethics, 27*(6), 1396–1407. https://doi.org/10.1177/0969733020919137

Trueland, J. (2019). Understanding patients' human rights helps you weigh ethical dilemmas: A human rights approach to practice ensures nursing care is person-centered and respects individual autonomy. *Nursing Standard, 34*(11), 56–58. https://doi.org/10.7748/ns.34.11.56.s19

Williams, P. (2020). *Basic geriatric nursing* (7th ed.). Elsevier.

1st edition 1992; revised 2004, 2024

Peer Review   7700

Definition: Systematic evaluation of a peer's performance compared with professional standards of practice

Activities:

- Develop and use policies to guide function of the peer review committee and review process, as necessary
- Participate in establishment of protocols and standards for professional practice
- Participate in committee meetings, as appropriate
- Coordinate evaluation process, as necessary
- Observe peer during performance of service as required for evaluation
- Focus evaluation on quality, safety, and patient satisfaction outcomes
- Consider the nurse's developmental stage (novice to expert) when conducting the evaluation
- Identify performance requiring support of peers
- Provide input in areas of strength and development needs, as indicated
- Review credentials of selected peer, as necessary
- Recommend promotion or clinical advancement, as appropriate
- Provide supervision and counseling, as appropriate
- Provide opportunity for feedback
- Develop shared responsibility for change or improvement, as necessary
- Coordinate appropriate continuing education and training, as necessary
- Participate in grievance proceedings, as needed

2nd edition 1996; revised 2018

Background Evidence:

George, V., & Haag-Heitman, B. (2011). Nursing peer review: The manager's role. *Journal of Nursing Management, 19*(2), 254–259.

Haag-Heitman, B., & George, V. (2011). Nursing peer review: Principles and practice. *American Nurse Today, 6*(9), 48–53.

Haag-Heitman, B., & George, V. (2011). *Peer review in nursing: Principles for successful practice.* Jones & Bartlett.

Morby, S. K., & Skalla, A. (2010). A human care approach to nursing peer review. *Nursing Science Quarterly, 23*(4), 297–300.

Pelvic Muscle Exercise   0560

Definition: Strengthening and training the levator ani and urogenital muscles through voluntary, repetitive contraction to decrease stress, urge, or mixed types of urinary incontinence

Activities:

- Determine ability to recognize urge to void
- Instruct to tighten then relax ring of muscle around urethra and anus, as if trying to prevent urination or bowel movement
- Instruct to avoid contracting abdomen, thighs, and buttocks, holding breath, or straining down during exercise
- Ensure that individual can differentiate between desired drawing up-and-in muscle contraction and non-desired bearing down effort
- Instruct female individual to identify levator ani and urogenital muscles by placing finger in vagina and squeezing
- Instruct individual to tighten pelvic floor muscles and hold for count of 10 and relax muscles completely for count of 10; instruct to do 8 to 12 repetitions, three to five times a day (i.e., morning, afternoon, and night).
- Inform individual that it takes 8 to 12 weeks for exercises to be effective
- Provide positive feedback for doing exercises as prescribed
- Instruct to monitor response to exercise by attempting to stop urine flow no more often than once per week
- Incorporate biofeedback or electrical stimulation for selected individuals when assistance indicated to identify correct muscles to contract and elicit desired strength of muscle contraction
- Provide written instructions describing intervention and recommended number of repetitions
- Discuss daily record of continence with individual to provide reinforcement
- Encourage, as appropriate and under supervision, bridge and squat exercises
- Use teach-back to ensure understanding

2nd edition 1996; revised 2000, 2004, 2024

Background Evidence:

Jacomo, R. H., Nascimento, T. R., Lucena da Siva, M., Salata, M. C., Alves, A. T., da Cruz, P. R. C., & Batista de Sousa, J. (2020). Exercise regimens other than pelvic floor muscle training cannot increase pelvic muscle strength: A systematic review. *Journal of Bodywork & Movement Therapies, 24*(4), 568–574. https://doi.org/10.1016/j.jbmt.2020.08.005

Jebakani, B., & Sameul, R. (2017). Effectiveness of pelvic floor exercises for stress urinary incontinence among the postpartum women. *Indian Journal of Physiotherapy & Occupational Therapy, 11*(3), 46–50. https://doi.org/10.5958/0973-5674.2017.00071.5

Okechukwu, C. E. (2021). Supervised pelvic floor muscle exercise for the treatment of female urinary incontinence. *Journal of Nursing & Midwifery Sciences, 8*(1), 66.

Robson, M. (2017). The squeezy pelvic floor muscle exercise app: User satisfaction survey. *Journal of Pelvic, Obstetric & Gynaecological Physiotherapy, 121,* 64–68.

Romero-Franco, N., Molina-Mula, J., Bosch-Donate, E., & Casado, A. (2021). Therapeutic exercise to improve pelvic floor muscle function in a female sporting population: a systematic review and meta-analysis. *Physiotherapy, 113,* 44–52. https://doi.org/10.1016/j.physio.2021.04.006

Sacomori, C., Berghmans, B., de Bie, R., Mesters, I., & Cardoso, F. L. (2020). Predictors for adherence to a home-based pelvic floor muscle exercise program for treating female urinary incontinence in Brazil. *Physiotherapy Theory & Practice, 36*(1), 186–195.

Perineal Care   1750

P

Definition: Maintenance of perineal skin integrity and relief of perineal discomfort

Activities:

- Assist with hygiene
- Keep the perineum dry
- Provide cushion for chair, as appropriate
- Inspect condition of incision or tear(s) (e.g., episiotomy, laceration, circumcision)
- Apply cold pack, as appropriate
- Apply a heat cradle or heat lamp, as appropriate
- Instruct patient on rationale and use of sitz baths
- Provide and assist with sitz baths, as necessary
- Clean the perineum thoroughly at regular intervals
- Maintain patient in comfortable position
- Apply absorbent pads to absorb drainage, as appropriate
- Apply protective barrier (e.g., zinc oxide, petrolatum), as appropriate
- Apply prescribed medication (e.g., antibacterial, antifungal), as appropriate
- Document characteristics of drainage, as appropriate
- Provide scrotal support, as appropriate
- Provide pain medications, as appropriate
- Instruct patient or significant other, as appropriate, regarding inspection of perineum for pathology (e.g., infection, skin breakdown, rash, abnormal discharge)

1st edition 1992; revised 2013

Background Evidence:

Albers, L. L., & Borders, N. (2007). Minimizing genital tract trauma and related pain following spontaneous vaginal birth. *Journal of Midwifery & Women's Health, 52*(3), 246–253.

Driver, D. S. (2007). Perineal dermatitis in critical care patients. *Critical Care Nurse, 27*(4), 42–47.

Gray, M., Ratliff, C., & Donovan, A. (2002). Protecting perineal skin integrity. Incontinent patients present unique challenges to successful skin care management. *Nursing Management, 33*(12), 61–63.

Leventhal, L. C., de Oliveira, S. M., Nobre, M. R., & da Silva, F. M. (2011). Perineal analgesia with an ice pack after spontaneous vaginal birth: A randomized controlled trial. *Journal of Midwifery & Women's Health, 56*(2), 141–146.

Nix, D., & Ermer-Seltun, J. (2004). A review of perineal skin care protocols and skin barrier product use. *Ostomy Wound Management, 50*(12), 59–67.

Potter, P. A., & Perry, A. G. (2009). *Fundamentals of nursing* (7th ed.). Mosby.

Ward, S. L., & Hisley, S. M. (2009). *Maternal-child nursing care: Optimizing outcomes for mothers, children, and families* (pp. 472–473). F.A. Davis. 487, 576, 843.

Peripheral Sensation Management   2660

Definition: Prevention or minimization of injury or discomfort in the patient with altered sensation

Activities:

- Monitor sharp or dull and hot or cold discrimination
- Monitor for paresthesia (e.g., numbness, tingling, hyperesthesia, hypoesthesia, and level of pain), as appropriate
- Encourage patient to use the unaffected body part to determine temperature of food, liquids, bathwater, etc.
- Encourage patient to use the unaffected body part to identify location and texture of objects
- Instruct patient or family to monitor position of body parts when bathing, sitting, lying, or changing position
- Instruct patient or family to examine skin daily for alteration in skin integrity
- Monitor fit of bracing devices, prosthesis, shoes, and clothing
- Instruct patient or family to use thermometer to test water temperature
- Encourage use of thermal insulated mitts when handling cooking utensils
- Encourage use of gloves or other protective clothing over affected body part when body part is in contact with objects that may be potentially hazardous because of their thermal, textural, or other inherent characteristics
- Avoid or carefully monitor use of heat or cold, such as heating pads, hot water bottles, and ice packs
- Encourage patient to wear well-fitting, low-heeled, soft shoes
- Place cradle over affected body parts to keep bed clothes off affected areas
- Check shoes, pockets, and clothing for wrinkles or foreign objects
- Instruct patient to use timed intervals rather than presence of discomfort as a signal to alter position
- Use pressure-relieving devices, as appropriate
- Protect body parts from extreme temperature changes
- Immobilize the head, neck, and back, as appropriate
- Monitor ability to void or defecate
- Establish a means of voiding, as appropriate
- Establish a means of bowel evacuation, as appropriate
- Administer analgesics, corticosteroids, anticonvulsants, tricyclic antidepressants, or local anesthesias, as necessary
- Monitor for thrombophlebitis and venous thromboembolism
- Discuss or identify causes of abnormal sensations or sensation changes
- Instruct patient to visually monitor position of body parts if proprioception is impaired

1st edition 1992; revised 2013

Background Evidence:

Bader, M. E., & Littlejohns, L. R. (Eds.). (2004). *AANN Core curriculum for neuroscience nursing* (4th ed.). W.B. Saunders.

Barker, E. (2008). *Neuroscience nursing: A spectrum of care* (3rd ed.). Mosby Elsevier.

Gore, M., Brandenburg, N. A., Dukes, E., Hoffman, D. L., Tai, K., & Stacey, B. (2005). Pain severity in diabetic peripheral neuropathy is associated with patient functioning, symptom levels of anxiety and depression, and sleep. *Journal of Pain and Symptom Management, 30*(4), 374–385.

Hickey, J. (2009). *The clinical practice of neurological and neurosurgical nursing* (6th ed.). Lippincott Williams & Wilkins.

Paice, J. A. (2009). Clinical challenges: Chemotherapy-induced peripheral neuropathy. *Seminars in Oncology Nursing, 25*(2 Suppl. 1), S8–S19.

Pugh, S., Mathiesen, C., Meighan, M., Summer, D., & Zrelak, P. (2008). *Guide to the care of the hospitalized patient with ischemic stroke* (pp. 5–38) (2nd ed.). American Association of Neuroscience Nurses.

Ratliff, C., Tomaselli, N., Goldberg, M., Bonham, P., Crawford, P., Flemister, B., Johnson, J., Kelechi, T., & Varnado, M. (2010). *Guideline for prevention and management of pressure ulcers.* Wound, Ostomy, and Continence Nurses Society.

Smith, C. M., & Cotter, V. (2008). Age-related changes in health. In E. Capezuti, D. Zwicker, M. Mezey, & T. Fulmer (Eds.), *Evidence-based geriatric nursing protocols for best practice* (3rd ed., pp. 431–458). Springer.

Peritoneal Dialysis Therapy   2150

Definition: Administration and monitoring of dialysis solution into and out of the peritoneal cavity

Activities:

- Explain the selected peritoneal dialysis procedure and purpose
- Warm the dialysis fluid before instillation
- Assess patency of catheter, noting difficulty in inflow/outflow
- Maintain record of inflow/outflow volumes and individual/cumulative fluid balance
- Have patient empty bladder before peritoneal catheter insertion
- Avoid excess mechanical stress on peritoneal dialysis catheters (e.g., coughing, dressing change, infusing large volumes)
- Monitor blood pressure, pulse, respirations, temperature, and patient response during dialysis
- Ensure aseptic handling of peritoneal catheter and connections
- Draw laboratory samples and review blood chemistries (e.g., blood urea nitrogen, serum creatinine, and serum Na, K, and PO_4 levels)
- Obtain cell count cultures of peritoneal effluent, if indicated
- Record baseline vital signs: weight, temperature, pulse, respirations, and blood pressure
- Measure and record abdominal girth
- Measure and record daily weight
- Anchor connections and tubing securely
- Check equipment and solutions, according to protocol

- Administer dialysis exchanges (inflow, dwell, and outflow), according to protocol
- Monitor for signs of infection (e.g., peritonitis and exit site inflammation/drainage)
- Monitor for signs of respiratory distress
- Monitor for bowel perforation or fluid leaks
- Work collaboratively with patient to adjust length of dialysis, diet regulations, and pain and diversion needs to achieve optimal benefit of the treatment
- Teach patient to monitor self for signs and symptoms that indicate need for medical treatment (e.g., fever, bleeding, respiratory distress, irregular pulse, cloudy outflow, and abdominal pain)
- Teach procedure to patient requiring home dialysis

1st edition 1992; revised 1996, 2004

Background Evidence:

Fearing, M. O., & Hart, L. K. (1992). Dialysis therapy. In G. M. Bulechek & J. C. McCloskey (Eds.), *Nursing interventions: Essential nursing treatments* (2nd ed., pp. 587–601). W.B. Saunders.

Smeltzer, S. C., & Bare, B. G. (2004). Management of patients with upper or lower urinary tract dysfunction (10th ed.) *Brunner & Suddarth's textbook of medical surgical nursing* (Vol. 2, pp. 1271–1308). Lippincott Williams & Wilkins.

Pessary Management   0630

Definition: Placement and monitoring of a vaginal device for treating stress urinary incontinence, uterine retroversion, genital prolapse, or incompetent cervix

Activities:
- Review history for contraindications for pessary therapy (e.g., pelvic infections, lacerations, space-occupying lesions, noncompliance, endometriosis)
- Determine estrogen requirements, as appropriate
- Discuss maintenance regimen before fitting pessary (i.e., fit is trial and error; frequent follow-up visits are required; cleaning procedures)
- Discuss sexual activity needs before selecting pessary
- Review manufacturer's directions regarding specific type of pessary
- Select type of pessary, as appropriate
- Instruct to empty bladder and rectum
- Perform speculum examination to visualize status of vaginal mucosa
- Perform pelvic examination
- Insert pessary according to manufacturer's instructions
- Ask to change positions (e.g., stand, squat, walk, bear down slightly)
- Perform second examination in upright position to verify fit
- Instruct on method for pessary removal, as appropriate
- Instruct on contraindications for intercourse or douching based upon pessary type
- Instruct to report discomfort, dysuria, changes in color, consistency, or frequency of vaginal discharge
- Prescribe medication to reduce irritation, as appropriate
- Determine ability to perform self-care of pessary
- Schedule appointment to recheck pessary fit at 24 hours and 72 hours and then as appropriate
- Recommend semi-annual Pap examinations, as appropriate
- Determine therapeutic response to pessary use
- Observe for presence of abnormal vaginal discharge, odor, itching, or vaginal color change
- Palpate placement of pessary
- Remove pessary, as appropriate
- Inspect vagina for excoriation, laceration, or ulceration
- Clean and inspect pessary per manufacturer's directions
- Replace or refit pessary, as appropriate
- Schedule ongoing practitioner follow-up at intervals of 1 to 3 months
- Recommend vaginal hygiene with water and mild soap
- Apply topical estrogen to reduce inflammation, as needed
- Recommend pelvic floor strengthening exercises, as appropriate
- Provide space to express doubts and questions about use of pessary
- Determine impact of pessary on sexual health
- Use teach-back to ensure understanding

3rd edition 2000; revised 2024

Background Evidence:

Dwyer, L., Kearney, R., & Lavender, T. (2019). A review of pessary for prolapse practitioner training. *British Journal of Nursing, 28*(9), S18–S24. https://doi.org/10.12968/bjon.2019.28.9.S18

Hooper, G. L. (2018). Person-Centered care for patients with pessaries. *The Nursing Clinics of North America, 53*(2), 289–301. https://doi.org/10.1016/j.cnur.2018.01.006

Rantell, A. (2019). Vaginal pessaries for pelvic organ prolapse and their impact on sexual function. *Sexual Medicine Reviews, 7*(4), 597–603. https://doi.org/10.1016/j.sxmr.2019.06.002

Smeltzer, S. C., & Bare, B. G. (2017). Management of patients with female reproductive disorders (14th ed.) *Brunner & Suddarth's textbook of medical surgical nursing* (Vol. 2, pp. 1478–1492). Lippincott Williams & Wilkins.

Vasconcelos, C., Silva Gomes, M. L., Ribeiro, G. L., Oriá, M., Geoffrion, R., & Vasconcelos Neto, J. A. (2020). Women and healthcare providers' knowledge, attitudes and practice related to pessaries for pelvic organ prolapse: A systematic review. *European Journal of Obstetrics, Gynecology, and Reproductive Biology, 247*, 132–142. https://doi.org/10.1016/j.ejogrb.2020.02.016

Wu, Y. M., & Welk, B. (2019). Revisiting current treatment options for stress urinary incontinence and pelvic organ prolapse: A contemporary literature review. *Research and Reports in Urology, 11*, 179–188. https://doi.org/10.2147/RRU.S191555

Phlebotomy: Arterial Blood Sample 4232

Definition: Obtaining a blood sample from an artery to assess oxygen and carbon dioxide levels, and acid-base balance

Activities:
- Determine if drawing blood from artery or arterial line
- Explain procedure and expectations
- Palpate radial, brachial, or femoral artery for pulse
- Perform Allen test before radial artery puncture
- Obtain syringe with anti-clot medication
- Cleanse skin area with appropriate solution
- Position extremity appropriately for access (e.g., hand hyperextended over rolled cloth; extremity hyper-abducted and externally rotated)
- Palpate artery proximal to needle entry with non-dominant hand
- Stabilize artery by pulling skin taut
- Insert needle at a 45–60 degree angle into artery with dominant hand until blood flash appears
- Allow syringe to fill to appropriate level; avoid pulling back on plunger
- Pull syringe back slightly and reposition needle if arterial flow lost
- Obtain specimen of blood
- Withdraw needle and immediately apply pressure to puncture site with sterile gauze
- Apply pressure until hemostasis achieved, per policy
- Apply pressure bandage over site, as appropriate
- Expel all air from syringe by holding sample upright and gently tapping
- Roll syringe between hands slowly
- Label specimen, according to agency protocol
- Arrange for immediate transport of specimen to laboratory
- Place syringe in ice if delay in transport
- Dispose of materials and all personal protective equipment appropriately
- Record temperature, oxygen percent, delivery method, site of puncture, and circulatory assessment after puncture

2nd edition, 1996; revised 2004, 2024

Background Evidence:

Brown, J. M. (2021). Arterial puncture. In American Association of Critical Care Nurses & D. L. Weigand (Eds.), *AACN Procedure Manual for High Acuity, Progressive, and Critical Care* (7th ed.). Elsevier.

Markewitz, B. A. (2018). Improved success rate of arterial puncture for blood gas analysis through standardization. *Labmedicine, 49*(2), 175–178. https://doi.org/10.1093/labmed/lmx082

Vahedian-Azimi, A., Rahimi-Bashar, F., Pourhoseingholi, M., Salesi, M., Shamsizadeh, M., Jamialahmadi, T., Gohari-Moghadam, K., & Sahebkar, A. (2021). Effect of the specific training course for competency in doing arterial blood gas sampling in the Intensive Care Unit: Developing a standardized learning curve according to the procedure's time and socio-professional predictors. *BioMed Research International, 2021*(2), 1–10.

Phlebotomy: Blood Acquisition 4234

Definition: Procuring blood and blood components from donors

Activities:
- Adhere to agency protocol for donor screening and acceptance (e.g., drug abuse, HIV status, tattoos)
- Obtain demographical information and written consent from donor
- Determine risks related to venipuncture (e.g., anticoagulation therapy, bleeding disorders)
- Ensure that donor has eaten 4 to 6 hours before donating
- Determine hemoglobin and hematocrit levels, weight, and vital signs
- Ensure availability of emergency equipment
- Ensure appropriate site (i.e., avoid arm on mastectomy side or hemodialysis shunt)
- Determine presence of allergies to tape, latex, or cleansing agents
- Ensure skin at site of venipuncture free of lesions
- Maintain strict aseptic technique
- Assemble equipment
- Place donor in semi-recumbent position during donation process
- Provide privacy and confidentiality
- Cleanse skin before venipuncture, according to agency protocol
- Ensure blood products collected in bag mixed with correct additive
- Maintain continuous flow of blood product
- Instruct to elevate arm and apply firm pressure for 2 to 3 minutes after completion of blood or blood product donation process
- Place pressure bandage or dressing over venipuncture site, as appropriate
- Instruct to remain recumbent per agency policy after donation, or longer if faintness or weakness experienced
- Encourage to remain seated after donation per agency policy
- Instruct to eat and drink immediately after donation, with increased fluid intake for next few days
- Label and store blood, according to agency protocol
- Stay with donor during and immediately after collection of blood
- Instruct to keep pressure bandage on and dry for several hours after donation
- Instruct to avoid strenuous activity or heavy lifting for several hours after donation
- Instruct to lie down with feet up if lightheaded, until feeling passes
- Instruct if bleeding after removing bandage to put pressure on site and raise arm until bleeding stops
- Instruct if bruising occurs to apply cold pack to area periodically during first 24 hours
- Recommend adding iron-rich foods to diet to replace iron lost with blood donation
- Use teach-back to determine understanding

2nd edition 1996; revised 2004, 2024

Background Evidence:

Garza, D., & Becan-McBride, K. (2018). *Phlebotomy handbook: Blood collection essentials* (10th ed.). Pearson.

Muegge, S. (2017). Stick to procedure when performing phlebotomy. *AAACN Viewpoint, 39*(3), 1–11.

Perry, A. G., Potter, P. A., Ostendorf, W. R., & Laplante, N. (2018). *Clinical nursing skills and techniques* (9th ed.). Elsevier.

Skarparis, K., & Ford, C. (2018). Venipuncture in adults. *British Journal of Nursing, 27*(22), 1312–1315. https://doi.org/10.12968/bjon.2018.27.22.1312

Phlebotomy: Venous Blood Sample   4238

Definition: Removal of a sample of venous blood from an uncannulated vein

Activities:

- Provide private environment
- Review order for sample to be drawn
- Verify correct identification
- Minimize anxiety by explaining procedure and rationale, as appropriate
- Review previous venipuncture experiences and preferences for venipuncture site
- Select vein, considering amount of blood needed, mental status, comfort, age, availability and condition of blood vessels, and presence of arteriovenous fistulas or shunts
- Determine possible risks associated with venipuncture (e.g., anticoagulant therapy, bleeding disorders)
- Determine presence of allergies to tape, latex, or cleansing agents
- Avoid areas prone to nerve injury
- Select appropriate blood specimen tube, size, and type of needle
- Position targeted extremity lower than level of heart
- Promote vessel dilation through use of tourniquet, gravity, application of heat, milking vein, or fist clenching and relaxation
- Avoid tourniquet application time of greater than 1 minute to minimize hemolysis of sample
- Cleanse area with appropriate solution, per agency protocol
- Cleanse site with circular motion, starting at point of anticipated venipuncture and moving in outward circle
- Maintain strict aseptic technique
- Ask to hold still when performing venipuncture
- Insert needle in direction of venous blood return
- Observe for blood return in needle
- Withdraw sample of blood
- Remove needle from the vein and apply pressure and dressing
- Advise to leave dressing in place for at least 1 hour
- Verify specimens has correct name, date, and time of collection, per agency protocol
- Send labeled specimen to appropriate laboratory
- Dispose of equipment properly

2nd edition 1996; revised 2018, 2024

Background Evidence:

Garza, D., & Becan-McBride, K. (2018). *Phlebotomy handbook: Blood collection essentials* (10th ed.). Pearson.

Muegge, S. (2017). Stick to procedure when performing phlebotomy. *AAACN Viewpoint, 39*(3), 1–11.

Perry, A. G., Potter, P. A., Ostendorf, W. R., & Laplante, N. (2018). *Clinical nursing skills and techniques* (9th ed.). Elsevier.

Skarparis, K., & Ford, C. (2018). Venipuncture in adults. *British Journal of Nursing, 27*(22), 1312–1315. https://doi.org/10.12968/bjon.2018.27.22.1312

Phototherapy: Mood Regulation   6926

P

Definition: Administration of doses of bright light to elevate mood and adjust circadian rhythm

Activities:

- Obtain provider prescription for phototherapy including frequency, distance, intensity, and duration, as appropriate
- Instruct about treatment (e.g., indications for use, treatment procedure)
- Assist in obtaining appropriate light source for treatment, including correct brightness, intensity, lux, and filtering of ultraviolet light (i.e., fluorescent bulbs emitting white light are preferred source)
- Increase treatment times for lower lux light sources
- Assist to set up prescribed light source in preparation for treatment, including correct distance and intensity
- Encourage use of treatment
- Monitor mood level (e.g., prolonged sadness, loss of energy, change in sleep pattern, irritability)
- Supervise as needed during treatment
- Monitor for side effects of treatment (e.g., headache, eyestrain, nausea, insomnia, hyperactivity)
- Ensure familiarity with baseline symptoms to discern whether therapy exacerbating symptoms and adverse effects
- Terminate treatment if develops side effects
- Notify provider of side effects
- Modify treatment, as ordered, to decrease or eliminate side effects
- Consider increasing dosage or adding evening does to regimen, if symptoms have not improved within 2 to 4 weeks
- Document treatment and response

4th edition 2004; revised 2024

Background Evidence:

D'Agostino, A., Ferrara, P., Terzoni, S., Ostinelli, E. G., Carrara, C., Prunas, C., Gambini, O., & Destrebecq, A. (2020). Efficacy of triple chronotherapy in unipolar and bipolar depression: A systematic review of the available evidence. *Journal of Affective Disorders, 276,* 297–304. https://doi.org/10.1016/j.jad.2020.07.026

Keltner, N. L., & Steele, D. (2019). *Psychiatric nursing* (8th ed.). Elsevier.

Leahy, L. G. (2017). Overcoming seasonal affective disorder. *Journal of Psychosocial Nursing & Mental Health Services, 55*(11), 10–14. https://doi.org/10.3928/02793695-20171016-03

Mitolo, M., Tonon, C., La, M. C., Testa, C., Carelli, V., & Lodi, R. (2018). Effects of light treatment on sleep, cognition, mood, and behavior in Alzheimer's Disease: A systematic review. *Dementia & Geriatric Cognitive Disorders, 46*(5/6), 371–384. https://doi.org/10.1159/000494921

Varcarolis, E. M., & Fosbre, C. D. (2021). *Essentials of psychiatric-mental health nursing* (4th ed.). Elsevier.

Phototherapy: Neonate 6924

Definition: Use of light therapy to reduce bilirubin levels in newborns

Activities:

- Review maternal and infant history for risk factors for hyperbilirubinemia (e.g., Rh or ABO incompatibility, polycythemia, sepsis, prematurity, malpresentation)
- Monitor for signs of jaundice
- Order serum bilirubin levels, as appropriate per protocol or primary practitioner request
- Report laboratory values to primary practitioner
- Place infant in isolette or radiant warmer
- Instruct family on phototherapy procedures and care
- Apply patches to cover both eyes, avoiding excessive pressure
- Remove eye patches every 4 hours or when lights are off, for parental contact and feeding
- Monitor eyes for edema, drainage, and color
- Place phototherapy lights above infant at appropriate height
- Check radiance of lights daily
- Monitor vital signs every 3 hours, per protocol or as needed
- Check temperature every 3 hours or as needed
- Change infant position every 3 hours or per protocol
- Monitor serum bilirubin levels, per protocol or practitioner request
- Evaluate neurological status every 4 hours or per protocol
- Monitor signs of dehydration (e.g., depressed fontanels, poor skin turgor, loss of weight)
- Weigh daily
- Encourage eight feedings per day
- Encourage family to participate in light therapy
- Instruct family on home phototherapy, as appropriate

2nd edition 1996; revised 2000, 2024

Background Evidence:

Chu, L., Qiao, J., & Xu, C. (2020). Home-based phototherapy versus hospital-based phototherapy for treatment of neonatal hyperbilirubinemia: A systematic review and meta-analysis. *Clinical Pediatrician, 59*(6), 588–595. https://doi.org/10.1177/0009922820916894

Faulhaber, F. R. S., Procianoy, R. S., & Silveira, R. C. (2019). Side effects of phototherapy on neonates. *American Journal of Perinatology, 36*(3), 252–257. https://doi.org/10.1055/s-0038-1667379

Hockenberry, M. J., Rodgers, C. C., & Wilson, D. (2022). *Wong's essentials of pediatric nursing*. Elsevier.

Itoh, S., Okada, H., Kuboi, T., & Kusaka, T. (2017). Phototherapy for neonatal hyperbilirubinemia. *Pediatrics International, 59*(9), 959–966. https://doi.org/10.1111/ped.13332

Matson, S., & Smith, J. E. (2016). *Core curriculum for maternal-newborn nursing*. Elsevier.

Mitra, S., & Rennie, J. (2017). Neonatal jaundice: Etiology, diagnosis and treatment. *British Journal of Hospital Medicine, 78*(12), 699–704. https://doi.org/10.12968/hmed.2017.78.12.699

Phototherapy: Skin 3510

Definition: Administration of doses of light to treat chronic or complex skin disorders or control inflammation

Activities:

- Determine type of condition to be treated
- Obtain provider prescription for phototherapy including frequency, distance, intensity, and duration, as appropriate
- Instruct about treatment (e.g., indications for use, treatment procedure, preparation of area to be treated)
- Test small area of skin initially with prescribed light source
- Increase treatment times as tolerated and per protocol
- Supervise as needed during treatment
- Monitor for side effects of treatment (e.g., increased areas of irritation, signs or symptoms of infection)
- Ensure familiarity with baseline skin condition to discern whether therapy effective
- Ensure availability for scheduled treatments (e.g., once weekly, two or three times weekly, monthly)
- Terminate or modify treatment if develops untoward side effects, as ordered
- Reduce treatment in incremental stages after desired effect achieved
- Educate related to care of treatment area between visits
- Use teach-back to ensure understanding
- Document treatment and response

8th edition 2024

Background Evidence:

Bell, A. (2018). Ensuring adherence to the British Association of Dermatologists' service guidance and standards for phototherapy units. *Dermatological Nursing, 17*(4), 39–42.

Grove, J. (2017). The use of intense pulsed light therapy in the treatment of acne vulgaris. *Journal of Aesthetic Nursing, 6*(8), 400–405.

Torres, A. E., Lyons, A. B., Hamzavi, I. H., & Lim, H. W. (2021). Role of phototherapy in the era of biologics. *Journal of the American Academy of Dermatology, 84*(2), 479–485. https://doi.org/10.1016/j.jaad.2020.04.095

Zhang, P., & Wu, M. X. (2018). A clinical review of phototherapy for psoriasis. *Lasers in Medical Science, 33*(1), 173–180. https://doi.org/10.1007/s10103-017-2360-1

P

Physical Accompaniment 6576

Definition: Escorting a person deemed a safety risk, to activities or diagnostic testing

Activities:

- Review each situation individually, ensuring accompaniment when necessary
- Determine number and type of personnel and equipment required
- Determine safety strategies required
- Ensure adequate means of communication among all involved
- Explain need for accompaniment and roles of involved individuals
- Ensure safety of individuals and personnel at all times
- Monitor equipment continuously as indicated
- Follow agency policies regarding accompaniment
- Document accompaniment including destination and persons attending

8th edition 2024

Background Evidence:

Evans, S. (2021). Accompaniment as a form of patient care. *Cardiopulmonary Physical Therapy Journal, 32*(2), 38–40. https://doi.org/10.1097/CPT.000 0000000000175

Frauenfelder, F. (2019). Psychiatric adult inpatient nursing described in the NANDA-I and NIC: Frauenfelder, F. (2019). *Psychiatric adult inpatient nursing described in the NANDA-I and NIC: A systematic evaluation of nursing classifications* [Doctoral dissertation. Radbound University] Radbound Repository. https://repository.ubn.ru.nl/handle/2066/203856

American Psychiatric Nurses Association. (2014). *Scope and standards of psychiatric-mental health nursing* (2nd ed.).

Keltner, N. L., & Steele, D. (2019). *Psychiatric nursing* (8th ed.). Elsevier.

Rebar, C. R., Gersch, C., & Heimgartner, N. M. (2020). *Psychiatric nursing made incredibly easy* (3rd ed.). Wolters Kluwer.

University of Iowa Hospitals and Clinics. (2018). Patient accompaniment. *Policy and Procedure Manual.*

Varcarolis, E. M., & Fosbre, C. D. (2021). *Essentials of psychiatric-mental health nursing* (4th ed.). Elsevier.

Physical Distance Facilitation 6594

Definition: Facilitation of distance between people and reduction in the number of times people come in close contact with each other to prevent the spread of a contagious disease

Activities:

- Determine need for social distancing (e.g., infected person, required excursions from home during contagious disease outbreak)
- Determine presence of risk factors for contagion (e.g., age, disabled, low socioeconomic class, crowded housing with poor ventilation, respiratory illness) or increased mortality (e.g., comorbidities, chronic respiratory disease, elderly)
- Instruct to find and follow guidance from local public health authorities before going out of home (e.g., restrictions on travel, leaving home, physical distancing requirements)
- Encourage avoidance of close physical contact between non-cohabiting persons when outside home or with infected persons in home (i.e., maintain distance between people per established guidelines)
- Minimize contact time with non-cohabiting persons or with infected persons
- Encourage use of PPE when outside home or in contact with infected person (e.g., masks, gloves)
- Encourage use of other everyday preventive actions (e.g., avoiding touching face with unwashed hands, frequently washing hands with soap and water for at least 20 seconds, using hand sanitizer)
- Instruct to cover nose and mouth with tissue during coughing or sneezing, dispose of tissue and perform hand hygiene after contact with respiratory secretions
- Encourage avoidance of unnecessary touching of items without proper hand hygiene
- Encourage avoidance of unnecessary excursions outside home and to limit opportunities to encounter persons outside home
- Model healthy social distancing in all interactions (e.g., per established guidelines)
- Instruct to consider available social distancing options to travel safely when running errands or commuting to and from work (i.e., distance ability with walking, bicycling, wheelchair rolling, or using public transit, rideshares, or taxis)
- Encourage to arrange to work from home where possible
- Encourage to avoid unnecessary use of public transportation
- Instruct when using public transit, maintain distance from other passengers or transit operators per established guidelines (e.g., waiting at bus station, seat selection on bus, ride share or train)
- Instruct to avoid pooled rides when using rideshares or taxis
- Instruct to sit in back seat in larger rideshare vehicles to keep appropriate distance from driver
- Instruct to maintain distance when meeting others in person per established guidelines
- Instruct to avoid crowded places and gatherings where distancing difficult
- Allow other people appropriate space when passing by them in both indoor and outdoor settings
- Instruct to only visit stores in person for household essentials when absolutely needed
- Instruct to maintain appropriate distance from others while shopping and in lines
- Instruct to follow physical guides to assist with maintaining proper distancing (e.g., use of masks, tape markings on floors, signs on walls)
- Instruct to use drive-thru, curbside pick-up, or delivery services to limit face-to-face contact with others whenever possible

P

- Instruct to wear masks and maintain physical distance between self and delivery service providers during exchanges
- Encourage to stay home and away from other people, staying appropriate distance away from other people in home if infected
- Restrict movements of infected person in household to single room with private bathroom, if possible
- Avoid sharing items like towels and utensils when infected
- Instruct on frequent hand hygiene
- Encourage to stay socially and spiritually connected via technology
- Encourage to visit loved ones by electronic devices where possible
- Encourage choice of safe social activities (e.g., call, video chat, social media connections)
- Encourage to remain active while socially distanced (e.g., walk, bike ride, wheelchair roll in neighborhood where distance can be maintained)

8th edition 2024

Background Evidence:

Centers for Disease Control and Prevention. (2020). *Social distancing.* https://www.cdc.gov/coronavirus/2019-ncov/prevent-getting-sick/social-distancing.html

Curran, E. (2020, June 16). Social distancing—do they mean us? *Nursing Times.* https://www.nursingtimes.net/opinion/social-distancing-do-they-mean-us-16-06-2020/

Maragakis, L. L. (2020). *Coronavirus, social and physical distancing and self-quarantine.* John Hopkins Website: Health. https://www.hopkinsmedicine.org/health/conditions-and-diseases/coronavirus/coronavirus-social-distancing-and-self-quarantine

Mukherji, A., Gupta, T., & Agarwal, J. P. (2020). Time, distance, shielding and ALARA; drawing similarities between measures for radiation protection and Coronavirus disease pandemic response. *Indian Journal of Cancer, 57*(2), 221–223.

Nicola, M., O'Neill, N., Sohrabi, C., Khan, M., Agha, M., & Agha, R. (2020). Evidence based management guideline for the COVID-19 pandemic. *International Journal of Surgery, 77,* 206–216.

Purba, A. K. (2020). How should the role of the nurse change in response to Covid-19? *Nursing Times, 116*(6), 25–28.

Wee, L., Sim, X., Conceicao, E., Aung, M., Tan, K., Ko, K., Wong, H., Wijaya, L., Tan, B., Venkatachalam, I., & Ling, M. (2020). Containing COVID-19 outside the isolation ward: The impact of an infection control bundle on environmental contamination and transmission in a cohorted general ward. *American Journal of Infection Control, 48*(9), 1056–1061.

Physical Restraint   6580

Definition: Application, monitoring, and removal of mechanical restraining devices or manual restraints used to limit physical mobility of patient

Activities:

- Obtain a physician's order or confer with a physician within 1 hour after the restraint is initiated
- Renew orders for physical restraint according to state rules and regulations and professional standards of care
- Ensure face to face evaluation is conducted by an appropriately credentialed provider within 1 hour of initiating use of physical restraints
- Evaluate the need for restraint hourly
- Provide patient with a private, yet adequately supervised, environment in situations in which a patient's sense of dignity may be diminished by the use of physical restraints
- Provide sufficient staff to assist with safe application of physical restraining devices or manual restraints
- Designate one nursing staff member to direct staff and communicate with the patient during the application of physical restraints
- Use appropriate hold when manually restraining patient in emergency situations or during transport
- Identify for patient and significant others those behaviors that necessitated the intervention
- Explain procedure, purpose, and time period of the intervention to patient and significant others in understandable and nonpunitive terms
- Explain to patient and significant others the behaviors necessary for termination of the intervention
- Monitor the patient's response to procedure
- Do not tie restraints to side rails of bed
- Secure restraints out of patient's reach
- Provide appropriate level of supervision to monitor patient and to allow for therapeutic actions, as needed
- Provide for patient's psychological comfort, as needed
- Provide diversional activities (e.g., television, read to patient, visitors, mobiles) to facilitate patient cooperation with the intervention, when appropriate
- Administer PRN medications for anxiety or agitation
- Monitor skin condition at restraint sites
- Monitor color, temperature, and sensation frequently in restrained extremities
- Provide for movement and exercise, according to patient's level of self-control, condition, and abilities
- Position patient to facilitate comfort and prevent aspiration and skin breakdown
- Provide for movement of extremities in patient with multiple restraints by rotating the removal and reapplication of one restraint at a time as safety permits
- Assist with periodic changes in body position
- Provide the dependent patient with a means of summoning help (e.g., bell or call light) when caregiver is not present
- Assist with needs related to nutrition, elimination, hydration, and personal hygiene
- Evaluate, at regular intervals, patient's need for continued restrictive intervention
- Involve patient in activities to improve strength, coordination, judgment, and orientation
- Involve patient in making decisions to move to a more or less restrictive form of intervention, when appropriate
- Remove restraints gradually (i.e., one at a time if in four-point restraints) as self-control increases
- Monitor patient's response to removal of restraints
- On termination of the restrictive intervention, process with the patient and staff the circumstances that led to the use of the intervention, as well as any patient concerns about the intervention itself
- Provide the next appropriate level of restrictive action (e.g., area restriction or seclusion), as needed
- Implement alternatives to restraints, such as sitting in a geri-chair or close observation, as appropriate
- Inform family about the risks and benefits of restraints and restraint reduction

- Document the rationale for use of restrictive intervention, patient's response to the intervention, patient's physical condition, nursing care provided throughout the intervention, and rationale for terminating the intervention

1st edition 1992; revised 1996, 2018

Background Evidence:

American Nurses Association. (2012). *Position statement: Reduction of patient restraints and seclusion in health care settings.* http://www.nursingworld.org/ MainMenuCategories/EthicsStandards/Ethics-Position-Statements/ Reduction-of-Patient-Restraint-and-Seclusion-in-Health-Care-Settings.pdf

Bradas, C., Sandhu, S., & Mion, L. (2012). Physical restraints and side rails in acute and critical care settings. In M. Boltz, E. Capezuti, T. Fulmer, & D. Zwicker (Eds.), *Evidence-based geriatric nursing protocols for best practice* (4th ed., pp. 229–245). Springer.

The Joint Commission. (2010). *The comprehensive accreditation manual for hospitals: The official handbook.* Joint Commission Resources.

Townsend, M. C. (2014). *Essentials of psychiatric mental health nursing: Concepts of care in evidence-based practice* (6th ed.). F.A. Davis.

Phytotherapy 2420

Definition: Use of active ingredients or substances contained in medicinal plants to maintain health or treat illness

Activities:

- Use health history to determine the suitability of herbal or flower essence therapy
- Verify health history for allergies
- Instruct the patient about therapeutic use of herbs or flower essences (e.g., background, philosophy, modes of action, contraindications)
- Select variety of plant indicated in relation to the individual's state of health
- Obtain medicinal substances from reputable source
- Consider using prepared stock flower essences such as the Bach collection of 38 flower essences
- Prepare medicinal herbs or flowers (e.g., gather, wash, cut, cook), as indicated
- Determine the form in which the medicinal plant or plant part is prepared (e.g., infusion, decoction, maceration)
- Store preparations out of direct sunlight in a moderate environment
- Determine dose and guidelines for the administration of herbal products
- Assist the patient on the correct use of herbal products (e.g., preparation, time of administration, method of administration)
- Explain the effects of interaction with other prescribed medicines, if necessary
- Monitor for the expected response or potential adverse effects
- Record in the clinical history the action and response to phytotherapy

Background Evidence:

Brendler, T., Gruenwald, J., Ulbricht, C., & Basch, E. (2006). Devil's claw (harpagophytum procumbens DC): An evidence-based systematic review by the natural standard research collaboration. *Journal of Herbal Pharmacotherapy, 6*(1), 89–126.

Bunchorntavakul, C., & Reddy, K. R. (2013). Review article: Herbal and dietary supplement hepatotoxicity. *Alimentary Pharmacology and Therapeutics, 37*(1), 3–17.

Dwyer, A. V., Whitten, D. L., & Hawrelak, J. A. (2011). Herbal medicines, other than St. John's Wort, in the treatment of depression: A systematic review. *Alternative Medicine Review, 16*(1), 40–49.

Lakhan, S., & Vieira, K. (2010). Nutritional and herbal supplements for anxiety and anxiety-related disorders: Systematic review. *Nutrition Journal, 9*(42). https://doi.org/10.1186/1475-2891-9-42

Sánchez, M. T. (2012). Phytotherapy for the treatment of chronic venous insufficiency. The buckeye. *Revista Internacional De Ciencias Podológicas, 6*(1), 31–37.

Sarris, J., Panossian, A., Schweitzer, I., Stough, C., & Scholey, A. (2011). Herbal medicine for depression, anxiety, and insomnia: A review of psychopharmacology and clinical evidence. *European Neuropsychopharmacology, 21*(12), 841–860.

Scheffer, M. (2009). *Bach flowers for crisis care: Remedies for emotional and psychological well-being.* Healing Arts Press.

7th edition 2018

P

Pneumatic Tourniquet Management 2865

Definition: Care of the patient undergoing pneumatic tourniquet-assisted procedures

Activities:

- Confirm the need for pneumatic tourniquet use in the physician's or anesthesia professional's plan of care
- Verify that the entire tourniquet system is complete, clean, and functioning according to the manufacturer's instructions for use
- Select a tourniquet cuff of appropriate width and length for extremity (e.g., as wide as possible without inhibiting surgical site exposure; use contoured cuffs for patient extremities that taper between the upper and lower edge of the cuff; cuff length should provide bladder overlap on limb and full engagement of hook-and-loop fasteners)
- Instruct patient about purpose of tourniquet and sensations expected (e.g., tingling, numbness, dull ache), as appropriate
- Evaluate patient for considerations related to tourniquet use (e.g., planned location of the tourniquet, condition of skin under and distal to the planned cuff site, size and shape of the extremity, peripheral pulses and sensation distal to the planned cuff site, ability to move digits in the involved extremity)

- Screen for potential contraindications for tourniquet use (e.g., risk factors for deep vein thrombosis, ischemic extremities)
- Assure that tourniquet tubing and connectors are incompatible with other tubing (e.g., IV tubing, vacuum system) or labeled to clearly identify that they are part of the tourniquet system
- Label tourniquet tubing clearly to indicate that tubing belongs to which cuff and which is associated with which components of the tourniquet system(s) during procedures involving tourniquet control on two extremities
- Position cuff tubing on or near the lateral aspect of the extremity
- Verify the correct surgical site before application of tourniquet cuff
- Wrap a low-lint, soft padding (e.g., limb protection sleeve, two layers of stockinet, cotton roll) around extremity under site of tourniquet cuff, ensuring that padding is wrinkle-free and does not pinch skin
- Apply and secure tourniquet cuff snugly around the extremity, avoiding neurovascular sites and ensuring that skin is not pinched
- Protect patient skin under the tourniquet cuff to prevent fluid accumulation (e.g., skin prep solutions, irrigation)
- Protect reusable tourniquet cuffs from contamination by fluid, blood, and other potentially infectious material during surgery
- Apply tourniquet protectors (e.g., U-shaped drapes, adhesive drapes, tourniquet covers) to minimize soiling, as indicated
- Set the tourniquet pressure to maintain the minimum effective pressure as instructed by physician, anesthesia professional, or per agency policy and based on patient's systolic blood pressure and limb circumference
- Alert anesthesia professional before wrapping the extremity
- Exsanguinate extremity by elevating and wrapping with an elastic bandage before cuff inflation
- Inflate the cuff under the direction of physician or anesthesia professional
- Monitor patient continuously during use and on deflation of tourniquet for physiological responses to tourniquet cuff inflation
- Assure that activation indicators and pressure displays are visible and audible alarms sufficiently loud to be heard over other sounds in the operating room
- Assure pneumatic tourniquet inflation time kept to a minimum
- Inform physician of tourniquet inflation time at regular, established intervals
- Confer with the surgeon and anesthesia professional about deflating the tourniquet for 10 to 15 minutes to allow tissue reperfusion when the duration of tourniquet inflation is longer than 2 hours
- Verify the tourniquet inflation pressure during the time-out process

- Avoid overheating patient when the tourniquet cuff is inflated, particularly in pediatric patients
- Verify tourniquet pressure and cuff inflation periodically during use
- Monitor tourniquet equipment and pressure continuously when used for an IV block
- Deflate the tourniquet cuff under the direction of the physician and anesthesia professional
- Deflate the tourniquet cuff used for an IV block incrementally
- Confirm sequence and timing of deflation of each tourniquet when tourniquets are used on two extremities
- Remove the tourniquet cuff
- Inspect skin under the tourniquet cuff after removal of cuff
- Evaluate the strength of peripheral pulses, sensation, and ability to move digits after deflation or removal of the cuff
- Document tourniquet equipment identification number, cuff site, pressure, inflation and deflation times, condition of skin under cuff, and peripheral circulatory and neurological evaluation, as per agency policy
- Provide a report on pressure settings, duration of the pneumatic tourniquet inflation, and patient outcomes when transferring the care of the patient to other caregivers
- Monitor patient for systemic responses and blood loss after cuff has been deflated
- Report complications to the physician and anesthesia professional and to other caregivers when the patient care is transferred
- Inspect and clean pneumatic tourniquet after use and according to manufacturer's written instructions
- Clean reusable cuffs and bladders using a U.S. Environmental Protection Agency registered hospital disinfectant, per agency policy

7th edition 2018

Background Evidence:

Association of Operating Room Nurses. (2013). RP summary: Recommended practices for care of patients undergoing pneumatic tourniquet-assisted procedures. *AORN Journal, 98*(4), 397–400.

Association of Operating Room Nurses. (2014). *Perioperative standards and recommended practices*.

Hicks, R. W., & Denholm, B. (2013). Implementing AORN recommended practices for care of patients undergoing pneumatic tourniquet-assisted procedures. *AORN Journal, 98*(4), 382–396.

O'Connor, C., & Murphy, S. (2007). Pneumatic tourniquet use in the perioperative environment. *Journal of Perioperative Practice, 17*(8), 391–397.

Point of Care Testing

7610

Definition: Performance of laboratory tests at the site of patient care

Activities:

- Obtain adequate training or orientation before performing testing
- Participate in color blindness testing, as needed for particular test and as required by institution
- Participate in proficiency testing programs as required by institution
- Follow institutional procedures for specimen collection and preservation, as appropriate

- Label specimens immediately to minimize sample mix-ups, as appropriate
- Use appropriate specimen for the test being performed
- Perform testing on collected specimens in a timely manner
- Use universal precautions when handling specimens for testing
- Store reagents according to manufacturer's requirements or as stated in institution's procedure manual
- Check expiration date of any reagent preparation, including test strips and contents of commercial kits to avoid using expired reagents

P

- Follow manufacturer guidelines and institutional procedures for instrument calibration
- Document instrument calibration as required
- Perform quality control checks according to manufacturer recommendation or as stated in institution procedure
- Document quality control checks as required
- Perform test according to manufacturer directions or as stated in institutional procedures
- Ensure accurate timing with testing that requires prescribed times
- Document results of tests, according to institutional procedure
- Verify the results of the point of care test with use of a central laboratory when a critical clinical decision is to be made
- Report abnormal or critical results to physician, as appropriate
- Perform cleaning and maintenance of instruments according to manufacturer guidelines or as stated in institutional procedure
- Document cleaning and maintenance as required
- Establish a multidisciplinary team including representation from relevant laboratory groups to oversee appropriate resources (e.g., equipment, space available, documentation needs) and training of personnel, as needed in particular setting
- Establish operational teams to oversee day to day operations, including training, proficiency testing, quality assurance, stock management, computer needs and Internet connectivity, and safety, as needed in particular setting
- Report test results to patient, as appropriate

2nd edition 1996; revised 2018

Background Evidence:

Academy of Medical Laboratory Science, Association of Clinical Biochemists in Ireland, Irish Medicines Board & RCPI Faculty of Pathology. (2007). *Guidelines for safe and effective management and use of point of care testing.* http://www.rcpi.ie/content/docs/000001/370_5_media.pdf

Dunning, M., & Fischbach, F. (2010). *Nurse's quick reference to common laboratory and diagnostic tests* (5th ed.). Lippincott Williams & Wilkin.

Robertson-Malt, S. (2008). Nursing role in point of care testing. *The Journal of Near-Patient Testing and Technology, 7*(4), 246–247.

Positioning   0840

Definition: Arranging of body to promote therapeutic benefit, physiological, and psychological well-being

Activities:

- Place on appropriate therapeutic mattress or bed
- Provide firm mattress
- Explain procedure of turning, as appropriate
- Encourage involvement in position changes, as appropriate
- Monitor oxygenation status before and after position change
- Premedicate before turning, as appropriate
- Place in designated therapeutic position
- Monitor neutral alignment, without extreme lateral rotation or hyperextension, as appropriate
- Incorporate preferred sleeping position into plan of care if not contraindicated
- Position in proper body alignment
- Immobilize or support affected body part, as appropriate
- Elevate affected body part, as appropriate
- Position to alleviate dyspnea (e.g., semi-Fowler position), as appropriate
- Provide support to edematous areas (e.g., pillow under arms, scrotal support), as appropriate
- Position to facilitate ventilation or perfusion matching (i.e., "good lung down"), as appropriate
- Encourage active or passive range-of-motion exercises, as appropriate
- Encourage joint goals to reduce risk of injury or other complications of immobility
- Identify number of professionals needed for passive positioning
- Provide appropriate support for neck
- Avoid placing in positions that increase pain
- Avoid placing amputation stump in flexion position
- Avoid changing positioning right after meals
- Minimize friction and shearing forces when positioning or turning
- Apply footboard to bed if indicated
- Turn using log roll technique
- Position to promote urinary drainage, as appropriate
- Position to avoid placing tension on wounds, as appropriate
- Prop with backrest, as appropriate
- Elevate affected limb higher than level of heart to improve venous return, as appropriate
- Instruct how to use good posture and good body mechanics when performing any activity
- Monitor traction devices for proper setup
- Maintain position and integrity of traction
- Elevate head of bed, as appropriate
- Turn as indicated by skin condition
- Develop written schedule for repositioning, as appropriate
- Turn immobilized person at least every 2 hours according to specific schedule, as appropriate
- Use appropriate devices to support limbs (e.g., hand roll, trochanter roll)
- Place call light and frequently used objects within reach
- Place bed-positioning switch within easy reach
- Document passive positioning time and procedure

1st edition 1992; revised 2000, 2024

Background Evidence:

Berman, A., Snyder, S. J., & Frandsen, G. (2018). *Kozier and Erb's Fundamentals of nursing: Concepts, process and practice* (10th ed.). Pearson.

Katz, S., Arish, N., Rokach, A., Zaltzman, Y., & Marcus, E. L. (2018). The effect of body position on pulmonary function: A systematic review. *BMC Pulmonary Medicine, 18*(1), 159–175.

Perry, A. G., Potter, P. A., Ostendorf, W. R., & Laplante, N. (2022). *Clinical Nursing Skills and Techniques* (10th ed.). Elsevier.

Schutt, S. C., Tarver, C., & Pezzani, M. (2017). Pilot study: Assessing the effect of continual position monitoring technology on compliance with patient turning protocols. *Nursing Open, 5*(1), 21–28.

Williams, P. (2020). *Basic geriatric nursing* (7th ed.). Elsevier.

P

Positioning: Intraoperative   0842

Definition: Placement of the patient or body part to promote surgical exposure while reducing or eliminating the risk of discomfort and complications

Activities:

- Determine length and type of procedure, anesthesia requirements, patient's age, body weight, and current medication regime
- Note nutritional status, presence of chronic illness, comorbidities, pre-existing pressure ulcers, and at-risk conditions (e.g., obesity, diabetes, anemia, advanced age, demineralizing bone conditions, pediatric patients)
- Identify high risk surgical situations (e.g., procedure greater than 2 hours, morbidly obese patients, vascular surgeries, excessive sustained pressure to certain body areas, cool environment with exposure of large body surfaces)
- Determine patient's range of motion, stability of joints, or presence of prostheses or implants
- Check peripheral circulation and neurological status
- Check skin integrity
- Document specific risk factors that may predispose patient to position-related injuries
- Check operating room table before patient transfer to ensure it is functioning, locked, and properly prepared with correct padded attachments
- Assure all needed equipment is clean and in good working order
- Assure a minimum of four persons to assist with transferring patient to the operating room table
- Lock wheels of stretcher and operating room bed during transfer of patient
- Document mode of operating room table transfer and number of persons assisting
- Check with anesthesia before moving an anesthetized patient
- Maintain body mechanics and employ ergonomic theory to prevent injury to self
- Move patients slowly and gently
- Provide warmth, privacy, and reassurance, as needed
- Protect all tubes, drains, lines, breathing circuits, and other devices
- Use assistive devices for immobilization, securing patient to operating room bed without compromising circulation underneath any restraining straps
- Employ restraining straps to prevent slippage of extremities
- Support the head and neck during transfer
- Coordinate transfer and positioning with stage of anesthesia or level of consciousness
- Support all body parts and maintain body alignment when moving an anesthetized patient
- Avoid pulling or dragging patients during transfers
- Protect the eyes, as appropriate
- Use assistive devices to support extremities and head
- Immobilize or support any body part, as appropriate
- Maintain patient's proper body alignment at all times

- Place on an appropriate therapeutic mattress or pad, as indicated
- Position patient for comfort whether asleep or awake
- Assure operative field adequately exposed
- Assure no awkward position, undue pressure on a body part, or use of stirrups or traction will obstruct the vascular supply to any body part
- Assure that respirations are not impeded by pressure of arms on the chest or by patient gown constricting neck or chest
- Employ padded shoulder braces to prevent irreparable nerve injury when Trendelenburg position employed
- Place in the proper surgical position for specific surgery (e.g., supine, prone, lateral chest, lithotomy, Kraske jackknife position)
- Elevate extremities, as appropriate
- Apply padding to bony prominences
- Apply padding or position patient to avoid pressure to superficial nerves
- Apply safety strap and arm restraint, as needed
- Adjust operating bed, as appropriate
- Monitor physiological effects of positioning and traction devices, as appropriate
- Monitor patient's position intraoperatively
- Intervene in situations in which position compromises patient outcomes
- Ensure access to airway, intravenous catheters, and monitoring devices
- Ensure that equipment or personnel do not create or impose pressure on patient during the procedure
- Monitor position, straps, and padding to assure placement is maintained throughout procedure
- Record position and devices used, including padding and safety measures
- Document all intraoperative assessments related to positioning and safety measures
- Reposition patient slowly at procedure end to allow for adequate hemodynamic accommodation

2nd edition 1996; revised 2018

Background Evidence:

Dybec, R. B. (2004). Intraoperative positioning and care of the obese patient. *Plastic Surgical Nursing, 24*(3), 118–122.

Graling, P., & Tea, C. (2006). Preventing intraoperative positioning injuries. *Nursing Management, 37*(7), 9–10.

Perry, A., Potter, P., & Ostendorf, W. (Eds.). (2014). *Clinical nursing skills and techniques* (8th ed.). Elsevier Mosby.

Rothrock, J. C. (Ed.). (2015). *Alexander's care of the patient in surgery* (15th ed.). Elsevier Mosby.

P

Positioning: Neurologic 0844

Definition: Achievement of optimal, appropriate body alignment for the patient experiencing or at risk for spinal cord injury or vertebral irritability

Activities:

- Immobilize or support the affected body part, as appropriate
- Place in the designated therapeutic position
- Refrain from applying pressure to the affected body part
- Support the affected body part
- Provide appropriate support for the neck
- Use appropriate body mechanics when positioning patient
- Provide a firm mattress
- Place on airflow bed, if possible
- Provide the patient with an adapted call system (e.g., low pressure, voice control, sip-and-puff straw like switch, chin movement switch) depending on level of motor function
- Maintain proper body alignment
- Position with head and neck in alignment
- Use heel boots to maintain ankles in neutral position
- Avoid positioning patient on bone flap removal site
- Position the head of bed as low as possible (measured by pulmonary function) to increase the surface area of the body and decrease pressure on bony prominences
- Turn using the log roll technique every 2 hours or more frequently, as indicated
- Stabilize the spine during position changes by keeping the spine in anatomical alignment (e.g., zero rotation)
- Monitor brain tissue oxygen and intracranial pressure in critically ill patients during positioning changes, as appropriate
- Apply an orthosis collar
- Instruct on orthosis collar care, as needed
- Monitor self-care ability when in orthosis collar or bracing device
- Apply and maintain a splinting or bracing device
- Monitor skin integrity under bracing device or orthosis collar
- Instruct on bracing device care, as needed
- Place a hand roll under the fingers
- Instruct the patient how to use good posture and good body mechanics when performing any activity
- Instruct on pin site care, as needed
- Monitor traction pin insertion site
- Perform traction or orthosis device pin insertion site care
- Monitor traction device setup
- Brace traction weights when moving patient
- Monitor for skin breakdown over bony prominences (e.g., sacrum, ischial tuberosities, heels)
- Provide passive range of motion to affected limbs as determined by rehabilitation staff
- Instruct family members on how to assist patient to turn in bed and how to provide range of motion, as appropriate
- Encourage patient to participate in position changes (i.e., remind staff when it is time to be turned) as feasible
- Instruct on ways (e.g., tilt, recline) to provide pressure relief to decrease potential for skin breakdown when using a wheelchair
- Monitor for orthostatic hypotension when transferring to a sitting position in wheelchair
- Use a slide board to assist transfer to a chair or wheel chair for those patients with fair balance

1st edition 1992; revised 2013

Background Evidence:

Fries, J. M. (2005). Critical rehabilitation of the patient with spinal cord injury. *Critical Care Nursing Quarterly, 28*(2), 179–187.

Ledwith, M. B., Bloom, S., Maloney-Wilensky, E., Coyle, B., Polomano, R., & LeRoux, P. D. (2010). Effect of body position on cerebral oxygenation and physiologic parameters in patients with acute neurological conditions. *Journal of Neuroscience Nursing, 42*(5), 280–287.

National Spinal Cord Injury Statistical Center. (2006). *The 2006 NSCISC statistical annual report for the model spinal cord injury care systems.*

Smeltzer, S. C., & Bare, B. G. (2004). Management of patients with neurologic trauma (10th ed.) *Brunner & Suddarth's textbook of medical surgical nursing* (Vol. 2, pp. 1910–1941). Lippincott Williams & Wilkins.

Sprigle, S., Maurer, C., & Sorenblum, S. E. (2010). Load redistribution in variable position wheelchairs in people with spinal cord injury. *Journal of Spinal Cord Medicine, 33*(1), 58–64.

P

Positioning: Prone 3330

Definition: Assisting ventilated persons into the prone position

Activities:

- Consider clinical criteria for positioning (e.g., ratio of partial pressure arterial oxygen and fraction of inspired oxygen less than 150 mmHg) and contraindications for positioning (e.g., spinal instability, facial or pelvic fractures, open chest or unstable chest wall, uncontrolled intracranial pressure, severe hemodynamic instability)
- Use institutional policies and procedures to standardize prone positioning (e.g., checklist, protocol, guidelines, work instructions about nursing care)
- Explain rationale and procedure for prone position, including risks and benefits
- Ensure adequate number of professionals for positioning with pre-assigned roles (e.g., respiratory therapist, nurses, physical therapist)
- Ensure stability and positioning of medical devices during positioning (e.g., orotracheal tube, chest drain, enteral feeding, bladder catheter)
- Record baseline vitals, hemodynamic data, and anterolateral aspects of skin
- Apply foam dressing to areas at risk for pressure injury (e.g., forehead, chin, sternum, shoulders, knees, anterior iliac crests)
- Pause enteral feedings for 1 hour prior to proning, then resume
- Ensure emergency intubation equipment at bedside
- Provide for adequate sedation
- Perform eye care (i.e., apply lubricant or ointments, tape lids closed)
- Position team members on both sides of bed (i.e., three on each side and head supported)

- Move person up in bed so head off bed during turn and head supported by team member
- Place arms either in swimmer's position or along sides of body
- Evaluate vital signs and blood gas analysis in first hour after maneuver and after every 4 or 6 hours, or as indicated
- Continuously monitor peripheral oxygen saturation and oxygen saturation values to be at levels of 92% to 96%
- Monitor for respiratory distress
- Return to supine position if hemodynamic instability occurs (e.g., unscheduled extubation, endotracheal tube obstruction, hemoptysis, SpO_2 <85% or PaO_2 <55 mmHg for more than five minutes, cardiac arrest, heart rate below 30 bpm, systolic blood pressure below 60 mmHg for more than 5 minutes)
- Check position of orotracheal tube after maneuver to avoid injuries to labial commissure and accidental extubation
- Rotate arms and head positions every 2 hours
- Recalibrate invasive equipment
- Record pronation time
- Record tolerance of procedure

8th edition 2024

Background Evidence:

Binda, F., Marelli, F., Galazzi, A., Pascuzzo, R., Adamini, I., & Laquintana, D. (2021). Nursing management of prone positioning in patients with COVID-19. *Critical Care Nurse*, 41(2), 27–35. https://doi.org/10.4037/ccn2020222

Gordon, A., Rabold, E., Thirumala, R., Husain, A. A., Patel, S., & Cheema, T. (2019). Prone positioning in ARDS. *Critical Care Nursing Quarterly*, 42(4), 371–375. https://doi.org/10.1097/CNQ.0000000000000277

Guérin, C., Albert, R. K., Beitler, J., Gattinoni, L., Jaber, S., Marini, J. J., Munshi, L., Papazian, L., Pesenti, A., Vieillard-Baron, A., & Mancebo, J. (2020). Prone position in ARDS patients: Why, when, how and for whom. *Intensive Care Medicine*, 46(12), 2385–2396. https://doi.org/10.1007/s00134-020-06306-w

Montanaro, J. (2021). Using in situ simulation to develop a prone positioning protocol for patients with ARDS. *Critical Care Nurse*, 41(1), 12–24. https://doi.org/10.4037/ccn2020830

Elharrar, X., Trigui, Y., Dols, A. M., Touchon, F., Martinez, S., Prud'homme, E., & Papazian, L. (2020). Use of prone positioning in non-intubated persons with COVID-19 and hypoxemic acute respiratory failure. *Journal of the American Medical Association (JAMA)*, 323(22), 2336–2338. https://doi.org/10.1001/jama.2020.8255

Jiang, L. G., LeBaron, J., Bodnar, D., Caputo, N. D., Chang, B. P., Chiricolo, G., & Sharma, M. (2020). Conscious proning: An introduction of a proning protocol for non-intubated, awake, hypoxic emergency department COVID-19 persons. *Academic Emergency Medicine*, 27(suppl 7), 566–569. https://doi.org/10.1111/acem.14035

Zaretsky, J., Corcoran, J. R., Savage, E., Berke, J., Herbsman, J., Fischer, M., Kmita, D., Laverty, P., Sweeney, G., & Horwitz, L. I. (2022). Increasing rates of prone positioning in acute care patients with COVID-19. *Joint Commission Journal on Quality and Patient Safety*, 48(1), 53–60. https://doi.org/10.1016/j.jcjq.2021.09.005

Positioning: Wheelchair   0846

Definition: Placement of a patient in a properly selected wheelchair to enhance comfort, promote skin integrity, and foster independence

Activities:

- Select the appropriate wheelchair for the patient (e.g., standard adult, semi reclining, fully reclining, amputee, extra wide, narrow)
- Select a wheelchair with seat low to floor for patient who will get around using foot propelling
- Select a cushion tailored to the patient's needs
- Use appropriate body mechanics when positioning patient
- Check patient's position in the wheelchair when patient sits on selected pad and wears proper footwear
- Position the pelvis in the middle and as far back on the seat as possible
- Check that the iliac crests are level and aligned from side to side
- Ensure that there is at least 2 to 3 inches of clearance on each side of the chair
- Ensure that wheelchair allows at least 2 to 3 inches of clearance from the back of knee to front of sling seat
- Check that footrests have at least 2 inches of clearance from the floor
- Maintain the angle of the hips at 100 degrees, the knees at 105 degrees, and the ankles at 90 degrees, with the heel resting flat on the footrests
- Measure the distance from the cushion to just under the elbow, add 1 inch, and adjust the armrests to this height
- Adjust the backrest to provide the amount of support required, usually 10 to 15 degrees from vertical
- Incline the seat 10 degrees toward the back
- Position legs so they are 20 degrees from vertical
- Monitor for patient's inability to maintain correct posture in wheelchair
- Monitor for effects of prolonged sitting (e.g., pressure ulcers, skin tears, bruises, contractures, discomfort, incontinence, social isolation, falls)
- Provide modifications or appliances to wheelchair to correct for patient problems or muscle weakness
- Provide padding and other enhancements (e.g., contoured padded backs, padded leg rest panels, arm troughs, padded trays) for patients with special needs
- Facilitate small shifts of body weight frequently
- Determine appropriate time frame for patient to remain in wheelchair based on health status
- Instruct patient on how to transfer from bed to wheelchair, as appropriate
- Provide trapeze or slide board to assist with transfer, as appropriate
- Instruct patient on how to operate wheelchair, as appropriate
- Instruct patient on exercises to increase upper body strength, as appropriate

1st edition 1992; revised 2013

Background Evidence:

Gavin-Dreschnack, D. (2004). Effects of wheelchair posture on patient safety. *Rehabilitation Nursing*, 29(6), 221–226.

Gavin-Dreschnack, D., Nelson, A., Fitzgerald, S., Harrow, J., Sanchez-Anguiano, A., Ahmed, S., & Powell-Cope, G. (2005). Wheelchair-related falls: Current evidence and directions of improved quality of care. *Journal of Nursing Care Quality, 20*(2), 119–127.

Kozier, B., Erb, G., Berman, A., & Snyder, S. (2004). Activity and exercise. In *Fundamentals of nursing: Concepts, process, and practice* (pp. 1058–1112) (7th ed.). Prentice Hall.

Mayall, J. K., & Desharnais, G. (1995). *Positioning in a wheelchair* (2nd ed.). Slack.

Nelson, A. L., Groer, S., Palacious, P., Mitchell, D., Sabharwal, S., Kirby, R. L., Gavin-Dreschnack, D., & Powell-Cope, G. (2010). Wheelchair-related falls in veterans with spinal cord injury residing in the community: A prospective cohort study. *Archives of Physical Medicine Rehabilitation, 91*(8), 1166–1173.

Postanesthesia Care 2870

Definition: Monitoring and management of the patient who has recently undergone general or regional anesthesia

Activities:

- Review patient's allergies, including allergy to latex
- Determine airway and circulatory adequacy
- Administer oxygen, as appropriate
- Monitor oxygenation
- Ventilate, as appropriate
- Monitor quality and number of respirations
- Encourage patient to deep breathe and cough
- Obtain handoff report from the operating room nurse and anesthetist or anesthesiologist
- Clarify any postoperative orders to be initiated in the post anesthesia care unit
- Monitor and record vital signs, including pain assessment, every 15 minutes or more often, as appropriate
- Monitor temperature
- Administer warming measures (e.g., warm blankets, convection blanket), as needed
- Monitor urinary output
- Provide nonpharmacological and pharmacological pain relief measures, as needed
- Administer antiemetic as ordered
- Administer narcotic antagonists per agency protocol, as appropriate
- Contact anesthetist, as appropriate
- Monitor intrathecal anesthetic level
- Monitor return of sensorium and motor function
- Monitor neurological status
- Monitor level of consciousness
- Provide for patient safety needs

- Provide warm blankets, as appropriate
- Interpret diagnostic tests, as appropriate
- Check patient's hospital record to determine baseline vital signs, as appropriate
- Compare current status with previous status to detect improvements and deterioration in patient's condition
- Provide verbal or tactile stimulation, as appropriate
- Administer IV medication to control shivering, as per agency protocol
- Monitor surgical site, as appropriate
- Restrain patient, as appropriate
- Adjust the bed, as appropriate
- Provide privacy, as appropriate
- Provide emotional support to the patient and family, as appropriate
- Determine patient's status for discharge
- Provide patient report to the postoperative nursing unit
- Discharge patient to next level of care

2nd edition 1996; revised 2004, 2018

Background Evidence:

American Society of Peri-Anesthesia Nurses. (2012). *2012–2014 Perianesthesia Nursing: Standards, practice recommendations and interpretive statements.*

Conner, R., Spruce, L., & Burlingame, B. (2013). *Perioperative standards and recommended practices.* Association of periOperative Registered Nurses.

Rothrock, J. C. (Ed.). (2015). *Alexander's care of the patient in surgery* (15th ed.). Elsevier Mosby.

P

Postmortem Care 1770

Definition: Provision of care to the deceased patient and family

Activities:

- Remove external objects from body (e.g., clothing, tubes, monitors), as needed
- Cleanse the body
- Place incontinent pad under buttocks and between legs
- Raise the head of the bed slightly to prevent pooling of fluids in head or face
- Place dentures in mouth, if possible
- Close the eyes
- Maintain proper body alignment
- Notify various departments and personnel, according to policy
- Label and secure personal belongings
- Notify clergy if requested by family

- Avoid restricting number of visitors
- Arrange for photographs
- Facilitate and support the family's viewing of the body
- Respect the family's religious beliefs and rituals
- Provide privacy and support for family members
- Answer questions concerning organ donation
- Answer questions concerning autopsy
- Label the body, according to policy, after the family has left
- Transfer the body to the morgue
- Notify mortician
- Notify coroner, as appropriate

1st edition 1992; revised 2013

Background Evidence:

Ackerman, M. J. (2009). State of postmortem genetic testing known as the cardiac channel molecular autopsy in the forensic evaluation of unexplained sudden cardiac death in the young. *Pacing & Clinical Electrophysiology, 32*(Suppl. 2), S86–S89.

De Lisle-Porter, M., & Podruchny, A. M. (2009). The dying neonate: Family-centered end-of-life care. *Neonatal Network, 28*(2), 75–83.

Kozier, B., Erb, G., Berman, A., & Snyder, S. (2004). Loss, grieving, and death. In *Fundamentals of nursing: Concepts, process, and practice* (pp. 1032–1058) (7th ed.). Prentice Hall.

Perry, A. G., & Potter, P. A. (2006). *Clinical nursing skills and techniques* (6th ed.). Elsevier Mosby.

Smith, T., Basa, E., Ewert-Flanagan, P., & Tilley, C. (2009). Incorporating spirituality into end-of-life and postmortem care. *Oncology Nursing Forum, 36*(3), 18.

Postpartal Care 6930

Definition: Providing care to a woman during the 6-week time period beginning immediately after childbirth

Activities:

- Monitor vital signs
- Monitor lochia for color, amount, odor, and presence of clots
- Have patient empty bladder before postpartum check and frequently
- Monitor fundal location, height, and tone, being sure to support the lower uterine segment during palpation
- Gently massage fundus until firm, as needed
- Monitor perineum or surgical incision and surrounding tissue (i.e., monitor for redness, edema, ecchymosis, discharge, and approximation of wound edges)
- Encourage early and frequent ambulation, assisting patient, when needed
- Encourage the postoperative patient to perform respiratory exercises, assisting patient, when needed
- Monitor patient's pain
- Comfort the patient experiencing shaking chills (i.e., provide warm blankets and offer beverages)
- Administer analgesics, as needed
- Instruct patient on non-pharmacological relief of pain (e.g., sitz baths, ambulation, massage, imagery, ice packs, witch hazel pads, and distraction)
- Instruct patient on perineal care to prevent infection and reduce discomfort
- Perform or assist with perineal care (i.e., apply ice pack, encourage patient to take sitz baths, and apply dry heat)
- Monitor breasts for temperature and color and nipple condition
- Instruct patient on breast changes
- Monitor bladder, including intake and output (e.g., emptying of bladder, palpable, color, odor, input, and output)
- Facilitate return to normal urinary functioning (i.e., assist with sitz baths, promote hydration, pour warm water on perineum, and encourage ambulation)
- Monitor bowels (e.g., date and time of last bowel movement, bowel sounds, presence of flatus)
- Facilitate return to normal bowel functioning (i.e., administer stool softener or laxative, instruct patient to increase consumption of fluids and fiber, encourage ambulation)
- Provide measures to reduce likelihood of deep vein thrombosis development (e.g., leg exercises and compression boot application)
- Monitor legs for Homans' sign and arrange for further testing, if needed
- Monitor patient's emotional status
- Encourage mother to discuss her labor and delivery experience
- Offer reassurance to patient on her ability to care for self and infant
- Provide information about mood changes (e.g., postpartum "blues," depression, and psychosis), including symptoms warranting further evaluation and treatment
- Monitor for symptoms of postpartum depression or psychosis
- Provide anticipatory guidance on physiological and psychological changes and their management
- Discuss activity and rest needs
- Discuss sexuality and contraceptive choices
- Monitor parent-infant attachment behaviors
- Facilitate optimal parent-infant attachment
- Instruct patient on nutritional needs, including the importance of a balanced diet and supplements, if indicated
- Instruct patient on infant's nutritional needs
- Provide adequate education and support on chosen feeding method
- Refer patient to lactation consultant, if indicated
- Instruct patient on danger signs that warrant immediate reporting (e.g., fever, depression)
- Administer Rh immune globulin and Rubella vaccine, if indicated
- Assist parent in scheduling newborn examination and postpartal examination
- Refer to appropriate resources for community support or follow-up care

1st edition 1992; revised 2013

Background Evidence:

Brockington, I. (2004). Postpartum psychiatric disorders. *The Lancet, 363*(9405), 303–310.

Morten, A., Kohl, M., O' Mahoney, P., & Pelosi, K. (1991). Certified nurse-midwifery care of the postpartum client: A descriptive study. *Journal of Nurse-Midwifery, 36*(5), 276–288.

Ward, S. L., & Hisley, S. M. (2009). Caring for the postpartal woman and her family. In *Maternal-child nursing care: Optimizing outcomes for mothers, children, & families* (pp. 469–509). F.A. Davis.

P

Preceptor: Employee   7722

Definition: Assisting and supporting a new or transferred employee through a planned orientation to a specific clinical area

Activities:

- Introduce new person to staff members
- Describe clinical focus of the unit and agency
- Communicate goals of the unit and agency
- Display an accepting attitude to individual assigned to the unit and agency
- Discuss the objectives of the orientation period
- Provide orientation checklist, as appropriate
- Tailor orientation to needs of new employee
- Discuss clinical ladder and types of care providers and their specific responsibilities
- Review skills needed to fulfill clinical role
- Review fire and disaster plans, as appropriate
- Review emergency code procedures, as appropriate
- Discuss use of policy and procedure manuals, as appropriate
- Instruct in use of clinical forms and other records, as appropriate
- Provide information and standards for universal precautions, as appropriate
- Discuss unit protocols, as appropriate
- Share work responsibilities during orientation, as appropriate
- Assist with locating needed supplies
- Orient to computer system, as appropriate
- Assist with new procedures, as appropriate
- Shape expectations for workload and scheduling
- Be aware of own personality and how that affects teaching style
- Be alert as to how generational differences may influence work attitudes and relationships
- Answer questions and discuss concerns, as appropriate
- Identify clinical specialists available for consultation, as appropriate
- Provide feedback on performance at specific intervals
- Share clinical stories and lessons learned to help shape clinical judgment
- Provide emotional support, especially during highly stressful times
- Include in unit social functions, as appropriate

2nd edition 1996; revised 2018

Background Evidence:

Garneau, A. Z. (2012). Mentorship and preceptorship. In J. Zerwekh & A. Garneau (Eds.), *Nursing today: Transitions and trends* (7th ed., pp. 47–60). Elsevier Saunders.

Grossman, S. (2013). *Mentoring in nursing: A dynamic and collaborative process* (2nd ed.). Springer.

Horton, C. D., DePaoli, S., Hertach, M., & Bower, M. (2012). Enhancing the effectiveness of nurse preceptors. *Online Journal for Nurses in Professional Development*, 28(4), E1–E7.

Twibell, R., St., Pierre, J., Johnson, D., Barton, D., Davis, C., Kidd, M., & Rook, G. (2012). Tripping over the welcome mat: Why new nurses don't stay and what the evidence says we can do about it. *American Nurse Today*, 7(6), 357–365.

Ulrich, B., Krozek, C., Early, S., Ashlock, D. H., Africa, L. M., & Carman, M. L. (2010). Improving retention, confidence, and competence of new graduate nurses; results from a 10-year longitudinal database. *Nursing Economic$*, 28(6), 36.

Preceptor: Student   7726

Definition: Assisting and supporting learning experiences for a student

Activities:

- Introduce students to staff members and patients
- Describe clinical focus of the unit and agency
- Communicate goals of the unit and agency
- Orient students to the unit and agency
- Display an accepting attitude to student assigned to the unit and agency
- Recognize the importance of your behavior as a role model
- Discuss the objectives of the experience, as appropriate
- Encourage open communication between the staff and students
- Make recommendations for patient assignments or potential learning experiences available for students, considering course objectives and student's level of skill, as appropriate
- Ensure patient's acceptance of students as caregivers
- Determine student's knowledge and skill level before delegating a task
- Provide as many opportunities as possible to practice complex skills (e.g., IV insertion, catheter insertion, leading team meetings, presentations to staff)
- Assist students to use policy and procedure manuals
- Ensure that students know and understand fire and disaster policies and emergency procedures
- Assist students to locate needed supplies
- Provide information and standards for universal precautions
- Discuss care plan for assigned patients, as appropriate
- Guide students in the application of the nursing process
- Include students in care planning conferences, as appropriate
- Facilitate student's communication with physicians and giving of patient reports
- Discuss any problems with students with the clinical instructor as soon as possible, as appropriate
- Provide observational experiences for activities beyond student's skill level
- Provide feedback to clinical instructor about student performance, as appropriate
- Establish and use electronic technologies (e.g., e-mail, text messages, social networks) to keep in touch with faculty member and students, as appropriate
- Provide constructive feedback to the student, when appropriate
- Assist student with new procedures, as appropriate

P

- Discuss issues in nursing practice with students based on specific patient situations, as appropriate
- Cosign charting with students, as appropriate
- Involve students in research activities, as appropriate
- Support student leadership experiences, as appropriate
- Serve as role model for developing collaborative relationships with other health care providers
- Inform clinical instructor of any changes in agency policy, as appropriate
- Orient to computer system, as appropriate
- Encourage student to work same days and same hours as preceptor
- Discourage use of multiple preceptors per student

Background Evidence:

Carlson, E., Pilhammar, E., & Wann-Hansson, C. (2010). "This is nursing": Nursing roles as mediated by precepting nurses during clinical practice. *Nurse Education Today*, 30(8), 763–767.

Koontz, A. M., Mallory, J. L., Burns, J. A., & Chapman, S. (2010). Staff nurses and students: The good, the bad, and the ugly. *MEDSURG Nursing*, 19(4), 240–246.

Luhanga, F., Myrick, F., & Yonge, O. (2010). The preceptor experience: An examination of ethical and accountability issues. *Journal of Professional Nursing*, 26(5), 264–271.

Sedgwick, M., & Harris, S. (2012). A critique of the undergraduate nursing preceptorship model. *Nursing Research and Practice*. https://doi.org/10.1155/2012/248356

2nd edition 1996; revised 2018

Preconception Counseling   5247

Definition: Providing therapeutic support to individuals of childbearing age before pregnancy to promote health and reduce risks

Activities:

- Ensure privacy and confidentiality
- Establish therapeutic, trusting relationship
- Review health history, including prenatal and obstetrical history, developmental history, and past and present health status related to confirmed or suspected genetic risk factors
- Review environment for possible risk factors (e.g., potential teratogen and carcinogen exposures)
- Review lifestyle for possible risk factors (e.g., tobacco, alcohol, prescription medication, drug use)
- Develop preconception, pregnancy-oriented, health risk profile based on history, prescription medication use, ethnic background, occupational and household exposures, diet, specific genetic disorders, and lifestyle
- Explore readiness for pregnancy with both partners
- Inquire about physical abuse, as indicated
- Obtain thorough sexual history, including frequency and timing of intercourse, use of spermicidal lubricants, and postcoital habits such as douching
- Investigate possible causes of infertility in couples who have not been able to get pregnant for more than 1 year
- Refer women with chronic medical conditions for a pre-pregnancy management plan
- Provide information related to risk factors
- Refer for genetic counseling for genetic risk factors
- Refer for prenatal diagnostic tests as needed for genetic, medical, or obstetrical risk factors
- Evaluate for hemoglobin or hematocrit levels, Rh status, urine dipstick, toxoplasmosis, sexually transmitted diseases, rubella, hepatitis, and genetic defects
- Advise partners to test to identify risks as needed
- Support decision making about advisability of pregnancy based on identified risk factors
- Counsel about avoiding pregnancy until appropriate treatment has been given (e.g., rubella vaccine, Rho(D) immune globulin, immune serum globulin, antibiotics)
- Evaluate need for screening mammogram based on age and desire for prolonged breastfeeding
- Encourage dental examination during preconception to minimize exposure to x-ray examinations and anesthetics
- Instruct about relationships among early fetal development and personal habits, medication use, teratogens, and self-care requisites (e.g., prenatal vitamins, folic acid)
- Educate about ways to avoid teratogens (e.g., handling cat litter, smoking cessation, alcohol substitutes)
- Refer to teratogens information service to locate specific information about environmental agents
- Advise use of folic acid for both partners at least 3 months before conception
- Discuss specific ways to prepare for pregnancy, including social, financial, and psychological demands of childbearing and childrearing
- Identify real or perceived barriers to family planning services and prenatal care and ways of overcoming barriers
- Discuss available methods of reproductive assistance and technology, as appropriate
- Encourage contraception until prepared for pregnancy, as appropriate
- Discuss timing of cessation of contraception to maximize accurate pregnancy dating
- Discuss methods of identifying fertility, signs of pregnancy, and ways to confirm pregnancy
- Discuss need for early registration and compliance with prenatal care, including specific high-risk programs that may be appropriate
- Encourage attendance at early pregnancy and parenting classes
- Encourage women to learn details of health insurance coverage, including waiting periods and available provider options
- Recommend self-care needed during preconception period
- Provide education and referrals to appropriate community resources
- Encourage participation in support groups for couples trying to get pregnant
- Provide copy of written plan of care for both persons
- Provide or recommend follow-up as needed
- Use teach-back to ensure understanding

2nd edition 1996; revised 2000, 2024

Background Evidence:

Fowler, J. R., Mahdy, H., & Jack, B. W. (2021). Preconception counseling. In *StatPearls*. StatPearls Publishing. https://pubmed.ncbi.nlm.nih.gov/28722910/

Henning, P. A., Burgess, C. K., Jones, H. E., & Norman, W. V. (2017). The effects of asking a fertility intention question in primary care settings: A systematic review protocol. *Systematic Reviews, 6*(1), 11. https://doi.org/10.1186/s13643-017-0412-z

Hubberd, A. L., Watson, N. A., Cobb, E., Wardian, J. L., Morrow, C. C., & Sauerwein, T. J. (2020). Preconception counseling for women with diabetes. *Clinical Diabetes: A Publication of the American Diabetes Association, 38*(1), 98–100. https://doi.org/10.2337/cd18-0109

Murugesu, L., Hopman, M. E., Van Voorst, S. F., Rosman, A. N., & Fransen, M. P. (2019). Systematic development of materials for inviting low health-literate individuals to participate in preconception counseling. *International Journal of Environmental Research and Public Health, 16*(21), 4223. https://doi.org/10.3390/ijerph16214223

Smith, A., Barr, W. B., Bassett-Novoa, E., & LeFevre, N. (2018). Maternity care update: Preconception care. *FP essentials, 467*, 11–16.

Pregnancy Termination Care   6950

Definition: Management of the physical and psychological needs of the woman undergoing a spontaneous or elective abortion

Activities:

- Prepare patient physically and psychologically for abortion procedure
- Explain sensations patient might experience
- Instruct on signs to report (e.g., increased bleeding, increased cramping, and passage of clots or tissue)
- Provide analgesics or antiemetics, as appropriate
- Perform back rub, as needed
- Administer medication to terminate pregnancy, per protocol
- Monitor patient for bleeding and cramping
- Initiate intravenous line, as appropriate
- Observe for signs of spontaneous abortion (e.g., cessation of cramping, increased pelvic pressure, and loss of amniotic fluid)
- Perform vaginal examination, as appropriate
- Assist delivery, as appropriate, depending on gestational age of fetus
- Weigh blood loss, as appropriate
- Monitor vital signs
- Observe for signs of shock
- Save all passed tissue
- Administer oxytocics after delivery, as appropriate
- Provide teaching for procedures (e.g., suction curettage, dilation and curettage, and uterine evacuation)
- Administer Rho(D) immune globulin for Rh-negative status
- Instruct patient about postabortion self-care and monitoring of side effects
- Provide anticipatory guidance about grief reaction to fetal death
- Encourage significant other to support patient before, during, or after abortion, if desired or with consent from the patient
- Provide information for referral to support groups (e.g., Resolve through Sharing, Compassionate Friends, SHARE Pregnancy and Infant Loss Support)
- Refer for psychological support or counseling, as needed
- Consider cultural and religious beliefs and values
- Refer for religious support, as desired
- Inform about "anniversary phenomenon"
- Complete delivery record and report of death, as appropriate
- Obtain specimens for genetic studies or autopsy, as appropriate

1st edition 1992; revised 1996, 2018

Background Evidence:

Gilbert, E. S. (2011). *Manual of high-risk pregnancy and delivery* (pp. 318–328) (5th ed.). Mosby Elsevier.

Mattson, S., & Smith, J. (Eds.). (2011). *Core curriculum for maternal-newborn nursing* (4th ed.). Saunders Elsevier.

Perry, S., Hockenberry, M., Lowdermilk, D., & Wilson, D. (Eds.). (2014). *Maternal child nursing care* (5th ed.). Elsevier Mosby.

Pillitteri, A. (2014). Nursing care for the family in need of reproductive life planning. In *Maternal & child health nursing: Care of the childbearing & childrearing family* (pp. 108–137) (7th ed.). Lippincott Williams & Wilkins.

Yonke, N., & Leeman, L. M. (2013). First-trimester surgical abortion techniques. *Obstetrics and Gynecology Clinics of North America, 40*(4), 647–670.

P

Premenstrual Syndrome (PMS) Management   1440

Definition: Alleviation or attenuation of physical or behavioral symptoms occurring during the luteal phase of the menstrual cycle

Activities:

- Instruct in prospective identification of major premenstrual symptoms (e.g., bloating, cramping, irritability), use of prospective calendar check list or symptom log, and recording of timing and severity of each symptom
- Review symptom log or check list
- Collaborate to prioritize most problematic symptoms
- Discuss complexity of management and need for stepwise approach to alleviate individual symptoms
- Collaborate to select and institute stepwise approach to eliminating symptoms
- Provide information about symptom specific self-care measures (e.g., exercise, calcium supplementation)
- Prescribe symptom specific medication (e.g., NSAIDs, hormone therapy) as appropriate to practice level
- Monitor changes in symptoms
- Encourage to participate in PMS support group if available
- Refer to specialist, as appropriate
- Encourage physical exercise, cognitive behavior therapy, and dietary changes

- Offer information about alternative or complementary therapies (e.g., supplements of calcium, vitamin D, *Vitex agnus-castus*, *Ginkgo biloba*)
- Explore non-pharmacological strategies to reduce pain (e.g., warm compress, hot bath, lie down ventrally and place pillows in abdominal region)
- Promote strategies to reduce stress and anxiety

4th edition 2004; revised 2024

Background Evidence:

Chin, L. N., & Nambiar, S. (2017). Management of premenstrual syndrome. *Obstetrics, Gynaecology & Reproductive Medicine, 27*(1), 1–6.

Gnanasambanthan, S., & Datta, S. (2019). Premenstrual syndrome. *Obstetrics, Gynaecology & Reproductive Medicine, 29*(10), 281–285.

Gudipally, P. R., & Sharma, G. K. (2020). Premenstrual syndrome. In *StatPearls*. StatPearls Publishing. https://www.ncbi.nlm.nih.gov/books/NBK560698/

Heydari, N., Abootalebi, M., Jamalimoghadam, N., Kasraeian, M., Emamghoreishi, M., & Akbarzaded, M. (2018). Evaluation of aromatherapy with essential oils of Rosa damascena for the management of premenstrual syndrome. *International Journal of Gynecology & Obstetrics, 142*(2), 156–161.

Simsek Kucukkelepce, D., Unver, H., Nacar, G., & Tashan, S. T. (2021). The effects of acupressure and yoga for coping with premenstrual syndromes on premenstrual symptoms and quality of life. *Complementary Therapies in Clinical Practice, 42*, 101282. https://doi.org/10.1016/j.ctcp.2020.101282

Prenatal Care   6960

Definition: Provision of health care during the course of pregnancy

Activities:

- Identify individual needs, concerns, and preferences, foster involvement in decision making, and identify and address barriers to care
- Discuss importance of participating in prenatal care throughout entire pregnancy and encourage involvement of patient's partner or other family member
- Encourage prenatal class attendance
- Monitor weight gain
- Monitor for hypertensive disorder (e.g., blood pressure, edematous ankles, hands, and face, and proteinuria)
- Monitor fetal heart tones
- Measure fundal height and compare with gestational age
- Monitor fetal movement
- Instruct patient on quickening and importance of monitoring fetal activity
- Monitor fetal presentation
- Review with patient changes noted on fetal growth and status
- Instruct patient on danger signs that warrant immediate reporting
- Discuss nutritional needs and concerns (e.g., balanced diet, folic acid, food safety, and supplements)
- Instruct patient on effects of exposure to or ingestion of harmful substances (e.g., alcohol, illicit drugs, teratogens, medications, herbs, and tobacco)
- Discuss activity level with patient (e.g., appropriate exercise, activities to avoid, and importance of rest)
- Provide genetic counseling and testing if indicated
- Instruct patient on routine laboratory testing to occur throughout pregnancy (e.g., urinalysis, hemoglobin level, ultrasound, gestational diabetes, and HIV)
- Instruct patient on nonroutine tests and treatments (e.g., nonstress test, biophysical profile, Rh-immune globulin, and stripping of membranes), if needed
- Review results of testing with patient
- Discuss oral health care
- Discuss sexuality
- Monitor psychosocial status of patient and patient's partner
- Monitor for risk factors affecting patient or fetal health status (e.g., mental health disorder and intimate partner violence)
- Offer support and counsel to the patient presenting with an unplanned or unwanted pregnancy
- Offer anticipatory guidance about physiological and psychological changes and discomforts (e.g., nausea, vomiting, musculoskeletal changes, fears, and breast tenderness)
- Assist patient in identifying strategies to cope with changes and relieve discomforts associated with pregnancy
- Discuss changing body image with patient
- Review safety precautions to be taken during pregnancy (e.g., seat belt use, avoidance of hot tubs and saunas, and travel restrictions)
- Provide accurate information pertaining to risks, benefits, contraindications, and side effects of immunizations, if needed
- Assist patient in preparing for labor and delivery (i.e., discuss pain management options, review labor signs and symptoms, discuss special circumstances requiring medical intervention, and encourage planned involvement of patient's partner or family)
- Offer anticipatory guidance on infant care and considerations (e.g., circumcision, feeding, and selection of pediatric health care provider)
- Discuss postpartal concerns and considerations (e.g., family planning and contraception, returning to work or school, and physiological and psychological changes)
- Provide referral to appropriate service (e.g., supplemental food program, drug dependency treatment, and mental health counseling), if needed

1st edition 1992; revised 2013

Background Evidence:

Department of Health and Human Services. (1989). *Caring for our future, the content of prenatal care: A report of the Public Health Service Expert Panel on the content of prenatal care.* Public Health Service.

Hanson, L., VandeVusse, L., Roberts, J., & Forristal, A. (2009). A critical appraisal of guidelines for antenatal care: Components of care and priorities in prenatal education. *Journal of Midwifery & Women's Health, 54*(6), 458–468.

Novick, G. (2009). Women's experience of prenatal care: An integrative review. *Journal of Midwifery & Women's Health, 54*(3), 226–237.

Pillitteri, A. (2007). *Maternal and child health nursing: Care of the childbearing and childrearing family* (5th ed.). Lippincott Williams & Wilkins.

P

Preoperative Coordination   2880

Definition: Facilitating preadmission diagnostic testing and preparation of the surgical patient

Activities:
- Review planned surgery
- Explain procedures in a way that the patient can understand
- Obtain client history, as appropriate
- Complete a physical assessment, as appropriate
- Review physician's orders
- Order or coordinate diagnostic testing, as appropriate
- Describe and explain preadmission treatments and diagnostic tests
- Interpret diagnostic test results, as appropriate
- Obtain blood specimens, as appropriate
- Obtain urine specimen, as needed
- Communicate any concerns (e.g., abnormal laboratory or diagnostic test results, issues related to the patient's understanding of the planned procedure) to the surgeon
- Inform patient and significant other of the date and time of surgery, time of arrival, and admission procedure
- Inform the patient and significant other of the location of receiving unit, surgery, and the waiting area
- Determine the patient's expectations about the surgery
- Involve patient in decisions related to surgery
- Reinforce information provided by other health care providers, as appropriate
- Obtain consent for treatment, as appropriate

- Provide time for the patient and significant other to ask questions and voice concerns
- Obtain financial clearance from third-party payers, as necessary
- Discuss postoperative discharge plans
- Assure that patient has significant other for postoperative needs, such as transportation home as indicated
- Determine ability of caretakers
- Telephone the patient to verify planned surgery

2nd edition 1996; revised 2000, 2018

Background Evidence:

Association of periOperative Registered Nurses. (2015). *Guidelines for perioperative practice.*

Kozier, B., Erb, G., Berman, A., & Snyder, S. (2015). Perioperative nursing. In A. Berman, S. Snyder, & G. Frandsen (Eds.), *Kozier & Erb's fundamentals of nursing: Concepts, process, and practice* (10th ed., pp. 959–998). Prentice Hall.

Potter, P., Perry, A., Stockert, P., & Hall, A. (Eds.). (2013). *Fundamentals of nursing* (8th ed.). Elsevier Mosby.

Rothrock, J. C. (Ed.). (2015). *Alexander's care of the patient in surgery* (15th ed.). Elsevier Mosby.

Preparatory Sensory Information   5580

Definition: Describing in concrete and objective terms the typical sensory experiences and events associated with an upcoming stressful health care procedure or treatment

Activities:
- Ensure readiness for explanations or descriptions
- Describe upcoming sequence of events and environment associated with procedure or treatment
- Describe typical sensations associated with procedure or treatment (e.g., see, feel, smell, taste, hear)
- Present descriptions of experiences prior to experience
- Provide person in emergent situations to explain procedures with rationales as they occur, where possible
- Present sensations and procedural or treatment events in sequence experienced
- Provide descriptions in specific language, using interpreter as needed
- Use age-appropriate tools as needed for pediatric persons (e.g., puppets, colorful toys)
- Describe sensations using descriptive words and length of time
- Avoid evaluative adjectives that reflect degree of sensation or emotional response
- Link sensations to their cause when it may not be self-evident
- Provide opportunity for questions and clarification of misunderstandings

1st edition 1992; revised 2000, 2024

Background Evidence:

Association of PeriOperative Registered Nurses. (2021). 2021 Guidelines for perioperative practice.

Hall, A. (2021). Patient education. In P. A. Potter, A. G. Perry, P. A. Stockert, & A. M. Hall. (Eds.), *Fundamentals of nursing* (10th ed., pp. 328–348). Elsevier.

Nguyen, M. H., Smets, M. A., Bol, N., Loos, E. F., Hanneke, W., Geijsen, D., Henegouwen, M., Tytgat, K., & van Weert, J. (2019). Tailored web-based information for younger and older patients with cancer: Randomized controlled trial of a preparatory educational intervention on patient outcomes. *Journal of Medical Internet research, 21*(10), e14407. https://doi.org/10.2196/14407

Perry, A. G., Potter, P. A., Ostendorf, W. R., & Laplante, N. (2018). *Clinical nursing skills and techniques.* Elsevier.

Rebar, C., & Bashaw, M. (2021). Concepts of care for perioperative patients. In D. D. Ignatavicius, M. L. Workman, C. Rebar, & N. M. Heimgartner (Eds.), *Medical-Surgical nursing: Concepts for interprofessional collaborative care* (10th ed., pp. 417–500). Elsevier.

Reid-Searl, K., O'Neill, B., Dwyer, T., & Crowley, K. (2017). Using a procedural puppet to teach pediatric nursing procedures. *Clinical Simulation in Nursing, 13*(1), 15–23.

Rothrock, J., & McEwen, D. R. (2019). *Alexander's care of the patient in surgery* (16th ed.). Elsevier.

P

Prescribing: Diagnostic Testing 8080

Definition: Ordering a diagnostic test to identify or monitor a health problem

Activities:
- Evaluate signs and symptoms of current health problem
- Consider the status of the existing chronic health condition
- Review past medical history, medications, allergies, past diagnostic testing pertinent to the presenting condition
- Evaluate the diagnostic utility of the test in addressing the specific clinical question (i.e., understand sensitivity and specificity of the diagnostic test for the presenting condition)
- Consult with accepted evidence-based practice guidelines, specialists, and other health care professionals, as appropriate
- Provide the patient or family members with the rationale for the proposed testing, including how the information would benefit clinical decision making or continued monitoring
- Allow for discussion and questions of the testing
- Provide alternatives to diagnostic testing, as appropriate
- Consider the availability and cost of the diagnostic testing and include the patient and family in the discussion
- Instruct the patient and family on what to expect of the diagnostic test
- Have a system in place to ensure test results are received when expected
- Identify a method that ensures accurate communication of test date, time, and location to the patient or caregiver
- Instruct the patient and family on the test date, time, location, and how to expect test results to be reported
- Employ a system that provides for the timely return of diagnostic test results and assurance that missing or delayed reports are noted and pursued
- Monitor for adverse effects of the diagnostic test
- Maintain knowledge of diagnostic testing used in practice (e.g., sensitivity or specificity, rationale, alternatives, standards of care, evidence based practice, side effects, monitoring and state regulations or policy issues)

6th edition 2013

Background Evidence:
Buppert, C. (2008). *Nurse practitioner's business practice and legal guide* (3rd ed.). Jones & Bartlett.

Chase, S. (2004). *Clinical judgment and communication in nurse practitioner practice*. F.A. Davis.

Dains, J. E., Baumann, L. C., & Scheibel, P. (2007). *Advanced health assessment & clinical diagnosis in primary care* (3rd ed.). Mosby Elsevier.

Prescribing: Nonpharmacologic Treatment 8086

Definition: Ordering nonpharmacologic treatment for a health problem

Activities:
- Determine signs and symptoms of current health problem
- Review past medical history, medications, allergies, and past diagnostic testing pertinent to the presenting condition
- Review past and current therapeutic treatments tried for the health problem, including the reasons for stopping treatment
- Document the effects of other treatments on the health problem
- Identify nonpharmacological treatments (e.g., exercise, diet, physical therapy, occupational therapy, heat and cold treatment) that are indicated for current health problems
- Consult with accepted evidence-based practice guidelines, specialists, and other health care professionals, as appropriate
- Consider the availability and cost of the recommended treatment and include the patient and family in the discussion
- Provide the patient and family members with the rationale for the proposed treatment, expected outcome, and duration of the treatment
- Allow for questions and discussion related to the diagnosis and treatment and provide alternatives to the treatment
- Refer to appropriate service provider
- Monitor for adverse effects of the treatment
- Ensure for follow up to assess response to treatment
- Maintain knowledge of treatments commonly used in practice, including rationale, alternatives, standards of care, evidence-based practice, side effects, monitoring, and state regulations or policy issues

6th edition 2013

Background Evidence:
Buppert, C. (2008). *Nurse practitioner's business practice and legal guide* (3rd ed.). Jones and Bartlett.

Chase, S. (2004). *Clinical judgment and communication in nurse practitioner practice*. F.A. Davis.

Dains, J. E., Baumann, L. C., & Scheibel, P. (2007). *Advanced health assessment & clinical diagnosis in primary care* (3rd ed.). Mosby Elsevier.

Dunphy, L. M., Winland-Brown, J. E., Porter, B. O., & Thomas, D. J. (2007). *Primary care: The art and science of advanced practice* (2nd ed.). F.A. Davis.

P

Presence   5340

Definition: Being with another, both physically and psychologically, during times of need

Activities:

- Establish intention to convey unconditional positive regard toward person and their situation
- Cultivate and communicate caring, empathy, compassion, and understanding
- Be sensitive to cultural traditions, beliefs, and practices
- Strive to know person as unique human being
- Convey sense of knowing that allows person to feel valued and understood
- Convey openness, authenticity, and genuineness
- Listen intently and actively to concerns
- Use silence, when appropriate
- Offer gentle touch judiciously to express concern, as appropriate
- Be physically available to offer assistance when needed
- Remain physically present without expecting interactional responses
- Provide privacy, as needed
- Offer to remain with person, as needed
- Inform availability
- Promote safety and reduce fear
- Reassure and assist parents in their supportive role with significant others

- Offer to contact other support persons, as appropriate

1st edition 1992; revised 1996, 2000, 2024

Background Evidence:

Lazenby, M. (2018). *Caring matters most: The ethical significance of nursing.* Oxford University Press.

Martin, N. M. (2021). Practicing presence with authenticity. *Journal of Christian Nursing, 38*(4), 259. https://doi.org/10.1097/CNJ.0000000000 0008

Maniago, J. D. (2017). Therapeutic presencing in nursing. *IARS' International Research Journal, 7*(2). https://doi.org/10.51611/iars.irj.v7i2.2017.81

Newman, M. (2008). *Transforming presence: The difference nursing makes.* F.A. Davis.

Parse, R. (2021). *The human becoming paradigm: An everchanging horizon.* A Discovery International.

Schaffer, M., & Norlander, L. (2009). *Being present: A nurse's resource for end-of-life communication.* Sigma Theta Tau International.

Watson, J. (2021). *Caring science as sacred science (revised ed.).* Lotus Library.

Pressure Injury Care   3520

Definition: Facilitation of healing in pressure injuries

Activities:

- Describe characteristics of pressure injury at regular intervals, including size (e.g., length, width, depth), stage (I–IV), location, exudate, granulation or necrotic tissue, and epithelization
- Monitor color, temperature, moisture, and appearance of surrounding skin
- Apply moist heat to pressure injury, as prescribed
- Cleanse skin with mild soap and water, as indicated
- Cleanse with appropriate nontoxic solution
- Note characteristics of drainage
- Apply permeable adhesive membrane to pressure injury, as prescribed
- Apply saline soaks, ointments, and dressings, as prescribed
- Provide adequate pain control (e.g., medication, music therapy, distraction, massage)
- Monitor for signs and symptoms of infection
- Position every 1 to 2 hours or more frequently, as appropriate
- Use specialty beds and mattresses, as appropriate
- Use protective devices
- Monitor nutritional status ensuring adequate dietary intake
- Consult dietitian
- Consult Wound Ostomy Continence Nurse (WOCN), as appropriate
- Instruct about signs of skin breakdown, as appropriate
- Instruct on wound care procedures (e.g., debridement, electrical stimulation)
- Use teach-back to ensure understanding

Background Evidence:

Atkinson, R. A., & Cullum, N. A. (2018). Interventions for pressure ulcers: A summary of evidence for prevention and treatment. *Spinal Cord, 56*(3), 186–198. https://doi.org/10.1038/s41393-017-0054-y

Berman, A., Snyder, S. J., & Frandsen, G. (2018). *Kozier and Erb's fundamentals of nursing: Concepts, process and practice* (10th ed.). Pearson.

Craven, R. F., Hirnle, C. J., & Henshaw, C. J. (2021). *Fundamentals of nursing: Human health and function* (8th ed.). Wolters-Kluwer.

Meier, C., Boes, S., Armin, G., Gmünder, H. P., Kamran, K., Metzger, S., Schaefer, D. J., Schmitt, K., Wolfram, S., Reto, W., & Scheel-Sailer Anke, (2019). Treatment and cost of pressure injury stage III or IV in four patients with spinal cord injury: The basel decubitus concept. *Spinal Cord Series and Cases, 5*(1), 1–9. https://doi.org/10.1038/s41394-019-0173-0

Potter, P. A., Perry, A. G., Stockert, P. A., & Hall, A. M. (2021). *Fundamentals of nursing* (10th ed.). Elsevier.

Segalla, G. V., Teixeira, S. T., & Rogero, M. M. (2021). Nutritional therapy and wound healing in pressure injury situations: An integrative review. *Nutrire, 46*(2). https://doi.org/10.1186/s41110-021-00147-3

Trisnaningtyas, W., Retnaningsih, R., & Rochana, N. (2021). Effects and interventions of pressure injury prevention bundles of care in critically ill patients: A systematic review. *Nurse Media: Journal of Nursing, 11*(2), 154–176. https://doi.org/10.14710/nmjn.v11i2.28881

P

1st edition 1992; revised 2000, 2004, 2024

Pressure Injury Prevention 3540

Definition: Prevention of localized damage to skin due to pressure or friction

Activities:

- Complete comprehensive inspection of skin
- Identify risk factors (e.g., diabetes, depressed immune system, vascular disease, nutritional deficiencies, smoking, immobility)
- Document any previous incidences of pressure injury
- Document skin status on admission, daily and per agency protocol
- Use established risk assessment tool to monitor risk factors (e.g., Braden, Norton scale)
- Use established guidelines or agency protocol for specific preventive activities (e.g., bundles)
- Use methods of measuring skin temperature to determine risk, per agency protocol
- Monitor vital signs with focus on MAP
- Monitor any areas of concern closely
- Inspect skin under medical devices regularly (e.g., face masks, nasal cannulas, feeding tubes, catheters, neck braces, tracheostomy tubes)
- Remove excessive moisture on skin (e.g., perspiration, wound drainage, feces, urine)
- Apply protective barriers (e.g., creams, moisture-absorbing pads), as prescribed
- Turn every 1 to 2 hours or more frequently, as appropriate
- Avoid friction when turning to prevent injury to fragile skin.
- Encourage frequent shifts of body weight
- Post turning schedule at bedside, as appropriate
- Use positioning and protective devices, as appropriate
- Avoid massaging over bony prominences
- Keep bed linens clean, dry, and wrinkle free
- Provide adequate pain control (e.g., medication, music therapy, distraction, massage)
- Utilize specialty beds and mattresses, as appropriate
- Monitor mobility and activity
- Ensure adequate dietary intake, especially protein, vitamins B and C, iron, and calories, using supplements, as appropriate
- Consult dietitian, as appropriate
- Consult Wound Ostomy Continence Nurse (WOCN) and skin champions as appropriate
- Instruct on signs of skin breakdown, as appropriate
- Use teach-back to ensure understanding

1st edition 1992; revised 1996, 2000, 2004, 2024

Background Evidence:

Agency for Healthcare Research and Quality. (2017, October). Pressure injury prevention in hospitals training program. https://www.ahrq.gov/patient-safety/settings/hospital/resource/pressure-injury/index.html

Alderden, J. G., Shibily, F., & Cowan, L. (2020). Best practice in pressure injury prevention among critical care patients. *Critical Care Nursing Clinics of North America*, 32(4), 489–500. https://doi.org/10.1016/j.cnc.2020.08.001

Berman, A., Snyder, S. J., & Frandsen, G. (2018). *Kozier and Erb's fundamentals of nursing: Concepts, process and practice* (10th ed.). Pearson.

Craven, R. F., Hirnle, C. J., & Henshaw, C. J. (2021). *Fundamentals of nursing: Human health and function* (8th ed.). Wolters-Kluwer.

Kottner, J., Cuddigan, J., Carville, K., Balzer, K., Berlowitz, D., Law, S., Litchford, M., Mitchell, P., Moore, Z., Pittman, J., Sigaudo-Roussel, D., Yee, C. Y., & Haesler, E. (2019). Prevention and treatment of pressure ulcers/injuries: The protocol for the second update of the international Clinical Practice Guideline 2019. *Journal of Tissue Viability*, 28(2), 51–58. https://doi.org/10.1016/j.jtv.2019.01.001

Moore, Z., Patton, D., Avsar, P., McEvoy, N. L., Curley, G., Budri, A., Nugent, L., Walsh, S., & O'Connor, T. (2020). Prevention of pressure ulcers among individuals cared for in the prone position: Lessons for the COVID-19 emergency. *Journal of Wound Care*, 29(6), 312–320. https://doi.org/10.12968/jowc.2020.29.6.312

Pittman, J., Beeson, T., Dillon, J., Yang, Z., Mravec, M., Malloy, C., & Cuddigan, J. (2021). Hospital-acquired pressure injuries and acute skin failure in critical care: A case-control study. *Journal of Wound, Ostomy, and Continence Nursing: Official Publication of The Wound, Ostomy and Continence Nurses Society*, 48(1), 20–30. https://doi.org/10.1097/WON.0000000000000734

Tayyib, N., Asiri, M. Y., Danic, S., Sahi, S. L., Lasafin, J., Generale, L. F., Malubay, A., Viloria, P., Palmere, M. G., Parbo, A., Aguilar, K. E., Licuanan, P. M., & Reyes, M. (2021). The effectiveness of the SKINCARE bundle in preventing medical-device related pressure injuries in critical care units: A clinical trial. *Advances in Skin & Wound Care*, 34(2), 75–80.

Procedural Support: Infant 6965

Definition: Providing strategies to minimize pain and stress while maximizing the infant's ability to cope with and recover from painful clinical procedures

Activities:

- Ensure the presence of a person dedicated to provide support to the infant
- Evaluate the need for painful procedures
- Separate the number and grouping of laboratory and diagnostic procedures according to infant's tolerance
- Avoid painful procedures at the same time as nonemergency routine care
- Use minimal amounts of tape or adhesives
- Use skin barrier whenever possible
- Use noninvasive monitoring devices whenever possible
- Instruct parents about signs and symptoms of pain and the comfort that they can provide
- Reduce light and noise whenever possible during painful procedures
- Use facilitated tucking (i.e., hand swaddle to hold extremities flexed and contained close to the trunk)
- Use blanket swaddling after a painful procedure
- Use nonnutritive sucking with a pacifier
- Use sucrose solution with pacifier before and throughout painful procedures
- Facilitate breastfeeding or feed breast milk during painful procedures

P

- Facilitate kangaroo care (i.e., skin-to-skin contact) with parent during painful procedures, when possible
- Facilitate holding by parent, when possible

7th edition 2018

Background Evidence:

Harrison, D., Yamada, J., & Stevens, B. (2010). Strategies for the prevention and management of neonatal and infant pain. *Current Pain and Headache Reports, 14*(2), 113–123.

McNair, C., Yeo, M. C., & Johnston, C. (2013). Nonpharmacological management of pain during common needle puncture procedures in infants: Current research evidence and practical considerations. *Clinics in Perinatology, 40*(3), 493–508.

Riddell, R., Racine, N., Turcotte, K., Uman, L., Horton, R., Osmun, L., Kohut, S., Stuart, J., Stevens, B., & Gerwitz-Stern, A. (2011). Nonpharmacological management of infant and young child procedural pain (review). *Cochrane Database of Systematic Reviews, 10*, CD006275. https://doi.org/10.1002/14651858.CD006275.pub2

Verklan, M., & Walden, M. (Eds.). (2010). *Core curriculum for neonatal intensive care nursing* (4th ed.). Saunders Elsevier.

Product Evaluation   7760

Definition: Determining the effectiveness of new products or equipment

Activities:

- Identify need for a new product or a change in a current product
- Assemble a multidisciplinary product selection and evaluation team if change will affect other providers
- Gather information on use of the existing product that is being replaced
- Establish criteria for product selection
- Decide on a disposable versus a reusable product
- Strive for standardization of inventory when within and across facilities, when possible
- Select product for evaluation
- Select a product that has an uncomplicated user interface
- Define perspective of analysis (benefit to patient or provider)
- Identify product efficacy and safety issues
- Contact other agencies using the product for additional information
- Define the objective of the evaluation
- Write trial criteria to be used during the evaluation
- Target appropriate areas in which to try a new product
- Conduct staff education needed to implement trial
- Complete trial evaluation forms
- Solicit input from other health care providers (e.g., biomedical engineers, pharmacists, physicians, other agencies), as needed
- Obtain patient evaluation of product, as appropriate
- Determine costs for new product implementation, including training, additional supplies, and maintenance agreements
- Determine whether a higher cost product achieves better patient outcomes
- Make recommendations to the appropriate committee or individual coordinating the evaluation
- Participate in ongoing monitoring of product use and effectiveness
- Report significant medical device adverse events to the FDA (Food and Drug Administration) as well as to the manufacturer

2nd edition 1996; revised 2018

Background Evidence:

Goodbody, J., & Gallo, M. (2010). Ensuring reusable equipment meets patients' needs and infection prevention guidelines. *Nursing Times, 106* (27), 15. 17.

Oman, K. S., Makic, M. B., Fink, R., Schraeder, N., Hulett, T., Keech, T., & Wald, H. (2012). Nurse-directed interventions to reduce catheter-associated urinary tract infections. *American Journal of Infection Control, 40*(6), 548–553.

Pyrek, K.M. (2012). Product evaluation and purchasing advice for perioperative nurses and infection preventionists. *Infection Control Today*. http://www.infectioncontroltoday.com/articles/2012/08/product-evaluation-and-purchasing-advice-for-perioperative-nurses-and-infection-preventionists.aspx

U.S. Food and Drug Administration. (2015). Medical device reporting (MDR). http://www.fda.gov/medicaldevices/safety/reportaproblem/default.htm

World Health Organization. (2010). *Increasing complexity of medical technology and consequences for training and outcome of care*. http://apps.who.int/medicinedocs/en/m/abstract/Js17699en/

Professional Development Facilitation   7770

Definition: Assisting with continuing education to enhance life-long learning

Activities:

- Encourage self-evaluation to include career interest, knowledge, and skills
- Assist in creating career plan with measurable goals, objectives, and actionable strategies
- Ensure plan includes balance of professional and personal life
- Identify opportunities to improve knowledge and skills (e.g., communication, technology)
- Prioritize continuing education opportunities to increase knowledge and skills
- Offer guidance in seeking advanced education (e.g., bachelor's, master's, doctorate)
- Encourage participation in professional organizations
- Encourage reading professional journals
- Recommend pursuing recognized specialty board certifications
- Encourage participation in quality improvement, safety, or decision-making teams
- Recommend participation in evidence-based practice initiatives
- Pursue organizational career advancement plans (e.g., clinical ladders), as appropriate

P

- Participate in peer review activities, as appropriate
- Collaborate with interdisciplinary team
- Recommend opportunities to advance role (e.g., charge RN, preceptor, leader)
- Encourage volunteer activities
- Assist in creating professional portfolio, curriculum vitae, or resume
- Provide guidance to conduct periodic review of goals, objectives, and strategies

8th edition 2024

Background Evidence:

Biedermann, N. (2022). Professional portfolio development: Personally, and professionally rewarding and satisfying. *Australian Nursing & Midwifery Journal, 27*(6), 41.

Bodine, J. L. (2021). Nursing professional development practitioners in leadership roles. *Journal for Nurses in Professional Development, 37*(6), 51–352. https://doi.org/10.1097/NND.0000000000000812

Brunt, B. A., & Bogdan, B. A. (2021). Nursing professional development leadership. In *StatPearls*. StatPearls Publishing. https://www.ncbi.nlm.nih.gov/books/NBK519064/

Harper, M. G., Maloney, P., & Shinners, J. (2017). Looking back and looking forward through the lens of the nursing professional development: Scope and standards of practice, 3rd edition. *Journal of Nursing Professional Development, 33*(6), 329–332.

Mlambo, M., Silén, C., & McGrath, C. (2021). Lifelong learning and nurses' continuing professional development: A metasynthesis of the literature. *BMC Nursing, 20*(1), 1–13. https://doi.org/10.1186/s12912-021-00579-2

Niesen, C. R., Kraft, S. J., & Meiers, S. J. (2018). Use of motivational interviewing by nurse leaders: Coaching for performance, development, and career goal setting. *The Health Care Manager, 37*(2), 183–192.

Smith, C. M., & Johnson, C. S. (2018). Preparing nurse leaders in nursing professional development: Developing a nursing professional development department plan. *Journal for Nurses in Professional Development, 34*(5), 283–285. https://doi.org/10.1097/NND.0000000000000460

Woolforde, L. (2018). Nursing professional development: Our spheres of expansion. *Journal of Nursing Professional Development, 4*(4), 237–238.

Program Development   8700

Definition: Planning, implementing, and evaluating a coordinated set of activities for a group or community

Activities:
- Identify significant health needs or problems
- Use available resources to determine need or priority (e.g., Community Health Needs Assessment tool)
- Convene task force to examine priority need or problem
- Educate stakeholders regarding process
- Identify alternative approaches to address need or problem
- Evaluate cost, resource needs, feasibility, and required activities
- Develop goals and objectives to address need or problem
- Describe methods, activities, and time frame for implementation
- Identify resources for and constraints on implementing program
- Gain acceptance for program by target group, providers, and related groups
- Hire personnel to implement and manage program, as appropriate
- Procure equipment and supplies, as appropriate
- Market program to intended stakeholders
- Facilitate adoption of program
- Monitor progress of program implementation
- Evaluate program for relevance, efficiency, and cost-effectiveness
- Modify and refine program

3rd edition 2000; revised 2024

Background Evidence:

Abbott, S., & Bryar, R. (2022). Nurse-led projects for people experiencing homelessness and other inclusion health groups: a realist evaluation. *British Journal of Community Nursing, 27*(1), 32–39. https://doi.org/10.12968/bjcn.2022.27.1.32

Chambers, R. S. (2021). Developing a peer support program to mitigate compassion fatigue in health care: A quality improvement project. *Nebraska Nurse, 54*(1), 4–5.

Moura, S., Nguyen, P., Benea, A., & Townsley, C. (2022). The development and implementation of the After Cancer Treatment Transition (ACTT) Program for survivors of cancer. *Canadian Oncology Nursing Journal, 32*(1), 3–21. https://doi.org/10.5737/23688076321311

Pirozzi, M., & Strigari, L. (2021). Project management for healthcare: The case of the translational research. *PM World Journal, 10*(4), 1–9.

Springer, M. L. (2019). *Project and program management: A competency-based approach* (4th ed.). Purdue University Press.

Progressive Muscle Relaxation   1460

Definition: Facilitating the tensing and releasing of successive muscle groups while attending to the resulting differences in sensation

Activities:
- Explain the purpose and process of the technique to the patient
- Instruct patient to wear comfortable, unrestricted clothing
- Screen for neck or back orthopedic injuries to which hyperextension of the upper spine would add discomfort and complications
- Screen for increased intracranial pressure, capillary fragility, bleeding tendencies, severe acute cardiac difficulties with hypertension, or other conditions in which tensing muscles might produce greater physiological injury and modify the technique, as appropriate
- Choose a quiet, comfortable setting
- Subdue the lighting
- Take precautions to prevent interruptions
- Ask patient to loosen any tight clothing
- Instruct the patient to sit in a reclining chair or lie down on a comfortable surface

P

- Instruct the patient to assume a passive attitude by focusing on achieving relaxation in specific body muscles and refrain from focusing on any other thoughts
- Instruct the patient to take a deep breath through the abdomen and hold for a few seconds and then exhale slowly
- Have the patient repeat the deep breathing several times, asking the patient to imagine the tension being released from the body with each exhale
- Have the patient tense systematically, for 5 to 10 seconds, each of 8 to 16 major muscle groups progressively from head to toe
- Instruct patient to focus on the sensations in the muscles when he/she is tense
- Instruct patient to focus on the sensations in the muscles when he/she is relaxed
- Begin by asking the patient to take a deep breath and tighten the muscles in the forehead by raising the eyebrows as high as possible for 5 to 10 seconds and then release the tension, focusing on the feeling of the muscles relaxing as he/she exhales
- Check periodically with the patient to ensure that the muscle group is relaxed
- Have the patient tense the muscle group again, if relaxation is not experienced
- Pause for 10 seconds before moving on to the next muscle group
- Monitor for indicators of nonrelaxation such as movement, uneasy breathing, talking, and coughing

- Instruct the patient to breathe deeply and to slowly let the breath and tension out
- Develop a personal relaxation "patter" that helps the patient to focus and feel comfortable
- Terminate the relaxation session gradually
- Allow time for the patient to express feelings concerning the intervention
- Encourage the patient to practice between regular sessions with the nurse

1st edition 1992; revised 1996, 2018

Background Evidence:

Anselmo, J. (2016). Relaxation. In B. M. Dossey & L. Keegan (Eds.), *Holistic nursing: A handbook for practice* (7th ed., pp. 239–268). Jones & Bartlett.

Freeman, L. (2009). Relaxation therapy. In *Mosby's complementary and alternative medicine: A research-based approach* (3rd ed., pp. 129–157). Mosby Elsevier.

Olpin, M., & Hesson, M. (2013). Progressive relaxation. In *Stress management for life: A research-based experiential approach* (3rd ed., pp. 294–303). Wadsworth.

Seaward, B. L. (2012). Progressive muscular relaxation. In *Managing stress: Principles and strategies for health and well-being* (7ed ed., pp. 477–486). Jones & Bartlett.

Prompted Voiding   0640

Definition: Promotion of urinary continence using timed verbal toileting reminders and positive social feedback for successful toileting

Activities:

- Determine ability to recognize urge to void
- Keep continence specification record for 3 days to establish voiding pattern and determine likelihood of success
- Establish interval of initial prompted voiding schedule based upon voiding pattern
- Establish beginning and ending time for prompted voiding schedule if not for 24 hours
- Approach within 15 minutes of prescribed prompted voiding intervals
- Allow time to self-initiate request for toileting assistance
- Determine awareness of continence status by asking if wet or dry
- Determine accuracy of response by physically checking clothing or linens, as appropriate
- Give positive feedback for accuracy of continence status response and success of maintaining continence between scheduled toileting times
- Use respectful communication in all requests for voiding
- Prompt for maximum of three times, to use toilet or substitute regardless of continence status
- Offer assistance with toileting regardless of continence status
- Provide privacy for toileting
- Give positive feedback by praising desired toileting behavior
- Refrain from commenting on incontinence or refusal to toilet

- Inform of time of next toileting session
- Instruct to consciously hold urine between toileting sessions, if not cognitively impaired
- Instruct to self-initiate requests to toilet in response to urge to void
- Document outcomes of toileting sessions in clinical record
- Discuss continence record with staff to provide reinforcement and encourage compliance with prompted voiding schedule on weekly basis and as needed
- Provide regular training for staff to ensure adequate comfort level with intervention

3rd edition 2000; revised 2024

Background Evidence:

Lai, C. K. Y., & Wan, X. J. (2017). Using prompted voiding to manage urinary incontinence in nursing homes: Can it be sustained? *Journal of the American Medical Directors Association, 18*(6), 509–514.

Newman, D. K. (2019). Evidence-based practice guideline: Prompted voiding for individuals with urinary incontinence. *Journal of Gerontological Nursing, 45*(2), 14–26. https://doi.org/10.3928/00989134-20190111-03

Rosenberg, K. (2017). Prompted voiding offers long-term benefits to nursing home residents. *AJN, American Journal of Nursing, 117*(11), 61. https://doi.org/10.1097/01.NAJ.0000526751.14668.e6

P

Pruritus Management 3550

Definition: Preventing and treating sensation to itch skin

Activities:

- Determine cause (e.g., dermatologic, systemic, medications, psychogenic)
- Perform full body physical examination to assist in identifying cause (e.g., location, onset, duration, rash, lesions, systemic symptoms)
- Consider laboratory and radiologic diagnostic testing, as indicated
- Treat or remove cause (e.g., insect infestation, infections, dry skin, allergic reaction) as indicated
- Provide comfort measures as indicated (e.g., cold applications, medications, emollients)
- Encourage use of complete emollient therapies (e.g., dermatological bath oils, soap substitutes, moisturizers), as indicated
- Instruct to avoid perfumed products (e.g., bubble baths, soaps, oils)
- Instruct to avoid bath soaps and shower gels that increase dry skin areas
- Apply dressings or splints to hand or elbow during sleep to limit uncontrollable scratching, as appropriate
- Apply medicated creams and lotions, as appropriate
- Administer anti-pruritics, as indicated
- Administer opiate antagonists, as indicated
- Apply antihistamine cream, as appropriate
- Apply cold to relieve irritation
- Consider complementary and alternative therapies for qualifying persons (e.g., acupressure, aromatherapy, acupuncture)
- Instruct to run humidifier in home
- Instruct not to wear tight-fitting clothing and wool or synthetic fabrics
- Instruct to keep fingernails trimmed short
- Instruct to minimize sweating by avoiding warm or hot environments
- Instruct to limit bathing to once or twice per week and no longer than 20 minutes in bath water, as appropriate
- Instruct to bathe in lukewarm water, pat skin dry, and avoid vigorous rubbing of skin to dry
- Instruct to apply emollients after bathing to seal in water absorbed from bath
- Encourage use of non-slip bathmat if oils and emollients used in bathing
- Instruct to use palm of hand to rub over wide area of skin or pinch skin gently between thumb and index finger to relieve itching
- Instruct persons with casts not to insert objects in cast to scratch skin
- Use teach-back to ensure understanding

3rd edition 2000; revised 2024

Background Evidence:

Bouya, S., Ahmadidarehsima, S., Badakhsh, M., Balouchi, A., & koochakzai, M. (2018). Effect of aromatherapy interventions on hemodialysis complications: A systematic review. *Complementary Therapies in Clinical Practice, 32*, 130–138. https://doi.org/10.1016/j.ctcp.2018.06.008

Campbell, P., Moss, J., Mulder, M., Roach, L., Wilson, N., Jacob, A., & Miles, H. (2020). The effectiveness of complementary and alternative medicine in the symptom management of pruritus in patients with end-stage kidney disease: A systematic review. *Renal Society of Australasia Journal, 16*(2), 58–68.

Golpanian, R., Gonzalez, J., & Yosipovitch, G. (2020). Practical approach for the diagnosis and treatment of chronic pruritus. *Journal for Nurse Practitioners, 16*, 590–596.

Pereira, M., & Ständer, S. (2017). Chronic pruritus: Current and emerging treatment options. *Drugs, 77*(9), 999–1007. https://doi.org/10.1007/s40265-017-0746-9

Ragazzo, J., Cesna, A., & Battistella, M. (2017). Uremic Pruritis. *Canadian Association of Nephrology Nurses and Technologists, 28*(1), 28–33.

Song, J., Xian, D., Yang, L., Xiong, X., Lai, R., & Zhong, J. (2018). Pruritus: Progress toward pathogenesis and treatment. *BioMed Research International, 2018*, 1–12. https://doi.org/10.1155/2018/9625936

P

Quality Monitoring   7800

Definition: Systematic collection and analysis of an organization's quality indicators

Activities:

- Identify patient care problems or opportunities to improve care
- Participate in selection and development of quality indicators appropriate to clinical setting and patient population
- Include structure, process, and outcome quality indicators
- Incorporate standards from appropriate professional groups
- Use preestablished criteria when collecting data
- Interview patients, families, and staff, as appropriate
- Promote and use electronic health records for collection, exchange, and analysis of data
- Review patient care record for documentation of care, as needed
- Conduct data analysis, as appropriate
- Compare results of data collected with preestablished norms
- Consult with nursing staff or other health professionals to develop action plans, as appropriate
- Negotiate solutions cognizant of local work loads
- Recommend changes in practice based on findings
- Report findings at staff meetings
- Review and revise standards, as appropriate

- Participate on evidence-based practice and quality improvement committees, as appropriate
- Provide orientation about quality improvement for new employees at the unit level
- Participate on intradisciplinary and interdisciplinary problem-solving teams

2nd edition 1996; revised 2018

Background Evidence:

Castle, N. G., & Ferguson, J. C. (2010). What is nursing home quality and how is it measured? *The Gerontologist, 50*(4), 426–442.

Cipriano, P. F. (2011). The future of nursing and health IT: The quality elixir. *Nursing Economic$, 29*(5), 282, 286–289.

Muller, A. C., Hujcs, M., Dubendorf, P., & Harrington, P. T. (2010). Sustaining excellence: Clinical nurse specialist practice and magnet designation. *Clinical Nurse Specialist, 24*(5), 252–259.

Stanhope, M., & Lancaster, J. (2014). *Public health nursing: Population-centered health care in the community* (8th ed.). Elsevier Mosby.

Quarantine Facilitation   6596

Definition: Providing care for persons needing to quarantine

Activities:

- Seek confirmation of need to quarantine
- Notify of need to quarantine based on recommendations from local, state, or national health institutions
- Provide detailed information about expected length of quarantine
- Educate to monitor for symptoms of communicable infectious disease to which they were exposed
- Provide rationale for necessity of quarantine
- Identify if resides alone or with others
- Provide recommendations to quarantine away from others living in home, as applicable
- Instruct on infection prevention practices
- Inform individual of quarantine restrictions specific to their communicable infectious disease (e.g., do not go to grocery store, do not interact with neighbors)
- Provide community resources, as available, to support individual while in quarantine
- Ensure access to basic human needs including food, water, household and medical supplies, and psychological support
- Promote physical activity based on overall health status, while in quarantine
- Evaluate nutritional, well-being, weight, and cardiovascular effects of quarantine if required for extended period of time
- Provide documentation to support job protection (e.g., Family and Medical Leave Act documentation)
- Instruct to continue current medication and health regimens, as appropriate
- Monitor for increased anxiety and depression

- Recommend appropriate interventions to promote mental and physical wellness during quarantine
- Provide written list of communication methods for contact with health care provider
- Offer telehealth appointments, as appropriate, for physical and mental health needs
- Use teach-back to ensure understanding
- Advocate for consistency in local, state, and national quarantine and isolation laws and policies

8th edition 2024

Background Evidence:

Ferreira, L. N., Pereira, L. N., da Fe Bras, M., & Ilchuk, K. (2021). Quality of life under the COVID-19 quarantine. *Quality of Life Research, 30*, 1389–1405. https://doi.org/10.1007/s11136-020-02724-x

Katz, R., Vaught, A., Formentos, A., & Capizola, J. (2018). Raising the yellow flag: State variation in quarantine laws. *Journal of Public Health Management and Practice, 24*(4), 380–384.

Kilic, R., Ataman Hatipoglu, C., & Gunes, C. (2020). Quarantine and its legal dimension. *Turkish Journal of Medical Sciences, 50*, 544–548. https://doi.org/10.3906/sag-2004-153

Mattioli, A. V., Puviani, M. B., Nasi, M., & Farinetti, A. (2020). COVID-19 pandemic: The effects of quarantine on cardiovascular risk. *European Journal of Clinical Nutrition, 74*, 852–855. https://doi.org/10.1038/s41430-020-0646-z

Sundwall, D. N. (2019). Quarantine in the 21st century: To be effective, public health policies must be inclusive. *American Journal of Public Health, 109*(9), 1184–1185. https://doi.org/10.2105/AJPH.2019.305224

Q

Radiation Therapy Management 6600

Definition: Assisting the patient to understand and minimize the side effects of radiation treatments

Activities:

- Monitor pretreatment workups for patients at risk for earlier onset, longer duration, and more distressing side effects
- Promote activities to modify the identified risk factors
- Monitor for side effects and toxic effects of treatment
- Provide information to patient and family regarding radiation effect on malignant cells
- Utilize recommended radiation precautions in the management of patients with cardiac pacemakers
- Monitor for alterations in skin integrity and treat appropriately
- Avoid use of adhesive tapes and other skin-irritating substances
- Provide special skin care to tissue folds that are prone to infection (e.g., buttocks, perineum, and groin)
- Avoid application of deodorants and aftershave lotions to treated areas
- Discuss the need for skin care, such as maintenance of dye markings, avoidance of soap, and other ointments, and protection during sunbathing or heat application
- Assist patient in planning for hair loss by teaching about available alternatives, such as wigs, scarves, hats, and turbans, as appropriate
- Teach patient to gently wash and comb hair and to sleep on a silk pillowcase to prevent further hair loss, as appropriate
- Reassure patient that hair will grow back after treatment is terminated, as appropriate
- Monitor for indications of infection of oral mucous membranes
- Encourage good oral hygiene with use of dental cleansing devices, such as unwaxed non-shredding floss, sonic toothbrushes, or water pics, as appropriate
- Initiate oral health restoration activities, such as use of artificial saliva, saliva stimulants, non–alcohol-based mouth sprays, sugarless mints, and fluoride treatments, as appropriate
- Teach patient on self-assessment of oral cavity, including signs and symptoms to report for further evaluation (e.g., burning, pain, and tenderness)
- Teach patient need for frequent dental follow-up care as dental caries can form rapidly
- Monitor for anorexia, nausea, vomiting, changes in taste, esophagitis, and diarrhea, as appropriate
- Promote adequate fluid and nutritional intake
- Promote therapeutic diet to prevent complications
- Discuss potential aspects of sexual dysfunction, as appropriate
- Teach implications of therapy on sexual function, including the time frame for contraceptive use, as appropriate
- Administer medications to control side effects (e.g., antiemetics for nausea and vomiting), as needed
- Monitor fatigue level by soliciting the patient's description of fatigue
- Teach patient and family techniques of energy management, as appropriate
- Assist patient in managing fatigue by planning frequent rest periods, spacing of activities, and limiting daily demands, as appropriate
- Encourage rest immediately after treatments
- Assist patient in achieving adequate comfort levels through the use of pain management techniques that are effective and acceptable to the patient
- Force fluids to maintain renal and bladder hydration, as appropriate
- Monitor for indications of urinary tract infection
- Teach patient and family about the effects of therapy on bone marrow functioning, as appropriate
- Instruct patient and family on ways to prevent infection, such as avoiding crowds, using good hygiene, and handwashing techniques, as appropriate
- Monitor for signs and symptoms of systemic infection, anemia, and bleeding
- Institute neutropenic and bleeding precautions, as indicated
- Facilitate patient's discussion of feelings about radiation therapy equipment, as appropriate
- Facilitate expression of fears about prognosis or success of treatments
- Provide concrete objective information related to the effects of therapy to reduce patient uncertainty, fear, and anxiety about treatment-related symptoms
- Instruct long-term survivors and their families of the possibility of second malignancies and the importance of reporting increased susceptibility to infection, fatigue, or bleeding
- Initiate and maintain protection according to agency protocol for patient receiving internal radiation treatment (e.g., gold seed placement or radiopharmaceutical agents)
- Explain protection protocols to patient, family, and visitors
- Offer diversional activities while patient is in radiation protection
- Limit visitor time in room, as appropriate
- Limit staff time in the room if patient is isolated for radiation precautions
- Distance oneself from the radiation sources while giving care (e.g., stand at the head of the bed of patient with uterine implants), as appropriate
- Shield oneself using a lead apron/shield while assisting with procedures involving radiation

1st edition 1992; revised 2008

Background Evidence:

Barsevick, A. M., Whitmer, K., Sweeney, C., & Nail, L. M. (2002). A pilot study examining energy conservation for cancer treatment-related fatigue. *Cancer Nursing, 25*(5), 333–341.

Brooks-Brunn, J. A. (2000). Esophageal cancer: An overview. *MEDSURG Nursing, 9*(5), 248–254.

Bruce, S. D. (2004). Radiation-induced xerostomia: How dry is your patient? *Clinical Journal of Oncology Nursing, 8*(1), 61–67.

Christman, N. J., & Cain, L. B. (2004). The effects of concrete objective information and relaxation on maintaining usual activity during radiation therapy. *Oncology Nursing Forum, 31*(2), E39–E45.

Colella, J., & Scrofine, S. (2004). High-dose brachytherapy for treating prostate cancer: Nursing considerations. *Urologic Nursing, 24*(1), 39–44, 52.

D'Haese, S., Bate, T., Claes, S., Boone, A., VanVoorden, V., & Efficace, F. (2005). Management of skin reactions during radiotherapy: A study of nursing practice. *European Journal of Cancer Care, 14*(1), 28–42.

Hogle, W. P. (2001). Pacing the standard of nursing practice in radiation oncology. *Clinical Journal of Oncology Nursing, 5*(6), 253–256, 267–268.

Itano, J. K., & Taoka, K. T. (Eds.). (2005). *Core curriculum for oncology nursing* (4th ed.). Elsevier Saunders.

R

Magnan, M. A., & Mood, D. W. (2003). The effects of health state, hemoglobin, global symptom distress, mood disturbance, and treatment site on fatigue onset, duration, and distress in patients receiving radiation therapy. *Oncology Nursing Forum, 30*(2), E33–E39.

Nail, L. M. (2002). Fatigue in patients with cancer. *Oncology Nursing Forum, 29*(3), 537–546.

Smith, M., Casey, L., Johnson, D., Gwede, C., & Riggin, O. Z. (2001). Music as a therapeutic intervention for anxiety in patients receiving radiation therapy. *Oncology Nursing Forum, 28*(5), 855–862.

Yarbro, C. H., Frogge, M. H., & Goodman, M. (2005). *Cancer nursing: Principles and practice* (6th ed.). Jones and Bartlett.

Rapid Sequence Induction and Intubation   3340

Definition: Coordination of prompt sedation and intubation while minimizing aspiration in life-threatening injuries or illnesses

Activities:

- Determine clinical indications for induction
- Verify identity
- Explain procedure and rationale if indicated
- Assemble appropriate equipment
- Determine landmarks on anatomy and absence of obstruction (e.g., foreign body, epiglottitis, edema) to facilitate endotracheal tube placement
- Preoxygenate with mask and bag for 3 minutes minimally
- Pre-medicate as indicated to mitigate physiological response of body to intubation (e.g., lidocaine, atropine, fentanyl)
- Give sedative (e.g., propofol, ketamine, etomidate) and paralytic (e.g., vecuronium, rocuronium, succinylcholine) at same time or quickly after induction
- Place in proper intubation position (e.g., towels under head, align ears with suprasternal notch) after sedation and paralysis
- Insert endotracheal tube and inflate cuff, no more than 1 minute after sedation and paralysis
- Mark level of insertion at teeth and secure tube
- Obtain confirmation of proper tube placement
- Document care, including tube type, medications used, and tolerance of procedure

8th edition 2024

Background Evidence:

Gooch, M. D., & Roberts, E. (2017). Changing the Emergency Department's practice of rapid sequence intubation to reduce the incidence of hypoxia. *Advanced Emergency Nursing Journal, 39*(4), 266–279. https://doi.org/10.1097/TME.0000000000000164

Macksey, L. F. (2018). *Nurse anesthesia pocket guide* (3rd ed.). Jones & Bartlett Learning.

Smith, T. L., & Van Meter, J. (2018). Maximizing success with rapid sequence intubations. *Advanced Emergency Nursing Journal, 40*(3), 183–193. https://doi.org/10.1097/TME.0000000000000204

Ureden, L. D., Stacy, K. M., & Lough, M. E. (2022). Pulmonary therapeutic management. In *Critical care nursing: Diagnosis and management* (pp. 502–503) (9th ed.). Elsevier.

Wahlen, B. M., El-Menyar, A., Asim, M., & Al-Thani, H. (2019). Rapid sequence induction (RSI) in trauma patients: Insights from healthcare providers. *World Journal of Emergency Medicine, 10*(1), 19–26. https://doi.org/10.5847/wjem.j.1920-8642.2019.01.003

Readmission Prevention   7470

Definition: Reducing repeated admissions to acute care institutions for high-risk persons

Activities:

- Identify persons at high risk for readmission based on condition, previous hospitalizations, emergency department visits, and social determinants of health (e.g., LACE criteria [**L**ength of stay during index admission, **A**cute [emergent admissions], **C**harlson comorbidity index, **E**D visits])
- Initiate ongoing flexible plan for discharge throughout care continuum
- Determine home resources including family or caregiver availability, as early as possible
- Encourage early involvement in all interactions related to home care and discharge needs
- Elicit goals for discharge
- Ensure that primary provider discharge goals and person goals coincide
- Focus discharge planning efforts at multiple points during the pre-discharge and post-discharge periods, assuring ongoing family or caregiver involvement
- Evaluate readiness for discharge as ongoing process
- Develop discharge plan that considers health literacy, health care, social, cultural, and financial needs
- Assist in planning for supportive environment necessary to provide posthospital care
- Provide description of possible signs and symptoms of condition post-discharge including helpful interventions
- Review what to do if problem arises at home
- Determine degree of understanding of overall discharge plan, including medications, dietary orders, treatments, and outpatient care, as indicated
- Instruct on specific areas needed to prevent readmission (e.g., medication adherence and management, dietary needs, monitoring and reporting symptoms, staying physically active)
- Provide medication calendar that lists brand and generic medication names and when and how to take medication
- Encourage to bring medication calendar during provider follow-up

R

- Elicit beliefs as to what constitutes an emergency
- Instruct on what to do in cases of emergency (i.e., when to dial 911 versus call private health care provider)
- Review any areas of poor understanding during instructions
- Provide written copies of all information in preferred language
- Provide appropriate contact numbers or provider or institution contact information with discharge instructions
- Develop action plan to know when need to alert provider about decline in health
- Report to provider any areas of concern for discharge teaching or planning, prior to discharge
- Place discharge instructions in electronic portal for easy access, if appropriate
- Ensure appropriate discharge care setting for at-risk persons
- Involve appropriate health care team for select high-risk persons (i.e., pharmacy for persons with greater than 15 medications, social services for homeless persons)
- Consider post-discharge visits for medication reconciliation and adherence check for at-risk persons (e.g., heart failure with high LACE scores)
- Enroll qualifying persons in 30-day readmission prevention program or transitional care program
- Ensure ongoing adequate information flow with primary care providers and interdisciplinary care team
- Ensure designated discharge advocate to coordinate with interdisciplinary team and at-risk person, if indicated
- Compile comprehensive and accurate discharge summary
- Expedite transmission of discharge summary to clinicians accepting care of person
- Plan for follow-up results from lab tests or labs pending at discharge
- Organize post-discharge outpatient services and health care equipment
- Advocate for home health assistance or health coaching for persons with areas of concern
- Provide telephone reinforcement of discharge plan within 48 hours of discharge
- Provide positive feedback via telephone during contacts to reinforce confidence and ability
- Coordinate with home health agencies to increase discharge information, follow-up, or after-hospital care, as indicated
- Consider home monitoring techniques for at-risk, qualifying persons (e.g., telemanagement, wireless sensors, video visits, audio and auscultation monitoring)
- Determine need for palliative care or hospice referral, if indicated
- Use teach-back to ensure understanding
- Document readmission prevention plan and updates, per institutional policy

8th edition 2024

Background Evidence:

Agency for Healthcare Research and Quality. (2017). *Preventing avoidable readmissions: Improving the hospital discharge process.* https://www.ahrq.gov/professionals/quality-patient-safety/patient-safety-resources/resources/impptdis/index.html

Bell, J. F., Whitney, R. L., Reed, S. C., Poghosyan, H., Lash, R. S., Kim, K. K., Davis, A., Bold, R. J., & Joseph, J. G. (2017). Systematic review of hospital readmissions among patients with cancer in the United States. *Oncology Nursing Forum, 44*(2), 176–191.

Bradley, D. M. (2019). A day in the life of a readmission prevention nurse. *Home Healthcare Now, 37*(4), 236.

Lodhi, M. K., Ansari, R., Yao, Y., Keenan, G. M., Wilkie, D., & Khokhar, A. A. (2017). Predicting hospital re-admissions from nursing care data of hospitalized patients. *Advances in Data Mining: Applications and Theoretical Aspects, 10357*, 181–193.

Ingles, A. (2020). Heart failure nurse navigator program interventions based on LACE scores reduce inpatient heart failure readmission rates. *Heart & Lung, 49*(2), 219.

Mafouz, E. M. (2019). Prevention of early readmission after acute decompensated heart failure. *International Journal of Cardiology, 255*, 202–203.

Savoy, M., Davis, J., & Bittner-Fagan, H. (2017). Improving patient safety: Prevention of hospital readmission. *Family Practice Essentials, 463*, 21–26.

Teh, R., & Janus, E. (2018). Identifying and targeting patients with predicted 30-day hospital readmissions using the revised LACE index score and early post-discharge intervention. *International Journal of Evidence-Based Healthcare, 16*(3), 174–181.

Reality Orientation 4820

R

Definition: Promotion of patient's awareness of personal identity, time, and environment

Activities:

- Address patient by name when initiating interaction
- Approach patient slowly and from the front
- Use a calm and unhurried approach when interacting with the patient
- Use a consistent approach (e.g., kind firmness, active friendliness, passive friendliness, matter-of-fact, and no demands) that reflects the particular needs and capabilities of the patient
- Speak in a distinct manner with an appropriate pace, volume, and tone
- Ask questions one at a time
- Avoid frustrating the patient by demands that exceed capacity (e.g., repeated orientation questions that cannot be answered, abstract thinking when patient can think only in concrete terms, activities that cannot be performed, decision making beyond preference or capacity)
- Inform patient of person, place, and time, as needed
- Present reality in manner that preserves the patient's dignity (e.g., provides an alternate explanation, avoids arguing, and avoids attempts to convince the patient)
- Repeat patient's last expressed thought, as appropriate
- Interrupt confabulation by changing the subject or responding to the feeling or theme rather than the content of the verbalization
- Give one simple direction at a time
- Use gestures and objects to increase comprehension of verbal communications
- Engage patient in concrete "here and now" activities (e.g., ADLs) that focus on something outside self that is concrete and reality oriented
- Provide physical prompting and posturing (e.g., moving patient's hand through necessary motions to brush teeth), as necessary for task completion

- Encourage use of aids that increase sensory input (e.g., eyeglasses, hearing aids, and dentures)
- Recommend patient wear personal clothing and assist, as needed
- Provide objects that symbolize gender identity (e.g., purse or cap), as appropriate
- Use picture cues to promote appropriate use of items
- Avoid unfamiliar situations, when possible
- Prepare patient for upcoming changes in usual routine and environment before their occurrence
- Provide for adequate rest and sleep, including short-term, daytime naps, as needed
- Provide caregivers who are familiar to the patient
- Encourage family to participate in care based on abilities, needs, and preferences
- Provide a consistent physical environment and daily routine
- Provide access to familiar objects, when possible
- Label items in environment to promote recognition
- Modulate human and environmental sensory stimuli (e.g., visiting sessions, sights, sounds, lighting, smells, and tactile stimulation) based on patient's needs
- Use environmental cues (e.g., signs, pictures, clocks, calendars, and color coding of environment) to stimulate memory, reorient, and promote appropriate behavior
- Remove stimuli (e.g., pictures on the wall and television) that create misperception in a particular patient, when possible.
- Provide access to current news events (e.g., television, newspapers, radio, and verbal reports), when appropriate
- Involve patient in a reality orientation group setting/class when appropriate and available
- Provide psychoeducation to family and significant others regarding promotion of reality orientation

- Monitor for changes in orientation, cognitive and behavioral functioning, and quality of life

1st edition 1992; revised 2008

Background Evidence:

Bates, J., Boote, J., & Beverley, C. (2004). Psychosocial interventions for people with a milder dementing illness: A systematic review. *Journal of Advanced Nursing, 45*(6), 644–658.

Cacchione, P. Z., Culp, K., Laing, J., & Tripp-Reimer, T. (2003). Clinical profile of acute confusion in the long-term care setting. *Clinical Nursing Research, 12*(2), 145–158.

Foreman, M. D., Mion, L. C., Trygstad, L., & Fletcher, K. (2003). Delirium: Strategies for assessing and treating. In M. Mezey, T. Fulmer, I. Abraham, & D. Zwicker (Eds.), *Geriatric nursing protocols for best practice* (2nd ed., pp. 116–140). Springer.

Hewitt, J. (2002). Psycho-affective disorder in intensive care units: A review. *Journal of Clinical Nursing, 11*(5), 575–584.

Minardi, H., & Hayes, N. (2003). Nursing older adults with mental health problems: Therapeutic interventions—part 2. *Nursing Older People, 15*(7), 20–24.

Onder, G., Zanetti, O., Giacobini, E., Frisoni, G. B., Bartorelli, L., Carbone, G., Lambertucci, P., Silveri, M. C., & Bernabei, R. (2005). Reality orientation therapy combined with cholinesterase inhibitors in Alzheimer's disease: Randomised control trial. *The British Journal of Psychiatry, 187*(5), 450–455.

Thomas, H., Feyz, M., LeBlanc, J., Brosseau, J., Champoux, M.-C., Christopher, A., Desrmeaux, N., Dorais, L., & Lin, H. (2003). North Star project: Reality orientation in an acute care setting for patients with traumatic brain injuries. *Journal of Head Trauma Rehabilitation, 18*(3), 292–302.

Videbeck, S. L. (2006). *Psychiatric mental health nursing* (3rd ed.). Lippincott Williams & Wilkins.

Recreation Therapy 5360

Definition: Purposeful use of recreational activities to enhance independent function and social skills as well as reduce or eliminate the effects of illness or disability

Activities:

- Identify any deficits that may limit participation in recreational activities (e.g., mobility, cognitive, economic)
- Assist patient to identify meaningful recreational activities (e.g., sports, drama, games, arts and crafts)
- Assist to explore the personal meaning of favorite recreational activities
- Include patient in the planning of recreational activities
- Assist patient to choose recreational activities consistent with physical, psychological, and social capabilities
- Assist in obtaining resources required for the recreational activity
- Provide safe recreational equipment
- Observe safety precautions
- Supervise recreational sessions, as appropriate
- Monitor patient's physical and mental capacities while participating in recreational activities
- Provide new recreational activities that are age and ability appropriate
- Provide recreational activities aimed at reducing anxiety (e.g., cards or puzzles)
- Assist in obtaining transportation to recreational activities
- Provide positive reinforcement for participation in activities

- Monitor emotional, physical, and social response to recreational activity

1st edition 1992; revised 1996, 2018

Background Evidence:

Bauer, C., Victorson, D., Rosenbloom, S., Borocas, J., & Silver, R. (2010). Alleviating distress during antepartum hospitalization: A randomized controlled trial of music and recreation therapy. *Journal of Women's Health, 19*(3), 523–531.

Caldwell, L. (2005). Leisure and health: Why is leisure therapeutic? *British Journal of Guidance & Counselling, 33*(1), 7–26.

Pressman, S. D., Matthews, K. A., Cohen, S., Martire, L. M., Scheier, M., Baum, A., & Schulz, R. (2009). Association of enjoyable leisure activities with psychological and physical well-being. *Psychosomatic Medicine, 71*(7), 725–732.

Yang, H., & An, D. (2011). Health people 2020: Implications for recreation therapy. *American Journal of Recreation Therapy, 10*(4), 17–23.

Zanca, J. M., & Dijkers, M. P. (2014). Describing what we do: A qualitative study of clinicians' perspectives on classifying rehabilitation interventions. *Archives of Physical Medicine and Rehabilitation, 95*(Suppl. 1), S55–S65.e2.

R

Rectal Prolapse Management 0490

Definition: Prevention and/or manual reduction of rectal prolapse

Activities:

- Identify patients with history of rectal prolapse
- Encourage avoidance of straining at stool, lifting, and excessive standing
- Instruct patient to regulate bowel function through diet, exercise, and medication, as appropriate
- Assist patient to identify specific activities that have triggered rectal prolapse episodes in the past
- Monitor for bowel incontinence
- Monitor status of rectal prolapse
- Position patient on left side with knees raised toward chest when rectum is prolapsed
- Place a warm water or saline soaked cloth over the protruding bowel to protect it from drying
- Encourage patient to remain in side-lying position to facilitate return of bowel into rectum naturally
- Manually reduce rectal prolapse with lubricated, gloved hand, gently applying pressure to prolapse until it returns to a normal position, as necessary
- Check rectal area 10 minutes after manual reduction to ensure that prolapse is in correct position
- Identify frequency of occurrence of rectal prolapse
- Notify physician of change in frequency of occurrence or inability to manually reduce prolapse, as appropriate
- Assist in preoperative workup, as appropriate, helping to explain the tests and reduce anxiety for the patient who will undergo surgical repair

2nd edition 1996; revised 2018

Background Evidence:

Fox, A., Tietze, P. H., & Ramakrishnan, K. (2014). Anorectal conditions: Rectal prolapse. *Family Physicians Essentials, 419*, 28–34.

Fry, R., Mahmoud, N., Maron, D., & Bleir, J. (2012). Colon and rectum. In C. Jr. Townsend, R. Beauchamp, B. Evers, & K. Mattox (Eds.), *Sabiston textbook of surgery: The biological basis of modern surgical practice* (19th ed., pp. 1294–1380). Elsevier Saunders.

Lembo, A., & Ullman, S. (2010). Constipation. In M. Feldman, L. Friedman, & L. Brandt (Eds.), *Sleisinger & Fordtran's gastrointestinal and liver disease: Pathophysiology/diagnosis/management* (9th ed, pp. 259–284). Saunders Elsevier.

Varma, M., Rafferty, J., & Buie, W. (2011). Practice parameters for the management of rectal prolapse. *Diseases of the Colon & Rectum, 54*(11), 1339–1346.

Referral 8100

Definition: Arrangement for services by another care provider or agency

Activities:

- Perform ongoing monitoring to determine the need for referral
- Identify preference for referral agency
- Identify health care providers' recommendation for referral, as needed
- Identify care required
- Determine whether appropriate supportive care is available in the home or community
- Determine whether rehabilitation services are available for use in the home
- Evaluate strengths and weaknesses of family and significant others for responsibility of care
- Evaluate accessibility of environmental needs for the patient in the home or community
- Determine appropriate equipment for use after discharge, as necessary
- Determine patient's financial resources for payment to another provider
- Arrange for appropriate home care services, as needed
- Inform patient of appropriate Internet sites for use after discharge
- Encourage an assessment visit by receiving agency or other care provider, as appropriate
- Contact appropriate agency or health care provider
- Minimize time between discharge and appointment with next provider
- Complete appropriate written referral
- Send written referral and patient's plan of care electronically, as appropriate
- Provide patient or family member with a copy of the referral information, as appropriate
- Arrange mode of transportation
- Discuss patient's plan of care with next health care provider

1st edition 1992; revised 2013

Background Evidence:

Berta, W., Barnsley, J., Bloom, J., Cockerill, R., Davis, D., Jaakkimainen, L., Mior, A., Talbot, Y., & Vayda, E. (2008). Enhancing continuity of information: Essential components of a referral document. *Canadian Family Physician, 54*(10), 1432–1433.

Cummings, E., Showell, C., Roehrer, E., Churchill, B., Turner, B., Yee, K. C., Wong, M. C., & Turner, P. (2010). *A structured evidence-based literature review on discharge, referral and admission. University of Tasmania.* Australia: ehealth Services Research Group.

Edwards, N., Davies, B., Ploeg, J., Virani, T., & Skelly, J. (2007). Implementing nursing best practice guidelines: Impact on patient referrals. *Online BMC Nursing, 6*(4). https://doi.org/10.1186/1472-6955-6-4

Heimly, V. (2009). Electronic referrals in healthcare: A review. In K. Adlassnig, B. Blobel, J. Mantas, & I. Masic (Eds.), *Medical informatics in a united and healthy Europe: Proceedings of MIE 2009* (pp. 321–331). Amsterdam, Netherlands: IOS Press.

Kim, Y., Chen, A. H., Keith, E., Yee, H. F., Jr., & Kushel, M. B. (2009). Not perfect, but better: Primary care providers' experiences with electronic referrals in a safety net health system. *Journal of General Internal Medicine, 24*(5), 614–619.

R

Reiki   1520

Definition: Using a specific sequence of hand positions and symbols to channel the universal life force for recharging, realigning, and rebalancing the human energy field

Activities:

- Create a calm and comfortable environment
- Use aroma or gentle music to create a healing atmosphere
- Wash your hands
- Ask about the chief complaints, such as the presence of pain in certain areas or the presence of a particular illness
- Have the Reiki receiver sit comfortably or lay down on a massage table, fully clothed, in a supine position
- Limit any unnecessary distractions
- Relax your mind and take a few deep breaths to focus yourself
- Remember: the Reiki does the work, not the practitioner
- Begin by sending Reiki from about 3 feet away as a gentle way of beginning the session, if possible
- Follow a specific series of hand placements: over eyes, over ears, one hand on forehead and one hand on top of head, hands under head, over the neck, upper chest, upper abdomen, lower abdomen, thighs (one at a time), knees (one at a time), lower legs, ankles, feet, bottoms of feet, have client roll over on to stomach, shoulders, waist area, lower back, backs of legs, and front of legs
- Draw or visualize Reiki symbols (e.g., power, mental or emotional, distance) as guided by your intuition
- Allow your intuition to guide your movements by placing hands on (or a few inches over) the part of the body that most requires healing
- Stay in each area for 5 to 15 minutes or until you feel the energy flow more slowly or your intuition informs you it is time to move hand position
- Ask for specific permission during the session to work on sexual organs or parts of the body that would be considered inappropriate, if so guided
- Move one hand at a time so that you maintain contact as much as possible
- Note whether the patient has experienced a relaxation response and any related changes

6th edition 2013

Background Evidence:

Lee, M. S., Pittler, M. H., & Ernst, E. (2008). Effects of Reiki in clinical practice: A systematic review of randomised clinical trials. *International Journal of Clinical Practice, 62*(6), 947–954.

Lubeck, W., Petter, F. A., & Rand, W. L. (2001). *The spirit of Reiki: The complete handbook of the Reiki system*. Twin Lakes, WI: Lotus Press.

Miles, P., & True, G. (2003). Reiki—Review of a biofield therapy history, theory, practice, and research. *Alternative Therapies in Health and Medicine, 9*(2), 62–72.

Ring, M. E. (2009). Reiki and changes in pattern manifestations. *Nursing Science Quarterly, 22*(3), 250–258.

Shore, A. G. (2004). Long-term effects of energetic healing on symptoms of psychological depression and self-perceived stress. *Alternative Therapies in Health and Medicine, 10*(3), 42–48.

Vitale, A. (2007). An integrative review of Reiki touch therapy research. *Holistic Nursing Practice, 21*(4), 167–179.

Wardell, D. W., & Engebretson, J. (2001). Biological correlates of Reiki touch healing. *Journal of Advanced Nursing, 33*(4), 439–445.

Relapse Prevention   5235

Definition: Reduce risk of recurrence of behaviors, signs, and symptoms of a mental health condition during the maintenance, stabilization, or recovery period

Activities:

- Identify nature and severity of signs and symptoms, as needed
- Determine current level of knowledge of treatment, illness, self-care, and resources available
- Establish physical, mental, and cognitive capacity to carry out recovery process independently
- Determine willingness to participate in treatment plan
- Explore past lapses or relapse episodes and relapse dreams or fantasies, as needed
- Explore perception, awareness and attitudes toward illness, and attitudes and motivation toward changing health
- Identify ethnic and cultural background, and community support, social environment, accommodation, religion, spiritual beliefs, and lifestyle factors
- Explore personal protectors (e.g., coping mechanisms, self-efficacy in high-risk situations), and environmental protectors and potentiators, as needed
- Explore personal vulnerability factors, high-risk behaviors, and cognitive factors (e.g., negative thinking, self-destructive patterns, rationalization, denial, desire for immediate gratification)
- Identify situations, stressors, and crisis events (e.g., developmental, situational, adventitious) that may lead to relapse
- Determine unrealistic expectancies in high-risk situations (i.e., expects substance use to help cope with negative emotions)
- Explore warning signs for relapse as needed
- Explain relapse process, as needed
- Examine extent of social network, readiness, and actual capabilities to participate in symptom recognition plan and any characteristic of network (e.g., level of expressed emotion)
- Establish relapse prevention plan with person, family, and social network (e.g., information, early detection, collaboration, agreements, actions, monitoring, realistic objectives for short, medium and long term), as needed
- Use specific intervention strategies to enhance coping with high-risk situations (e.g., enhance self-efficacy, relapse management, cognitive restructuring)
- Consider recommending participation in evidence-based self-management program with service users
- Focus specific interventions on enhancing cognitive, emotional, and behavioral self-awareness

R

- Promote participation in disease prevention, health promotion, treatment, and rehabilitation programs, as appropriate
- Perform psychoeducation to persons, families, or social network (e.g., course of disease, early signs of relapse, comorbidities, treatment, sleep, coping skills, managing relationships), as needed
- Administer medication, as appropriate
- Use interdisciplinary approach, promoting coordination between different levels of care
- Offer crisis resolution and home-treatment teams as first-line service if severity of episode or level of risk to self or others exceeds capacity of services or other community teams
- Provide home care and monitoring, as needed
- Maintain contact and follow-up, as needed
- Avoid blaming or using value judgments
- Facilitate hope for the future, as needed
- Perform family intervention, as needed
- Encourage manifestation of feelings, perceptions, and fears, as needed
- Facilitate expression of difficulties for adherence to treatment and therapeutic plan, as needed
- Encourage to assume responsibility for ADLs and self-care
- Encourage healthy lifestyle (e.g., practice of physical exercise adapted to condition, healthy diet, participation in leisure activities, sleep hygiene), as needed
- Promote treatment concordance, as needed.
- Discuss effects of alcohol, tobacco, prescription and non-prescription drugs, and illicit drugs and their possible interference with treatment
- Promote sustained abstinence from substance use over time
- Discuss any non-prescribed therapies including complementary therapies (e.g., safety and efficacy of therapies, possible interference with therapeutic effects of prescribed medication, psychological interventions)
- Promote use of adequate coping strategies in high-risk situations (i.e., behavioral strategy such as leaving the situation; cognitive strategy such as positive self-talk or self-reassurance), as appropriate
- Provide communication and problem-solving skills training, as needed

- Instruct to recognize and monitor warning signals (e.g., stress, lack of lifestyle balance, strong positive expectancies)
- Instruct family and social network regarding monitoring of early warning signals, as needed
- Instruct and encourage in techniques for anxiety and stress management (e.g., mindfulness-based techniques, relaxation techniques, stimulus control techniques), as needed
- Instruct and encourage in motivational techniques, as needed
- Assist to identify and use strengths and abilities
- Link with community resources, as needed
- Link with self-care or support groups, as needed
- Monitor vital signs, as needed
- Monitor serum, urine, and expired air levels, as needed
- Perform pharmacological monitoring, as needed
- Monitor occasional lapses that may precipitate relapse, as needed
- Monitor regularly for signs and symptoms of relapse (e.g., intensifying behaviors, medications modified or discontinued), especially when early warning signs are already present
- Use teach-back to ensure understanding

8th edition 2024

Background Evidence:

Johansen, K. K., Hounsgaard, L., Frandsen, T. F., Fluttert, F. A. J., & Hansen, J. P. (2021). Relapse prevention in ambulant mental health care tailored to patients with schizophrenia or bipolar disorder. *Journal of Psychiatric and Mental Health Nursing, 28*(4), 549–577. https://doi.org/10.1111/jpm.12716

Menon, J., & Kandasamy, A. (2018). Relapse prevention. *Indian Journal of Psychiatry, 60*(Suppl 4), S473–S478. https://doi.org/10.4103/psychiatry.IndianJPsychiatry_36_18

Moriarty, A. S., Coventry, P. A., Hudson, J. L., Cook, N., Fenton, O. J., Bower, P., Lovell, K., Archer, J., Clarke, R., Richards, D. A., Dickens, C., Gask, L., Waheed, W., Huijbregts, K. M., van der Feltz–Cornelis, C., Ali, S., Gilbody, S., & McMillan, D. (2020). The role of relapse prevention for depression in collaborative care: A systematic review. *Journal of Affective Disorders, 265*, 618–644. https://doi.org/10.1016/j.jad.2019.11.105

Sharpe, L., Jones, E., Ashton-James, C. E., Nicholas, M. K., & Refshauge, K. (2020). Needed components of psychological treatment in pain management programs: A Delphi study. *European Journal of Pain, 24*(6), 1160–1168. https://doi.org/10.1002/ejp.1561

Relaxation Therapy 6040

Definition: Use of techniques to encourage and elicit relaxation for the purpose of decreasing undesirable signs and symptoms such as pain, muscle tension, or anxiety

Activities:

- Describe the rationale for relaxation and the benefits, limits, and types of relaxation available (e.g., music, meditation, rhythmic breathing, jaw relaxation, and progressive muscle relaxation)
- Screen for current decreased energy level, inability to concentrate, or other concurrent symptoms that may interfere with cognitive ability to focus on relaxation technique
- Determine whether any relaxation intervention in the past has been useful
- Consider the individual's willingness to participate, ability to participate, preference, past experiences, and contraindications, before selecting a specific relaxation strategy
- Provide detailed description of chosen relaxation intervention

- Create a quiet, non-disrupting environment with dim lights and comfortable temperature, when possible
- Suggest that the individual assume a comfortable position with unrestricted clothing and eyes closed
- Individualize the content of the relaxation intervention (e.g., by asking for suggestions of changes)
- Elicit behaviors that are conditioned to produce relaxation, such as deep breathing, yawning, abdominal breathing, or peaceful imaging
- Invite the patient to relax and let the sensations happen
- Use soft tone of voice with a slow, rhythmical pace of words
- Demonstrate and practice the relaxation technique with the patient

- Encourage return demonstrations of techniques, if possible
- Anticipate the need for the use of relaxation
- Provide written information about preparing and engaging in relaxation techniques
- Encourage frequent repetition or practice of technique(s) selected
- Provide undisturbed time because patient may fall asleep
- Encourage control of when the relaxation technique is performed
- Regularly evaluate individual's report of relaxation achieved, and periodically monitor muscle tension, heart rate, blood pressure, and skin temperature, as appropriate
- Develop a tape of the relaxation technique for the individual to use, as appropriate
- Use relaxation as an adjuvant strategy with pain medication or in conjunction with other measures, as appropriate
- Evaluate and document the response to relaxation therapy

Background Evidence:

Benson, H., & Klipper, M. Z. (2000). *The relaxation response.* HarperTorch.

Herr, K. A., & Mobily, P. R. (1999). Pain management. In G. M. Bulechek & J. C. McCloskey (Eds.), *Nursing interventions: Effective nursing treatments* (3rd ed., pp. 149–171). W. B. Saunders.

Mandle, C. L., Jacobs, S. C., Arcari, P. M., & Domar, A. D. (1996). The efficacy of relaxation response interventions with adult patients: A review of the literature. *Journal of Cardiovascular Nursing, 10*(3), 4–26.

McCaffery, M., & Pasero, C. (1999). Practical nondrug approaches to pain. In M. McCaffery & C. Pasero (Eds.), *Pain: Clinical manual* (2nd ed., pp. 399–427). Mosby.

Snyder, M. (1998). Progressive muscle relaxation. In M. Snyder & R. Lindquist (Eds.), *Complementary/alternative therapies in nursing* (3rd ed., pp. 1–13). Springer.

1st edition 1992; revised 2008

Religious Addiction Therapy   5422

Definition: Promoting healthy religious lifestyle

Activities:

- Identify excessive dependence upon religious leaders and practice
- Recognize cultural and background influences on religious dependence
- Seek guidance from those knowledgeable of culture or religious background
- Examine religious practices in terms of balanced relationships and beliefs
- Encourage behaviors that contribute to growth and faith development, consistent with culture or belief system
- Explore various elements of religious addiction
- Explore freedom for beneficial religious formations
- Instruct on methods to defend from religious or other addictive processes
- Offer to pray for healthy, life-giving relationships with self, God or Higher Power, and others, as appropriate
- Explore process of ongoing faith development with individual
- Educate about dangers of using religion to control other persons
- Promote formation of self-help groups or support groups that are relevant to individual, to develop religious balance
- Identify and share resources of groups and professional counseling services within community
- Use teach-back to ensure understanding

Background Evidence:

American Psychiatric Nurses Association. (2014*). Psychiatric-mental health Nursing: Scope and Standards of Practice.* (2nd ed.).

Holtzhausen, L. (2017). Addiction – a brain disorder or a spiritual disorder. *Mental Health and Addiction Research, 2*(1). https://doi.org/10.15761/MHAR.1000128

Jones, C. L. C. (2020). Spiritual well-being in older adults: A Concept Analysis. *Journal of Christian Nursing, 37*(4), E31–E38. https://doi.org/10.1097/CNJ.0000000000000770

Keltner, N. L., & Steele, D. (2019). *Psychiatric nursing* (8th ed.). Elsevier.

Rebar, C. R., Gersch, C., & Heimgartner, N. M. (2020). *Psychiatric nursing made incredibly easy.* Wolters Kluwer.

Rousselet, M., Duretete, O., Hardouin, J. B., & Grall-Bronnec, M. (2017). Cult membership: What factors contribute to joining or leaving? *Psychiatry Research, 257,* 27–33. https://doi.org/10.1016/j.psychres.2017.07.018

Timmins, F., & Caldeira, S. (2017). Understanding spirituality and spiritual care in nursing. *Nursing Standard, 31*(22), 50–57.

Varcarolis, E. M., & Fosbre, C. D. (2021). *Essentials of psychiatric-mental health nursing* (4th ed.). Elsevier.

Weinandy, J. T. G., & Grubbs, J. B. (2021). Religious and spiritual beliefs and attitudes towards addiction and addiction treatment: A scoping review. *Addictive Behaviors Reports, 14,* 100393. https://doi.org/10.1016/j.abrep.2021.100393

R

3rd edition 2000, revised 2024

Religious Ritual Enhancement   5424

Definition: Facilitating participation in preferred religious practices

Activities:

- Treat individual with dignity and respect
- Provide opportunities for discussion of various belief systems
- Encourage discussion about religious concerns
- Encourage participation in religious rituals or practices that are not detrimental to health or safety
- Identify desires regarding religious expression (e.g., lighting candles, fasting, circumcision ceremonies, food practices)
- Provide access to pastoral care or religious advisor of choice
- Offer quiet or sacred space for person and visitors when possible
- Provide access to relevant items of religious participation (e.g., Bible, Quran, prayer rug, rosary, chador, veil, kippah, prayer shawl)

- Demonstrate respect when religious items are displayed or given
- Encourage ritual planning, participation, and attendance, as appropriate
- Coordinate or provide transportation to worship site, when practical
- Provide video or audio access to religious services, as available
- Coordinate or provide healing services, communion, meditation, or prayer in place of residence or other setting
- Explore alternatives for worship
- Encourage to reflect on significant past spiritual experiences
- Develop sense of timing for prayer or ritual to avoid interruptions
- Assist with making desired changes

3rd edition 2000; revised 2004, 2024

Background Evidence:

American Psychiatric Nurses Association. (2014*). Psychiatric-mental health Nursing: Scope and Standards of Practice.* (2nd ed.).

Ayyari, T., Salehabadi, R., Rastaghi, S., & Rad, M. (2020). Effects of spiritual interventions on happiness level of the female elderly residing in nursing home. *Journal of Evidence-based Care, 10*(1), 36–43.

Jones, C. L. C. (2020). Spiritual well-being in older adults: A concept analysis. *Journal of Christian Nursing, 37*(4), E31–E38. https://doi.org/10.1097/CNJ.0000000000000770

Keltner, N. L., & Steele, D. (2019). *Psychiatric nursing* (8th ed.). Elsevier.

Lopes de Souza, P. T., de Araújo Ferreira, J., Cassia Silva de Oliveira, E., Alves de Lima, N. B., da Rocha Cabral, J., & de Oliveira, R. C. (2019). Basic human needs in intensive care. *Revista de Pesquisa: Cuidado e Fundamental, 11*(4), 1011–1016. https://doi.org/10.9789/2175-5361.2019.v11i4.1011-1016

Rebar, C. R., Gersch, C., & Heimgartner, N. M. (2020). *Psychiatric nursing made incredibly easy* (rd ed.). Wolters Kluwer.

Timmins, F., & Caldeira, S. (2017). Understanding spirituality and spiritual care in nursing. *Nursing Standard, 31*(22), 50–57.

Varcarolis, E. M., & Fosbre, C. D. (2021). *Essentials of psychiatric-mental health nursing* (4th ed.). Elsevier.

Relocation Stress Reduction 5350

Definition: Assisting the individual to prepare for and cope with movement from one environment to another

Activities:

- Inform person of need to move
- Answer all questions promptly and completely
- Present optimistic attitude by pointing out positive aspects of relocation
- Explore context of relocation including age and gender of person, previous relocations, perception of relocation, ability to adjust
- Include in relocation plans, as appropriate
- Explore what most important in person's life (e.g., family, friends, personal belongings)
- Examine thoroughly all needs and preferences and include all available options for relocating
- Encourage individual and family to discuss concerns regarding relocation
- Allow time to think and provide opportunities to ask questions or state concerns
- Validate and acknowledge positive and negative feelings surrounding transition
- Assist to grieve and work through losses associated with relocation
- Listen attentively and respond honestly
- Resolve concerns promptly, where possible
- Be aware of transfer anxiety related to loss of close monitoring, secure environment, and dedicated staff when in acute care settings
- Evaluate for psychological symptoms of relocation stress syndrome (e.g., anxiety, confusion, helplessness, loneliness, withdrawal, anorexia, ongoing worry, pessimism, anorexia, depression, increased demands)
- Monitor for physiological symptoms of relocation (e.g., weight change, change in vital signs, decreased cognitive ability, inability to sleep)
- Support during relocation process
- Ensure personal agency over transition with respect to individual preferences
- Support shared decision-making between family and individual
- Encourage to participate in preparations for transition to reduce uncertainty
- Facilitate communication and coordination of event prior to relocation
- Select ideal time and date for transition
- Plan for personal items to be in place before relocating
- Create personal space and sense of home
- Establish routines that are preferred by person
- Avoid extreme disruptions in routine
- Encourage individual and family to discuss concerns regarding relocation
- Evaluate available support systems (e.g., extended family, community involvement, religious affiliations)
- Consider mental health, finances, personal history, and cultural background when making decisions
- Encourage individual and family to seek counseling, as appropriate
- Avoid negative assumptions on function and cognitive status of person
- Avoid patronization of person
- Provide diversional activities (e.g., involvement in hobbies, usual activities)
- Facilitate social integration and encourage pursuit of new relationships (e.g., assign a "buddy" to help acquaint to new environment)
- Facilitate visitations during first week of relocation
- Facilitate maintenance of relationships between person and friends and family
- Ensure access to technology to support communication connections (e.g., phones, tablets, computers, internet)
- Evaluate effect of disruption of lifestyle, loss of home, and adaptation to new environment
- Educate all staff related to relocation stress syndrome and its treatments

- Ensure policies established on when to transfer from acute care areas, such as avoiding nighttime or premature transfer where possible
- Arrange for adequate staff available to ensure smooth transition
- Document response to relocation

4th edition 2004; revised 2024

Background Evidence:

Johnson, J. L., Beard, J., & Evans, D. (2017). Caring for refugee youth in the school setting. *NASN School Nurse*, 32(2), 122–128. https://doi.org/10.1177/1942602X16672310

Lee, S., Oh, H. S., Suh, Y. O., & Seo, W. S. (2017). A tailored relocation stress intervention programme for family caregivers of patients transferred from a surgical intensive care unit to a general ward. *Journal of Clinical Nursing*, 26(5-6), 784–794.

Richardson, A., Blenkinsopp, A., Downs, M., & Lord, K. (2019). Stakeholder perspectives of care for people living with dementia moving from hospital to care facilities in the community: A systematic review. *BMC Geriatrics*, 19(202), 1–12.

Ryman, F. V. M., Erisman, J. C., Darvey, L. M., Osborne, J., Swartsenburg, E., & Syurina, E. V. (2019). Health effects of the relocation of patients with dementia: A scoping review to inform medical and policy decision making. *The Gerontologist*, 59(6), e647–e682.

Varcarolic, E. M., & Halter, M. J. (2018). *Foundations of psychiatric mental health nursing*. Saunders/Elsevier.

Williams, P. (2020). *Basic geriatric nursing* (7th ed.). Elsevier.

Won, M. H., & Youn-Jung, S. (2020). Development and psychometric evaluation of the relocation stress syndrome scale-short form for patients transferred from adult intensive care units to general wards. *Intensive & Critical Care Nursing*, 58. https://doi.org/10.1016/j.iccn.2020.102800

Young, J. A., Lind, C., & Orange, J. B. (2021). A qualitative systematic review of experiences of persons with dementia regarding transition to long-term care. *Dementia*, 20(1), 5–27.

Reminiscence Therapy   4860

Definition: Using the recall of past events, feelings, and thoughts to facilitate pleasure, quality of life, or adaptation to present circumstances

Activities:
- Choose a comfortable setting
- Set aside adequate time
- Identify, with the patient, a theme for each session (e.g., work life)
- Select an appropriately small number of participants for group reminiscence therapy
- Utilize effective listening and attending skills
- Determine which method of reminiscence (e.g., taped autobiography, journal, structured life review, scrapbook, open discussion, and storytelling) is most effective
- Introduce props (e.g., music for auditory, photo albums for visual, perfume for olfactory), addressing all five senses to stimulate recall
- Encourage verbal expression of both positive and negative feelings of past events
- Observe body language, facial expression, and tone of voice to identify the importance of recollections to the patient
- Ask open-ended questions about past events
- Encourage writing of past events
- Maintain focus of sessions, more on the process than on an end product
- Provide support, encouragement, and empathy for participant(s)
- Use culturally sensitive props, themes, and techniques
- Assist the person to address painful, angry, or other negative memories
- Use the patient's photo albums or scrapbooks to stimulate memories
- Assist the patient in creating or adding to a family tree, or to write his/her oral history
- Encourage the patient to write to old friends or relatives
- Use communication skills such as focusing, reflecting, and restating to develop the relationship
- Comment on the affective quality accompanying the memories in an empathetic manner
- Use direct questions to refocus back to life events, as necessary
- Inform family members about the benefits of reminiscence
- Gauge the length of the session by the patient's attention span
- Give immediate positive feedback to cognitively impaired patients
- Acknowledge previous coping skills
- Repeat sessions weekly or more often over prolonged period
- Gauge the number of sessions by the patient's response and willingness to continue

1st edition 1992; revised 1996, 2000, 2004

Background Evidence:

Brady, E. M. (1999). Stories at the hour of our death. *Home Healthcare Nurse*, 17(3), 176–180.

Burnside, I., & Haight, B. (1992). Reminiscence and life review: Analysing each concept. *Journal of Advanced Nursing*, 17(7), 855–862.

Burnside, I., & Haight, B. (1994). Reminiscence and life review: Therapeutic interventions for older people. *Nurse Practitioner*, 19(4), 55–61.

Coleman, P. G. (1999). Creating a life story: The task of reconciliation. *The Gerontologist*, 39(2), 133–139.

Haight, B. K. (2001). Life reviews: Helping Alzheimer's patients reclaim a fading past. *Reflections on Nursing Leadership*, 27(1), 20–22.

Hamilton, D. (1992). Reminiscence therapy. In G. Bulechek & J. McCloskey (Eds.), *Nursing interventions: Treatments for nursing diagnoses* (pp. 292–303). W. B. Saunders.

Harrand, A. G., & Bollstetter, J. J. (2000). Developing a community-based reminiscence group for the elderly. *Clinical Nurse Specialist*, 14(1), 17–22.

Johnson, R. A. (1999). Reminiscence therapy. In G. M. Bulechek & J. C. McCloskey (Eds.), *Nursing interventions: Effective nursing treatments* (3rd ed., pp. 371–384). W. B. Saunders.

Puentes, W. J. (2000). Using social reminiscence to teach therapeutic communication skills. *Geriatric Nursing*, 21(6), 315–318.

R

Reproductive Technology Management 7886

Definition: Assisting a patient through the steps of complex infertility treatment

Activities:

- Provide education about various treatment modalities (e.g., intrauterine insemination, in vitro fertilization-embryo transfer (IVF-ET), gamete intrafallopian transfer (GIFT), zygote intrafallopian transfer (ZIFT), donor sperm, donor oocytes, gestational carrier, and surrogacy)
- Discuss ethical dilemmas before initiating a particular treatment modality
- Explore feelings about assisted reproductive technology (e.g., known vs. anonymous oocyte or sperm donors, cryopreserved embryos, selective reduction, and use of a host uterus)
- Refer for preconception counseling, as needed
- Instruct patient about ovulation prediction and detection techniques (e.g., basal temperature and urine testing)
- Instruct patient about administration of ovulatory stimulants
- Schedule tests based on the menstrual cycle, as needed
- Coordinate activities of the multidisciplinary team for treatment process
- Assist out-of-town individuals in locating housing while participating in the program
- Provide education to gamete donors and their partners
- Collaborate with in vitro fertilization team in screening and selecting gamete donors
- Explore psychosocial issues involving gamete donation before administering medications for comfort
- Coordinate synchronization of donor and recipient hormonal cycles
- Draw specimens for endocrine determination
- Perform ultrasound examinations to ascertain follicular growth
- Participate in team conferences to correlate test results for evaluating oocyte maturity
- Set up equipment for oocyte retrieval
- Assist with freezing and preservation of embryos, as indicated
- Assist with fertilization procedures
- Prepare patient for embryo transfer
- Provide anticipatory guidance about typical emotional reactions, including extremes of anguish and joy
- Discuss risks, including the likelihood of miscarriage, ectopic pregnancy, and ovarian hyperstimulation
- Inform about ectopic pregnancy precautions
- Inform about symptoms of ovarian hyperstimulation to report
- Perform pregnancy tests
- Provide support for grieving when implantation fails to occur
- Schedule follow-up medication, tests, and ultrasound examinations
- Assist with hormonal and ultrasound monitoring of early pregnancy
- Refer for genetic counseling related to maternal age at conception, as needed
- Refer to infertility support groups, as needed
- Follow up with patients who have stopped treatment because of pregnancy, adoption, or the decision to remain childfree
- Assist patients to focus on life areas of success unrelated to fertility status
- Discuss methods of securing workplace support for necessary absences during treatment
- Provide counseling about financial and insurance issues
- Participate in reporting data about treatment outcomes to national registry

2nd edition 1996; revised 2018

Background Evidence:

Burns, L. (2012). Dealing with emotional distress following failed IVF. In K. Sharif & A. Coomarasamy (Eds.), *Assisted reproduction techniques: Challenges and management options* (pp. 417–420). West Sussex, United Kingdom: Wiley-Blackwell.

Hoffman, B., Schorge, J., Schaffer, J., Halvorson, L., Bradshaw, K., & Cunningham, F. (2012). Treatment of the infertile couple. In *Williams gynecology* (pp. 529–553) (2nd ed.). McGraw-Hill.

Lobo, R. (2012). Infertility. In G. Lentz, R. Lobo, D. Gershenson, & V. Katz (Eds.), *Comprehensive gynecology* (6th ed., pp. 869–895). Elsevier Mosby.

Wright, P., & Johnson, J. (2008). Infertility. In R. Gibbs, B. Karlan, A. Haney, & I. Nygaard (Eds.), *Danforth's obstetrics and gynecology* (10th ed., pp. 705–715). Lippincott Williams & Wilkins.

R

Research Protocol Management 8130

Definition: Implementation and coordination of research protocol

Activities:

- Ensure completion of informed consent and Institutional Review Board (IRB) approval
- Review implementation of study protocol as specified
- Confirm participants' understanding of risks and benefits of research
- Perform activities per routine while participants under study observation
- Document data according to procedure and study protocol
- Provide private space for conducting interviews or data collection as needed
- Assist to complete study questionnaires or other data collection tool, according to study protocol
- Obtain summary of study results for participating staff and interested study participants
- Communicate regularly with researcher about progress of data collection, as appropriate
- Monitor amount of participation in research studies
- Monitor participants response to research protocol
- Inform investigator of any adverse events

8th edition 2024

Background Evidence:

American Nurses Association. (2015). *Code of ethics for nurses with interpretive statements.*

American Nurses Association. (2021). *Nursing: Scope and standards of practice* (4th ed.).

Guido, G. W. (2020). *Legal and ethical issues in nursing* (7th ed.). Pearson.

Polit, D. F., & Beck, C. T. (2019). *Nursing research: Generating and assessing evidence for nursing practice* (11th ed.). Wolters Kluwer.

Resilience Promotion   8340

Definition: Facilitating development, use, and strengthening of coping strategies for environmental and societal stressors

Activities:

- Determine current coping strategies
- Facilitate increased use of positive coping strategies
- Encourage practice of mindfulness (e.g., journaling, yoga, meditation) and resources to manage stress (e.g., tranquility room)
- Promote positive lifestyle (e.g., proper nutrition, ample sleep, hydration, regular exercise) for body wellness, to adapt to stress and reduce toll of emotions like anxiety or depression
- Foster avoidance of negative outlets (i.e., masking pain with alcohol, drugs, or harmful substances)
- Facilitate development of meaningful, healthy relationships with empathetic and understanding people
- Encourage development of routines and traditions (e.g., birthdays, holidays)
- Facilitate acceptance of support from concerned persons
- Encourage regular connections and interactions with support persons (e.g., counselors, employee assistance, chaplains)
- Encourage active involvement in groups, faith-based communities, or other local organizations
- Facilitate use of healthy personal goals, using past experiences
- Encourage to seek help with progress toward goals
- Encourage to accept and embrace change
- Assist in developing interpersonal skills, as needed
- Provide role models, as needed
- Assist in developing optimism for the future
- Assist in identifying resources for advice and support
- Encourage family group activities
- Assist family in providing atmosphere conducive to learning
- Encourage positive health-seeking behaviors
- Educate on age-appropriate expectations
- Encourage family to establish rules
- Assist in acquiring assertiveness skills
- Assist in role playing decision-making skills
- Encourage participation in services or activities
- Use teach-back to determine understanding

3rd edition 2000; revised 2024

Background Evidence:

American Psychological Association. (2020). *Building your resilience*. http://www.apa.org/helpcenter/road-resilience.aspx

Coffield, C., Michael, S., & Srinivasavaradan, D. (2021). Building resilience: Resources to help families grow from challenging times. *Exceptional Parent, 51*(1), 33–38.

Cooper, A. L., Brown, J. A., & Leslie, G. D. (2021). Nurse resilience for clinical practice: An integrative review. *Journal of Advanced Nursing, 77*(6), 2623–2640. https://doi.org/10.1111/jan.14763

Duncan, J. M., Garrison, M. E., & Killian, T. S. (2021). Measuring family resilience: Evaluating the Walsh Family Resilience questionnaire. *Family Journal, 29*(1), 80–85. https://doi.org/10.1177/1066480720956641

Gomes de Medeiros, A. P., Pinheiro de Carvalho, M. A., Araújo de Medeiros, J. R., Dias Dantas, G., Carvalho do Nascimento, A. Q. I., Silva Pimentel, E. R., da Silva Pascoal, F. F., & Porfirio Souza, G. (2019). Resilient characteristics of families in dealing with psychic suffering. *Journal of Nursing UFPE / Revista de Enfermagem UFPE, 13*, 38–44. https://doi.org/10.5205/1981-8963.2019.236727

Luo, D., Eicher, M., & White, K. (2020). Individual resilience in adult cancer care: A concept analysis. *International Journal of Nursing Studies, 102*, 103467. https://doi.org/10.1016/j.ijnurstu.2019.103467

McKinley, C. E., & Theall, K. P. (2021). Weaving Healthy Families Program: Promoting resilience while reducing violence and substance use. *Research on Social Work Practice, 31*(5), 476–492. https://doi.org/10.1177/1049731521998441

Silva, D. J., Petrilla, C. M., Matteson, D., Mannion, S., & Huggins, S. L. (2020). Increasing resilience in youth and families: YAP's Wraparound Advocate Service Model. *Child & Youth Services, 41*(1), 51–82. https://doi.org/10.1080/0145935X.2019.1610870

Stacey, G., & Cook, G. (2019). A scoping review exploring how the conceptualisation of resilience in nursing influences interventions aimed at increasing resilience. *International Practice Development Journal, 9*(1), 1–16. https://doi.org/10.19043/ipdj.91.009

Wakhid, A., & Hamid, A. Y. S. (2020). Family resilience minimizes posttraumatic stress disorder: A systematic review. *Enfermería Clínica, 30*, 1–5. https://doi.org/10.1016/j.enfcli.2020.01.002

Resilience Promotion: Community   8720

R

Definition: Facilitating use of assets to strengthen public health and healthcare systems to improve physical, behavioral, and social health

Activities:

- Determine presence of unemployment, homelessness, educational attainment, incarceration, and mental and physical health issues in population or community
- Use available documents to identify community priorities (e.g., Community Health Needs Assessment)
- Promote development of adequate community services to assist in decreasing areas of concern (i.e., promote access to public health, health care and social services, unemployment services, behavioral health services, housing)
- Strengthen access to public health, health care, and social services
- Ensure community members know how to access care and are not limited by real or perceived barriers to services
- Promote access to physical and psychological health care
- Provide community members with regular educational events and resources to know what to do to care for themselves and others in both routine and emergency situations
- Encourage individuals to strengthen health and resilience (e.g., develop healthy lifestyles, maintain connections to meaningful groups, create evacuation and disaster response plans for self and family)
- Encourage social connectedness in which community members are regularly involved in each other's lives

- Provide at-risk individuals with programs that serve them (e.g., counselors, social services, employee assistance) and allow them to take active part in protecting their health
- Urge programs that serve at-risk individuals to develop robust disaster and continuity of operations plans
- Promote development of health and wellness groups, faith-based communities, or other local organizations
- Build networks that include social services (e.g., behavioral health services, community organizations, businesses, academia, at-risk individuals, and faith-based stakeholders in addition to traditional public health, health care, and emergency management partners)
- Support ongoing educational programs related to public health and behavioral health measures, emergency preparedness, and community health resilience interventions

8th edition 2024

Background Evidence:

American Psychological Association. (2020). *Resilience*. https://www.apa.org/topics/resilience

Crowe, L. (2017). Tips on building resilience and improving well-being. *Emergency Nurse, 24*(10), 14. https://doi.org/10.7748/en.24.10.14.s16

Ellis, W., Dietz, W. H., & Chen, K.-L. D. (2022). Community resilience: A dynamic model for public health 3.0. *Journal of Public Health Management & Practice, 28*, S18–S26. https://doi.org/10.1097/PHH.0000000000001413

Gerhardstein, B., Tucker, P. G., Rayman, J., & Reh, C. M. (2019). A fresh look at stress and resilience in communities affected by environmental contamination. *Journal of Environmental Health, 82*(4), 36–38.

Jewett, R. L., Mah, S. M., Howell, N., & Larsen, M. M. (2021). Social cohesion and community resilience during COVID-19 and pandemics: A rapid scoping review to inform the United Nations Research Roadmap for COVID-19 Recovery. *International Journal of Health Services, 51*(3), 325–336. https://doi.org/10.1177/0020731421997092

Mann, G., Cafer, A., Kaiser, K., & Gordon, K. (2020). Community resilience in a rural food system: Documenting pathways to nutrition solutions. *Public Health, 186*, 157–163. https://doi.org/10.1016/j.puhe.2020.06.041

Teodorczuk, A., Thomson, R., Chan, K., & Rogers, G. D. (2017). When I say... resilience. *Medical Education, 51*(12), 1206–1208. https://doi.org/10.1111/medu.13368

U.S. Department of Health and Human Services. (2020). *Community resilience.* https://www.phe.gov/Preparedness/planning/abc/Pages/community.aspx

---

Respiratory Monitoring 3350

Definition: Collection and analysis of patient data to ensure airway patency and adequate gas exchange

Activities:

- Monitor rate, rhythm, depth, and effort of respirations
- Note chest movement, watching for symmetry, use of accessory muscles, and supraclavicular and intercostal muscle retractions
- Monitor for noisy respirations, such as crowing or snoring
- Monitor breathing patterns (e.g., bradypnea, tachypnea, hyperventilation, Kussmaul respirations, Cheyne-Stokes respirations, apneustic, Biot's respiration, ataxic patterns)
- Monitor oxygen saturation levels continuously in sedated patients (e.g., SaO_2, SvO_2, SpO_2), per agency policy and as indicated
- Provide for noninvasive continuous oxygen sensors (e.g., finger, nose, or forehead devices) with appropriate alarm systems in patients with risk factors (e.g., morbidly obese, confirmed obstructive sleep apnea, history of respiratory problems requiring oxygen therapy, extremes of age), per agency policy and as indicated
- Palpate for equal lung expansion
- Percuss anterior and posterior thorax from apices to bases bilaterally
- Note location of trachea
- Monitor for diaphragmatic muscle fatigue, as indicated by paradoxical motion
- Auscultate breath sounds, noting areas of decreased or absent ventilation and presence of adventitious sounds
- Determine the need for suctioning by auscultating for crackles and rhonchi over major airways
- Auscultate lung sounds after treatments to note results
- Monitor PFT values, particularly vital capacity, maximal inspiratory force, forced expiratory volume in 1 second (FEV_1), and FEV_1/FVC, as available
- Monitor mechanical ventilator readings, noting increases in inspiratory pressures and decreases in tidal volume, as appropriate
- Monitor for increased restlessness, anxiety, and air hunger
- Note changes in SaO_2, SvO_2, end tidal CO_2, and ABG values, as appropriate
- Monitor patient's ability to cough effectively
- Note onset, characteristics, and duration of cough
- Monitor patient's respiratory secretions
- Provide frequent intermittent monitoring of respiratory status in at-risk patients (e.g., opioid therapy, newborn, mechanical ventilation, facial or chest burns, neuromuscular disorders)
- Monitor for dyspnea and events that improve and worsen it
- Monitor for hoarseness and voice changes every hour in patients with facial burns
- Monitor for crepitus, as appropriate
- Monitor chest x-ray reports
- Open the airway using the chin lift or jaw thrust technique, as appropriate
- Place the patient on side to prevent aspiration; log roll if cervical aspiration suspected, as indicated
- Institute resuscitation efforts, as needed
- Institute respiratory therapy treatments (e.g., nebulizer), as needed

1st edition 1992; revised 2013

Background Evidence:

Becker, D. E., & Casabianca, A. B. (2009). Respiratory monitoring: Physiological and technical considerations. *Anesthesia Progress, 56*(1), 14–22.

Bodin, D. A. (2003). Telemetry: Beyond the ICU. *Nursing Management, 34*(8), 46–50.

Carbery, C. (2008). Basic concepts in mechanical ventilation. *Journal of Perioperative Practice, 18*(3), 106–114.

Fetzer, S. J. (2011). Vital signs. In P. A. Potter, A. G. Perry, P. Stockert, & A. Hall (Eds.), *Basic nursing* (7th ed., pp. 278–280). Mosby Elsevier.

Hutchinson, D., & Whyte, K. (2008). Neuromuscular disease and respiratory failure. *Practical Neurology, 8*(4), 229–237.

Maddox, R. R., Williams, C. K., Oglesby, H., Butler, B., & Colclasure, B. (2006). Clinical experience with patient-controlled analgesia using continuous respiratory monitoring and a smart infusion system. *American Journal of Health-System Pharmacy, 63*(2), 157–164.

Pratt, E. S. (2011). Oxygenation. In P. A. Potter, A. G. Perry, P. Stockert, & A. Hall (Eds.), *Basic nursing* (7th ed., pp. 800–813). Mosby Elsevier.

R

Respite Care   7260

Definition: Provision of short-term care to provide relief for family caregiver

Activities:

- Establish a therapeutic relationship with patient and family
- Monitor endurance of caregiver
- Inform patient and family of available state funding for respite care
- Arrange for residential respite care
- Coordinate volunteers for in-home services, as appropriate
- Coordinate community support services (i.e., meals, day care, summer camp)
- Arrange for substitute caregiver
- Monitor skill level of respite care provider
- Follow usual routine of care
- Provide care, such as exercises, ambulation, and hygiene, as appropriate
- Provide a program of suitable activities, as appropriate
- Obtain emergency telephone numbers
- Determine how to contact usual caregiver
- Provide emergency care, as necessary
- Maintain normal home environment
- Provide a report to usual caregiver on return

1st edition 1992; revised 2013

Background Evidence:

Barnard-Brak, L., & Thomson, D. (2009). How is taking care of caregivers of children with disabilities related to academic achievement? *Child Youth Care Forum, 38*(2), 91–102.

Barrett, M., Wheatland, B., Haselby, P., Larson, A., Kristjanson, L., & Whyatt, D. (2009). Palliative respite services using nursing staff reduces hospitalization of patients and improves acceptance among carers. *International Journal of Palliative Nursing, 15*(8), 389–395.

Cowen, P. S., & Reed, D. A. (2002). Effects of respite care for children with developmental disabilities: Evaluation of an intervention for at risk families. *Public Health Nursing, 19*(4), 272–283.

Donath, C., Winkler, A., & Grassel, E. (2009). Short-term residential care for dementia patients: Predictors for utilization and expected quality from a family caregiver's point of view. *International Psychogeriatrics, 21*(4), 703–710.

Molzahn, A. E., Gallagher, E., & McNulty, V. (2009). Quality of life associated with adult day centers. *Journal of Gerontological Nursing, 35*(8), 37–46.

Perry, J., & Bontinen, K. (2001). Evaluation of a weekend respite program for persons with Alzheimer disease. *Canadian Journal of Nursing Research, 33*(1), 81–95.

Salin, S., Kaunonen, M., & Astedt-Kurki, P. (2009). Informal carers of older family members: How they manage and what support they receive from respite care. *Journal of Clinical Nursing, 18*(4), 492–501.

Resuscitation   6320

Definition: Administering emergency measures to sustain life

Activities:

- Evaluate unresponsiveness to determine appropriate action
- Call for help if no breathing or no normal breathing and no response
- Call a code, according to agency standard
- Obtain the automated external defibrillator (AED)
- Attach the AED and implement specified actions
- Assure rapid defibrillation, as appropriate
- Perform cardiopulmonary resuscitation that focuses on chest compressions in adults and compressions with breathing efforts for children, as appropriate
- Initiate 30 chest compressions at specified rate and depth, allowing for complete chest recoil between compressions, minimizing interruptions in compressions, and avoiding excessive ventilation
- Assure patient's airway is open
- Provide two rescue breaths after initial 30 chest compressions completed
- Minimize the interval between stopping chest compressions and delivering a shock, if indicated
- Tailor rescue actions to the most likely cause of arrest (e.g., cardiac or respiratory arrest)
- Monitor the quality of CPR provided
- Monitor patient response to resuscitation efforts
- Use either the head tilt or jaw thrust maneuver to maintain an airway
- Clear oral, nasal, and tracheal secretions when possible and without interfering with chest compressions, as appropriate
- Administer manual ventilation when possible and without interfering with chest compressions, as appropriate
- Call for physician assistance, as needed
- Connect the person to an ECG monitor if needed when defibrillation is completed
- Initiate an IV line and administer IV fluids, as indicated
- Check that electronic equipment is working properly
- Provide standby equipment
- Provide appropriate medications
- Apply cardiac or apnea monitor
- Obtain electrocardiogram
- Interpret ECG and deliver cardioversion or defibrillation, as needed
- Evaluate changes in chest pain
- Assist with insertion of endotracheal tube (ET), as indicated
- Assess lung sounds after intubation for proper ET position
- Assist with performing chest x-ray examination after intubation
- Assure organized post cardiac arrest care (e.g., safe transport to appropriate nursing care unit)
- Offer family members opportunities to be present during resuscitation when in the best interests of the patient
- Support family members who are present during resuscitation (e.g., ensure safe environment, provide explanations and commentary, allow appropriate communication with patient, continually assess needs, provide opportunities to reflect on resuscitation efforts after event)
- Provide opportunities for team members to be involved in team debriefings or reflect on resuscitation efforts after event
- Document sequence of events

1st edition 1992; revised 2013

R

Background Evidence:

Boucher, M. (2010). Family-witnessed resuscitation. *Emergency Nurse*, *18*(5), 10–14.

Carlson, K. (Ed.). (2009). *Advanced critical care nursing*. Saunders Elsevier.

Field, J., Hazinski, M., Sayre, M., Chameides, L., Schexnayder, S., Hemphill, R., Samson, R. A., Kattwinkel, J., Berg, R. A., Bhanji, F., Cave, D. M., Jauch, E. C., Kudenchuk, P. J., Neumar, R. W., Peberdy, M. A., Perlman, J. M., Sinz, E., Travers, A. H., Berg, M. D., Billi, J. E., & Hoek, T. L. V. (2010). Part 1: Executive summary: 2010 American Heart Association guidelines for cardiopulmonary resuscitation and emergency cardiovascular care. *Circulation*, *122*(18 Suppl. 3), S640–S656.

Hazinski, M. F. (Ed.). (2010). *Highlights of the 2010 American Heart Association guidelines for CPR and ECC*. American Heart Association.

Urden, L., Stacy, K. M., & Lough, M. E. (2010). *Critical care nursing: Diagnosis and management* (6th ed.). Mosby Elsevier.

Wiegand, D. (Ed.). (2011). *AACN procedure manual for critical care* (6th ed.). Elsevier Saunders.

Resuscitation: Fetus 6972

Definition: Administering emergency measures to improve placental perfusion or correct fetal acid-base status

Activities:

- Monitor fetal vital signs using auscultation and palpation or electronic fetal monitor, as appropriate
- Observe for non-reassuring (abnormal) fetal heart rate signs (e.g., bradycardia, tachycardia, nonreactivity, variable decelerations, late decelerations, prolonged decelerations, decreased long-term or short-term variability, sinusoidal pattern)
- Include mother and support person in explanation of measures needed to enhance fetal oxygenation
- Use universal precautions
- Discontinue syntocinon to decrease uterine activity
- Reposition mother to left lateral or hands-and-knees position
- Reevaluate fetal heart rate
- Apply oxygen at 10 to 15 L/min if positioning is ineffective in correcting non-reassuring (abnormal) pattern of fetal heart rate
- Initiate intravenous line, as appropriate
- Give a bolus of 1 L crystalloid IV fluid
- Monitor maternal vital signs
- Administer IV vasopressor if blood pressure is low
- Perform a vaginal examination with fetal scalp stimulation
- Apprise midwife or physician about outcome of resuscitation measures
- Document strip interpretation, activities performed, fetal outcome, and maternal response
- Apply internal monitors once the amniotic membranes are ruptured to obtain more information about the fetal heart rate response to uterine activity
- Use fetal scalp electrode if fetal heart rate tracing is suboptimal
- Reassure and calm mother and support person(s)
- Administer tocolytic medication to reduce contractions, as appropriate
- Perform amnioinfusion for non-reassuring (abnormal) variable decelerations in fetal heart rate or meconium-stained amniotic fluid
- Turn to left-lateral position for pushing during second-stage labor to improve placental perfusion
- Coach to decrease pushing efforts for non-reassuring (abnormal) fetal heart signs to allow reestablishment of placental perfusion
- Consult with obstetrician to obtain fetal blood sample, as appropriate
- Anticipate requirements for mode of delivery and neonatal support, based on fetal responses to resuscitation techniques

---

2nd edition 1996; revised 2018

Background Evidence:

Kither, H., & Monaghan, S. (2013). Intrauterine fetal resuscitation. *Anaesthesia & Intensive Care Medicine*, *14*(7), 287–290.

Macones, G. (2015). Management of intrapartum category I, II, and III fetal heart rate tracings. In V. A. Barss (Ed.), *UpToDate*. http://www.uptodate.com/contents/management-of-intrapartum-category-i-ii-and-iii-fetal-heart-rate-tracings

Velayudhareddy, S., & Kirankumar, H. (2010). Management of foetal asphyxia by intrauterine foetal resuscitation. *Indian Journal of Anaesthesia*, *54*(5), 394–399.

Resuscitation: Neonate 6974

Definition: Administering emergency measures to support newborn adaptation to extrauterine life

Activities:

- Set up equipment for resuscitation before birth
- Test resuscitation bag, suction, and oxygen flow to ensure proper function
- Place newborn under the radiant warmer
- Insert laryngoscope to visualize the trachea to suction for meconium-stained fluid, as appropriate
- Intubate with an endotracheal tube to remove meconium from the lower airway, as appropriate
- Reintubate and suction until the return is clear of meconium
- Use mechanical suction to remove meconium from lower airway
- Dry with a prewarmed blanket to remove amniotic fluid, to reduce heat loss, and to provide stimulation
- Position the newborn on back, with neck slightly extended to open airway
- Open the airway by slightly extending the neck, placing in the "sniffing" position
- Suction secretions from nose and mouth with a bulb syringe
- Provide tactile stimulation by rubbing the soles of the feet or rubbing the infant's back
- Monitor respirations
- Monitor heart rate
- Monitor oxygen saturations by placing an oximeter probe on the right wrist
- Initiate positive-pressure ventilation for apnea, gasping, or heart rate lower than 100 beats per minute

- Set oxygen blender at 21% at 5 to 8 L to fill resuscitation bag and titrate based on oxygen saturations, as necessary
- Adjust bag to fill correctly
- Obtain a tight seal with a mask that covers the chin, mouth, and nose
- Ventilate at a rate of 40 to 60 breaths per minute using 20 to 40 cm of water for initial breaths and 15 to 20 cm of water for subsequent pressures
- Auscultate to ensure adequate ventilation
- Check heart rate after 15 to 30 seconds of ventilation
- Give chest compression for heart rate of less than 60 beats per minute or if greater than 80 beats per minute with no increase
- Compress sternum 0.5 to 0.75 inches using a 3:1 ratio for delivering 90 compressions and 30 breaths per minute
- Check heart rate after 30 seconds of compressions
- Continue compressions until heart rate is greater than or equal to 60 beats per minute
- Continue ventilations until adequate spontaneous respirations begin and color becomes pink
- Insert endotracheal tube for prolonged ventilation or poor response to bag and mask ventilation
- Auscultate bilateral breath sounds for confirmation of endotracheal tube placement

- Observe for rise of chest without gastric distention to check placement
- Secure airway to face with tape
- Insert an orogastric catheter if ventilation is given for more than 2 minutes
- Prepare medications (e.g., narcotic antagonists, epinephrine, volume expanders, and sodium bicarbonate), as needed
- Administer medications per order
- Document time, sequence, and neonatal responses to all steps of resuscitation
- Provide explanation to parents, as appropriate
- Assist with neonatal transfer or transport, as appropriate

2nd edition 1996; revised 2018

Background Evidence:

American Academy of Pediatrics, & American College of Obstetricians and Gynecologists. (2012). *Guidelines for perinatal care* (7th ed.). American Academy of Pediatrics.

American Heart Association, & American Academy of Pediatrics. (2011). *Textbook of neonatal resuscitation* (6th ed.). American Academy of Pediatrics.

Risk Identification 6610

Definition: Analysis of potential risk factors, determination of health risks, and prioritization of risk reduction strategies for an individual or group

Activities:

- Review past health history and documents for evidence of existing or previous medical and nursing diagnoses and treatments
- Review data derived from routine risk assessment measures
- Determine availability and quality of resources (e.g., psychological, financial, education level, family and other social, and community)
- Identify agency resources to assist in decreasing risk factors
- Maintain accurate records and statistics
- Identify biological, environmental, and behavioral risks and their interrelationships
- Identify typical coping strategies
- Determine past and current level of functioning
- Determine status of basic living needs
- Determine community resources appropriate for basic living and health needs
- Determine compliance with medical and nursing treatments
- Instruct on risk factors and plan for risk reduction
- Use mutual goal setting, as appropriate
- Consider criteria useful in prioritizing areas for risk reduction (e.g., awareness and motivation level, effectiveness, cost, feasibility, preferences, equity, stigmatization, and severity of outcomes if risks remain unaddressed)
- Discuss and plan for risk reduction activities in collaboration with individual or group
- Implement risk reduction activities
- Initiate referrals to health care personnel and/or agencies, as appropriate
- Plan for long-term monitoring of health risks
- Plan for long-term follow-up of risk reduction strategies and activities

1st edition 1992; revised 2013

Background Evidence:

Doll, L. S., Bonzo, S. E., Mercy, J. A., & Sleet, D. A. (Eds.). (2007). *Handbook of injury and violence prevention [E. N. Haas, Managing].* Springer.

Kutcher, S., & Chehil, S. (2007). *Suicide risk management: A manual for health professionals.* Oxford: Blackwell.

Stanhope, M., & Lancaster, J. (2008). *Public health nursing: Population-centered health care in the community* (7th ed.). Mosby Elsevier.

R

Risk Identification: Childbearing Family 6612

Definition: Identification of an individual or family likely to experience difficulties in parenting, and prioritization of strategies to prevent parenting problems

Activities:

- Determine age of mother
- Determine developmental stage of parent
- Determine parity of mother

- Determine economic status of family
- Determine educational status of mother
- Determine marital status of mother

- Determine residential status of mother (e.g., place of residence, homelessness, living with someone, immigration status)
- Determine literacy
- Determine outcomes of all prior pregnancies
- Determine whether previous children born to mother are still in her care
- Ascertain understanding of English or other language used in community
- Determine prior involvement with social services
- Determine prior history of abuse and violence
- Determine prior history of depression or other mental illness
- Determine health and immunization status of siblings
- Monitor behaviors that may indicate a problem with attachment
- Review prenatal and intrapartal records for documented signs of prenatal attachment
- Review prenatal history for factors that predispose patient to complications
- Review, update, and complete information as pregnancy develops and at intrapartum, postpartum, and neonatal admissions, as needed
- Note medications that mother received during prenatal period
- Review prenatal history for possible stressors affecting neonatal glucose stores (e.g., diabetes, pregnancy-induced hypertension, and cardiac or renal disorders)
- Review history for abnormal prenatal growth patterns as detected by ultrasonography or fundal changes
- Review maternal history of chemical dependency, noting duration, type of drugs used (including alcohol), and time and strength of last dose before delivery
- Determine the patient's feelings about an unplanned pregnancy
- Determine whether unplanned pregnancy is approved of by the family
- Determine whether unplanned pregnancy is supported by the family
- Document psychosocial adaptation to pregnancy by the patient, the father, other children and adults in the household, family members, and others in close relationship to the pregnant woman
- Note presence of multiple gestation and consider challenges of raising multiples
- Note any medications (e.g., sedative, anesthetic, or analgesic) administered to mother during intrapartal period
- Note maternal morbidities that could delay attachment (e.g., prolonged labor, infection, sedating medications)
- Note fetal and neonatal morbidities (e.g., fetal distress, hypoxia, oligohydramnios or polyhydramnios, hyperglycemia or hypoglycemia) that could delay its ability to interact with caretakers

- Identify reason for separation from newborn after birth
- Monitor parent-infant interactions, noting behaviors thought to indicate attachment
- Note attachment behaviors to multiples (e.g., twins, triplets)
- Promote family attachment through patient education
- Implement activities that promote attachment
- Evaluate behavioral assessment of neonates during early pediatric visits for possible indications of parenting adjustment problems
- Promote a postpartum maternal follow-up at 2 to 6 weeks to a qualified health care professional
- Promote newborn follow-up at 2 and 6 weeks by a qualified health care professional
- Prioritize areas for risk reduction in collaboration with the individual or family
- Plan for risk reduction activities in collaboration with the individual or family
- Promote newborn safety by requiring newborn discharge into an approved car seat
- Refer to the appropriate community agency for follow-up if risk of parenting problems or a lag in attachment has been identified

1st edition 1992; revised 2013

Background Evidence:

Fouquier, K. F. (2011). The concept of motherhood among three generations of African American women. *Journal of Nursing Scholarship, 43*(2), 145–153.

Lutz, K. F., Anderson, L. S., Pridham, K. A., Riesch, S. K., & Becker, P. T. (2009). Furthering the understanding of parent-child relationships: A nursing scholarship review series. Part 1: Introduction. *Journal for Specialists in Pediatric Nursing, 14*(4), 256–261.

Lutz, K. F., Anderson, L. S., Riesch, S. K., Pridham, K. A., & Becker, P. T. (2009). Furthering the understanding of parent-child relationships: A nursing scholarship review series. Part 2: Grasping the early parenting experience—The insider view. *Journal for Specialists in Pediatric Nursing, 14*(4), 262–283.

Taubman-Ben-Ari, O., Findler, L., & Kuint, J. (2010). Personal growth in the wake of stress: The case of mothers of preterm twins. *Journal of Psychology, 144*(2), 185–204.

Underdown, A., & Barlow, J. (2011). Interventions to support early relationships: Mechanisms identified within infant massage programmes. *Community Practitioner, 84*(4), 21–26.

Ward, S. L., & Hisley, S. M. (2009). *Maternal-child nursing care: Optimizing outcomes for mothers, children, & families.* F. A. Davis.

Risk Identification: Genetic   6614

Definition: Identification and analysis of potential genetic risk factors in an individual, family, or group

Activities:
- Ensure privacy and confidentiality
- Explore confirmed or suspected genetic risk factors to determine level of understanding
- Review complete health history, including prenatal and obstetrical history, developmental history, and past and present health status related to confirmed or suspected genetic risk factors

- Review environment for possible risk factors (e.g., potential teratogen and carcinogen exposures)
- Review lifestyle for possible risk factors (e.g., tobacco, alcohol, prescription medication, drug use)
- Determine presence and quality of support systems, and previous coping skills
- Obtain comprehensive family history and construct at least three-generation pedigree

R

- Obtain documented diagnosis of affected family members
- Review options for diagnostic testing that may confirm or predict presence of genetic disorder, such as biochemical or radiographic studies, chromosome analysis, linkage analyses, or direct DNA testing
- Provide information about diagnostic procedures
- Discuss advantages, risks, and financial costs of diagnostic options
- Discuss insurance and possible job discrimination issues as relevant
- Discuss issues in testing other family members as relevant
- Initiate genetic counseling intervention based upon risk identification, as appropriate
- Refer to genetic health care specialists for genetic counseling, as needed
- Provide written summary of risk identification counseling, as indicated

3rd edition 2000; revised 2024

Background Evidence:

Kin,g E., Mahon, S. M. (2017). Genetic testing: Challenges and changes in testing for hereditary cancer syndromes. *Clinical Journal of Oncology Nursing*, *21*(5), 589–598. https://doi.org/10.1188/17.CJON.589-598

McEwen, A., & Jacobs, C. (2021). Who we are, what we do, and how we add value: The role of the genetic counseling 'philosophy of practice' statement in a changing time. *Journal of Genetic Counseling*, *30*(1), 114–120. https://doi.org/10.1002/jgc4.1308

McReynolds, K., & Lewis, S. (2017). Genetic counseling for hereditary cancer: A primer for NPs. *Nurse Practitioner Journal*, *42*(7), 22–28. https://doi.org/10.1097/01.NPR.0000520422.06782.65

Mendes, Á., Metcalfe, A., Paneque, M., Sousa, L., Clarke, A. J., & Sequeiros, J. (2018). Communication of information about genetic risks: Putting families at the center. *Family Process*, *57*(3), 836–846. https://doi.org/10.1111/famp.12306

Patch, C., & Middleton, A. (2018). Genetic counselling in the era of genomic medicine. *British Medical Bulletin*, *126*(1), 27–36. https://doi.org/10.1093/bmb/ldy008

Sharma, S., Khanna, G., & Gangane, S. D. (2019). *Textbook of pathology and genetics for nurses*. India: Elsevier.

Risk Identification: Infectious Disease   6620

Definition: Analysis of potential risk factors, determination of health risks, and prioritization of risk reduction strategies for individuals with infectious diseases

Activities:

- Determine risk factors using the appropriate agency guidelines (e.g., World Health Organization, Centers for Disease Control and Prevention)
- Review recent travel history to determine exposure
- Determine immunization status
- Determine exposure to groups of people and need for contact tracing (e.g., daycare, university residence halls, long-term care facility, hospital)
- Maintain privacy when contact tracing for identification of other individuals who may have been exposed
- Determine if high-risk behaviors are present (e.g., unprotected sex, close contact with at-risk people for more than 15 minutes)
- Recommend appropriate testing, treatment, and quarantine procedures for individuals with known exposure
- Isolate from others if concern for droplet or airborne spread while waiting for testing confirmation
- Instruct on appropriate methods to prevent spread
- Follow prescribed treatment regimen
- Inform care takers, as applicable, on symptoms that may signify transmission
- Initiate appropriate preventative measures in various settings
- Report communicable infectious diseases, as required by law, to the appropriate public health departments on the local, state, and national level

8th edition 2024

Background Evidence:

Centers for Disease Control and Prevention, National Center for Emerging and Zoonotic Infectious Diseases (NCEZID), Division of Healthcare Quality Promotion (DHQP) (2019). Infection control in healthcare personnel: Infrastructure and routine practices for occupational infection prevention and control services. Accessed at https://www.cdc.gov/infectioncontrol/guidelines/healthcare-personnel/assessment.html

Johansson, M. A., Quandelacy, T. M., Kada, S., Prasad, P. V., Steele, M., Brooks, J. T., Slayton, R. B., Biggerstaff, M., & Butler, J. C. (2021). SARS-CoV-2 transmission from people without COVID-19 symptoms. *JAMA Network Open*, *4*(1). https://doi.org/10.1001/jamanetworkopen.2020.35057

Levy, S. B., Gunta, J., & Edemekong, P. (2019). Screening for sexually transmitted diseases. *Primary Care: Clinics in Office Practice*, *46*, 157–173. https://doi.org/10.1016/j.pop.2018.10.013

Martin, G., & Boland, M. (2018). Planning and preparing for public health threats at airports. *Globalization and Health*, *14*(28), 1–5. https://doi.org/10.1186/s12992-018-0323-3

Saurabh, S., & Prateek, S. (2017). Role of contact tracing in containing the 2014 Ebola outbreak: A review. *African Health Sciences*, *17*(1), 225–236. https://doi.org/10.4314/ahs.v17i1.28

United States Preventative Services Task Force. (n.d.). *Recommendations*. https://www.uspreventiveservicestaskforce.org/uspstf/topic_search_results

World Health Organization. (2021). *Considerations for implementing and adjusting public health and social measures in the context of COVID-19*. Accessed at https://www.who.int/publications/i/item/considerations-in-adjusting-public-health-and-social-measures-in-the-context-of-covid-19-interim-guidance

R

Role Enhancement 5370

Definition: Assisting a patient, significant other, and/or family to improve relationships by clarifying and supplementing specific role behaviors

Activities:

- Assist patient to identify various roles in life cycle
- Assist patient to identify usual role in family
- Assist patient to identify role transition periods throughout the lifespan
- Assist patient to identify role insufficiency
- Assist patient to identify behaviors needed for role development
- Assist patient to identify specific role changes required due to illness or disability
- Assist adult children to accept elderly parent's dependency and the role changes involved, as appropriate
- Encourage patient to identify a realistic description of change in role
- Assist patient to identify positive strategies for managing role changes
- Facilitate discussion of role adaptations of family to compensate for ill member's role changes
- Assist patient to imagine how a particular situation might occur and how a role would evolve
- Facilitate role rehearsal by having patient anticipate others' reactions to enactment
- Facilitate discussion of how siblings' roles will change with newborn's arrival, as appropriate
- Provide rooming-in opportunities to help clarify parents' roles, as appropriate
- Facilitate discussion of role adaptations related to children's leaving home (empty nest syndrome), as appropriate
- Serve as role model for learning new behaviors, as appropriate
- Facilitate opportunity for patient to role play new behaviors
- Facilitate discussion of expectations between patient and significant other in reciprocal role
- Teach new behaviors needed by patient/parent to fulfill a role
- Facilitate reference group interactions as part of learning new roles

1st edition 1992; revised 2008

Background Evidence:

Bunten, D. (2001). Normal changes with aging. In M. Maas, K. Buckwalter, M. Hardy, T. Tripp-Reimer, M. Titler, & J. Specht (Eds.), *Nursing care of older adults: Diagnoses, outcomes, & interventions* (pp. 518–520). Mosby.

Ebersole, P., Hess, P., Touhy, T., & Jett, K. (2005). *Gerontological nursing & healthy aging* (2nd ed.). Elsevier Mosby.

Larsen, P. D., Lewis, P. R., & Lubkin, I. M. (2006). Illness behavior and roles. In I. M. Lubkin & P. D. Larsen (Eds.), *Chronic illness: Impact and interventions* (pp. 23–44). Jones and Bartlett.

Mercer, R. T. (2004). Becoming a mother versus maternal role attainment. *Journal of Nursing Scholarship*, 36(3), 226–232.

Miller, J. F. (2000). *Coping with chronic illness: Overcoming powerlessness* (3rd ed.). F. A. Davis.

Moorhead, S. A. (1985). Role supplementation. In G. M. Bulechek & J. C. McCloskey (Eds.), *Nursing interventions: Treatments for nursing diagnoses* (pp. 152–159). W. B. Saunders.

R

Safety Huddle 7810

Definition: Focused, brief, interprofessional communication exchange of concerns, hazards, essential care needs, organizational information, and recognition of performance

Activities:

- Plan scheduled meetings with consistent time and location
- Foster interprofessional participation
- Use structured communication tool to organize topics
- Review follow-up safety issues and proactively identify safety concerns for current day (e.g., high-risk fall, high-risk medication infusions, sitters, video monitoring, indwelling central venous or urinary catheter days, persons with similar names)
- Give every team member opportunity to contribute
- Encourage sharing of positive observations and concerns (e.g., what works, what does not)
- Include discussion of issues with equipment and room concerns
- Direct concerns raised during huddles to appropriate person or groups for resolution
- Keep huddle meetings brief (i.e., 5–10 minutes)
- Use visual management board to provide information on huddle agenda, current safety issues and performance metrics, if available
- Provide for privacy of information shared (i.e., avoid using protective health information [PHI] limit detail written on visual management board)
- Use designated team member to note issues for follow-up
- Provide updates on recent or upcoming relevant safety announcements and initiatives, (e.g., changes to high-alert medications, adherence to standardized checklists)
- Evaluate process periodically and revise as indicated

Background Evidence:

Agency for Healthcare Research and Quality. (2017). *Daily Huddles* (AHRQ Publication No. 16[17]-0019-4-EF).

Agency for Healthcare Research and Quality. (2019). *TeamSTEPPS 2.0 Fundamentals*. https://www.ahrq.gov/teamstepps/instructor/fundamentals/index.html

Fiveash, J. M., Smith, M. L., Moore, A. K., Jandarov, R., & Sopirala, M. M. (2021). Build upon basics: An intervention utilizing safety huddles to achieve near-zero incidence of catheter associated urinary tract infection at a department of Veterans Affairs long-term care facility. *American Journal of Infection Control, 49*(11), 1419–1422. https://doi.org/10.1016/j.ajic.2021.03.017

Foster, S. (2017). Implementing safety huddles. *British Journal of Nursing, 26*(16), 953. https://doi.org/10.12968/bjon.2017.26.16.953

Gray, T. (2020). Safety huddle in a community nursing setting. *British Journal of Community Nursing, 25*(9), 446–450. https://doi.org/10.12968/bjcn.2020.25.9.446

Peet, J., Theobald, K. A., & Douglas, C. (2022). Building safety cultures at the frontline: An emancipatory Practice Development approach for strengthening nursing surveillance on an acute care ward. *Journal of Clinical Nursing (John Wiley & Sons, Inc.), 31*(5/6), 642–656. https://doi.org/10.1111/jocn.15923

Stapley, E., Sharples, E., Lachman, P., Lakhanpaul, M., Wolpert, M., & Deighton, J. (2018). Factors to consider in the introduction of huddles on clinical wards: perceptions of staff on the SAFE programme. *International Journal of Quality Health Care, 30*(1), 44–49.

8th edition 2024

Seclusion 6630

Definition: Solitary containment in a fully protective environment with close surveillance by nursing staff for purposes of safety or behavior management

Activities:

- Obtain a physician's order, if required by institutional policy, to use a physically restrictive intervention
- Designate one nursing staff member to communicate with the patient and to direct other staff
- Identify for patient and significant others those behaviors that necessitated the intervention
- Explain procedure, purpose, and time period of the intervention to patient and significant others in understandable and nonpunitive terms
- Explain to patient and significant others the behaviors necessary for termination of the intervention
- Contract with patient (as patient is able) to maintain control of behavior
- Instruct on self-control methods, as appropriate
- Assist in dressing in clothing that is safe and in removing jewelry and eyeglasses
- Remove all items from seclusion area that patient might use to harm self or others
- Assist with needs related to nutrition, elimination, hydration, and personal hygiene

- Provide food and fluids in unbreakable containers
- Provide appropriate level of supervision and surveillance to monitor patient and to allow for therapeutic actions, as needed
- Inform patient of video surveillance, as appropriate
- Explain reasons for the video monitoring
- Give careful consideration to who is responsible for watching the video monitor for changes in patient status
- Reassure patient of safety within the seclusion area during monitoring
- Distinguish direct visual inspection from checks performed through video monitoring and document appropriately
- Acknowledge your presence to patient periodically
- Administer PRN medications for anxiety or agitation
- Provide for patient's psychological comfort, as needed
- Monitor seclusion area for temperature, cleanliness, and safety
- Reduce sensory stimuli around the seclusion area
- Arrange for routine cleaning of seclusion area
- Evaluate, at regular intervals, patient's need for continued restrictive intervention
- Involve patient in making decisions to move to a more or less restrictive intervention, when appropriate

S

- Determine patient's need for continued seclusion
- Document rationale for restrictive intervention, patient's response to intervention, patient's physical condition, nursing care provided throughout intervention, and rationale for terminating the intervention
- Process with the patient and staff, on termination of the restrictive intervention, the circumstances that led to the use of the intervention, as well as any patient concerns about the intervention itself
- Provide the next appropriate level of restrictive intervention (e.g., physical restraint or area restriction), as needed

1st edition 1992; revised 2013

Background Evidence:

Byatt, N., & Glick, R. (2008). Safety in the psychiatric emergency service. In R. L. Glick, J. S. Berlin, A. B. Fishkind, & S. L. Zeller (Eds.), *Emergency psychiatry: Principles and practice* (pp. 33–44). Lippincott Williams & Wilkins.

Happell, B., & Koehan, S. (2010). Attitudes to the use of seclusion: Has contemporary mental health policy made a difference? *Journal of Clinical Nursing, 19*(21–22), 3208–3217.

Harper-Jaques, S., & Reimer, M. (2005). Management of aggression and violence. In M. A. Boyd (Ed.), *Psychiatric nursing: Contemporary practice* (3rd ed., pp. 802–822). Lippincott Williams & Wilkins.

Hyde, S., Fulbrook, P., Fenton, K., & Kilshaw, M. (2009). A clinical improvement project to develop and implement a decision-making framework for the use of seclusion. *International Journal of Mental Health Nursing, 18*(6), 398–408.

Needham, H., & Sands, N. (2010). Post-seclusion debriefing: A core nursing intervention. *Perspectives in Psychiatric Care, 46*(3), 221–233.

Olsen, D. P. (1998). Ethical considerations of video monitoring of psychiatric patients in seclusion and restraint. *Archives of Psychiatric Nursing, 12*(2), 90–94.

Sedation Management 2260

Definition: Provision of necessary physiological support during the administration of medications that alter consciousness

Activities:

- Review health history and results of diagnostic tests to determine whether meets agency criteria for conscious sedation by registered nurse
- Ask about any previous experiences with conscious sedation
- Check for drug allergies
- Determine last food and fluid intake
- Review medications and verify absence of contraindications for sedation
- Instruct about effects of sedation
- Review informed written consent
- Evaluate level of consciousness and protective reflexes before administering sedation
- Obtain baseline vital signs, oxygen saturation, EKG, height, and weight
- Ensure emergency resuscitation equipment readily available, specifically source to deliver 100% oxygen, emergency medications, and defibrillator
- Initiate IV line
- Administer medication as per health care provider order or protocol, titrating carefully according to response
- Monitor level of consciousness, airway, vital signs, oxygen saturation, ET CO_2, and EKG, as per agency protocol during procedure
- Monitor for adverse effects of medication after administration (e.g., agitation, respiratory depression, hypotension, undue somnolence, hypoxemia, arrhythmias, apnea, exacerbation of pre-existing condition)
- Use sedation scale to determine LOC (e.g., Ramsay scale)
- Ensure availability of and administer antagonists as appropriate, per health care provider order or protocol
- Determine whether meets discharge criteria (e.g., Aldrete scale)
- Document actions and response, as per agency policy
- Discharge or transfer, as per agency protocol
- Provide written discharge instructions, as per agency protocol

2nd edition 1996; revised 2000, 2004, 2024

Background Evidence:

American Society of Anesthesiologists Task Force on Moderate Procedural Sedation and Analgesia. (2018). Practice guidelines for moderate procedural sedation and analgesia. *Anesthesiology, 128,* 437–479. https://doi.org/10.1097/ALN.0000000000002043

Croke, L. (2021). Guideline for care of the patient receiving moderate sedation/analgesia. *AORN Journal, 113*(6), P4–P6. https://doi.org/10.1002/aorn.13436

Czarnecki, M. L., & Turner, H. N. (2018). *Core curriculum for pain management nursing.* Elsevier.

DiNisco, S. M. (2021). *Advanced practice nursing: Essential knowledge for the profession* (4th ed.). Jones & Bartlett.

Mohr, N. M., Stoltze, A., Ahmed, A., Kiscaden, E., & Shane, D. (2018). Using continuous quantitative capnography for emergency department procedural sedation: a systematic review and cost-effectiveness analysis. *Internal & Emergency Medicine, 13*(1), 75–85. https://doi.org/10.1007/s11739-016-1587-3

Schick, L., & Windle, (2017). *Perianesthesia nursing core curriculum* (4th ed.). American Society of Perianesthesia Nurses.

Seizure Management 2680

Definition: Care of a patient during a seizure and the postictal state

Activities:

- Maintain airway
- Turn onto side
- Guide movements to prevent injury
- Monitor direction of head and eyes during seizure
- Loosen clothing
- Remain with patient during seizure
- Establish IV access, as appropriate
- Apply oxygen, as appropriate
- Monitor neurological status
- Monitor vital signs
- Reorient after seizure

- Record length of seizure
- Record seizure characteristics (e.g., body parts involved, motor activity, and seizure progression)
- Document information about seizure
- Administer medication, as appropriate
- Administer anticonvulsants, as appropriate
- Monitor antiepileptic drug levels, as appropriate
- Monitor postictal period duration and characteristics

1st edition 1992; revised 2013

Background Evidence:

American Association of Neuroscience Nurses. (2009). *Care of the patient with seizures. AANN Clinical Practice Guidelines Series* (2nd ed. rev.).

Clore, E. (2010). Seizure precautions for pediatric bedside nurses. *Pediatric Nursing, 36*(4), 191–194.

Fitzsimmons, B., & Bohan, E. (2009). Common neurosurgical and neurological disorders. In P. Morton & D. Fontaine (Eds.), *Critical care nursing: A holistic approach* (9th ed., pp. 873–918). Lippincott Williams & Wilkins.

French, J., Kanner, A., Bautista, J., Abou-Kalil, B., Browne, T., Harden, C., Theodore, W. H., Bazil, C., Stern, J., Schachter, S. C., Bergen, D., Hirtz, D., Montouris, D., Nespeca, M., Gidal, B., Marks, W. J., Jr., Turk, W. R., Fischer, J. H., Bourgeois, B., Wilner, A., & Glauser, T. A. (2004). Efficacy and tolerability of the new antiepileptic drugs I: Treatment of new onset epilepsy. *Neurology, 62*(8), 1252–1260.

Smeltzer, S., Bare, B., Hinkle, J., & Cheever, K. (2010). Management of patients with neurological dysfunction. In *Brunner & Suddarth's textbook of medical-surgical nursing* (12th ed., pp. 1881–1888). Lippincott Williams & Wilkins.

Seizure Precautions 2690

Definition: Prevention or minimization of potential injuries sustained by a patient with a known seizure disorder

Activities:

- Provide low-height bed, as appropriate
- Escort patient during off-ward activities, as appropriate
- Monitor drug regimen
- Monitor compliance in taking antiepileptic medications
- Have patient or significant other keep record of medications taken and occurrence of seizure activity
- Instruct patient not to drive
- Instruct patient about medications and side effects
- Instruct family or significant other about seizure first aid
- Monitor antiepileptic drug levels, as appropriate
- Instruct patient to carry medication alert card
- Remove potentially harmful objects from the environment
- Keep suction at bedside
- Keep Ambu bag at bedside
- Keep oral or nasopharyngeal airway at bedside
- Use padded side rails
- Keep side rails up
- Instruct patient on potential precipitating factors
- Instruct patient to call if aura occurs

1st edition 1992; revised 2013

Background Evidence:

American Association of Neuroscience Nurses. (2009). *Care of the patient with seizures. AANN Clinical Practice Guidelines Series* (2nd ed. rev.).

Clore, E. (2010). Seizure precautions for pediatric bedside nurses. *Pediatric Nursing, 36*(4), 191–194.

Fitzsimmons, B., & Bohan, E. (2009). Common neurosurgical and neurological disorders. In P. Morton & D. Fontaine (Eds.), *Critical care nursing: A holistic approach* (9th ed., pp. 873–918). Lippincott Williams & Wilkins.

French, J., Kanner, A., Bautista, J., Abou-Kalil, B., Browne, T., Harden, C., Theodore, W. H., Bazil, C., Stern, J., Schachter, S. C., Bergen, D., Hirtz, D., Montouris, D., Nespeca, M., Gidal, B., Marks, W. J., Jr., Turk, W. R., Fischer, J. H., Bourgeois, B., Wilner, A., & Glauser, T. A. (2004). Efficacy and tolerability of the new antiepileptic drugs I: Treatment of new onset epilepsy. *Neurology, 62*(8), 1252–1260.

Smeltzer, S., Bare, B., Hinkle, J., & Cheever, K. (2010). Management of patients with neurological dysfunction. In *Brunner & Suddarth's textbook of medical-surgical nursing* (12th ed., pp. 1881–1888). Lippincott Williams & Wilkins.

Self-Awareness Enhancement 5390

S

Definition: Assisting a patient to explore and understand his/her thoughts, feelings, motivations, and behaviors

Activities:

- Encourage patient to recognize and discuss thoughts and feelings
- Assist patient to realize that everyone is unique
- Assist patient to identify the values that contribute to self-concept
- Assist patient to identify usual feelings about self
- Share observation or thoughts about patient's behavior or response
- Facilitate patient's identification of usual response patterns to various situations
- Assist patient to identify life priorities
- Assist patient to identify the effect of illness on self-concept
- Verbalize patient's denial of reality, as appropriate
- Confront patient's ambivalent (angry or depressed) feelings
- Make observation about patient's current emotional state
- Assist patient to accept dependency on others, as appropriate
- Assist patient to change view of self as victim by defining own rights, as appropriate
- Assist patient to be aware of negative self-statements
- Assist patient to identify guilty feelings
- Help patient identify situations that precipitate anxiety
- Explore with patient the need to control
- Assist patient to identify positive attributes of self
- Assist patient/family to identify reasons for improvement
- Assist patient to identify abilities and learning styles
- Assist patient to reexamine negative perceptions of self

- Assist patient to identify source of motivation
- Assist patient to identify behaviors that are self-destructive
- Facilitate self-expression with peer group
- Assist patient to recognize contradictory statements

1st edition 1992; revised 2004

Background Evidence:

Craven, R. F., & Hirnle, C. J. (2003). *Fundamentals of nursing: Human health and function* (4th ed.). Lippincott Williams & Wilkins.

Stuart, G. W., & Laraia, M. T. (2005). *Principles and practice of psychiatric nursing* (8th ed.). Mosby.

Self-Care Assistance   1800

Definition: Assisting another to perform activities of daily living

Activities:

- Determine level of assistance needed with self-care activities or instrumental activities of daily living (e.g., shopping, cooking, housekeeping, laundry, use of transportation, managing money, managing medications, use of communication, use of time)
- Consider culture and age when promoting self-care activities
- Determine needs for safety-related changes in home (e.g., wider door frames to allow for wheelchair access to bathroom, removal of scatter-rugs)
- Determine needs for home enhancements (e.g., laundry and other facilities located on main floor, side rails in hallways, grab-bars in bathrooms)
- Determine financial resources and personal preferences regarding modifications to home or care
- Verify presence of safety equipment in home (e.g., smoke detectors, carbon monoxide detectors, fire extinguishers)
- Verify adequacy of lighting throughout house, especially in working areas (e.g., kitchen, bathroom) and at night (e.g., appropriately placed nightlights)
- Provide tools to assist in daily activities (e.g., extenders to reach items in cupboards, in closets, on countertops, on stovetops, and in refrigerator; specialized knobs to operate household equipment such as stoves or microwaves)
- Provide cognitive enhancing techniques (e.g., up-to-date calendars, clearly legible and understandable lists for medication times, easy-to-see clocks)
- Provide visual safety devices or techniques (e.g., painting edges of steps bright yellow, clear pathway through walkways of house, non-skid surfaces installed in showers and bathtubs)
- Establish routine for self-care activities and assist with activities as needed
- Determine whether physical or cognitive ability stable or declining, and respond to changes accordingly
- Consult with occupational or physical therapist to collaborate on self-care needs
- Assist in establishing methods and routines for cooking, cleaning, and shopping
- Instruct to wear clothing with short or tight-fitting sleeves when cooking
- Assist in setting-up tasks so person can complete task (e.g., chop food, place clothing in easy-to-reach place, unpack groceries)
- Monitor ability for independent self-care
- Monitor need for adaptive devices for personal hygiene, dressing, grooming, toileting, and eating
- Provide therapeutic environment by ensuring warm, relaxing, private, and personalized experience
- Provide desired personal articles (e.g., deodorant, toothbrush, bath soap)
- Provide assistance until fully able to assume self-care
- Assist in accepting dependency needs

- Use consistent repetition of health routines as means of establishing them
- Encourage to perform normal activities of daily living to level of ability
- Encourage independence, but intervene when unable to perform
- Instruct family to encourage independence, to intervene only when unable to perform
- Provide methods of contacting for support and assistance (e.g., lifeline, list of nonemergent numbers for police, fire, poison control, utility companies)
- Instruct on alternative methods of transportation (e.g., buses and bus schedules, taxis, city or county transportation for disabled people)
- Obtain transportation enhancements to offset disabilities (e.g., hand controls on cars, wide rear-view mirror), as appropriate
- Instruct not to smoke in bed, while reclining, or after taking mind-altering medication
- Instruct individual and caregiver on what to do if experiences fall or other injury (e.g., what to do, how to gain access to emergency services, how to prevent further injury)
- Provide appropriate container for used sharps, as appropriate
- Instruct on appropriate and safe storage for medications
- Instruct on appropriate use of monitoring equipment (e.g., glucose-monitoring device, lancets)
- Instruct on appropriate methods of dressing wounds and appropriate disposal of soiled dressings
- Verify ability to open medication containers
- Refer to family and community services as needed
- Use teach-back to ensure understanding

1st edition 1992; revised 2008, 2024

Background Evidence:

Berman, A., Snyder, S. J., & Frandsen, G. (2018). In *Kozier and Erb's Fundamentals of nursing: Concepts, process and practice* (10th ed.). Pearson.

Craven, R. F., Hirnle, C. J., & Henshaw, C. J. (2021). Self-care and hygiene. In *Fundamentals of nursing: Human health and function* (8th ed.). Wolters-Kluwer.

Hockenberry, M. J., Rodgers, C. C., & Wilson, D. (2022). *Wong's essentials of pediatric nursing* (11th ed.). Elsevier.

Perry, A. G., Potter, P. A., Ostendorf, W. R., & LaPlante, N. (2021). *Clinical nursing skills and technique* (10th ed.). Mosby.

Potter, P. A., Perry, A. G., Stockert, P. A., & Hall, A. M. (2021). *Fundamentals of Nursing* (10th ed.). Elsevier.

Selbera, L. M., Boyd, L. D., Vineyard, J., & Smallidge, D. L. (2021). Impact of oral health education on the knowledge, behaviors, attitudes, and self-efficacy of caregivers for individuals with intellectual and developmental disabilities. *Journal of Dental Hygiene, 95*(2), 21–27.

Williams, P. (2020). *Basic geriatric nursing* (7th ed.). Elsevier.

Self-Care Assistance: Toileting 1804

Definition: Assisting another with elimination

Activities:
- Consider the culture of the patient when promoting self-care activities
- Consider age of patient when promoting self-care activities
- Remove essential clothing to allow for elimination
- Assist patient to toilet/commode/bedpan/fracture pan/urinal at specified intervals
- Consider patient's response to lack of privacy
- Provide privacy during elimination
- Facilitate toilet hygiene after completion of elimination
- Replace patient's clothing after elimination
- Flush toilet/cleanse elimination utensil (commode, bedpan)
- Institute a toileting schedule, as appropriate
- Instruct patient/appropriate others in toileting routine
- Institute bathroom rounds, as appropriate and needed
- Provide assistive devices (e.g., external catheter or urinal), as appropriate
- Monitor patient's skin integrity

1st edition 1992; revised 2008

Background Evidence:

Kozier, B., Erb, G., Berman, A., & Snyder, S. (2004). *Fundamentals of nursing: Concepts, process, and practice* (7th ed.). Prentice Hall.

Perry, A. G., & Potter, P. A. (2006). *Clinical nursing skills and techniques* (6th ed.). Elsevier Mosby.

Smith, S. F., Duell, D. J., & Martin, B. C. (2004). *Clinical nursing skills: Basic to advanced skills* (6th ed.). Prentice Hall.

Self-Care Assistance: Transfer 1806

Definition: Assisting a patient with limitation of independent movement to learn to change body location

Activities:
- Review chart for activity orders
- Determine current ability of patient to transfer self (e.g., mobility level, limitations of movement, endurance, ability to stand and bear weight, medical or orthopedic instability, level of consciousness, ability to cooperate, ability to comprehend instructions)
- Select transfer technique that is appropriate for patient
- Instruct patient in all appropriate techniques with the goal of reaching the highest level of independence
- Instruct individual on techniques for transfer from one area to another (e.g., bed to chair, wheelchair to vehicle)
- Instruct individual in use of ambulatory aids (e.g., crutches, wheelchairs, walkers, trapeze bars, cane)
- Identify methods to prevent injury during transfer
- Provide assistive devices (e.g., bars attached to walls, ropes attached to headboard or footboard for help in moving to center or edge of bed) to help individual transfer independently, as appropriate
- Make sure equipment works before using it
- Demonstrate technique, as appropriate
- Determine amount and type of assistance needed
- Assist patient in receiving all necessary care (e.g., personal hygiene, gathering belongings) before performing the transfer, as appropriate
- Provide privacy, avoid drafts, and preserve the patient's modesty
- Use proper body mechanics during movements
- Keep patient's body in proper alignment during movements
- Raise and move patient with a hydraulic lift as necessary
- Move patient using a transfer board as necessary
- Use a belt to assist a patient who can stand with assistance, as appropriate
- Assist patient to ambulate using your body as a human crutch, as appropriate
- Maintain traction devices during move, as appropriate
- Evaluate patient at end of transfer for proper body alignment, nonocclusion of tubes, wrinkled linens, unnecessarily exposed skin, adequate patient level of comfort, raised side rails, and call bell within reach
- Provide encouragement to patient as he/she learns to transfer independently
- Document progress, as appropriate

4th edition 2004; revised 2008

Background Evidence:

Lewis, S. M., Hetkemper, M. M., & Dirksen, S. R. (2003). *Medical-surgical nursing: Assessment and management of clinical problems.* Mosby.

Perry, A. G., & Potter, P. A. (2004). *Fundamentals of nursing* (6th ed.). Mosby.

Perry, A. G., & Potter, P. A. (2006). *Clinical nursing skills and techniques* (6th ed.). Elsevier Mosby.

Smeltzer, S. C., & Bare, B. G. (2004). *Brunner & Suddarth's textbook of medical-surgical nursing* (10th ed.). Lippincott Williams and Wilkins.

S

Self-Efficacy Enhancement 5395

Definition: Strengthening an individual's confidence in his/her ability to perform a health behavior

Activities:
- Explore individual's perception of his/her capability to perform the desired behavior
- Explore individual's perception of benefits of executing the desired behavior
- Identify individual's perception of risks of not executing the desired behavior
- Identify barriers to changing behavior
- Provide information about the desired behavior
- Assist individual to commit to a plan of action for changing behavior

- Reinforce confidence in making behavior changes and taking action
- Provide an environment supportive to learning knowledge and skills needed to carry out the behavior
- Use teaching strategies that are culturally and age appropriate (e.g., games, computer-assisted instruction, or conversation maps)
- Model/demonstrate desired behavior
- Engage in role play to rehearse behavior
- Provide positive reinforcement and emotional support during the learning process and while implementing the behavior
- Provide opportunities for mastery experiences (e.g., successful implementation of the behavior)
- Use positive persuasive statements regarding the individual's ability to carry out the behavior
- Encourage interaction with other individuals who are successfully changing their behavior (e.g., support group or group education participation)
- Prepare individual for the physiological and emotional states that may be experienced during initial attempts to carry out a new behavior

5th edition 2008

Background Evidence:
Bandura, A. (1997). *Self-efficacy: The exercise of control*. W. H. Freeman.
Fisher, K. (2006). School nurses' perceptions of self-efficacy in providing diabetes care. *Journal of School Nursing, 22*(4), 223–228.
Lau-Walker, M. (2006). A conceptual care model for individualized care approach in cardiac rehabilitation—combining both illness representation and self-efficacy. *British Journal of Health Psychology, 11*(pt. 1), 103–117.
Litarowsky, J. A., Murphy, S. O., & Canham, D. L. (2004). Evaluation of an anaphylaxis training program for unlicensed assistive personnel. *Journal of School Nursing, 20*(5), 279–284.
Long, J. D., & Stevens, K. R. (2004). Using technology to promote self-efficacy for healthy eating in adolescents. *Journal of Nursing Scholarship, 36*(2), 34–139.
Pender, N. J., Murdaugh, C. L., & Parsons, M. A. (2002). *Health promotion in nursing practice* (4th ed.). Prentice Hall.

Self-Esteem Enhancement   5400

Definition: Assisting a patient to increase his or her personal judgment of self-worth

Activities:

- Monitor patient's statements of self-worth
- Determine patient's locus of control
- Determine patient's confidence in own judgment
- Encourage patient to identify strengths
- Assist patient to find self-acceptance
- Encourage eye contact in communicating with others
- Reinforce the personal strengths that patient identifies
- Encourage patient to engage in self-talk and to verbalize positive affirmations daily to self
- Provide experiences that increase patient's autonomy, as appropriate
- Assist patient to identify positive responses from others
- Refrain from negatively criticizing
- Assist the patient to cope with bullying or teasing
- Convey confidence in patient's ability to handle situation
- Assist in setting realistic goals to achieve higher self-esteem
- Assist patient to accept dependence on others, as appropriate
- Assist patient to reexamine negative perceptions of self
- Encourage increased responsibility for self, as appropriate
- Assist patient to identify the effect of peer group on feelings of self-worth
- Explore previous achievements of success
- Explore reasons for self-criticism or guilt
- Encourage the patient to evaluate own behavior
- Encourage patient to accept new challenges
- Reward or praise patient's progress toward reaching goals
- Facilitate an environment and activities that will increase self-esteem
- Assist patient to identify significance of culture, religion, race, gender, and age on self-esteem
- Instruct parents on the importance of their interest and support in their children's development of a positive self-concept
- Instruct parents to set clear expectations and to define limits with their children
- Instruct parents to recognize children's accomplishments
- Monitor frequency of self-negating verbalizations
- Monitor lack of follow-through in goal attainment
- Monitor levels of self-esteem over time, as appropriate
- Make positive statements about patient

1st edition 1992; revised 2013

Background Evidence:
Bode, C., van der Heij, A., Taal, E., & van de Laar, M. A. (2010). Body-self unity and self-esteem in patients with rheumatic diseases. *Psychology, Health & Medicine, 15*(6), 672–684.
Bunten, D. (2001). Normal changes with aging. In M. Maas, K. Buckwalter, M. Hardy, T. Tripp-Reimer, M. Titler, & J. Specht (Eds.), *Nursing care of older adults: Diagnoses, outcomes, & interventions* (pp. 518–520). Mosby.
Lai, H., Lu, C., Jwo, J., Lee, P., Chou, W., & Wen, W. (2009). The effects of a self-esteem program incorporated into health and physical education classes. *Journal of Nursing Research, 17*(4), 233–240.
Lim, J., Kim, M., Kim, S., Kim, E., Lee, J., & Ko, Y. (2010). The effects of a cognitive-behavioral therapy on career attitude maturity, decision making style, and self-esteem of nursing students in Korea. *Nurse Education Today, 30*(8), 731–736.
Weber, S., Puskar, K., & Ren, D. (2010). Relationships between depressive symptoms and perceived social support, self-esteem, & optimism in a sample of rural adolescents. *Issues in Mental Health Nursing, 31*(9), 584–588.

S

Self-Hypnosis Facilitation   5922

Definition: Teaching and monitoring the use of a self-initiated hypnotic state for therapeutic benefit

Activities:

- Determine whether the patient is an appropriate candidate for self-hypnosis
- Utilize self-hypnosis as an adjunct to other treatment modalities (e.g., individual hypnotherapy by a therapist, individual psychotherapy, group therapy, family therapy, etc.)
- Introduce the patient to the concept of self-hypnosis as a therapeutic modality
- Identify with the patient those problems/issues that are amenable to treatment with self-hypnosis
- Obtain history of the problem to be treated by self-hypnosis
- Determine goals for self-hypnosis with patient
- Determine patient's receptivity about using self-hypnosis
- Correct myths and misconceptions of self-hypnosis
- Ensure the patient has accepted the treatment
- Evaluate the suitability of the patient by assessing his or her hypnotic suggestibility
- Provide the patient with an individualized procedure for the process of self-hypnosis that reflects his/her specific needs and goals
- Assist the patient to identify appropriate induction techniques (e.g., Chevreul's pendulum illusion, relaxation, imagining walking down a staircase, eye closure, arm levitation, simple muscle relaxation, visualization exercises, attention to breathing, repetition of key words/phrases, and others)
- Assist the patient to identify appropriate deepening techniques (e.g., movement of a hand to the face, imagery escalation technique, fractionation, and others)
- Encourage the patient to become proficient at self-hypnosis by practicing the technique
- Contract for a practice schedule with the patient, if needed
- Monitor the patient's response to self-hypnosis on an ongoing basis
- Solicit the patient's feedback regarding his/her comfort with the procedure and experience of self-hypnosis
- Assist the patient to process and interpret what occurs as a result of the self-hypnosis sessions
- Recommend modifications in the patient's practice of self-hypnosis (frequency, intensity, specific techniques) based on his/her response and level of comfort
- Assist the patient to evaluate progress made toward therapy goals

4th edition 2004; revised 2008

Background Evidence:

Fontaine, K. L. (2005). Hypnotherapy and guided imagery. In K. L. Fontaine (Ed.), *Complementary & alternative therapies for nursing practice* (2nd ed., pp. 301–338). Prentice Hall.

Freeman, L. (Ed.). (2004). Hypnosis. In *Mosby's complementary & alternative medicine: A research-based approach* (2nd ed., pp. 237–274). Mosby.

Fromm, E., & Kahn, S. (1990). *Self-hypnosis. The Chicago paradigm.* The Guilford Press.

Lynn, S. J., & Kirsch, I. (2006). *Essentials of clinical hypnosis: An evidence-based approach.* Washington, DC: American Psychological Association.

Rankin-Box, D. (2001). Hypnosis. In D. Rankin-Box (Ed.), *The nurse's handbook of complementary therapies* (2nd ed., pp. 208–214). Edinburgh: Bailliere Tindall.

Sanders, S. (1991). *Clinical self-hypnosis: The power of words and images.* The Guilford Press.

Zahourek, R. P. (1985). *Clinical hypnosis and therapeutic suggestion in nursing.* Grune & Stratton.

Zarren, J. I., & Eimer, B. N. (2002). *Brief cognitive hypnosis: Facilitating the change of dysfunctional behavior.* Springer.

Self-Modification Assistance   4470

Definition: Reinforcement of self-directed change initiated by the patient to achieve personally important goals

Activities:

- Encourage the patient to examine personal values and beliefs and his or her satisfaction with them
- Appraise the patient's reasons for wanting to change
- Assist the patient in identifying a specific goal for change
- Assist the patient in identifying target behaviors that need to change to achieve the desired goal
- Assist the patient in identifying the target behaviors' effects on social and environmental surroundings
- Appraise the patient's present knowledge and skill level in relationship to the desired change
- Assist the patient in identifying the stages of change: precontemplation, contemplation, preparation, action, maintenance, and termination
- Appraise the patient's social and physical environment for extent of support of desired behaviors
- Explore with the patient potential barriers to change behavior
- Identify with the patient the most effective strategies for behavior change
- Explain to the patient the importance of self-monitoring in attempting behavior change
- Assist the patient in identifying the frequency with which specific behaviors occur
- Assist the patient in developing a portable, easy-to-use coding sheet to aid in recording behaviors (may be a graph or chart)
- Instruct the patient to record the incidence of behaviors for at least 3 days but up to 2 to 3 weeks
- Encourage the patient to identify appropriate, meaningful reinforcers and rewards
- Encourage the patient to choose a reinforcer or reward that is significant enough to sustain the behavior
- Assist the patient in developing a list of valued extrinsic and intrinsic rewards
- Encourage the patient to begin with extrinsic rewards and progress to intrinsic rewards
- Instruct the patient that reward list may include manners in which the nurse, family, or friends can assist the patient in behavior change

S

- Assist the patient in formulating a systematic plan for behavior change
- Encourage the patient to identify steps that are manageable in size and able to be accomplished in a set amount of time
- Foster moving toward primary reliance on self-reinforcement instead of family or nurse for rewards
- Instruct the patient on how to move from continuous reinforcement to intermittent reinforcement
- Assist the patient in evaluating progress by comparing records of previous behavior with present behavior
- Encourage the patient to develop a visual measure of changes in behavior (e.g., a graph)
- Foster flexibility during the shaping plan, promoting complete mastery of one step before advancing to the next
- Encourage the patient to adjust the shaping plan to enhance behavior change (e.g., size of steps or reward), if needed
- Assist the patient in identifying the circumstances or situations in which the behavior occurs (e.g., cues, triggers)
- Assist the patient in identifying even small successes
- Explain to the patient the function of cues and triggers in producing behavior
- Assist the patient in appraising the physical, social, and interpersonal settings for the existence of cues and triggers
- Encourage the patient to develop a "cue analysis sheet" that illustrates links between cues and behaviors
- Instruct the patient on the use of "cue expansion," increasing the number of cues that prompt a desired behavior
- Instruct the patient on the use of "cue restriction or limitation," decreasing the frequency of cues that elicit an undesirable behavior
- Assist the patient in identifying methods of controlling behavioral cues
- Assist the patient in identifying existent behaviors that are habitual or automatic (e.g., brushing teeth and tying shoes)
- Assist the patient in identifying existing paired stimuli and habitual behavior (e.g., eating a meal and brushing teeth afterward)

- Encourage the patient to pair a desired behavior with an existing stimulus or cue (e.g., exercising after work every day)
- Encourage the patient to continue pairing desired behavior with existing stimuli until it becomes automatic or habitual
- Explore with the patient the option of using a technological device in organizing coding sheets, change data, cue analysis, and visual measures of change (e.g., computer, smart phone)
- Explore with the patient the potential use of imagery, meditation, or progressive relaxation in attempting behavior change
- Explore with the patient the possibility of using role playing to clarify behaviors

1st edition 1992; revised 2013

Background Evidence:

Antony, M. M. (2005). Cognitive behavior therapy. In M. Hersen (Ed.), *Encyclopedia of behavior modification and cognitive behavior therapy* (pp. 186–195). Sage.

Franklin, P. D., Farzanfar, R., & Thompson, D. D. (2009). E-health strategies to support adherence. In S. A. Shumaker, J. K. Ockene, & K. A. Riekert (Eds.), *Handbook of health behavior change* (3rd ed., pp. 169–190). Springer.

Karoly, P. (2005). Self-control. In M. Hersen & J. Rosqvist (Eds.), *Encyclopedia of behavior modification and cognitive behavior therapy* (pp. 504–508). Sage.

Karoly, P. (2005). Self-monitoring. In M. Hersen & J. Rosqvist (Eds.), *Encyclopedia of behavior modification and cognitive behavior therapy* (pp. 521–525). Sage.

Prochaska, J. O., Johnson, S., & Lee, P. (2008). The transtheoretical model of behavior change. In S. A. Shumaker, J. K. Ockene, & K. A. Riekert (Eds.), *Handbook of health behavior change* (3rd ed., pp. 59–84). Springer.

Stuart, G. W. (Ed.). (2009). *Principles and practice of psychiatric nursing* (9th ed.). Mosby Elsevier.

Watson, D. L., & Tharp, R. G. (2007). *Self-directing behavior: Self-modification for personal adjustment* (9th ed.). Wadsworth.

Self-Responsibility Facilitation 4480

Definition: Encouraging a patient to assume more responsibility for own behavior

Activities:

- Hold patient responsible for own behavior
- Discuss with patient the extent of responsibility for present health status
- Determine whether patient has adequate knowledge about health care condition
- Encourage verbalizations of feelings, perceptions, and fears about assuming responsibility
- Assist patients to identify areas in which they could readily assume more responsibility
- Encourage goal setting
- Facilitate the patient and family to make choices concerning their care, as appropriate
- Encourage independence, but assist patient when unable to perform
- Ensure patients and family members have the appropriate resources to assume more responsibility
- Discuss consequences of not dealing with own responsibilities
- Provide opportunities for self-evaluation and self-reflection
- Monitor level of responsibility that patient assumes

- Provide positive constructive feedback for accepting additional responsibility for behavior change
- Encourage admission of wrongdoing, as appropriate
- Set limits on manipulative behaviors
- Refrain from arguing or bargaining about the established limits with the patient
- Encourage patient to take as much responsibility as possible for own self-care
- Assist parents in identifying age-appropriate tasks for which a child could be responsible, as appropriate
- Encourage parents to clearly communicate expectations for responsible behavior in child, as appropriate
- Encourage parents to follow through on expectations for responsible behavior in child, as appropriate
- Facilitate family support for new level of responsibility sought or attained by patient
- Assist with creating a timetable to guide increased responsibility in the future

1st edition 1992; revised 1996, 2018

Background Evidence:

Betancourt, J. R., & Quinlan, J. (2007). Personal responsibility versus responsible options: Health care, community health promotion, and the battle against chronic disease. *Preventing Chronic Disease*, *4*(3). http://www.cdc.gov/pc/issues/2007/jul/07_0017.htm

Fortinash, K., & Worret, P. (2012). *Psychiatric mental health nursing* (5th ed.). Elsevier Mosby.

Horton, S. (2014). What is personal health responsibility? *ABNF Journal*, *25*(1), 5–9.

Schmidt, H. (2009). Just health responsibility. *Journal of Medical Ethics*, *35*(1), 21–26.

Snelling, P. C. (2012). Say something interesting about responsibility for health. *Nursing Philosophy*, *13*(3), 161–178.

Sexual Assault Trauma Care   6300

Definition: Provision of emotional and physical support immediately following a reported sexual assault

Activities:
- Provide support individual to stay with person
- Contact Sexual Assault Nurse Examiners (SANEs), forensically trained nurses, Sexual Assault Response Teams (SART), Sexual Assault Forensic Examiners (SAFEs), or Sexual Assault Examiners (SAEs) to conduct examination, as available in organization
- Inform person about availability of sexual assault crisis counsellor
- Contact sexual assault crisis counsellor upon request of person
- Explain legal proceedings available
- Explain sexual assault protocol and obtain consent to proceed
- Document whether showered, douched, or bathed after incident
- Document mental state, physical state (e.g., clothing, dirt, debris), history of incident, evidence of violence, and prior gynecological history
- Determine presence of cuts, bruises, bleeding, lacerations, or other signs of physical injury
- Implement sexual assault protocol (i.e., label and save soiled clothing, vaginal secretions, fingernail scraping, vaginal hair combings)
- Secure samples for legal evidence
- Offer medication to prevent pregnancy, as appropriate
- Offer prophylactic antibiotic medication against STI
- Offer hepatitis B vaccination
- Inform patient of HIV testing, as appropriate
- Give clear, written instructions about medication use, crisis support services, and legal support
- Provide with sexual assault crisis center phone number
- Document according to agency and sexual assault collection policy
- Secure all collection evidence in locked area and hold for law enforcement

1st edition 1992; revised 2000, 2024

Background Evidence:

American Nursing Association. (2017). *Forensic nursing: Scope and standards of practice* (2nd ed.).

Boyd, M. R. (2018). Caring for abused persons. In M. A. Boyd (Ed.), *Psychiatric nursing: Contemporary practice* (6th ed.). Wolters Kluwer.

Cochran, C. B. (2019). An evidence-based approach to suicide risk assessment after sexual assault. *Journal of Forensic Nursing*, *15*(2), 84–92. https://doi.org/10.1097/JFN.0000000000000241

Delgadillo, D. C. (2017). When there is no sexual assault nurse examiner: Emergency nursing care for female adult sexual assault patients. *JEN: Journal of Emergency Nursing*, *43*(4), 308–315. https://doi.org/10.1016/j.jen.2016.11.006

Dworkin, E. R. (2020). Risk for mental disorders associated with sexual assault: A meta-analysis. *Trauma, Violence & Abuse*, *21*(5), 1011–1028.

Grundy-Bowers, M., & Read, M. (2020). Developing cultural competence in caring for LGBTQI+ patients. *Nursing Standard*, *35*(2), 29–34. https://doi.org/10.7748/ns.2019.e11390

Nathan, S., & Ferrara, M. (2020). An innovative trauma-informed curriculum for sexual assault care. *Journal of Nursing Education*, *59*(6), 336–340. https://doi.org/10.3928/01484834-20200520-07

U.S. Department of Justice. (2018). *National Training Standards for Sexual Assault Medical Forensic Examiners* (2nd ed.).

Sexual Counseling   5248

Definition: Use of an interactive process focusing on the need to make adjustments in sexual practice or to enhance coping with a sexual event or disorder

Activities:
- Establish a therapeutic relationship based on trust and respect
- Establish the length of the counseling relationship
- Provide privacy and ensure confidentiality
- Inform patient early in the relationship that sexuality is an important part of life and that illness, medications, and stress (or other problems and events patient is experiencing) often alter sexual functioning
- Encourage patient to verbalize fears and to ask questions about sexual functioning
- Preface questions about sexuality with a statement that tells the patient that many people experience sexual difficulties
- Begin with the least sensitive topics and proceed to the more sensitive
- Collect the client's sexual history paying close attention to normal patterns of functioning and the terms used by the patient to describe sexual function
- Determine the duration of sexual dysfunction and potential causes
- Monitor for stress, anxiety, and depression as possible causes of sexual dysfunction
- Determine the knowledge level of the patient and understanding about sexuality in general
- Provide information about sexual functioning, as appropriate

S

- Discuss the effect of the health and illness on sexuality
- Discuss the effect of medications and supplements on sexuality, as appropriate
- Discuss the effect of changes in sexuality on significant other
- Discuss necessary modifications in sexual activity, as appropriate
- Help patient to express grief and anger about alterations in body functioning or appearance, as appropriate
- Avoid displaying aversion to an altered body part
- Introduce patient to positive role models who have successfully conquered a similar problem, as appropriate
- Provide factual information about sexual myths and misinformation that patient may verbalize
- Discuss alternative forms of sexual expression that are acceptable to patient, as appropriate
- Instruct the patient on use of medication(s) and devices to enhance ability to perform sexually, as appropriate
- Determine amount of sexual guilt associated with the patient's perception of the causative factors of illness
- Avoid prematurely terminating discussion of guilt feelings, even when these seem unreasonable
- Include the significant other in the counseling as much as possible, as appropriate
- Use humor and encourage patient to use humor to relieve anxiety or embarrassment, being careful to use humor that is appropriate to the situation, tactful, and respectful of patient beliefs and cultural background
- Provide reassurance that current and new sexual practices are healthy, as appropriate
- Provide reassurance and permission to experiment with alternative forms of sexual expression, as appropriate
- Provide referral or consultation with other members of the health care team, as appropriate
- Refer the patient to a sex therapist, as appropriate

1st edition 1992; revised 2013

Background Evidence:

Barton-Burke, M., & Gustason, C. J. (2007). Sexuality in women with cancer. *Nursing Clinics of North America, 42*(4), 531–554.

Brassil, D. F., & Keller, M. (2002). Female sexual dysfunction: Definitions, causes, and treatment. *Urologic Nursing, 22*(4), 237–244, 284.

Clayton, A., & Ramamurthy, S. (2008). The impact of physical illness on sexual dysfunction. *Advances in Psychosomatic Medicine, 29*, 70–88.

Ginsberg, T. B., Pomerantz, S. C., & Kramer-Feeley, V. (2005). Sexuality in older adults: Behaviours and preferences. *Age and Ageing, 34*(5), 475–480.

Jaarsma, T., Steinke, E. E., & Gianotten, W. L. (2010). Sexual problems in cardiac patients: How to assess, when to refer. *Journal of Cardiovascular Nursing, 25*(2), 159–164.

Lewis, L. J. (2004). Examining sexual health discourses in a racial/ethnic context. *Archives of Sexual Behavior, 33*(3), 223–234.

Schwarz, E. R., Kapur, V., Bionat, S., Rastogi, S., Gupta, R., & Rosanio, S. (2008). The prevalence and clinical relevance of sexual dysfunction in women and men with chronic heart failure. *International Journal of Impotence Research, 20*(1), 85–91.

Steinke, E. E. (2005). Intimacy needs and chronic illness. *Journal of Gerontological Nursing, 31*(5), 40–50.

Steinke, E. E., & Jaarsma, T. (2008). Impact of cardiovascular disease on sexuality. In D. Moser & B. Riegel (Eds.), *Cardiac nursing: A companion to Braunwald's heart disease* (pp. 241–253). Saunders Elsevier.

Shock Management   4250

Definition: Facilitation of the delivery of oxygen and nutrients to systemic tissue with removal of cellular waste products in a patient with severely altered tissue perfusion

Activities:

- Monitor vital signs, orthostatic blood pressure, mental status, and urinary output
- Position the patient for optimal perfusion
- Institute and maintain airway patency, as appropriate
- Monitor pulse oximetry, as appropriate
- Administer oxygen and/or mechanical ventilation, as appropriate
- Monitor ECG, as appropriate
- Utilize arterial line monitoring to improve accuracy of blood pressure readings, as appropriate
- Draw arterial blood gases and monitor tissue oxygenation
- Monitor trends in hemodynamic parameters (e.g., CVP, MAP, pulmonary capillary/artery wedge pressure)
- Monitor determinants of tissue oxygen delivery (e.g., PaO_2, SaO_2, hemoglobin levels, CO), if available
- Monitor sublingual carbon dioxide levels and/or gastric tonometry, as appropriate
- Monitor for symptoms of respiratory failure (e.g., low PaO_2, elevated $PaCO_2$ levels, respiratory muscle fatigue)
- Monitor laboratory values (e.g., CBC with differential, coagulation profile, ABG, lactate level, cultures, and chemistry profile)
- Insert and maintain large bore IV access
- Administer IV fluid challenge while monitoring hemodynamic pressures and urinary output, as appropriate
- Administer crystalloid or colloid intravenous fluids, as appropriate
- Administer packed red blood cells, fresh frozen plasma, and/or platelets, as appropriate
- Monitor for hyperdynamic state of septic shock post fluid resuscitation (e.g., increased CO, decreased SVR, flushed skin, or increased temperature)
- Administer vasopressors, as appropriate
- Administer antiarrhythmic agents, as appropriate
- Initiate early administration of antimicrobial agents and closely monitor their effectiveness, as appropriate
- Administer antiinflammatory agents and/or bronchodilators, as appropriate
- Monitor serum glucose and treat abnormal levels, as appropriate
- Monitor fluid status, including daily weights, hourly urine output, I&O
- Monitor renal function (e.g., BUN, Cr levels, creatinine clearance)
- Administer diuretics, as appropriate
- Administer continuous renal replacement therapy or hemodialysis, as appropriate
- Insert nasogastric tube to suction and monitor secretions, as appropriate
- Administer thrombolytics, as appropriate
- Administer recombinant activated protein C, as appropriate
- Administer low dose vasopressin, as appropriate
- Administer corticosteroids, as appropriate

S

- Administer inotropes, as appropriate
- Administer venodilators, as appropriate
- Administer DVT and stress ulcer prophylaxis, as appropriate
- Offer emotional support to the patient and family, encouraging realistic expectations

1st edition 1992; revised 2004, 2008

Background Evidence:

Ahrens, T., & Tuggle, D. (2004). Surviving sever sepsis: Early recognition and treatment. *Critical Care Nurse, 24*(Suppl. 2), 2–15.

Albright, T. N., Zimmerman, M. A., & Selzman, C. H. (2002). Vasopressin in the cardiac surgery intensive care unit. *American Journal of Critical Care, 11*(4), 326–330.

American Heart Association. (2005). 2005 American Heart Association guidelines for cardiopulmonary resuscitation and emergency cardiovascular care. *Circulation, 112*(Suppl. 24), IV-1–IV-211.

Bridges, E. J., & Dukes, S. (2005). Cardiovascular aspects of septic shock: Pathophysiology, monitoring, and treatment. *Critical Care Nurse, 25*(2), 14–40.

Dellinger, R. P., Carlet, J. M., Masur, H., Gerlach, H., Calandra, T., Cohen, J., Gea-Banacloche, J., Keh, D., Marshall, J. C., Parker, M. M., Ramsay, G., Zimmerman, J. L., Vincent, J.-L., & Levy, M. (2004). Surviving sepsis campaign guidelines for management of severe sepsis and septic shock. *Critical Care Medicine, 32*(3), 858–873.

Flynn, M. B., & McLeskey, S. (2005). Shock, systemic inflammatory response syndrome, and multiple organ dysfunction syndrome. In P. G. Morton, D. K. Fontaine, C. M. Hudak, & B. M. Gallo (Eds.), *Critical care nursing: A holistic approach* (8th ed., pp. 1152–1178). Lippincott Williams & Wilkins.

Porth, C. M. (2004). *Essentials of pathophysiology: Concepts of altered health states*. Lippincott Williams & Wilkins.

Smeltzer, S. C., & Bare, B. G. (2004). *Brunner & Suddarth's textbook of medical-surgical nursing* (10th ed.). Lippincott Williams & Wilkins.

Tazbir, J. (2004). Sepsis and the role of activated protein C. *Critical Care Nurse, 24*(6), 40–45.

Shock Management: Cardiac   4254

Definition: Promotion of adequate tissue perfusion for a patient with severely compromised pumping function of the heart

Activities:

- Monitor for signs and symptoms of decreased cardiac output
- Auscultate lung sounds for crackles or other adventitious sounds
- Note signs and symptoms of decreased cardiac output
- Monitor for inadequate coronary artery perfusion (ST changes on EKG, elevated cardiac enzymes, angina), as appropriate
- Monitor coagulation studies, including prothrombin time (PT), partial thromboplastin time (PTT), fibrinogen, fibrin degradation/split products, and platelet counts, as appropriate
- Monitor and evaluate indicators of tissue hypoxia (mixed venous oxygen saturation, central venous oxygen saturation, serum lactate levels, sublingual capnometry)
- Administer supplemental oxygen, as appropriate
- Maintain optimal preload by administering IV fluids or diuretics, as appropriate
- Prepare patient for cardiac revascularization (percutaneous coronary intervention or coronary artery bypass graft)
- Administer positive inotropic/contractility medications, as appropriate
- Promote afterload reduction (e.g., with vasodilators, angiotensin converting enzyme inhibitors, or intraaortic balloon pumping), as appropriate
- Promote optimal preload while minimizing afterload (e.g., administer nitrates while maintaining pulmonary artery occlusion pressure within prescribed range), as appropriate
- Promote adequate organ system perfusion (with fluid resuscitation and/or vasopressors to maintain mean arterial pressure greater than or equal to 60 mm Hg, as appropriate

1st edition 1992; revised 2008

Background Evidence:

Antman, E., Anbe, D., Armstrong, P., Bates, E., Green, L., Hand, M., Hockman, J. S., Krumholz, H. M., Kushner, F. G., Lamas, G. A., Mullany, C. J., Ornato, J. P., Pearle, D. L., Sloan, M. A., Smith, S. C., Antman, E. M., Smith, S. C., Alpert, J. S., Anderson, J. L., Faxon, D. P., & Ornato, J. (2004). ACC/AHA guidelines for the management of patients with ST-elevation myocardial infarction—Executive summary. *Circulation, 110*(5), 588–636.

Bridges, E. J., & Dukes, S. (2005). Cardiovascular aspects of septic shock: Pathophysiology, monitoring, and treatment. *Critical Care Nurse, 25*(2), 14–40.

Hollenberg, S., Ahrens, T., Annane, D., Astiz, M., Chalfin, D., Dasta, J., Heard, S., Martin, C., Napolitano, L., Susla, G., Totaro, R., Vincent, J.-L., & Zanotti-Cavazzoni, S. (2004). Practice parameters for hemodynamic support of sepsis in adult patients: 2004 update. *Critical Care Medicine, 32*(9), 1928–1948.

Irwin, R. S., & Rippe, J. M. (Eds.). (2003). *Irwin and Rippe's intensive care medicine* (5th ed.). Lippincott Williams & Wilkins.

McCance, K. L., & Huether, S. E. (2002). *Pathophysiology: The biologic basis for disease in adults and children* (4th ed.). Mosby.

S

Shock Management: Sepsis   4255

Definition: Promotion of adequate tissue perfusion for a person with a life-threatening organ dysfunction and an overreactive systemic response to infection

Activities:

- Determine sepsis risk level
- Use appropriate screening tools once risk level established (e.g., Sequential Organ Failure Assessment [SOFA], quick SOFA [qSOFA], Systemic Inflammatory Response Syndrome [SIRS] Criteria)
- Identify presence of at-risk conditions (e.g., age, debilitated and immunocompromised persons, recent illness, trauma, invasive procedures, chronic conditions, change in cognition and affect)
- Evaluate vital signs and laboratory values using prescribed criteria from screening tools
- Use real time surveillance screening

- Identify possible causes (e.g., recent exposure to infection)
- Remove any potential source of infections (e.g., inflamed IV lines, urinary catheters with cloudy output)
- Follow protocol for sepsis care bundle for all persons with positive screening results and confirmed infections, in prescribed time frames (i.e., 1-hour resuscitation bundle started within 1 hour of person presentation of sepsis or septic shock; may not necessarily complete all bundle elements within 1 hour of recognition)
- Monitor lactate levels continuously when >2 mmol/L
- Obtain blood cultures as quickly as possible and prior to administering antibiotics
- Administer broad spectrum IV antibiotics within first hour, as prescribed
- Administer IV crystalloid for hypotension (MAP <65 mm Hg) or lactate ≥4 mmol/L, per protocol and facility policy
- Apply vasopressors if remains hypotensive (MAP <65 mmHg) during or after fluid resuscitation, as prescribed
- Use vasopressors to maintain MAP ≥65 mmHg
- Reexamine volume status and tissue perfusion after initial fluid administration if persistent hypotension (MAP <65 mmHg) or if initial lactate was ≥4 mmol/L
- Ensure all bundle criteria achieved within prescribed time frames (i.e., less than 1 hour but no more than 6 hours)
- Apply bundle criteria time frames with clock start when person meets screening criteria, or in ER, clock begins at presentation to triage
- Document all reassessments and ongoing bundle or resuscitation measures
- Perform focused exam after initial fluid resuscitation, including at least two of the following: CVP, SvO$_2$, bedside cardiovascular ultrasound, dynamic assessment of fluid responsiveness with passive leg raises or fluid challenge
- Maintain ongoing screening for SIRS criteria in at-risk persons (e.g., fever, HR, respiratory rate, PaCO$_2$, laboratory values)
- Maintain ongoing screening for SOFA criteria in qualifying at-risk persons (e.g., blood pressure, respiratory rate, any change in mental status)
- Maintain ongoing screening for qSOFA criteria in qualifying at-risk persons (e.g., oxygen levels, laboratory values, hypotension requiring vasopressor support, Glasgow Coma Scale score, urine output)
- Ensure ongoing screening for septic shock in persons meeting sepsis criteria (e.g., significantly decreased urine output, abrupt change in mental status, decrease in platelet count, difficulty breathing, abnormal heart pumping function, abdominal pain)
- Communicate sepsis status in handoff reports
- Use aseptic technique with all at-risk and immunocompromised persons
- Ensure that all catheters and IVs are discontinued as soon as possible
- Monitor for early detection indicators (e.g., increased serum lactate level, normal or low WBC count, decreased segmented WBC level, increased immature WBC level)

- Instruct on signs of infection, how to monitor temperature, need to take all prescribed antibiotics to completion, and time matters with severe infections
- Educate about underlying medical conditions and potential hazards
- Instruct on need for vaccinations (e.g., influenza, pneumonia)
- Instruct on need to prevent infections by cleaning all wounds carefully
- Instruct to refrigerate foods properly and avoid eating undercooked meats
- Use teach-back to ensure understanding

8th edition 2024

Background Evidence:

Centers for Medicare and Medicaid Services. (2019). *Process of care measures reported under the Hospital Inpatient Quality Reporting (IQR) and Outpatient Quality Reporting (OQR) programs.* https://medicare.gov/hospitalcompare/Data/Measures.html

Colorafi, K. J., Ferrell, K., D'Andrea, A., & Colorafi, J. (2019). Influencing outcomes with automated time zero for sepsis through statistical validation and process improvement. *mHealth, 5,* 36. https://doi.org/10.21037/mhealth.2019.09.04

Cooper, A. (2020). Corticosteroids for treating sepsis in children and adults. *Critical Care Nurse, 40*(4), 83–84.

Delawder, J., & Hutton, L. (2020). An interdisciplinary code sepsis team to improve sepsis-bundle compliance: A quality improvement project. *Journal of Emergency Nursing, 46*(1), 91–98.

Flynn-Makic, M. B., & Bridges, E. (2018). Managing sepsis and septic shock: Current guidelines and definitions. *American Journal of Nursing, 118*(2), 34–39.

Kalantari, A., & Rezaie, S. R. (2019). Challenging the one-hour sepsis bundle. *The Western Journal of Emergency Medicine, 20*(2), 185–190.

Ladha, E., House-Kokan, M., & Gillespie, M. (2019). The ABCs of sepsis: A framework for understanding the pathophysiology of sepsis. *Canadian Journal of Critical Care Nursing, 30*(4), 12–21.

Levy, M., Evans, L., & Rhodes, A. (2018). The Surviving Sepsis Campaign bundle: 2018 update. *Intensive Care Medicine, 44,* 925–928.

Rhodes, A., Evans, L. E., Alhazzani, W., Levy, M. M., Antonelli, M., Ferrer, R., Kumar, A., Sevransky, J. E., Sprung, C. L., Nannally, M. E., Rochwerg, B., Rubenfeld, G. D., Angus, D. C., Annane, D., Beale, R. J., Belinghan, G. J., Bernard, G. R., Chiche, J.-D., Coopersmith, C., De Backer, D. P., … Dellinger, R. P. (2017). Surviving Sepsis Campaign: International guidelines for management of sepsis and septic shock: 2016. *Critical Care Medicine, 45*(3), 486–552.

Roney, J. K., Whitley, B. E., & Long, J. D. (2020). Implementation of a MEWS-Sepsis screening tool: Transformational outcomes of a nurse-led evidence-based practice project. *Nursing Forum, 55,* 144–148.

Seckel, M. (2019). Updating your sepsis practice. *Critical Care Nurse, 39*(4), 72.

Smith, S., & Zolotorofe, I. (2018). Sepsis screening for ambulatory care nursing. *AAACN Viewpoint, 40*(3), 3–7.

Worapratya, P., & Wuthisuthimethawee, P. (2019). Septic shock in the ER: Diagnostic and management challenges. *Open Access Emergency Medicine: OAEM, 11,* 77–86.

Shock Management: Vasogenic 4256

Definition: Promotion of adequate tissue perfusion for a patient with severe loss of vascular tone

Activities:
- Monitor for physiological changes related to loss of vascular tone (e.g., note decreased BP, bradycardia, tachypnea, reduced pulse pressure, anxiety, oliguria)

- Place patient in a supine position with legs elevated to increase preload, as appropriate
- Consider Trendelenburg position if head injury has been ruled out

- Administer high flow oxygen, as appropriate
- Administer epinephrine via SQ, IV, or ET routes for anaphylaxis, if appropriate
- Assist in early endotracheal intubation, as appropriate
- Monitor ECG
- Administer atropine for bradycardia, as appropriate
- Utilize transcutaneous pacing, as appropriate
- Monitor pneumatic antishock garment, as appropriate
- Maintain two large-bore intravascular access sites
- Administer isotonic crystalloids as bolus doses, keeping systolic pressure at 90 mm Hg or more, as appropriate
- Administer antihistamine and/or corticosteroid, as appropriate
- Administer vasopressors
- Treat overdoses with appropriate reversal agent
- Insert NG tube and administer charcoal lavage, as appropriate
- Monitor body temperature
- Avoid hypothermia with warming blankets
- Treat hyperthermia with antipyretic drugs, a cooling mattress, or a sponge bath
- Prevent or control shivering with medication or by wrapping the extremities
- Monitor trends in hemodynamic parameters (e.g., CVP, MAP, PAWP, or PCWP wedge pressure)
- Administer antibiotics, as appropriate
- Administer anti-inflammatory medications, as appropriate
- Avoid stimuli that will precipitate neurogenic reaction (e.g., skin stimulation, distended bladder, or constipation)
- Monitor coagulation studies, including prothrombin time (PT), partial thromboplastin time (PTT), fibrinogen, fibrin degradation/split products, and platelet counts, as appropriate

1st edition 1992; revised 2008

Background Evidence:

Ahrens, T., & Tuggle, D. (2004). Surviving severe sepsis: Early recognition and treatment. *Critical Care Nurse, 24*(Suppl. 2), 2–15.

American Heart Association. (2005). 2005 American Heart Association guidelines for cardiopulmonary resuscitation and emergency cardiovascular care. *Circulation, 112*(Suppl. 24), IV-1–IV-211.

Bridges, E. J., & Dukes, S. (2005). Cardiovascular aspects of septic shock: Pathophysiology, monitoring, and treatment. *Critical Care Nurse, 25*(2), 14–40.

Dellinger, R. P., Carlet, J. M., Masur, H., Gerlach, H., Calandra, T., Cohen, J., Gea-Banacloche, J., Keh, D., Marshall, J. C., Parker, M. M., Ramsay, G., Zimmerman, J. L., Vincent, J.-L., & Levy, M. (2004). Surviving sepsis campaign guidelines for management of severe sepsis and septic shock. *Critical Care Medicine, 32*(3), 858–873.

Flynn, M. B., & McLeskey, S. (2005). Shock, systemic inflammatory response syndrome, and multiple organ dysfunction syndrome. In P. G. Morton, D. K. Fontaine, C. M. Hudak, & B. M. Gallo (Eds.), *Critical care nursing: A holistic approach* (8th ed., pp. 1152–1178). Lippincott Williams & Wilkins.

Hollenberg, S., Ahrens, T., Annane, D., Astiz, M., Chalfin, D., Dasta, J., Heard, S., Martin, C., Napolitano, L., Susla, G., Totaro, R., Vincent, J.-L., & Zanotti-Cavazzoni, S. (2004). Practice parameters for hemodynamic support of sepsis in adult patients: 2004 update. *Critical Care Medicine, 32*(9), 1928–1948.

Smeltzer, S. C., & Bare, B. G. (2004). *Brunner & Suddarth's textbook of medical-surgical nursing* (10th ed.). Lippincott Williams & Wilkins.

Shock Management: Volume   4258

Definition: Promotion of adequate tissue perfusion for a patient with severely compromised intravascular volume

Activities:

- Monitor for sudden loss of blood, severe dehydration, or persistent bleeding
- Check all secretions for frank or occult blood
- Prevent blood volume loss (e.g., apply pressure to site of bleeding)
- Monitor for fall in systolic blood pressure to less than 90 mm Hg or a fall of 30 mm Hg in hypertensive patients
- Monitor sublingual carbon dioxide levels
- Monitor for signs/symptoms of hypovolemic shock (e.g., increased thirst, increased HR, increased SVR, decreased urine output, decreased bowel sounds, decreased peripheral perfusion, altered mental status, or altered respirations)
- Position the patient for optimal perfusion
- Insert and maintain large-bore IV access
- Administer IV fluids such as isotonic crystalloids or colloids, as appropriate
- Administer warmed IV fluids and blood products, as indicated
- Administer oxygen and/or mechanical ventilation, as appropriate
- Draw arterial blood gases and monitor tissue oxygenation
- Monitor hemoglobin/hematocrit level
- Administer blood products (e.g., packed red blood cells, platelets, or fresh frozen plasma), as appropriate
- Monitor coagulation studies, including prothrombin time (PT), partial thromboplastin time (PTT), fibrinogen, fibrin degradation/split products, and platelet counts, as appropriate
- Monitor laboratory studies (e.g., serum lactate, acid-base balance, metabolic profiles, and electrolytes)

1st edition 1992; revised 2008

Background Evidence:

American Heart Association. (2005). 2005 American Heart Association guidelines for cardiopulmonary resuscitation and emergency cardiovascular care. *Circulation, 112*(Suppl. 24), IV-1–IV-211.

Flynn, M. B., & McLeskey, S. (2005). Shock, systemic inflammatory response syndrome, and multiple organ dysfunction syndrome. In P. G. Morton, D. K. Fontaine, C. M. Hudak, & B. M. Gallo (Eds.), *Critical care nursing: A holistic approach* (8th ed., pp. 1152–1178). Lippincott Williams & Wilkins.

Kuhlman, D. K. (Ed.). (2003). *Resuscitation: Fluid therapy. Congress Review: Cutting edge therapeutics.* 32nd Critical Care Congress 2003 in San Antonio, TX: Society of Critical Care Medicine.

Porth, C. M. (2004). *Essentials of pathophysiology: Concepts of altered health states.* Lippincott Williams & Wilkins.

Smeltzer, S. C., & Bare, B. G. (2004). *Brunner & Suddarth's textbook of medical-surgical nursing* (10th ed.). Lippincott Williams & Wilkins.

S

Shock Prevention 4260

Definition: Detecting and treating a patient at risk for impending shock

Activities:

- Monitor for early compensatory shock responses (e.g., normal blood pressure, narrowed pulse pressure, mild orthostatic hypotension [15 to 25 mm Hg], slight delayed capillary refill, pale/cool skin or flushed skin, slight tachypnea, nausea and vomiting, increased thirst, or weakness)
- Monitor for early signs of systemic inflammatory response syndrome (e.g., increased temperature, tachycardia, tachypnea, hypocarbia, leukocytosis, or leucopenia)
- Monitor for early signs of allergic reactions (e.g., rhinitis, wheezing, stridor, dyspnea, itching, hives and wheals, cutaneous angioedema, GI upset, abdominal pain, diarrhea, anxiety, and restlessness)
- Monitor for early signs of cardiac compromise (e.g., declining CO and urinary output, increasing SVR and PCWP, crackles in the lungs, S_3 and S_4 heart sounds, and tachycardia)
- Monitor possible sources of fluid loss (e.g., chest tube, wound, and nasogastric drainage; diarrhea; vomiting; and increasing abdominal and extremity girth, hematemesis, or hematochezia)
- Monitor circulatory status (e.g., blood pressure, skin color, skin temperature, heart sounds, heart rate and rhythm, presence and quality of peripheral pulses, and capillary refill)
- Monitor for signs of inadequate tissue oxygenation (e.g., apprehension, increased anxiety, changes in mental status, agitation, oliguria, and cool, mottled periphery)
- Monitor pulse oximetry
- Monitor temperature and respiratory status
- Monitor EKG
- Monitor daily weights, intake, and output
- Monitor laboratory values, especially Hgb and Hct levels, clotting profile, ABG, lactate level, electrolyte levels, cultures, and chemistry profile
- Monitor invasive hemodynamic parameters (e.g., CVP, MAP, and central/mixed venous oxygen saturation), as appropriate
- Monitor sublingual CO_2 or gastric tonometry, as appropriate
- Note bruising, petechiae, and condition of mucous membranes
- Note color, amount, and frequency of stools, vomitus, and nasogastric drainage
- Test urine for blood, and protein, as appropriate
- Monitor for signs/symptoms of ascites and abdominal or back pain
- Place patient in supine, legs elevated position (volume, vasogenic) or supine, head and shoulders elevated (cardiogenic), as appropriate
- Institute and maintain airway patency, as appropriate
- Administer IV and/or oral fluids, as appropriate
- Insert and maintain large-bore IV access, as appropriate
- Administer IV fluid challenge while monitoring hemodynamic pressures and urinary output, as appropriate
- Administer antiarrhythmics, diuretics, and/or vasopressors, as appropriate
- Administer packed red blood cells, fresh frozen plasma, and/or platelets, as appropriate
- Initiate early administration of antimicrobial agents and closely monitor their effectiveness, as appropriate
- Administer oxygen and/or mechanical ventilation, as appropriate
- Administer anti-inflammatory agents and/or bronchodilators, as appropriate
- Monitor blood glucose and administer insulin therapy, as appropriate
- Administer IV, intraosseous, or endotracheal epinephrine, as appropriate
- Teach patient to avoid known allergens and how to use an anaphylaxis kit, as appropriate
- Perform skin testing to determine agents causing anaphylaxis and/or allergic reactions, as appropriate
- Advise patients at risk for severe allergic reactions to undergo desensitization therapy
- Advise patients at risk to wear or carry medical alert information
- Instruct patient and/or family on precipitating factors of shock
- Instruct patient and family about signs/symptoms of impending shock
- Instruct patient and family about steps to take with onset of shock symptoms

1st edition 1992; revised 2008

Background Evidence:

Ahrens, T., & Tuggle, D. (2004). Surviving severe sepsis: Early recognition and treatment. *Critical Care Nurse, 24*(Suppl. 2), 2–15.

American Heart Association. (2005). 2005 American Heart Association guidelines for cardiopulmonary resuscitation and emergency cardiovascular care. *Circulation, 112*(Suppl. 24), IV-1–IV-211.

Flynn, M. B., & McLeskey, S. (2005). Shock, systemic inflammatory response syndrome, and multiple organ dysfunction syndrome. In P. G. Morton, D. K. Fontaine, C. M. Hudak, & B. M. Gallo (Eds.), *Critical care nursing: A holistic approach* (8th ed., pp. 1152–1178). Lippincott Williams & Wilkins.

Porth, C. M. (2004). *Essentials of pathophysiology: Concepts of altered health states.* Lippincott Williams & Wilkins.

Smeltzer, S. C., & Bare, B. G. (2004). *Brunner & Suddarth's textbook of medical-surgical nursing* (10th ed.). Lippincott Williams & Wilkins.

S

Sibling Support 7280

Definition: Assisting a child to cope with a brother or sister's illness, chronic condition, or disability

Activities:

- Explore knowledge about clinical condition
- Evaluate stress related to condition
- Explore coping processes
- Facilitate family members' awareness of sibling's feelings
- Provide information about common responses
- Assume advocacy role as indicated (i.e., in life-threatening situations when anxiety high and parents or other family members unable to perform role)
- Recognize that each child responds differently

- Encourage care of young sibling in own home if possible
- Assist to maintain or modify usual routines and activities of daily living as necessary
- Promote communication between siblings
- Value each child individually, avoiding comparisons
- Help child to see differences and similarities between self and sibling with special needs
- Encourage visits to affected brother or sister
- Explain care of affected brother or sister
- Encourage participation in care of affected brother or sister, as appropriate
- Instruct on strategies to interact with affected sister or brother
- Permit siblings to settle own difficulties
- Recognize and respect when not emotionally ready to visit affected sibling
- Respect well child's reluctance to be with or to include sibling with special needs in activities
- Encourage maintenance of parental or family interactional patterns
- Assist to clarify, explore, and expose concerns and fears
- Use drawings, puppetry, and dramatic play to see how perceives events
- Clarify concern for contracting illness of affected sibling and develop strategies for coping with concern
- Instruct related to pathology of disease, according to developmental stage and learning style
- Use concrete substitutes for sibling unable to visit affected brother or sister (e.g., pictures, videos)
- Explain that they are not cause of illness
- Instruct on strategies for meeting own emotional and developmental needs
- Praise when has patience, has sacrificed, or has been particularly helpful

- Acknowledge personal strengths and abilities to cope with stress successfully
- Provide referral to peer sibling group, as appropriate
- Provide community resource referrals, as necessary
- Communicate situation to school nurse to promote support in accord with parental wishes
- Encourage parents to have individual moments with siblings

1st edition 1992; revised 2000, 2024

Background Evidence:

Aita, M., Héon, M., Savanh, P., De Clifford-Faugère, G., & Charbonneau, L. (2021). Promoting family and siblings' adaptation following a preterm birth: A quality improvement project of a family-centered care nursing educational intervention. *Journal of Pediatric Nursing, 58*, 21–27. https://doi.org/10.1016/j.pedn.2020.11.006

Havill, N., Fleming, L. K., & Knafl, K. (2019). Well siblings of children with chronic illness: A synthesis research study. *Research in Nursing & Health, 42*(5), 334–348. https://doi.org/10.1002/nur.21978

Hill, K., & Brenner, M. (2019). Well siblings' experiences of living with a child following a traumatic brain injury: A systematic review protocol. *Systematic Reviews, 8*(1), 81. https://doi.org/10.1186/s13643-019-1005-9

Hockenberry, M. J., & Wilson, D. M. S. (Eds.). (2018). *Wong's nursing care of infants and children* (11th Ed.). Elsevier.

Leane, M. (2019). Siblings caring for siblings with intellectual disabilities: Naming and negotiating emotional tensions. *Social Science & Medicine, 230*, 264–270. https://doi.org/10.1016/j.socscimed.2019.04.022

Wakimizu, R., Fujioka, H., Nishigaki, K., & Matsuzawa, A. (2020). Quality of life and associated factors in siblings of children with severe motor and intellectual disabilities: A cross-sectional study. *Nursing & Health Sciences, 22*(4), 977–987. https://doi.org/10.1111/nhs.12755

Skin Care: Absorbent Products   3570

Definition: Prevention of skin complications in adults when using permeable, protective fabrics, or materials

Activities:

- Establish type of incontinence (e.g., slight or light incontinence, moderate to heavy incontinence, fecal or urinary incontinence) or excessive skin fold sweat
- Use assessment tool or standardized scale to identify persons at risk for skin breakdown (e.g., Braden Scale, International Consultation on Incontinence Questionnaire - Short Form [ICIQ-SF])
- Determine personal needs (e.g., odor control, prevention of clothing stains, self-application, skin breakdown or friction areas, aesthetic audio or visual qualities, price, bariatric size)
- Determine expectations for product use (e.g., skin fold moisture protection, swimming wear, day wear, night wear, travel wear, wet bed prevention, urinary or fecal incontinence coverage, reusable or washable)
- Consider product attributes (e.g., cloth backing, perineal pads, panty liners, padded diapers, waistband products, overnight briefs, day briefs, removable, reusable, pull-ups, reusable tabs)
- Adjust product robustness as indicated by time of need (i.e., use light perineal pads for slight leakage, change to heavier briefs for night coverage)
- Avoid exceeding product guidelines for change of product (e.g., change every 3 hours)

- Match product to skin care needs (i.e., avoid snug plastic products if risk for skin breakdown)
- Fit product to anatomy (i.e., use hip measurements and ensure leg and waist openings are snug, avoid too tight or too loose fittings, use product sizing charts where available, cut skin fold protectors to desired size before applying)
- Avoid cutting precut skinfold sheets
- Fold precut skinfold sheet in half during application for better fit if indicated
- Change precut skinfold sheet daily or when wet
- Choose product that fits clothing (e.g., less absorbent, smaller product, avoid colored adhesives or designs under light clothing)
- Choose product with ease of use as indicated by needs
- Ensure product odor neutralization capabilities as indicated by preference
- Consider product needs when administering medications with incontinence effects (e.g., laxatives, diuretics)
- Inspect skin area with every product change or toileting occurrence
- Inspect skin and mucous membranes for redness, extreme warmth, edema, drainage or signs of pressure buildup (i.e., reddened skin that does not blanch)

S

- Apply topical preventative skin treatments as indicated
- Avoid reusing soiled products, even with minimal soil apparent
- Instruct on product types, usage, indications, and contraindications
- Determine ability to select products and include in planning, where appropriate
- Instruct about signs of skin breakdown and potential changes in product required for breakdown occurrences
- Instruct about skin care while using products
- Monitor skin for rashes and abrasions and change product as indicated when rash or abrasion present
- Change product if causing tightness or restrictive movement
- Document skin condition every eight hours or as indicated

8th edition 2024

Background Evidence:

Berman, A., Snyder, S. J., & Frandsen, G. (2021). Hygiene. In *Kozier and Erb's fundamentals of nursing: Concepts, process and practice* (11th ed., pp. 669–685). Pearson.

Craven, R. F., Hirnle, C. J., & Henshaw, C. M. (2021). Hygiene and self-care. In *Fundamentals of nursing: Human health and function* (8th ed., pp. 604–634). Wolters-Kluwer.

Doty, S. K., & Engels, D. (2021). Containment methods for incontinence. *Nursing made incredibly easy! 19*(5), 30–38. https://doi.org/10.1097/01. NME.0000767248.48860.3e

Hockenberry, M. J., Rodgers, C. C., & Wilson, D. (2022). *Wong's essentials of pediatric nursing* (11th ed.). Elsevier.

Kanerva Rice, S., Pendrill, L., Petersson, N., Nordlinder, J., & Farbrot, A. (2018). Rationale and design of a novel method to assess the usability of body-worn absorbent incontinence care products by caregivers. *Journal of Wound, Ostomy & Continence Nursing, 45*(5), 456–464. https://doi.org/10.1097/WON.0000000000000462

Perry, A. G., Potter, P. A., Ostendorf, W. R., & LaPlante, N. (2021). *Clinical nursing skills and technique* (10th ed.). Mosby.

Potter, P. A., Perry, A. G., Stockert, P. A., & Hall, A. M. (2021). *Fundamentals of nursing* (10th ed.). Elsevier.

Schwartz, D., Magen, Y. K., Levy, A., & Gefen, A. (2018). Effects of humidity on skin friction against medical textiles as related to prevention of pressure injuries. *International Wound Journal, 15*(6), 866–874.

Voegeli, D. (2019). Prevention and management of moisture-associated skin damage. *Nursing Standard, 34*(2), 77–82. https://doi.org/10.7748/ns.2019.e11314

Williams, P. (2020). *Basic geriatric nursing* (7th ed). Elsevier.

Skin Care: Donor Site   3582

Definition: Prevention of wound complications and promotion of healing at the donor site

Activities:

- Inspect donor site dressing at least daily, as per agency protocol
- Change dressing as per agency protocol
- Provide adequate pain control (e.g., medication, music therapy, distraction, massage)
- Apply medications to wound site per agency protocol
- Monitor for signs of infection (e.g., fever, pain) and other post-operative complications
- Keep skin donor site clean, dry, and free from pressure
- Instruct individual to keep healed skin donor site soft and pliable
- Instruct to apply pressure for excessive bleeding and notify health care provider if application of pressure not resulting in decreased bleeding
- Instruct individual to avoid exposing skin donor site to extremes in temperature, external trauma, and sunlight
- Instruct on signs and symptoms to report to health care provider immediately
- Use teach-back to ensure understanding

4th edition 2004, revised 2024

Background Evidence:

American Nurses Association & International Society of Plastic and Aesthetic Nurses. (2020). *Plastic and aesthetic nursing: Scope and standards of practice* (3rd ed.).

Myers, B. A. (2020). *Wound management: Principles and practice* (4th ed.). Pearson.

Nicol, N. H. (2016). *Dermatological nursing essentials: A core curriculum* (3rd ed.). Wolters Kluwer.

Rebar, C. R., & Bidigare, C. (2021). Concepts of care for patients with skin problems. In D. Ignativicius, M. L. Workman, C. R. Rebar, & N. M. Heimgartner (Eds.), *Medical-Surgical nursing: Concepts for interprofessional collaborative care* (10th ed., pp. 1101–1188). Elsevier.

Uoya, Y., Ishii, N., Sakai, S., Kiuchi, T., Uno, T., & Kishi, K. (2021). A novel technique to achieve rapid wound healing of donor site wounds in split-thickness skin grafts of a patient undergoing anticoagulation therapy. *International Journal of Lower Extremity Wounds, 20*(2), 162–166. https://doi.org/10.1177/1534734620938169

Skin Care: Graft Site   3583

Definition: Prevention of wound complications and promotion of graft site healing

Activities:

- Apply dressings, as per agency protocol
- Provide adequate pain control (e.g., medication, music therapy, distraction, massage)
- Follow agency protocol for treatment of graft site (e.g., elevate graft site, needle aspiration, bleb treatment)
- Avoid friction and shearing forces at new graft site
- Instruct on allowed activities until graft adheres
- Instruct to keep affected part immobilized during healing
- Inspect dressing daily, as per agency protocol
- Monitor color, warmth, capillary refill, and turgor of graft
- Monitor for signs of infection (e.g., fever, pain) and other complications

- Prevent development of complications of immobility (e.g., pneumonia, pulmonary emboli, pressure injury)
- Provide emotional support, understanding, and consideration
- Instruct on care of graft site area (e.g., compression stocking, dressing, avoidance of sun light and heating pad, no smoking), as prescribed
- Use teach-back to ensure understanding

4th edition 2004, revised 2024

Background Evidence:

American Nurses Association & International Society of Plastic and Aesthetic Nurses. (2020). *Plastic and aesthetic nursing: Scope and standards of practice* (3rd ed.).

Myers, B. A. (2020). *Wound management: Principles and practice* (4th ed.). Pearson.

Nicol, N. H. (2016). *Dermatological nursing essentials: A core curriculum* (3rd ed.). Wolters Kluwer.

Rebar, C. R., & Bidigare, C. (2021). Concepts of care for patients with skin problems. In D. Ignativicius, M. L. Workman, C. R. Rebar, & N. M. Heimgartner (Eds.), *Medical-Surgical nursing: Concepts for interprofessional collaborative care* (10th ed., pp. 1101–1188). Elsevier.

Uoya, Y., Ishii, N., Sakai, S., Kiuchi, T., Uno, T., & Kishi, K. (2021). A novel technique to achieve rapid wound healing of donor site wounds in split-thickness skin grafts of a patient undergoing anticoagulation therapy. *International Journal of Lower Extremity Wounds, 20*(2), 162–166. https://doi.org/10.1177/1534734620938169

Skin Care: Topical Treatment 3584

Definition: Application of topical substances or manipulation of devices to promote skin integrity and minimize breakdown

Activities:

- Inspect skin daily for persons at risk of breakdown
- Institute measures to reduce risk for skin or tissue breakdown (e.g., reduce frequency of complete bathing, keep skin free from waste or exudate, use mild soaps, use emollients, turn or reposition frequently)
- Rate any lesions or areas of breakdown using standardized tool or scale (e.g., Braden Scale)
- Apply topical treatment to affected area (e.g., antibiotic, anti-inflammatory, emollient, anti-fungal, debriding agent), as appropriate
- Apply clear occlusive dressing to affected areas as needed
- Paint or spray skin warts with liquid nitrogen, as appropriate
- Refrain from giving local heat applications
- Document degree of skin breakdown
- Avoid using rough-textured bed linens and keep linens clean, dry, free of wrinkles and foreign objects
- Clean with antibacterial soap, as appropriate
- Refrain from using alkaline soap on skin
- Use plain water to cleanse and avoid drying skin where possible (e.g., newborn)
- Rinse skin carefully and completely to avoid drying effects of soap
- Soak in colloidal bath to enhance skin moisture, as appropriate
- Dry skin thoroughly
- Provide toilet hygiene as needed
- Wash skin and supply clean, dry linens after episodes of incontinence
- Keep skin dry after episodes of diaphoresis
- Check skin surfaces where moisture caused by perspiration can be trapped
- Apply drying powders to deep skinfolds or dust skin with medicated powder, as appropriate
- Remove adhesive tape and debris
- Provide support to edematous areas (e.g., pillow under arms, scrotal support), as appropriate
- Apply lubricant to moisten lips and oral mucosa as needed
- Administer back rub or neck rub, as appropriate
- Change condom catheter, as appropriate
- Apply incontinence underwear loosely, as appropriate
- Place on incontinence pads, as appropriate
- Massage around affected areas of dryness or redness, as appropriate
- Apply appropriately fitting ostomy appliance, as needed
- Initiate consultation of specialty services, as needed
- Dress in nonrestrictive clothing
- Encourage adults at risk for skin tears to wear long sleeves, long trousers, or knee-high socks
- Cover hands with mittens to avoid excessive scratching or tearing at skin, as appropriate
- Use devices on bed and chair (e.g., pads) that protect person
- Apply heel protectors, as appropriate
- Turn person on bedrest or immobilized person at least every 2 hours, using specific schedule
- Provide appropriate pads, cushions, mattresses, or beds that are designed to reduce pressure for persons on bedrest
- Provide thorough foot care
- Provide dental hygiene
- Instruct older adults who have been using baking soda or salt for tooth cleansing to avoid ingesting due to high sodium content
- Provide sunscreen in recommended SPF for exposure
- Add moisture to environment with a humidifier as needed
- Institute measures to promote adequate healing (i.e., provide adequate rest, food and fluids, check wounds and skin daily, avoid skin tears from adhesive tapes)

1st edition 1992; revised 1996, 2000, 2024

Background Evidence:

Awank, B., Dayang, A., Avsar, P., Patton, D., O'Connor, T., Budri, A., Nugent, L., & Moore, Z. (2021). What is the impact of topical preparations on the incidence of skin tears in older people? A systematic review. *Wounds UK, 17*(2), 33–43.

S

Colwell, J. C. (2021). Skin integrity and wound care. In A. Perry, P. Potter, P. Stockert, & A. Hall (Eds.), *Fundamentals of Nursing* (10th ed., pp. 1235–1299). Elsevier.

Cooke, A., Bedwell, C., Campbell, M., McGowan, L., Ersser, S. J., & Lavender, T. (2018). Skin care for healthy babies at term: A systematic review of the evidence. *Midwifery, 56*, 29–43.

Pather, P., Hines, S., Kynoch, K., & Coyer, F. (2017). Effectiveness of topical skin products in the treatment and prevention of incontinence-associated

dermatitis: A systematic review. *JBI Database of Systematic Reviews & Implementation Reports, 15*(5), 1473–1496.

Potter, P.A., Ostendorf, W.R., & LaPlante, N. (2018). *Clinical nursing skills and techniques* (9th ed.) Personal hygiene and bedmaking. (pp. 445-481). Mosby.

Williams, P. (2020). Care of aging skin and mucous membranes: *Basic geriatric nursing* (7th ed., pp. 272–291). Elsevier.

Skin Surveillance 3590

Definition: Collection and analysis of patient data to maintain skin and mucous membrane integrity

Activities:

- Inspect skin and mucous membranes for redness, extreme warmth, edema, or drainage
- Observe extremities for color, warmth, swelling, pulses, texture, edema, and ulcerations
- Inspect condition of surgical incision, as appropriate
- Use an assessment tool to identify patients at risk for skin breakdown (e.g., Braden Scale)
- Monitor skin color and temperature
- Monitor skin and mucous membranes for areas of discoloration, bruising, and breakdown
- Monitor skin for rashes and abrasions
- Monitor skin for excessive dryness and moistness
- Monitor for sources of pressure and friction
- Monitor for infection, especially of edematous areas
- Inspect clothing for tightness
- Document skin or mucous membrane changes
- Institute measures to prevent further deterioration (e.g., overlay mattress, repositioning schedule)
- Instruct family member/caregiver about signs of skin breakdown, as appropriate

1st edition 1992; revised 2008

Background Evidence:

McCance, K. L., & Huether, S. E. (2006). *Pathophysiology: The biologic basis for disease in adults and children* (5th ed.). Mosby.

Perry, A. G., & Potter, P. A. (2006). *Clinical nursing skills and techniques* (6th ed.). Elsevier Mosby.

Potter, P. A., & Perry, A. G. (2005). *Fundamentals of nursing* (6th ed.). Mosby.

Taylor, C., Lillis, C., LeMone, P., & Lynn, P. (2008). *Fundamentals of nursing: The art and science of nursing care* (6th ed.). Lippincott Williams and Wilkins.

Titler, M., Pettit, D., Bulechek, G., McCloskey, J., Craft, M., Cohen, M., Crossley, J. D., Denehy, J. A., Glick, O. J., Kruckeberg, T. W., Maas, M. L., Prophet, C. M., & Tripp-Reimer, T. (1991). Classification of nursing interventions for care of the integument. *Nursing Diagnosis, 2*(2), 45–56.

Urden, L. D., Stacy, K. M., & Lough, M. E. (2006). *Thelan's critical care nursing: Diagnosis and management* (5th ed.). Mosby Elsevier.

Sleep Enhancement 1850

Definition: Facilitation of regular sleep and wake cycles

S

Activities:

- Determine sleep and activity pattern
- Approximate regular sleep and wake cycle in planning care
- Explain importance of adequate sleep during various stages and occurrences in life (e.g., pregnancy, illness, psychosocial stresses)
- Determine effects of medications on sleep pattern
- Monitor and record sleep pattern and number of sleep hours
- Monitor sleep pattern and note physical (e.g., sleep apnea, obstructed airway, pain or discomfort, urinary frequency) and psychological (e.g., fear, anxiety) circumstances that interrupt sleep
- Instruct to monitor sleep patterns
- Monitor participation in fatigue-producing activities during wakefulness to prevent overtiredness
- Adjust environment (e.g., light, noise, temperature, mattress, bed) to promote sleep
- Instruct to limit use of electronic devices (e.g., phone, Internet, television)
- Decrease or eliminate routine, non-essential nighttime cares
- Encourage to establish bedtime routine to facilitate transition from wakefulness to sleep
- Facilitate maintenance of usual bedtime routines, pre-sleep cues or props, and familiar objects (e.g., for children—a favorite blanket or toy, rocking, pacifier, story; for adults—a book to read, warm bath), as appropriate
- Assist to eliminate stressful situations before bedtime
- Monitor bedtime food and beverage intake for items that facilitate or interfere with sleep
- Instruct to avoid bedtime foods and beverages that interfere with sleep (e.g., caffeinated beverages, food with high sugar content, gas-forming foods)
- Assist to limit daytime sleep by providing activity that promotes wakefulness, as appropriate
- Instruct on autogenic muscle relaxation or other non-pharmacological forms of sleep inducement
- Initiate comfort measures of massage, positioning, and affective touch

- Encourage sleep enhancement devices and apps, as appropriate
- Provide non-pharmacological sleep enhancements (e.g., aromatherapy, decreased light intensity)
- Consider combinations of devices, comfort measures, non-pharmacological enhancements
- Promote increase in number of hours of sleep, if needed
- Provide for naps during day, if indicated, to meet sleep requirements
- Group care activities to minimize number of awakenings and to allow for sleep cycles of at least 90 minutes
- Adjust medication administration schedule to support sleep and wake cycle
- Instruct about factors (e.g., physiological, psychological, lifestyle, frequent work shift changes, rapid time zone changes, excessively long work hours, other environmental factors) that contribute to sleep pattern disturbances
- Guide in developing sleep hygiene protocol (e.g., follow regular sleep schedule, get out of bed when cannot sleep, do not spend too much time in bed, avoid excessive tasks in bed, make bedroom comfortable)
- Consider sleep medications
- Encourage use of sleep medications that do not contain REM sleep suppressor(s) (e.g., melatonin)
- Regulate environmental stimuli to maintain normal day-night cycles, as indicated
- Discuss sleep-enhancing techniques
- Provide written information about sleep enhancement techniques

- Document instructions and responses
- Use teach-back to ensure understanding

1st edition 1992; revised 2004, 2024

Background Evidence:

Bion, V., Lowe, A. S., Puthucheary, Z., & Montgomery, H. (2018). Reducing sound and light exposure to improve sleep on the adult intensive care unit: An inclusive narrative review. *Journal of the Intensive Care Society, 19*(2), 138–146. https://doi.org/10.1177/1751143717740803

Capezuti, E., Sagha Zadeh, R., Pain, K., Basara, A., Jiang, N. Z., & Krieger, A. C. (2018). A systematic review of non-pharmacological interventions to improve nighttime sleep among residents of long-term care settings. *BMC Geriatrics, 18*(1), 1–18.

Jun, J., Kapella, M. C., & Hershberger, P. E. (2021). Non-pharmacological sleep interventions for adult patients in intensive care units: A systematic review. *Intensive and Critical Care Nursing, 67*, 103124. https://doi.org/10.1016/j.iccn.2021.103124

Sullan, M. J., Patel, B. B., Bauer, R. M., & Jaffee, M. S. (2021). Impact of a sleep enhancement protocol on nighttime room entries in an inpatient rehabilitation facility. *Rehabilitation Nursing, 46*(4), 232–243. https://doi.org/10.1097/RNJ.0000000000000291

Whitman, E. (2017). Using music to stabilize NICU babies—as well as their parents. *Modern Healthcare, 47*(17), 0028.

Williams, R., Jacques, K. K., Mirza, S., Matters, L., & Guerrier, L. D. (2021). Care square. *Nursing, 51*(9), 66–70. https://doi.org/10.1097/01.NURSE.0000769884.72964.d9

Smoking Cessation Assistance   4490

Definition: Helping another to stop smoking

Activities:

- Record current smoking status and smoking history at every visit, including vaping
- Identify factors for nicotine dependence (e.g., impulsivity, likelihood of withdrawal, environmental stressors) using screening tool, as indicated
- Determine readiness to learn about smoking cessation
- Monitor readiness to attempt to quit smoking
- Discuss presence of smoking related illnesses
- Offer tobacco cessation treatment in hospital to all current smokers and at discharge
- Offer follow-up to persons who are attempting to quit smoking, if possible
- Give clear, strong, and consistent advice to quit smoking
- Provide special counseling and psychosocial intervention to pregnant smokers
- Help identify reasons to stop smoking
- Help identify barriers to stop smoking
- Help motivated persons to set quit date
- Discuss risks and consequences of continuing smoking or vaping, and rewards and benefits of cessation
- Provide motivational interventions to stimulate future quit attempts
- Instruct on physical symptoms of nicotine withdrawal (e.g., headache, dizziness, nausea, irritability, insomnia)
- Monitor smoking abstinence symptoms during treatment
- Explain physical withdrawal symptoms from nicotine are temporary
- Investigate possible challenges to remain abstinent

- Inform about dangers of vaping as alternative method (e.g., same nicotine health issues, vaping addictive, nicotine concentration stronger)
- Inform about nicotine replacement products (e.g., patch, gum, nasal spray, inhaler) to help reduce physical withdrawal symptoms
- Assist to identify psychosocial aspects (e.g., positive and negative feelings associated with smoking) that influence smoking behavior
- Assist in developing smoking cessation plan that addresses psychosocial aspects that influence smoking behavior
- Assist to recognize cues that prompt to smoke (e.g., being around others who smoke, frequenting places where smoking allowed)
- Assist to develop practical methods to resist cravings (e.g., spend time with nonsmoking friends, frequent places where smoking not allowed, relaxation exercises)
- Encourage self-rewards at specific intervals of smoke-free living (e.g., 1 week, 1 month, 6 months)
- Provide encouragement to maintain smoke-free lifestyle
- Encourage to attend smoking cessation support group
- Assist with any self-help methods
- Help plan specific coping strategies and resolve problems that result from quitting
- Advise to avoid dieting while trying to give up smoking as can undermine chances of quitting
- Advise to work out plan to cope with others who smoke and avoid being around them
- Inform that dry mouth, cough, scratchy throat, and feeling on edge are symptoms that may occur after quitting; patch or gum may help with cravings

S

- Advise to avoid smokeless tobacco, dipping, and chewing as these can lead to addiction and health problems, including oral cancer, gum problems, loss of teeth, and heart problems
- Manage medications for tobacco dependence, such as nicotine replacement therapy and bupropion, as appropriate
- Arrange for follow-up contacts with person to acknowledge that withdrawal difficult, to reinforce importance of remaining abstinent, and to offer congratulations on progress
- Provide social support during smoking cessation treatment
- Promote policies that establish and enforce smoke-free environment
- Advise to keep journal for relapses or near relapses, what causes them, and what can be learned from them
- Help person deal with lapses
- Offer referral to other services, as appropriate
- Contact national and local resource organizations for resource materials

1st edition 1992; revised 2000, 2004, 2024

Background Evidence:

Barua, R. S., Rigotti, N. A., Benowitz, N. L., Cummings, K. M., Jazayeri, M. A., Morris, P. B., Ratchford, E. V., Sarna, L., Stecker, E. C., & Wiggins, B. S. (2018). 2018 ACC expert consensus decision pathway on tobacco cessation treatment: A report of the American College of Cardiology Task Force on Clinical Expert Consensus Documents. *Journal of the American College of Cardiology, 72*(25), 3332–3365. https://doi.org/10.1016/j.jacc.2018.10.027

Corvalán, B., María Paz, Véjar M., Leonardo, Bambs S., Claudia, Pavié G., Juana, Zagolin B., & Mónica, & Cerda L., Jaime. (2017). Clinical practice guidelines for smoking cessation. *Revista médica de Chile, 145*(11), 1471–1479. https://doi.org/10.4067/s0034-98872017001101471

The Royal Australian College of General Practitioners. (2019). *Supporting smoking cessation: A guide for health professionals* (2nd ed.). RACGP.

US Preventive Services Task Force, Krist, A. H., Davidson, K. W., Mangione, C. M., Barry, M. J., Cabana, M., Caughey, A. B., Donahue, K., Doubeni, C. A., Epling, J. W., Jr, Kubik, M., Ogedegbe, G., Pbert, L., Silverstein, M., Simon, M. A., Tseng, C. W., & Wong, J. B. (2021). Interventions for tobacco smoking cessation in adults, including pregnant persons: US Preventive Services Task Force Recommendation Statement. *JAMA, 325*(3), 265–279. https://doi.org/10.1001/jama.2020.25019

Verbiest, M., Brakema, E., van der Kleij, R., Sheals, K., Allistone, G., Williams, S., McEwen, A., & Chavannes, N. (2017). National guidelines for smoking cessation in primary care: A literature review and evidence analysis. *NPJ Primary Care Respiratory Medicine, 27*, 2. https://doi.org/10.1038/s41533-016-0004-8

World Health Organization. (2014). *Toolkit for delivering the 5A's and 5R's brief tobacco interventions in primary care.* https://apps.who.int/iris/bitstream/handle/10665/112835/9789241506953_eng.pdf;jsessionid=B0B8CEF43A471878B490FAF8BE2E3EB7?sequence=1

Social Justice Facilitation

8740

Definition: Engaging in practices designed to promote optimal health care environments that embrace concepts of diversity, equity, and inclusion

Activities:

- Identify social inequities and determine how they contribute to disparities in health outcomes
- Evaluate how processes of social exclusion (e.g., history of colonialism, misrecognition, disrespect, stigma, fear of difference, dominance, oppression) contribute to health care disparities
- Evaluate how upstream factors (e.g., low educational status or opportunity, income disparities, discrimination, social marginalization) impede positive health outcomes in broad and inequitable way
- Evaluate how midstream factors (e.g., homelessness, food insecurity, trauma) contribute to individual factors and social needs that may affect health
- Use postcolonial and intersectional perspectives to understand how structural inequities and structural violence result in health disparities
- Recognize health inequities as outcomes of race, class, and gender discrimination
- Collaborate with persons directly affected by social injustices
- Adopt inclusive approach
- Convey respect for human dignity for all
- Convey respect and unconditional positive regard for individual and group differences since valued recognition is foundational condition for human dignity
- Refrain from making judgments based on gender, race, class, sexual orientation, abilities, age, or circumstances
- Recognize biases, assumptions, prejudicial attitudes, stereotypes that contribute to social injustices and health care inequalities when relating to persons
- Promote social solidarity by creating opportunities designed to promote sense of belonging and safety
- Establish working non-hierarchical partnerships mindful of human dignity, caringly honest and tactful
- Create and participate in community meetings, town meetings, citizen salons, and intergroup programs for dialogue to explore issues of culture, politics, racism, geographic location, violence, and religion and their contribution to health inequalities
- Work with partnerships to discover social, environmental, educational, and economic conditions associated with injustices that influence well-being
- Identify specific social and structural changes required to correct social and institutional injustices that sustain inequalities and perpetuate advantages for some and disadvantages for others
- Tailor care toward individual and groups with greatest needs to provide more resources and support
- Identify existing positive strengths and traits of persons, families, communities, and populations affected by unjust situations
- Develop collaborative strategies to rectify oppressive power dynamics and dehumanizing conditions that interfere with human flourishing
- Collaborate with other nurses, health care professionals and interested stakeholders (e.g., politicians, business owners, philanthropists, teachers, community organizers, clergy, attorneys, engineers) to develop multipronged strategies to dismantle social, political, or economic structures responsible for social and health inequities
- Facilitate access to health services for individuals, families, and communities to settings where nurses work including federally qualified health centers (FQHCs), retail clinics, home health and home visiting, telehealth, school nursing, and school-based health centers, and nurse-managed health centers

S

- Develop and use strategies (e.g., care management, person-centered care, cultural humility) to overcome barriers to quality care, structural inequities, and implicit bias
- Use principles of transcultural nursing to provide care to diverse communities that are culturally respectful and appropriate
- Advocate and speak out against racism, discrimination, and injustice
- Promote health equity by working with public policy makers and organizational leaders to transform health-related public policies, which contribute to health disparities

8th edition 2024

Background Evidence:

Chinn, P. L., & Kramer, M. (2021). Integrated theory and knowledge development in nursing: *Chapter 3. Emancipatory knowledge development* (11th ed.). Elsevier.

da Silva, K. L., Moura Rabelo, A. R., Gandra, E. C., Siqueira Costa Schreck, R., Assunção Guimarães, R., Marques, M. F., & Belga, S. (2021). Social inequalities in Brazilian nursing discourse: Social commitment and hegemonic struggle. *Revista de Enfermagem Referência, 5*, 1–7. https://doi.org/10.12707/RV20089

Falk-Rafael, A., & Betker, C. (2012). Witnessing social injustice downstream and advocating for health equity upstream: "The trombone slide" of nursing. *Advances in Nursing Science, 35*(2), 98–112.

National Academies of Sciences, Engineering, and Medicine. (2021). *The Future of Nursing 2020–2030: Charting a Path to Achieve Health Equity.* The National Academies Press. https://doi.org/10.17226/25982

Nemetchek, B. (2019). A concept analysis of social justice in global health. *Nursing Outlook, 67*(3), 244–251.

Sadarangani, T. R. (2020). The nurse's role in promoting health equity and improving racial justice in older adults through elimination of unconscious bias. *Geriatric Nursing, 41*(6), 1025–1027.

Stonehouse, D. P. (2021). Understanding nurses' responsibilities in promoting equality and diversity. *Nursing Standard, 27*–33. https://doi.org/10.7748/ns.2021.e11531

Yanicki, S. M., Kushner, K. E., & Reutter, L. (2015). Social inclusion/exclusion as matters of social (in)justice: A call for nursing action. *Nursing Inquiry, 22*, 121–133.

Social Marketing   8750

Definition: Use of marketing principles to influence the health beliefs, attitudes, and behaviors to benefit a target population

Activities:

- Maintain focus on the target audience through all activities
- Cultivate partnerships with the target audience and appropriate professionals
- Identify the overall goal to be achieved in collaboration with the target audience
- Identify the key formal, social, and governmental groups involved
- Conduct a needs assessment of the environment, identifying target audience desires
- Conduct organization or group assessment
- Identify appropriate quantitative and qualitative research to provide information, support, and indicators of success
- Design a plan of action based on mutually agreed-upon goals
- Nurture the voluntary basis of the planned social change
- Identify the product (behavior change), the price (consumer's actions), and the place (how the product reaches the consumer)
- Consider the financial resources necessary and available
- Identify specific activities for each goal, including naming of appropriate participants
- Implement the plan in collaboration with the target population
- Control the plan through monitoring of assigned tasks
- Provide appropriate reports on a timely basis
- Evaluate the plan for achievement of goals with consideration of sustainability and affordability
- Modify the plan, as needed

5th edition 2008

Background Evidence:

Brown, K. M., Bryant, C., Forthofer, M., Perrin, K., Quinn, G., Wolper, M., & Lindenberger, J. (2000). Florida cares for women social marketing campaign: A case study. *American Journal of Health Behavior, 24*(1), 44–52.

Grier, S., & Bryant, C. (2005). Social marketing in public health. *Annual Review of Public Health, 26*, 319–339.

Kotler, P., & Roberto, E. (1989). *Social marketing: Strategies for changing public behavior.* Free Press.

Pirani, S., & Reizes, T. (2005). The turning point social marketing national excellence collaborative: Integrating social marketing into routine public health practice. *Journal of Public Health Management and Practice, 11*(2), 131–138.

Smith, W. (2000). Social marketing: An evolving definition. *American Journal of Health Behavior, 24*(1), 11–17.

Szydlowski, S., Chattopadhyay, S., & Babela, R. (2005). Social marketing as a tool to improve behavioral health services for underserved populations in transition. *The Health Care Manager, 24*(1), 12–20.

S

Socialization Enhancement   5100

Definition: Facilitation of another person's ability to interact with others

Activities:

- Encourage enhanced involvement in already established relationships
- Encourage patience in developing relationships
- Promote relationships with persons who have common interests and goals
- Encourage social and community activities
- Promote sharing of common problems with others
- Encourage honesty in presenting oneself to others
- Promote involvement in totally new interests
- Encourage respect for the rights of others
- Facilitate the use of sensory deficit aids, such as eyeglasses and hearing aids
- Encourage participation in group and/or individual reminiscence activities
- Facilitate patient participation in storytelling groups

- Refer patient to interpersonal skills group or program in which understanding of transactions can be increased, as appropriate
- Allow testing of interpersonal limits
- Give feedback about improvement in care of personal appearance or other activities
- Help patient increase awareness of strengths and limitations in communicating with others
- Use role playing to practice improved communication skills and techniques
- Provide role models who express anger appropriately
- Confront patient about impaired judgment, when appropriate
- Request and expect verbal communication
- Give positive feedback when patient reaches out to others
- Encourage patient to change environment, such as going outside for walks or to movies
- Facilitate patient input and planning of future activities
- Encourage small group planning for special activities
- Explore strengths and weaknesses of current network of relationships

1st edition 1992; revised 2000, 2004, 2008

Background Evidence:

Frisch, N. (2006). Group therapy. In N. Frisch & L. Frisch (Eds.), *Psychiatric mental health nursing* (3rd ed., pp. 756–769). Delmar.

Hawkins, J., Kosterman, R., Catalano, R., Hill, K., & Abbott, R. (2005). Promoting positive adult functioning through social development intervention in childhood. *Archives of Pediatric and Adolescent Medicine, 159*(1), 25–31.

Kopelowicz, A., & Liberman, R. (2003). Integrating treatment with rehabilitation for persons with major mental illnesses. *Psychiatric Services, 54*(11), 1491–1498.

Resnick, B., & Fleishell, A. (2002). Developing a restorative care program: A five-step approach that involves the resident. *American Journal of Nursing, 102*(7), 91–95.

Swanson, E., & Drury, J. (2001). Sensory/perceptual alterations. In M. Maas, K. Buckwalter, M. Hardy, T. Tripp-Reimer, M. Titler, & J. Specht (Eds.), *Nursing care of older adults: Diagnoses, outcomes and interventions* (pp. 476–491). Mosby.

Varcarolis, E. (2006). Mood disorders/depression. In E. Varcarolis, V. Carson, & N. Shoemaker (Eds.), *Foundations of psychiatric/mental health nursing: A clinical approach* (pp. 326–358). Saunders Elsevier.

Waterman, J., Blegen, M., Clinton, P., & Specht, J. (2001). Social isolation. In M. Maas, K. Buckwalter, M. Hardy, T. Tripp-Reimer, M. Titler, & J. Specht (Eds.), *Nursing care of older adults: Diagnoses, outcomes, & interventions* (pp. 651–663). Mosby.

Weiss, S. (2004). Children. In C. Kneisl, H. Wilson, & E. Trigoboff (Eds.), *Contemporary psychiatric-mental health nursing* (pp. 589–614). Prentice Hall.

Specimen Management 7820

Definition: Obtaining, preparing, and preserving a specimen for a laboratory test

Activities:

- Obtain required sample, according to protocol
- Instruct patient how to collect and preserve specimen, as appropriate
- Provide specimen container required
- Apply special specimen collection devices for infants, toddlers, or impaired adults, as needed
- Assist with the biopsy of a tissue or organ, as appropriate
- Assist with aspiration of fluid from a body cavity, as appropriate
- Store specimen collected over time, according to protocol
- Seal all specimen containers to prevent leakage or contamination
- Label specimen with appropriate data before leaving the patient
- Place specimen in appropriate container for transport
- Arrange transport of the specimen to the laboratory
- Order specimen-related routine laboratory tests, as appropriate

1st edition 1992; revised 2008

Background Evidence:

Perry, A. G., & Potter, P. A. (2006). *Clinical nursing skills and techniques* (6th ed.). Elsevier Mosby.

Potter, P. A., & Perry, A. G. (2005). *Fundamentals of nursing* (6th ed.). Mosby.

Taylor, C., Lillis, C., LeMone, P., & Lynn, P. (2008). *Fundamentals of nursing: The art and science of nursing care* (6th ed.). Lippincott Williams and Wilkins.

Spiritual Growth Facilitation 5426

Definition: Facilitation of growth in person or family's capacity to identify, connect with, and call upon the source of meaning, purpose, comfort, strength, and hope in their life

Activities:

- Recognize own spiritual beliefs regarding relationship with greater power
- Convey engagement, interest, and compassion
- Build trusting relationship
- Demonstrate caring presence and comfort by spending time with person, their family, or significant others
- Model healthy relating and reasoning skills
- Provide environment that fosters meditative or contemplative attitude for self-reflection
- Encourage conversation that assists person in sorting out spiritual concerns and beliefs
- Determine unique, expressed spiritual needs
- Assist person with identifying barriers and attitudes that hinder growth, self-discovery, or ability to achieve personal spiritual needs
- Encourage examination of spiritual commitment based on beliefs and values
- Assist exploring beliefs as related to healing of body, mind, and spirit

- Offer prayer support, as appropriate
- Nurture faith in higher power during spiritual care encounters through use of devotions, prayers, physical touch, scripture, or music, as appropriate
- Take initiative in prayers, monitoring readiness, openness, and comfort level with praying or being prayed for, as indicated
- Encourage participation in devotional services, retreats, and special prayer or study programs
- Promote relationships with others for fellowship and service
- Encourage use of spiritual celebration and rituals
- Refer to support groups, mutual self-help, or other spiritually based programs, as appropriate
- Refer for pastoral care or primary spiritual caregiver, as indicated
- Refer for additional guidance and support in body, mind, and spirit connection, as needed

3rd edition 2000; revised 2024

Background Evidence:

Burkhardt, M. A., & Nagai-Jacobson, M. C. (2022). Spirituality and health. In M. A. Blaszko Helming, D. A. Shields, K. M. Avino, & W. E. Rosa (Eds.), *Dossey & Keegan's Holistic nursing handbook: A handbook for practice* (8th ed., pp. 121–143). Jones & Bartlett.

Cone, P. H., & Giske, T. (2018). Integrating spiritual care into nursing education and practice: Strategies utilizing Open Journey Theory. *Nurse Education Today, 71*, 22–25.

Hawthorne, D. M., & Gordon, S. C. (2020). The invisibility of spiritual nursing care in clinical practice. *Journal of Holistic Nursing, 38*(1), 147–155.

Johnston-Taylor, E. (2020). What can I do when my manager says I cannot give spiritual care: Part 2? *Journal of Christian Nursing, 37*(3), 191.

Mamier, I., Talor, E. J., & Winslow, B. W. (2019). Nurse spiritual care: Prevalence and correlates. *Western Journal of Nursing Research, 41*(4), 537–554.

Mcharo, S. K. (2018). T.R.U.S.T. model for inclusive spiritual care. *Journal of Holistic Nursing, 36*(3), 282–290.

Spiritual Support   5420

Definition: Assisting the person or family to feel balance and connection with a greater power

Activities:

- Recognize own spiritual beliefs regarding relationship with greater power
- Convey engagement, interest, and compassion
- Use therapeutic communications to establish trust and empathic caring
- Use tools to monitor and evaluate spiritual well-being, as appropriate (e.g., formal spiritual assessments; admission statements related to religion, nationality, language; statements related to illness)
- Ensure adequate time available for therapeutic interaction
- Begin conversations with concrete and easily discussed questions and prompts while being open to when or if person or family member wants to talk about more personal beliefs
- Treat with dignity and respect
- Ask if thinks of self as spiritual or religious and use response to determine if conversation should continue
- Allow person or family to steer conversation (i.e., have maximal control over discourse)
- Determine importance of faith or beliefs for person or family (e.g., regular attendance at religious services; scheduled prayer sessions; adherence to religious rituals)
- Encourage review of past life and focus on events and relationships that provided spiritual strength and support
- Encourage life review through reminiscence
- Be open to expressions of concern, loneliness, or powerlessness
- Be available to listen to feelings and express empathy
- Ensure that nurse will be available to support individual in times of suffering
- Encourage to be open to feelings about illness and death
- Assist to properly express and relieve anger in appropriate ways
- Provide opportunities for discussion of various belief systems and world views
- Use values clarification techniques to help clarify beliefs and values, as appropriate
- Share own beliefs about meaning and purpose, as appropriate
- Share own spiritual perspective, as appropriate

- Facilitate use of meditation, prayer, and other religious traditions and rituals
- Listen carefully to communication, and develop sense of timing for prayer or spiritual rituals
- Provide privacy and quiet times for spiritual activities
- Instruct about methods of relaxation, meditation, and guided imagery, as appropriate
- Provide spiritual music, literature, radio, or television programs if indicated
- Take initiative in prayers for individuals, families or groups, monitoring readiness, openness and comfort level with praying or being prayed for, as indicated
- Pray with person or family, if requested
- Be aware of religious rules, celebrations, and customs that may affect nursing or spiritual care (e.g., dietary laws, fasting, blood transfusions, free-flowing water for cleansing)
- Adapt nursing care to accommodate person's spiritual or religious rituals, where possible
- Arrange visits by spiritual advisor or clergy, if indicated
- Encourage participation in spiritual or religious interactions with family members, friends, and others
- Determine if person would like to be able to attend religious services
- Accommodate attendance at services where possible (e.g., live-streamed television services)
- Encourage participation in support groups
- Encourage religious service attendance, if desired
- Encourage use of spiritual resources, if desired
- Provide desired spiritual articles, according to individual preferences
- Refer to spiritual advisor of individual's choice, if possible and appropriate
- Refer for additional guidance and support in body, mind, and spirit connection, as needed

1st edition 1992; revised 2004; 2024

S

Background Evidence:

Burkhardt, M. A., & Nagai-Jacobson, M. C. (2022). Spirituality and health. In M. A. Blaszko Helming, D. A. Shields, K. M. Avino, & W. E. Rosa (Eds.), *Dossey & Keegan's Holistic nursing handbook: A handbook for practice* (8th ed., pp. 121–143). Jones & Bartlett.

Cone, P. H., & Giske, T. (2018). Integrating spiritual care into nursing education and practice: Strategies utilizing Open Journey Theory. *Nurse Education Today, 71*, 22–25.

Fowler, J. (2017). From staff nurse to nurse consultant: Spiritual care part 9 Judaism. *British Journal of Nursing, 26*(22), 1262.

Fowler, J. (2017). From staff nurse to nurse consultant: Spiritual care part 7 Islam. *British Journal of Nursing, 26*(19), 1082.

Fowler, J. (2017). From staff nurse to nurse consultant: Spiritual care part 6 Hinduism. *British Journal of Nursing, 26*(17), 996.

Fowler, J. (2017). From staff nurse to nurse consultant: Spiritual care part 4 Christianity. *British Journal of Nursing, 26*(14), 834.

Hawthorne, D. M., & Gordon, S. C. (2020). The invisibility of spiritual nursing care in clinical practice. *Journal of Holistic Nursing, 38*(1), 147–155.

Johnston-Taylor, E. (2020). What can I do when my manager says I cannot give spiritual care: Part 2? *Journal of Christian Nursing, 37*(3), 191.

Mamier, I., Taylor, E. J., & Winslow, B. W. (2019). Nurse spiritual care: Prevalence and correlates. *Western Journal of Nursing Research, 41*(4), 537–554.

Mcharo, S. K. (2018). T.R.U.S.T. model for inclusive spiritual care. *Journal of Holistic Nursing, 36*(3), 282–290.

Splinting 0910

Definition: Stabilization, immobilization, and protection of an injured body part with a supportive appliance

Activities:

- Monitor circulation (e.g., pulse, capillary refill, and sensation) in injured body part
- Monitor movement distal to injury site
- Monitor for bleeding at injury site
- Cover open wound with dressing and control bleeding before applying splint
- Minimize movement of patient, especially injured body part
- Identify most appropriate splint material (e.g., rigid, soft, anatomical, or traction)
- Pad rigid splints
- Immobilize joint above and joint below injury site
- Support feet using a footboard
- Place injured hand or wrist in position of function
- Apply splint in position injured body part is found, using hands to support injury site, minimizing movement, and using the assistance of another health care team member when possible
- Apply a sling, as appropriate
- Monitor skin integrity under supportive appliance
- Encourage isometric exercises, as appropriate
- Instruct patient or family how to care for the splint

1st edition 1992; revised 2013

Background Evidence:

Pfeiffer, R. P., Thygerson, A., & Palmieri, N. F. (2009). In B. Gulli & E. W. Ossman, Medical (Eds.), *Sports first aid and injury prevention*. Jones & Bartlett.

Schottke, D. (2007). Injuries to muscles and bones. In A. N. Pollack (Ed.), *First responder: Your first response in emergency care* (4th ed., pp. 327–367). Jones & Bartlett.

Thygerson, A. (2005). Splinting extremities. In *American Academy of Orthopaedic Surgeons, First aid, CPR, and AED* (4th ed., pp. 239–254). Jones & Bartlett.

Staff Supervision 7830

Definition: Facilitating the delivery of high-quality patient care by others

Activities:

- Create a work environment that validates the importance of each employee to the organization
- Acknowledge an employee's area of expertise
- Ensure that staff members provide care within their approved scopes of practice
- Ensure that staff members have current licensure, as appropriate
- Select a management style appropriate to the work situation and employee characteristics
- Encourage open communication
- Identify opportunities for participation in decision making
- Provide a job description for all new employees
- Provide clear expectations for job performance
- Share evaluation methods used with employee
- Foster teamwork and a sense of purpose for the work group
- Set goals for staff, as appropriate
- Consider employee growth in work assignments
- Share information about the organization and future plans
- Listen to employee concerns and suggestions
- Provide feedback on work performance at regular intervals
- Provide coaching and encouragement
- Reinforce good performance
- Facilitate employee opportunities to be "winners"
- Provide recognition for behavior that supports organizational goals
- Maintain an attitude of trust of others
- Seek advice from employees, as appropriate
- Use informal networks to accomplish goals
- Provide challenges and opportunities for employee growth
- Monitor quality of work performance
- Monitor quality of employee's relationships with other health care providers
- Incorporate understanding of generational differences when assigning and evaluating work

S

- Document strengths and weaknesses of employee
- Seek information on employee concerns for patient care and the work environment
- Seek feedback from patients concerning care provided
- Encourage staff to solve own problems
- Initiate disciplinary action, as appropriate, adhering to policies and procedures
- Counsel employee on how to improve performance, as appropriate
- Set time frames for needed behavior changes, as appropriate
- Provide reeducation to improve performance, as needed
- Complete evaluation forms at appropriate time intervals
- Discuss evaluation results privately

2nd edition 1996; revised 2018

Background Evidence:

Blanchard, K., Zigarmi, P., & Zigarmi, D. (2013). *Leadership and the one-minute manager: Increasing effectiveness through situational leadership II.* Harper Collins.

Gillen, P., & Graffin, S. (2010). Nursing delegation in the United Kingdom. *OJIN: The Online Journal of Issues in Nursing, 15*(2), Manuscript 6. https://doi.org/10.3912/OJIN.Vol15No02Man06

McCready, V. (2011). Generational issues in supervision and administration. *The ASHA Leader, 16*, 12–15. https://doi.org/10.1044/leader.FTRI.16052011.12

Yoder-Wise, P. (2011). *Leading and managing in nursing* (5th ed.). Elsevier Mosby.

Stem Cell Infusion   4266

Definition: Infusion of hematopoietic stem cells and monitoring of the patient's response

Activities:

- Ensure the product to be infused has been prepared, labeled, and classified according to institution protocol
- Explain the procedure and the aim of the infusion of hematopoietic stem cells to patients and caregivers
- Inform the patient and the family about the possible negative effects (e.g., transfusion reaction, volume overload, pulmonary embolism, changes in vital signs, and nausea/vomiting) that may appear during infusion
- Use peppermint oil or hard candy to counteract the offensive smell and taste of preservative
- Prepare infusion equipment without filter and other necessary materials (e.g., physiological serum 0.9%, venous pressure measurement systems, sphygmomanometer, phonendoscope, thermometer, and pulsometer)
- Verify that the infusion equipment has no filter and no infusion pumps to avoid cellular damage
- Use saline solution to flush the equipment
- Prepare emergency material and drugs to treat serious negative reactions, including anaphylaxis kit, oxygen administration equipment, and suction equipment
- Use gloves during the manipulation of the infusion product
- Ensure aseptic manipulation of equipment, connections, and product
- Administer prehydration solution according to the protocol
- Coordinate immediate administration of the defrosted infusion product
- Administer premedication prescribed according to the protocol of the institution
- Avoid irradiation and any type of mechanical or physical damage to the infusion product
- Make sure that the infusion product is received in optimal isolation and refrigeration conditions (1° to 24° C)
- Verify the labeling and the identification of both the bags and the patient (using patient name and hospital number) immediately before infusion
- Administer the infusion through a central venous catheter through the largest lumen available for ease of flow
- Infuse each bag at the rate, sequence, and time established in the protocol guidelines of the institution and according to the tolerance of the patient
- Monitor for possible adverse reactions (e.g., nausea, vomiting, abdominal cramps, diarrhea, facial flare, arrhythmia, dyspnea) and stop the infusion and call the physician, if necessary
- Irrigate the infusion catheter with saline solution after the infusion of each bag
- Irrigate the intravenous line with saline solution if syringes were used to infuse the product in order to reduce the loss of stem cells that could remain in the lumen of the catheter or infusion system
- Dispose of spare material and hazardous waste according to agency protocol
- Monitor vital signs according to institutional protocol during and after the procedure
- Record volume of stem cells and normal saline administered
- Monitor the elimination of urine, paying attention to volume, color, and osmolality
- Observe for signs and symptoms of circulatory overload
- Record the patient's response (e.g., tolerance and negative effects) according to the protocol of the institution
- Document adverse events according to agency protocol
- Provide patients and family with emotional support

6th edition 2013

Background Evidence:

Bevans, M., & Shelburne, N. (2004). Hematopoietic stem cell transplantation. *Clinical Journal of Oncology Nursing, 8*(5), 541–543.

Foundation for the Accreditation of Cellular Therapy. (2002). *Standards for hematopoietic progenitor cell collection, processing & transplantation* (2nd ed.).

Saria, M. G., & Gosselin-Acomb, T. K. (2007). Hematopoietic stem cell transplantation: Implications for critical care nurses. *Clinical Journal of Oncology Nursing, 11*(1), 53–63.

Sauer-Heilborn, A., Kadidlo, D., & McCullough, J. (2004). Patient care during infusion of hematopoietic progenitor cells. *Transfusion, 44*(6), 907–916.

S

Subarachnoid Hemorrhage Precautions 2720

Definition: Reduction of internal and external stimuli or stressors to minimize risk of rebleeding prior to surgery or endovascular procedure to secure ruptured aneurysm

Activities:
- Place patient in a private room
- Bed rest with bedside commode, as appropriate
- Maintain darkened room
- Decrease stimuli in patient's environment
- Restrict television, radio, and other stimulants
- Monitor response to visitors
- Limit visitors, if indicated
- Provide information to patient and family regarding need for environmental modifications and visiting limitations
- Give sedation, as needed
- Administer pain medications PRN
- Monitor neurological status
- Notify physician of neurological deterioration
- Monitor pulse and BP
- Maintain hemodynamic parameters within prescribed limits
- Monitor ICP and CPP if indicated
- Monitor CSF output and characteristics, if indicated
- Administer stool softeners
- Avoid rectal stimulation
- Instruct patient not to strain or perform Valsalva maneuver
- Implement seizure precautions
- Administer anticonvulsants, as appropriate

1st edition 1992; revised 2008

Background Evidence:

Ackerman, L. L. (1992). Interventions related to neurologic care. *Nursing Clinics of North America, 27*(2), 325–346.

Barker, E. (2002). Cranial surgery. In E. Barker (Ed.), *Neuroscience nursing— A spectrum of care* (2nd ed., pp. 303–349). Mosby.

Hickey, J. V., & Buckley, D. M. (2003). Cerebral aneurysms. In J. V. Hickey (Ed.), *The clinical practice of neurological and neurosurgical nursing* (5th ed., pp. 523–548). Lippincott Williams & Wilkins.

Hickle, J. L., Guanci, M. M., Bowman, L., Hermann, L., McGinty, L. B., & Rose, J. (2004). Cerebrovascular events of the nervous system. In M. K. Bader & L. R. Littlejohns (Eds.), *AANN core curriculum for neuroscience nursing* (4th ed., pp. 536–585). Saunders.

Lee, K. (1980). Aneurysm precautions: A physiologic basis for minimizing rebleeding. *Heart & Lung, 9*(2), 336–343.

Substance Use Prevention 4500

Definition: Deterrence of alcohol or drug abuse

Activities:
- Identify risk factors for substance use (e.g., maladaptive behaviors, negative life events, family conflict, child abuse, and neglect)
- Explain causes and consequences of substance misuse
- Counsel how to cope with increased levels of stress
- Assist individual to use anxiety reducing strategies
- Counsel how to prepare, cope, or avoid difficult or emotionally painful events, or irritating or frustrating situations
- Assist to reduce social isolation, as appropriate
- Encourage responsible decision making about lifestyle choices
- Engage in evidence-based substance abuse prevention programs (e.g., life skills training, social skills training, competence enhancement program, social resistance skills training)
- Encourage parents on importance of good role modeling
- Instruct parents and teachers in identification of signs and symptoms of addiction
- Support parents regarding development of parenting skills, nurturing behaviors, establishing clear boundaries or rules, and parental monitoring
- Instruct parents to support school policy that prohibits drug and alcohol consumption at extracurricular activities
- Encourage parents to participate in children's activities beginning in preschool through adolescence
- Recommend responsible changes in alcohol and drug curricula for primary grades
- Encourage school programs on avoidance of drugs and alcohol as recreational activities
- Support or organize community groups to reduce injuries associated with alcohol
- Promote media campaigns on substance use issues
- Survey students on use of alcohol and drugs and alcohol-related behaviors, if indicated
- Assist in organizing activities for teenagers after functions like prom and homecoming
- Facilitate coordination of efforts between various community groups concerned with substance use
- Involve families in prevention programs
- Support religious beliefs, practices, and participation in spiritual programs inspired by faith

1st edition 1992; revised 2000, 2024

Background Evidence:

American Nurses Association and International Nursing Society on Addictions. (2013). *Addictions nursing: Scope and standards of practice.* American Nurses Association.

Boyd, M. A. (2021). *Psychiatric nursing: Contemporary practice* (7th ed.). Wolters Kluwer.

Grim, B. J., & Grim, M. E. (2019). Belief, behavior, and belonging: how faith is indispensable in preventing and recovering from substance abuse. *Journal of Religion and Health, 58*(5), 1713–1750. https://doi.org/10.1007/s10943-019-00876-w

Hines, C. B., & Owings, C. R. (2021). Opioids: Understanding how acute actions impact chronic consequences. *Dimensions of Critical Care Nursing, 40*(5), 268–274. https://doi.org/10.1097/DCC.0000000000000487

Pfister, A., Koschmieder, N., & Wyss, S. (2020). Limited access to family-based addiction prevention services for socio-economically deprived families in Switzerland: A grounded theory study. *International Journal*

S

for Equity in Health, 19(1), 194. https://doi.org/10.1186/s12939-020-01305-1

Ryan, S. A., Kokotailo, P., & Committee on Substance Use and Prevention. (2019). Alcohol use by youth. Pediatrics, 144(1), e20191357. https://doi.org/10.1542/peds.2019-1357

Substance Abuse and Mental Health Services Administration. (2019). Substance Abuse and Mental Health Services Administration: Substance misuse prevention for young adults. National Mental Health and Substance Use Policy Laboratory.

Tierney, M., Finnell, D. S., Naegle, M., Mitchell, A. M., & Pace, E. M. (2020). The future of nursing: Accelerating gains made to address the continuum of substance use. Archives of Psychiatric Nursing, 34(5), 297–303. https://doi.org/10.1016/j.apnu.2020.07.010

Substance Use Treatment   4510

Definition: Care of patient and family members demonstrating dysfunction as a result of substance abuse or dependence

Activities:

- Foster a trusting relationship while setting clear limits (i.e., provide gentle but firm evidence of dysfunction, stay focused on substance abuse or dependency, and inspire hope)
- Consider presence of comorbidity, or cooccurring psychiatric or medical disorder, making changes in treatment accordingly
- Assist patient in understanding disorder as a disease related to several factors (e.g., genetic, psychological, and situational circumstances)
- Inform patient that the volume and frequency of substance use leading to dysfunction varies greatly between people
- Instruct patient on effects of substance used (e.g., physical, psychological, and social)
- Discuss treatment needs for associated medical, psychological, social, vocational, housing, and legal difficulties
- Encourage or praise patient efforts to accept responsibility for substance use-related dysfunction and treatment
- Provide symptom management during the detoxification period
- Administer medications (e.g., disulfiram, acamprosate, methadone, naltrexone, nicotine patches or gum, or buprenorphine), as indicated
- Instruct patient or family about medications used for treatment
- Provide therapy (e.g., cognitive therapy, motivational therapy, counseling, family support, family therapy, or adolescent community reinforcement approach), as indicated
- Establish multidisciplinary programs (e.g., short-term inpatient residential therapy, detoxification program, or residential therapeutic community treatment), if appropriate
- Encourage patient to participate in self-help support program during and after treatment (e.g., 12-step programs, Women for Sobriety, or Rational Recovery)
- Discuss importance of abstaining from substance use, identifying most appropriate treatment goal (e.g., complete abstinence, day-by-day sobriety, or use of substance in moderation)
- Coordinate and facilitate group confrontation strategy to address use of and role defenses play in substance use (e.g., denial)
- Instruct patient on stress management techniques (e.g., exercise, meditation, and relaxation therapy)
- Assist patient in developing healthy, effective coping mechanisms
- Identify and address dysfunctional relationship patterns in patient's familial or other social ties (e.g., codependency and enabling)
- Assist in identifying and facilitating connections with supportive persons
- Assist in resocialization, rebuilding relationships, and decreasing self-centeredness

- Monitor for substance use during treatment (e.g., urine screens and breath analysis)
- Monitor for infectious disease (e.g., HIV/AIDS, hepatitis B and C, and tuberculosis), treating and providing assistance to modify behaviors, if necessary
- Assist patient in developing self-worth, encouraging positive efforts and motivation
- Encourage patient to keep a detailed chart of substance use to evaluate progress
- Assist the patient to evaluate the amount of time spent using the substance and the usual patterns within the day
- Participate in efforts to remain abreast of available programs, resources, and legislation aimed at education, prevention, and treatment of substance use disorders
- Instruct patient on symptoms or behaviors that increase chances of relapse (e.g., exhaustion, depression, dishonesty, and complacency)
- Develop plan for relapse prevention (e.g., contracting, identify resources for various needs in stressful situation, and identify health promoting activities to take place of substance use)
- Instruct family on substance use disorder and related dysfunction and include in treatment planning and activities
- Encourage family to participate in recovery efforts
- Provide referral

1st edition 1992; revised 2013

Background Evidence:

Essau, C. A. (Ed.). (2008). Adolescent addiction: Epidemiology, assessment, and treatment. Academic Press.

Jacobson, S. A., Pies, R. W., & Katz, I. R. (2007). Treatment of substance-related disorders. In Clinical manual of geriatric psychopharmacology (pp. 403–475). American Psychiatric.

Lickteig, M. (2009). Substance use disorders. In W. K. Mohr (Ed.), Psychiatric-mental health nursing: Evidence-based concepts, skills, and practices (7th ed., pp. 607–650). Wolters Kluwer Health/Lippincott Williams & Wilkins.

Trigoboff, E. (2009). Substance-related disorders. In C. R. Kneisl & E. Trigoboff (Eds.), Contemporary psychiatric-mental health nursing (2nd ed., pp. 323–369). Pearson Prentice Hall.

World Health Organization, Department of Mental Health and Substance Abuse. (2009). Guidelines for the psychosocially assisted pharmacological treatment of opioid dependence.

S

Substance Use Treatment: Alcohol Withdrawal 4512

Definition: Care of the person experiencing sudden cessation of alcohol consumption

Activities:
- Determine level of alcohol consumption, mental, and physical condition
- Monitor blood alcohol concentration and useful markers such as CBC, urea, electrolytes, and liver function tests
- Monitor severity of withdrawal syndrome with validated scales (e.g., Clinical Institute Withdrawal Assessment of Alcohol Scale - Revised [CIWA -AR])
- Encourage fluids (e.g., water, electrolyte drinks)
- Create low-stimulation environment for detoxification
- Monitor vital signs during withdrawal
- Monitor for delirium tremens
- Provide reality orientation, as appropriate
- Administer medications for management of alcohol dependence or relapse prevention, as appropriate
- Medicate to relieve physical discomfort as needed
- Approach abusive behavior in neutral manner
- Address hallucinations in therapeutic manner
- Maintain adequate nutrition and fluid intake
- Administer vitamin therapy, as appropriate
- Monitor for covert alcohol consumption during detoxification
- Listen to person and family concerns about alcohol withdrawal
- Instruct about signs and symptoms that may occur during withdrawal (e.g., fatigue, depression)

- Provide psychosocial interventions such as motivational interviewing and brief counseling, as appropriate
- Provide emotional support to person and family, as appropriate
- Recommend follow-up with proper counseling

1st edition 1992; revised 2000, 2024

Background Evidence:

American Nurses Association and International Nursing Society on Addictions. (2013). *Addictions nursing: Scope and standards of practice.* American Nurses Association.

Boyd, M. A. (2021). *Psychiatric nursing: Contemporary practice* (7th ed.). Wolters Kluwer.

Duong, T., Vytialingam, R., & O'Regan, R. (2018). *A brief guide to the management of alcohol and other drug withdrawal.* Perth, Western Australia: Mental Health Commission.

Manning, V., Arunogiri, S., Frei, M., Ridley, K., Mroz, K., Campbell, S., & Lubman, D. (2018). *Alcohol and other drug withdrawal: Practice guidelines* (3rd ed.). Turning Point.

Substance Abuse and Mental Health Services Administration and National Institute on Alcohol Abuse and Alcoholism. (2015). *Medication for the treatment of alcohol use disorder: A brief guide.* Substance Abuse and Mental Health Services Administration.

Substance Use Treatment: Drug Withdrawal 4514

Definition: Care of patient experiencing drug detoxification

Activities:
- Monitor vital signs
- Monitor respiratory and cardiac systems (e.g., hypertension, tachycardia, and bradypnea)
- Monitor for changes in level of consciousness
- Monitor intake and output
- Monitor for suicidal tendencies
- Implement precautions for patient at risk for suicide
- Monitor withdrawal symptoms (e.g., fatigue, sensory disturbances, irritability, violence, depression, panic attacks, cravings, insomnia, agitation, muscle pain, appetite changes, yawning, weakness, headache, runny nose, dilated pupils, chills, anxiety, sweating, nausea, vomiting, tremors, psychosis, and ataxia)
- Provide symptom management
- Administer medications (e.g., benzodiazepines, chlorpromazine, diazepam, nicotine replacement, phenobarbital, clonidine, trazodone, methadone, alpha-2 adrenergic agonists, and antipsychotics), remaining aware of cross-tolerance
- Implement precautions for patient at risk for seizures
- Provide adequate nutrition (e.g., small amounts of fluids frequently and high-calorie foods)
- Assist with activities of daily living
- Implement precautions for patient at risk for falling
- Maintain low-stimulation environment (e.g., talk in a low, calm voice; provide reassurance about safety; and ensure a comfortable, darkened, quiet, and nonthreatening environment)
- Reorient patient to reality

- Encourage patient to participate in follow-up support (e.g., peer group therapy, individual or family counseling, and drug recovery educational programs)
- Offer supportive assistance (e.g., provision of food and shelter, structured psychotherapy)
- Provide referral
- Facilitate support by family and significant others
- Provide support to family or significant others, as appropriate
- Instruct patient and family on process of drug use and dependency

1st edition 1992; revised 2013

Background Evidence:

Lickteig, M. (2009). Substance use disorders. In W. K. Mohr (Ed.), *Psychiatric-mental health nursing: Evidence-based concepts, skills, and practices* (7th ed., pp. 607–650). Wolters Kluwer Health/Lippincott Williams & Wilkins.

Trigoboff, E. (2009). Substance-related disorders. In C. R. Kneisl & E. Trigoboff (Eds.), *Contemporary psychiatric-mental health nursing* (2nd ed., pp. 323–369). Pearson: Prentice Hall.

World Health Organization, Department of Mental Health and Substance Abuse. (2009). *Guidelines for the psychosocially assisted pharmacological treatment of opioid dependence.*

S

Substance Use Treatment: Overdose   4516

Definition: Care of a patient demonstrating toxic effects as a result of consuming one or more drugs

Activities:

- Create or maintain an open airway
- Monitor respiratory, cardiac, gastrointestinal, renal, and neurological status
- Monitor vital signs
- Place patient in most appropriate position (e.g., semi-Fowler's position if patient is awake; left lateral recumbent position if patient is unresponsive)
- Provide safe environment (i.e., pad side rails, keep bed in lowest position, remove dangerous objects, and position safety officer near patient's room)
- Establish rapport with patient or family (i.e., use nonjudgmental approach; do not reprimand)
- Perform necessary toxicology screening and system function tests (e.g., urine and serum drug screening, arterial blood gases, electrolyte levels, liver enzymes, blood urea nitrogen, and creatinine)
- Contact poison control center for assistance in determining definitive treatment
- Establish intravenous access, administering infusions, as prescribed
- Monitor for symptoms specific to drug consumed (e.g., constricted pupils, hypotension, and bradycardia for opiate overdose; nausea, vomiting, diaphoresis, and right upper quadrant pain 48 to 72 hours after acetaminophen overdose; and dilated pupils, tachycardia, seizures, and chest pain for cocaine overdose)
- Administer agents specific to substance consumed and patient symptoms (e.g., antiemetics, naloxone, thiamine, glucose, flumazenil, calcium, vasopressors, antiarrhythmics, and inotropics)
- Administer agents or perform procedures to impair drug absorption and increase drug excretion (e.g., ipecac, activated charcoal, gastric lavage, hemodialysis, cathartics, exchange transfusion, altering urine and serum pH, and whole-bowel irrigation)
- Communicate with patient, providing reassurance, addressing hallucinations or delusions, and conveying understanding of fears or other feelings
- Monitor intake and output
- Treat hyperthermia (i.e., apply ice packs for fever caused by amphetamine or cocaine intoxication)
- Provide emotional support to patient and family
- Monitor for suicidal tendencies
- Provide instruction on proper use of drug
- Assist patient in identifying ways to minimize potential for accidental overdose (e.g., store medications in original container, address issues with confusion or memory, and store medications out of children's reach)
- Instruct family or caregiver on patient's need for follow-up care
- Instruct family or caregiver on aspiration and seizure precautions
- Provide referral (e.g., home health agency, social worker, psychiatry, or drug use treatment program)

1st edition 1992; revised 2013

Background Evidence:

Johnson, J. M. (2008). Over-the-counter overdoses: A review of ibuprofen, acetaminophen, and aspirin toxicity in adults. *Advanced Emergency Nursing Journal, 30*(4), 369–378.

Smeltzer, S. C., Bare, B. G., Hinkle, J. L., & Cheever, K. H. (2008). Emergency nursing. In *Brunner & Suddarth's textbook of medical-surgical nursing* (11th ed., pp. 2516–2557). Lippincott Williams & Wilkins.

Sturt, P. A. (2005). Toxicologic conditions. In J. Fultz & P. A. Sturt (Eds.), *Mosby's emergency nursing reference* (3rd ed., pp. 643–681). Elsevier Mosby.

Suicide Prevention   6340

Definition: Reducing the risk for self-inflicted harm with intent to end life

Activities:

- Determine presence of suicidal risk using valid suicide assessment scale
- Determine if has suicide plan
- Determine whether has available means to follow through with suicide plan
- Consider hospitalization of anyone at serious risk for suicidal behavior
- Treat and manage any psychiatric illness or symptoms that may be placing person at risk for suicide (e.g., mood disorder, hallucinations, delusions, panic, substance abuse, grief, personality disorder, organic impairment, crisis)
- Administer medications to decrease anxiety, agitation, or psychosis and to stabilize mood, as appropriate
- Advocate for quality of life and pain control issues
- Conduct mouth checks after medication administration to ensure that person is not "cheeking" medications for later overdose attempt
- Provide small amounts of prescriptive medications that may be lethal to those at risk, to decrease opportunity for suicide, as appropriate
- Monitor for medication side effects and desired outcomes
- Involve in planning own treatment, as appropriate
- Instruct in coping strategies (e.g., assertiveness training, impulse control, progressive muscle relaxation), as appropriate
- Interact at regular intervals to convey caring and openness and to provide an opportunity to talk about feelings
- Use direct, non-judgmental approach in discussing suicide
- Encourage to seek out care providers to talk as urge to harm self occurs
- Avoid repeated discussion of past suicide history by keeping discussions focused on present and future
- Discuss plans for dealing with suicidal ideation in future (e.g., precipitating factors, who to contact, where to go for help, ways to alleviate feelings of self-harm)
- Assist to identify network of support persons and resources (e.g., clergy, family, providers)

S

- Initiate suicide precautions (i.e., ongoing observation and monitoring of person, provision of protective environment) when at serious risk of suicide
- Place in least restrictive environment that allows for necessary level of observation
- Continue regular assessment of suicidal risk (at least daily) to adjust suicide precautions appropriately
- Consult with treatment team before modifying suicide precautions
- Search newly hospitalized person and personal belongings for weapons or potential weapons during inpatient admission procedure, as appropriate
- Search environment routinely and remove dangerous items to maintain as hazard free
- Limit access to windows, unless locked and shatterproof, as appropriate
- Limit use of potential weapons (e.g., sharps, ropelike objects)
- Monitor during use of potential weapons (e.g., razor)
- Use protective interventions (e.g., area restrictions, seclusion, physical restraints) if lacks restraint to refrain from harming self as needed
- Communicate risk and relevant safety issues to other care providers
- Assign to room located near nursing station for ease in observation, as appropriate
- Increase surveillance at times when staffing predictably low (e.g., staff meetings, change of shift report, staff mealtimes, nights, weekends, times of chaos on nursing unit)
- Consider strategies to decrease isolation and opportunity to act on harmful thoughts (e.g., use of sitter)
- Observe, record, and report any change in mood or behavior that may signify increasing suicidal risk
- Document results of regular surveillance checks
- Explain suicide precautions and relevant safety issues (e.g., purpose, duration, behavioral expectations, behavioral consequences)
- Facilitate support by family and friends
- Involve family in discharge planning (e.g., illness and medication teaching, recognition of increasing suicidal risk, plan for dealing with thoughts of harming self, community resources)

- Refer to mental health care provider (e.g., psychiatrist, psychiatric or mental health advanced practice nurse) for evaluation and treatment of suicide ideation and behavior as needed
- Provide information about available community resources and outreach programs
- Use teach-back to determine understanding
- Improve access to mental health services
- Increase public's awareness of suicide as preventable health problem

1st edition 1992; revised 2000, 2004, 2024

Background Evidence:

American Psychiatric Nurses Association. (2014). *Scope and standards of psychiatric-mental health nursing* (2nd ed.).

Butcher, H. K., & Ingram, T. (2018). Secondary suicide prevention in later life. *Journal of Gerontological Nursing, 44*(11), 20–32.

Chauliac, N., Leaune, E., Gardette, V., Poulet, E., & Duclos, A. (2020). Suicide prevention interventions for older people in nursing homes and long-term care facilities: A systematic review. *Journal of Geriatric Psychiatry & Neurology, 33*(6), 307–315. https://doi.org/10.1177/0891988719892343

Keltner, N. L., & Steele, D. (2019). *Psychiatric nursing* (8th ed.). Elsevier.

Kinsley, K., & Pritchett, W. (2021). Ambulatory Care Nurses: Suicide causes and prevention. *AAACN Viewpoint, 43*(2), 13–15.

Lindstrom, A. C., & Earle, M. (2021). Improving suicidal ideation screening and suicide prevention strategies on adult nonbehavioral health units. *Journal of Doctoral Nursing Practice, 14*(2), 122–129.

Manister, N. N., Murray, S., Burke, J. M., Finegan, M., & McKiernan, M. E. (2017). Effectiveness of nursing education to prevent inpatient suicide. *Journal of Continuing Education in Nursing, 48*(9), 413–419. https://doi.org/10.3928/00220124-20170816-07

Navin, K., Kuppili, P. P., Menon, V., & Kattimani, S. (2019). Suicide prevention strategies for general hospital and psychiatric inpatients: A narrative review. *Indian Journal of Psychological Medicine, 41*(5), 403–412.

Varcarolis, E. M., & Fosbre, C. D. (2021). *Essentials of psychiatric-mental health nursing* (4th ed.). Elsevier.

Supply Chain Management　　7840

Definition: Ensuring acquisition and maintenance of appropriate items for providing patient care

Activities:

- Identify items commonly used for patient care
- Determine stock level needed for each item
- Add new items to inventory list, as appropriate
- Work with physicians and others to standardize the specifications for products and reduce total number of supplies
- Check items for expiration dates at specific intervals
- Inspect integrity of sterile packages
- Ensure that supply area is cleaned regularly
- Avoid stockpiling expensive items
- Assist in the automation and upkeep of the inventory list to avoid overstocking and overspending
- Order new or replacement equipment, as necessary
- Coordinate purchases with other departments to reduce costs, as appropriate
- Work with suppliers and vendors to ensure best product at lowest cost, as needed

- Ensure that maintenance requirements on special equipment are completed
- Order patient education materials, as appropriate
- Have supplies shipped directly to patient's home, as appropriate
- Order specialty items for patient, as appropriate
- Charge patient for supplies, as appropriate
- Mark unit and agency equipment for identification, as appropriate
- Review supply budget and inventory costs, as appropriate
- Participate in the value analysis process to determine whether it is the "right product" at the "right price"
- Participate in the governing agency's integrated supply chain management process, as appropriate
- Understand how the use of GS1 Global Traceability Standard to identify items and locations can improve patient safety and reduce costs of supplies

2nd edition 1996; revised 2018

Background Evidence:

Dudas, J. (2010). Keeping an eye on the big picture: Mayo Clinic's integrated supply chain management. In *GS1 Healthcare Reference Book 201 0–2011* (pp. 21–24). Brussels, Belgium: GS1 Global Office.

GS1. (2012). *GS1 standards document: Business process and system requirements for full supply chain traceability* (Issue 1.3.0). http://www.gs1.org/docs/gsmp/traceability/Global_Traceability_Standard.pdf

Jarousse, L. (2011). Strategic supply chain management. *Hospitals and Health Networks.* http://www.hhnmag.com/articles/4522-strategic-supply-chain-management

Milburn, A. B., Mason, J., & Spicer, J. (2012). Characterizing the home health care supply chain. *Home Healthcare Management & Practice, 24*(6), 267–275.

Support Group   5430

Definition: Use of a group environment to provide emotional support and health-related information for members

Activities:

- Determine level and appropriateness of patient's present support system
- Use a support group during transitional stages to help patient adjust to a new lifestyle
- Determine purpose of the group and nature of the group process
- Determine the most appropriate venue for the group's meeting (e.g., face to face or online)
- Identify faith-based groups as available options for clients, as appropriate
- Create a relaxed, accepting atmosphere
- Clarify early on the goals of the group and the members' and leader's responsibilities
- Use a coleader, as appropriate
- Use a written contract, if deemed appropriate
- Choose members who can contribute to and benefit from group interaction
- Form a group of optimal size (e.g., 5 to 12 members)
- Address the issue of mandatory attendance
- Address the issue of whether new members can join at any time
- Establish a time and place for the group meeting
- Meet in 1- to 2-hour sessions, as appropriate
- Begin and end on time and expect participants to remain until the conclusion
- Arrange chairs in a circle in close proximity
- Schedule a limited number of sessions (e.g., 6 to 12) in which the work of the group will be accomplished
- Publicize membership policies to avoid problems that may arise as the group progresses
- Monitor and direct active involvement of group members
- Encourage expression and sharing of experiential knowledge
- Encourage expression of mutual aid

- Encourage appropriate referrals to professionals for information
- Emphasize personal responsibility and control
- Maintain positive pressure for behavior change
- Emphasize the importance of active coping
- Identify topic themes that occur in the group discussion
- Do not allow group to become a nonproductive social gathering
- Assist the group to progress through the stages of group development, from orientation through cohesiveness to termination
- Attend to the needs of the group as a whole, as well as the needs of individual members
- Refer the patient to other specialist, as appropriate

1st edition 1992; revised 2013

Background Evidence:

American Psychiatric Nurses Association. (2007). *Psychiatric-mental health nursing: Scope and standards of practice.*

Cincinnati Children's Hospital Medical Center. (2009). *Best evidence statement (BESt) inpatient support groups for families of children with intractable epilepsy.*

Dundon, E. (2006). Adolescent depression: A metasynthesis. *Journal of Pediatric Health Care, 20*(6), 384–392.

Kurlowicz, L., & Harvath, T. (2008). Depression. In E. Capezuti, D. Zwicker, M. Mezey, & T. Fulmer (Eds.), *Evidence-based geriatric nursing protocols for best practice* (3rd ed., pp. 57–82). Springer.

McQueen, K., Montgomery, P., Lappan-Gracon, S., Evans, M., & Hunter, J. (2008). Evidence-based recommendations for depressive symptom in postpartum women. *Journal of Obstetric, Gynecologic and Neonatal Nursing, 37*(2), 127–136.

Percy, C. A., Gibbs, T., Potter, L., & Boardman, S. (2009). Nurse-led peer support group: Experiences of women with polycystic ovary syndrome. *Journal of Advanced Nursing, 65*(10), 2046–2055.

Support System Enhancement   5440

Definition: Facilitation of support to patient by family, friends, and community

Activities:

- Identify psychological response to situation and availability of support system
- Determine adequacy of existing social networks
- Identify degree of family support, financial support, and other resources
- Determine barriers to unused and underused support systems
- Monitor current family situation and the support network
- Encourage the patient to participate in social and community activities

- Encourage relationships with persons who have common interests and goals
- Refer to a self-help group or Internet-based resource, as appropriate
- Identify community resource strengths and weaknesses and advocate for change, when appropriate
- Refer to a community-based prevention or treatment program, as appropriate
- Provide services in a caring and supportive manner

S

- Involve family/significant other(s) and friends in the care and planning
- Identify available resources for caregiver support
- Explain to concerned others how they can help

1st edition 1992; revised 2013

Background Evidence:

Commission on Social Determinants of Health. (2008). *Closing the gap in a generation: Health equity through action on the social determinants of health.* World Health Organization.

Dossey, B. M., & Keegan, L. (2009). *Holistic nursing: A handbook for practice* (5th ed.). Jones & Bartlett.

Häggman-Laitila, A., Tanninen, H. M., & Pietilä, A. M. (2010). Effectiveness of resource-enhancing family-oriented intervention. *Journal of Clinical Nursing, 19*(17-18), 2500–2510.

Hudson, D. B., Campbell-Grossman, C., Keating-Lefler, R., & Cline, P. (2008). New mothers' network: The development of an internet-based social support intervention for African American mothers. *Issues in Comprehensive Pediatric Nursing, 31*(1), 23–35.

Stuart, G. W. (Ed.). (2009). Prevention and mental health promotion. In *Principles and practice of psychiatric nursing* (9th ed., pp. 172–183). Mosby Elsevier.

Surgical Assistance   2900

Definition: Assisting the surgeon or dentist with operative procedures and care of the surgical patient

Activities:

- Perform surgical hand antisepsis in accordance with the hospital protocol or rules
- Don a sterile gown and gloves using aseptic technique
- Assist the surgical team while they don gown and gloves
- Adopt a position that allows you to keep the surgical field in sight throughout the surgery
- Anticipate and provide needed supplies and instruments throughout the procedure
- Ensure that appropriate instruments, supplies, and equipment are sterile and in good working order
- Transfer the scalpel or dermatographic pencil to the surgeon, as appropriate
- Provide the instruments in an appropriate safe manner
- Grasp tissue, as appropriate
- Dissect tissue, as appropriate
- Irrigate and suction surgical wound, as appropriate
- Protect tissue, as appropriate
- Provide hemostasis, as appropriate
- Maintain the sterility of the surgical field throughout the procedure, disposing of contaminated elements, and taking measures to preserve surgical integrity and asepsis
- Remove soiled sponges and deposit them in an appropriate place, replacing them with clean ones
- Clean the incision site and drains of blood, secretions, and residual skin antiseptic
- Assist in the closing of the surgical wound
- Dry the skin at the incision site and drains
- Apply reinforcement bands, dressings, or bandages to the surgical wound
- Assist in estimating blood loss
- Connect the drains to their collection systems, attach them, and keep them in the appropriate position
- Prepare and care for specimens, as appropriate
- Communicate information to the surgical team, as appropriate
- Communicate patient status and progress to family, as appropriate
- Arrange for equipment needed immediately after surgery
- Assist in transferring patient to the cart or bed and transport to appropriate postanesthesia or postoperative area
- Report to the post-anesthesia or postoperative nurse pertinent information about the patient and procedure performed
- Document information, as per agency policy

2nd edition 1996; revised 2013

Background Evidence:

Association of periOperative Registered Nurses. (2010). *Perioperative standards and recommended practices.*

Fuller, J. (2008). *Surgical technology: Principles and practice* (4th ed.). Panamericana.

Phippen, M., Ulmer, B. C., & Wells, M. M. (2009). *Competency for safe patient care during operative and invasive procedures.* Competency & Credentialing Institute.

Rothrock, J. C. (Ed.). (2011). *Alexander's care of the patient in surgery* (14th ed.). Elsevier Mosby.

Rothrock, J. C., & Siefert, P. C. (Eds.). (2009). *Assisting in surgery: Patient centered care.* Competency & Credentialing Institute.

Surgical Instrumentation Management   2910

Definition: Managing the requirements for materials, instruments, equipment, and sterility of the surgical field

Activities:

- Consult surgical schedules, check operating room assignments, and obtain information on the surgical procedure and anesthetic technique
- Determine the equipment, instruments, and supplies needed for care of the patient in surgery and make arrangements for availability
- Assemble equipment, instruments, and supplies for the surgery
- Change into the scrubs, footwear, cap, and mask specific to the surgical area before entering the operating room
- Place tables containing instruments and equipment in the appropriate areas
- Check instruments and arrange in order of use
- Keep sharp and pointed objects (e.g., scalpel blades and needles) separate from other objects in order to avoid injuries during preparation

- Verify the safety and proper operation of the equipment and instruments required for patient care (e.g., surgical table, perfusion pumps, temperature regulating equipment, electric scalpels)
- Prepare supplies, drugs, and solutions for use, as indicated
- Obtain the sterile supplies and materials appropriate to the surgery, observing aseptic technique
- Confirm the integrity of the packages or wrappings, expiration dates, and sterility controls, and follow the traceability of the materials in keeping with hospital regulations
- Prepare the consumable clothing and supplies appropriate to the type of surgery
- Turn on and position lights
- Drape the instrument tables, Mayo tables, and auxiliary tables with sterile cloth or impermeable fields, as appropriate
- Establish a safety perimeter around the tables and materials with regard to other professional and nonsterile areas
- Provide towels/pads for the surgical team to dry their hands on
- Secure devices in the surgical field (e.g., cables, circuit cameras, aspirators)
- Remove instruments and supplies from the surgical table once the surgery is finished
- Remove field forceps, aspirator tube, electric scalpel, and other elements from the surgical field after the conclusion of the operation
- Roll up the fields, sheets, and surgical drapes used in the surgery, avoiding the spread and contamination of the air, and dispose of them in an appropriate container
- Remove scalpel blades from their handles, needles, sharp and pointed objects and deposit them in appropriate containers
- Separate the clean materials and instruments from the dirty or highly contaminated ones to facilitate cleaning, disinfection, and later sterilization
- Coordinate and assist in the cleaning and preparation of the operating room for the next patient (i.e., collect and put away machines, supports, and other supplies)

6th edition 2013

Background Evidence:

Association of periOperative Registered Nurses. (2010). *Perioperative standards and recommended practices.*

Fuller, J. (2008). *Surgical technology: Principles and practice* (4th ed.). Madrid: Panamericana.

Gruendemann, B. J., & Mangum, S. S. (2001). *Infection prevention in surgical settings.* W. B. Saunders.

Phippen, M., Ulmer, B. C., & Wells, M. M. (2009). *Competency for safe patient care during operative and invasive procedures.* Competency & Credentialing Institute.

Rothrock, J. C. (Ed.). (2011). *Alexander's care of the patient in surgery* (14th ed.). Elsevier Mosby.

Rothrock, J. C., & Siefert, P. C. (Eds.). (2009). *Assisting in surgery: Patient centered care.* Competency & Credentialing Institute.

Surgical Precautions   2920

Definition: Minimizing the potential for iatrogenic injury to the patient related to a surgical procedure

Activities:

- Check ground isolation monitor
- Arrange the oxygenation and artificial ventilation equipment and material (e.g., laryngoscopes, tubes, aspirator, masks, Magill forceps, stiffening wires, phonendoscope)
- Verify the correct functioning of equipment
- Monitor the accessories specific to the required surgical position (e.g., supports, stirrups, fasteners)
- Check suction for adequate pressure and complete assembly of canisters, tubing, and catheters
- Remove any unsafe equipment
- Verify consent for surgery and other treatments, as appropriate
- Participate in a preoperative briefing with others, as per agency policy
- Welcome the patient, establishing a relationship of trust and offering counsel
- Verify with the patient or appropriate others the procedure and surgical site
- Verify that patient's identification band and blood band are correct
- Ask patient or appropriate other to state patient's name and birth date
- Participate in the preoperative "time out" to verify correct patient, procedure, and site, as per agency policy
- Ensure documentation and communication of any allergies
- Assist in the transfer of the patient to the surgical table while monitoring devices
- Preserve the patient's privacy, avoiding unnecessary exposure or chills
- Count sponges, sharps, and instruments before, during, and after surgery, as per agency policy
- Record results of counts, as per agency policy
- Remove and store prostheses appropriately
- Provide a sterile container for depositing sharp objects
- Provide an electrosurgical unit, grounding pad, and active electrode, as appropriate
- Verify integrity of electrical cords
- Verify proper functioning of electrosurgical unit
- Verify absence of cardiac pacemaker, other electrical implant, or metal prostheses contraindicating use of electrosurgical cautery
- Verify that the patient is not touching metal
- Inspect the patient's skin at the site of grounding pad
- Apply grounding pad to dry, intact skin with minimal hair, over large muscle mass, and as close to the operative site as possible
- Verify that prep solutions are nonflammable or that flammable prep agents have evaporated before draping
- Remove residual flammable prep agents before the start of surgery
- Evacuate oxygen from under surgical drapes
- Take precautions before the surgery starts against ionizing radiation or use protective equipment in situations that require it
- Protect grounding pad from prep and irrigation solutions and damage
- Apply and use holster to store active electrode during surgery
- Adjust coagulation and cutting currents as instructed by physician or agency policy
- Inspect the patient's skin for injury after use of electrosurgery
- Deposit waste materials in the appropriate containers
- Assist in the transfer of the patient, verifying the proper position of tubes, catheters, and drains, and adopting the position appropriate to the surgery performed
- Cover the patient to avoid unnecessary exposure and loss of heat

S

- Document appropriate information on the operative record
- Participate in a postoperative debriefing, as per agency policy

2nd edition 1996; revised 2013

Background Evidence:

Association of periOperative Registered Nurses. (2010). *Perioperative standards and recommended practices*.

Emergency Care Research Institute (ECRI). (2007). Electrosurgery. In *Healthcare Risk Control Risk Analysis* (*Vol. 4*).

Fuller, J. (2008). *Surgical technology: Principles and practice* (4th ed.). Madrid: Panamericana.

Gruendemann, B. J., & Mangum, S. S. (2001). *Infection prevention in surgical settings*. W. B. Saunders.

Phippen, M., Ulmer, B. C., & Wells, M. M. (2009). *Competency for safe patient care during operative and invasive procedures*. Competency & Credentialing Institute.

Rothrock, J. C. (Ed.). (2011). *Alexander's care of the patient in surgery* (14th ed.). Elsevier Mosby.

Rothrock, J. C., & Siefert, P. C. (Eds.). (2009). *Assisting in surgery: Patient centered care*. Competency & Credentialing Institute.

World Alliance for Patient Safety. (2008). *Surgical safety checklist and implementation manual*. World Health Organization.

Surgical Preparation   2930

Definition: Providing care to a patient immediately prior to surgery and determining that the required procedures and tests are documented in the clinical record

Activities:

- Identify patient's level of anxiety or fear concerning the surgical procedure
- Reinforce preoperative teaching information
- Explain procedures in a way that the patient can understand
- Complete preoperative checklist
- Ensure patient is NPO, as appropriate
- Ensure that a completed history and physical is recorded in the chart
- Verify that the surgical consent form is properly signed
- Assure that the surgical site is marked with a permanent marker by the surgeon, as indicated
- Involve the patient in marking the surgical site, as indicated
- Verify that the required laboratory and diagnostic test results are in the chart
- Verify that blood transfusions are available, as appropriate
- Verify that an ECG has been completed, as appropriate
- List allergies on the front of the chart
- Communicate any concerns (e.g., abnormal laboratory or diagnostic test results, issues related to the patient's understanding of the planned procedure) to the surgeon
- Communicate special care considerations such as blindness, hearing loss, or handicap to operating room staff, as appropriate
- Determine whether patient's wishes about health care are known (e.g., advance directives, organ donor cards)
- Verify that patient identification band, allergy band, and blood bands are readable and in place
- Remove jewelry and tape rings in place, as appropriate
- Remove nail polish, makeup, and hairpins, as appropriate
- Remove dentures, glasses, contacts, or other prostheses, as appropriate
- Ensure that money or valuables are in a safe place, as appropriate
- Administer bowel preparation medications, as appropriate
- Explain preoperative medications that will be used, as appropriate
- Administer and document preoperative medications, as appropriate
- Start IV therapy, as directed
- Send required medications or equipment with patient to the operating room, as appropriate
- Insert NG tube or Foley catheter, as appropriate
- Explain tubing and equipment associated with preparation activities
- Administer surgical shave, scrub, shower, enema, or douche, as appropriate
- Apply antiembolism stockings, as appropriate
- Apply sequential compression device sleeves, as appropriate
- Instruct patient to void immediately before preoperative medications, as appropriate
- Check that patient is in proper attire based on institutional policy
- Support patient with high anxiety or fear level
- Assist patient onto cart for transport, as appropriate
- Provide time for family members to speak with patient before transport
- Encourage parents to accompany child to the operating room, as appropriate
- Provide information to family concerning waiting areas and visiting times for surgical patients
- Support family members, as appropriate
- Prepare room for patient's return postoperative

1st edition 1992; revised 2000, 2018

Background Evidence:

Association of periOperative Registered Nurses. (2015). *Guidelines for perioperative practice*.

Kozier, B., Erb, G., Berman, A., & Snyder, S. (2015). Perioperative nursing. In A. Berman, S. Snyder, & G. Frandsen (Eds.), *Kozier & Erb's fundamentals of nursing: Concepts, process, and practice* (10th ed., pp. 959–998). Prentice Hall.

Potter, P., Perry, A., Stockert, P., & Hall, A. (Eds.). (2013). *Fundamentals of nursing* (8th ed.). Elsevier Mosby.

Rothrock, J. C. (Ed.). (2015). *Alexander's care of the patient in surgery* (15th ed.). Elsevier Mosby.

S

Surveillance   6650

Definition: Purposeful, ongoing in-person monitoring, acquisition, interpretation, and synthesis of information

Activities:
- Determine health risks and perceptions of health status, including information about normal behavior and routines, as appropriate
- Ask about recent signs, symptoms, or problems
- Select appropriate indices for ongoing monitoring based on condition
- Adjust frequency of data collection and interpretation as indicated by condition
- Provide continuous monitoring for unstable or critically ill persons
- Continuously monitor for presence of trigger areas for immediate response (e.g., low oxygenation levels, low or elevated heart rates, low or elevated blood pressure, bed alarm)
- Activate rapid response team if indicated by presence of trigger areas, per agency protocol
- Monitor coping strategies
- Monitor current status with previous status to detect improvements and deterioration in condition (e.g., behavior patterns, bleeding tendency, neurological status, oxygenation status, vital signs)
- Facilitate acquisition and interpretation of diagnostic tests including laboratory data, as appropriate
- Monitor equipment to enhance acquisition of reliable data
- Notify health care provider of significant changes
- Initiate or change health care treatment to maintain parameters within limits ordered by health care provider, using established or standing protocols
- Prioritize actions based on condition
- Obtain health care provider consult when data indicate needed change in health care therapy
- Analyze health care provider orders in conjunction with condition to ensure safety
- Obtain consultation from appropriate health care worker to initiate new treatment or change existing treatments
- Provide proper environment for desirable outcomes (e.g., match nurse competency to care needs, provide required person to nurse ratio, provide adequate auxiliary staffing, ensure continuity of care)
- Explain diagnostic test results to person and families
- Involve person and family in monitoring activities, as appropriate
- Facilitate acquisition of interdisciplinary services, as appropriate

1st edition 1992; revised 2004, 2013, 2024

Background Evidence:

Jahrsdoerfer, M. (2019). Clinical Surveillance, a concept analysis: Leveraging real-time data and advanced analytics to anticipate patient deterioration. Bringing theory in practice. *Online Journal of Nursing Informatics (OJNI) HIMSS*, *23*(1). https://www.himss.org/resources/clinical-surveillance-concept-analysis-leveraging-real-time-data-and-advanced-analytics-anticipate

Milhomme, D., Gagnon, J., & Lechasseur, K. (2018). The clinical surveillance process as carried out by expert nurses in a critical care context: A theoretical explanation. *Intensive & Critical Care Nursing, 44*, 24–30. https://doi.org/10.1016/j.iccn.2017.07.010

Moreira, A. P. A., Escudeiro, C. L., Christovam, B., Silvino, Z. R., de Carvalho, M. F., & da Silva, R., Carlos Lyra. (2017). Use of technologies in intravenous therapy: Contributions to a safer practice. *Revista Brasileira De Enfermagem, 70*(3), 623–629, 595–601. https://doi.org/10.1590/0034-7167-2016-0216

Peet, J., Theobald, K. A., & Douglas, C. (2022). Building safety cultures at the frontline: An emancipatory Practice Development approach for strengthening nursing surveillance on an acute care ward. *Journal of Clinical Nursing (John Wiley & Sons, Inc.), 31*(5/6), 642–656. https://doi.org/10.1111/jocn.15923

Stotts, J. R., Lyndon, A., Chan, G. K., Bekmezian, A., & Rehm, R. S. (2020). Nursing surveillance for deterioration in pediatric patients: An integrative review. *Journal of Pediatric Nursing, 50*, 59–74. https://doi.org/10.1016/j.pedn.2019.10.008

Sun, C., & Cato, K. (2020). How much time do nurses spend using electronic devices at work. *Nursing Management (Springhouse), 51*(3), 22–29. https://doi.org/10.1097/01.NUMA.0000651184.19361.4e

Urden, L. D., Stacy, K. M., & Lough, M. E. (2018). *Critical care nursing* (8th ed.). Elsevier. ISBN: 9780323447522.

Surveillance: Community   6652

Definition: Purposeful, ongoing monitoring, acquisition, interpretation, reporting and synthesis of data for decision making in the community

Activities:
- Identify purpose, procedure, and reporting mechanisms for required and voluntary health data reporting systems
- Focus surveillance on community needs as identified by local agencies and health care providers (i.e., community health needs assessment)
- Collect data needing to be reported related to health events, such as diseases and injuries
- Engage community members in collecting health information for people who have limited access or barriers to healthcare services
- Establish frequency of data collection and analysis
- Report data to appropriate agency using standard reporting mechanisms
- Follow up on reports to ensure accuracy and usefulness of information
- Use reports to recognize need for additional data collection, analysis, and interpretation
- Adapt tools and approaches for data collection, reporting, and communication
- Instruct on importance of follow-up of contagious disease treatment
- Participate in program development (e.g., teaching, policy making, lobbying) as associated with community data collection and reporting

S

- Provide regular training, supervision, and incentives to promote sustainability
- Reinforce community surveillance for sustainability
- Establish mechanism for information feedback and communication with community
- Provide regular reports concerning observable benefits to community

3rd edition 2000, revised 2024

Background Evidence:

Pusey-Reid, E., Quinn, L., & Foley, C. A. (2021). Review of COVID-19 for nurses. *MEDSURG Nursing, 30*(5), 297–333.

Rector, C. & Stanley, M.J. (2022). Community and public health nursing: Promoting the public's health (10th ed.). Wolter Kluwer.

Smolinski, M., Crawley, A., Olsen, J., Jayaraman, T., & Libel, M. (2017). Participatory disease surveillance: Engaging communities directly in reporting, monitoring, and responding to health threats. *Journal of Medical Internet Research: Public Health Surveillance, 3*(4), e62. https://doi.org/10.2196/publichealth.7540

St. John, J., Mayfield-Johnson, S. L., & Hernandez-Gordon, W. D. (2021). *Promoting the health of the community: Community health workers describing their roles, competencies and practice.* Springer.

Taylor, M. (2021). Advancing disease surveillance: Public Health Nursing and infectious disease epidemiology. *DNA Reporter, 46*(3), 14.

Technical Contributors to the June 2018 WHO meeting. (2019). A definition for community-based surveillance and a way forward: Results of the WHO global technical meeting, France, 26 to 28 June 2018. *Euro Surveillance, 24*(2). https://doi.org/10.2807/1560-7917.ES.2019.24.2.1800681

Tehrani, N., & Anderson-Cole, L. (2021). Screening and surveillance. *Occupational Health & Wellbeing, 73*(4), 18–21.

Surveillance: Late Pregnancy 6656

Definition: Purposeful and ongoing acquisition, interpretation, and synthesis of maternal-fetal data for treatment, observation, or admission

Activities:

- Review obstetrical history if available
- Determine maternal-fetal health risks through patient interview
- Establish gestational age by reviewing history or calculating expected date of confinement (EDC) from last menstrual period
- Monitor maternal and fetal vital signs
- Monitor behavior of patient and support person
- Implement electronic fetal monitoring, as appropriate
- Inquire about presence and quality of fetal movement
- Monitor for signs of premature labor (e.g., less than 4 contractions per hour, backache, cramping, show, and pelvic pressure from 20 to 37 weeks of gestation), as appropriate
- Monitor for signs of pregnancy-induced hypertension (e.g., hypertension, headache, blurred vision, nausea, vomiting, visual alterations, hyperreflexia, edema, and proteinuria), as appropriate
- Monitor elimination patterns, as appropriate
- Monitor for signs of urinary tract infection, as appropriate
- Facilitate acquisition of diagnostic tests, as appropriate
- Interpret results of diagnostic tests, as appropriate
- Retrieve and interpret laboratory data and contact physician, as appropriate
- Explain diagnostic test results to patient and family
- Initiate interventions for IV therapy, fluid resuscitation, and medication administration, as needed
- Provide comfort measures, as needed
- Monitor nutritional status, as appropriate
- Monitor changes in sleep patterns, as appropriate
- Obtain history of sexually transmitted diseases and frequency of intercourse, as appropriate
- Monitor uterine activity (e.g., frequency, duration, and intensity of contractions)
- Perform Leopold's maneuver to determine fetal position
- Note type, amount, and onset of vaginal drainage
- Perform speculum examination for diagnosis of spontaneous rupture of amniotic membranes unless there is evidence of frank bleeding
- Test amniotic fluid (e.g., nitrazine, ferning, and pooling), as appropriate
- Obtain cervical cultures, as appropriate (e.g., history of beta-streptococcal infection, herpes, or prolonged rupture of membranes)
- Examine cervix for dilatation, effacement, softening, position, and station
- Perform ultrasonography to determine fetal presentation or placental position, as appropriate
- Institute appropriate treatment using standing protocols
- Prioritize actions based on patient status (e.g., treat, continue to observe, admit, or discharge)

2nd edition 1996; revised 2018

Background Evidence:

American College of Nurse-Midwives. (2012). *Core competencies for basic midwifery practice.* http://www.midwife.org/ACNM/files/ACNMLibraryData/UPLOADFILENAME/000000000050/Core%20Comptencies%20Dec%202012.pdf

Berghella, V., Baxter, J. K., & Chau, S. P. (2009). Evidence-based labor and delivery management. *American Journal of Obstetrics and Gynecology, 199*(5), 445–454.

Davidson, M., London, M., & Ladewig, P. (2012). *Old's maternal-newborn nursing and women's health across the lifespan* (9th ed.). Pearson.

S

Surveillance: Remote Monitoring   6658

Definition: Collection, transmission, and evaluation of an individual's health data using technology

Activities:

- Determine reasons for monitoring with health care provider
- Ensure appropriate data collection permissions and authorizations are obtained
- Advise person of any risks from remote surveillance method used
- Limit access to monitoring equipment and person's data to trained and authorized personnel
- Ensure technology equipment assembled and connected by authorized, trained personnel
- Ensure comfort level with use of technology
- Instruct on use of equipment if indicated (e.g., wearable devices, mobile devices, smartphone apps)
- Establish frequency of data collection and interpretation as indicated
- Instruct person or caregiver on role in data gathering (e.g., applying equipment, answering questions, recording data same time daily)
- Ensure understanding of importance of data transmission
- Ensure data obtained from person wherever possible (i.e., avoid caregiver speaking for person or reporting data, if appropriate)
- Monitor incoming data for validity and reliability
- Determine health risks from data interpretation (e.g., vital signs, glucose readings, ECGs), as appropriate
- Obtain information about usual behavior and routines
- Monitor condition to detect improvements or deterioration
- Collaborate and consult with primary caregiver as necessary
- Initiate or change treatment as prescribed by primary care provider
- Analyze primary caregiver orders in conjunction with current person status to ensure safety
- Explain test results and interventions
- Troubleshoot all equipment and systems to enhance acquisition of reliable data
- Coordinate placement, replacement, or set-up of equipment and supplies
- Obtain consultation from appropriate health care worker to initiate new treatment or change existing treatments, as indicated
- Maintain confidentiality and security of data
- Provide individual with access to own data, as appropriate
- Document assessments, advice, instructions, or other information given to individual according to specified guidelines
- Determine how person or family member can be reached for future surveillance, as appropriate
- Identify or aggregate data that has programmatic or population implications

3rd edition 2000, revision 2024

Background Evidence:

Jahrsdoerfer, M. (2019). Clinical surveillance, a concept analysis: Leveraging real-time data and advanced analytics to anticipate patient deterioration. Bringing theory in practice. *Online Journal of Nursing Informatics (OJNI) HIMSS*, *23*(1). https://www.himss.org/resources/clinical-surveillance-concept-analysis-leveraging-real-time-data-and-advanced-analytics-anticipate

Kay, R., Rosen, M., & Ron, R. (2020). Digitally-enabled remote care for cancer patients: Here to stay. *Seminars in Oncology Nursing, 36*, 1–6.

Lambe, C. (2020). Providing safe virtual health care: Nurses must be fully aware of how to maintain patient safety and confidentiality when providing health care via a virtual platform. *Kai Tiaki Nursing New Zealand, 26*(9), 37.

Nieman, C. L., & Oh, E. S. (2020). Connecting with older adults via telemedicine. *Annals of Internal Medicine, 173*(10), 831–832. https://doi.org/10.7326/M20-1322

Speyer, R., Denman, D., Wilkes-Gillan, S., Chen, Y., Bogaardt, H., Kim, J., Heckathorn, D., & Cordier, R. (2018). Effects of telehealth by allied health professionals and nurses in rural and remote areas: A systematic review and meta-analysis. *Journal of Rehabilitative Medicine, 50*, 225–235.

Surveillance: Video Monitoring   6660

Definition: Continuous visual monitoring of activity to enhance safety

Activities:

- Determine reasons for surveillance with health care providers
- Instruct on purpose, process, and risks for video monitoring
- Obtain written consent
- Limit access to monitoring equipment and data to trained and authorized persons
- Ensure technology equipment assembled and connected by authorized, trained personnel
- Ensure all video technicians and caregivers have training in equipment and in responses to observed activities
- Provide report to video technicians prior to start of each shift
- Ensure video technician understands purpose for monitoring (e.g., fall risk, cognitive impairment, elopement risk, potential for seizure, substance withdrawal, behavioral issues)
- Respond to reports from video technician regarding unsafe activity
- Notify video technicians not to communicate with person via video microphone but instead contact nurse first, when individuals have communication difficulties, confusion, or delirium
- Instruct video technicians to notify nurse whenever they observe an at-risk activity
- Provide privacy (e.g., turn off monitoring when providing care, request non-recorded monitoring where possible, limit number of video technicians)
- Document video monitoring use per agency policy
- Determine need for continued monitoring every shift and discontinue when no longer needed

8th edition 2024

S

Background Evidence:

Abbe, J. R., & O'Keeffe, C. (2021). Continuous video monitoring: Implementation strategies for safe patient care and identified best practices. *Journal of Nursing Care Quality*, 36(2), 137–142. https://doi.org/10.1097/NCQ.0000000000000502

Canfield, C., & Galvin, S. (2018). Bedside nurse acceptance of intensive care unit telemedicine presence. *Critical Care Nurse*, 8(6), e1–e4.

Kroll, D., Stanghellini, E., DesRoches, S., Lydon, C., Webster, A., O'Reilly, M., Hurwitz, S., Aylward, P., Cartright, J., McGrath, E., Delaporta, L., Meyer, A., Kristan, M., Falaro, L., Murphy, C., Karno, J., Pallin, D., Schaffer, A., Shah, S., & Lakatos, B. (2020). Virtual monitoring of suicide risk in the general hospital and emergency department. *General Hospital Psychiatry*, 63, 33–38.

Lambe, C. (2020). Providing safe virtual health care: Nurses must be fully aware of how to maintain patient safety and confidentiality when providing health care via a virtual platform. *Kai Tiaki Nursing New Zealand*, 26(9), 37.

Silven, A. V., Petrus, A., Villalobos-Quesada, M., Dirikgil, E., Oerlemans, C. R., Landstra, C. P., Boosman, H., van Os, H., Blanker, M. H., Treskes, R. W., Bonten, T. N., Chavannes, N. H., Atsma, D. E., & Teng, Y. (2020). Telemonitoring for patients with COVID-19: Recommendations for design and implementation. *Journal of Medical Internet Research*, 22(9), e20953. https://doi.org/10.2196/20953

Sustenance Support   7500

Definition: Helping an individual/family in need to locate food, clothing, or shelter

Activities:

- Determine adequacy of patient's financial situation
- Determine adequacy of food supplies in home
- Inform individual/families about how to access local food pantries and free lunch programs
- Inform individual/families about how to access low-rent housing and subsidy programs
- Inform about rental laws and protections
- Inform individual/families of available emergency housing shelter programs
- Arrange transportation to emergency housing shelter
- Discuss with the individual/families available job service agencies
- Arrange for individual/families transportation to job services, if necessary
- Inform individual/families of agency providing clothing assistance
- Arrange transportation to agency providing clothing assistance as necessary
- Inform individual/families of agency programs for support, such as Red Cross and Salvation Army, as appropriate
- Discuss with the individual/families financial aid support available
- Assist individual/families to complete forms for assistance, such as forms for housing and financial aid
- Inform individual/families of available free health clinics
- Assist individual/families to reach free health clinics
- Inform individual/families of eligibility requirements for food stamps
- Inform individual/families of available schools and/or day care centers, as appropriate

1st edition 1992; revised 2004, 2008

Background Evidence:

Brush, B. L., & Powers, E. M. (2001). Health and service utilization patterns among homeless men in transition: Exploring the need for on-site, shelter-based nursing care. *Scholarly Inquiry for Nursing Practice*, 15(2), 143–154.

Green, D. M. (2005). History, discussion, and review of a best practices model for service delivery for the homeless. *Social Work in Mental Health*, 3(4), 1–16.

Mulroy, E. A., & Lauber, H. (2004). A user-friendly approach to program evaluation and effective community interventions for families at risk of homelessness. *Social Work*, 49(4), 573–586.

Strehlow, A. J., & Amos-Jones, T. (1999). The homeless as a vulnerable population. *Nursing Clinics of North America*, 34(2), 261–274.

Suturing   3620

Definition: Approximating edges of a wound using sterile suture material and a needle

Activities:

- Identify patient allergies to anesthetics, suture materials, sterile adhesive strips, tape, and povidone-iodine or other topical solutions
- Identify history of keloid formation, as appropriate
- Refer deep, facial, joint, or potentially infected wounds to a physician
- Immobilize a frightened child or confused adult, as appropriate
- Shave hair from the immediate wound site using proper technique
- Cleanse the surrounding skin with soap and water or other mild antiseptic solution
- Use sterile technique during suture procedure
- Administer a topical or injectable anesthetic to the area, as appropriate
- Allow sufficient time for the anesthetic to numb the area
- Select an appropriate gauge suture needle and suturing material
- Determine method of suturing (continuous or interrupted) most appropriate for the wound
- Position the needle so that it enters and exits perpendicular to the skin surface
- Pull the needle through, following the line or curve of the needle itself
- Pull the suture tight enough to avoid buckling the skin
- Secure the suture line with square knots
- Apply sterile adhesive strips to enhance wound closure (e.g., place perpendicular to incision line; place across suture ends to prevent slippage or excessive pulling), as appropriate
- Cleanse the sutured area before applying an antiseptic or dressing

- Apply a dressing, as appropriate
- Instruct patient concerning care of the suture line or sterile adhesive strips, including signs and symptoms of infection
- Instruct patient on sutures or sterile adhesive strips removal
- Remove sutures within 1 to 2 weeks of their placement, depending on the anatomical location (on the face, remove in 5 to 7 days; on the neck, 7 days; on the scalp, 10 days; on the trunk and upper extremities, 10 to 14 days; and on the lower extremities, 14–21 days), as indicated
- Use proper technique in removing sutures (i.e., gently elevate with forceps, cut, grasp by knot pull toward suture line)
- Schedule return visit, as appropriate

1st edition 1992; revised 1996, 2018

Background Evidence:

Dockery, G. D. (2008). Scar prevention: Proper surgical technique, suturing, and dressing can help minimize postoperative skin complications. *Podiatry Management*, 27(5), 153–154, 156, 158, 160–162. (Excerpted from Dockery, G. L., & Crawford, M. E., Eds., Lower extremity soft tissue & cutaneous plastic surgery, Chapter 26: Scars, 2006, Saunders, Elsevier).

Mackay-Wiggan, J., & Elston, D.M. (2014). *Suturing techniques*. http://emedicine.medscape.com/article/1824895-overview#a15

Perry, A., Potter, P., & Ostendorf, W. (Eds.). (2014). *Clinical nursing skills and techniques* (8th ed.). Elsevier Mosby.

Rothrock, J. C. (Ed.). (2011). *Alexander's care of the patient in surgery* (14th ed.). Elsevier Mosby.

Swallowing Therapy   1860

Definition: Facilitating swallowing and preventing complications of impaired swallowing

Activities:

- Determine type of difficulty with swallowing (e.g., inflammation, stricture, neurological dysfunction)
- Collaborate with other members of interprofessional health care team (e.g., occupational therapist, speech pathologist, dietitian) to provide continuity in rehabilitative plan
- Determine ability to focus attention on learning and performing eating and swallowing tasks
- Remove distractions from environment before starting exercises
- Provide privacy as desired or indicated
- Position self so person can see and hear directions
- Explain rationale of swallowing regimen
- Collaborate with speech therapist to instruct about swallowing exercise regimen
- Provide and use assistive devices, as appropriate
- Avoid use of drinking straws
- Assist to sit in erect position (i.e., as close to 90 degrees as possible) for feeding or swallowing exercise
- Assist to position head in forward flexion in preparation for swallowing (e.g., "chin tuck")
- Assist to maintain sitting position for 30 minutes after completing meal
- Instruct to open and close mouth in preparation for food manipulation
- Instruct not to talk during eating if appropriate
- Guide in phonating staccato sounds to promote soft palate elevation if appropriate
- Use jaw, tongue, and swallow exercises to build strength as indicated
- Provide a lollipop to suck on to enhance tongue strength if appropriate
- Assist hemiplegic person to sit with affected arm forward on table
- Assist to place food at back of mouth and on unaffected side
- Monitor for signs and symptoms of aspiration
- Monitor tongue movements while eating
- Monitor for sealing of lips during eating, drinking, and swallowing
- Monitor for signs of fatigue during eating, drinking, and swallowing
- Provide rest period before eating or exercise to prevent excessive fatigue
- Check mouth for pocketing of food after eating
- Instruct to reach for particles of food on lips or chin with tongue
- Assist to remove food particles from lips and chin if unable to extend tongue
- Monitor consistency of food and liquid based on findings of swallowing study
- Consult with therapist and provider to gradually advance consistency of food
- Assist to maintain adequate caloric and fluid intake
- Monitor body weight
- Monitor body hydration (e.g., intake, output, skin turgor, mucous membranes)
- Provide mouth care as needed
- Instruct caregivers on how to position, feed, and monitor
- Instruct on nutritional requirements and dietary modifications in collaboration with dietitian
- Instruct on emergency measures for choking
- Instruct how to check for pocketed food after eating
- Provide written instructions, as appropriate
- Provide scheduled practice sessions for family or caregiver as needed
- Use teach-back to ensure understanding

1st edition 1992; revised 2000, 2024

Background Evidence:

Craven, R. F., Hirnle, C. J., & Henshaw, C. J. (2021). Self-care and hygiene. In *Fundamentals of nursing: Concepts and competencies for practice* (9th ed.). Wolters-Kluwer.

Kondwani, J. B., Chu, H., Kao, C. C., Voss, J., Chiu, H. J., Chang, P. C., Chen, R., & Chou, K. R. (2021). Swallowing exercises for head and neck cancer patients: A systematic review and meta-analysis of randomized control trials. *International Journal of Nursing Studies*, 114, 103827. https://doi.org/10.1016/j.ijnurstu.2020.103827

Malhi, H. (2018). Diagnosing and managing dysphagia in the acute setting. *British Journal of Nursing*, 27(22), 1294–1297.

Perlow, H. K., Ramey, S. J., Farnia, B., Silver, B., Kwon, D., Chinea, F. M., Sotnick, S. C., Klein, L. B., Elsayyad, N., Samuels, M. A., Freedman, L., Yechieli, R., & Samuels, S. E. (2018). Nutrition and swallowing therapy in head and neck cancer: Utilization of care and preventative efficacy. *Nutrition & Cancer*, 70(8), 1290–1298.

Perry, A. G., Potter, P. A., Ostendorf, W. R., & LaPlante, N. (2021). *Clinical nursing skills and technique* (10th ed.). Mosby.

Potter, P. A., Perry, A. G., Stockert, P. A., & Hall, A. M. (2021). *Fundamentals of nursing* (10th ed.). Elsevier.

Williams, P. (2020). *Basic geriatric nursing* (7th ed). Elsevier.

S

Teaching: Adolescent Development 12–21 Years   5670

Definition: Instruction on appropriate activities to promote the physical, cognitive, and social development for an adolescent

Activities:

- Provide with written materials appropriate to identified needs
- Instruct parent to establish family rules and to remain consistent on enforcement
- Instruct parent to maintain open lines of communication with adolescent
- Encourage regular physical activity
- Instruct parent to monitor and discourage excessive screen time (e.g., video games, TV, computer, phone)
- Encourage to sleep 9 to 10 hours per night
- Guide parents to remove media devices from bedroom, as appropriate
- Instruct parent to encourage and praise for accomplishments
- Instruct parent to promote positive body image and self-esteem
- Educate about expected pubertal changes and encourage honest, age-appropriate discussion with reassurance
- Educate about safe sex practices and potential risks and encourage honest, age-appropriate discussion
- Guide parent to provide privacy in home, as appropriate
- Instruct parent to promote selection of good friends and healthy relationships
- Instruct parent to continue to model moral behavior and citizenship
- Instruct parent to encourage goal setting and assist adolescent to begin planning for future
- Instruct parent to teach strategies to balance commitments (e.g., school, job, social life)
- Reinforce communication skills, anger management, and conflict resolution
- Encourage competence, independence, and self-responsibility
- Instruct parent to establish adolescent responsibilities and privileges
- Encourage healthy hobbies or activities
- Include adolescents and parents together in instructions as needed
- Use teach-back to ensure understanding

8th edition 2024

Background Evidence:

Garzon Maaks, D. L., Barber Starr, N., Brady, M. A., Gaylord, N. M., Driessnack, M., & Duderstadt, K. (2021). *Burns' pediatric primary care* (7th ed.). Elsevier.

Hagan, J. F., Shaw, J. S., & Duncan, P. M. (2017). *Bright futures: Guidelines for health supervision of infants, children, and adolescents* (4th ed.). American Academy of Pediatrics.

Hockenberry, M. J., Wilson, D., & Rodgers, C. (2019). *Wong's nursing care of infants and children* (11th ed.). Elsevier.

Perry, S. E., Hockenberry, M. J., Lowdermilk, D. L., & Wilson, D. (2018). *Maternal child nursing care* (6th ed.). Elsevier.

Richardson, B. (2020). *Pediatric primary care: Practice guidelines for nurses* (4th ed.). Jones & Bartlett Learning.

Teaching: Adolescent Nutrition 12–21 Years   5672

Definition: Instruction on nutrition and feeding practices for adolescents

Activities:

- Provide with written materials appropriate to identified needs
- Encourage parents to role model healthy eating habits
- Involve in food selection and preparation
- Instruct to continue to eat meals as a family, as able
- Encourage variety of healthy foods
- Reinforce importance of healthy eating and drinking water
- Discourage excessive caffeine, high sugar foods and beverages, and energy drinks
- Encourage to brush teeth with fluoridated toothpaste twice per day
- Instruct parents to promote dental exams twice per year
- Instruct parents to encourage adolescent to practice good dental hygiene
- Educate on dangers of dieting for weight loss and eating disorders
- Monitor supplement use if indicated
- Include adolescents and parents together in instructions as needed
- Use teach-back to ensure understanding

8th edition 2024

Background Evidence:

Garzon Maaks, D. L., Barber Starr, N., Brady, M. A., Gaylord, N. M., Driessnack, M., & Duderstadt, K. (2021). *Burns' pediatric primary care* (7th ed.). Elsevier.

Hagan, J. F., Shaw, J. S., & Duncan, P. M. (2017). *Bright futures: Guidelines for health supervision of infants, children, and* (4th ed.). American Academy of Pediatrics.

Hockenberry, M. J., Wilson, D., & Rodgers, C. (2019). *Wong's nursing care of infants and children* (11th ed.). Elsevier.

Perry, S. E., Hockenberry, M. J., Lowdermilk, D. L., & Wilson, D. (2018). *Maternal child nursing care* (6th ed.). Elsevier.

Richardson, B. (2020). *Pediatric primary care: Practice guidelines for nurses* (4th ed.). Jones & Bartlett Learning.

T

Teaching: Adolescent Safety 12–21 Years   5674

Definition: Instruction on safety promotion for adolescents

Activities:
- Provide with written materials appropriate to identified needs
- Encourage parents to maintain open lines of communication with adolescent
- Educate parents to establish clear family rules and to remain consistent on enforcement
- Guide parents to establish curfew
- Instruct parents to model motor vehicle safety and discuss common adolescent risky behaviors (e.g., distracted driving, speeding, car surfing, night-time driving, non-use of vehicle restrains)
- Encourage to establish motor vehicle safety plan
- Instruct parents to remove guns from home or store ammunition and guns separately in locked boxes
- Encourage parents to emphasize healthy relationships (e.g., adolescent peer group friends, romantic relationships) and beware of bullying
- Encourage proper safety equipment for motorized or nonmotorized activities and while engaging in sports
- Encourage water safety (i.e., do not swim alone, do not use substances while swimming, enter water of unknown depths feet first)
- Instruct parents to monitor for signs of high-risk behaviors (e.g., substance abuse, unsafe relationships, self-harm practices, eating disorders, disordered mood, depression)
- Instruct parents to be knowledgeable about adolescent social media activity and reinforce safe usage
- Include adolescents and parents together in instructions as needed
- Use teach-back to ensure understanding

8th edition 2024

Background Evidence:
Garzon Maaks, D. L., Barber Starr, N., Brady, M. A., Gaylord, N. M., Driessnack, M., & Duderstadt, K. (2021). *Burns' pediatric primary care* (7th ed.). Elsevier.

Hagan, J.F., Shaw, J.S., & Duncan, P.M. (2017). Bright futures: Guidelines for health supervision of infants, children, and (4th ed.). American Academy of Pediatrics.

Hockenberry, M. J., Wilson, D., & Rodgers, C. (2019). *Wong's nursing care of infants and children* (11th ed.). Elsevier.

Perry, S. E., Hockenberry, M. J., Lowdermilk, D. L., & Wilson, D. (2018). *Maternal child nursing care* (6th ed.). Elsevier.

Richardson, B. (2020). *Pediatric primary care: Practice guidelines for nurses* (4th ed.) Jones & Bartlett Learning.

Teaching: Disease Process   5602

Definition: Assisting a person to understand information related to a specific disease process

Activities:
- Determine current level of knowledge related to specific disease process
- Determine optimal methods of learning
- Explain pathophysiology of disease and relationship to anatomy and physiology, at person's level of understanding
- Describe common signs and symptoms of disease, as appropriate
- Explain what has already been done to manage symptoms
- Describe disease process, as appropriate
- Identify possible etiologies, as appropriate
- Provide information about condition, as appropriate
- Identify changes in physical condition for person
- Avoid empty reassurances
- Provide actual information about prognosis and condition, as appropriate
- Provide family and significant others with information about progress, as appropriate
- Provide information about available diagnostic measures, as appropriate
- Discuss lifestyle changes that may be required to prevent future complications or control disease process
- Discuss therapy and treatment options
- Describe rationale behind management, therapy, or treatment recommendations
- Encourage to explore options or get second opinion, as appropriate or indicated
- Describe possible chronic complications, as appropriate
- Encourage self-management and behavioral changes to improve disease symptoms and health outcomes
- Instruct on measures to control or minimize symptoms, as appropriate
- Explore possible resources and support, as appropriate
- Refer to local community agencies and support groups, as appropriate
- Instruct on signs and symptoms to report to health care provider, as appropriate
- Provide phone numbers to call if complications occur
- Reinforce information provided by other health care team members, as appropriate
- Use teach-back to ensure understanding

1st edition 1992; revised 2000, 2004, 2024

Background Evidence:
Bastable, S. B. (2020). *Nurse as educator: Principles of teaching and learning for nursing practice* (5th ed.). Jones & Bartlett Publishers.

Browne, K., Divilly, D., McGarry, M., Sweeney, C., & Kelly, M. E. (2017). Chronic disease management—The patient's perspective. *Irish Medical Journal, 110*(2), 511.

Brady, T. J., Ledsky, R., Lafontant, B., & Baker, T. N. (2018). Marketing self-management education: Lessons on messaging and framing. *American Journal of Health Behavior, 42*(5), 3–20. https://doi.org/10.5993/AJHB.42.5.1

Lam, C. K., Copel, L. C., & Deveneau, L. (2021). Nurse faculty experiences teaching chronic illness self-management concepts. *Nursing Education Perspectives, 32*(4). https://doi.org/10.1097/01.NEP.0000000000000808

Poghosyan, L., Norful, A. A., Liu, J., & Friedberg, M. W. (2018). Nurse practitioner practice environments in primary care and quality of care for chronic diseases. *Medical Care, 56*(9), 791–797. https://doi.org/10.1097/MLR.0000000000000961

T

Teaching: Early Childhood Development 1–5 Years   5680

Definition: Instruction on appropriate activities to promote development for toddlers and preschoolers

Activities:

- Provide with written materials appropriate to identified knowledge needs
- Instruct to provide opportunity for play among children of similar age
- Educate to offer choices, as appropriate
- Direct to encourage child to express self through providing positive rewards or feedback for attempts
- Instruct to assist each child to become aware of importance as individual
- Educate to be consistent and structured with behavior management or modification strategies
- Instruct to talk, read, sing to child
- Encourage to describe what is happening (i.e., let's wash your hands)
- Direct to help child learn to express emotions
- Educate to limit rules, but consistently enforce them
- Encourage to minimize screen time
- Instruct to have misbehaving child take breaks or "time outs"
- Educate to provide reassurance to child
- Direct to limit use of word "No" but redirect attention, when needed
- Instruct to provide opportunity for large and fine motor activities
- Educate to establish consistent bedtime routine
- Inform on signs of toilet training readiness and training strategies
- Instruct to teach and role model table manners
- Instruct to encourage child to interact with others by role modeling interaction skills
- Educate to self-help skills (e.g., feeding, toileting, brushing teeth, washing hands, dressing)
- Direct to teach child how to seek help from others when needed
- Instruct to assist child with sharing and taking turns
- Instruct to facilitate role playing or imaginative play
- Use teach-back to ensure understanding

8th edition 2024

Background Evidence:

Garzon Maaks, D. L., Barber Starr, N., Brady, M. A., Gaylord, N. M., Driessnack, M., & Duderstadt, K. (2021). *Burns' pediatric primary care* (7th ed.). Elsevier.

Hagan, J. F., Shaw, J. S., & Duncan, P. M. (2017). *Bright futures: Guidelines for health supervision of infants, children, and adolescents* (4th ed.). American Academy of Pediatrics.

Hockenberry, M. J., Wilson, D., & Rodgers, C. (2019). *Wong's nursing care of infants and children* (11th ed.). Elsevier.

Perry, S. E., Hockenberry, M. J., Lowdermilk, D. L., & Wilson, D. (2018). *Maternal child nursing care* (6th ed.). Elsevier.

Richardson, B. (2020). *Pediatric primary care: Practice guidelines for nurses* (4th ed.). Jones & Bartlett Learning.

Teaching: Early Childhood Nutrition 1–5 Years   5682

Definition: Instruction on nutrition and feeding practices for toddlers and preschoolers

Activities:

- Provide with written materials appropriate to identified needs
- Guide to role model healthy eating habits
- Inform to provide structured mealtime environment as family
- Educate to offer cup and utensils at mealtime
- Instruct to allow toddler to self-feed and to provide finger foods
- Instruct to provide nutritious meals and snacks at regularly scheduled times to avoid grazing
- Inform to anticipate appetite slumps and continue to offer healthy food options
- Educate to offer choices and allow experimentation
- Instruct to feed child while calm in seated position
- Guide to limit sugary foods and beverages
- Inform to introduce whole milk from 1 to 2 years, followed by reduced fat milk
- Educate to avoid bottles in bed
- Instruct to avoid choking hazards (e.g., popcorn, hotdogs, hard foods, gum, whole grapes)
- Guide to brush child's teeth with fluoridated toothpaste
- Use teach-back to ensure understanding

8th edition 2024

Background Evidence:

Garzon Maaks, D. L., Barber Starr, N., Brady, M. A., Gaylord, N. M., Driessnack, M., & Duderstadt, K. (2021). *Burns' pediatric primary care* (7th ed.). Elsevier.

Hagan, J. F., Shaw, J. S., & Duncan, P. M. (2017). *Bright futures: Guidelines for health supervision of infants, children, and adolescents* (4th ed.). American Academy of Pediatrics.

Hockenberry, M. J., Wilson, D., & Rodgers, C. (2019). *Wong's nursing care of infants and children* (11th ed.). Elsevier.

Perry, S. E., Hockenberry, M. J., Lowdermilk, D. L., & Wilson, D. (2018). *Maternal child nursing care* (6th ed.). Elsevier.

Richardson, B. (2020). *Pediatric primary care: Practice guidelines for nurses* (4th ed.). Jones & Bartlett Learning.

T

Teaching: Early Childhood Safety 1–5 Years   5684

Definition: Instruction on safety for toddlers and preschoolers

Activities:

- Provide with written materials appropriate to identified needs
- Instruct to have child sit calmly while eating
- Educate to avoid having child eat in car
- Instruct to avoid choking hazards (e.g., popcorn, hotdogs, hard foods, whole grapes, gum, large chunks of raw fruits or vegetables)
- Instruct on recommended car seat practices
- Instruct to never leave child alone outdoors or in vehicle
- Guide to remove or lock firearms in safe place in home
- Encourage to teach and reinforce "good touch, bad touch" and stranger safety
- Instruct to apply sunscreen often to prevent sunburn
- Guide to maintain child-proof living and play environment
- Educate to teach and reinforce water safety
- Guide never to leave child unattended near water
- Instruct to have child wear helmet while riding toys with wheels
- Use teach-back to ensure understanding

Background Evidence:

Garzon Maaks, D. L., Barber Starr, N., Brady, M. A., Gaylord, N. M., Driessnack, M., & Duderstadt, K. (2021). *Burns' pediatric primary care* (7th ed.). Elsevier.

Hagan, J. F., Shaw, J. S., & Duncan, P. M. (2017). *Bright futures: Guidelines for health supervision of infants, children, and adolescents* (4th ed.). American Academy of Pediatrics.

Hockenberry, M. J., Wilson, D., & Rodgers, C. (2019). *Wong's nursing care of infants and children* (11th ed.). Elsevier.

Perry, S. E., Hockenberry, M. J., Lowdermilk, D. L., & Wilson, D. (2018). *Maternal child nursing care* (6th ed.). Elsevier.

Richardson, B. (2020). *Pediatric primary care: Practice guidelines for nurses* (4th ed). Jones & Bartlett Learning.

8th edition 2024

Teaching: Group   5604

Definition: Development, implementation, and evaluation of a teaching program for a group of individuals experiencing the same health condition

Activities:

- Establish need for program
- Provide environment conducive to learning
- Include family or significant others, as appropriate
- Determine administrative support and budget
- Coordinate resources within facility to form planning or advisory committee, which can contribute to positive outcomes for program and provide forum for ensuring commitment to program
- Utilize community resources, as appropriate
- Define potential target populations
- Write program goals and outline major content areas with learning objectives
- Write job description for coordinator responsible for education
- Select coordinator
- Establish ground rules for behavior at meetings
- Determine optimal methods of learning for group members
- Preview available educational materials
- Develop new educational materials, as appropriate
- List possible teaching strategies, educational materials, and learning activities
- Train teaching personnel, as appropriate
- Educate staff about teaching program, as appropriate
- Provide written schedule, including dates, times, and places of teaching sessions or classes, to staff and individuals, as appropriate
- Determine appropriate days and times to reach maximum number of participants
- Prepare announcements or memos to publicize outcomes, as appropriate
- Manage size and competencies of group, as appropriate
- Orient persons to educational program and objectives to accomplish
- Provide for special needs of learners (e.g., ease of access, portable oxygen), as appropriate
- Tailor educational methods or materials to group's learning needs or characteristics, as appropriate
- Provide group instruction
- Evaluate progress in program and mastery of content
- Document progress on permanent health care record, if indicated
- Revise teaching strategies and learning activities to increase learning, if necessary
- Provide forms for evaluation of program
- Provide for further individual instruction, as appropriate
- Evaluate extent to which program goals were attained
- Communicate evaluation of program's goal attainment to planning or advisory committee
- Hold summative evaluation sessions for planning or advisory committee to revamp program, as appropriate
- Document number who have attained learning objectives
- Refer persons to other specialists or agencies to meet learning objectives, as appropriate

1st edition 1992; revised 2000, 2024

Background Evidence:

Bastable, S. B. (2020). *Nurse as educator: Principles of teaching and learning for nursing practice* (5th ed.). Jones & Bartlett.

T

Fereidouni, Z., Sabet Sarvestani, R., Hariri, G., Kuhpaye, S. A., Amirkhani, M., & Kalyani, M. N. (2019). Moving into action: The master key to patient education. *The Journal of Nursing Research: JNR*, 27(1), 1–8. https://doi.org/10.1097/jnr.0000000000000280

Iriarte-Roteta, A., Lopez-Dicastillo, O., Mujika, A., Ruiz-Zaldibar, C., Hernantes, N., Bermejo-Martins, E., & Pumar-Méndez, M. J. (2020). Nurses' role in health promotion and prevention: A critical interpretive synthesis. *Journal of Clinical Nursing*, 29(21-22), 3937–3949. https://doi.org/10.1111/jocn.15441

Ross, A., Yang, L., Wehrlen, L., Perez, A., Farmer, N., & Bevans, M. (2019). Nurses and health-promoting self-care: Do we practice what we preach? *Journal of Nursing Management*, 27(3), 599–608. https://doi.org/10.1111/jonm.12718

Teaching: Individual 5606

Definition: Planning, implementation, and evaluation of a teaching program designed to address a patient's particular needs

Activities:
- Establish rapport
- Establish teacher credibility, as appropriate
- Determine the patient's learning needs
- Determine patient readiness to learn
- Appraise the patient's current level of knowledge and understanding of content
- Appraise the patient's educational level
- Appraise the patient's cognitive, psychomotor, and affective abilities or disabilities
- Determine the patient's ability to learn specific information (e.g., developmental level, physiological status, orientation, pain, fatigue, unfulfilled basic needs, emotional state, and adaptation to illness)
- Determine the patient's motivation to learn specific information (e.g., health beliefs, past noncompliance, bad experiences with health care or learning, and conflicting goals)
- Enhance the patient's readiness to learn, as appropriate
- Set mutual, realistic learning goals with the patient
- Identify learning objectives necessary to reach goals
- Determine the sequence for presenting the information
- Appraise the patient's learning style
- Select appropriate teaching methods and strategies
- Select appropriate educational materials
- Provide instructional pamphlets, videos, and online resources, when appropriate
- Tailor the content to the patient's cognitive, psychomotor, and affective abilities or disabilities
- Adjust instruction to facilitate learning, as appropriate
- Provide an environment conducive to learning
- Instruct the patient, when appropriate
- Evaluate the patient's achievement of the stated objectives
- Reinforce behavior, as appropriate
- Correct misinterpretations of information, as appropriate
- Provide time for the patient to ask questions and discuss concerns
- Select new teaching methods or strategies, if previous ones were ineffective
- Refer the patient to other specialists or agencies to meet the learning objectives, as appropriate
- Document the content presented, the written materials provided, and the patient's receptivity to and understanding of the information, or patient behaviors that indicate learning on the permanent medical record
- Include the family, as appropriate

1st edition 1992; revised 2013

Background Evidence:
Falvo, D. R. (2011). *Effective patient education: A guide to increased adherence.* Jones & Bartlett.

Friedman, A. J., Cosby, R., Boyko, S., Hatton-Bauer, J., & Turnbull, G. (2011). Effective teaching strategies and methods of delivery for patient education: A systematic review and practice guideline recommendations. *Journal of Cancer Education*, 26(1), 12–21.

Garvey, N., & Noonan, B. (2011). Providing individualized education to patients post myocardial infarction: A literature review. *British Journal of Cardiac Nursing*, 6(2), 73–79.

Potter, P. A., & Perry, A. G. (2009). *Fundamentals of nursing* (7th ed.). Mosby Elsevier.

Teaching: Infant Development 0–3 Months 5655

Definition: Instruction on appropriate sensory activities to promote infant development through the first three months of life

Activities:
- Describe normal infant development
- Assist to identify infant readiness cues and responses to stimulation
- Protect infant from overstimulation
- Assist to set up routine for infant stimulation
- Instruct to perform activities that encourage movement or provide sensory stimulation
- Have demonstrate techniques learned during teaching
- Instruct to promote face-to-face interaction with infant
- Educate to talk, sing, and smile at infant while giving care
- Inform to praise infant for all efforts to respond to stimulation
- Instruct to tell infant his or her name frequently
- Guide to whisper to baby
- Instruct to encourage touching and hugging infant frequently
- Encourage to respond to crying by holding, rocking, singing, talking, walking, repositioning, rubbing or massaging back, and wrapping, as appropriate
- Educate to rock infant in either upright position or cradle position
- Guide to sponge or tub bathe using various massaging strokes with soft wash cloth or sponge and pat dry with soft towel
- Inform to massage infant by rubbing lotion in gentle but firm strokes
- Instruct to rub soft toys on infant's body
- Educate to encourage infant to feel different textures and identify them for infant

- Guide to blow air in circles on alert infant's arms, legs, and tummy
- Inform to encourage infant to grasp soft toys or caregiver's fingers
- Encourage to promote shaking of rattles, encouraging auditory following of sounds
- Instruct parents to provide opportunities for infant to reach for objects
- Educate to encourage visual following of objects
- Guide to reposition infant every hour unless sleeping
- Inform to place infant on tummy while awake to encourage head lifting
- Educate to position infant on back under cradle gym
- Guide to show brightly colored pictures, such as in board books
- Instruct to encourage infant to look in mirror
- Use teach-back to ensure understanding

5th edition 2008; revised 2024

Background Evidence:

Garzon Maaks, D. L., Barber Starr, N., Brady, M. A., Gaylord, N. M., Driessnack, M., & Duderstadt, K. (2021). *Burns' pediatric primary care* (7th ed.). Elsevier.

Hagan, J. F., Shaw, J. S., & Duncan, P. M. (2017). *Bright futures: Guidelines for health supervision of infants, children, and adolescents* (4th ed.). American Academy of Pediatrics.

Hockenberry, M. J., Wilson, D., & Rodgers, C. (2019). *Wong's nursing care of infants and children* (11th ed.). Elsevier.

Perry, S. E., Hockenberry, M. J., Lowdermilk, D. L., & Wilson, D. (2018). *Maternal child nursing care* (6th ed.). Elsevier.

Richardson, B. (2020). *Pediatric primary care: Practice guidelines for nurses* (4th ed.) Jones & Bartlett Learning.

Teaching: Infant Development 4–6 Months   5658

Definition: Instruction on appropriate sensory activities to promote infant development from the fourth through the sixth months of life

Activities:
- Describe normal infant development
- Assist to identify infant readiness cues and responses to stimulation
- Protect infant from overstimulation
- Assist to set up routine for infant stimulation
- Inform to perform activities that encourage movement or provide sensory stimulation
- Instruct to encourage infant to lie on back and kick with feet
- Educate to place toys just outside infant reach
- Instruct to offer toys to encourage infant to grasp
- Instruct to lay infant on back or tummy and help to roll over
- Educate to provide opportunity for infant to explore cloth or soft plastic books
- Instruct to encourage infant to use toys for teething
- Instruct to encourage infant to bang toys together and hand transfer toys
- Instruct to support infant in sitting position
- Instruct to spoon feed infant
- Educate to talk and sing to infant
- Instruct to play song and motion games (e.g., pat-a-cake) with infant
- Use teach-back to ensure understanding

8th edition 2024

Background Evidence:

Garzon Maaks, D. L., Barber Starr, N., Brady, M. A., Gaylord, N. M., Driessnack, M., & Duderstadt, K. (2021). *Burns' pediatric primary care* (7th ed.). Elsevier.

Hagan, J. F., Shaw, J. S., & Duncan, P. M. (2017). *Bright futures: Guidelines for health supervision of infants, children, and adolescents* (4th ed.). American Academy of Pediatrics.

Hockenberry, M. J., Wilson, D., & Rodgers, C. (2019). *Wong's nursing care of infants and children* (11th ed.). Elsevier.

Perry, S. E., Hockenberry, M. J., Lowdermilk, D. L., & Wilson, D. (2018). *Maternal child nursing care* (6th ed.). Elsevier.

Richardson, B. (2020). *Pediatric primary care: Practice guidelines for nurses* (4th ed.) Jones & Bartlett Learning.

Teaching: Infant Development 7–9 Months   5656

Definition: Instruction on appropriate sensory activities to promote infant development from the seventh month through the ninth month of life

Activities:
- Describe normal infant development
- Assist to identify infant readiness cues and responses to stimulation
- Protect infant from overstimulation
- Assist to set up routine for infant stimulation
- Educate to perform activities that encourage movement or provide sensory stimulation
- Instruct to place infant on abdomen, putting palms on soles of infant's feet and pushing gently forward
- Instruct to stand infant on lap, swaying side to side
- Educate to introduce infant to body parts
- Guide to play hide-and-seek and peek-a-boo with infant
- Educate to place infant in high chair, encouraging infant to feel food and feed self
- Instruct to allow infant to hold spoon and cup
- Encourage to dance with infant while holding infant upright
- Use teach-back to ensure understanding

5th edition 2008, revised 2024

T

Background Evidence:

Garzon Maaks, D. L., Barber Starr, N., Brady, M. A., Gaylord, N. M., Driessnack, M., & Duderstadt, K. (2021). *Burns' pediatric primary care* (7th ed.). Elsevier.

Hagan, J. F., Shaw, J. S., & Duncan, P. M. (2017). *Bright futures: Guidelines for health supervision of infants, children, and adolescents* (4th ed.). American Academy of Pediatrics.

Hockenberry, M. J., Wilson, D., & Rodgers, C. (2019). *Wong's nursing care of infants and children* (11th ed.). Elsevier.

Perry, S. E., Hockenberry, M. J., Lowdermilk, D. L., & Wilson, D. (2018). *Maternal child nursing care* (6th ed.). Elsevier.

Richardson, B. (2020). *Pediatric primary care: Practice guidelines for nurses* (4th ed) Jones & Bartlett Learning.

Teaching: Infant Development 10–12 Months   5657

Definition: Instruction on appropriate sensory activities to promote infant development from the tenth month through the twelfth month of life

Activities:

- Describe normal infant development
- Assist to identify infant readiness cues and responses to stimulation
- Protect infant from overstimulation
- Assist to set up routine for infant stimulation
- Educate to perform activities that encourage movement or provide sensory stimulation
- Guide to pull infant to standing, holding onto hands for stabilization
- Instruct to guide infant to walk holding infant by hands or wrists with arms above head
- Educate to encourage ball play (e.g., rolling, grasping, stopping, retrieving)
- Instruct to wave bye-bye to infant while encouraging infant to imitate
- Educate to take infant on house tour, identifying objects and rooms
- Instruct to play follow-the-leader, practicing imitation of infant noises, animals, or songs
- Instruct to say words to infant, encouraging infant to say them back
- Educate to demonstrate how to remove and replace objects from container
- Instruct to demonstrate stacking objects
- Use teach-back to ensure understanding

5th edition 2008; revised 2024

Background Evidence:

Garzon Maaks, D. L., Barber Starr, N., Brady, M. A., Gaylord, N. M., Driessnack, M., & Duderstadt, K. (2021). *Burns' pediatric primary care* (7th ed.). Elsevier.

Hagan, J. F., Shaw, J. S., & Duncan, P. M. (2017). *Bright futures: Guidelines for health supervision of infants, children, and adolescents* (4th ed.). American Academy of Pediatrics.

Hockenberry, M. J., Wilson, D., & Rodgers, C. (2019). *Wong's nursing care of infants and children* (11th ed.). Elsevier.

Perry, S. E., Hockenberry, M. J., Lowdermilk, D. L., & Wilson, D. (2018). *Maternal child nursing care* (6th ed.). Elsevier.

Richardson, B. (2020). *Pediatric primary care: Practice guidelines for nurses* (4th ed) Jones & Bartlett Learning.

Teaching: Infant Nutrition 0–3 Months   5640

Definition: Instruction on nutrition and feeding practices through the first three months of life

Activities:

- Provide written materials appropriate to identified needs
- Instruct to feed only breastmilk or formula for first year (i.e., avoid replacing formula or breast milk with milk)
- Instruct to always hold infant upright in semi-reclined position when giving bottle
- Inform to burp infant during and after feeding
- Instruct on proper formula or breastmilk preparation and storage
- Instruct to never prop bottle or give bottle in bed
- Inform to avoid putting cereal in bottle, only formula or breastmilk
- Instruct to limit water intake to ½ oz to 1 oz at a time, 4 oz daily
- Instruct to avoid use of honey or corn syrup
- Guide to allow nonnutritive sucking
- Instruct to discard leftover formula and clean bottle after every feeding
- Instruct to administer vitamin D supplement as appropriate
- Use teach-back to ensure understanding

5th edition 2008; revised 2024

Background Evidence:

Garzon Maaks, D. L., Barber Starr, N., Brady, M. A., Gaylord, N. M., Driessnack, M., & Duderstadt, K. (2021). *Burns' pediatric primary care* (7th ed.). Elsevier.

Hagan, J. F., Shaw, J. S., & Duncan, P. M. (2017). *Bright futures: Guidelines for health supervision of infants, children, and adolescents* (4th ed.). American Academy of Pediatrics.

Hockenberry, M. J., Wilson, D., & Rodgers, C. (2019). *Wong's nursing care of infants and children* (11th ed.). Elsevier.

Perry, S. E., Hockenberry, M. J., Lowdermilk, D. L., & Wilson, D. (2018). *Maternal child nursing care* (6th ed.). Elsevier.

Richardson, B. (2020). *Pediatric primary care: Practice guidelines for nurses* (4th ed) Jones & Bartlett Learning.

T

Teaching: Infant Nutrition 4–6 Months 5641

Definition: Instruction on nutrition and feeding practices from the fourth month through the sixth month of life

Activities:
- Provide written materials appropriate to identified needs
- Instruct to introduce solids without added salt or sugar when infant demonstrates readiness cues
- Instruct to introduce iron-rich foods
- Instruct to introduce one new food at a time
- Instruct to avoid giving juice or sweetened drinks
- Instruct to feed from spoon only
- Use teach-back to ensure understanding

5th edition 2008; revised 2024

Background Evidence:
Garzon Maaks, D. L., Barber Starr, N., Brady, M. A., Gaylord, N. M., Driessnack, M., & Duderstadt, K. (2021). *Burns' pediatric primary care* (7th ed.). Elsevier.

Hagan, J. F., Shaw, J. S., & Duncan, P. M. (2017). *Bright futures: Guidelines for health supervision of infants, children, and adolescents* (4th ed.). American Academy of Pediatrics.

Hockenberry, M. J., Wilson, D., & Rodgers, C. (2019). *Wong's nursing care of infants and children* (11th ed.). Elsevier.

Perry, S. E., Hockenberry, M. J., Lowdermilk, D. L., & Wilson, D. (2018). *Maternal child nursing care* (6th ed.). Elsevier.

Richardson, B. (2020). *Pediatric primary care: Practice guidelines for nurses* (4th ed.). Jones & Bartlett Learning.

Teaching: Infant Nutrition 7–9 Months 5642

Definition: Instruction on nutrition and feeding practices from the seventh month through the ninth month of life

Activities:
- Provide written materials appropriate to identified needs
- Instruct to introduce finger foods when infant can sit up
- Instruct to introduce cup when infant can sit up
- Instruct to have infant join family at meal times
- Instruct to expect mess
- Instruct to observe for cues of satiation
- Instruct to let infant begin self-feedings and observe to avoid choking
- Instruct to offer fluids after solids
- Instruct to avoid sugary food or drinks (e.g., flavored milks, soda)
- Instruct to offer variety of foods according to the food pyramid
- Instruct to avoid juice
- Explain it may take several offerings before infant accepts new food
- Use teach-back to ensure understanding

5th edition 2008; revised 2024

Background Evidence:
Garzon Maaks, D. L., Barber Starr, N., Brady, M. A., Gaylord, N. M., Driessnack, M., & Duderstadt, K. (2021). *Burns' pediatric primary care* (7th ed.). Elsevier.

Hagan, J. F., Shaw, J. S., & Duncan, P. M. (2017). *Bright futures: Guidelines for health supervision of infants, children, and adolescents* (4th ed.). American Academy of Pediatrics.

Hockenberry, M. J., Wilson, D., & Rodgers, C. (2019). *Wong's nursing care of infants and children* (11th ed.). Elsevier.

Perry, S. E., Hockenberry, M. J., Lowdermilk, D. L., & Wilson, D. (2018). *Maternal child nursing care* (6th ed.). Elsevier.

Richardson, B. (2020). *Pediatric primary care: Practice guidelines for nurses* (4th ed.). Jones & Bartlett Learning.

Teaching: Infant Nutrition 10–12 Months 5643

Definition: Instruction on nutrition and feeding practices from the tenth month through the twelfth month of life

Activities:
- Provide with written materials appropriate to identified needs
- Instruct to offer three meals and healthy snacks
- Instruct to begin to wean from bottle to cup
- Instruct to avoid sugary food or drinks (e.g., flavored milks, soda)
- Instruct to begin table foods
- Instruct to allow infant to feed self with spoon
- Instruct that child may begin whole milk at 1 year of age
- Use teach-back to ensure understanding

5th edition 2008; revised 2024

Background Evidence:
Garzon Maaks, D. L., Barber Starr, N., Brady, M. A., Gaylord, N. M., Driessnack, M., & Duderstadt, K. (2021). *Burns' pediatric primary care* (7th ed.). Elsevier.

Hagan, J. F., Shaw, J. S., & Duncan, P. M. (2017). *Bright futures: Guidelines for health supervision of infants, children, and adolescents* (4th ed.). American Academy of Pediatrics.

Hockenberry, M. J., Wilson, D., & Rodgers, C. (2019). *Wong's nursing care of infants and children* (11th ed.). Elsevier.

Perry, S. E., Hockenberry, M. J., Lowdermilk, D. L., & Wilson, D. (2018). *Maternal child nursing care* (6th ed.). Elsevier.

Richardson, B. (2020). *Pediatric primary care: Practice guidelines for nurses* (4th ed.) Jones & Bartlett Learning.

Teaching: Infant Safety 0–3 Months   5645

Definition: Instruction on safety through the first three months of life

Activities:

- Provide written materials appropriate to identified needs
- Instruct to install and use car seat according to manufacturer's recommendations
- Instruct to place infant alone on back to sleep and keep loose bedding, pillows, and toys out of crib
- Guide parents on dress for proper infant temperature regulation
- Instruct to only use cribs that meet current safety standards
- Instruct to avoid use of jewelry or cords or chains on infant
- Instruct to use and maintain all equipment properly (e.g., swings, strollers, playpens, port-a-cribs)
- Inform to avoid holding infant while smoking or drinking hot liquids
- Instruct to hold infant when feeding, avoid propping of bottle, and test formula temperature
- Instruct to monitor experienced and trained childcare providers
- Inform how to prevent falls
- Instruct to test water temperature of bath
- Instruct not to leave baby unattended near pets or siblings
- Instruct to verify smoke detectors are installed and functioning in home
- Inform on proper precautions against sun exposure
- Instruct to avoid feeding solids until 4 to 6 months
- Encourage to complete CPR training
- Instruct never to shake, toss, or swing infant in the air
- Use teach-back to ensure understanding

5th edition 2008; revised 2024

Background Evidence:

Garzon Maaks, D. L., Barber Starr, N., Brady, M. A., Gaylord, N. M., Driessnack, M., & Duderstadt, K. (2021). *Burns' pediatric primary care* (7th ed.). Elsevier.

Hagan, J. F., Shaw, J. S., & Duncan, P. M. (2017). *Bright futures: Guidelines for health supervision of infants, children, and adolescents* (4th ed.). American Academy of Pediatrics.

Hockenberry, M. J., Wilson, D., & Rodgers, C. (2019). *Wong's nursing care of infants and children* (11th ed.). Elsevier.

Perry, S. E., Hockenberry, M. J., Lowdermilk, D. L., & Wilson, D. (2018). *Maternal child nursing care* (6th ed.). Elsevier.

Richardson, B. (2020). *Pediatric primary care: Practice guidelines for nurses* (4th ed.) Jones & Bartlett Learning.

Teaching: Infant Safety 4–6 Months   5646

Definition: Instruction on safety from the fourth month through the sixth month of life

Activities:

- Provide written materials appropriate to identified needs
- Instruct to avoid use of walkers or jumpers due to danger of injury and detrimental effects on muscle development
- Instruct never to leave infant unattended in bath, grocery cart, high chair, or on sofa
- Instruct to evaluate hanging crib toys
- Instruct to use safe high chair when infant able to sit
- Instruct to feed only soft or mashed foods
- Instruct to remove small objects from infant's reach
- Instruct to avoid sunscreen until 6 months old
- Use teach-back to ensure understanding

5th edition 2008; revised 2024

Background Evidence:

Garzon Maaks, D. L., Barber Starr, N., Brady, M. A., Gaylord, N. M., Driessnack, M., & Duderstadt, K. (2021). *Burns' pediatric primary care* (7th ed.). Elsevier.

Hagan, J. F., Shaw, J. S., & Duncan, P. M. (2017). *Bright futures: Guidelines for health supervision of infants, children, and adolescents* (4th ed.). American Academy of Pediatrics.

Hockenberry, M. J., Wilson, D., & Rodgers, C. (2019). *Wong's nursing care of infants and children* (11th ed.). Elsevier.

Perry, S. E., Hockenberry, M. J., Lowdermilk, D. L., & Wilson, D. (2018). *Maternal child nursing care* (6th ed.). Elsevier.

Richardson, B. (2020). *Pediatric primary care: Practice guidelines for nurses* (4th ed.) Jones & Bartlett Learning.

Teaching: Infant Safety 7–9 Months   5647

Definition: Instruction on safety from the seventh month through the ninth month of life

Activities:

- Provide written materials appropriate to identified needs
- Instruct to avoid sources of lead poisoning
- Instruct to keep dangerous items out of infant's reach
- Instruct to provide barriers to dangerous areas
- Instruct to supervise infant's activity at all times

- Instruct to maintain smoke-free environment
- Instruct to keep number for poison control on hand
- Use teach-back to ensure understanding

5th edition 2008; revised 2024

Background Evidence:

Garzon Maaks, D. L., Barber Starr, N., Brady, M. A., Gaylord, N. M., Driessnack, M., & Duderstadt, K. (2021). *Burns' pediatric primary care* (7th ed.). Elsevier.

Hagan, J. F., Shaw, J. S., & Duncan, P. M. (2017). *Bright futures: Guidelines for health supervision of infants, children, and adolescents* (4th ed.). American Academy of Pediatrics.

Hockenberry, M. J., Wilson, D., & Rodgers, C. (2019). *Wong's nursing care of infants and children* (11th ed.). Elsevier.

Perry, S. E., Hockenberry, M. J., Lowdermilk, D. L., & Wilson, D. (2018). *Maternal child nursing care* (6th ed.). Elsevier.

Richardson, B. (2020). *Pediatric primary care: Practice guidelines for nurses* (4th ed). Jones & Bartlett Learning.

Teaching: Infant Safety 10–12 Months   5648

Definition: Instruction on safety from the tenth month through the twelfth month of life

Activities:

- Provide written materials appropriate to identified needs
- Instruct to provide protection from glass furniture, sharp edges, unstable furniture, and appliances
- Instruct to store all cleaning supplies, medications, and personal care products out of infant's reach
- Instruct to use childproof latches on cupboards
- Instruct to prevent infant's access to upper story windows, balconies, and stairs
- Instruct to keep infant away from ponds, pools, toilets, and all containers with liquid to prevent drowning
- Instruct to select toys according to manufacturer's age recommendations
- Instruct to ensure multiple barriers to pool or hot tub area
- Instruct to monitor car seat for weight limit and consider toddler rear-facing seat
- Instruct to never leave infant alone while outside or in vehicle
- Use teach-back to ensure understanding

Background Evidence:

Garzon Maaks, D. L., Barber Starr, N., Brady, M. A., Gaylord, N. M., Driessnack, M., & Duderstadt, K. (2021). *Burns' pediatric primary care* (7th ed.). Elsevier.

Hagan, J. F., Shaw, J. S., & Duncan, P. M. (2017). *Bright futures: Guidelines for health supervision of infants, children, and adolescents* (4th ed.). American Academy of Pediatrics.

Hockenberry, M. J., Wilson, D., & Rodgers, C. (2019). *Wong's nursing care of infants and children* (11th ed.). Elsevier.

Perry, S. E., Hockenberry, M. J., Lowdermilk, D. L., & Wilson, D. (2018). *Maternal child nursing care* (6th ed.). Elsevier.

Richardson, B. (2020). *Pediatric primary care: Practice guidelines for nurses* (4th ed.). Jones & Bartlett Learning.

5th edition 2008; revised 2024

Teaching: Infection Control   5649

Definition: Instruction to minimize or eliminate the acquisition and transmission of infectious agents

Activities:

- Determine current level of knowledge related to acquisition and transmission of infectious agents
- Instruct about preexisting conditions that increase infection risk
- Determine current infection prevention practices
- Instruct to use soap and water or alcohol-based sanitizer for cleansing hands
- Avoid rinsing off or wiping off hands after using hand sanitizer
- Encourage to ask about hand hygiene for those caring for them (i.e., has caregiver washed their hands upon entering room or home)
- Instruct when to wash hands to protect self at home and in healthcare settings (e.g., before, during, and after food preparation, before eating, after using toilet, after contact with pets or pet products or pet waste, after contact with garbage, before and after contact with someone who is sick)
- Encourage to perform hand hygiene under observation to ensure proper technique and understanding
- Advise to avoid close contact with people who are sick
- Advise to stay home and avoid traveling when sick
- Advise not to share or reuse cups, dishes, or utensils without washing them with hot and soapy water
- Advise not to drink water that has been sitting out more than 15 minutes
- Advise to use masks and social distancing (i.e., keeping at least 3–6 feet away from others not in immediate household) during periods of increased respiratory infection activity in community
- Instruct to cover mouth and nose with tissue when coughing or sneezing
- Instruct to use nearest waste receptacle to dispose of tissue after use
- Instruct to perform hand hygiene after having contact with respiratory secretions and contaminated objects or materials

T

- Instruct frail and at-risk persons and family members to avoid crowds and gatherings when social distancing not possible
- Instruct as indicated for routine bodily hygiene (e.g., bathe daily, wash armpits, groin, genitals and rectal area twice per day)
- Instruct to clean toothbrush twice per week
- Advise to avoid touching eyes, nose, or mouth as much as possible
- Advise to clean and disinfect frequently touched surfaces at home, work or school, especially when someone is ill
- Encourage deep breathing and coughing, as appropriate
- Promote appropriate nutritional and fluid intake
- Promote safe food preservation and preparation
- Encourage fluid intake, as appropriate
- Encourage rest
- Instruct to take antibiotics as prescribed and until finished
- Instruct about signs and symptoms of infection and when to contact health care provider
- Instruct how to avoid infections
- Instruct to self-isolate if contagious with infectious agent, per local public health guidelines
- Instruct to quarantine when exposed to persons with confirmed infectious agents, per local public health guidelines
- Encourage to obtain vaccinations for infectious diseases

8th edition 2024

Background Evidence:

Carrico, R. M., Garrett, H., Balcom, D., & Burton-Glowicz, J. (2019). Infection prevention and control core practices: A roadmap for nursing practice. *The Nurse Practitioner, 44*(3), 50–55.

Cochrane, J., & Jersby, M. (2019). When to wear personal protective equipment to prevent infection. *British Journal of Nursing, 28*(15), 982–984.

Munoz-Figueroa, G. P., & Ojo, O. (2018). The effectiveness of alcohol-based gel for hand sanitizing in infection control. *British Journal of Nursing, 27*(7), 382–388.

Patel, P. K., Popovich, K. J., Collier, S., Lassiter, S., Mody, L., Ameling, J. M., & Meddings, J. (2019). Foundational elements of infection prevention in the STRIVE curriculum. *Annals of Internal Medicine, 171*(7), S10–S19.

Perry, A. G., Potter, P. A., Ostendorf, W., & Laplante, N. (2021). *Clinical nursing skills and techniques* (10th ed.). Elsevier.

Prior, M., Delac, K., Melone, D., & Laux, L. (2020). Determining nursing education needs during a rapidly changing COVID-19 environment. *Critical Care Nursing Quarterly, 43*(4), 428–450.

Ridley, N. (2020). Effective hand hygiene: Wash your hands and reduce the risk. *British Journal of Nursing, 29*(1), 10.

Wilson, B. J., Zitella, L. J., Erb, C. H., Foster, J., Peterson, M., & Wood, S. K. (2018). Prevention of infection: A systematic review of evidence-based practice interventions for management in patients with cancer. *Clinical Journal of Oncology Nursing, 22*(2), 157–168.

Windle, M. (2018). Pretty please, wash your hands!. *Med-Surg Matters, 27*(3), 9–10.

Teaching: Middle Childhood Development 6–12 Years   5650

Definition: Instruction on appropriate activities to promote physical, cognitive, and social development for school-aged children

Activities:

- Provide with written materials appropriate to identified needs
- Guide to establish family rules and remain consistent on enforcement
- Educate to avoid physical punishment
- Instruct to minimize screen time to 1 to 2 hour per day
- Inform to encourage 1 hour or more of physical activity per day
- Instruct to read stories and encourage child to read aloud
- Encourage to maintain consistent bedtime
- Instruct to keep electronics out of child's bedroom to promote sleep (i.e., TV, cell phone, computer)
- Encourage praise for accomplishments
- Instruct to promote positive body image and self-esteem
- Educate to role model moral and social behaviors
- Inform to teach conflict resolution and anger management skills
- Guide to facilitate and encourage fantasy and imaginative play
- Encourage to educate child about puberty and encourage honest, age-appropriate discussion
- Instruct to educate child about sex and encourage honest, age-appropriate discussion
- Guide to foster cooperation, not competition, among children
- Educate to encourage competence, independence, and self-responsibility
- Instruct to assign age-appropriate chores, responsibilities, and privileges
- Inform to encourage healthy hobbies and activities that promote fitness and motor skill development
- Use teach-back to ensure understanding

8th edition 2024

Background Evidence:

Garzon Maaks, D. L., Barber Starr, N., Brady, M. A., Gaylord, N. M., Driessnack, M., & Duderstadt, K. (2021). *Burns' pediatric primary care* (7th ed.). Elsevier.

Hagan, J. F., Shaw, J. S., & Duncan, P. M. (2017). *Bright futures: Guidelines for health supervision of infants, children, and adolescents* (4th ed.). American Academy of Pediatrics.

Hockenberry, M. J., Wilson, D., & Rodgers, C. (2019). *Wong's nursing care of infants and children* (11th ed.). Elsevier.

Perry, S. E., Hockenberry, M. J., Lowdermilk, D. L., & Wilson, D. (2018). *Maternal child nursing care* (6th ed.). Elsevier.

Richardson, B. (2020). *Pediatric primary care: Practice guidelines for nurses* (4th ed). Jones & Bartlett Learning.

T

Teaching: Middle Childhood Nutrition 6–12 Years   5652

Definition: Instruction on nutrition and feeding practices for school-aged children

Activities:
- Provide written materials appropriate to identified needs
- Guide to role model healthy eating habits
- Instruct to continue to eat meals as family, as able
- Educate to encourage variety of healthy foods
- Guide to teach importance of healthy eating and drinking water
- Encourage to discourage or limit sugary foods and beverages
- Inform to anticipate appetite to vary at times (i.e., growth spurts, changes in activity level)
- Guide to allow child to respond to internal cues of satiety
- Encourage to involve child in meal planning, grocery shopping, including reading food labels, and food preparation
- Educate to encourage child to brush teeth with fluoridated toothpaste twice per day
- Instruct on the dangers of dieting for weight loss
- Use teach-back to ensure understanding

8th edition 2024

Background Evidence:

Garzon Maaks, D. L., Barber Starr, N., Brady, M. A., Gaylord, N. M., Driessnack, M., & Duderstadt, K. (2021). *Burns' pediatric primary care* (7th ed.). Elsevier.

Hagan, J.F., Shaw, J.S., & Duncan, P.M. (2017). Bright futures: Guidelines for health supervision of infants, children, and adolescents (4th ed.). American Academy of Pediatrics.

Hockenberry, M. J., Wilson, D., & Rodgers, C. (2019). *Wong's nursing care of infants and children* (11th ed.). Elsevier.

Perry, S. E., Hockenberry, M. J., Lowdermilk, D. L., & Wilson, D. (2018). *Maternal child nursing care* (6th ed.). Elsevier.

Richardson, B. (2020). *Pediatric primary care: Practice guidelines for nurses* (4th ed). Jones & Bartlett Learning.

Teaching: Middle Childhood Safety 6–12 Years   5654

Definition: Instruction on safety promotion for school-aged children

Activities:
- Provide with written materials appropriate to identified needs
- Instruct on proper motor vehicle restraint use, and that child must ride in back seat
- Educate to practice and reinforce firearm safety
- Guide to reinforce "good touch, bad touch" and teach "just say no" concepts
- Encourage to discuss how to ask for help
- Instruct to use sunscreen when outdoors
- Educate to reinforce water safety and encourage swimming lessons
- Guide to reinforce use of proper safety equipment, such as helmet while riding bike or other nonmotorized activities, discourage motorized vehicles use (e.g., ATVs, mopeds, snowmobiles)
- Educate to encourage proper safety equipment during sports (e.g., mouth guard, helmet, eye protection)
- Instruct to have fire safety plan, practice regular fire drills
- Guide to provide adequate supervision, as should not be left alone
- Encourage to monitor for signs of high-risk behaviors (e.g., substance abuse, unsafe relationships)
- Inform to be knowledgeable about child digital and social media activity, keep computer in central area of the house, and teach social media safety
- Use teach-back to ensure understanding

8th edition 2024

Background Evidence:

Garzon Maaks, D. L., Barber Starr, N., Brady, M. A., Gaylord, N. M., Driessnack, M., & Duderstadt, K. (2021). *Burns' pediatric primary care* (7th ed.). Elsevier.

Hagan, J.F., Shaw, J.S., & Duncan, P.M. (2017). Bright futures: Guidelines for health supervision of infants, children, and adolescents (4th ed.). American Academy of Pediatrics.

Hockenberry, M. J., Wilson, D., & Rodgers, C. (2019). *Wong's nursing care of infants and children* (11th ed.). Elsevier.

Perry, S. E., Hockenberry, M. J., Lowdermilk, D. L., & Wilson, D. (2018). *Maternal child nursing care* (6th ed.). Elsevier.

Richardson, B. (2020). *Pediatric primary care: Practice guidelines for nurses* (4th ed). Jones & Bartlett Learning.

T

Teaching: Preoperative   5610

Definition: Assisting a patient to understand and mentally prepare for surgery and the postoperative recovery period

Activities:
- Inform the patient and family of the scheduled date, time, and location of surgery
- Inform the patient and family how long the surgery is expected to last
- Determine the patient's previous surgical experiences, background, culture, and level of knowledge related to surgery
- Appraise the patient's and family's anxiety relating to surgery
- Provide time for the patient to ask questions and discuss concerns
- Describe the preoperative routines (e.g., anesthesia, diet, bowel preparation, tests/labs, voiding, skin preparation, IV therapy, clothing, family waiting area, transportation to operating room), as appropriate

- Describe any preoperative medications, the effects these will have on the patient, and the rationale for using them
- Inform the family of the location to wait for the results of the surgery, as appropriate
- Conduct a tour of the postsurgical unit and waiting area, as appropriate
- Introduce the patient to the staff who will be involved in the surgery and postoperative care, as appropriate
- Reinforce the patient's confidence in the staff involved, as appropriate
- Provide information on what will be heard, smelled, seen, tasted, or felt during the event
- Discuss possible pain-control measures
- Explain the purpose of frequent postoperative assessments
- Describe the postoperative routines and equipment (e.g., medications, respiratory treatments, tubes, machines, support hose, surgical dressings, ambulation, diet, family visitation) and explain their purpose
- Instruct the patient on the technique of getting out of bed, as appropriate
- Evaluate the patient's ability to demonstrate getting out of bed, as appropriate
- Instruct the patient on the technique of splinting, coughing, and deep breathing
- Evaluate the patient's ability to demonstrate splinting incision, coughing, and deep breathing
- Instruct the patient on how to use the incentive spirometer
- Evaluate the patient's ability to demonstrate proper use of the incentive spirometer
- Instruct the patient on the technique of leg exercises
- Evaluate the patient's ability to demonstrate leg exercises
- Stress the importance of early ambulation and pulmonary care

- Inform the patient how to assist in recuperation
- Reinforce information provided by other health care team members, as appropriate
- Determine the patient's expectations of the surgery
- Correct unrealistic expectations of the surgery, as appropriate
- Provide time for the patient to rehearse events that will happen, as appropriate
- Instruct the patient to use coping techniques directed at controlling specific aspects of the experience (e.g., relaxation, imagery), as appropriate
- Instruct patient in regard to smoking cessation, as appropriate
- Instruct in a way that matches the patient's style of learning, including the use of holistic approaches and educational materials, as appropriate
- Document teaching, including patient's response to teaching

1st edition 1992; revised 2013

Background Evidence:

deWit, S. C. (2009). *Medical-surgical nursing: Concepts & practice.* Saunders Elsevier.

Kruzik, N. (2009). Benefits of preoperative education for adult elective surgery patients. *AORN Journal, 90*(3), 381–387.

Lewis, S., Dirksen, S., Heitkemper, M., Bucher, L., & Camera, I. (2011). *Medical-surgical nursing: Assessment and management of clinical problems* (8th ed.). Elsevier Mosby.

Potter, P. A., Perry, A. G., Stockert, P. A., & Hall, A. M. (2013). *Fundamentals of nursing* (8th ed.). Elsevier Mosby.

Selimen, D., & Andsoy, II. (2011). The importance of a holistic approach during the perioperative period. *AORN Journal, 93*(4), 482–490.

Teaching: Prescribed Diet   5614

Definition: Preparing a patient to correctly follow a prescribed diet

Activities:

- Appraise the patient's current level of knowledge about prescribed diet
- Appraise the patient's current and past eating patterns as well as preferred foods and current eating habits
- Determine the patient's and family's perspectives, cultural backgrounds, and other factors that may affect the patient's willingness to follow prescribed diet
- Determine any financial limitations that may affect food purchases
- Instruct the patient on the proper name of the prescribed diet
- Explain the purpose of diet adherence to overall health
- Inform the patient about how long the diet should be followed
- Instruct the patient about how to keep a food diary, as appropriate
- Instruct the patient on allowed and prohibited foods
- Inform the patient of possible drug and food interactions, as appropriate
- Assist the patient to accommodate food preferences into the prescribed diet
- Assist the patient in substituting ingredients to conform favorite recipes to the prescribed diet
- Instruct the patient about how to read labels and select appropriate foods
- Observe the patient's selection of foods appropriate to prescribed diet
- Instruct the patient about how to plan appropriate meals

- Provide written meal plans, as appropriate
- Recommend a cookbook that includes recipes consistent with the diet, as appropriate
- Reinforce information provided by other health care team members, as appropriate
- Reinforce the importance of continued monitoring and changing needs that may require further alteration of dietary plan of care
- Refer patient to dietitian, as appropriate
- Include the family, as appropriate

1st edition 1992; revised 2013

Background Evidence:

deWit, S.C. (2009). Medical-surgical nursing: Concepts and practice. Saunders Elsevier.

Dossey, B. M., & Keegan, L. (2009). *Holistic nursing: A handbook for practice* (5th ed.). Jones & Bartlett.

Dudek, S. G. (2007). *Nutrition essentials for nursing practice* (5th rev ed.). Lippincott Williams & Wilkins.

Lewis, S., Dirksen, S., Heitkemper, M., Bucher, L., & Camera, I. (2011). *Medical-surgical nursing: Assessment and management of clinical problems* (8th ed.). Elsevier Mosby.

Potter, P. A., Perry, A. G., Stockert, P. A., & Hall, A. M. (2013). *Fundamentals of nursing* (8th ed.). Elsevier Mosby.

Teaching: Prescribed Exercise   5612

Definition: Preparing a patient to achieve or maintain a prescribed level of exercise

Activities:

- Appraise the patient's current level of exercise and knowledge of prescribed exercise
- Monitor the patient for physiological and psychological limitations, as well as background and culture
- Inform the patient of the purpose for, and the benefits of, the prescribed exercise
- Assist the patient in setting goals for slow, steady increase in exercise
- Instruct patient regarding use of pain medication and alternative methods of pain control before exercise, as needed
- Instruct the patient how to perform the prescribed exercise
- Instruct the patient how to monitor tolerance of the exercise
- Instruct the patient how to keep an exercise diary, as appropriate
- Inform the patient what activities are appropriate based on physical condition
- Caution the patient on the dangers of overestimating capabilities, as appropriate
- Warn the patient of the effects of extreme heat and cold, as appropriate
- Instruct the patient on methods to conserve energy, as appropriate
- Instruct the patient about how to properly stretch before and after exercise and the rationale for doing so, as appropriate
- Instruct the patient how to warm up and cool down before and after exercise and the importance of doing so, as appropriate
- Instruct the patient on good posture and body mechanics, as appropriate
- Instruct patient to report signs of possible problems, (e.g., pain, dizziness, and swelling) to health care provider
- Observe the patient perform the prescribed exercise
- Provide information on available assistive devices that may be used to facilitate performance of the required skill, as appropriate
- Instruct the patient on the assembly, use, and maintenance of assistive devices, as appropriate
- Assist the patient to incorporate exercise regimen into daily routine
- Assist the patient to properly alternate periods of rest and activity
- Refer the patient to physical therapist, occupational therapist, or exercise physiologist, as appropriate
- Reinforce information provided by other health care team members, as appropriate
- Provide written information or diagrams for continued reference
- Provide frequent feedback to prevent bad habits from forming
- Include the family, as appropriate
- Provide information on available community resources and support groups to increase the patient's compliance with exercise, as appropriate
- Refer the patient to a rehabilitation center, as appropriate

1st edition 1992; revised 2013

Background Evidence:

Berman, A., Snyder, S., Kozier, B., & Erb, G. (2008). Activity and exercise. In *Kozier & Erb's fundamentals of nursing: Concepts, processes, and practice* (8th ed., pp. 1104–1162). Prentice Hall.

deWit, S. C. (2009). *Medical-surgical nursing: Concepts & practice.* Saunders Elsevier.

Perme, C., & Chandrashekar, R. (2009). Early mobility and walking program for patients in intensive care units: Creating a standard of care. *American Journal of Critical Care, 18*(3), 212–221.

Potter, P. A., Perry, A. G., Stockert, P. A., & Hall, A. M. (2013). *Fundamentals of nursing* (8th ed.). Elsevier Mosby.

Pryor, J. (2009). Coaching patients to self-care: A primary responsibility of nursing. *International Journal of Older People Nursing, 4*(2), 79–88.

Teaching: Prescribed Medication   5616

Definition: Preparing a person to safely take prescribed medications and monitor for effects

Activities:

- Use standardized tool to elicit all medication information, including prescribed medications, non-prescription medications, and dietary and herbal supplements
- Provide individualized approach to instructions, using visual aids, instructional booklets written in simple language or person's language, or videos, as appropriate
- Begin instruction as soon as possible to allow for addition instructional sessions, as appropriate
- Ensure information accommodates level of health literacy
- Use problem scenarios to increase learning (e.g., side effects, contaminated syringe)
- Provide professional interpreters rather than family or friends during instruction, as needed
- Provide information about use of non-prescription medications and how they may influence existing condition
- Determine if using culturally based home health remedies
- Provide information about possible effects of home health remedies on use of non-prescription and prescribed medications
- Instruct to recognize distinctive characteristics of medications, as appropriate
- Inform of both generic and brand names of each medication
- Instruct on purpose and action of each medication
- Explain how health care providers choose most appropriate medication
- Instruct on dosage, route, and duration of each medication
- Instruct on proper administration or application of each medication
- Review knowledge of medications
- Acknowledge knowledge of medications
- Evaluate ability to self-administer medications
- Instruct to perform needed procedures before taking medication (e.g., check pulse, glucose), as appropriate
- Inform what to do if dose of medication missed

T

- Instruct on criteria to use when deciding to alter medication dosage or schedule, as appropriate
- Inform of consequences of not taking or abruptly discontinuing medications, as appropriate
- Instruct on specific precautions to observe when taking medications (e.g., no driving, no using power tools), as appropriate
- Instruct on possible adverse side effects of each medication
- Instruct how to relieve or prevent certain side effects, as appropriate
- Instruct on appropriate actions to take if side effects occur
- Instruct on signs and symptoms of overdosage and underdosage
- Inform of possible medication or food interactions, as appropriate
- Provide information on process of medication administration when sick
- Instruct how to properly store medication
- Instruct on proper care of devices used for administration
- Instruct on proper disposal of needles and syringes at home and where to dispose of sharps container in community, as appropriate
- Provide written information about action, purpose, side effects, and needed material related to medications
- Assist to develop written medication schedule
- Determine if adherence or memory cue needed (e.g., medication dose containers organized by hours and days of week)
- Instruct to carry documentation of prescribed medication regimen
- Instruct how to fill prescriptions, as appropriate
- Inform of possible changes in appearance or dosage when filling generic medication prescriptions
- Warn of risks associated with taking expired medication
- Caution against giving prescribed medication to others
- Determine ability to obtain required medications

- Provide information on medication reimbursement, as appropriate
- Provide information on cost savings programs or organizations to obtain medications and devices, as appropriate
- Provide information on medication alert devices and how to obtain them
- Reinforce accurate information provided by other health care team members, as appropriate
- Use teach-back to ensure understanding

1st edition 1992; revised 1996, 2004, 2024

Background Evidence:

Berman, A., Snyder, S. J., & Frandsen, G. (2018). Medications. In *Kozier and Erb's Fundamentals of nursing: Concepts, process and practice* (10th ed., pp. 750–829). Pearson.

Craven, R. F., Hirnle, C. J., & Henshaw, C. J. (2021). Medication administration (Chapter 20). In *Fundamentals of nursing: Human health and function* (8th ed.). Wolters-Kluwer.

Potter, P. A., Ostendorf, W. R., & LaPlante, N. (2018). Safe medication preparation. In *Clinical nursing skills and techniques* (9th ed., pp. 501–522). Mosby.

Sanoski, C. A., & Vallerand, A. H. (2021). *Davis's drug guide for nurses* (17th ed.). F.A. Davis.

Tomlinson, J., Cheong, V., Fylan, B., Silcock, J., Smith, H., Karban, K., & Blenkinsopp, A. (2020). Successful care transitions for older people: A systematic review and meta-analysis of the effects of interventions that support medication continuity. *Age and Ageing, 49*(4), 558–569. https://doi-org.ezp.waldenulibrary.org/10.1093/ageing/afaa002

Williams, P. (2020). Medications and older adults. In *Basic geriatric nursing* (7th ed., pp. 132–149). Elsevier.

Teaching: Procedures or Treatments   5618

Definition: Preparing a person to understand and mentally prepare for a prescribed procedure or treatment

Activities:

- Determine optimal methods of learning
- Inform when and where procedure or treatment will take place, as appropriate
- Inform about how long procedure or treatment expected to last
- Inform about who will be performing procedure or treatment
- Reinforce confidence in staff involved, as appropriate
- Determine previous experiences and level of knowledge related to procedure or treatment
- Explain purpose of procedure or treatment
- Describe pre-procedure or treatment activities
- Explain procedure or treatment
- Review informed consent for procedure or treatment according to agency policy, as appropriate
- Instruct how to cooperate and participate during procedure or treatment, as appropriate
- Encourage child's participation in procedure or treatment
- Conduct tour of procedure or treatment room and waiting area, as appropriate
- Introduce person to staff involved in procedure or treatment, as appropriate
- Explain need for certain equipment (e.g., monitoring devices) and function
- Discuss need for special measures during procedure or treatment, as appropriate

- Provide information on what will be heard, smelled, seen, tasted, or felt during event
- Describe post-procedure or post-treatment assessments or activities and rationale
- Inform how person can aid in recuperation
- Reinforce information provided by other health care team members, as appropriate
- Provide time for person to rehearse events that will happen, as appropriate
- Instruct to use coping techniques directed at controlling specific aspects of experience (e.g., relaxation, imagery), as appropriate
- Provide distraction for child that will divert attention away from procedure
- Provide information on when and where results will be available and who will explain them
- Determine expectations of procedure or treatment
- Correct unrealistic expectations of procedure or treatment, as appropriate
- Discuss alternative treatments, as appropriate
- Encourage to share doubts, fears, and perceptions about treatment or procedure
- Include family and significant others, as appropriate
- Use teach-back to ensure understanding

1st edition 1992; revised 2000, 2024

Background Evidence:

Bastable, S. B. (2020). *Nurse as educator: Principles of teaching and learning for nursing practice (5th ed.)*. Jones & Bartlett.

Cutilli, C. C. (2020). Excellence in patient education: Evidence-based education that "sticks" and improves patient outcomes. *The Nursing Clinics of North America, 55*(2), 267–282. https://doi.org/10.1016/j.cnur.2020.02.007

Fereidouni, Z., Sabet Sarvestani, R., Hariri, G., Kuhpaye, S. A., Amirkhani, M., & Kalyani, M. N. (2019). Moving into action: The master key to patient education. *The Journal of Nursing Research: JNR, 27*(1), 1–8. https://doi.org/10.1097/jnr.0000000000000280

Keçeci, A., Toprak, S., & Kiliç, S. (2019). How effective are patient education materials in educating patients? *Clinical Nursing Research, 28*(5), 567–582. https://doi.org/10.1177/1054773817740521

Kozier, B., Erb, G., Berman, A., & Snyder, S. (2020). Teaching. In *Fundamentals of nursing: Concepts, process, and practice* (11th ed., pp. 295–318). Pearson Education.

Pinchera, B., DelloIacono, D., & Lawless, C. A. (2018). Best practices for patient self-management: Implications for nurse educators, patient educators, and program developers. *Journal of Continuing Education in Nursing, 49*(9), 432–440. https://doi.org/10.3928/00220124-20180813-09

Teaching: Psychomotor Skill   5620

Definition: Preparing a patient to perform a psychomotor skill

Activities:

- Establish rapport
- Establish teacher credibility, as appropriate
- Determine the patient's learning needs
- Determine patient readiness to learn
- Establish level of patient ability in performing skill
- Adjust teaching methodology to accommodate patient age and ability, as needed
- Demonstrate the skill for the patient
- Give clear, step-by-step directions
- Instruct the patient to perform the skill one step at a time
- Inform the patient of the rationale for performing the skill in the specified manner
- Guide patients' bodies so that they can experience the physical sensations that accompany the correct motions, as appropriate
- Provide written information or diagrams, as appropriate
- Provide practice sessions (spaced to avoid fatigue, but often enough to prevent excessive forgetting), as appropriate
- Provide adequate time for task mastery
- Observe patient return demonstrate the skill
- Provide frequent feedback to patients on what they are doing correctly and incorrectly, so that bad habits are not formed
- Provide information on available assistive devices that may be used to facilitate performance of the required skill, as appropriate
- Instruct the patient on the assembly, use, and maintenance of assistive devices, as appropriate
- Include the family, as appropriate

1st edition 1992; revised 2013

Background Evidence:

Falvo, D. R. (2011). *Effective patient education: A guide to increased adherence.* Jones and Bartlett.

Friedman, A. J., Cosby, R., Boyko, S., Hatton-Bauer, J., & Turnbull, G. (2011). Effective teaching strategies and methods of delivery for patient education: A systematic review and practice guideline recommendations. *Journal of Cancer Education, 26*(1), 12–21.

Potter, P. A., Perry, A. G., Stockert, P. A., & Hall, A. M. (2013). *Fundamentals of nursing* (8th ed.). Elsevier Mosby.

Teaching: Safe Sex   5622

Definition: Providing instruction concerning protection during sexual activity

Activities:

- Obtain sexual history, including number of past sexual partners, frequency of intercourse, and past occurrences of and treatments for sexually transmitted infections (STIs)
- Instruct patient on anatomy and physiology of human reproduction
- Instruct patient on STI and conception, as necessary
- Instruct patient on factors that increase risk of STI (e.g., unprotected sexual intercourse, increased genital mucosal surface area, increased number of sexual contacts, presence of genital sores, advanced illness, and sexual intercourse during menstruation)
- Discuss patient's knowledge, understanding, motivation, and commitment level regarding various sexual protection methods
- Discuss methods of sexual protection for sexual intercourse and oral sex (e.g., medication-free, barrier, vaccination, hormonal, intrauterine device, abstinence, and sterilization), including effectiveness, side effects, contraindications, and signs and symptoms that warrant reporting to a health care professional
- Discuss religious, cultural, developmental, socioeconomical, and individual considerations pertaining to sexual protection choice
- Provide accurate information pertaining to the implications of having multiple sexual partners
- Instruct patient on low-risk sexual practices, such as those which avoid bodily penetration or the exchange of body fluids
- Instruct patient on the importance of good hygiene, using a water-soluble lubricant, and voiding after intercourse to decrease the susceptibility to infections
- Instruct patient on proper use of condoms (e.g., how to choose, keep intact, apply, and remove)
- Provide patient with sexual protection products (e.g., condoms and dental dams)
- Encourage patient to obtain routine examinations and report signs and symptoms of STIs to a health care provider
- Encourage patient to discuss sexual histories and safe sex practices with partner

T

- Discuss with patient importance of sexual partner notification when diagnosed with STI
- Consider population-based factors affecting safe sex education (e.g., culturally tailored interventions, ethnically matched providers)
- Use social networks (e.g., Internet, phone) to reach marginalized or geographically isolated populations

1st edition 1992; revised 2013

Background Evidence:

Paranjape, A., Bernstein, L., St., George, D. M., Doyle, J., Henderson, S., & Corbie-Smith, G. (2006). Effect of relationship factors on safer sex decisions in older inner-city women. *Journal of Women's Health, 15*(1), 90–97.

Vergidis, P. I., & Falagas, M. E. (2009). Meta-analyses on behavioral interventions to reduce the risk of transmission of HIV. *Infectious Disease Clinics of North America, 23*(2), 309–314.

Ward, S. L., & Hisley, S. M. (2009). *Maternal-child nursing care: Optimizing outcomes for mothers, children, & families.* F.A. Davis.

Wilson, T. E., Hogben, M., Malka, E. S., Liddon, N., McCormack, W. M., Rubin, S. R., & Augenbraun, M. A. (2009). A randomized controlled trial for reducing risks for sexually transmitted infections through enhanced patient-based partner notification. *American Journal of Public Health, 99*(Suppl. 1), S104–S110.

Teaching: Sexuality   5624

Definition: Assisting individuals to understand physical and psychosocial dimensions of sexual growth and development

Activities:

- Create an accepting, nonjudgmental atmosphere
- Explain human anatomy and physiology of the male and female body
- Explain the anatomy and physiology of human reproduction
- Discuss signs of fertility (related to ovulation and menstrual cycle)
- Explain emotional development during childhood and adolescence
- Facilitate communication between the child, adolescent, and parent
- Support parents' role as the primary sexuality educator of their children
- Educate parents on sexual growth and development through the life span
- Provide parents with a bibliography of sexuality education materials
- Discuss what values are, how we obtain them, and their effect on our choices in life
- Facilitate the child's and adolescent's awareness of family, peer, societal, and media influence on values
- Use appropriate questions to assist the child and adolescent to reflect on what is important personally
- Discuss peer and social pressures to sexual activity
- Explore the meaning of sexual roles
- Discuss sexual behavior and appropriate ways to express one's feelings and needs
- Inform children and adolescents of the benefits to postponing sexual activity
- Educate children and adolescents on the negative consequences of early childbearing (e.g., poverty and loss of education and career opportunities)
- Educate about sexually transmitted diseases and AIDS
- Promote responsibility for sexual behavior
- Discuss benefits of abstinence
- Inform about effective contraceptives, as appropriate
- Instruct accessibility of contraceptives and how to obtain them
- Assist in choosing an appropriate contraceptive, as appropriate
- Facilitate role playing where decision making and assertive communication skills may be practiced to resist peer and social pressures of sexual activity
- Enhance self-esteem through peer role modeling and role playing
- Discuss how aging changes (e.g., medications, medical conditions, chronic illness) may affect sexual desires and actions, as appropriate
- Identify helpful resources on the Internet provided by responsible organizations (e.g., Center for Parent Education and Resources, Health World Education, National Association of School Nurses, Planned Parenthood of Northern New England)

2nd edition 1996; revised 2018

Background Evidence:

Center for Parent Information and Resources. (2016). *Sexuality education for students with disabilities.* http://www.parentcenterhub.org/respository/sexed/

Kazer, M. W. (2012). Issues regarding sexuality. In M. Boltz, E. Capezuti, T. Fulmer, & D. Zwicker (Eds.), *Evidence-based geriatric nursing protocols for best practice* (4th ed., pp. 500–515). Springer.

McLaughlin, L., & Broer, E. (2014). Effectiveness of sexual health promotion in adolescents. *RN Journal.* http://rn-journal.com/journal-of-nursing/effectiveness-of-sexual-health-promotion-in-adolescents

Steinke, E., Jaarsma, T., Barnason, S., Byrne, M., Doherty, S., Dougherty, C., Fridlund, B., Kautz, D. D., Mårtensson, J., Mosack, V., Moser, D. K., & Moser, D. (2013). Sexual counseling for individuals with cardiovascular disease and their partners. *European Heart Journal, 34*(41), 3217–3235.

Teaching: Sports-Injury Prevention   6648

Definition: Instruction on the prevention of sports-related injury

Activities:

- Provide written materials appropriate to identified needs
- Instruct on general fitness as prerequisite
- Educate about modifying game rules according to age and ability of participants
- Explore options in finding sport that fits with interests and abilities
- Set realistic goals
- Educate on appropriate matching of competitors by age, weight, and stage of physical maturation

T

- Instruct on safety rules, training guidelines, and correct biomechanics
- Educate on safe playing conditions
- Educate on proper use and condition of safety equipment
- Instruct on need for appropriate supervision when training for recreational and competitive events
- Instruct on need for physical exam before participation
- Inform importance of warm-up and cool-down activities
- Instruct on use of protective and supportive garments for all sports, and ensuring players without protective garments are not placed into contact situations
- Recommend use of certified athletic trainers for competitive sports
- Instruct on need for health care coverage at competitive sporting events, as appropriate
- Develop emergency plan in case of serious injury
- Recommend use of preseason seminars for athletes, families, and coaches, to increase awareness of injury prevention
- Collaborate with other professionals in planning programs related to injury prevention
- Instruct parents and athletes of steps they can take to prevent injuries
- Educate on signs and symptoms of overuse injuries, dehydration, heat exhaustion, use of performance enhancing drugs, eating disorders, menstrual dysfunction, and stress
- Instruct to collect data on injury type, rate, treatment, and referrals
- Instruct to monitor long-term health of athletes and return of injured athletes to participation to prevent reinjury
- Educate to provide emotional support for athletes experiencing injury
- Encourage coaches to get annual CPR and first aid training, with emphasis on recognizing head injuries
- Communicate importance of emphasizing "fun" in sports with coaches
- Ensure coaches are well informed of normal development and physical, emotional, and social needs of athlete
- Communicate information about special health care concerns of individual athletes, as appropriate

- Develop oversight groups to ensure education of school and volunteer coaches
- Educate parents on qualifications and behavior expected of coaches
- Encourage parents to become involved in their children's sports programs
- Instruct on importance of monitoring athletes for signs and symptoms of stress
- Provide referrals for athletes with emotional or psychosocial concerns
- Educate on relaxation techniques and coping strategies for athletes, coaches, and parents
- Use teach-back to ensure understanding

3rd edition 2000; revised 2024

Background Evidence:

Ercan, S., & Önal, Ö. (2021). Development, validity and reliability of the Sports Injury Prevention Awareness Scale. *Spor Hekimligi Dergisi/Turkish Journal of Sports Medicine*, *56*(3), 138–145. https://doi.org/10.47447/tjsm.0546

Knapik, J. J., Hoedebecke, B. L., Rogers, G. G., Sharp, M. A., & Marshall, S. W. (2019). Effectiveness of mouthguards for the prevention of orofacial injuries and concussions in sports: Systematic review and meta-analysis. *Sports Medicine*, *49*(8), 1217–1232. https://doi.org/10.1007/s40279-019-01121-w

Nyland, J., Cecil, A., Singh, R., & Raj Pandey, C. (2020). Protective and supportive garments and bracing to enhance extreme sport performance and injury prevention. *Muscles, Ligaments & Tendons Journal (MLTJ)*, *10*(2), 325–332. https://doi.org/10.32098/mltj.02.2020.18

Rebmann, T., Weaver, N. L., Elliott, M. B., DeClue, R. W., Patel, N. J., & Schulte, L. (2018). Factors related to injury prevention programming by Missouri school nurses. *Journal of School Nursing*, *34*(4), 292–3001.

Robinson, M. L. (2021). Management of patients with musculoskeletal trauma. In J. L. Hinkle, K. H. Cheever, K. Overbaugh, Brunner & Suddarth's (Eds.), *Textbook of Medical Surgical Nursing* (15th ed). Wolters Kluwer.

Teaching: Toddler Nutrition 13–18 Months   5660

Definition: Instruction on nutrition and feeding practices from the thirteenth month through the eighteenth month of life

Activities:

- Provide parents with written materials appropriate to identified knowledge needs
- Instruct parent/caregiver to discontinue bottle feeding
- Instruct parent/caregiver to offer textured solids
- Instruct parent/caregiver to continue use of spoon and self-feeding
- Instruct parent/caregiver to introduce dairy products
- Instruct parent/caregiver to provide healthy snacks
- Instruct parent/caregiver to offer small portions and frequent feedings
- Instruct parent/caregiver to avoid "diet" food/drinks (e.g., non-fat milk, diet soda)
- Instruct parent/caregiver to avoid force feeding as there is decreased appetite

Background Evidence:

Barness, L. A. (Ed.). (1993). *Pediatric nutrition handbook* (3rd ed.). American Academy of Pediatrics.

California Department of Health Services WIC Supplemental Nutrition Branch. (1998). *Feeding your baby 1-3 years old* [brochure].

Formon, S. J. (1993). *Nutrition of normal infants*. Mosby.

Hockenberry, M. J., & Wilson, D. (Eds.). (2007). *Wong's nursing care for infants and children* (8th ed.). Elsevier Mosby.

Hockenberry, M. J., Wilson, D., & Winkelstein, M. (Eds.). (2005). *Wong's essentials of pediatric nursing* (7th ed.). Elsevier Mosby.

Pillitteri, A. (2007). *Maternal and child health nursing: Care of the childbearing and childrearing family* (5th ed.). Lippincott Williams & Wilkins.

Satter, E., & Sharkey, P. B. (1997). *Ellyn Satter's nutrition and feeding for infants and children: Handout masters*. Ellen Satter Associates.

5th edition 2008

T

Teaching: Toddler Nutrition 19–24 Months   5661

Definition: Instruction on nutrition and feeding practices from the nineteenth month through the twenty-four month of life

Activities:

- Provide parents with written materials appropriate to identified knowledge needs
- Instruct parent/caregiver to encourage drinking water for thirst
- Instruct parent/caregiver to limit fluids before meals
- Instruct parent/caregiver to offer foods high in iron and protein
- Instruct parent/caregiver to have regular mealtimes and eat as a family
- Instruct parent/caregiver to increase or decrease foods, as appropriate
- Instruct parent/caregiver to avoid fruit drinks and flavored milk
- Instruct parent/caregiver to read the labels for nutritive content
- Instruct parent/caregiver to discontinue bottle feeding

Background Evidence:

Barness, L. A. (Ed.). (1993). *Pediatric nutrition handbook* (3rd ed.). American Academy of Pediatrics.

California Department of Health Services WIC Supplemental Nutrition Branch. (1998). *Feeding your baby 1-3 years old* [brochure].

Formon, S. J. (1993). *Nutrition of normal infants.* Mosby.

Hockenberry, M. J., & Wilson, D. (Eds.). (2007). *Wong's nursing care for infants and children* (8th ed.). Elsevier Mosby.

Hockenberry, M. J., Wilson, D., & Winkelstein, M. (Eds.). (2005). *Wong's essentials of pediatric nursing* (7th ed.). Elsevier Mosby.

Pillitteri, A. (2007). *Maternal and child health nursing: Care of the childbearing and childrearing family* (5th ed.). Lippincott Williams & Wilkins.

Satter, E., & Sharkey, P. B. (1997). *Ellyn Satter's nutrition and feeding for infants and children: Handout masters.* Ellen Satter Associates.

5th edition 2008

Teaching: Toddler Nutrition 25–36 Months   5662

Definition: Instruction on nutrition and feeding practices from the twenty-fifth month through the thirty-sixth month of life

Activities:

- Provide parents with written materials appropriate to identified knowledge needs
- Instruct parent/caregiver to give child healthy food choices
- Instruct parent/caregiver to encourage raw/cooked vegetables
- Instruct parent/caregiver to provide healthy snacks between meals
- Instruct parent/caregiver to be creative in food preparation for picky eater
- Instruct parent/caregiver to offer small portions of food
- Instruct parent/caregiver to limit fat content in foods
- Instruct parent/caregiver to have child participate in food preparation
- Instruct parent/caregiver to offer iron-fortified cereals, avoiding high-sugar cereals
- Instruct parent/caregiver to increase protein foods
- Instruct parent/caregiver to include all food groups
- Instruct parent/caregiver to avoid use of food as rewards

Background Evidence:

Barness, L. A. (Ed.). (1993). *Pediatric nutrition handbook* (3rd ed.). American Academy of Pediatrics.

California Department of Health Services WIC Supplemental Nutrition Branch. (1998). *Feeding your baby 1-3 years old* [brochure].

Formon, S. J. (1993). *Nutrition of normal infants.* Mosby.

Hockenberry, M. J., & Wilson, D. (Eds.). (2007). *Wong's nursing care for infants and children* (8th ed.). Elsevier Mosby.

Hockenberry, M. J., Wilson, D., & Winkelstein, M. (Eds.). (2005). *Wong's essentials of pediatric nursing* (7th ed.). Elsevier Mosby.

Pillitteri, A. (2007). *Maternal and child health nursing: Care of the childbearing and childrearing family* (5th ed.). Lippincott Williams & Wilkins.

Satter, E., & Sharkey, P. B. (1997). *Ellyn Satter's nutrition and feeding for infants and children: Handout masters.* Ellen Satter Associates.

5th edition 2008

Teaching: Toddler Safety 13–18 Months   5665

Definition: Instruction on safety from the thirteenth month through the eighteenth month of life

Activities:

- Provide parents with written materials appropriate to identified knowledge needs
- Instruct parent/caregiver to supervise child outdoors
- Instruct parent/caregiver to educate child about dangers of throwing and hitting
- Instruct parent/caregiver to prevent access to electrical outlets, cords, and electrical equipment/appliances/tools
- Instruct parent/caregiver to store weapons and weapon-like items under lock and key
- Instruct parent/caregiver to educate child about safe ways of interacting with pets
- Instruct parent/caregiver to secure doors/gates to prevent child's access to dangerous areas (e.g., street, driveway, pool)
- Instruct parent/caregiver to dispose of and/or remove the doors to unused refrigerators, ice chests, and other air-tight containers

- Instruct parent/caregiver to use back burners of the stove, install knob covers, and/or restrict child's access to kitchen
- Instruct parent/caregiver to set home water heater temperature to between 120 degrees and 130 degrees Fahrenheit

5th edition 2008

Background Evidence:

American Academy of Pediatrics. (1994a). *1 to 2 years: Safety for your child* [brochure].

American Academy of Pediatrics. (1994b). *2 to 4 years: Safety for your child* [brochure].

California Center for Childhood Injury Prevention. (1997). *Safe home assessment program.*

California Department of Health Services Childhood Lead Poisoning Prevention Branch. (1994). *Lead: Simple things that you can do to prevent childhood lead poisoning* [brochure].

Hockenberry, M. J., & Wilson, D. (Eds.). (2007). *Wong's nursing care for infants and children* (8th ed.). Elsevier Mosby.

Hockenberry, M. J., Wilson, D., & Winkelstein, M. (Eds.). (2005). *Wong's essentials of pediatric nursing* (7th ed.). Elsevier Mosby.

Pillitteri, A. (2007). *Maternal and child health nursing: Care of the childbearing and childrearing family* (5th ed.). Lippincott Williams & Wilkins.

Teaching: Toddler Safety 19–24 Months   5666

Definition: Instruction on safety from the nineteenth month through the twenty-fourth month of life

Activities:

- Provide parents with written materials appropriate to identified knowledge needs
- Instruct parent/caregiver to install car seat and use it according to manufacturer's recommendations
- Instruct parent/caregiver to store sharp objects, appliances, and kitchen items out of child's reach
- Instruct parent/caregiver to instruct child on dangers of the street
- Instruct parent/caregiver to store all cleaning supplies, medications, and personal care products out of child's reach
- Instruct parent/caregiver to ensure multiple barriers to pool/hot tub area

5th edition 2008

Background Evidence:

American Academy of Pediatrics. (1994a). *1 to 2 years: Safety for your child* [brochure].

American Academy of Pediatrics. (1994b). *2 to 4 years: Safety for your child* [brochure].

California Center for Childhood Injury Prevention. (1997). *Safe home assessment program.*

California Department of Health Services Childhood Lead Poisoning Prevention Branch. (1994). *Lead: Simple things that you can do to prevent childhood lead poisoning* [brochure].

Hockenberry, M. J., & Wilson, D. (Eds.). (2007). *Wong's nursing care for infants and children* (8th ed.). Elsevier Mosby.

Hockenberry, M. J., Wilson, D., & Winkelstein, M. (Eds.). (2005). *Wong's essentials of pediatric nursing* (7th ed.). Elsevier Mosby.

Pillitteri, A. (2007). *Maternal and child health nursing: Care of the childbearing and childrearing family* (5th ed.). Lippincott Williams & Wilkins.

Teaching: Toddler Safety 25–36 Months   5667

Definition: Instruction on safety from the twenty-fifth month through the thirty-sixth month of life

Activities:

- Provide parents with written materials appropriate to identified knowledge needs
- Instruct parent/caregiver to instruct child on dangers of weapons
- Instruct parent/caregiver to select toys according to manufacturer's age recommendations
- Instruct parent/caregiver to provide supervision and instruct about safe use of large climbing and riding toys
- Instruct parent/caregiver to store matches/lighters out of child's reach and instruct child about the dangers of fire and fire starters
- Instruct parent/caregiver to always supervise child around swimming pools, ponds, and hot tubs
- Instruct parent/caregiver to instruct child about stranger danger and good touch/bad touch
- Instruct parent/caregiver to provide an approved helmet for bike riding and instruct child to always wear it
- Instruct parent/caregiver to prevent child's access to upper story windows, balconies, and stairs
- Instruct parent/caregiver to closely supervise child when out in public settings
- Instruct parent/caregiver to instruct child how to get adult help when he or she feels scared or in danger

5th edition 2008

Background Evidence:

American Academy of Pediatrics. (1994). *2 to 4 years: Safety for your child* [brochure].

California Center for Childhood Injury Prevention. (1997). *Safe home assessment program.*

California Department of Health Services Childhood Lead Poisoning Prevention Branch. (1994). *Lead: Simple things that you can do to prevent childhood lead poisoning* [brochure].

Hockenberry, M. J., & Wilson, D. (Eds.). (2007). *Wong's nursing care for infants and children* (8th ed.). Elsevier Mosby.

Hockenberry, M. J., Wilson, D., & Winkelstein, M. (Eds.). (2005). *Wong's essentials of pediatric nursing* (7th ed.). Elsevier Mosby.

Pillitteri, A. (2007). *Maternal and child health nursing: Care of the childbearing and childrearing family* (5th ed.). Lippincott Williams & Wilkins.

T

Teaching: Toilet Training 5634

Definition: Instruction on determining the child's readiness and strategies to assist the child to learn independent toileting skills

Activities:

- Instruct parent about how to determine the child's physical readiness for toilet training (e.g., child is at least 18- to 24 months of age; shows evidence of being able to hold urine before void; recognizes urge to go or that he or she has just voided or defecated; shows some regularity in elimination patterns; is able to navigate to the toilet/potty, sit on it, and get off when completed; is able to remove and replace clothing before and after elimination; is able to wipe self and wash hands after elimination)
- Instruct parent about how to determine the child's psychosocial readiness for toilet training (e.g., child expresses interest in and desire to participate/cooperate in toileting; has vocabulary to communicate need to eliminate; is anxious to please parents; imitates the behaviors of others)
- Instruct parent about how to determine parental/family readiness for toilet training: (e.g., parent has knowledge and time to devote to training process; parent/family is experiencing no major transitions during or shortly after the process such as change of job or residence, divorce, birth of another child; has realistic expectations about child development and the time and energy needed to successfully complete the process; understands child may regress during times of stress or illness)
- Provide information on strategies to promote toilet training
- Provide information on how to dress the child in loose, easy-to-remove clothing
- Provide information on how to agree on vocabulary to be used during training process
- Provide information on opportunities for child to observe others during the toileting process
- Provide information on how to take the child to the potty to introduce him or her to the equipment and process
- Provide information on how to take the child to the potty on a regular basis and encourage him or her to sit
- Provide information on how to reinforce the child's success with any part of the process
- Provide information on how to consider the child's temperament or behavior style when planning strategies
- Provide information on how to expect and ignore accidents
- Provide information on how to communicate strategies, expectations, and progress to other care providers
- Support parents throughout this process
- Encourage parents to be flexible and creative in developing and implementing training strategies
- Provide additional information, as requested or needed

4th edition 2004; revised 2008

Background Evidence:

Brazelton, T. B., Christophersen, E. R., Frauman, A. C., Gorski, P. A., Poole, J. M., Stradtler, A. C., & Wright, C. D. (1999). Instruction, timelines, and medical influences affecting toilet training. *Pediatrics, 103*(6), 1353–1358.

Doran, J., & Lister, A. (1998). Toilet training: Meeting the needs of children and parents. *Community Practitioner, 71*(5), 179–180.

Hockenberry, M. J., & Wilson, D. (Eds.). (2007). *Wong's nursing care for infants and children* (8th ed.). Elsevier Mosby.

Hockenberry, M. J., Wilson, D., & Winkelstein, M. (Eds.). (2005). *Wong's essentials of pediatric nursing* (7th ed.). Elsevier Mosby.

Kinservik, M. A., & Friedhoff, M. M. (2000). Control issues in toilet training. *Pediatric Nursing, 26*(3), 267–274.

Pillitteri, A. (2007). *Maternal and child health nursing: Care of the childbearing and childrearing family* (5th ed.). Lippincott Williams & Wilkins.

Stadtler, A. C., Gorski, P. A., & Brazelton, T. B. (1999). Toilet training methods, clinical interventions, and recommendations. *Pediatrics, 103*(6 pt. 2), 1359–1361.

Technology Management 7880

Definition: Managing health care technology to provide care or sustain life

Activities:

- Determine reasons for equipment use with health care provider
- Ensure appropriate data collection permissions and authorizations are obtained where indicated
- Advise any risks from equipment used as needed
- Ensure that recommended equipment has appropriate decision-making support capabilities
- Change or replace equipment, per protocol
- Maintain equipment in good working order
- Correct or replace malfunctioning equipment
- Zero and calibrate equipment, as appropriate
- Keep emergency equipment in appropriate and readily accessible place
- Ensure proper grounding of electronic equipment
- Plug life-sustaining equipment into electrical outlets connected to an emergency power source
- Have equipment checked by bioengineering on routine maintenance schedule, as appropriate
- Recharge batteries in portable equipment
- Set alarm limits on equipment, as appropriate
- Respond to equipment alarms appropriately
- Consult with other health care team members and recommend equipment or devices
- Use data for reassessment
- Verify data entry from biomedical devices to electronic health record
- Display clinical summaries and trend analysis of pertinent data
- Manually assess condition when machine-derived data conflicts with nurse's perception
- Place bedside equipment strategically to maximize access and prevent tripping over tubes and cords
- Become knowledgeable of equipment and proficient in use
- Instruct person and family how to operate equipment, as appropriate
- Inform person and family of expected outcomes and side effects associated with using equipment

T

- Facilitate ethical decision making related to use of life-sustaining and life-support technologies, as appropriate
- Demonstrate to family members how to communicate with person on life-support equipment
- Facilitate interaction between family members and person receiving life-support therapy
- Monitor effect of equipment use on physiological, psychological, and social functioning of person and family
- Monitor effectiveness of technology on outcomes

1st edition 1992; revised 2013, 2024

Background Evidence:

Ben Hassen, D. (2020). Mobile-aided diagnosis systems are the future of health care. *Eastern Mediterranean Health Journal, 26*(9), 1135–1141.

Borum, C. (2018). Barriers for hospital-based nurse practitioners utilizing clinical decision support systems. *CIN: Computers Informatics Nursing, 36*(4), 177–182.

Chahal, A., & Rudnick, A. (2019). Selecting digital health technologies for validation and piloting by healthcare providers: A decision-making perspective from Ontario. *International Journal of Technology Assessment in Health Care, 35*, 1–4. https://doi.org/10.1017/S0266462318003720

Esmaeilzadeh, P. (2020). Use of AI-based tools for healthcare purposes: A survey study from consumers' perspectives. *BMC Medical Informatics and Decision Making, 20*, 170–189.

Genies, M. C., Biondi, E. A., & Berenholtz, S. M. (2019). Leveraging health information technology in the quest to improve health care value. *Quality Management in Health Care, 28*(1), 63–64.

Shinners, L., Aggar, C., Grace, S., & Smith, S. (2020). Exploring healthcare professionals' understanding and experiences of artificial intelligence technology use in the delivery of healthcare: An integrative review. *Health Informatics Journal, 26*(2), 1225–1236.

Sittig, D. F., Wright, A., Coiera, E., Magrabi, F., Ratwani, R., Bates, D. W., & Singh, H. (2020). Current challenges in health information technology–related patient safety. *Health Informatics Journal, 26*(1), 181–189.

Telecommunication Consultation   8180

> *Definition:* Eliciting information, listening, providing support, or teaching remotely in response to stated concerns, between different sites

Activities:

- Identify self with name and credentials, organization; let person know if call recorded (e.g., for quality monitoring), using voice to create therapeutic relationship
- Determine if person would like to proceed via phone or video conference, as available
- Inform person about call purpose and process
- Obtain consent, if indicated
- Confirm person's telephone number or method of reconnection if interrupted (e.g., email address, chat room number)
- Request person to move to quiet location or consider wearing headphones to minimize background noise where possible
- Identify concerns about health status
- Establish level of knowledge and source of that knowledge
- Determine ability to understand telephone teaching or instructions (e.g., hearing deficits, confusion, language barriers)
- Review pertinent information about purpose of contact (e.g., medical diagnoses if any, past health history, current treatment regimen, results of tests)
- Speak slowly and clearly and avoid raising voice volume
- Be aware of visual or audio cues that information not understood
- Consider cultural and socioeconomic aspects to person's response
- Provide means of overcoming any identified barrier to learning or use of support systems
- Identify actual or potential problems related to implementation of self-care regimen
- Make recommendations about regimen changes as appropriate, using established guidelines as needed and available
- Consult with primary care provider about changes in treatment regimen as necessary
- Inquire about related complaints or symptoms, according to standard protocol as needed and available
- Obtain data related to effectiveness of current treatments
- Determine psychological response to situation and availability of support system
- Identify degree of family support and involvement in care
- Involve family or significant others in care and planning, as indicated
- Determine any safety risks to caller and others
- Determine whether concerns require further evaluation, using standard protocol as needed and if necessary
- Use screening tools when identifying individuals who may need more comprehensive, in-person assessment
- Provide clear instruction on how to access needed care, if concerns
- Provide information about treatment regimen and resultant self-care responsibilities according to scope of practice and established guidelines, as necessary
- Provide information about prescribed therapies and medications, as appropriate
- Provide information about health promotion or health education, as appropriate
- Provide information about community resources, educational programs, support groups, and self-help groups, as indicated
- Provide services in calm, caring, and supportive manner
- Answer questions
- Determine understanding of information provided
- Use teach-back to ensure understanding
- Maintain confidentiality, as indicated
- Document any assessments, advice, instructions, or other information provided according to specified organizational guidelines
- Follow guidelines for investigating or reporting suspected child, geriatric, or spousal abuse situations
- Follow up to determine disposition
- Document disposition and person's intended actions
- Determine need and time intervals for further intermittent assessment, as appropriate
- Determine how person or family member can be reached for return contact, as appropriate
- Document permission for return call and identify persons able to receive call information

T

- Discuss and resolve problem contact with supervisory or collegial help

---

2nd edition 1996; revised 2000, 2024

Background Evidence:

American Academy of Ambulatory Care Nursing. (2018). *Scope and standards of practice for professional telehealth nursing* (6th ed.).

Chernitzer, D., & Gustin, T. S. (2020). Evaluating advanced practice nurses' knowledge and use of electronic consultations. *The Journal for Nurse Practitioners*, *16*(2), 151–153. https://doi.org/10.1016/j.nurpra.2019.11.023

Fiona Imlach, F., McKinlay, E., Middleton, L., Kennedy, J., Pledger, M., Russell, L., Churchward, M., Cumming, J., & McBride-Henry. (2020). Telehealth consultations in general practice during a pandemic lockdown: Survey and interviews on patient experiences and preferences. *BMC Family Practice*, *21*, 269–282.

Nieman, C. L., & Oh, E. S. (2020). Connecting with older adults via telemedicine. *Annals of Internal Medicine*, *173*, 831–832.

Rutledge, C., Kott, K., Schweickert, P. A., Poston, R., Fowler, C., & Haney, T. S. (2017). Telehealth and eHealth in nurse practitioner training: current perspectives. *Advances in Medical Education and Practice*, *8*, 399–409.

Seehusen, D. A., & Azrak, A. (2019). The effectiveness of outpatient telehealth consultations. *American Family Physician*, *100*(9), 575–577.

Sitton-Kent, L., Humphreys, C., & Miller, P. (2018). Supporting the spread of health technology in community services. *British Journal of Community Nursing*, *23*(3), 118–122.

Temperature Regulation 3900

Definition: Attaining or maintaining normothermia

Activities:

- Determine cause of temperature alteration (e.g., excessive heat exposure, volume depletion, exertional, drug-induced, radiation, evaporation, conduction, convection, infection)
- Monitor laboratory values for serum electrolytes, urinalysis, blood cultures, and complete blood count
- Institute continuous core temperature monitoring device, as appropriate
- Monitor temperature per guidelines for body temperature readings (i.e., normothermia by monitoring every 30 minutes twice then per protocol, hypothermia and hyperthermia treat by continuous monitoring per core temperature monitoring device), as appropriate
- Monitor blood pressure, pulse, and respirations, as appropriate
- Monitor skin color and temperature
- Report signs and symptoms of hypothermia and hyperthermia
- Treat hyperthermia per protocol (e.g., cooling blankets, cooled IV fluids, fan, cold packs, place in cooled water)
- Use cooling mattress, water-circulating blankets, tepid baths, icepack or gel-pad application, and intravascular cooling catheterization to lower body temperature, as appropriate
- Treat hypothermia per protocol (e.g., warming blankets, warmed IV fluids, warmed oxygen therapy)
- Use warming mattress, warm blankets, and warm ambient environment to raise body temperature, as appropriate
- Adjust environmental temperature to person needs
- Give appropriate medication to prevent or control shivering
- Administer antipyretic medication, as appropriate
- Administer antibiotics, as appropriate
- Monitor for complications (e.g., renal impairment, acid-base imbalance, coagulopathy, pulmonary edema, cerebral edema, multiple organ dysfunction syndrome)
- Promote adequate fluid and nutritional intake, if appropriate
- Instruct how to prevent heat exhaustion and heat stroke
- Discuss importance of thermoregulation and possible negative effects of excess chilling, as appropriate
- Instruct about actions to prevent hypothermia from cold exposure
- Inform of indications of heat exhaustion and appropriate emergency treatment, as appropriate
- Inform about indications of hypothermia and appropriate emergency treatment, as appropriate
- Use teach-back to ensure understanding

1st edition 1992; revised 2013, 2024

Background Evidence:

Barwood, M. J., Goodall, S., & Bateman, J. (2018). The effect of hot and cold drinks on thermoregulation, perception, and performance: The role of the gut in thermoreception. *European Journal of Applied Physiology*, *118*(12), 2643–2654. https://doi.org/10.1007/s00421-018-3987-8

Craven, R. F., Hirnle, C. J., & Henshaw, C. J. (2021). *Fundamentals of nursing: Human health and function* (8th ed.). Wolters-Kluwer.

Hill, B., & Mitchell, A. (2021). Tympanic thermometers support fast and accurate temperature monitoring in acute and alternative care. *British Journal of Nursing*, *30*(5), 288–295. https://doi.org/10.12968/bjon.2021.30.5.288

Kenney, W. L., Wolf, S. T., Dillon, G. A., Berry, C. W., & Alexander, L. M. (2021). Temperature regulation during exercise in the heat: Insights for the aging athlete. *Journal of Science & Medicine in Sport*, *24*(8), 739–746. https://doi.org/10.1016/j.jsams.2020.12.007

Perry, A. G., Potter, P. A., Ostendorf, W. R., & LaPlante, N. (2021). *Clinical nursing skills and technique* (10th ed.). Mosby.

Potter, P. A., Perry, A. G., Stockert, P. A., & Hall, A. M. (2021). *Fundamentals of Nursing* (10th ed.). Elsevier.

Saqe-Rockoff, A., Schubert, F. D., Ciardiello, A., & Douglas, E. (2018). Improving thermoregulation for trauma patients in the Emergency Department: An evidence-based practice project. *Journal of Trauma Nursing*, *25*(1), 14–E2. https://doi.org/10.1097/JTN.0000000000000336

Williams, P. (2020). *Basic geriatric nursing* (7th ed.). Elsevier.

Temperature Regulation: Newborn 3910

Definition: Attaining or maintaining normothermia from birth to extrauterine life and subsequent period of stabilization

Activities:

- Monitor temperature at least every 30 minutes until stable, as appropriate
- Institute continuous core temperature monitoring device, as appropriate
- Monitor blood pressure, pulse, and respirations, as appropriate
- Monitor skin color and temperature
- Monitor for and report signs and symptoms of hypothermia and hyperthermia
- Promote adequate fluid and nutritional intake
- Wrap infant immediately after birth to prevent heat loss
- Wrap low birthweight infant in plastic (e.g., polyethylene, polyurethane) immediately after birth while still covered with amniotic fluid, as appropriate and according to agency protocol
- Apply stockinette cap to prevent heat loss
- Place in isolette or under warmer, as needed
- Maintain humidity at 50% or greater in incubator to reduce evaporative heat loss
- Prewarm items (e.g., blankets, snugglies) placed next to infant in incubator
- Adjust environmental temperature to infant needs
- Instruct parents on methods to maintain adequate infant body temperature
- Use teach-back to ensure understanding

8th edition 2024

Background Evidence:

Dixon, K. L., Carter, B., Harriman, T., Doles, B., Sitton, B., & Thompson, J. (2021). Neonatal thermoregulation: A golden hour protocol update. *Advances in Neonatal Care, 21*(4), 280–288. https://doi.org/10.1097/ANC.0000000000000799

Donnellan, D., Moore, Z., Patton, D., O'Connor, T., & Nugent, L. (2020). The effect of thermoregulation quality improvement initiatives on the admission temperature of premature/very low birth-weight infants in neonatal intensive care units: A systematic review. *Journal for Specialists in Pediatric Nursing, 25*(2), 1–13. https://doi.org/10.1111/jspn.12286

Gardner, S. L., Cater, B. S., Enzman-Hines, M., & Niermeyer, S. (2021). *Merenstein & Gardner's handbook of neonatal intensive care: An interprofessional approach* (9th ed.). Elsevier.

Gest, C. D. (2021). A web-based nursing education for thermoregulation. *Journal for Nurses in Professional Development, 37*(4), 249–256. https://doi.org/10.1097/NND.0000000000000755

Langan, M., Watson, C., O'Connor, T., Moore, Z., & Patton, D. (2020). What is the effectiveness of combining warming mattresses and plastic bags versus plastic bags only for thermoregulation in preterm infants? A systematic review. *Journal of Neonatal Nursing, 26*(1), 30–36. https://doi.org/10.1016/j.jnn.2019.09.006

Thakur, S., Kumar, Y., & Chand, S. (2018). Effectiveness of cling wrap in terms of maintenance of body temperature and weight of neonates. *International Journal of Nursing Education, 10*(3), 106–108. https://doi.org/10.5958/0974-9357.2018.00077.6

Temperature Regulation: Perioperative 3902

Definition: Attaining and maintaining desired body temperature throughout the surgical event

Activities:

- Identify and discuss type of anesthesia planned for patient with surgical team
- Identify patient risk factors for experiencing abnormalities in body temperature (e.g., general or major regional anesthesia, age, major trauma, burns, low body weight, personal or familial risk for malignant hyperthermia)
- Prewarm the patient with active warming device (e.g., forced-air warming) for at least 15 minutes before start of anesthesia, as appropriate
- Transport patient using warming device (e.g., heated isolette), as appropriate
- Apply and regulate active warming device (e.g., forced-air warming)
- Adjust ambient room temperature to minimize the risk of hypothermia (i.e., in addition to forced-air warming, when large surface areas are exposed, maintain room temperature at or above 73.4 degrees Fahrenheit or 23 degrees Celsius)
- Minimize exposure of patient during surgical prepping and procedure, when possible
- Provide warm or cool irrigating solutions, as appropriate
- Monitor the temperature of irrigating solutions
- Warm or cool intravenous fluids, as appropriate
- Provide and regulate blood warmer
- Provide or assist in provision of heated, humidified anesthetic gases, as appropriate
- Provide heated intraperitoneal gases (e.g., carbon dioxide) for laparoscopy
- Discontinue active warming activities (e.g., forced air warming), when appropriate
- Monitor vital signs, including continuous core body temperature
- Monitor for abnormal or unintentional increases or decreases in body temperature
- Monitor electrocardiography results
- Monitor expired carbon dioxide (capnography)
- Monitor laboratory results (e.g., arterial blood gases, electrolytes)
- Ensure active warming equipment and supplies are in place and in good working order
- Maintain emergency equipment and supplies for malignant hyperthermia, per protocol, including dantrolene sodium, in perioperative and perianesthesia areas
- Initiate malignant hyperthermia protocol, as appropriate
- Prepare or administer dantrolene sodium
- Provide handoff communication regarding patient risk of abnormalities in temperature (e.g., personal or familial risk for malignant hyperthermia)
- Ensure proper body temperature until patient is awake and alert

2nd edition 1996; revised 2013

Background Evidence:

Association of periOperative Registered Nurses. (2011). Recommended practices for the prevention of unplanned perioperative hypothermia. In *Perioperative standards and recommended practices for inpatient and ambulatory settings*, 307–320.

Hooper, V. D., Chard, R., Clifford, T., Fetzer, S., Fossum, S., Godden, B., Martinez, E. A., Noble, K., O'Brien, D., Odem-Forren, J., Peterson, C., & Ross, J. (2009). ASPAN's evidence-based clinical practice guideline for the promotion of perioperative normothermia. *Journal of PeriAnesthesia Nursing*, 24(5), 271–287.

Hopkins, P. M. (2011). Malignant hyperthermia: Pharmacology of triggering. *British Journal of Anaesthesia*, 107(1), 48–56.

Malignant Hyperthermia Association. (2010). *Transfer of care guidelines.*

Sessler, D. I. (2008). Temperature monitoring and perioperative thermoregulation. *Anesthesiology*, 109(2), 318–338.

Therapeutic Play   4430

Definition: Purposeful and directive use of toys or other materials to assist children in communicating their perception and knowledge of their world and to help in gaining mastery of their environment

Activities:

- Provide a quiet environment that is free from interruptions
- Provide sufficient time to allow for effective play
- Structure play session to facilitate desired outcome
- Communicate the purpose of play session to child and parent
- Discuss play activities with family
- Set limits for therapeutic play session
- Provide safe play equipment
- Provide developmentally appropriate play equipment
- Provide play equipment that stimulates creative, expressive play
- Provide play equipment that stimulates role playing
- Provide real or simulated hospital operating-room medical equipment to encourage expression of knowledge and feelings about hospitalization, treatments, or illness
- Supervise therapeutic play sessions
- Encourage child to manipulate play equipment
- Encourage child to share feelings, knowledge, and perceptions
- Validate child's feelings expressed during the play session
- Communicate acceptance of feelings, both positive and negative, expressed through play
- Observe the child's use of play equipment
- Monitor child's reactions and anxiety level throughout play session
- Identify child's misconceptions or fears through comments made during hospital role-play session
- Continue play sessions on a regular basis to establish trust and reduce fear of unfamiliar equipment or treatments, as appropriate
- Record observations made during play session

1st edition 1992; revised 2000

Background Evidence:

Hart, R., Mather, P. L., Slack, J. L., & Powell, M. A. (1992). *Therapeutic play activities for hospitalized children.* Mosby Year Book.

Raphel, S., & Bennett, C. F. (2005). Child psychiatric nursing. In G. W. Stuart & M. T. Laraia (Eds.), *Principles and practice of psychiatric nursing* (8th ed., pp. 728–752). Mosby.

Snyder, M. (1992). Play. In M. Snyder (Ed.), *Independent nursing interventions* (2nd ed., pp. 287–293). Delmar.

Tiedeman, M. E., Simon, K. A., & Clatworthy, S. (1990). Communication through therapeutic play. In M. J. Craft & J. A. Denehy (Eds.), *Nursing interventions for infants and children* (pp. 93–110). W.B. Saunders.

Vessey, J. A., & Mahon, M. M. (1990). Therapeutic play and the hospitalized child. *Journal of Pediatric Nursing*, 5(5), 328–333.

Therapeutic Touch   5465

Definition: Attuning to the universal energy field by seeking to act as a healing influence using the natural sensitivity of hands and passing them over the body to gently focus, direct, and modulate the human energy field

Activities:

- Create a comfortable environment without distractions
- Determine willingness to experience the intervention
- Identify mutual goals for the session
- Advise the patient to ask questions whenever they arise
- Place patient in either a comfortable sitting or supine position
- Center self by focusing awareness on the inner self
- Focus on the intention to facilitate wholeness and healing at all levels of consciousness
- Place hands with palms facing the patient 3 to 5 inches from the patient's body
- Begin the 1- to 2-minute assessment by moving the hands slowly and steadily over as much of the patient as possible, from head to toe and front to back
- Move the hands in very gentle downward movements through the patient's energy field, thinking of the patient as a unitary whole and facilitating an open and balanced energy flow
- Note the overall pattern of the energy flow, especially any areas of disturbance such as congestion or unevenness, which may be perceived through very subtle cues in the hands (e.g., temperature change, tingling, or other subtle feelings of movement)
- Focus intention on facilitating symmetry and healing in disturbed areas
- Continue the treatment by very gently facilitating the flow of healing energy into areas of disturbance
- Finish when it is judged that the appropriate amount of change has taken place (i.e., for an infant, 1–2 minutes; for an adult, 5–10 minutes), keeping in mind the importance of gentleness
- Encourage the patient to rest for 20 minutes or more after treatment
- Note whether the patient has experienced a relaxation response and any related changes

1st edition 1992; revised 2000, 2013

Background Evidence:
Coakley, A. B., & Duffy, M. E. (2010). The effect of therapeutic touch on postoperative patients. *Journal of Holistic Nursing, 28*(3), 193–200.
Engle, V. F., & Graney, M. J. (2000). Biobehavioral effects of therapeutic touch. *Journal of Nursing Scholarship, 32*(3), 287–293.
Krieger, D. (1993). *Accepting your power to heal: The personal practice of therapeutic touch.* Bear & Company.
Krieger, D. (2002). *Therapeutic touch: As transpersonal healing.* Lantern Books.
Monroe, C. M. (2009). The effects of therapeutic touch on pain. *Journal of Holistic Nursing, 27*(2), 85–92.

O'Mathuna, D. P. (2000). Evidence-based practice and reviews of therapeutic touch. *Journal of Nursing Scholarship, 32*(3), 279–285.
Peters, R. M. (1999). The effectiveness of therapeutic touch: a meta-analytic review. *Nursing Science Quarterly, 12*(1), 52–61.
Sayre-Adams, J., & Wright, S. (1995). The essentials of practice. In J. Sayre-Adams & S. Wright (Eds.), *The theory and practice of therapeutic touch* (pp. 75–110). Elsevier.
Winstead-Fry, P., & Kijek, J. (1999). An integrative review and meta-analysis of therapeutic touch research. *Alternative Therapies in Health & Medicine, 5*(6), 58–67.

Therapy Group   5450

Definition: Application of psychotherapeutic techniques to a group, including the utilization of interactions between members of the group

Activities:

- Determine the purpose of the group (e.g., maintenance of reality testing, facilitation of communication, examination of interpersonal skills, and support) and the nature of the group process
- Form a group of optimal size: 5 to 12 members
- Create specific group rules and guidelines (e.g., confidentiality, respectful communication and behavior, attendance, socialization of members outside the group, participation) to ensure that all members are compliant
- Provide an individualized orientation session for each new member of the group before first group session
- Provide a manual that includes the group rules and guidelines for all group members
- Choose group members who are willing to participate actively and take responsibility for own problems
- Determine whether level of motivation is high enough to benefit from group therapy
- Use a coleader, as appropriate
- Address the issue of mandatory attendance
- Address the issue of whether new members can join at any time
- Establish a time and place for the group meeting
- Meet in 1- to 2-hour sessions, as appropriate
- Begin and end on time and expect participants to remain until the conclusion
- Arrange chairs in a circle in close proximity
- Move the group to the working stage as quickly as possible
- Assist the group in forming therapeutic norms
- Help the group to work through their resistance to change
- Give the group a sense of direction that enables them to identify and resolve each step of development
- Use the technique of "process illumination" to encourage exploration of the significant meaning of the message
- Encourage self-disclosure and discussion of the past only as it relates to the function and goals of the group
- Use the technique of "here-and-now activation" to move the focus from the generic to the personal, from the abstract to the specific
- Encourage members to share things they have in common with each other
- Encourage members to share their anger, sadness, humor, mistrust, and other feelings with each other
- Assist members in the process of exploration and acceptance of any anger felt toward the group leader and others
- Confront behaviors that threaten group cohesion (e.g., tardiness, absences, disruptive socialization, subgrouping, and scapegoating)
- Provide social reinforcement (e.g., verbal and nonverbal) for desired behaviors/responses
- Provide structured group exercises, as appropriate, to promote group function and insight
- Use role playing and problem solving, as appropriate
- Help members provide feedback to each other, so that they develop insights into their own behavior
- Incorporate leaderless sessions, when appropriate to the goals and function of the group
- Conclude session with a summary of the proceedings
- Meet individually with the member who desires premature termination to examine rationale for this
- Assist member to terminate from the group, if appropriate
- Assist group to review the past and a member's relationship with the group when someone leaves
- Recruit new members, as appropriate, to maintain the integrity of the group

1st edition 1992; revised 1996, 2018

Background Evidence:

Boyd, M. A. (2015). Group interventions. In M. A. Boyd (Ed.), *Psychiatric nursing: Contemporary practice* (5th ed., pp. 186–194). Lippincott Williams & Wilkins.
Jung, X. T., & Newton, R. (2009). Cochran reviews of non-medication-based psychotherapeutic and other interventions for schizophrenia, psychosis, and bipolar: A systematic literature review. *International Journal of Mental Health Nursing, 18*(4), 239–249.
Puskar, K., McClure, E., & McGinnis, K. (2007). Advanced practice nurse's role in alcohol abuse group therapy. *Australian Journal of Advanced Nursing, 25*(1), 64–69.
Stuart, G. W. (2013). Therapeutic groups. In *Principles and practice of psychiatric nursing* (10th ed., pp. 617–627). Mosby.
Yalom, I. D., & Leszcz, M. (2005). *The theory and practice of group psychotherapy* (5th ed.). Basic Books.

T

Thermoregulation Management 3920

Definition: Alleviation of symptoms and related conditions associated with an increase in body temperature resulting from a disruption in body regulatory mechanisms

Activities:
- Determine cause of increased body temperature (e.g., poikilothermia, malignant hyperthermia, spinal cord injury above T6, extreme physical exertion)
- Ensure patent airway and administer cooled oxygen as needed
- Monitor vital signs and neurological status
- Discontinue any presumed causative medication if experiencing neuroleptic malignant syndrome (e.g., selective serotonin reuptake inhibitors [SSRI], monoamine oxidase inhibitors [MAOI], or tricyclic antidepressants)
- Establish IV access
- Discontinue physical activity and place into cooler environment
- Loosen or remove clothing
- Apply external cooling methods (e.g., cold packs to neck, chest, abdomen, scalp, armpits, and groin; cooling blanket), as appropriate
- Place in cooled water, as tolerated, but avoid causing shivering
- Avoid alcohol sponge bath
- Provide oral rehydrating solution (e.g., sports drink) or other cold fluid if tolerated
- Do not offer food or liquid by mouth if neurological impairment
- Do not administer salt tablets
- Administer IV fluids, using cooled solutions, as appropriate
- Apply internal cooling methods (e.g., iced gastric, bladder, peritoneal, or thoracic lavage), as appropriate
- Administer pharmacological agents as needed
- Do not administer aspirin or other antipyretic if suspect damage to thermoregulation centers (e.g., hypothalamus)
- Insert nasogastric tube, as appropriate
- Insert urinary catheter
- Discontinue cooling activities when core body temperature reaches 39° C
- Monitor for abnormalities in mental status (e.g., confusion, bizarre behavior, anxiety, loss of coordination, agitation, seizure, coma)
- Monitor core body temperature using appropriate device (e.g., rectal or esophageal probe)
- Obtain laboratory values for serum electrolytes, urinalysis, cardiac enzymes, liver enzymes, blood cultures, and complete blood count and monitor results
- Monitor urine output
- Monitor arterial blood gases
- Monitor for hypoglycemia
- Monitor electrocardiography results
- Monitor for complications (e.g., renal impairment, acid-base imbalance, coagulopathy, pulmonary edema, cerebral edema, multiple organ dysfunction syndrome)
- Provide transportation to hospital for further treatment if needed
- Instruct on risk factors for heat-related illness (e.g., high environmental temperature, high humidity, dehydration, physical exertion, obesity, extremes of age, certain drugs, heart disease)
- Instruct on measures to prevent heat-related illness (e.g., prevent sun overexposure; ensure adequate intake of nutritious foods and fluids before, during, and after physical activity; seek settings in which air conditioning available; wear lightweight, light-colored, and loose-fitting clothing)
- Instruct on early signs and symptoms of heat-related illness and when to seek assistance from health care professional
- Use teach-back to ensure understanding

8th edition 2024

Background Evidence:
LaPierre, L., & Mondor, E. E. (2017). The ups and downs of fever: Where are we at with targeted temperature management in the ICU? *Canadian Journal of Critical Care Nursing, 28*(2), 39.

Moreda, M., Beacham, P. S., Reese, A., & Mulkey, M. A. (2021). Increasing the effectiveness of targeted temperature management. *Critical Care Nurse, 41*(5), 59–63. https://doi.org/10.4037/ccn2021637

Rodway, G. W., & Suether, S. E. (2019). Pain, temperature, sleep, and sensory function. In S. E. Huether & K. L. McCance (Eds.), *Understanding pathophysiology*. Elsevier.

Schell-Chaple, H. (2018). Fever suppression in patients with infection. *Nursing Critical Care, 13*(5), 6–13. https://doi.org/10.1097/01.CCN.0000534921.93547.1a

Souza, M. V., Damião, E. B. C., Buchhorn, S. M. M., & Rossato, L. M. (2021). Non-pharmacological fever and hyperthermia management in children: an integrative review. *Acta Paul Enferm, 34*, eAPE00743.

Turan, N., Çulha, Y., Aydın, G. Ö., & Kaya, H. (2020). Persistent fever and nursing care in neurosurgical patients. *Journal of Neurological & Neurosurgical Nursing, 2*, 80–85. https://doi.org/10.15225/PNN.2020.9.2.6

T

Thrombolytic Therapy Management 4270

Definition: Collection and analysis of patient data to expedite safe, appropriate provision of an agent that dissolves a thrombus

Activities:
- Verify patient's identity
- Obtain history of present illness and medical history
- Perform physical examination (e.g., general appearance, heart rate, blood pressure, respiratory rate, temperature, pain level, height, and weight)
- Explain all procedures to the patient and significant other(s)
- Allow significant other(s) at patient's bedside, if possible
- Obtain pulse oximetry and apply oxygen, as appropriate
- Perform targeted assessment of the system that is indicated by the history of present illness
- Obtain 12-lead ECG, as appropriate

- Initiate intravenous line and obtain blood samples for laboratory tests
- Obtain stat computerized tomography head scan, as appropriate
- Obtain V/Q scan, as appropriate
- Consider guidelines for candidacy (e.g., therapy inclusion and exclusion criteria)
- Determine whether the patient will receive the therapy
- Obtain informed consent
- Prepare for thrombolytic therapy, if indicated
- Obtain additional intravenous access site
- Avoid arterial sampling to prevent bleeding complications
- Prepare thrombolytic agents, per facility protocol
- Administer thrombolytic agents, according to specific guidelines for administration
- Administer additional medications, as ordered
- Continually monitor cardiac rhythm, vital signs, level of pain, heart and lung sounds, level of consciousness, peripheral perfusion, intake and output, change in neurological status, and resolution of symptoms, as indicated
- Observe for signs of bleeding

- Obtain additional radiological tests (e.g., chest x-ray), as indicated
- Prepare to initiate basic and advanced life support measures, if indicated
- Prepare to transfer for definitive care (e.g., cardiac catheterization lab, ICU)

5th edition 2008

Background Evidence:

Emergency Nurses Association. (1994). *Standards of emergency nursing practice* (4th ed.). W.B. Saunders.

Emergency Nurses Association. (2000). *Emergency nursing core curriculum* (5th ed.). W.B. Saunders.

Hazinski, M. F., Cummins, R. O., & Field, J. M. (Eds.). (2002). *2000 handbook of emergency cardiovascular care for healthcare providers*. Dallas, TX: American Heart Association.

Lacy, C. F., Armstrong, L. L., Goldman, M. P., & Lance, L. L. (2005). *Drug information handbook* (13th ed.). Lexi-Comp.

Total Parenteral Nutrition (TPN) Administration   1200

Definition: Delivery of nutrients intravenously and monitoring of patient response

Activities:

- Assure placement of proper intravenous line related to duration of nutrients to be infused (e.g., centrally placed line preferred; peripheral lines only in well-nourished individuals expecting to need TPN for less than 2 weeks)
- Use central lines only for infusion of high caloric nutrients or hyperosmolar solutions (e.g., 10% dextrose, 2% amino acids with standard additives)
- Assure TPN solutions infused in a noncentral catheter are limited to osmolarity less than 900 mOsm/L
- Insert peripheral intravenous central catheter, per agency protocol
- Ascertain correct placement of intravenous central catheter by x-ray examination
- Maintain central line patency and dressing, per agency protocol
- Monitor for infiltration, infection, and metabolic complications (e.g., hyperlipidemia, elevated triglycerides, thrombocytopenia, platelet dysfunction)
- Check the TPN solution to ensure that correct nutrients are included, as ordered
- Maintain sterile technique when preparing and hanging TPN solutions
- Provide regular, aseptic, and meticulous care of the central venous catheter, particularly the catheter exit site, to assure prolonged, safe, and complication-free use
- Avoid use of the catheter for purposes other than delivery of TPN (e.g., blood transfusions and blood sampling)
- Use an infusion pump for delivery of TPN solutions
- Maintain a constant flow rate of TPN solution
- Avoid rapid replacement of TPN solution when interrupted for supplemental infusions
- Monitor daily weight
- Monitor intake and output

- Monitor serum albumin, total protein, electrolyte, lipid profiles, glucose levels, and chemistry profile
- Monitor vital signs, as indicated
- Monitor urine glucose for glycosuria, acetone, and protein
- Maintain a small oral nutritional intake during TPN, whenever possible
- Encourage a gradual transition from parenteral to enteral feeding, if indicated
- Administer insulin, as ordered, to maintain serum glucose level in the designated range, as appropriate
- Report abnormal signs and symptoms associated with TPN to the physician and modify care accordingly
- Maintain universal precautions
- Instruct patient and family about care of and indications for TPN
- Assure patient and family comprehension and competency before discharge home with ongoing TPN

1st edition 1992; revised 2013

Background Evidence:

American Society for Parenteral and Enteral Nutrition (ASPEN) Board of Directors. (2009). Clinical guidelines for the use of parenteral and enteral nutrition in adult and pediatric patients. *Journal of Parenteral & Enteral Nutrition*, 33(3), 255–259.

Kerner, J. A., Jr., Hurwitz, M., Duggan, C., Watkins, J., & Walker, W. A. (2008). Parenteral nutrition. In C. Duggan, J. Watkins, & W. A. Walker (Eds.), *Nutrition in pediatrics: Basic science & clinical applications* (4th ed., pp. 777–793). BC Decker.

Pittiruti, M., Hamilton, H., Biffi, R., MacFie, J., & Pertkiewicz, M. (2009). ESPEN guidelines on parenteral nutrition: Central venous catheters. *Clinical Nutrition*, 28(4), 365–377.

T

Touch 5460

Definition: Providing comfort and communication through purposeful tactile contact

Activities:

- Evaluate one's own personal comfort in using touch with patients and family members
- Evaluate the readiness of the patient when offering touch
- Evaluate the environmental context before offering touch
- Determine which body part is best to touch and the length of touch that produces the most positive responses in the recipient
- Observe cultural taboos about touch
- Hug reassuringly, when appropriate
- Put arm around patient's shoulders, as appropriate
- Hold patient's hand to provide emotional support
- Apply gentle pressure at wrist, hand, or shoulder of seriously ill patient
- Rub back in synchrony with patient's breathing, as appropriate
- Stroke body part in slow, rhythmical fashion, as appropriate
- Massage around painful area, as appropriate
- Elicit from parents common actions used to soothe and calm their child
- Hold infant or child firmly and snugly
- Encourage parents to touch newborn or ill child
- Surround premature infant with blanket rolls (nesting)
- Swaddle infant snugly in a blanket to keep arms and legs close to the body
- Place infant on mother's body immediately after birth
- Encourage mother to hold, touch, and examine the infant while umbilical cord is being severed
- Encourage parents to hold infant
- Encourage parents to massage infant
- Demonstrate quieting techniques for infants
- Provide appropriate pacifier for nonnutritive sucking in newborns
- Provide oral stimulation exercises before tube feedings in premature infants
- Evaluate the effect when using touch

1st edition 1992; revised 2008

Background Evidence:

Gleeson, M., & Timmins, F. (2005). A review of the use and clinical effectiveness of touch as a nursing intervention. *Clinical Effectiveness in Nursing*, 9(1-2), 69–77.

Molsberry, D., & Shogan, M. G. (1990). Communicating through touch. In M. J. Craft & J. A. Denehy (Eds.), *Nursing interventions for infants & children* (pp. 127–150). W.B. Saunders.

Rombalski, J. J. (2003). A personal journey in understanding physical touch as a nursing intervention. *Journal of Holistic Nursing*, 21(1), 73–80.

Snyder, M., & Nojima, Y. (1998). Purposeful touch. In M. Snyder & R. Lindquist (Eds.), *Complementary/alternative therapies in nursing* (3rd ed., pp. 149–158). Springer.

Weiss, S. J. (1988). Touch. In J. Fitzpatrick, R. Taunton, & J. Benoliel (Eds.), *Annual Review of Nursing Research* (Vol. 6, pp. 3–27). Springer.

Weiss, S. J. (1991). The tactile environment of caregiving: Implications for health science and health care. *The Science of Caring*, 3(2), 33–40.

Traction/Immobilization Care 0940

Definition: Management of a patient who has traction and/or a stabilizing device to immobilize and stabilize a body part

Activities:

- Position in proper body alignment
- Maintain proper body alignment in bed to enhance traction
- Ensure that proper weights are being applied (e.g., traction and countertraction measures)
- Ensure that the ropes and pulleys are working properly and hang freely off the floor
- Ensure that the pull of ropes and weights remains along the axis of the fractured bone
- Brace traction weights while moving patient
- Maintain traction at all times
- Monitor traction system at least once per shift
- Monitor self-care ability while in traction
- Monitor external fixation device
- Monitor pin insertion sites
- Remove skin traction devices at least daily for skin inspection and cleansing of skin
- Monitor skin and bony prominences for signs of skin breakdown
- Monitor circulation, movement, and sensation of affected extremity
- Monitor for complications of immobility (e.g., deep vein thrombosis, chest infection, muscle wasting, foot drop)
- Provide adequate pain-relief measures
- Perform pin insertion site care at least daily
- Administer appropriate skin care at friction points
- Provide trapeze for movement in bed, as appropriate
- Instruct on bracing device care, as needed
- Instruct on external fixation device care, as needed
- Instruct on pin site care, as needed
- Instruct in importance of adequate nutrition for bone healing
- Monitor for body image disturbances and need for counseling

1st edition 1992; revised 1996, 2018

Background Evidence:

Clarke, S., & Santy-Tomlinson, J. (2014). *Orthopaedic and trauma nursing: An evidence-based approach to musculoskeletal care*. John Wiley and Sons.

Halstead, J., & Stoten, S. (2010). *Orthopedic nursing: Caring for patients with musculoskeletal disorders* (2nd ed.). Brockton, MA: Western Schools.

Harvey, C., David, J., Eckhouse, D., Kurkowski, T., Mains, C., & Roberts, D. (2013). The National Association of Orthopaedic Nurses (NAON) scope and standards of orthopaedic nursing practice, 3rd edition. *Orthopedic Nursing*, 32(3), 139–152.

Whiteing, N. (2008). Fractures: Pathophysiology, treatment and nursing care. *Nursing Standard*, 23(2), 49–57.

T

Transcutaneous Electrical Nerve Stimulation (TENS) 1540

Definition: Stimulation of skin and underlying tissue with controlled, low-voltage electrical pulses

Activities:
- Discuss the rationale for limits and potential problems of TENS with the patient and family
- Determine whether a recommendation for TENS is appropriate
- Do not use TENS if the patient has a pacemaker
- Discuss therapy with provider and obtain prescription for TENS, if appropriate
- Verify that the TENS unit has full battery charge
- Inspect the wires for first signs of wear, replacing wires, as needed
- Select stimulation site, considering alternate sites when direct application is not possible (e.g., adjacent to, distal to, bracketing the site, between affected areas and the brain, and contralateral to the pain)
- Apply disposable or reusable electrodes to the site of stimulation
- Apply wires to electrodes and TENS unit, making sure wires are securely plugged into connections
- Determine therapeutic amplitude, rate, and pulse width
- Adjust the amplitude, rate, and pulse width to predetermined settings indicated
- Maintain stimulation for predetermined interval (e.g., continuous or intermittent)
- Secure TENS unit to the patient (e.g., on patient's belt or waistband of pants), if continuous application is necessary
- Discontinue use when sensation is strong yet tolerable
- Adjust the site and settings to achieve the desired response based on individual tolerance
- Inspect sites of electrodes for possible skin irritation at every application or at least every 12 hours
- Provide verbal and written instruction on the use of TENS and its operation
- Use TENS alone or in conjunction with other measures, as appropriate
- Document the effectiveness of TENS

1st edition 1992; revised 2013

Background Evidence:
DeSantana, J. M., Walsh, D. M., Vance, C., Rakel, B. A., & Sluka, K. A. (2008). Effectiveness of transcutaneous electrical nerve stimulation for treatment of hyperalgesia and pain. *Current Rheumatology Reports, 10*(6), 492–499.

Herr, K. A., & Kwekkeboom, K. L. (2003). Assisting older clients with pain management in the home. *Home Health Care Management and Practice, 15*(3), 237–250.

Lynn, P. (2011). *Taylor's clinical nursing skills: A nursing process approach* (3rd ed.). Wolters Kluwer Health/Lippincott Williams & Wilkins.

Sluka, K. S., & Walsh, D. M. (2003). Transcutaneous nerve stimulation: Basic science mechanisms and clinical effectiveness. *Journal of Pain, 4*(3), 109–121.

Transfer 0970

Definition: Moving a patient with limitation of independent movement

Activities:
- Review chart for activity orders
- Determine mobility level and limitations of movement
- Determine level of consciousness and ability to cooperate
- Plan type and method of move
- Determine amount and type of assistance needed
- Make sure equipment works before using it
- Discuss need for relocation with patient and/or family
- Discuss with patient and helpers how the move will be done
- Assist patient in receiving all necessary care (e.g., personal hygiene, gathering belongings) before performing the transfer, as appropriate
- Provide privacy, avoid drafts, and preserve the patient's modesty
- Make sure the new location of the patient is ready
- Adjust equipment to working heights and lock all wheels, as needed
- Raise side rail on opposite side of nurse to prevent patient from falling out of bed
- Use proper body mechanics during movements
- Keep patient body in proper alignment during movements
- Raise and move patient with hydraulic lift, as necessary
- Move patient using transfer board, as necessary
- Transfer patient from a bed to stretcher, or vice versa, using a turning sheet, as appropriate
- Use a transfer board, as appropriate
- Use a belt to assist a patient who can stand with assistance, as appropriate
- Use an incubator, stretcher, or bed to move a weak, injured, or surgical patient from one area to another
- Use a wheelchair to move a patient unable to walk
- Cradle and carry an infant or small child
- Assist patient to ambulate, using your body as a human crutch, as appropriate
- Maintain traction devices during move, as appropriate
- Evaluate patient at end of transfer for proper body alignment, nonocclusion of tubes, wrinkle-free linens, unnecessarily exposed skin, adequate patient level of comfort, raised side rails, and call bell within reach

5th edition 2008

Background Evidence:
Craven, R., & Hirnle, C. (2007). *Fundamentals of nursing: Human health and function* (5th ed.). Lippincott Williams & Wilkins.

Perry, A. G., & Potter, P. A. (2004). *Fundamentals of nursing* (6th ed.). Mosby.

Perry, A. G., & Potter, P. A. (2006). *Clinical nursing skills and techniques* (6th ed.). Mosby.

Stahl, L. (1996). Working with people: How to transfer patients to other units. *American Journal of Nursing, 96*(8), 57–58.

T

Transgender Hormone Therapy 2430

Definition: Providing care for person seeking to physically change their bodies to match sense of gender identity

Activities:

- Counsel about known risks and benefits of exogenous hormone therapy
- Confirm informed consent to hormone therapy
- Explore acute, active mental health complaints that may be adversely affected by hormone therapy
- Discuss with family about teenagers on hormone therapy
- Determine family's level of support and understanding of hormone treatment and gender acceptance
- Explore and provide psychosocial supports and referrals, as indicated
- Communicate assessment and findings to health care provider who will be prescribing hormone therapy
- Examine person's goals and understanding of hormone therapy to ensure concordance with general nature and purpose of hormone therapy
- Examine understanding of physical, mental health, and social benefits and risks of hormone therapy
- Discuss alternatives to hormone therapy, when applicable
- Discuss alternative surgical referrals, if person intends to continue with sexual re-assignment
- Counsel person on psychoactive effects of hormones (i.e., some mood and mental health problems such as depression and anxiety)
- Gather information about mood and mental health for purpose of forecasting symptoms that may be intensified by hormone therapy
- Guide to discuss these symptoms with health care provider who will be prescribing hormone therapy.
- Explore social transition needs (e.g., peer support, psychotherapy, documentation changes, care coordination, legal advocacy)
- Confirm use of medications as prescribed
- Encourage to talk about doubts, fears, and acceptance of hormone therapy
- Monitor bodily changes and adverse effects every 3 months for first year, then every 6 to 12 months
- Request for transgender men dosage of serum testosterone at follow-up visits with practical target in male range (300–1000 ng/dL)
- Request for transgender women dosage of serum testosterone and estradiol at follow-up visits with a practical target in the female range (testosterone 30–100 ng/dL; estradiol <200 ng/mL)
- Monitor transgender men hormone levels, hematocrit, and lipid profile before starting hormones and at follow-up visits
- Monitor transgender women hormone levels, prolactin, and triglycerides before starting hormones and at follow-up visits
- Perform, according to health care prescription, bone mineral density screening before starting hormones for persons at risk for osteoporosis
- Instruct about cancer risks (e.g., transgender men's cervix or breasts, transgender women's breasts and prostate)
- Instruct about hormone level risks (e.g., too high dangerous, low level reverses sex)
- Ensure follow-up counseling related to social effect of transgender change
- Use teach-back to ensure understanding

8th edition 2024

Background Evidence:

Baker, K. E., Wilson, L. M., Sharma, R., Dukhanin, V., McArthur, K., & Robinson, K. A. (2021). Hormone therapy, mental health, and quality of life among transgender people: A systematic review. *Journal of the Endocrine Society*, 5(4), bvab011. https://doi.org/10.1210/jendso/bvab011

Clark, B. A., Marshall, S. K., & Saewyc, E. M. (2020). Hormone therapy decision-making processes: Transgender youth and parents. *Journal of Adolescence*, 79, 136–147. https://doi.org/10.1016/j.adolescence.2019.12.016

Joseph, A., Cliffe, C., Hillyard, M., & Majeed, A. (2017). Gender identity and the management of the transgender patient: A guide for non-specialists. *Journal of the Royal Society of Medicine*, 110(4), 144–152. https://doi.org/10.1177/0141076817696054

Klein, D. A., Paradise, S. L., & Goodwin, E. T. (2018). Caring for transgender and gender-diverse persons: What clinicians should know. *American Family Physician*, 98(11), 645–653.

Radix, A. (2019). Hormone therapy for transgender adults. *The Urologic Clinics of North America*, 46(4), 467–473. https://doi.org/10.1016/j.ucl.2019.07.001

Souza Santos, R., Frank, A. P., Nelson, M. D., Garcia, M. M., Palmer, B. F., & Clegg, D. J. (2017). Sex, gender, and transgender: Metabolic impact of cross hormone therapy. *Advances in Experimental Medicine and Biology*, 1043, 611–627. https://doi.org/10.1007/978-3-319-70178-3_27

T

Transport: Interfacility 7890

Definition: Moving a patient from one facility to another

Activities:

- Assure that a medical screening examination has been performed and documented
- Assure that the patient has been stabilized within the capabilities of the transferring facility or has met the conditions under which unstable patients may be transferred under the Emergency Treatment and Labor Act (EMTALA)
- Determine need for transfer of patient, ensuring that the patient requires treatment at the receiving facility and the benefits of the transfer outweigh the risks
- Obtain written order from physician to transport patient
- Identify preference of patient or significant other(s) for receiving facility and physician, as appropriate
- Document that the receiving facility will accept the patient and has the necessary equipment and staff to handle the clinical situation
- Obtain written consent for transfer from patient or significant other(s)
- Obtain written consent for transfer of minors, as appropriate
- Obtain written consent for release of patient information to receiving facility

- Facilitate the contact of receiving physician by attending physician, as indicated per EMTALA laws, and document this contact
- Arrange for required type of transport
- Provide a nurse-to-nurse clinical report about the patient to the receiving facility and document this contact
- Mobilize and provide necessary personnel, transfer equipment, and pharmaceuticals
- Copy medical records for receiving facility, including current record of events
- Assure that the medical records accompany the patient to the receiving facility
- Complete the certification for transfer that is signed, timed, and dated by the physician
- Document the medical reason for transfer, as well as the medical benefits and risks of the transfer, as indicated per EMTALA laws
- Document all information pertaining to patients refusing transfer
- Attempt to secure written statement of refusal to transfer from patient, if indicated
- Continue to treat patients refusing transfer within the capability of the facility

5th edition 2008

Background Evidence:

Bowen, S. L. (2004). Neonatal transport. In M. T. Verklan & M. Walden (Eds.), *Core curriculum for neonatal intensive care nursing.* W.B. Saunders.

Casaubon, D. (2001). EMTALA: Practical application with an algorithm. *Journal of Emergency Nursing, 27*(4), 364–368.

Gilstrap, L. C., Oh, W., Greene, M. F., & Lemons, J. A. (Eds.). (2002). Interhospital care of the perinatal patient. In *Guidelines for perinatal care* (5th ed., pp. 57–71). American Academy of Pediatrics & American College of Obstetricians and Gynecologists.

Glass, D. L., Rebstock, J., & Handberg, E. (2004). Emergency Treatment and Labor Act (EMTALA): Avoiding the pitfalls. *Journal of Perinatal and Neonatal Nursing, 18*(2), 103–114.

Society of Critical Care Medicine. (1993). Guidelines for the transfer of critically ill patients. *Critical Care Medicine, 21*(6), 931–937.

Warren, J., Fromm, R. E., Jr., Orr, R. A., Rotello, L. C., & Horst, H. M. (2004). Guidelines for the inter- and intrahospital transport of critically ill patients. *Critical Care Medicine, 32*(1), 256–262.

Transport: Intrafacility   7892

Definition: Moving a patient from one area of a facility to another

Activities:
- Facilitate pre-transport coordination and communication
- Obtain physician order before transport, as appropriate
- Determine amount and type of assistance needed
- Provide appropriate personnel to assist in transport
- Provide appropriate equipment to assist in transport
- Discuss need for relocation with patient and significant other(s)
- Assist patient in receiving all necessary care (e.g., personal hygiene, gathering belongings) before performing the transfer, as appropriate
- Make sure the new location for the patient is ready
- Move patient using required equipment, as necessary
- Use an incubator, stretcher, or bed to move a weak, injured, or surgical patient from one area to another
- Use a wheelchair to move a patient unable to walk
- Cradle and carry an infant or small child
- Assist patient to ambulate, using your body as a human crutch, as appropriate
- Provide escort during transport, as needed
- Monitor, as appropriate, during transport
- Provide a clinical report about patient to the receiving location, as appropriate
- Document pertinent information related to transport
- Evacuate patients in emergencies such as fire, hurricane, or tornado according to agency disaster plan

5th edition 2008

Background Evidence:

Craven, R. F., & Hirnle, C. J. (2003). *Fundamentals of nursing: Human health and function* (4th ed.). Philadelphia, PA: Lippincott Williams & Wilkins.

Perry, A. G., & Potter, P. A. (2001). *Fundamentals of nursing* (5th ed.). Mosby.

Perry, A. G., & Potter, P. A. (2006). *Clinical nursing skills and techniques* (6th ed.). Elsevier Mosby.

Stahl, L. (1996). Working with people: How to transfer patients to other units. *American Journal of Nursing, 96*(8), 57–58.

Warren, J., Fromm, R. E., Jr., Orr, R. A., Rotello, L. C., & Horst, H. M. (2004). Guidelines for the inter- and intrahospital transport of critically ill patients. *Critical Care Medicine, 32*(1), 256–262.

T

Trauma Therapy: Child   5410

Definition: Use of an interactive helping process to resolve a trauma experienced by a child

Activities:
- Teach specific stress-management techniques before trauma exploration to restore a sense of control over thoughts and feelings
- Explore the trauma and its meaning to the child
- Use developmentally appropriate language to ask about the trauma
- Use relaxation and desensitization procedures to assist the child to describe the event
- Establish trust, safety, and the right to gain access to carefully guarded trauma material by monitoring reactions to the disclosure
- Proceed with therapy at the child's own pace

- Establish a signal the child can give if the trauma-focused work becomes overwhelming
- Focus therapy on self-regulation and rebuilding a sense of security
- Use art and play to promote expression
- Involve the parents or caretakers in therapy, as appropriate
- Educate the parents about their child's response to the trauma and to the process of therapy
- Assist parents in resolving their own emotional distress about the trauma
- Assist appropriate others to provide support
- Avoid involving parents or caretakers if they are the cause of the trauma
- Assist the child to reconsider assumptions made about the traumatic event with step-by-step analysis of any perceptive and cognitive distortions
- Explore and correct inaccurate attributions regarding the trauma, including omen formation and survivor's guilt
- Help identify and cope with feelings
- Explain the grief process to the child and parent(s), as appropriate
- Assist the child to examine any distorted assumptions and conclusions

- Assist child in reestablishing a sense of security and predictability in his or her life
- Assist child to integrate the restructured trauma events into history and life experience
- Address posttrauma role functioning in family life, peer relationships, and school performance

4th edition 2004

Background Evidence:

Boyd, M. R. (2005). Caring for abused persons. In M. A. Boyd (Ed.), *Psychiatric nursing: Contemporary practice* (3rd ed., pp. 823–856). Lippincott Williams & Wilkins.

Clark, C. C. (1997). Posttraumatic stress disorder: How to support healing. *American Journal of Nursing, 97*(8), 27–33.

DiPalma, L. M. (1997). Integrating trauma theory into nursing practice and education. *Clinical Nurse Specialist, 11*(3), 102–107.

Pifferbaum, B. (1997). Posttraumatic stress disorder in children: A review of the past 10 years. *Journal of the American Academy of Child and Adolescent Psychiatry, 36*(11), 1503–1511.

Triage: Community Disaster   6362

Definition: Establishing priorities of care for urgent treatment at event site while allocating scarce resources

Activities:

- Acquire current information about nature of event (e.g., number of victims, severity of injuries, area involved)
- Communicate with central authority (i.e., Command Center)
- Ensure proper personnel alerted (e.g., nursing leadership, ER leadership, administration leadership)
- Consider resources available
- Contact supplementary health care workers (e.g., surgeons, dentists, veterinarians, hospice nurses, retired clinicians, volunteers), as indicated
- Set up reception and triage staging areas with decontamination resources near event location, as indicated
- Notify acute care facilities in area to expect transfers
- Use hallways, parking areas, lobbies, lawns, or rooftops for health care, as needed
- Increase security staff to keep order and protect physical facilities
- Determine risk from contact with victims (e.g., poisonous gas, radiation, biohazard)
- Obtain PPE and ensure all co-workers are protected, if indicated
- Alert all personnel of possibility of victims accessing health care system without prior health care contact (e.g., walking wounded)
- Ensure proper triage and contamination measures used with walking wounded
- Initiate steps to obtain additional resources (e.g., PPE, health care equipment)
- Obtain additional personnel for care of victims once triage completed
- Assign personnel to assist at event site if indicated
- Participate in prioritization of persons for treatment
- Evaluate critical persons from the field first
- Identify person's chief complaint
- Obtain information about medical history
- Check for medical alert tags, as appropriate
- Conduct primary survey of all body systems, as appropriate

- Monitor for and treat life-threatening injuries or acute needs
- Use color-coded signage to assist with communication, assuring rapid categorization of all persons
- Use triage tag priority system as indicated by person status (e.g., red for immediate care, yellow for delay, green for minor, black for unlikely to survive)
- Consider relocating persons with minor injuries
- Consider palliative care measures for persons unlikely to survive (e.g., notify clergy)
- Establish morgue
- Evacuate or transport injured requiring higher-level care
- Initiate appropriate emergency measures for each person after triage completed for all, as indicated
- Perform secondary body system survey after triage completed for all, as appropriate
- Ensure that all personnel are allowed to debrief with peers or counsellors after event
- Evaluate response to event including input from key personnel involved (e.g., after-action report)
- Conduct annual disaster drills for emergency room staff
- Conduct regular community disaster drills for training assistive personnel

3rd edition 2000; revised 2024

Background Evidence:

Emergency Nurses Association. (2019). *Trauma nursing core course* (8th ed.).

Ghanbari, V., Ardalan, A., Zareiyan, A., Nejati, A., Hanfling, D., Bagheri, A., & Rostamnia, L. (2021). Perceptions on principle of priority setting in disaster triage: A Q-method study. *International Emergency Nursing, 59*, N.PAG. https://doi.org/10.1016/j.ienj.2021.101064

Ram-Titkin, E. (2017). Ethical considerations of triage following natural disasters: The IDF experience in Haiti as a case study. *Bioethics, 31*(6), 467–475.

T

Sharma, S. K., & Sharma, N. (2020). Hospital preparedness and resilience in public health emergencies at district hospitals and community health centers. *Journal of Health Management, 22*(2), 146–156. https://doi.org/10.1177/0972063420935539

Sheek-Hussein, M., Abu-Zidan, F. M., & Stip, E. (2021). Disaster management of the psychological impact of the COVID-19 pandemic. *International Journal of Emergency Medicine, 14*(1), 1–10. https://doi.org/10.1186/s12245-021-00342-z

Sweet, V., & Foley, A. (2020). *Sheehy's emergency nursing: Principles and practice.* Elsevier.

Sweet, V. (2018). *Emergency nursing core curriculum.* Elsevier.

Whiteside, T., Kane, E., Aljohani, B., Alsamman, M., & Pourmand, A. (2020). Redesigning emergency department operations amidst a viral pandemic. *American Journal of Emergency Medicine, 38*(7), 1448–1453.

Triage: Emergency Center   6364

Definition: Establishing priorities and initiating treatment for persons in an emergency center

Activities:

- Ensure use of personal protective equipment (PPE), if indicated
- Use pre-triage evaluation during infectious disease outbreaks
- Isolate pre-triage persons if indicated
- Perform brief, rapid, and accurate evaluation on all incoming persons, using institutional guidelines and standards of care
- Examine signs and symptoms simultaneously during rapid initial evaluation
- Use focused questions about symptoms, history of travel, and contacts at pre-triage stations
- Determine temperature using non-contact technology
- Obtain additional data on persons to determine acuity level (e.g., vital signs, pain level rating, physical examination, pertinent medical history, current medications)
- Assign emergency acuity rating using systematic standards (e.g., five-level acuity rating system, ABCD ratings)
- Move person to area determined by acuity rating and infection status
- Ensure care provided as indicated by acuity rating and infection status
- Provide information to receiving health care provider
- Evaluate and transfer women in labor
- Explain triage process to those presenting for service
- Ensure legal requirements are met (e.g., Emergency Medical Treatment and Active Labor Act [EMTALA])
- Provide medical screening examination (MSE) for all persons by independent licensed practitioner (i.e., triage not considered MSE)
- Perform crisis intervention, as appropriate
- Diffuse escalating violence, as appropriate
- Refer nonurgent persons to clinics, other primary care providers, or health department
- Monitor persons waiting to be seen
- Serve as liaison between health care team and persons in waiting area
- Answer questions and reassure persons and families
- Ensure psychological support to person and providers
- Control flow of persons including visitors

Background Evidence:

Awad, M. E., Rumley, J. C. L., Vazquez, J. A., & Devine, J. G. (2020). Perioperative considerations in urgent surgical care of suspected and confirmed covid-19 orthopaedic patients: Operating room protocols and recommendations in the current covid-19 pandemic. *Journal of the American Academy of Orthopaedic Surgeons, 28*(11), 451–463. https://doi.org/10.5435/JAAOS-D-20-00227

Benabbas, R., Shah, R., Zonnoor, B., Mehta, N., & Sinert, R. (2020). Impact of triage liaison provider on emergency department throughput: A systematic review and meta-analysis. *American Journal of Emergency Medicine, 38*(8), 1662–1670.

Briggs, J., & Grossman, V. (2019). *Emergency nursing 5-tier triage protocols.* Springer Publishing, Inc.

Burgess, L., Kynoch, K., & Hines, S. (2019). Implementing best practice into the emergency department triage process. *International Journal of Evidence-Based Healthcare, 17*(1), 27–35. https://doi.org/10.1097/XEB.0000000000000144

Mathew, R., Sinha, T. P., Sahu, A. K., Bhoi, S., & Galwankar, S. (2020). Coronavirus-19 pandemic: A two-step triage protocol for emergency department. *Journal of Emergency Trauma & Shock, 13*, 169–171.

Mendonça, A., de Carvalho Queluci, G., Rodrigues de Souza, V., Couto Dias, S., & da Silveira Jasmim, J. (2018). Nursing skills in emergency services: A systematic review. *Journal of Nursing, 12*(10), 2816–2824.

Moura, B. R. S., Oliveira, G. N., Medeiros, G., Vieira, A., de, S., Nogueira, L., & de, S. (2022). Rapid triage performed by nurses: Signs and symptoms associated with identifying critically ill patients in the emergency department. *International Journal of Nursing Practice, 28*(1), 1–10. https://doi.org/10.1111/ijn.13001

Sweet, V., & Foley, A. (2020). *Sheehy's emergency nursing: Principles and practice.* Elsevier.

Whiteside, T., Kane, E., Aljohani, B., Alsamman, M., & Pourmand, A. (2020). Redesigning emergency department operations amidst a viral pandemic. *American Journal of Emergency Medicine, 38*(7), 1448–1453.

3rd edition 2000; revised 2024

T

Triage: Telecommunication   6366

Definition: Using telecommunications to identify the nature and urgency of health issues problems

Activities:

- Identify self with name and credentials, organization
- Inform that call maybe recorded (e.g., for quality monitoring)
- Display willingness to help (e.g., "How may I help?")

- Obtain information about purpose of call (e.g., nature of crisis, symptoms, medical diagnosis, health history, current treatment regimen)
- Identify concerns about health status

- Speak directly to person whenever possible
- Listen for nonverbal symptoms (e.g., shortness of breath, wheezing, long pauses, slurring of speech)
- Use interpreter, as needed
- Evaluate cultural and socioeconomic barriers to person's response (e.g., language barriers, lack of health care insurance, lack of understanding of health care terms)
- Access person's electronic record for additional health history, as available
- Direct, facilitate, and calm caller by giving simple instructions for action, as needed
- Use standardized symptom-based guidelines or evidence-based nursing protocols to identify and evaluate significant data and classify urgency of symptoms
- Prioritize reported symptoms, determining highest possible risk using guidelines
- Obtain data related to effectiveness of current treatments, if any
- Determine whether concerns require further evaluation, applying standard guidelines
- Provide first-aid instructions or emergency directions for crises (e.g., CPR instructions, birthing instructions), using standard guidelines
- Stay connected while contacting emergency services, according to organization's protocol
- Provide clear directions for transport to hospital, as needed
- Advise on options for referral and intervention
- Provide information about treatment regimen and resultant self-care responsibilities, as necessary, according to scope of practice and established guidelines
- Confirm understanding of advice or directions through verbalization (i.e., ask to repeat what was discussed)
- Ask if anything would keep them from following advice or directions that were given
- Determine need and establish time intervals for further intermittent assessment
- Document any assessments, advice, instructions, or other information given to person, according to specified guidelines
- Determine how person or family member can be reached for return telephone calls, as appropriate

- Document permission for return call and identify persons able to receive call information
- Follow up to determine disposition and document disposition and person's intended action, as necessary
- Maintain confidentiality, as per state and legal guidelines (i.e., age of majority varies by state)
- Follow legal guidelines (i.e., traveling persons may be outside nurse's state of licensure)
- Discuss and resolve problem calls with supervisory or collegial help
- Use teach-back to ensure understanding

3rd edition 2000; revised 2024

Background Evidence:

American Academy of Ambulatory Care Nursing. (2018). Scope and standards of practice for professional telehealth nursing (6th ed.). Anthony J. Jannetti.

Erkelens, D. C., Rutten, F. H., Wouters, L. T., Dolmans, L. S., de Groot, E., Damoiseaux, R. A., & Zwart, D. L. (2020). Accuracy of telephone triage in patients suspected of transient ischemic attack or stroke: A cross-sectional study. *BMC Family Practice, 21*(1), 1–10. https://doi.org/10.1186/s12875-020-01334-3

Montandon, D., Souza-Junior, V., Almeida, R., Marchi-Alves, L., Mendes, I., & Godoy, S. (2019). How to perform prehospital emergency telephone triage: A systematic review. *Journal of Trauma Nursing, 26*(2), 104–110.

Owens, S. J. (2017). Telephone triage in ophthalmology settings. *Insight: The Journal of the American Society of Ophthalmic Registered Nurses, 42*(3), 26–29.

Pirschel, C. (2018). How oncology nurses provide quality care through telephone triage. *Oncology Nursing Society VOICE, 33*(11), 24–28.

Wouters, L. T., Zwart, D. L., Erkelens, D. C., Huijsmans, M., Hoes, A. W., Damoiseaux, R. A., Rutten, F. H., & Groot, E. (2020). Tinkering and overruling the computer decision support system: Working strategies of telephone triage nurses who assess the urgency of callers suspected of having an acute cardiac event. *Journal of Clinical Nursing, 29*(7/8), 1175–1186. https://doi.org/10.1111/jocn.15168

Truth Telling 5470

Definition: Use of whole truth, partial truth, or decision delay to promote the patient's self-determination and well-being

Activities:

- Clarify own values about the particular situation
- Clarify the values of the patient, family, health care team, and institution about the particular situation
- Clarify own knowledge base and communication skills about the situation
- Determine patient's desire and preference for truth in the situation
- Consult with the patient's family before telling the truth, as culturally appropriate
- Point out discrepancies between the patient's expressed beliefs and behaviors, as appropriate
- Collaborate with other health care providers about the choice of options (i.e., whole truth, partial truth, or decision delay) and their needed participation in the options
- Determine risks to patient and self, associated with each option
- Choose one of the options, based on the ethics of the situation and leaning more favorably toward the use of truth or partial truth

- Establish a trusting relationship
- Deliver the truth with sensitivity, warmth, and directness
- Make the time to deal with the consequences of the truth
- Refer to another if that person has better rapport, better knowledge and skills to deliver the truth, or more time and ability to deal with the consequences of telling the truth
- Prepare patients for truth telling by encouraging them to invite family or significant other(s) to be present
- Remain with the patient to whom you have told the truth and be prepared to clarify, support, and receive feedback
- Be physically present to communicate caring and support, if decision to withhold information has been made
- Choose decision delay when there is missing information, lack of knowledge, and lack of rapport
- Attend to verbal and nonverbal cues during the communication process
- Monitor the patient's and family's responses to the interaction, including alterations in pain, restlessness, anxiety, mood

change, involvement in care, ability to synthesize new information, ability to verbalize feelings, and reported satisfaction with care, as appropriate
- Document the patient's responses at various stages of the intervention

1st edition 1992; revised 2008

Background Evidence:
Collis, S. P. (2006). The importance of truth-telling in health care. *Nursing Standard, 20*(17), 41–45.

Glass, E., & Cluxton, D. (2004). Truth-telling: Ethical issues in clinical practice. *Journal of Hospice and Palliative Nursing, 6*(4), 232–242.

Hertogh, C. M., The, B. A., Miesen, B. M., & Eefsting, J. A. (2004). Truth telling and truthfulness in the care for patients with advanced dementia: An ethnographic study in Dutch nursing homes. *Social Science & Medicine, 59*(8), 1685–1693.

Jotkowitz, A. B., Clarifield, A. M., & Glick, S. (2005). The care of patients with dementia: A modern Jewish ethical perspective. *Journal of the American Geriatrics Society, 53*(5), 881–884.

Tuckett, A. G. (2004). Truth-telling in clinical practice and the arguments for and against: A review of the literature. *Nursing Ethics, 11*(5), 500–513.

Williamson, C. B., & Livingston, D. J. (1992). Truth telling. In G. M. Bulechek & J. C. McCloskey (Eds.), *Nursing interventions: Essential nursing treatments* (2nd ed., pp. 151–167). W.B. Saunders.

Wros, P. L., Doutrich, D., & Izumi, S. (2004). Ethical concerns: Comparison of values from two cultures. *Nursing & Health Sciences, 6*(2), 131–140.

Tube Care   1870

Definition: Management of a patient with an external drainage device exiting the body

Activities:
- Determine indication for the indwelling tube or catheter
- Use automatic stop orders and reminders to request an order to remove the device when the indication is resolved
- Maintain proper hand hygiene before, during, and after tube insertion or manipulation
- Maintain patency of tube, as indicated by tube type and manufacturer directions
- Keep the drainage container at the proper level
- Provide sufficiently long tubing to allow freedom of movement, as appropriate
- Secure tubing to prevent pressure and accidental removal
- Monitor patency of catheter and tube drainage device or system, noting any difficulty in drainage
- Monitor amount, color, and consistency of drainage from tube
- Empty the collection appliance, according to organizational policy, patient condition, and manufacturer instructions
- Ensure proper placement of the tube
- Assure functioning of tube and associated equipment
- Connect tube to suction or proper drainage device, as appropriate
- Check tube patency, as appropriate
- Irrigate tube to ensure patency, according to organizational policy, patient condition, and manufacturer instructions
- Change tube routinely, as indicated by agency protocol
- Inspect the area around the tube insertion site for redness and skin breakdown, as appropriate
- Administer skin care and dressing changes at the tube insertion site, as appropriate
- Assist the patient in securing tube(s) and drainage devices while walking, sitting, and standing, as appropriate
- Encourage periods of increased activity, as appropriate
- Clamp tubing to facilitate ambulation, if appropriate
- Monitor patient's and family members' responses to presence of external drainage devices
- Instruct patient and family about the purpose of the tube and how to care for it
- Provide emotional support to deal with long-term use of tubes and external drainage devices, as appropriate

1st edition 1992; revised 2013

Background Evidence:
Best, C., & Hitchings, H. (2010). Enteral tube feeding—from hospital to home. *British Journal of Nursing, 19*(3), 174–179.

Briggs, D. (2010). Nursing care and management of patients with intrapleural drains. *Nursing Standard, 24*(21), 47–56.

Foxley, S. (2011). Indwelling urinary catheters: accurate monitoring of urine output. *British Journal of Nursing, 20*(9), 564–569.

Herter, R., & Kazer, M. (2010). Best practices in urinary catheter care. *Home Healthcare Nurse, 28*(6), 342–349.

Mongardon, N., Tremey, B., & Marty, J. (2010). Thoracentesis and chest tube management in critical care medicine: a multicenter survey of current practice. *Chest, 138*(6), 1524–1525.

Nazarko, L. (2010). Effective evidence-based catheter management: an update. *British Journal of Nursing, 19*(15), 948–953.

Omorogieva, O. (2010). Managing patients on enteral feeding tubes in the community. *British Journal of Community Nursing, 15*(Suppl. 11), S6–S13.

Tube Care: Chest   1872

Definition: Management of a patient with an external device exiting the chest cavity

Activities:
- Determine indication for the indwelling chest tube (e.g., pneumothorax versus drainage of fluids)
- Maintain proper hand hygiene before, during, and after chest tube insertion or manipulation
- Monitor for audible air leaks after insertion, indicating improper insertion of tube requiring additional sutures or repositioning
- Assure familiarity with chest valve device (e.g., water-seal drainage, drainage valve, or flutter valve) and drainage equipment
- Follow manufacturer recommendations for care of chest valve device and drainage equipment
- Monitor for proper functioning of device, correct placement in the pleural space, and tube patency (i.e., respiratory swing or fluid oscillating as patient breathes, either in tube or at the fluid meniscus)

T

- Note presence of continuous bubbling during inspiration and expiration, indicating either potential worsening of patient condition or a breach in the closed drainage system
- Monitor for signs and symptoms of pneumothorax
- Monitor for symptoms of resolving pneumothorax (e.g., decrease in bubbling, respiratory swinging, or tidaling in underwater drainage seal device and tubing)
- Assess patient experiencing sudden changes in swinging, tidaling, or bubbling for emergent conditions
- Ensure that all tubing connections are securely attached and taped
- Assure use of one-way drainage device, usually an underwater seal drainage bottle
- Adhere to the recommended water seal level indicated on the underwater seal drainage bottle (i.e., too little water leads to pneumothorax, too much water results in ineffective drainage, or ineffective resolution of pneumothorax)
- Keep the external water seal drainage container below chest level
- Clamp chest tubes whenever external water seal drainage container is positioned above chest level for extended periods, assuring clamps are in place for as brief a time as possible
- Use only nontraumatic chest tube clamps
- Assure nontraumatic chest tube clamps are available for any accidental disconnection or damage to the drainage system or to the tubes (e.g., tape spare set of nontraumatic clamps to head of bed or to wall behind headboard)
- Provide sufficiently long tubing to allow freedom of movement, as appropriate
- Anchor the tubing securely
- Assure use of multi-chamber underwater seal drain devices that provide separate chambers for drainage, water seal, and suction, when indicated by patient condition
- Monitor x-ray reports for tube position
- Document chest tube tidaling, output, and air leaks
- Document bubbling of the suction chamber of the chest tube drainage system and tidaling in water-seal chamber
- Perform stripping and milking of tube only when indicated by patient condition (e.g., patient symptomatic and tube occluded), or as ordered by the physician

- Monitor for crepitus around chest tube site
- Observe for signs of intrapleural fluid accumulation
- Observe volume, shade, color, and consistency of drainage from lung, and record appropriately
- Observe for signs of infection
- Send questionable tube drainage for culture and sensitivity (e.g., cloudy or purulent drainage or patient with high temperature)
- Assist patient to cough, deep breathe, and turn every 2 hours
- Document patient response to cough, deep breath, and turn, including swinging, tidaling, and bubbling in chest tube and drainage system
- Clean around the tube insertion site, per agency protocol
- Change dressing around chest tube every 48 to 72 hours and as needed, per agency protocol
- Use petroleum jelly gauze for dressing change
- Ensure that chest tube drainage device is maintained in an upright position
- Change chest tube drainage bottles or multichamber drain devices to avoid overfilling or for infection control purposes, as needed
- Avoid occluding the drainage bottle or device when still attached to the patient, when changing the bottles or devices
- Instruct patient and family about proper chest tube care

1st edition 1992; revised 2013

Background Evidence:

Briggs, D. (2010). Nursing care and management of patients with intrapleural drains. *Nursing Standard, 24*(21), 47–56.

Halm, M. A. (2007). To strip or not to strip? Physiological effects of chest tube manipulation. *American Journal of Critical Care, 16*(6), 609–612.

Mongardon, N., Tremey, B., & Marty, J. (2010). Thoracentesis and chest tube management in critical care medicine: a multicenter survey of current practice. *Chest, 138*(6), 1524–1525.

Taubert, J., Bungay, S., Banaglorioso, C., Adams, A., Mathew, J., & Magana, E. (2008). An evidence-based approach in education of nurses and their role in care of the oncology patient with a chest tube. *Oncology Nursing Forum, 35*(3), 531–532.

Tube Care: Gastrointestinal   1874

Definition: Care of a person with a tube inserted in the gastrointestinal tract

Activities:

- Monitor for proper placement of tube by inspecting oral cavity, checking for residual (i.e., observe amount, color, and appearance of aspirate), and monitoring external length of tube, according to agency protocol
- Confirm tube placement before using or if concern regarding tube location, per agency protocol (e.g., x-ray examination, pH testing)
- Monitor reports of routine chest and abdominal radiographic films for reference to tube location
- Connect tube to suction, if indicated
- Secure tube to appropriate body part, with consideration for person comfort and skin integrity
- Mark tubing at point of exit to maintain proper placement and check regularly for movement, once placement confirmed by x-ray
- Irrigate tube, per agency protocol
- Avoid IV syringes when administering feedings or solutions into tubes to decrease chance of inadvertently accessing IV lines

- Perform appropriate abdominal assessments prior to initiating any feedings, irrigations, or medication administrations via tube
- Monitor for sensations of fullness, nausea, and vomiting
- Monitor bowel sounds
- Monitor for any signs of respiratory distress
- Monitor for diarrhea, nausea, cramping, or bloating
- Encourage chewing gum to avoid ileus, as appropriate
- Monitor fluid and electrolyte status
- Monitor amount, color, and consistency of nasogastric output
- Replace amount of gastrointestinal output with the appropriate IV solution, as ordered
- Provide nose and mouth care three to four times daily or as needed
- Provide hard candy or chewing gum to moisten mouth, as appropriate
- Initiate and monitor delivery of enteral tube feedings, per agency protocol
- Determine level of understanding related to tube purpose and care

- Instruct related to tube purpose and rationale for use
- Instruct person and family how to care for tube, when indicated
- Provide skin care around tube insertion site
- Remove tube, when indicated
- Document tube placement including tolerance of procedure, x-ray confirmation, depth of insertion

1st edition 1992; revised 2000, 2024

Background Evidence:

Berman, A., Snyder, S. J., & Frandsen, G. (2018). Nutrition. In *Kozier and Erb's fundamentals of nursing: Concepts, process and practice* (10th ed., pp. 1127–1167). Pearson.

Miller, T. (2021). Nutrition. In A. Perry, P. Potter, P. Stockert, & A. Hall (Eds.), *Fundamentals of nursing* (10th ed., pp. 1120–1147). Elsevier.

Potter, P. A., Ostendorf, W. R., & LaPlante, N. (2018). Enteral nutrition. In *Clinical nursing skills and techniques* (9th ed., pp. 830–860). Mosby.

Rebar, C. R. (2021). Concepts of care for patients with malnutrition: Undernutrition and obesity. In D. Ignativicius, M. L. Workman, C. R. Rebar, & N. M. Heimgartner (Eds.), *Medical-Surgical nursing: Concepts for interprofessional collaborative care* (10th ed., pp. 1205–1208). Elsevier.

Roveron, G., Antonini, M., Barbierato, M., Calandrino, V., Canese, G., Chiurazzi, L. F., Coniglio, G., Gentini, G., Marchetti, M., Minucci, A., Nembrini, L., Neri, V., Trovato, P., & Ferrara, F. (2018). Clinical Practice Guidelines for the nursing management of percutaneous endoscopic gastrostomy and jejunostomy (PEG/PEJ) in adult patients. *Journal of Wound, Ostomy & Continence Nursing, 45*(4), 326–334.

St. Onge, J. L. (2021). Nutrition. In R. F. Craven, C. J. Hirnle, & C. J. Henshaw (Eds.), *Fundamentals of nursing: Human health and function* (8th ed., pp. 410–471). Wolters-Kluwer.

Williams, P. (2020). Maintaining fluid balance and meeting nutritional needs. In *Basic geriatric nursing* (7th ed., pp. 104–130). Elsevier.

Tube Care: Umbilical Line   1875

Definition: Management of a newborn with an umbilical catheter

Activities:

- Assist with or insert umbilical catheter in neonates, as ordered or per protocol (e.g., birthweight greater than 1500 g, shock)
- Check position of catheter with x-ray examination
- Monitor and record depth of insertion
- Infuse medication and nutrients via umbilical venous line, as ordered or per protocol
- Avoid administration of any medications into arterial catheter
- Obtain venous or arterial pressures, as appropriate
- Obtain blood samples as appropriate, taking care to aspirate and flush slowly (1 mL/30 seconds) to prevent excessive fluctuations in arterial pressure
- Flush catheter with heparinized solution, as appropriate
- Change IV tubing and transducer no more than every 72 hours or per institution recommendations
- Change tubing for blood or lipids every 24 hours
- Use a central line maintenance bundle to prevent infections
- Cleanse connections with alcohol, as needed
- Stabilize catheter to abdomen using occlusive dressing or other securement device
- Provide calming support (e.g., pacifier, music, distraction, massage) to patient during procedure, as needed
- Avoid use of physical restraints whenever possible
- Position infant on back
- Document appearance of umbilical site and nurse actions
- Observe for signs requiring catheter removal (e.g., pulseless leg, darkening of toes, blanching of toes or leg, hypertension, redness around umbilicus, visible clots in catheter)
- Remove catheter, as appropriate per order or protocol, by withdrawing catheter slowly over 5 minutes
- Apply pressure to umbilicus for at least 5 minutes
- Leave umbilicus uncovered
- Observe for hemorrhage

2nd edition 1996; revised 2018

Background Evidence:

American Academy of Pediatrics & American College of Obstetricians and Gynecologists. (2012). *Guidelines for perinatal care* (7th ed.).

Karlsen, K. (2013). *The S.T.A.B.L.E. program instructor manual: Post-resuscitation/pre-transport stabilization care of sick infants—guidelines for neonatal healthcare providers* (6th ed.). Park City, UT: The S.T.A.B.L.E. Program.

The Joint Commission. (2012). *Preventing central line–associated bloodstream infections: A global challenge, a global perspective.* Joint Commission Resources.

Verklan, M. T., & Walden, M. (Eds.). (2010). *Core curriculum for neonatal intensive care nursing* (4th ed.). Saunders Elsevier.

T

Tube Care: Urinary   1876

Definition: Management of a patient with urinary drainage equipment

Activities:

- Determine indication for the indwelling urinary catheter
- Use automatic stop orders and reminders to request an order to remove the device when the indication is resolved
- Maintain proper hand hygiene before, during, and after catheter insertion or manipulation
- Maintain a closed, sterile, and unobstructed urinary drainage system
- Assure placement of drainage bag below level of bladder
- Avoid tilting urine bags or meters to empty or measure urine output (i.e., preventative measure for ascending contamination)
- Use urine bags or meters with emptying devices located at the bottom of the device
- Maintain patency of urinary catheter system

- Irrigate urinary catheter system using sterile technique, as appropriate
- Perform routine meatal care with soap and water during daily bathing
- Clean the urinary catheter externally at the meatus
- Cleanse surrounding skin area at regular intervals
- Change the urinary catheter at regular intervals, as indicated and per agency protocol
- Change the urinary drainage apparatus at regular intervals, as indicated and per agency protocol
- Note urinary drainage characteristics
- Clamp suprapubic or retention catheter, as ordered
- Position patient and urinary drainage system to promote urinary drainage (i.e., assure drainage bag is below level of bladder)
- Use a catheter securement device
- Empty urinary drainage apparatus at regular and specified intervals
- Empty the drainage bag before all patient transports
- Avoid placing the drainage bag between the patient's legs during transport
- Disconnect leg bag at night and connect to bedside drainage bag
- Check leg bag straps for constriction at regular intervals
- Maintain meticulous skin care for patients with a leg bag
- Cleanse urinary drainage equipment, per agency protocol
- Obtain urine specimen through closed urinary drainage system's port

- Monitor for bladder distention
- Assure catheter removal as soon as indicated by patient condition
- Explore elimination options to prevent reinsertion (e.g., bladder scanner, bedside commode, urinal, moisture-wicking underpads, nursing rounds)
- Instruct patient and family about proper catheter care

1st edition 1992; revised 2000, 2013

Background Evidence:

Foxley, S. (2011). Indwelling urinary catheters: accurate monitoring of urine output. *British Journal of Nursing, 20*(9), 564–569.

Herter, R., & Kazer, M. (2010). Best practices in urinary catheter care. *Home Healthcare Nurse, 28*(6), 342–349.

Hung, A., Giesbrecht, N., Pelingon, P., & Bissonnette, R. (2010). Sterile water versus antiseptic agents as a cleansing agent during periurethral catheterizations. *NENA Outlook, 33*(2), 18–21.

Makic, M. B., VonRueden, K. T., Rauen, C. A., & Chadwick, J. (2011). Evidence-based practice habits: Putting more sacred cows out to pasture. *Critical Care Nurse, 31*(2), 38–62.

Nazarko, L. (2010). Effective evidence-based catheter management: an update. *British Journal of Nursing, 19*(15), 948–953.

Newman, D. K., & Willson, M. M. (2011). Review of intermittent catheterization and current best practices. *Urologic Nursing, 31*(1), 28–48.

Tube Care: Ventriculostomy/Lumbar Drain   1878

Definition: Management of a patient with an external cerebrospinal fluid drainage system

Activities:

- Monitor drainage trends
- Monitor amount and rate of cerebrospinal fluid drainage
- Monitor CSF drainage characteristics: color, clarity, and consistency
- Record CSF drainage
- Change or empty drainage bag, as needed
- Administer antibiotics, as appropriate
- Monitor insertion site for infection
- Reinforce an insertion site dressing, as needed
- Restrain patient, as needed
- Explain and reinforce mobility restrictions to patient
- Monitor for CSF rhinorrhea and otorrhea
- Relevel the drainage apparatus, as needed

1st edition 1992; revised 2013

Background Evidence:

Arabi, Y., Memish, Z. A., Balkhy, H. H., Francis, C., Ferayanm, A., Shimemeri, A. A., & Almuneef, M. A. (2005). Ventriculostomy-associated infections: Incidence and risk factors. *American Journal of Infection Control, 33*(3), 137–143.

Arbour, R. (2004). Intracranial hypertension: Monitoring and nursing assessment. *Critical Care Nurse, 24*(5), 19–34.

Chi, H., Chang, K., Chang, H., Chiu, N., & Huang, F. (2010). Infections associated with indwelling ventriculostomy catheters in a teaching hospital. *International Journal of Infectious Diseases, 14*(3), e216–e219.

Overstreet, M. (2003). How do I manage a lumbar drain? *Nursing 2003, 33*(3), 74–75.

Robinet, K. (1985). Increased intracranial pressure: Management with an intraventricular catheter. *Journal of Neurosurgical Nursing, 17*(2), 95–104.

T

Ultrasonography: Bladder   0565

Definition: Performance of ultrasound exams to determine bladder function or structure

Activities:

- Determine indication for bladder ultrasound imaging (e.g., urinary retention, assessment of post-void residual volume, diagnostic examination)
- Instruct about examination indications, procedure, purpose, and limitations
- Apply appropriate protocol for bladder ultrasound evaluation (e.g., review of postoperative or postpartum assessment for urinary retention, evaluation of decrease in urinary output with or without bladder catheter, post-void residual volume measurement)
- Select adequate transducer for bladder examination
- Identify previous abdominal surgeries, scars, tumors, ascites, visceral distension, or other anatomical features with potential to confound bladder evaluation
- Apply ultrasound gel in suprapubic region or directly on transducer
- Position transducer properly just above pubic symphysis
- Obtain clear picture of bladder and centralize in monitor
- Perform bladder volume measurements, as appropriate
- Use colored Doppler function, as appropriate
- Identify position of distal tip of urinary catheter, catheter function, and balloon volume in ultrasound image, as appropriate
- Identify and measure residual post-void volume with ultrasound 10 to 20 minutes after emptying bladder
- Perform systematic ultrasound bladder assessment, if necessary
- Discuss bladder evaluation with primary practitioner, consultants and person, as appropriate
- Assist with removing gel, if appropriate
- Clean ultrasound device
- Document findings, including reason for bladder ultrasound, urinary volume measured, response to procedure and any unusual findings

8th edition 2024

Background Evidence:

Agency for Healthcare Research and Quality. (2020, October). Appendix C. Sample bladder scan policy. In *Toolkit for Reducing Catheter-Associated Urinary Tract Infections in Hospital Units: Implementation Guide*. https://www.ahrq.gov/hai/cauti-tools/impl-guide/implementation-guide-appendix-c.html

Berman, A., Snyder, S. J., & Frandsen, G. (2018). Urinary elimination. In *Kozier and Erb's fundamentals of nursing: Concepts, process and practice* (10th ed., pp. 1191–1199). Pearson

Ceratti, R. D. N., & Beghetto, M. G. (2021). Incidence of urinary retention and relations between patient's complaint, physical examination, and bladder ultrasound. *Revista Gaúcha de Enfermagem, 42*. https://doi.org/10.1590/1983-1447.2021.20200014

Chen, S. C., Chen, P. Y., Chen, G. C., Chuang, S. Y., Tzeng, I. S., & Lin, S. K. (2018). Portable bladder ultrasound reduces incidence of urinary tract infection and shortens hospital length of stay in patients with acute ischemic stroke. *The Journal of Cardiovascular Nursing, 33*(6), 551.

Potter, P. A., Ostendorf, W. R., & LaPlante, N. (2018). Urinary elimination. In *Clinical nursing skills and techniques* (9th ed., pp. 876–892). Mosby.

Schallom, M., Prentice, D., Sona, C., Vyers, K., Arroyo, C., Wessman, B., & Ablordeppey, E. (2020). Accuracy of measuring bladder volumes with ultrasound and bladder scanning. *American Journal of Critical Care, 29*(6), 458–467.

Sweeney, M., & Cerepani, M. J. (2021). Bladder scan misleading a vascular emergency as urinary retention. *Advanced Emergency Nursing Journal, 43*(1), 35–38.

Ultrasonography: Obstetric and Gynecologic   6982

Definition: Performance of ultrasound exams to determine ovarian, endometrial, uterine, or fetal status

Activities:

- Determine clinical indication for ultrasound imaging (e.g., obstetrical or gynecological)
- Set up equipment required for noninvasive or invasive procedure (e.g., transducer, vaginal transducer)
- Instruct patient and family about examination indications and procedure, its purpose and limitations
- Prepare patient physically and emotionally for procedure
- Apply appropriate protocol for ultrasound evaluation (e.g., evaluation of pregnancy, evaluation of postmenopausal bleeding, evaluation of specialized obstetrical procedures)
- Warm the transducer gel for patient comfort
- Instruct patient to empty bladder before transvaginal ultrasound
- Place transducer on abdomen or in vagina, as appropriate
- Allow patient to insert transvaginal probe, if desired by patient
- Obtain clear picture of anatomical structures on the monitor
- Identify uterine position, size, and endometrial thickness, as appropriate
- Identify ovarian location and size, as appropriate
- Monitor follicular growth throughout ovulation, as appropriate
- Monitor gestational sac growth and location
- Monitor fetal parameters, including number, size, cardiac activity, presentation, and position
- Identify placental location
- Observe for placental abnormalities, as appropriate
- Measure amniotic fluid indexes
- Monitor fetal breathing movements, gross movements, and tone
- Identify fetal structures to parents, as appropriate
- Provide picture of fetus, as appropriate
- Obtain multiple measurements of endometrial thickness from various angles for women presenting with postmenopausal bleeding
- Consider saline infusion sonohysterography as an additional method of evaluating a poorly defined endometrial echo for postmenopausal bleeding
- Discuss tests results with primary practitioner, consultants, and patient, as appropriate
- Schedule additional tests or procedures, as necessary

- Assist patient with removing gel and putting on clothes, as indicated
- Clean equipment
- Document findings per institutional policy, including that the patient was informed and acknowledged the findings
- Provide all documentation to the patient's primary health care provider

2nd edition 1996; revised 2018

Background Evidence:

Association of Women's Health, Obstetric and Neonatal Nurses (AWHONN). (2010). *Ultrasound examinations performed by nurses in obstetric,* *gynecologic, and reproductive medicine settings: Clinical competencies and educational guide* (3rd ed.).

Carr, S. (2011). Ultrasound for nurses in reproductive medicine. *Journal of Obstetric, Gynecologic & Neonatal Nursing, 40*(5), 638–653.

Grube, W., Ammon, T., & Killen, M. D. (2011). The role of ultrasound imaging in detecting endometrial cancer in postmenopausal women with vaginal bleeding. *Journal of Obstetric, Gynecologic & Neonatal Nursing, 40*(5), 632–637.

International Society of Ultrasound in Obstetrics and Gynecology (ISUOG). (2014). ISUOG Education Committee recommendations for basic training in obstetric and gynecological ultrasound. *Ultrasound in Obstetrics & Gynecology, 43*(1), 113–116.

Unilateral Neglect Management 2760

Definition: Protecting and safely reintegrating the affected part of the body while helping the patient adapt to disturbed perceptual abilities

Activities:

- Evaluate baseline mental status, comprehension, motor function, sensory function, attention span, and affective responses
- Monitor for abnormal responses to three primary types of stimuli: sensory, visual, and auditory
- Provide realistic feedback about patient's perceptual deficit
- Perform personal care in a consistent manner with thorough explanation
- Ensure that affected extremities are properly and safely positioned
- Adapt the environment to the deficit by focusing on the unaffected side during the acute period
- Supervise and assist in transferring and ambulating
- Touch unaffected shoulder when initiating conversation, as appropriate
- Place food and beverages within field of vision and turn plate, as necessary
- Rearrange the environment to use the right or left visual field, such as positioning personal items, television, or reading materials within view on unaffected side
- Give frequent reminders to redirect the patient's attention, cueing the patient to the environment
- Avoid rapid movement in the room
- Avoid moving objects in the environment
- Position bed in room, so that individuals approach and care for patient on unaffected side
- Keep side rail up on affected side, as appropriate
- Instruct patient to scan from left to right
- Provide range of motion and massage to affected side
- Encourage patient to touch and use affected body part
- Consult with occupational and physical therapists concerning timing and strategies to facilitate reintegration of neglected body parts and function
- Gradually focus patient's attention to the affected side, as patient demonstrates an ability to compensate for neglect
- Gradually move personal items and activity to affected side, as patient demonstrates an ability to compensate for neglect
- Stand on affected side when ambulating with patient, as patient demonstrates an ability to compensate for neglect
- Assist patient with activities of daily living from affected side, as patient demonstrates an ability to compensate for neglect
- Assist patient to bathe and groom affected side first, as patient demonstrates an ability to compensate for neglect
- Focus tactile and verbal stimuli on affected side, as patient demonstrates an ability to compensate for neglect
- Instruct caregivers on the cause, mechanisms, and treatment of unilateral neglect
- Include family in rehabilitation process to support the patient's efforts and assist with care, as appropriate

2nd edition 1996; revised 2018

Background Evidence:

Dai, C., Huang, Y., Chou, L., Wu, S., Wang, R., & Lin, L. (2013). Effects of primary caregiver participation in vestibular rehabilitation for unilateral neglect patients with right hemispheric stroke: A randomized controlled trial. *Neuropsychiatric Disease and Treatment, 9*, 477–484.

Klinke, M., Hafsteinsdóttir, T., Hjaltason, H., & Jónsdóttir, H. (2015). Ward-based interventions for patients with hemispatial neglect in stroke rehabilitation: A systematic literature review. *International Journal of Nursing Studies, 52*(8), 1375–1403.

National Institute for Health and Clinical Excellence. (2013). *Stroke rehabilitation: Long term rehabilitation after stroke.* London, England: National Collaborating Centre for Women's and Children's Health.

Woodward, S., & Mestecky, A. (Eds.). (2011). *Neuroscience nursing: Evidence-based practice.* Wiley-Blackwell.

U

Urinary Bladder Training   0570

Definition: Improving bladder function for those with urge incontinence by increasing the bladder's ability to hold urine and the person's ability to suppress urination

Activities:

- Determine ability to recognize urge to void
- Encourage to keep voiding diary
- Keep continence specification record for 3 days to establish voiding pattern
- Assist to identify patterns of incontinence
- Review voiding diary with person
- Establish interval of initial toileting schedule, based on voiding pattern
- Establish beginning and ending time for toileting schedule, if not for 24 hours
- Establish interval for toileting of not less than 1 hour and preferably not less than 2 hours
- Toilet person or remind to void at prescribed intervals
- Provide privacy for toileting
- Use power of suggestion (e.g., running water, flushing toilet) to assist to void
- Use peppermint essential oil on cotton ball or drop in toilet to assist to void
- Avoid leaving on toilet for more than 5 minutes
- Reduce toileting interval by 1/2 hour if more than three incontinence episodes in 24 hours
- Maintain toileting interval if three or less incontinence episodes in 24 hours
- Increase toileting interval by one half hour if unable to void at two or more scheduled toileting times
- Increase toileting interval by 1 hour if no incontinence episodes for 3 days until optimal 4-hour interval achieved
- Use bladder scanner as indicated
- Implement intermittent catheterization protocol as indicated
- Express confidence that incontinence can be improved
- Instruct to consciously hold urine until scheduled toileting time
- Discuss daily record of continence to provide reinforcement

2nd edition 1996; revised 2004, 2024

Background Evidence:

Berman, A., Snyder, S. J., & Frandsen, G. (2018). Urinary elimination. In *Kozier and Erb's fundamentals of nursing: Concepts, process and practice* (10ed. ed., pp. 1174–1200). Pearson.

Gaikwad, A. J., & Kanase, S. B. (2020). Effect of structured bladder training in urinary incontinence. *Indian Journal of Physiotherapy & Occupational Therapy, 14*(1), 30–36.

Jefferson, L. (2021). Urinary elimination. In P. A. Potter, A. G. Perry, P. A. Stockert, & A. M. Hall (Eds.), *Fundamentals of nursing* (10th ed., pp. 1150–1171). Elsevier.

Kopf-Klakken, S. (2021). Urinary elimination. In R. F. Craven, C. J. Hirnle, & C. J. Henshaw (Eds.), *Fundamentals of nursing: Human health and function* (9th ed., pp. 1096–1114). Wolters-Kluwer.

Lough, M. E. (2022). Kidney disorders and therapeutic management. In L. D. Urden, K. M. Stacy, & M. E. Lough (Eds.), *Critical care nursing: Diagnosis and management* (9th ed., pp. 655–668). Elsevier.

Newman, D. K. (2019). Evidence-based practice guideline: Prompted voiding for individuals with urinary incontinence. *Journal of Gerontological Nursing, 45*(2), 14–26. https://doi.org/10.3928/00989134-20190111-03

Perry, A. G., Potter, P. A., Ostendorf, W. R., & LaPlante, N. (2021). Urinary elimination. In *Clinical nursing skills and technique* (10th ed., pp. 870–880). Mosby.

Touhy, T. (2020). Elimination. In K. Jett & T. A. Touhy (Eds.), *Toward healthy aging* (10th ed., pp. 201–210). Elsevier.

Williams, P. (2020). *Basic geriatric nursing* (7th ed). Elsevier.

Urinary Catheterization   0580

Definition: Insertion of a catheter into the bladder for temporary or permanent drainage of urine

Activities:

- Determine clinical indications for indwelling or intermittent catheterization
- Verify identification and ensure absence of allergies to catheter materials
- Consider bladder ultrasonography evaluation before catheterization, if appropriate
- Explain procedure and rationale for catheterization
- Assemble appropriate equipment
- Ensure privacy and proper draping for modesty (i.e., only expose genitalia)
- Ensure correct lighting for proper visualization of anatomy
- Prefill catheter bulb to check patency and size, if recommended by catheter manufacturer
- Maintain strict aseptic technique
- Maintain proper hand hygiene before, during and after catheter insertion or manipulation
- Position appropriately (i.e., female on back with legs apart or on side with upper leg flexed at hip and knee, male on back)
- Cleanse area around urethral meatus with antibacterial solution, sterile saline, or sterile water, per agency protocol
- Use sterile lubricant in catheter tip or apply it directly in urethra, as appropriate
- Insert straight or retention catheter into bladder, as appropriate
- Use smallest size catheter, as appropriate
- Ensure that catheter inserted far enough into bladder to prevent trauma to urethral tissues with inflation of balloon
- Confirm position of catheter tip with bladder ultrasonography, if necessary
- Fill catheter bulb for indwelling catheter, adhering to age and body size manufacturer recommendations (e.g., 10 mL adult, 5 mL child)
- Obtain urine sample for analysis, if prescribed
- Connect retention catheter to bedside drainage bag or leg bag
- Secure catheter to skin, as appropriate

U

- Place drainage bag below level of bladder
- Maintain closed and unobstructed urinary drainage system
- Monitor intake and output
- Perform or instruct related to clean intermittent catheterization, when appropriate
- Perform post-void residual catheterization, as needed
- Document care, including catheter size, type, and bulb fill amount
- Ensure catheter removal as soon as indicated by condition
- Instruct on proper catheter care

1st edition 1992; revised 2013; 2024

Background Evidence:

Berman, A., Snyder, S. J., & Frandsen, G. (2018). Urinary elimination. In *Kozier and Erb's fundamentals of nursing: Concepts, process and practice* (10th ed., pp. 1191–1199). Pearson.

Engberg, S., Clapper, J., McNichol, L., Thompson, D., Welch, V. W., & Gray, M. (2020). Current evidence related to intermittent catheterization: A scoping review. *Journal of Wound Ostomy & Continence Nursing, 47*(2), 140–165.

Hinkle, J. L., & Cheever, K. H. (2018). *Brunner and Suddarth's textbook of medical-surgical nursing* (14th ed.). Wolters Kluwer.

Hillery, S. (2020). Intermittent self-catheterization: a person-centered approach. *British Journal of Nursing, 29*(15), 858–860.

Potter, P. A., Ostendorf, W. R., & LaPlante, N. (2018). Urinary elimination. In *Clinical nursing skills and techniques* (9th ed., pp. 876–892). Mosby.

Royal College of Nursing. (2019). Catheter care: RCN guidance for health care professionals.

Urinary Catheterization: External   0581

Definition: Placement of an external device for drainage of urine

Activities:

- Determine clinical indications for placement of drainage system
- Verify identification and ensure absence of allergies to catheter materials
- Explain procedure and rationale for catheterization
- Assemble appropriate equipment
- Set suction at 40 mm Hg continuous for female device
- Connect all tubing, collection cannister, and external catheter to suction and check to ensure functioning suction for female device
- Ensure privacy and proper positioning for modesty (i.e., only expose legs and genitalia)
- Ensure correct lighting for proper visualization of anatomy
- Cleanse perineal area with soap and water, avoiding use of barrier creams
- Perform inspection of skin to ensure skin intact before applying device
- Retract foreskin for uncircumcised male and cleanse shaft underneath and replace foreskin
- Clip hair from base of penis if needed
- Apply adhesive, adhesive tape, or protective coating to penile shaft per manufacturer directions
- Apply pre-rolled condom sheath to penis ensuring funnel area against glans but not rubbing it
- Adhere condom sheath to penis avoiding wrinkling or constriction of condom sheath around shaft
- Connect to drainage system or leg bag below level of bladder, as indicated
- Evaluate penis 30 minutes after application for adverse effects (e.g., edema, discoloration, absence of urine flow)
- Position female such that legs, gluteus, and labia can be easily separated for external catheter placement
- Tuck soft gauze side of device between separated labia and gluteus, ensuring top of gauze aligned with pubic bone
- Place legs together after positioning external catheter and assuring suction turned on
- Align bedpan for bowel movements such that catheter suction not compromised, as needed
- Document care, including catheter type and tolerance of procedure
- Maintain closed and unobstructed urinary drainage system
- Monitor intake and output
- Replace catheter per institutional policy (e.g., every 8–12 hours or if soiled with feces or blood)
- Remove catheter by fully separating legs, leaving suction on, and pulling catheter gently away from labia
- Change condom catheter per institutional policy
- Ensure catheter removal as soon as indicated by condition
- Instruct on proper catheter care

8th edition 2024

Background Evidence:

Berman, A., Snyder, S. J., & Frandsen, G. (2018). Urinary elimination. In *Kozier and Erb's Fundamentals of nursing: Concepts, process and practice* (10th ed., pp. 1191–1199). Pearson.

Craven, R. F., Hirnle, C. J., & Henshaw, C. J. (2021). Urinary elimination. In *Fundamentals of nursing: Human health and function* (8th ed.). Wolters-Kluwer.

Eckert, L., Mattia, L., Patel, S., Okumura, R., Reynolds, P., & Stuiver, I. (2020). Reducing the risk of indwelling catheter-associated urinary tract infection in female patients by implementing an alternative female external urinary collection device: A quality improvement project. *Journal of Wound Ostomy Continence Nursing, 47*(1), 50–53. https://doi.org/10.1097/won.0000000000000601

Glover, E., Bleeker, E., Bauermeister, A., Koehlmoos, A., & Van Whye, M. (2018). External catheters and reducing adverse effects in the female inpatient. Northwestern College Department of Nursing. https://nwcommons.nwciowa.edu/cgi/viewcontent.cgi?article=1026&context=celebrationofresearch

Potter, P. A., Ostendorf, W. R., & LaPlante, N. (2021). Urinary elimination. In *Clinical nursing skills and techniques* (10th ed., pp. 876–892). Mosby.

Root, N., Horigan, A. E., & Lough, M. E. (2021). External female urinary catheter: Implementation in the emergency department. *Journal of Emergency Nursing, 47*(1), 131–138. https://doi.org/10.1016/j.jen.2020.09.008

U

Warren, C., Fosnacht, J. D., & Tremblay, E. E. (2021). Implementation of an external female urinary catheter as an alternative to an indwelling urinary catheter. *American Journal of Infection Control, 49*(6), 764–768.

Williams, P. (2020). *Basic geriatric nursing* (7th ed.). Elsevier.

Urinary Catheterization: Intermittent   0582

Definition: Regular periodic use of a catheter to empty the bladder

Activities:
- Review comprehensive and individualized urinary assessment information focusing on causes of incontinence or retention (e.g., urinary output, urinary voiding pattern, cognitive function, preexistent urinary or uro-gynecologic problems)
- Verify identification and ensure absence of allergies to catheter materials
- Measure residual volume using bladder ultrasound or scanner, if appropriate
- Implement urinary catheterization protocol as appropriate
- Explain purpose, supplies, method, and rationale of intermittent catheterization
- Select catheter size small enough to reduce risk of trauma but large enough for drainage
- Place in appropriate position
- Cleanse meatus and surrounding area with antiseptic solution per agency protocol using sterile technique
- Use lubricant in catheter tip or apply directly in urethra, as appropriate
- Use sterile technique for catheterization
- Monitor color, odor, and clarity of urine
- Measure urine volume drained
- Collect routine urine tests, as needed
- Maintain detailed record of catheterization schedule, fluid intake, and output
- Instruct on signs and symptoms of urinary tract infection
- Educate on clean intermittent catheterization technique, if appropriate
- Explain importance of and demonstrate adequate hand hygiene
- Determine readiness and willingness to perform intermittent self-catheterization at home
- Demonstrate procedure and use teach-back to ensure understanding, as appropriate
- Determine catheterization schedule based on comprehensive and individualized urinary assessment
- Determine need for prophylactic antibacterial therapy
- Educate to catheterize before bedtime to reduce nocturia, if necessary
- Assist to develop social support network (e.g., family, friends, professionals, institutions) that can help with health condition
- Instruct designated staff how to monitor and support persons performing self-catheterization at community settings (e.g., daycare, school, nursing homes), if appropriate

1st edition 1992; revised 1996, 2000, 2024

Background Evidence:

Beauchemin, L., Newman, D. K., Le Danseur, M., Jackson, A., & Ritmiller, M. (2018). Best practices for clean intermittent catheterization. *Nursing2020, 48*(9), 49–54.

Berman, A., Snyder, S. J., & Frandsen, G. (2018). Urinary elimination. In *Kozier and Erb's Fundamentals of nursing: Concepts, process and practice* (10th ed., pp. 1191–1199). Pearson.

Collins, L. (2018). Use of intermittent self-catheterization for voiding dysfunction. *British Journal of Nursing, 27*(15), 866–868. https://doi.org/10.12968/bjon.2018.27.15.866

Engberg, S., Clapper, J., McNichol, L., Thompson, D., Welch, V. W., & Gray, M. (2020). Current evidence related to intermittent catheterization: A scoping review. *Journal of Wound Ostomy & Continence Nursing, 47*(2), 140–165.

Hinkle, J. L., & Cheever, K. H. (2018). *Brunner and Suddarth's textbook of medical-surgical nursing* (14th ed.). Wolters Kluwer.

Leek, H., Mansfeld, K. J., Reus, A., & Moore, K. H. (2019). Clean intermittent self-catheterization: A randomized controlled crossover trial of single-use versus multiple re-use of catheters. *Australian & New Zealand Continence Journal, 25*(3), 64–73.

Potter, P. A., Ostendorf, W. R., & LaPlante, N. (2018). Urinary elimination. In *Clinical nursing skills and techniques* (9th ed., pp. 876–892). Mosby.

Urinary Elimination Management   0590

Definition: Maintenance of an optimum urinary elimination pattern

Activities:
- Determine usual elimination pattern
- Determine ability to recognize urge to void
- Consider age when determining voiding patterns (i.e., enuresis and toilet training in toddlers and preschoolers, incontinence due to physiological changes in older adults)
- Consider cultural and social differences when providing care
- Monitor urinary elimination including frequency, consistency, odor, volume, and color, as appropriate
- Monitor functional status for any changes that might impact urinary elimination ability (e.g., ability to safely ambulate or stand, ability to follow directions, motivation to help in self-care activities)
- Identify factors that contribute to incontinence episodes (e.g., unable to get up quickly, not close to bathroom)
- Note time of last urinary elimination, as appropriate
- Use bladder scanner as indicated
- Implement intermittent catheterization protocol as indicated
- Instruct to record urinary output, as appropriate

- Ensure easy access to commode, urinal, or bathroom
- Instruct to respond immediately to urge to void, as appropriate
- Respond to requests for toileting assistance promptly
- Place call light within easy reach
- Offer help at regular intervals (e.g., morning after awakening, after meals, before bedtime)
- Assist with use of urinals or bedpans, as needed
- Provide personal hygiene as needed after urination
- Monitor for signs and symptoms of urinary retention, urinary tract infection, dehydration, or fluid overload
- Encourage adequate fluid intake, particularly with indwelling catheters
- Refer to health care provider if signs and symptoms of urinary tract infection occur
- Obtain midstream voided specimen for urinalysis, as appropriate
- Instruct to drink 8 ounces of liquid with meals, between meals, and in early evening
- Assist with development of toileting routine, as appropriate
- Instruct to empty bladder before relevant procedures
- Record time of first voiding following procedure, as appropriate
- Instruct on signs and symptoms of urinary tract infection and to monitor for urinary tract infection
- Educate to obtain midstream urine specimens at first sign of return of infection signs and symptoms
- Use teach-back to determine understanding

1st edition 1992; revised 2000, 2004, 2024

Background Evidence:

Berman, A., Snyder, S. J., & Frandsen, G. (2018). Urinary elimination. In *Kozier and Erb's Fundamentals of nursing: Concepts, process and practice* (10th ed., pp. 1174–1200). Pearson.

Jefferson, L. (2021). Urinary elimination. In P. A. Potter, A. G. Perry, P. A. Stockert, & A. M. Hall (Eds.), *Fundamentals of nursing* (10th ed., pp. 1150–1171). Elsevier.

Kopf-Klakken, S. (2021). Urinary elimination. In R. F. Craven, C. J. Hirnle, & C. J. Henshaw (Eds.), *Fundamentals of nursing: Human health and function* (8th ed.). Wolters-Kluwer.

Lough, M. E. (2022). Kidney disorders and therapeutic management. In L. D. Urden, K. M. Stacy, & M. E. Lough (Eds.), *Critical care nursing: Diagnosis and management* (9th ed., pp. 655–668). Elsevier.

Perry, A. G., Potter, P. A., Ostendorf, W. R., & LaPlante, N. (2021). Urinary elimination. In *Clinical nursing skills and technique* (10th ed., pp. 870–880). Mosby.

Touhy, T. (2020). Elimination. In K. Jett & T. A. Touhy (Eds.), *Toward healthy aging* (10th ed., pp. 201–210). Elsevier.

Williams, P. (2020). *Basic geriatric nursing* (7th ed.). Elsevier.

Urinary Habit Training   0600

Definition: Establishing an individualized toileting schedule to preempt involuntary bladder emptying for persons with limited cognitive or physical ability

Activities:

- Involve caregivers in the process of developing individualized toileting schedules
- Keep a continence specification record for 3 days to establish voiding pattern
- Use an electronic monitoring device to establish episodes of incontinence, as appropriate
- Establish interval of initial toileting schedule, based on voiding pattern and usual routine (e.g., eating, rising, and retiring)
- Establish beginning and ending time for the toileting schedule, if not for 24 hours
- Establish interval for toileting of preferably not less than 2 hours
- Assist patient to toilet and prompt to void at prescribed intervals
- Provide special toilet adaptations, such as a raised seat or a handrail, if needed
- Provide privacy for toileting
- Use power of suggestion (e.g., running water or flushing toilet) to assist patient to void
- Avoid leaving patient on toilet for more than 5 minutes
- Reduce toileting interval by one half hour if there are more than two incontinence episodes in 24 hours
- Maintain toileting interval if there are two or less incontinence episodes in 24 hours
- Increase the toileting interval by one half hour if patient has no incontinence episodes in 48 hours until optimal 4-hour interval is achieved

- Discuss daily record of continence with caregivers to provide reinforcement and encourage compliance with toileting schedule
- Maintain scheduled toileting to assist in establishing and maintaining voiding habit
- Give positive feedback or positive reinforcement (e.g., 5 minutes of social conversation) to patient when he or she voids at scheduled toileting times and make no comment when patient is incontinent

2nd edition 1996; revised 2018

Background Evidence:

Lewis, S., Dirksen, S., Heitkemper, M., Bucher, L., & Camera, I. (2011). *Medical-surgical nursing: Assessment and management of clinical problems* (8th ed., pp. 1150–1151). Elsevier Mosby.

Ostaszkiewicz, J., Chestney, T., & Roe, B. (2004, updated 2009). Habit retraining for the management of urinary incontinence in adults. *Cochrane Database of Systematic Reviews, 2004*(2). https://doi.org/10.1002/14651858.CD002801.pub2

U

Urinary Incontinence Care 0610

Definition: Assistance in promoting continence and maintaining perineal skin integrity

Activities:

- Identify multifactorial causes of incontinence (e.g., urinary output, voiding pattern, cognitive function, preexistent urinary problems, postvoid residual, and medications)
- Use DIAPPERS acronym (Delirium, Infection, Atrophic urethritis or vaginitis, Pharmacology, Psychological disorders, Endocrine disorders, Restricted mobility, Stool impaction) to identify possible causes of transient incontinence
- Provide privacy for elimination
- Explain etiology of problem and rationale for actions
- Include family members in management strategies, as appropriate
- Monitor urinary elimination, including frequency, consistency, odor, volume, and color
- Obtain urine for culture and sensitivity testing, as needed
- Discuss procedures and expected outcomes with patient
- Assist to develop and maintain a sense of hope
- Modify clothing and environment to provide easy access to toilet
- Assist to select appropriate incontinence garments or pads for short-term management while more definitive treatment is designed
- Provide protective garments or incontinence pads, as needed
- Cleanse genital skin area at regular intervals
- Provide positive feedback for any decrease in episodes of incontinence
- Limit fluids for 2 to 3 hours before bedtime, as appropriate
- Schedule diuretic administration to have least impact on lifestyle
- Instruct patient and family to record urinary output and pattern, as appropriate
- Implement programs of timed voiding (i.e., offer to help use toilet every 2 hours while awake) or prompted voiding (i.e., encourage patient to request help when urge to void is felt), as appropriate
- Instruct patient to drink a minimum of 1500 cc fluids a day
- Instruct in ways to avoid constipation or stool impaction
- Advise that even 5% to 10% of weight loss can help symptoms
- Instruct on how to perform Kegel exercises to strengthen pelvic floor muscles
- Limit ingestion of bladder irritants (e.g., colas, coffee, tea, chocolate, sugar substitutes, spicy foods, alcohol)
- Monitor effectiveness of surgical, medical, pharmacological, and self-prescribed treatments
- Monitor bowel habits
- Determine need for placement and continuation of an indwelling catheter, as complications increase the longer the catheter is in place
- Refer to urinary continence specialist, as appropriate

1st edition 1992; revised 1996, 2018

Background Evidence:

Blanchette, K. (2012). Exploration of nursing care strategies for the management of urinary incontinence in hospitalized women. *Urologic Nursing,* *32*(5), 256–259.

Hersh, L., & Salzman, B. (2013). Clinical management of urinary incontinence in women. *American Family Physician, 87*(9), 634–640.

Knott, L. (2013). *Urge incontinence.* https://patient.info/womens-health/lower-urinary-tract-symptoms-in-women-luts/urge-incontinence

Roe, B., Flanagan, L., Jack, B., Barrett, J., Chung, A., Shaw, C., & Williams, K. (2011). Systematic review of the management of incontinence and promotion of continence in older people in care homes: Descriptive studies with urinary incontinence as primary focus. *Journal of Advanced Nursing, 67*(2), 228–250.

Urinary Incontinence Care: Enuresis 0612

Definition: Promotion of urinary continence in children who are bedwetting past the usual age of control

Activities:

- Interview parent to obtain data about toilet-training history, voiding pattern, urinary tract infections, food sensitivities, and constipation
- Determine frequency, duration, and circumstances of enuresis
- Discuss effective and ineffective methods of prior treatment
- Monitor family's and child's level of frustration and stress
- Assist with diagnostic evaluation (e.g., physical exam, cystogram, cystoscopy, and lab tests) to rule out physical causation
- Discuss techniques to use in reducing enuresis (e.g., night light, restricted fluid intake 3 hours before bedtime, scheduled nocturnal bathroom trips, and use of alarm system)
- Discuss practical ways to reduce the impact of bedwetting (e.g., bed protections, washable and disposable products)
- Promote a diet rich in fiber with raw fruits and vegetables
- Encourage child to verbalize feelings
- Emphasize child's strengths
- Encourage parents to demonstrate love and acceptance at home to counteract peer ridicule
- Inform children and young people and their parents and caregivers that bedwetting is not their fault and that punitive measures should not be used
- Reassure parents and caregivers that many children under 5 years of age wet the bed about once a week
- Suggest a trial of at least 2 nights in a row without diapers or pull-ups for a child with bedwetting who is under 5 years and has been toilet trained by day for longer than 6 months
- Use positive awards for agreed-upon behavior (e.g., using the toilet before sleep, taking medication) rather than for dry nights
- Consider use of an alarm system when bedwetting has not responded to advice on fluids, toileting, or rewards

U

- Inform users and caregivers about the benefits of alarms combined with reward systems (e.g., waking up when the alarm goes off, going to the toilet after the alarm has gone off, returning to bed and resetting the alarm)
- Continue alarm treatment until a minimum of 3 weeks uninterrupted dry nights has been achieved
- Discuss psychosocial dynamics of enuresis with parents (e.g., familial patterns, family disruption, self-esteem issues)
- Administer medications for short-term control, as appropriate
- Refer those who have not responded to courses of treatment with an alarm or medication to a specialist

2nd edition 1996; revised 2018

Background Evidence:

American Society of Registered Nurses. (2010). Increase in bedwetting year-round. *The Journal of Advanced Nursing Practice*. https://www.asrn.org/journal-advanced-practice-nursing/812-increase-in-bedwetting-year-round.html

National Institute for Health and Clinical Excellence. (2010). *Nocturnal enuresis: The management of bedwetting in children and young people*. London, England: National Clinical Guideline Centre.

Wootton, J., & Norfolk, S. (2010). Nocturnal enuresis: assessing and treating children and young people. *Community Practitioner, 83*(12), 37–39.

Urinary Retention Care   0620

Definition: Assistance in relieving bladder distention

Activities:

- Determine amount and characteristics of urinary output (e.g., urinary voiding pattern, cognitive function, preexistent urinary problems)
- Monitor use and effects of pharmacological treatments that could alter bladder emptying
- Provide privacy for elimination
- Use the power of suggestion by running water or flushing the toilet
- Stimulate the reflex bladder by applying cold to the abdomen, stroking the inner thigh, or running water
- Provide enough time for bladder emptying (10 minutes)
- Use spirits of wintergreen in bedpan or urinal
- Provide Credé maneuver, as necessary
- Use double-voiding technique (i.e., wait a short time after emptying the bladder and then try again)
- Instruct patient or family member to record urinary output, as appropriate
- Instruct in ways to avoid constipation or stool impaction
- Monitor intake and output
- Monitor degree of bladder distention by palpation and percussion
- Assist with toileting at regular intervals, as appropriate
- Catheterize for residual, as appropriate
- Implement intermittent catheterization, as appropriate
- Insert and monitor use of indwelling urethral catheter, as necessary
- Determine need for continued use of an indwelling catheter, as complications increase the longer it is in place
- Be on the lookout for complications of catheterization (e.g., infection, blockage, encrustment, psychological effects)
- Refer to urinary continence specialist, as appropriate

1st edition 1992; revised 1996, 2018

Background Evidence:

Agency for Healthcare Research and Quality. (2013). *Chronic urinary retention (CUR) treatment*. http://effectivehealthcare.ahrq.gov/index.cfm/search-for-guides-reviews-and-reports/?productid=1539&pageaction=displayproduct

Blanchette, K. (2012). Exploration of nursing care strategies for the management of urinary incontinence in hospitalized women. *Urologic Nursing, 32*(5), 256–259.

Herter, R., & Kazer, M. W. (2010). Best practices in urinary catheter care. *Home Healthcare Nurse, 28*(6), 342–349.

Johansson, R. M., & Christensson, L. (2010). Urinary retention in older patients in connection with hip fracture surgery. *Journal of Clinical Nursing, 19*(15-16), 2110–2116.

Lewis, S., Dirksen, S., Heitkemper, M., Bucher, L., & Camera, I. (2011). *Medical-surgical nursing: Assessment and management of clinical problems* (8th ed., pp. 1150–1151). Elsevier Mosby.

U

Vaccination Management   6530

Definition: Facilitating access to vaccination, providing instructions, administering, and monitoring vaccination status

Activities:

- Implement team approach to provide person with vaccine information at multiple contact points within healthcare system
- Determine history and immunization status to decide appropriate vaccinations needs
- Identify conditions that increase risk for serious adverse reactions (i.e., anaphylactic reaction to previous vaccine, egg or gelatin allergy)
- Discuss conditions that might compromise ability of vaccine to produce immunity
- Identify pregnancy and breastfeeding status
- Instruct pregnant females about recommended vaccinations to promote immunity to neonate after delivery (e.g., tetanus, pertussis, influenza vaccines)
- Discuss vaccine recommendations including annual influenza and tetanus, diphtheria, and pertussis (TDaP) when pregnant or breastfeeding
- Provide education on vaccines not to receive during pregnancy (e.g., human papillomavirus [HPV], measles, mumps, rubella (MMR), varicella, certain travel-related vaccines)
- Instruct that health and well-being are significantly impacted by unmet immunization needs
- Instruct about recommended immunizations necessary for children (e.g., hepatitis B, hepatitis A, rotavirus, diphtheria, tetanus, pertussis, influenza, polio, measles, mumps, rubella, meningococcal serogroup A, C, W, Y, meningococcal serogroup B, varicella), route of medication administration, reasons and benefits of use, adverse reactions, and side effects schedule
- Inform about recommended ages and vaccine schedules for administration
- Inform about immunization protection against illness not presently required by law (e.g., influenza, pneumococcal, herpes zoster, human papillomavirus, hepatitis A, hepatitis B, COVID-19 vaccinations)
- Instruct about vaccinations available in event of special incidence or exposure (e.g., cholera, influenza, plague, rabies, Rocky Mountain spotted fever, smallpox, typhoid fever, typhus, yellow fever, tuberculosis)
- Provide vaccine information statements prepared by Centers for Disease Control and Prevention, endorsing vaccines using scientific-based facts
- Provide and update vaccine database and individual's medical record for recording date and type of immunizations
- Secure informed consent to administer vaccine
- Determine proper administration techniques, including simultaneous administration and latest recommendations regarding use of immunizations
- Check accuracy and completeness of each person medication administration record (MAR) prior to giving any medications
- Follow six rights of medication administration, including right person, time, vaccine and diluent, dosage, route, needle, technique, injection site and documentation
- Identify using at least two identifiers (e.g., name, birthdate)
- Determine knowledge of medication and understanding of method of administration
- Perform necessary pre-medication assessments (e.g., blood pressure, pulse)
- Administer injections to infants in anterolateral thighs, simultaneously when more than one injection, and with additional staff to assist, as appropriate
- Provide education on pain alleviating techniques available during vaccine administration, including age-appropriate comfort measures for children
- Incorporate desired pain management techniques to reduce immunization-associated pain
- Observe person for specified period after medication administration
- Document vaccination information per agency protocol (e.g., manufacturer, lot number, expiration date)
- Inform families which immunizations are required by law for entering preschool, kindergarten, junior high, high school, and college
- Schedule immunizations at appropriate time intervals
- Determine immunization status at every health care visit (including emergency room and hospital admission) and provide immunizations as needed
- Use visual aids, handouts, and recommendations from credible sources regarding vaccination safety
- Provide culturally sensitive and appropriate educational level communication on risks and benefits of vaccines
- Keep education brief and succinct
- Discuss importance, effectiveness, and necessity of vaccines requiring multiple doses or boosters
- Develop follow-up immunization plan if person has multiple immunization needs that prevent dual administration or temporary precautions
- Provide education on common and expected post-vaccine side effects
- Ensure availability of vaccine when providing education so vaccination can happen in succession
- Audit school immunization records for completeness on yearly basis
- Instruct about keeping immunizations current
- Follow healthcare agency guidelines (e.g., American Academy of Pediatrics, American Academy of Family Physicians, Centers for Disease Control and Prevention, U.S. Public Health Service) for immunization administration
- Inform travelers of vaccinations appropriate for travel to foreign countries
- Recognize that delay in series administration does not indicate restarting schedule
- Discuss costs associated with vaccine administration including local resources that provide coverage assistance for cost of immunizations, as appropriate
- Support with financial planning to pay for immunizations (e.g., insurance coverage, health department clinics)
- Identify providers who participate in free vaccination programs
- Advocate for programs and policies that provide free or affordable immunizations to all populations
- Support national registry to track immunization status
- Document vaccine education
- Document refusal of immunizations, as appropriate
- Follow up regularly with person to anticipate future vaccine needs

V

- Prepare, educate, and answer questions before immunizations are due
- Use teach-back to ensure understanding

1st edition 1992; revised 2000, 2004, 2024

Background Evidence:

Abdullahi, L. H., Kagina, B. M., Ndze, V. N., Hussey, G. D., & Wiysonge, C. S. (2020). Improving vaccination uptake among adolescents. *Cochrane Database of Systematic Reviews, 1*, CD011895. https://doi.org/10.1002/14651858.CD011895.pub2

American Academy of Pediatrics. (2020). *Immunizations: Vaccine administration.* https://www.aap.org/en-us/advocacy-and-policy/aap-health-initiatives/immunizations/Practice-Management/Pages/Vaccine-Administration.aspx

American Academy of Pediatrics. (2021). *Administering vaccines: Dose, route, site, and needle size.* https://www.immunize.org/catg.d/p3085.pdf

Centers for Disease Control and Prevention. (2021). Catch-up immunizations schedule for persons aged 4 months–18 years who start late or who are more than 1 month behind, United States 2021. https://www.cdc.gov/vaccines/schedules/hcp/imz/catchup.html#table-catchup

Centers for Disease Control and Prevention. (2021). *Recommended adult immunization schedule for ages 19 years and older.* https://www.cdc.gov/vaccines/schedules/downloads/adult/adult-combined-schedule.pdf

Centers for Disease Control and Prevention. (2021). *Recommended child and adolescent immunization schedule for ages 18 years or younger.* https://www.cdc.gov/vaccines/schedules/downloads/child/0-18yrs-child-combined-schedule.pdf

Cwynar, C. M., & Osborne, K. (2019). Immunization-associated pain: Taking research to the bedside. *Journal of Pediatric Health Care, 33*(4), 446–454. https://doi.org/10.1016/j.pedhc.2018.12.004

Heavey, E. (2020). Guiding patients to appropriate vaccination during pregnancy. *The Nurse Practitioner, 45*(6), 19–24. https://doi.org/10.1097/01.NPR.0000666180.07149.f6

Validation Therapy 6670

Definition: Use of a method of therapeutic communication with elderly persons with dementia that focuses on emotional rather than factual content

Activities:

- Determine the patient's stage of cognitive impairment (e.g., malorientation, time confusion, repetitive motions, or vegetation)
- Avoid using validation strategies when the confusion is due to acute, reversible causes, or in the vegetation stage of confusion
- Listen with empathy
- Refrain from correcting or contradicting the patient's perceptions and experiences
- Accept the client's reality
- Avoid using "feeling" words
- Ask nonthreatening factual questions (e.g., Who? What? Where? When? How?)
- Avoid asking "Why?"
- Rephrase statements, repeating the patient's key words, while picking up tempo
- Maintain eye contact while reflecting the look in patient's eyes
- Match and express the client's emotion (e.g., love, fear, grief)
- Sing and interact using music familiar to the patient
- Observe and mirror body movements
- Use supportive touch (gentle touch to cheek, shoulder, arm, or hand)
- Speak the client's language by listening carefully to the verbs the client uses, and use the client's preferred sense (auditory, visual, kinesthetic)
- Link behavior to needs such as love, safety, activity, and usefulness
- Reminisce with the patient by reviewing the past
- Help the person find a familiar coping method

5th edition 2008

Background Evidence:

Day, C. R. (1997). Validation therapy: A review of the literature. *Journal of Gerontological Nursing, 23*(4), 29–34.

Feil, N. (2002). *The validation breakthrough: Simple techniques for communicating with people with Alzheimer's type dementia* (2nd ed.). Health Professions Press.

Taft, L. B. (1998). Validation therapy. In M. Synder & R. Lindquist (Eds.), *Complementary/alternative therapies in nursing* (3rd ed., pp. 231–242). Springer.

Warner, M. (2000). Designs for validation therapy. *Nursing Homes: Long Term Care Management, 49*(6), 25–28.

Values Clarification 5480

Definition: Assisting another to clarify her/his own values in order to facilitate effective decision-making

Activities:

- Consider the ethical and legal aspects of free choice, given the particular situation, before beginning the intervention
- Create an accepting, nonjudgmental atmosphere
- Encourage consideration of issues
- Encourage consideration of values underlying choices and consequences of the choice
- Use appropriate questions to assist the patient in reflecting on the situation and what is important personally
- Assist patient to prioritize values
- Use a value sheet clarifying technique (written situation and questions), as appropriate
- Pose reflective, clarifying questions that give the patient something to think about
- Avoid use of cross-examining questions
- Encourage patient to make a list of what is important and not important in life and the time spent on each
- Encourage patient to list values that guide behavior in various settings and types of situations
- Develop and implement a plan with the patient to try out choices

V

- Evaluate the effectiveness of the plan with the patient
- Provide reinforcement for actions in the plan that support the patient's values
- Help patient define alternatives and their advantages and disadvantages
- Help patient evaluate how values are in agreement with or conflict with those of family members/significant other(s)
- Support the patient in communicating own values to others
- Avoid use of the intervention with persons with serious emotional problems

1st edition 1992; revised 2008

Background Evidence:

Clark, C. C. (1996). *Wellness practitioner: Concepts, research and strategies* (2nd ed.). Springer.

Craven, R., & Hirnle, C. (2007). *Fundamentals of nursing: Human health and function* (5th ed.). Lippincott Williams & Wilkins.

Seroka, A. M. (1994). Values clarification and ethical decision making. *Seminars for Nurse Managers, 2*(1), 8–15.

Wilberding, J. Z. (1992). Values clarification. In G. M. Bulechek & J. C. McCloskey (Eds.), *Nursing interventions: Essential nursing treatments* (2nd ed., pp. 315–325). W.B. Saunders.

Vehicle Safety Promotion 9050

Definition: Increasing awareness of measures to reduce unintentional injuries from motorized and nonmotorized vehicles

Activities:

- Determine current awareness of vehicular safety, as appropriate
- Identify safety needs of target audience
- Identify individuals and groups at high risk for vehicular injury
- Identify safety hazards in environment
- Eliminate safety hazards in environment, when possible
- Give information about risks associated with motorized or non-motorized vehicle use, as indicated
- Instruct high-risk populations about vehicular hazards and risks (e.g., drinking, risk-taking behaviors, noncompliance with laws)
- Collaborate with community agencies (e.g., schools, police, local health department, child safety coalitions) in educational efforts to promote vehicle safety
- Provide literature about importance of and methods to increase vehicle safety
- Educate about rules of road for drivers of motorized and non-motorized vehicles
- Educate about importance of proper and regular use of protective devices to decrease risk of injury (e.g., car seats, seat belts, helmets)
- Emphasize importance of always wearing seat belts
- Encourage drivers not to start automobile until all passengers restrained, and ensure car parked and turned off before passengers exit vehicle
- Encourage adult drivers to lock doors and trunk when vehicle not in use, and store keys out of reach of children
- Encourage adults to be role models in use of seat belts and safe driving practices
- Encourage adults to never leave children unattended in or around parked vehicles
- Provide information on how to properly dress child to achieve optimal safe fit in car seat
- Monitor temperature of seat belt buckle to prevent burns during hot weather
- Monitor caregivers' use of approved child safety seats and seat belts
- Instruct on proper installation of child safety seats following manufacture guidelines
- Instruct about car seat expiration and replacement recommendations
- Instruct caregivers to secure infants in child safety seats and children under 13 years of age in back seat of automobile
- Encourage caregivers to keep infants and toddler safety seat in rear facing position as long as possible, up to height and weight limit of seat per manufacturer
- Instruct caregivers to secure children in forward facing car safety seats with harness for as long as possible, up to weight or height limit allowed by seat manufacturer
- Educate caregivers that children whose weight or height above forward-facing limit for their car safety seat should use belt-positioning booster seat until vehicle lap and shoulder belt fits properly
- Instruct caregivers on proper use and positioning of vehicle shoulder strap and lap belt appropriate to child size
- Encourage caregivers to take child safety seats when traveling (e.g., airplane, train, bus)
- Demonstrate strategies caregivers can use to keep children occupied while restrained in seat belts or child safety seats
- Praise children and families for proper and regular use of safe practices in vehicles
- Instruct passengers to refrain from riding in vehicles beyond seating capacity or in areas without seats
- Provide child safety seats to all families through community resources
- Evaluate need for specialized car seats for safe transportation of low-birth-weight or preterm infants and children with special health care needs
- Communicate special care plan for any child with medical condition including what to do during transport if medical emergency occurs
- Educate about risks of distracted or impaired driving and methods to reduce incidence for motorized and non-motorized vehicles (e.g., texting, drug or alcohol use, limit number of passengers for young drivers, both hands on wheel or handlebars, secure loose items)
- Inform caregivers of importance of selecting bicycle that fits child properly and adjusting it periodically as child grows
- Encourage use of adaptive devices to increase bicycle visibility (e.g., mirrors, horns, reflective devices, lights)
- Stress importance of always wearing properly fit helmet and bright or reflective clothing on bicycles, motorcycles, and other motorized vehicles (e.g., all-terrain vehicles, snowmobiles)
- Emphasize importance of wearing shoes and protective clothing while on motorized and nonmotorized vehicles
- Instruct to refrain from sidewalk bicycle riding
- Instruct to ride in same direction as traffic and obey street signs and signals
- Encourage use of hand signals when riding non-motorized vehicle
- Monitor community injury rates to determine further educational need

V

- Support legislative initiatives that promote and enforce vehicular safety
- Use teach-back to ensure understanding

3rd edition 2000; revised 2024

Background Evidence:

Bull, M. J. & Engle, W. A. & The Committee on Injury, Violence, and Poison Prevention and the Committee on Fetus and Newborn (2009). Reaffirmed 2019. Safe transportation of preterm and low birth weight infants at hospital discharge, *Pediatrics*, 123(5), 1424–1429.https://doi.org/10.1542/peds.2009-0559

Davis, N. L., & Shah, N. (2018). Use of car beds for infant travel: A review of the literature. *Journal of Perinatology*, 38(10), 1287–1294. https://doi.org/10.1038/s41372-018-0195-7

Durbin, D. R., & Hoffman, B. D. (2018). Child passenger safety , & Council on Injury, Violence, and Poison Prevention. *Pediatrics*, *142*(5), e20182460. https://doi.org/10.1542/peds.2018-2460

Durbin, D. R., Hoffman, B. D., & Council on Injury, Violence, and Poison Prevention. (2018). Child passenger safety, *Pediatrics*, 142(5), e20182461.https://doi.org/10.1542/peds.2018-2461

O'Neil, J., Hoffman, B., Agran, P. F., Denny, S. A., Hirsh, M., Johnston, B., Lee, L. K., Monroe, K., Schachter, J., Tenenbein, M., Zonfrillo, R., & Quinlanm, K. (2019). Transporting Children with Special Health Care Needs. *Pediatrics*, *143*(5). https://doi.org/10.1542/peds.2019-0724

National Highway Traffic Safety Administration (n.d.). *Child Safety*. United States Department of Transportation. https://www.nhtsa.gov/road-safety/child-safety

---

Ventilation Assistance   3390

Definition: Promotion of an optimal spontaneous breathing pattern that maximizes oxygen and carbon dioxide exchange in the lungs

Activities:

- Maintain patent airway
- Position to alleviate dyspnea
- Position to facilitate ventilation and perfusion matching ("good lung down"), as appropriate
- Assist with frequent position changes, as appropriate
- Position to minimize respiratory efforts (e.g., elevate head of bed, provide overbed table to lean on)
- Monitor effects of position change on oxygenation (e.g., ABG, SaO_2, SvO_2, end-tidal CO_2, Qsp/Qt, A-aDO_2 levels)
- Encourage slow deep breathing, turning, and coughing
- Use fun techniques to encourage deep breathing for children (e.g., blow bubbles with bubble blower; blow on pinwheel, whistle, harmonica, balloons, party blowers; have blowing contest using ping-pong balls or feathers)
- Assist with incentive spirometer, as appropriate
- Provide chest physiotherapy with postural drainage (e.g., thoracic squeezing, expiratory rib cage compression, chest wall percussion) or arrange for provision, as indicated
- Suction as indicated
- Provide manual hyperinflation, as indicated
- Auscultate breath sounds, noting areas of decreased or absent ventilation and presence of adventitious sounds
- Monitor for respiratory muscle fatigue
- Initiate and maintain supplemental oxygen, as prescribed
- Administer appropriate pain medication to prevent hypoventilation
- Ambulate three to four times per day, as appropriate
- Encourage adequate hydration
- Provide humidified air as indicated
- Monitor respiratory and oxygenation status
- Administer medications (e.g., bronchodilators, inhalers) that promote airway patency and gas exchange
- Implement non-pharmacological breathing enhancement measures (e.g., acupressure, music therapy, hypnosis), as appropriate
- Instruct on pursed lip breathing techniques, as appropriate
- Instruct on breathing techniques and exercises (e.g., breathing control breaths, thoracic expansion exercises, forced expiration technique, breathing control breaths combined with huffs, deep-breathing exercises), as appropriate
- Initiate program of respiratory muscle strength or endurance training as early as possible, as appropriate
- Encourage to obtain vaccinations (e.g., pneumonia, annual influenza)
- Encourage to avoid smoke, pollutants, and persons with respiratory illnesses
- Use teach-back to ensure understanding

1st edition 1992; revised 2000, 2024

Background Evidence:

Boon, C. J. W. (2021). Oxygenation. In P. A. Potter, A. G. Perry, P. A. Stockert, & A. M. Hall (Eds.), *Fundamentals of nursing* (10th ed., pp. 930–935). Elsevier.

Bryant, R. (2022). The child with respiratory dysfunction. In Hockenberry, Rodgers&Wilson *Wong'sessentialsofpediatricnursing*(11thed.,pp.619–677). Elsevier.

Jett, K. (2020). Respiratory health and illness. In K. Jett & T. A. Touhy (Eds.), *Toward healthy aging* (10th ed., pp. 315–320). Elsevier.

Slang, R., Finsrud, L. T., & Olsen, B. F. (2020). Nursing interventions in intensive care unit patients with breathing difficulties: A scoping review of the evidence. *Nordic Journal of Nursing Research*, 40(4), 176–187. https://doi.org/10.1177/2057158520948834

Stacy, K. (2022). Pulmonary therapeutic management. In L. D. Urden, K. M. Stacy, & M. E. Lough (Eds.), *Critical care nursing: Diagnosis and management* (9th ed., pp. 499–532). Elsevier.

Williams, P. (2020). Activity and exercise. In *Basic geriatric nursing* (pp. 310–332) (7th ed). Elsevier.

V

Vision Screening 6675

Definition: Early detection of vision disorders

Activities:
- Inform parent or patient that screening does not take the place of an eye examination and that the screening will not detect all vision disorders or diseases
- Test all children in kindergarten, first, third, fifth, seventh, and ninth grades
- Test all new and transfer students, all hearing-impaired children (annually), children referred by a teacher, and any others according to state school health protocols
- Recognize that vision screenings at their best are only able to detect visual impairments that impact distance vision
- Plan vision screenings for a day that does not conflict with other school activities and ensure that it is announced on the school calendar
- Plan for a rescreening day within 30 days of the initial screenings
- Provide training for staff and volunteers, including record keeping and confidentiality, as needed
- Practice good sanitation, including washing hands before beginning screening
- Disinfect reusable eye occulars before use and after each individual is screened
- Take into account societal and cultural factors when conducting screenings; those who reside in lower socioeconomic areas are more susceptible to poverty, malnourishment, and negative visual health consequences
- Ensure that the screening room is well lit with no distractions or patterned wall or direct sunlight
- Observe the ABCs: Appearance of the eyes (e.g., crossed, wandering, red, watery, drooping eyelids); Behavior (e.g., squinting, blinking, rubbing eyes, turning head to use only one eye, tilting head, tripping); Complaints (e.g., headaches, eye pain, dizziness, itching eyes, blurred vision, unusual sensitivity to light)
- Use approved screening devices and tools to test for distance visual acuity, stereoacuity (i.e., discerning depth or distance of an object), and color deficiency, as recommended by an established professional health organization
- Use an eye chart-based vision test, appropriate for age and skill level, for those aged 3 years or older as the standard for determining distance acuity
- Begin by screening the right eye first so that if interrupted you know that you always start on the right eye
- Follow the administration and scoring directions provided with each test (e.g., Monocular Distance Visual Acuity, muscle balance using Alternate Cover Test, stereopsis screening using Random Dot E Test, Color Deficit)
- Recognize that poor vision in adults is associated with increased risk of falls and decreased quality of life
- Refer those children ages 6 years and up who score 20/30 and those ages 3 to 5 years who score 20/40 on the eye chart to an eye doctor
- Refer those unable to complete a vision test to an eye doctor
- Refer those with low vision, pink eye, dry eyes, floaters, flashes, contact lens infections, eye injury, and other eye abnormalities to eye doctor
- Ensure effective follow-up for individuals with detected vision disorders
- Clean and store vision tools and equipment after use
- Document all findings and referrals according to state department of health requirements

7th edition 2018

Background Evidence:
Ohio Department of Health. (2007). *Vision screening requirements and guidelines*.
Unite for Sight. (n.d.). *Challenges and failure of vision screenings*. http://www.uniteforsight.org/health-screenings/vision-screenings

Visitation Facilitation 7560

Definition: Promoting beneficial visits by family and friends

Activities:
- Determine patient's preferences for visitation and release of information
- Consider legal/ethical implications regarding patient and family visitation and information rights
- Determine need for limited visitation, such as too many visitors, patient's being impatient or tired, or physical status
- Determine need for more visits from family and friends
- Identify specific problems with visits, if any
- Establish flexible, patient-centered visiting policies, as appropriate
- Prepare the environment for visitation
- Discuss visiting policy with family members/significant other(s)
- Discuss policy for overnight stay of family members/significant other(s)
- Discuss family's understanding of patient's condition
- Negotiate responsibilities and activities of family/significant other(s) to assist patient, such as feeding
- Establish optimal times for family/significant other(s) to visit patient
- Provide rationale for limited visiting time
- Evaluate periodically with both the family and the patient whether visitation practices are meeting the needs of the patient/family, and revise accordingly
- Inform visitors, including children, what they may expect to see and hear before their first hospital visitation, as appropriate
- Explain procedure being done
- Encourage the family member to use touch, as well as verbal communication, as appropriate
- Provide a chair at the bedside
- Be flexible with visitation while facilitating periods of rest
- Monitor patient's response to family visitation
- Note patient's verbal and nonverbal cues regarding visitation
- Facilitate visitation of children, as appropriate
- Encourage use of the telephone to maintain contact with significant other(s), as appropriate

V

- Screen visitors, especially children, for communicable diseases before visitation
- Clarify the meaning of what the family member perceived during the visit
- Provide support and care for family members after visitation, as needed
- Provide family with unit telephone number to call when they go home
- Inform family that a nurse will call at home if significant change in patient status occurs
- Provide sleeping arrangements for relatives close to the unit, as appropriate
- Assist family members to find adequate lodging and meals
- Inform family of legislation that they may have the right to 12 weeks unpaid leave of absence from work
- Answer questions and give explanations of care in terms that visitors can understand
- Convey feelings of acceptance to the visitors
- Facilitate meeting/consultation with physician and other providers
- Debrief visitors, including children, after the visit
- Assist parents to plan for ongoing support of children after the visit
- Arrange animal visitation, as appropriate

1st edition 1992; revised 2000

Background Evidence:

Daly, J. M. (1999). Visitation facilitation. In G. M. Bulechek & J. C. McCloskey (Eds.), *Nursing interventions: Effective nursing treatments*. W.B. Saunders.

Halm, M. (1990). Effects of support groups on anxiety of family members during critical illness. *Heart & Lung, 19*(1), 62–71.

Kleiber, C., Davenport, T., & Freyenberger, B. (2006). Open bedside rounds for families with children in pediatric intensive care units. *American Journal of Critical Care, 15*(5), 492–496.

Kleiber, C., Montgomery, L. A., & Craft-Rosenberg, M. (1995). Information needs of the siblings of critically ill children. *Children's Health Care, 24*(1), 47–60.

Krapohl, G. L. (1995). Visiting hours in the adult intensive care unit: Using research to develop a system that works. *Dimensions of Critical Care Nursing, 14*(5), 245–258.

Lazure, L. L. (1997). Strategies to increase patient control of visiting. *Dimensions of Critical Care Nursing, 16*(1), 11–19.

Montgomery, L. A., Kleiber, C., Nicholson, A., & Craft-Rosenberg, M. (1997). A research-based sibling visitation program for the neonatal ICU. *Critical Care Nurse, 17*(2), 29–40.

Sims, J. M., & Miracle, V. A. (2006). A look at critical care visitation: The case for flexible visitation. *Dimensions of Critical Care Nursing, 25*(4), 175–180.

Titler, M. G., Cohen, M. Z., & Craft, M. J. (1991). Impact of adult critical care hospitalization: Perceptions of patients, spouses, children, and nurses. *Heart & Lung, 20*(2), 174–182.

Vital Signs Monitoring 6680

Definition: Collection and analysis of cardiovascular, respiratory, pain, and body temperature data

Activities:

- Monitor blood pressure, pulse, temperature, pain, and respiratory status, as appropriate
- Follow agency protocol for use of automatic vital signs monitoring systems
- Auscultate manual blood pressures in both arms and compare
- Compare manual blood pressure readings to automatic monitoring readings at least once daily
- Note trends and wide fluctuations in blood pressure
- Monitor blood pressure while person lying, sitting, and standing, before and after position changes, as appropriate
- Monitor blood pressure after person has taken cardiac medications, if possible
- Monitor blood pressure, pulse, and respirations before, during, and after activity, as appropriate
- Initiate appropriate method (e.g., axillary, rectal, oral, tympanic membrane) of temperature measurement considering condition and ability
- Initiate and maintain continuous temperature monitoring device, as appropriate
- Monitor for and report signs and symptoms of hypothermia and hyperthermia
- Monitor presence and quality of central and peripheral pulses
- Monitor pulse for rate, rhythm, volume, amplitude, and symmetry
- Take apical and radial pulses simultaneously and note difference, as appropriate
- Monitor for pulsus paradoxus
- Monitor for pulsus alternans
- Monitor for widening or narrowing pulse pressure
- Monitor cardiac rhythm and rate
- Monitor cardiac output
- Monitor heart tones
- Monitor respiratory rate and rhythm (e.g., depth, symmetry)
- Monitor lung sounds
- Monitor oxygen levels with pulse oximetry
- Monitor for abnormal respiratory patterns (e.g., Cheyne-Stokes, Kussmaul, orthopneic, paradoxical, Biot, apneustic, ataxic, excessive sighing)
- Monitor skin color, temperature, and moistness
- Monitor for central and peripheral cyanosis
- Monitor for clubbing of nail beds
- Monitor for presence of Cushing's triad (i.e., wide pulse pressure, bradycardia, and increase in systolic BP)
- Monitor pain using validated pain assessment scale
- Monitor pain before and after pain medication administration
- Identify possible causes of changes in vital signs
- Check accuracy of instruments used for acquisition of data routinely, preferably every 8 hours

1st edition 1992; revised 2004, 2024

Background Evidence:

Henshaw, C. M. (2021). Vital signs. In R. F. Craven, C. J. Hirnle, & C. M. Henshaw (Eds.), *Fundamentals of nursing: Human health and function* (9th ed., pp. 373–441). Wolters-Kluwer.

de Castro, C. C., Pereira, A. K., da, S., & Bastos, B. R. (2018). Implementation of the evaluation of pain as the fifth vital sign. *Journal of Nursing UFPE / Revista de Enfermagem UFPE, 12*(11), 3009–3014. https://doi.org/10.5205/1981-8963-v12i11a236994p3009-3014-2018

Downey, C. L., Chapman, S., Randell, R., Brown, J. M., & Jayne, D. G. (2018). The impact of continuous versus intermittent vital signs monitoring

V

in hospitals: A systematic review and narrative synthesis. *International Journal of Nursing Studies, 84*, 19–27.

Flack, J. M., & Adekola, B. (2020). Blood pressure and the new ACC/AHA hypertension guidelines. *Trends Cardiovascular Medicine, 30*(3), 160–164. https://doi.org/10.1016/j.tcm

Newman, S. (2017). Do not disturb: Vital sign monitoring as a predictor of clinical deterioration in monitored patients. *Kentucky Nurse, 65*(2), 15–17.

Perry, A. G., & Potter, P. A. (2020). *Fundamentals of nursing* (10th ed.). Elsevier.

Perry, A. G., Potter, P. A., Ostendorf, W., & LaPlante, N. (2021). *Clinical nursing skills and techniques (10th ed.)*. Elsevier.

Sapra, A., Malik, A., & Bhandari, P. (2020). Vital sign assessment. In *StatPerals*. StatPearls Publishing. https://www.ncbi.nlm.nih.gov/books/NBK553213/

Tucker, G., & Lusher, A. (2018). The use of early warning scores to recognize and respond to patient deterioration in district nursing. *British Journal of Community Nursing, 23*(2), 76–79. https://doi.org/10.12968/bjcn.2018.23.2.76

Vomiting Management   1570

Definition: Prevention and alleviation of vomiting

Activities:

- Perform comprehensive assessment of vomiting episodes to determine branch of emetic pathway involved (e.g., vestibular system, chemoreceptor trigger zone)
- Ascertain severity and intensity of symptoms using an assessment tool or scale (e.g., Self-Care Journal, Visual Analog Scales, Duke Descriptive Scales, Rhodes Index of Nausea and Vomiting (INV) Form 2)
- Determine emesis color, consistency, and for presence of blood
- Determine timing and force of emesis
- Measure or estimate emesis volume
- Review pre-treatment history, including dietary history with likes, dislikes, and cultural preferences
- Observe for nonverbal cues of discomfort, especially for infants, children, and those unable to communicate effectively, such as individuals with Alzheimer's disease
- Evaluate precipitating and relieving factors (e.g., movement, food, fluids, hunger, aromas), and characteristics (e.g., duration, frequency)
- Control environmental factors that may evoke vomiting (e.g., aversive smells, sound, unpleasant visual stimulation)
- Reduce or eliminate personal factors that precipitate or increase vomiting (e.g., anxiety, fear, lack of knowledge)
- Position to prevent aspiration during episodes
- Maintain oral airway during episodes
- Provide physical support during vomiting (e.g., assisting to bend over, support head)
- Maintain privacy and dignity during episodes
- Provide comfort (e.g., cool cloths to forehead, sponging face, providing clean dry clothes) during and after episodes
- Demonstrate acceptance of vomiting
- Collaborate with person when selecting vomiting control strategy
- Suggest carrying plastic bag for emesis containment
- Use oral hygiene to clean mouth and nose
- Clean up after episodes with special attention to removing odors
- Wait at least 30 minutes after episodes before offering fluids (assuming normal gastrointestinal tract and normal peristalsis)
- Begin fluids that are clear and free of carbonation
- Gradually increase fluids if no vomiting occurs over 30-minute period
- Monitor for damage to esophagus and posterior pharynx if vomiting and retching are prolonged
- Monitor fluid and electrolyte balance (e.g., skin turgor, laboratory results)
- Encourage rest
- Use nutritional supplements to maintain body weight, if necessary
- Weigh regularly
- Instruct on use of non-pharmacological techniques (e.g., biofeedback, hypnosis, relaxation, guided imagery, music therapy, distraction, acupressure, essential oils) to manage vomiting
- Encourage use of non-pharmacological techniques along with other vomiting control measures
- Inform other health care professionals and family members of any non-pharmacological strategies being used by person
- Assist person and family to seek and provide support for themselves
- Monitor effects of vomiting management
- Use teach back to ensure understanding

3rd edition 2000; revised 2024

Background Evidence:

Dilek, B., & Necmiye, C. (2020). Usage of aromatherapy in symptom management in cancer patients: A systematic review. *International Journal of Caring Sciences, 13*(1), 537–546.

Ford, C., & Park, L. (2020). Assessing and managing nausea and vomiting in adults. *British Journal of Nursing, 29*(11), 602–605.

Rothenberger, C. D. (2019). Hyperemesis gravidarum. *Med-Surg Matters, 28*(3), 4–6.

Walsh, D., Davis, M., Ripamonti, C., Bruera, E., Davies, A., & Molassiotis, A. (2017). 2016 Updated MASCC/ESMO consensus recommendations: Management of nausea and vomiting in advanced cancer. (Systematic Review). *Supportive Care in Cancer, 25*, 333–340.

Zorba, P., & Ozdemir, L. (2018). The preliminary effects of massage and inhalation aromatherapy on chemotherapy-induced acute nausea and vomiting: A quasi-randomized controlled pilot trial. *Cancer Nursing, 41*(5), 359–366.

V

Weight Gain Assistance 1240

Definition: Facilitating increase in body weight

Activities:
- Refer for diagnostic workup to determine cause of being underweight, as appropriate
- Weigh at specified intervals, as appropriate
- Discuss possible causes of low body weight
- Review medication history
- Monitor for nausea and vomiting
- Determine cause of nausea or vomiting, and treat appropriately
- Administer medications to reduce nausea and pain before eating, as appropriate
- Monitor daily calories consumed
- Monitor serum albumin, total proteins, lymphocyte, and electrolyte levels
- Encourage increased calorie intake
- Instruct on how to increase calorie intake
- Provide variety of high-calorie nutritious foods to select
- Consider food preferences, using personal choices and cultural and religious preferences
- Provide oral care before meals, as needed
- Provide rest periods, as needed
- Ensure in sitting position before eating or feeding
- Assist with eating or feed, as appropriate
- Provide appropriate foods as prescribed (e.g., general diet, mechanical soft, blended or commercial formula via nasogastric or gastrostomy tube, total parental nutrition)
- Create pleasant, relaxing environment at mealtime
- Serve food in pleasant, attractive manner
- Discuss socioeconomic factors contributing to inadequate nutrition
- Discuss perceptions or factors interfering with ability or desire to eat
- Refer to community agencies that can assist in acquiring food, as appropriate
- Instruct about meal planning, as appropriate
- Recognize that weight loss may be part of natural progression of terminal illness (e.g., cancer)
- Instruct on realistic expected outcomes regarding illness and potential for weight gain
- Determine food preferences regarding favorite foods, seasonings, and temperature
- Provide dietary supplements, as appropriate
- Create social setting for food consumption, as appropriate
- Instruct on how to buy low-cost, nutritious foods, as appropriate
- Reward for weight gain
- Chart weight gain progress and post in strategic location
- Encourage attendance at support groups, as appropriate
- Use teach-back to ensure understanding

1st edition 1992; revised 2004, 2024

Background Evidence:

Carl, R. (2019). Healthy weight practices for child and adolescent athletes. *Pediatric Annals, 48*(7), e286–e289. https://doi.org/10.3928/19382359-20190617-02

Conviser, J. H., Fisher, S. D., & McColley, S. A. (2018). Are children with chronic illnesses requiring dietary therapy at risk for disordered eating or eating disorders? A systematic review. *International Journal of Eating Disorders, 51*(3), 187–213. https://doi.org/10.1002/eat.22831

De Coen, J., Verbeken, S., & Goossens, L. (2021). Media influence components as predictors of children's body image and eating problems: A longitudinal study of boys and girls during middle childhood. *Body Image, 37*, 204–213. https://doi.org/10.1016/j.bodyim.2021.03.001

Fitzpatrick, S., MacDonald, D. E., McFarlane, T., & Trottier, K. (2019). An experimental comparison of emotion regulation strategies for reducing acute distress in individuals with eating disorders. *Canadian Journal of Behavioural Science, 51*(2), 90–99. https://doi.org/10.1037/cbs0000119

Helvaci, M. R., Algin, M. C., Abyad, A., & Pocock, L. (2018). Physical inactivity or an excessive eating habit. *Middle East Journal of Nursing, 12*(1), 14–18. https://doi.org/10.5742/MEJN.2018.93346

McCabe, M., Fuller-Tyszkiewicz, M., Mellor, D., & Maïano, C. (2020). Body image, disordered eating, higher weight, and their associated factors: Can we use the same scales to measure constructs across different countries? *Body Image, 35*, 316–319. https://doi.org/10.1016/j.bodyim.2020.09.017

Weight Management 1260

Definition: Facilitating maintenance of optimal body weight and percent body fat

Activities:
- Determine motivation for weight management
- Discuss relationship between food intake, exercise, weight gain, and weight loss
- Discuss health conditions that may affect weight
- Discuss habits, customs, cultural, and heredity factors that influence weight
- Discuss risks associated with being over- and underweight
- Determine motivation for changing eating habits
- Determine ideal body weight and ideal percent body fat
- Develop method to keep daily record of intake, exercise sessions, or changes in body weight
- Encourage to write down realistic weekly goals for food intake and exercise and display in location to review daily
- Encourage to chart weekly weights, as appropriate
- Encourage to consume adequate amounts of water daily
- Plan rewards to celebrate reaching short-term and long-term goals
- Inform about support groups availability
- Assist in developing well-balanced meal plans consistent with level of energy expenditure
- Use teach-back to ensure understanding

1st edition 1992; revised 2004, 2024

W

Background Evidence:

Alkhawaldeh, A., Khatatbeh, M., Al Bashtawy, M., Al-Awamreh, K., Al Qadire, M., Al Omari, O., Khasawneh, B., Al Bashtawy, B., Al Bashtawy, S., & Alshakh, H. (2017). Behavioural approaches to treating overweight and obesity in adolescents. *Nursing Children & Young People, 29*(9), 44–46. https://doi.org/10.7748/ncyp.2017.e918

Berman, A., Snyder, S. J., & Frandsen, G. (2018). *Kozier and Erb's Fundamentals of nursing: Concepts, process and practice* (10th ed.). Pearson.

Cheng, F. W., Garay, J. L., & Handu, D. (2021). Weight management interventions for adults with overweight or obesity: An evidence analysis center scoping review. *Journal of the Academy of Nutrition & Dietetics, 121*(9), 1855–1865. https://doi.org/10.1016/j.jand.2020.07.022

Coutts, A. (2021). The nurse's role in providing strategies and advice on weight management. *British Journal of Nursing, 30*(21), S20–S27. https://doi.org/10.12968/bjon.2021.30.21.S20

Craven, R. F., Hirnle, C. J., & Henshaw, C. J. (2021). *Fundamentals of nursing: Human health and function* (8th ed.). Wolters-Kluwer.

Ensign, A., & Couch, K. (2021). Improving effective weight management in a university health center. *Journal for Nurse Practitioners, 17*(10), 1183–1188. https://doi.org/10.1016/j.nurpra.2021.09.023

Greathouse, K. L., Faucher, M. A., & Hastings-Tolsma, M. (2017). The gut microbiome, obesity, and weight control in women's reproductive health. *Western Journal of Nursing Research, 39*(8), 1094–1119. https://doi.org/10.1177/0193945917697223

Potter, P. A., Perry, A. G., Stockert, P. A., & Hall, A. M. (2021). *Fundamentals of nursing* (10th ed.). Elsevier.

Suire, K. B., Kavookjian, J., Feiss, R., & Wadsworth, D. D. (2021). Motivational Interviewing for weight management among women: A meta-analysis and systematic review of RCTs. *International Journal of Behavioral Medicine, 28*(4), 403–416. https://doi.org/10.1007/s12529-020-09934-0

Williams, P. (2020). *Basic geriatric nursing* (7th ed.). Elsevier.

Weight Reduction Assistance — 1280

Definition: Facilitating loss of weight and/or body fat

Activities:

- Determine patient's desire and motivation to reduce weight or body fat
- Determine with the patient the amount of weight loss desired
- Use the terms "weight" or "excess" rather than "obesity," "fatness," and "excess fat"
- Set a realistic weekly goal for weight loss
- Post the weekly goal in a strategic location
- Weigh patient weekly
- Chart progress of reaching final goal and post in a strategic location
- Discuss setbacks to help patient overcome challenges and be more successful
- Reward patient when attaining goals
- Encourage use of internal reward systems when goals are accomplished
- Set a realistic plan with the patient to include reduced food intake and increased energy expenditure
- Encourage self-monitoring of dietary intake and exercise by having patient keep a paper or handheld electronic diary
- Assist patient to identify motivation for eating and internal and external cues associated with eating
- Encourage substitution of undesirable habits with favorable habits
- Post reminder and encouragement signs to do health-promotion behaviors, rather than eating
- Assist with adjusting diets to lifestyle and activity level
- Facilitate patient participation in at least one energy-expending activity three times a week
- Provide information about amount of energy expended with specific physical activities
- Assist in selection of activities according to amount of desired energy expenditure
- Plan an exercise program, taking into consideration the patient's limitations
- Advise to be active at home while doing household chores and find ways to move during day-to-day activities
- Administer medications for weight loss (e.g., sibutramine, orlistat), as prescribed
- Develop a daily meal plan with a well-balanced diet, reduced calories, and reduced fat, as appropriate
- Encourage the patient to emphasize fruits, vegetables, whole grains, fat-free or low-fat milk and milk products, lean meats, fish, beans, eggs, and meats
- Encourage use of sugar substitute, as appropriate
- Recommend adoption of diets that will lead to achievement of long-range goals for weight loss
- Encourage attendance at support groups for weight loss (e.g., Take Off Pounds Sensibly [TOPS], Weight Watchers)
- Refer to a community weight-control program, as appropriate
- Refer to an online weight-loss program (e.g., Weight-Control Information Network), as appropriate
- Instruct on how to read labels when purchasing food to control amount of fat and calorie density of food obtained
- Instruct on how to calculate percentage of fat in food products
- Instruct on food selection in restaurants and social gatherings that are consistent with planned calorie and nutrient intake
- Discuss with patient and family the influence of alcohol consumption on food ingestion

1st edition 1992; revised 2013

Background Evidence:

Kanekar, A., & Sharma, M. (2010). Pharmacological approaches for management of child and adolescent obesity. *Journal of Clinical Medicine Research, 2*(3), 105–111.

National Institute of Diabetes and Digestive and Kidney Diseases. (2005). *Talking with patients about weight loss: Tips for primary care professionals.* (Publication No. 05-5634).

National Institute of Diabetes and Digestive and Kidney Diseases. (2009). *Weight loss for life.* (Publication No. 04-3700).

National Institute of Diabetes and Digestive and Kidney Diseases. (2010). *Active at any size.* (NIH Publication No. 10-4352).

Shay, L. (2008). Self-monitoring and weight management. *Online Journal of Nursing Informatics, 12*(1). http://ojni.org/12_1/shay.html

Whitlock, E.P., O'Connor, E.A., Williams, S.B., Beil, T.L., & Lutz, K.W. (2008). *Effectiveness of weight management programs in children and adolescents.* Evidence Report/Technology Assessment No. 170 (Publication No. 08-E014). Agency for Healthcare Research and Quality.

W

Wound Care 3660

Definition: Prevention of complications and promotion of wound healing

Activities:

- Remove any existing dressing, adhesive, or clothing around wound
- Shave hair surrounding affected area, as needed
- Note characteristics of wound, including drainage, color, size, and odor
- Measure initially and with each dressing change or as ordered
- Remove embedded material (e.g., splinter, tick, glass, gravel, metal), as needed
- Cleanse with normal saline or non-cytotoxic cleanser including area around wound (e.g., peri-wound area)
- Place affected area in whirlpool bath, as appropriate
- Provide incision site care, as needed
- Apply appropriate topical treatment to skin or lesion, as prescribed
- Apply appropriate dressing (e.g., dry dressing, moist dressing, sterile dressing) that controls exudate but does not further desiccate wound
- Keep surrounding area dry while protecting wound
- Reinforce dressing, as needed
- Change dressing according to amount of exudate and drainage
- Change type of dressing as needed for proper advancement of wound healing
- Inspect wound with each dressing change
- Regularly compare and record any changes in wound
- Position to avoid placing tension on wound, as appropriate
- Reposition person at least every 2 hours, as appropriate
- Encourage fluids, as appropriate
- Refer to wound ostomy clinician, as appropriate
- Refer to dietitian, as appropriate
- Apply wound healing devices (e.g., TENS, wound vac), as prescribed
- Place pressure-relieving devices (e.g., low-air-loss, foam, or gel mattresses; heel or elbow pads; chair cushion), as appropriate
- Assist to obtain wound care supplies
- Consider caregiver time, ease of use, availability, and cost when selecting dressings for home use
- Instruct on storage and disposal of dressings and supplies
- Instruct about wound care procedures
- Instruct about signs and symptoms of infection
- Document wound location, size, and appearance with each wound care episode
- Use teach-back to ensure understanding

1st edition 1992; revised 2000, 2004, 2024

Background Evidence:

Boon, C. J. W. (2021). Skin integrity and wound care. In P. A. Potter, A. G. Perry, P. A. Stockert, & A. M. Hall (Eds.), *Fundamentals of nursing* (10th ed., pp. 1176–1206). Elsevier.

Craven, R. F., Hirnle, C. J., & Henshaw, C. J. (2021). *Fundamentals of nursing: Human health and function* (8th ed.). Wolters-Kluwer.

Dowsett, C., Bain, K., Hoffmann, C., Brennan, M. R., Greco, A., Karlsmark, T., Keast, D., Liberato de Moura, M. R., Lázaro-Martínez, J. L., Münter, K., Swanson, T., Vuagnat, H., & Bain, M. (2021). The Wound Care Pathway – An evidence-based and step-by-step approach towards wound healing. *Wounds International, 12*(3), 78–85.

Williams, M. (2021). Wound infections: An overview. *British Journal of Community Nursing, 26*(Sup6), S22–S25.

Wound Care: Burns 3661

Definition: Prevention of wound complications due to burns and facilitation of wound healing

Activities:

- Cool the burn with warm water (20° C) or saline solution at the time of injury, if possible
- Wash chemical wounds continuously for 30 minutes or longer to ensure the elimination of all burn agent
- Determine the area of entrance and exit of electrical burns to evaluate which organs might be involved
- Obtain an electrocardiogram (ECG) in all electrical burns
- Raise the temperature of the patient who has burns due to cold
- Keep the airway open to ensure ventilation
- Monitor the level of consciousness in patients with large burns
- Evaluate the mouth and nasal fossae of the patient to identify any possible lesion due to inhalation
- Evaluate the wound, examining its depth, extension, localization, pain, causative agent, exudation, granulation or necrotic tissue, epithelization, and signs of infection
- Administer tetanus toxoid, as appropriate
- Use physical isolation measures to prevent infection (e.g., mask, gown, sterile gloves, cap, and foot coverings)
- Inform the patient of the procedure to be followed to dress the wound
- Provide comfort measures before dressing change
- Set up a sterile field and maintain maximum asepsis throughout the whole process
- Take off outside bandage/dressing by cutting it and soaking with saline solution or water
- Perform debridement of wound, as appropriate
- Apply topical agents to the wound, as needed
- Place an occlusive dressing without exerting compression
- Position to preserve functionality of limbs and joints to avoid retraction
- Provide adequate pain control with pharmacological and non-pharmacological measures
- Provide skin care to donor and graft sites
- Ensure adequate nutritional and fluid intake
- Administer gamma-globulin to avoid fluid shifts, as needed
- Help the patient determine the true extent of the physical and functional changes
- Offer the patient cosmetic correction options
- Recommend methods to protect affected part
- Help the patient accept the physical changes and adapt to lifestyle (e.g., sexual, family, employment, and social relations)
- Provide acceptance and emotional support throughout care

5th edition 2008

Background Evidence:

Badger, J. M. (2001). Burns: the psychological aspects. *American Journal of Nursing, 101*(11), 38–42.

DeSanti, L. (2005). Pathophysiology and current management of burn injury. *Advances in Skin and Wound Care, 18*(6), 323–332.

Flynn, M. B. (2004). Nutritional support for the burn-injured patient. *Critical Care Nursing Clinics of North America, 16*(1), 139–144.

Kavanagh, S., & de Jong, A. (2004). Care of burn patients in the hospital. *Burns, 30*(Suppl. 8), A2–A6.

Pérez, M., Lara, J., Ibáñez, J., Cagigal, L., & León, C.M. (2006). *Guía de Actuación ante el paciente quemado. Málaga, España: Complejo Hospitalario Carlos*

Haya, Unidad de Enfermería de Quemados, Dirección de Enfermería (in Spanish).

Smeltzer, S. C., & Bare, B. G. (2004). *Brunner & Suddarth's textbook of medical-surgical nursing* (10th ed.). Lippincott Williams & Wilkins.

Thompson, J. T., Meredith, J. W., & Molnar, J. A. (2002). The effect of burn nursing units on burn wound infections. *Journal of Burn Care & Rehabilitation, 23*(4), 281–286.

Weddell, R. (2004). Improving pain management for patients in a hospital burns unit. *Nursing Times, 100*(11), 38–40.

Wound Care: Closed Drainage 3662

Definition: Maintenance of a pressure drainage system at the wound site

Activities:

- Gather necessary equipment and supplies at bedside (e.g., calibrated specimen cup, absorbent pad, and gloves)
- Assist patient to comfortable position
- Avoid transfer of microorganisms (i.e., wash hands and don clean disposable gloves)
- Expose catheter insertion site and tubing, placing drainage system on absorbent pad
- Check pump and catheter for patency, seal, and stability, being careful to avoid inadvertent removal of sutures, if present
- Monitor for signs of infection, inflammation, and discomfort around drain
- Notify appropriate health care provider of occluded catheter, signs of infection or discomfort, dislodged tubing, and full drainage system
- Remove plug or disconnect tubing, depending on drainage system type (e.g., Hemovac or Jackson-Pratt)
- Empty drainage into specimen cup, avoiding contamination of drainage spout
- Clean drainage spout using antiseptic swab

- Compress drainage system and hold tightly while reinserting plug or connecting tubing
- Position system appropriately (i.e., avoid kinking of tubing and secure to patient's clothing or bedding, as appropriate)
- Record the volume and characteristics of the drainage (e.g., color, consistency, and odor)
- Compress system to provide suction at regular time intervals, according to institutional policy
- Number the collection devices, if more than one exists
- Discard soiled items in an appropriate manner

1st edition 1992; revised 2013

Background Evidence:

Craven, R. F., & Hirnle, C. J. (2009). Skin integrity and wound healing. *In Fundamentals of nursing: Human health and function* (pp. 989–1032) (6th ed.). Lippincott Williams & Wilkins.

Smith, S. F., Duell, D. J., & Martin, B. C. (2008). Wound care and dressings. In *Clinical nursing skills: Basic to advanced skills* (pp. 874–938) (7th ed.). Pearson: Prentice Hall.

Wound Care: Nonhealing 3664

Definition: Palliative care and prevention of complications of a malignant or other wound that is not expected to heal

Activities:

- Provide adequate pain control (e.g., relaxation, distraction, analgesic therapy to be administered before and after dressing)
- Agree to take breaks while carrying out procedures on the ulcer
- Soak dressing pads in saline solution before removal, when appropriate
- Describe the characteristics of the ulcer, noting the size, location, discharge, color, bleeding, pain, odor, and any edema
- Record changes observed in the evolution of the ulcer
- Note signs and symptoms of wound infection
- Note signs of dermatitis in peri-ulcerous skin, using barrier creams, where appropriate
- Irrigate the ulcer with water or saline solution, avoiding excessive pressure
- Avoid wiping when cleansing
- Avoid the use of antiseptics
- Clean the ulcer, starting with the cleanest zone and moving toward the dirtiest
- Gently pat the peri-ulcerous skin dry

- Avoid chemical or mechanical tissue removal
- Apply topical medication (e.g., cytostatic, antibiotic, analgesic), as required
- Use activated carbon dressings, if appropriate
- Use highly absorbent dressings in cases of abundant discharge
- Install a drainage device, as needed
- Apply manual pressure on bleeding points or potential bleeding zones
- Discuss with the patient the most worrying aspect of the ulcer
- Ascertain the impact the ulcer is having on the patient's quality of life (e.g., sleep, appetite, activity, humor, relationships)
- Demonstrate to the patient or family members the procedure for caring for the ulcer, as appropriate
- Instruct the patient and family about the signs of infection
- Help the patient and family obtain the necessary dressing materials
- Demonstrate to the patient and family how to dispose of used dressings

W

- Demonstrate methods for protecting the wound from blows, pressure, and friction (e.g., use of pillows, cushions, pads)
- Encourage the patient to engage in social activities, exercise, and relaxation, as appropriate
- Encourage the patient to look at the body part that has undergone the change
- Provide the patient and family caregiver with emotional support
- Identify methods of reducing the impact caused by any disfigurement through the use of clothing, if appropriate
- Help the patient take greater responsibility with self-care, to the extent possible
- Encourage the patient and family to play an active role in treatment and rehabilitation, as appropriate

6th edition 2013

Background Evidence:

Carroll, M. C., Fleming, M., Chitambar, C. R., & Neuburg, M. (2002). Diagnosis workup and prognosis of cutaneous metastases of unknown primary origin. *Dermatologic Surgery, 28*(6), 533–535.

Cormio, G., Capotorto, M., Vagno, G., Cazzolla, A., Carriero, C., & Selvaggi, L. (2003). Skin metastases in ovarian carcinoma: A report of nine cases and a review of the literature. *Gynecologic Oncology, 90*(3), 682–685.

Emmons, K. R., & Lachman, V. D. (2010). Palliative wound care: A concept analysis. *Journal of Wound, Ostomy, and Continence Nursing, 37*(6), 639–644.

Ferris, F. D., Al Khateib, A., Fromantin, I., Hoplamazian, L., Hurd, T., Krasner, D., Maida, V., Price, P., & Rich-Vanderbij, L. (2007). Palliative wound care: Managing chronic wounds across life's continuum: A consensus statement from the International Palliative Wound Care Initiative. *Journal of Palliative Medicine, 10*(1), 37–39.

Langemo, D., Anderson, J., Hanson, D., Thompson, P., & Hunter, S. (2007). Understanding palliative wound care. *Nursing, 37*(1), 65–66.

Lookingbill, D. P., Spangler, N., & Helm, K. F. (1993). Cutaneous metastases in patients with metastatic carcinoma: A retrospective study of 4020 patients. *Journal of the American Academy of Dermatology, 29*(2 Pt 1), 228–236.

Lund-Nielsen, B., Müller, K., & Adamsen, L. (2005). Malignant wounds in women with breast cancer: Feminine and sexual perspectives. *Journal of Clinical Nursing, 14*(1), 56–64.

Seaman, S. (2006). Management of malignant fungating wounds in advanced cancer. *Seminars in Oncology Nursing, 22*(3), 185–193.

Wound Care: Protection 3670

Definition: Placement of dressing to cover or support a wound to immobilize, compress, prevent further harm, and promote healing

Activities:

- Determine type and size of covering needed (e.g., packing, dry, wet, abdominal, sling, elastic wrap)
- Explain procedure including purpose for dressing or bandage
- Administer analgesic 30 to 60 minutes prior to application, as indicated
- Place in appropriate position to apply dressing (e.g., supine for abdominal, sitting for sling or extremity wrap)
- Provide for adequate privacy
- Remove any previous bandages or wraps
- Cleanse area while avoiding contamination of wound and keeping surrounding area sterile
- Inspect condition of any wound, including size, location, exudate, or swelling
- Apply topical treatments, as prescribed
- Apply loose woven gauze as contact layer and add additional layers of gauze as needed, finishing with thicker woven pad
- Use split gauze around drains
- Pack damp fine mesh or open weave gauze into deep wounds assuring all wound surfaces are in contact with moist gauze; cover with loose woven gauze and thicker woven pad
- Apply adhesive over gauze and beyond dressing
- Use nonallergenic adhesive if necessary
- Use protective window of stoma adhesive or hydrocolloid pad as adhesive barrier, if indicated by skin irritation
- Use roller gauze or elastic net to secure extremity dressings
- Elevate dependent extremities for 15 minutes before applying elastic wrap
- Apply elastic wrap beginning at distal body part and wrap toward proximal boundary
- Wrap with appropriate binder or elastic wrap if needed to support wound healing
- Use triangle, recurrent, or cravat bandaging to secure or support dressings in unusually shaped areas (e.g., ear, crown of head, armpit, jaw, hip)
- Use figure of eight, spiral or circular wrap technique when wound pressure needed
- Check wrapped area frequently during application to ensure not too tight and remaining in proper alignment or splinting position
- Apply abdominal or breast binder by laying or rolling person onto dressing and wrapping from back to front
- Use body landmarks to ensure proper position of dressing (e.g., symphysis pubis, costal margins, joints)
- Use padding over bony prominences underneath dressings, as needed
- Evaluate distal circulation with extremity dressing application, at least twice more in next 8 hours, and then every 8 hours
- Evaluate ability to breathe deeply and cough effectively when abdominal or breast dressing application complete
- Reapply, adjust, or remove dressing or binders if any compromise to circulation or breathing noted
- Remove dressings to assess wound and circulation at least every 8 hours
- Label dressing with date, time, initials
- Document level of comfort, circulation status, appearance and size of wound, type of dressing applied, presence of swelling and range of motion, ability to ventilate properly, as applicable
- Instruct on care and application of dressings
- Use teach-back to ensure understanding

8th edition 2024

W

Background Evidence:

Berman, A., Snyder, S. J., & Frandsen, G. (2018). Skin integrity and wound care. In *Kozier and Erb's Fundamentals of nursing: Concepts, process and practice* (pp. 837–857) (10th ed.). Pearson.

Boon, C. J. W. (2021). Skin integrity and wound care. In P. A. Potter, A. G. Perry, P. A. Stockert, & A. M. Hall (Eds.), *Fundamentals of nursing* (10th ed., pp. 1176–1206). Elsevier.

Brock, G. (2018). The fine points of taping. *Canadian Journal of Rural Medicine, 23*(2), 52–55.

Craven, R. F., Hirnle, C. J., & Henshaw, C. J. (2021). *Fundamentals of nursing: Human health and function* (8th ed.). Wolters-Kluwer.

Dowsett, C., Bain, K., Hoffmann, C., Brennan, M. R., Greco, A., Karlsmark, T., Keast, D., Liberato de Moura, M. R., Lázaro-Martínez, J. L., Münter, K.,

Swanson, T., Vuagnat, H., & Bain, M. (2021). The Wound Care Pathway – An evidence-based and step-by-step approach towards wound healing. *Wounds International, 12*(3), 78–85.

Fulcher, E., & Gopee, N. (2020). Effect of different compression bandaging techniques on the healing rate of venous leg ulcers: a literature review. *British Journal of Community Nursing, 25*(Sup6), S20–S26.

Milne, C., Thomason, H., & Hughes, M. (2020). Managing highly exuding wounds: Removing the risk of infection. *Wounds International, 11*(3), 42–48.

Perry, A. G., Potter, P. A., Ostendorf, W. R., & LaPlante, N. (2021). *Clinical nursing skills and technique* (10th ed.). Mosby.

Williams, M. (2021). Wound infections: An overview. *British Journal of Community Nursing, 26*(Sup6), S22–S25.

Wound Irrigation   3680

Definition: Rinsing or washing out wound with solution

Activities:

- Gather necessary equipment and supplies at bedside (e.g., sterile irrigation set, waterproof pad, sterile basin, sterile irrigating solution, sterile gloves, and equipment for dressing change)
- Identify any allergies related to products used
- Explain the procedure to the patient
- Provide analgesics before wound care, as needed
- Assist patient to comfortable position, being sure solution will flow by gravity from least to most contaminated area into collection basin
- Place waterproof pad and bath blankets under patient
- Perform hand hygiene
- Don mask, goggles, and gown, if needed
- Remove dressing and inspect wound and surrounding tissue, reporting abnormalities to appropriate health care provider (e.g., infection and necrosis)
- Pour prescribed irrigating solution into sterile irrigation container, being sure to warm solution to body temperature
- Don sterile gloves
- Open irrigating syringe and place into container with solution
- Place sterile basin at distal end of wound
- Fill irrigating syringe with solution
- Avoid aspirating the solution back into the syringe
- Flush wound gently with solution until solution in bin runs clear, being sure to hold syringe tip 1 inch above wound and rinse from least to most contaminated area
- Attach sterile latex or silicone catheter to filled syringe, when necessary (to irrigate deep wounds)
- Avoid forcing the catheter into an abdominal wound to prevent perforation of the intestine
- Refill irrigation syringe with solution, maintaining sterility (i.e., when using catheter, disconnect catheter, fill syringe, and reconnect catheter)
- Open commercial cleaning solution package if using for irrigation and use according to instructions
- Cleanse and dry surrounding skin after procedure
- Institute appropriate care of wound or burn
- Apply sterile dressing
- Pack the wound with the appropriate type of sterile dressing
- Monitor patient's pain, tolerance, comfort, and anxiety levels during procedure
- Maintain a sterile field during procedure, as appropriate (e.g., use assistants to prevent child from moving and contaminating wound or sterile field and instruct child not to touch wound)
- Instruct patient or family performing procedure at home on appropriate technique and necessary modifications (e.g., stress importance of washing hands before and after irrigation when sterile technique not used)
- Discard items in an appropriate manner

1st edition 1992; revised 2013

Background Evidence:

Craven, R. F., & Hirnle, C. J. (2009). Skin integrity and wound healing. *In Fundamentals of nursing: Human health and function* (pp. 989–1032) (6th ed.). Lippincott Williams & Wilkins.

Smith, S. F., Duell, D. J., & Martin, B. C. (2008). Wound care and dressings. *In Clinical nursing skills: Basic to advanced skills* (pp. 874–938) (7th ed.). Pearson: Prentice Hall.

W

Yoga   6050

Definition: Guiding an individual or group to perform repetitive physical movements, postures, meditation, breathing, and relaxation techniques

Activities:

- Evaluate willingness and functional ability for engaging in yoga
- Screen for contraindications that limit or prohibit participation (e.g., deep vein thrombosis, spinal surgery, inflammation, areas with open lesions)
- Describe types of yoga including benefits, and limits of each type (e.g., Yin, hot, aerial, pre-natal, barre, ashtanga)
- Identify personal and mutual purpose or goal (e.g., increase awareness, flexibility, empathy, relaxation, reduction of stress)
- Select routine and style of yoga to achieve goals
- Select specific areas of body to be addressed by movements
- Create calm, comfortable, private space
- Provide yoga mat and appropriate music
- Limit unnecessary distractions (e.g., light, noise, visitors)
- Recommend comfortable clothes and absence of restricting items (e.g., belt, shoes)
- Avoid eating 2 hours before practice
- Avoid drinking water during practice
- Explain what foods can be eaten before practice if needed (e.g., easily digestible foods, whole grain carbohydrates, high protein foods)
- Allow for modification of poses and use of props (e.g., blankets, chairs) for those who would benefit from modifications (e.g., pregnant, older adults)
- Assist in attaining initial comfortable position with focus on balance
- Encourage to center self (e.g., focus with few deep breaths, focus awareness of inner self, relax mind and body, attune to earth's energy)
- Discuss basic components of yoga (e.g., initial breathing exercises, various poses for strengthening, flexibility and balance, final meditative period)
- Instruct on initial breathing exercises (e.g., awareness of current pattern, posture and relation to breathing, structural changes on inhalation, contraction of muscles during exhalation, smooth pattern, focus on breathing when attention wanders)
- Advise to stare at fixed point or close eyes
- Encourage concentration and breathing pattern focus to any region with pain or discomfort
- Instruct on pose techniques (e.g., ensure 15 minutes of poses, mix poses [standing, seated, kneeling, supine, prone], alternate with period of relaxation)
- Acknowledge some pain and discomfort often unavoidable during poses
- Encourage forward bends, back bends, side bends, twists, inversions, and balances during pose transitions
- End session using Savasana pose (i.e., laying on back, placing feet on mat in relaxed open position, relaxing arms a few inches away from body with palms facing upward, tuck chin half toward chest to lengthen back of neck, closing eyes, deep breathing with focus on letting go of energy expended)
- Determine ability to increase frequency and duration of practice and integrate into daily routines
- Encourage increase of meditation time by short interval each time of practice and integration into regular sessions
- Identify conditions that cause discomfort before and after (e.g., fatigue, alertness, stress, presence of other persons)
- Monitor physical, social, mental, emotional, and spiritual responses during session
- Provide feedback related to energetic work in understandable terms
- Encourage focus on what can be done, not deficiencies
- Use teach back to ensure understanding

8th edition 2024

Background Evidence:

Bukar, N. K., Eberhardt, L. M., & Davidson, J. (2019). East meets west in psychiatry: Yoga as an adjunct therapy for management of anxiety. *Archives of Psychiatric Nursing*, 33(4), 371–376.

Kupershmidt, S., & Barnable, T. (2019). Definition of a yoga breathing (Pranayama) protocol that improves lung function. *Holistic Nursing Practice*, 33(4), 197–203.

Malarvizhi, M., Maheshkumar, K., Bhavani, M., & Hariprasad, B. (2019). Effect of 6 months of yoga practice on quality of life among patients with asthma: A randomized control trial. *Advances in Integrative Medicine*, 6(4), 163–166. https://doi.org/10.1016/j.aimed.2018.12.001

Mascaro, J. S., Waller, A. V., Wright, L., Leonard, T., Haack, C., & Waller, E. K. (2019). Individualized, single session yoga therapy to reduce physical and emotional symptoms in hospitalized hematological cancer patients. *Integrative Cancer Therapies*, 18, 1–8. https://doi.org/10.1177/1534735419861692

Stephens, M. (2017). *Yoga therapy: Foundations, methods, and practices for common ailments*. North Atlantic Books.

Wiles, A. K., Van Puymbroeck, M., Crowe, B. M., & Schmid, A. A. (2021). An investigation into the use of yoga in recreational therapy practice. *Therapeutic Recreation Journal*, 55(1), 78–96. https://doi.org/10.18666/TRJ-2021-V55-I1-10145

Y

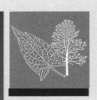

## PART FOUR

Core Interventions for Nursing Specialty Areas

Core Interventions For Nursing Specialty Areas

In this section, the core interventions for 57 specialty areas are listed alphabetically. Core interventions are defined as a limited, central set of interventions that define the nature of the specialty. A person reading the list of core interventions would be able to determine the area of specialty practice. The core set of interventions does *not* include all the interventions used by nurses in the specialty; rather, the set includes those interventions used frequently or predominantly by nurses in the specialty, or those that are critical to the role of the specialty nurse.

This list of specialty core interventions initially resulted from a survey to nurses belonging to specialty organizations who were asked to validate if appropriate for use. The research and an initial list of core interventions for 39 specialty areas were published in the third edition of Nursing Interventions Classification (NIC). New specialties as well as updates including new interventions were added in subsequent editions.

For this edition, each specialty list was reviewed and updated with new and missing core interventions, and four new specialties were added: Disaster Nursing, Informatics Nursing, Legal Nurse Consulting, and Travel Health Nursing. The entire list of 57 specialties for which core interventions are identified follows:

1. Addictions Nursing
2. Ambulatory Care Nursing
3. Burn Nursing
4. Camp Nursing
5. Child and Adolescent Psychiatric Nursing
6. College Health Nursing
7. Community Public Health Nursing
8. Correctional Care Nursing
9. Critical Care Nursing
10. Dermatology Nursing
11. Developmental Disability Nursing
12. Diabetes Nursing
13. Disaster Nursing
14. Domestic Violence Nursing
15. Emergency Nursing
16. Faith Community Nursing
17. Flight Nursing
18. Forensic Nursing
19. Gastroenterological Nursing
20. Genetics Nursing
21. Gerontological Nursing
22. HIV/AIDS Care Nursing
23. Holistic Nursing
24. Home Health Nursing
25. Hospice and Palliative Care Nursing
26. Infection Control and Epidemiology Nursing
27. Informatics Nursing
28. Infusion Nursing
29. Legal Nursing
30. Medical-Surgical Nursing
31. Midwifery Nursing
32. Neonatal Nursing
33. Nephrology Nursing
34. Neuroscience Nursing
35. Nurse Anesthesiology/Post Anesthesia Care Nursing
36. Obstetric Nursing
37. Occupational Health Nursing
38. Oncology Nursing
39. Ophthalmic Nursing
40. Orthopedic Nursing
41. Otorhinolaryngology and Head/Neck Nursing
42. Pain Management Nursing
43. Pediatric Nursing
44. Pediatric Hematology/Oncology Nursing
45. Perioperative Nursing
46. Plastic Surgery Nursing
47. Psychiatric/Mental Health Nursing
48. Radiology Nursing
49. Rehabilitation Nursing
50. School Nursing
51. Spinal Cord Injury Nursing
52. Transplant Nursing
53. Travel Health Nursing
54. Urologic Nursing
55. Vascular Nursing
56. Women's Health Nursing
57. Wound, Ostomy, and Continence Nursing

The identification of core interventions by specialty helps to communicate the nature of nursing in different practice areas. The listing of core interventions by specialty areas of practice is very useful in the development of nursing information systems, staff education programs, staff competency evaluations, referral networks, certification or licensing examinations, nursing school curricula, and research and theory construction. We encourage members of specialty organizations who are interested in building clinical databases to use the interventions contained in

NIC so that nurses can achieve the benefits inherent in a standardized language. We welcome the submission of new interventions as users see the need, as well as the submission of new specialty organizations as they arise.

Addictions Nursing

- Active Listening
- Anger Control Assistance
- Anticipatory Guidance
- Assertiveness Training
- Behavior Contracting
- Behavior Management
- Behavior Modification: Social Skills
- Body Search
- Capillary Blood Sample
- Chemical Restraint
- Commendation
- Conflict Mediation
- Coping Enhancement
- Counseling
- De-Escalation Management
- Delirium Management
- Discharge Planning
- Eating Disorders Management
- Elopement Precautions
- Environmental Management: Safety
- Family Therapy
- Fluid/Electrolyte Management
- Forgiveness Facilitation
- Guilt Work Facilitation
- Health Coaching
- Health Education
- Health Screening
- Hope Inspiration
- Impulse Control Training
- Journaling
- Life Skills Enhancement
- Limit Setting
- Medication Administration
- Medication Management
- Nutrition Management
- Pain Management: Chronic
- Recreation Therapy
- Referral
- Relapse Prevention
- Risk Identification
- Self-Awareness Enhancement
- Self-Esteem Enhancement
- Self-Responsibility Facilitation
- Smoking Cessation Assistance
- Socialization Enhancement
- Spiritual Support
- Substance Use Prevention
- Substance Use Treatment
- Substance Use Treatment: Alcohol Withdrawal
- Substance Use Treatment: Drug Withdrawal
- Substance Use Treatment: Overdose
- Support Group
- Teaching: Disease Process
- Teaching: Group
- Teaching: Safe Sex
- Therapy Group
- Vital Signs Monitoring

Ambulatory Care Nursing

- Anxiety Reduction
- Behavior Modification
- Capillary Blood Sample
- Case Management
- Coping Enhancement
- Decision-Making Support
- Delegation
- Discharge Follow-Up
- Documentation
- Documentation: Meetings
- Electronic Health Record Access Assistance
- Emotional Support
- Examination Assistance
- Health Care Provider Collaboration
- Health Coaching
- Health Education
- Health Literacy Enhancement
- Health Screening
- Health System Guidance
- IV Therapy
- Medication Administration: Intradermal
- Medication Administration: Intramuscular (IM)
- Medication Administration: Intravenous (IV)
- Medication Administration: Oral
- Medication Management
- Medication Prescribing
- Nutritional Counseling
- Point of Care Testing
- Prescribing: Diagnostic Testing
- Prescribing: Nonpharmacologic Treatment
- Referral
- Risk Identification
- Surveillance
- Staff Supervision
- Teaching: Adolescent Development
- Teaching: Adolescent Nutrition
- Teaching: Adolescent Safety
- Teaching: Disease Process
- Teaching: Early Childhood Development
- Teaching: Early Childhood Nutrition

- Teaching: Early Childhood Safety
- Teaching: Individual
- Teaching: Infant Development 0–3 Months
- Teaching: Infant Development 4–6 Months
- Teaching: Infant Development 7–9 Months
- Teaching: Infant Development 10–12 Months
- Teaching: Middle Childhood Development
- Teaching: Middle Childhood Nutrition
- Teaching: Middle Childhood Safety
- Teaching: Prescribed Diet
- Teaching: Prescribed Medication
- Teaching: Procedure or Treatment
- Telecommunication Consultation
- Transgender Hormone Therapy
- Transport: Interfacility
- Triage: Emergency Center
- Triage: Telecommunication
- Vaccination Management
- Vision Screening
- Vital Signs Monitoring
- Wound Care: Protection

Burn Nursing

- Bathing
- Bed Rest Care
- Body Image Enhancement
- Comfort Management
- Coping Enhancement
- Electrolyte Management
- Emotional Support
- Family Involvement Promotion
- Fluid Management
- Fluid Monitoring
- Grief Work Facilitation
- Hope Inspiration
- Infection Control
- Intravenous Therapy
- Medication Administration
- Medication Administration: Intravenous (IV)
- Medication Administration: Skin
- Medication Management
- Nutrition Therapy
- Pain Management: Acute
- Pain Management: Chronic
- Positioning
- Self-Care Assistance
- Shock Management: Sepsis
- Skin Care: Donor Site
- Skin Care: Graft Site
- Skin Surveillance
- Teaching: Procedure or Treatment
- Temperature Regulation
- Vital Signs Monitoring
- Wound Care
- Wound Care: Burns
- Wound Care: Protection

Camp Nursing

- Allergy Management
- Anxiety Reduction
- Behavior Modification: Social Skills
- Bleeding Reduction
- Conflict Mediation
- Counseling
- Documentation
- Emergency Care
- Emotional Support
- First Aid
- Heat/Cold Application
- Humor
- Hyperthermia Management
- Infection Control
- Life Skills Enhancement
- Limit Setting
- Medication Administration: Oral
- Medication Management
- Pain Management: Acute
- Referral
- Risk Identification
- Skin Surveillance
- Suicide Prevention
- Teaching: Adolescent Development
- Teaching: Adolescent Nutrition
- Teaching: Adolescent Safety
- Teaching: Middle Childhood Development
- Teaching: Middle Childhood Nutrition
- Teaching: Middle Childhood Safety
- Teaching: Sports-Injury Prevention
- Telecommunication Consultation
- Vital Signs Monitoring
- Wound Care

Child and Adolescent Psychiatric Nursing

- Abuse Protection Support: Child
- Activity Therapy
- Adolescent Care
- Art Therapy
- Behavior Management: Inattention and Hyperactivity
- Behavior Management: Self-Harm
- Behavior Management: Sexual
- Behavior Modification: Social Skills
- Body Search
- Bowel Incontinence Care: Encopresis
- Caring Interaction Development
- Case Management
- Child Care
- Conflict Mediation
- Dance Therapy
- De-Escalation Management
- Delusion Management
- Elopement Precautions
- Environmental Management: Community
- Family Involvement Promotion
- Family Mobilization
- Family Process Maintenance
- Family Therapy
- Guided Reflection
- Health Education
- Health Literacy Enhancement
- Human Trafficking Detection
- Impulse Control Training
- Life Skills Enhancement
- Medication Management
- Medication Prescribing
- Mood Management
- Multidisciplinary Care Conference
- Normalization Promotion
- Parenting Promotion
- Physical Accompaniment
- Resilience Promotion
- Staff Supervision
- Teaching: Adolescent Development
- Teaching: Adolescent Nutrition
- Teaching: Adolescent Safety
- Teaching: Early Childhood Development
- Teaching: Early Childhood Nutrition
- Teaching: Early Childhood Safety
- Teaching: Middle Childhood Development
- Teaching: Middle Childhood Nutrition
- Teaching: Middle Childhood Safety
- Teaching: Prescribed Medication
- Telecommunication Consultation
- Transgender Hormone Therapy
- Trauma Therapy: Child
- Urinary Incontinence Care: Enuresis

College Health Nursing

- Active Listening
- Anxiety Reduction
- Asthma Management
- Communicable Disease Management
- Coping Enhancement
- Counseling
- Crisis Intervention
- Decision-Making Support
- Eating Disorders Management
- Emotional Support
- First Aid
- Health Coaching
- Health Education
- Health Screening
- Health System Guidance
- Medication Administration: Subcutaneous
- Medication Management
- Medication Prescribing
- Nutrition Management
- Prescribing: Diagnostic Testing
- Prescribing: Nonpharmacologic Treatment
- Referral
- Self-Esteem Enhancement
- Sexual Assault Trauma Care
- Sexual Counseling
- Sleep Enhancement
- Smoking Cessation Assistance
- Substance Use Prevention
- Suicide Prevention
- Teaching: Individual
- Teaching: Safe Sex
- Teaching: Sexuality
- Teaching: Sports-Injury Prevention
- Vaccination Management
- Vehicle Safety Promotion
- Vision Screening
- Weight Management

Community Public Health Nursing

- Abuse Protection Support
- Bioterrorism Preparedness
- Case Management
- Collaboration Enhancement
- Community Disaster Preparedness
- Community Health Advocacy
- Community Health Development
- Consultation

- Cultural Care Negotiation
- Discharge Planning: Home Preparation
- Environmental Management: Community
- Environmental Management: Worker Safety
- Environmental Risk Protection
- Family Planning: Contraception
- Fiscal Resource Management
- Health Care Information Exchange
- Health Care Provider Collaboration
- Health Education
- Health Literacy Enhancement
- Health Policy Monitoring
- Health Screening
- Health System Guidance
- Home Maintenance Assistance
- Human Trafficking Detection
- Medication Administration
- Pandemic Precautions
- Parenting Promotion
- Program Development
- Quarantine Facilitation
- Readmission Prevention
- Referral
- Resilience Promotion: Community
- Risk Identification
- Risk Identification: Infectious Disease
- Social Justice Facilitation
- Social Marketing
- Surveillance: Community
- Sustenance Support
- Teaching: Adolescent Development
- Teaching: Adolescent Nutrition
- Teaching: Adolescent Safety
- Teaching: Early Childhood Development
- Teaching: Early Childhood Nutrition
- Teaching: Early Childhood Safety
- Teaching: Group
- Teaching: Infant Development 0–3 Months
- Teaching: Infant Development 4–6 Months
- Teaching: Infant Development 7–9 Months
- Teaching: Infant Development 10–12 Months
- Teaching: Infant Nutrition 0–3 Months
- Teaching: Infant Nutrition 4–6 Months
- Teaching: Infant Nutrition 7–9 Months
- Teaching: Infant Nutrition 10–12 Months
- Teaching: Infant Safety 0–3 Months
- Teaching: Infant Safety 4–6 Months
- Teaching: Infant Safety 7–9 Months
- Teaching: Infant Safety 10–12 Months
- Teaching: Middle Childhood Development
- Teaching: Middle Childhood Nutrition
- Teaching: Middle Childhood Safety
- Teaching: Safe Sex
- Teaching: Toddler Nutrition 13–18 Months
- Teaching: Toddler Nutrition 19–24 Months
- Teaching: Toddler Nutrition 25–36 Months
- Teaching: Toddler Safety 13–18 Months
- Teaching: Toddler Safety 19–24 Months
- Teaching: Toddler Safety 25–36 Months
- Vaccination Management
- Vehicle Safety Promotion

Correctional Care Nursing

- Active Listening
- Anger Control Assistance
- Area Restriction
- Behavior Contracting
- Body Search
- Caring Interaction Development
- Commendation
- Coping Enhancement
- Counseling
- Cultural Care Negotiation
- De-Escalation Management
- Emergency Care
- Emotional Support
- Environmental Management: Violence Prevention
- Environmental Risk Protection
- Family Integrity Promotion
- First Aid
- Forgiveness Facilitation
- Health Care Information Exchange
- Health Policy Monitoring
- Health Screening
- Hope Inspiration
- Humor
- Life Skills Enhancement
- Limit Setting
- Medication Administration
- Medication Management
- Nutrition Management
- Physical Accompaniment
- Presence
- Program Development
- Referral
- Relapse Prevention
- Skin Surveillance
- Substance Use Prevention
- Substance Use Treatment
- Substance Use Treatment: Alcohol Withdrawal
- Substance Use Treatment: Drug Withdrawal
- Substance Use Treatment: Overdose
- Suicide Prevention
- Surveillance
- Teaching: Group
- Teaching: Individual
- Teaching: Prescribed Medication
- Teaching: Safe Sex
- Wound Care

Critical Care Nursing

- Acid-Base Monitoring
- Advanced Care Planning
- Airway Management
- Airway Suctioning
- Analgesic Administration
- Anxiety Reduction
- Artificial Airway Management
- Bereavement Care
- Cardiac Care: Acute
- Cardiac Risk Management
- Caregiver Support
- Central Venous Access Management: Central Insertion
- Central Venous Access Management: Peripheral Insertion
- Circulatory Care: Mechanical Assist Device
- Code Management
- Decision-Making Support
- Defibrillator Management: External
- Defibrillator Management: Internal
- Delegation
- Discharge Planning
- Documentation
- Electrolyte Management
- Electrolyte Monitoring
- Emotional Support
- Endotracheal Extubation: Palliative
- Extracorporeal Membrane Oxygenation (ECMO) Therapy
- Family Involvement Promotion
- Family Presence Facilitation
- Fluid Management
- Fluid Monitoring
- Fluid/Electrolyte Management
- Health Care Provider Collaboration
- Hemodynamic Regulation
- Intracranial Pressure (ICP) Monitoring
- Intravenous (IV) Therapy
- Invasive Hemodynamic Monitoring
- Mechanical Ventilation Management: Invasive
- Mechanical Ventilation Management: Noninvasive
- Mechanical Ventilation Management: Pneumonia Prevention
- Mechanical Ventilatory Weaning
- Medication Administration
- Medication Administration: Intravenous (IV)
- Multidisciplinary Care Conference
- Nausea Management
- Neurologic Monitoring
- Oxygen Therapy
- Pacemaker Management: Permanent
- Pacemaker Management: Temporary
- Pain Management: Acute
- Pain Management: Chronic
- Patient Rights Protection
- Positioning
- Positioning: Prone
- Rapid Sequence Intubation
- Readmission Prevention
- Respiratory Monitoring
- Sedation Management
- Shock Management
- Shock Management: Sepsis
- Teaching: Procedure or Treatment
- Technology Management
- Temperature Regulation
- Thermoregulation Management
- Thrombolytic Therapy Management
- Transport: Interfacility
- Transport: Intrafacility
- Visitation Facilitation
- Vital Signs Monitoring
- Vomiting Management

Dermatology Nursing

- Behavior Modification
- Body Image Enhancement
- Coping Enhancement
- Decision-Making Support
- Documentation
- Emotional Support
- Environmental Management: Community
- Examination Assistance
- Health Care Provider Collaboration
- Health Education
- Health Screening
- Incision Site Care
- Infection Control
- Laser Precautions
- Learning Facilitation
- Medication Administration: Skin
- Phototherapy: Skin
- Pressure Injury Care
- Pruritus Management
- Self-Responsibility Facilitation
- Skin Care: Absorbent Products
- Skin Care: Donor Site
- Skin Care: Graft Site
- Skin Care: Topical Treatment
- Skin Surveillance
- Support System Enhancement
- Surgical Assistance
- Teaching: Disease Process
- Teaching: Prescribed Medication
- Teaching: Procedure or Treatment
- Telecommunication Consultation
- Wound Care
- Wound Irrigation

Developmental Disability Nursing

- Abuse Protection Support
- Adolescent Care
- Anxiety Reduction
- Aspiration Precautions
- Behavior Management
- Behavior Management: Self-Harm
- Behavior Modification: Social Skills
- Bowel Management
- Case Management
- Child Care
- Communication Enhancement: Hearing Deficit
- Communication Enhancement: Speech Deficit
- Communication Enhancement: Visual Deficit
- De-Escalation Management
- Developmental Enhancement: Infant
- Discharge Follow-Up
- Documentation
- Environmental Management: Safety
- Family Involvement Promotion
- Financial Resource Assistance
- Functional Ability Enhancement
- Health Coaching
- Health Education
- Health Literacy Enhancement
- Health Screening
- Incident Reporting
- Infection Control
- Life Skills Enhancement
- Medication Administration
- Medication Management
- Multidisciplinary Care Conference
- Normalization Promotion
- Nutrition Management
- Patient Rights Protection
- Relocation Stress Reduction
- Risk Identification: Genetic
- Seizure Management
- Seizure Precautions
- Self-Care Assistance
- Social Justice Facilitation
- Staff Supervision
- Teaching: Prescribed Medication
- Teaching: Safe Sex
- Telecommunication Consultation
- Weight Management

Diabetes Nursing

- Amputation Care
- Behavior Contracting
- Caregiver Support
- Case Management
- Decision-Making Support
- Discharge Follow-Up
- Exercise Promotion
- Family Involvement Promotion
- Financial Resource Assistance
- Foot Care
- Health Coaching
- Health Education
- Health Screening
- Health System Guidance
- Hyperglycemia Management
- Hyperlipidemia Management
- Hypertension Management
- Hypoglycemia Management
- Infection Control
- Lower Extremity Monitoring
- Medication Administration: Continuous Subcutaneous Infusion
- Medication Management
- Medication Management: Wearable Infusion Device
- Multidisciplinary Care Conference
- Mutual Goal Setting
- Nutrition Management
- Nutritional Counseling
- Nutritional Monitoring
- Pressure Injury Care
- Pressure Injury Prevention
- Risk Identification
- Skin Surveillance
- Smoking Cessation Assistance
- Support Group
- Teaching: Disease Process
- Teaching: Prescribed Diet
- Teaching: Prescribed Medication
- Teaching: Procedure or Treatment
- Telecommunication Consultation
- Weight Management
- Weight Reduction Assistance
- Wound Care: Nonhealing

Disaster Nursing

- Admission Care
- Bioterrorism Preparedness
- Calming Technique
- Community Disaster Preparedness
- Community Health Advocacy
- Community Health Development
- Coping Enhancement
- Counseling

- Crisis Intervention
- Emergency Care
- Emotional Support
- Environment Management: Community
- Environment Risk Protection
- Environmental Management: Safety
- Family Presence Facilitation
- First Aid
- Grief Work Facilitation
- Health Policy Monitoring
- Health Screening
- Hope Enhancement
- Pandemic Precautions
- Quarantine Facilitation
- Resilience Promotion: Community
- Risk Identification
- Social Justice Facilitation
- Spiritual Support
- Support Group
- Support System Enhancement
- Transfer
- Trauma Therapy Child
- Triage: Disaster
- Triage: Emergency Center
- Triage: Telecommunication

Domestic Violence Nursing

- Abuse Protection Support: Child
- Abuse Protection Support: Domestic Partner
- Abuse Protection Support: Elder
- Active Listening
- Anxiety Reduction
- Assertiveness Training
- Calming Technique
- Conflict Mediation
- Communicable Disease Management
- Consultation
- Coping Enhancement
- Counseling
- Crisis Intervention
- Decision-Making Support
- De-Escalation Management
- Deposition
- Documentation
- Emergency Care
- Emotional Support
- Environmental Management: Violence Prevention
- Family Integrity Promotion
- Family Therapy
- First Aid
- Forensic Data Collection
- Grief Work Facilitation
- Health Care Information Exchange
- Health Screening
- Health System Guidance
- Hope Inspiration
- Human Trafficking Detection
- Incident Reporting
- Life Skills Enhancement
- Patient Identification
- Sexual Assault Trauma Care
- Referral
- Resilience Promotion: Community
- Risk Identification
- Self-Esteem Enhancement
- Social Justice Facilitation
- Spiritual Support
- Substance Use Prevention
- Support Group
- Teaching: Individual
- Therapy Group
- Triage: Telecommunication

Emergency Nursing

- Abuse Protection Support: Child
- Abuse Protection Support: Domestic Partner
- Advanced Care Planning
- Airway Management
- Anaphylaxis Management
- Bioterrorism Preparedness
- Blood Products Administration
- Bereavement Care
- Cardiac Care: Acute
- Circulatory Care: Arterial Insufficiency
- Circulatory Care: Venous Insufficiency
- Code Management
- Crisis Intervention
- Defibrillator Management: External
- Defibrillator Management: Internal
- Documentation
- Dysrhythmia Management
- Electrolyte Management
- Emergency Care
- Endotracheal Extubation: Palliative
- Family Presence Facilitation
- First Aid
- Fluid/Electrolyte Management
- Fluid Resuscitation
- Forensic Data Collection
- Hyperthermia Management
- Hypovolemia Management
- Human Trafficking Detection
- Intravenous (IV) Insertion
- Intravenous (IV) Therapy
- Mechanical Ventilation Management: Noninvasive
- Medication Administration

- Neurologic Monitoring
- Oxygen Therapy
- Pacemaker Management: Temporary
- Pain Management: Acute
- Pandemic Precautions
- Patient Identification
- Phlebotomy: Venous Blood Sample
- Physical Distancing Facilitation
- Prescribing: Diagnostic Testing
- Quarantine Facilitation
- Rapid Sequence Intubation
- Readmission Prevention
- Respiratory Monitoring
- Resuscitation

- Risk Identification: Infectious Disease
- Seizure Management
- Sexual Assault Trauma Care
- Shock Management
- Shock Management: Sepsis
- Teaching: Individual
- Thrombolytic Therapy Management
- Transport: Interfacility
- Transport: Intrafacility
- Triage: Emergency Center
- Triage: Telecommunication
- Vital Signs Monitoring
- Wound Care

Faith Community Nursing

- Abuse Protection Support
- Active Listening
- Anticipatory Guidance
- Caregiver Support
- Coping Enhancement
- Crisis Intervention
- Cultural Care Negotiation
- Decision-Making Support
- Emotional Support
- Environmental Management: Community
- Family Integrity Promotion
- Family Support
- Forgiveness Facilitation
- Grief Work Facilitation
- Guilt Work Facilitation
- Health Care Information Exchange
- Health Education
- Health Literacy Enhancement
- Health System Guidance
- Hope Inspiration
- Humor

- Listening Visits
- Medication Management
- Presence
- Referral
- Religious Addiction Therapy
- Religious Ritual Enhancement
- Relocation Stress Reduction
- Resilience Promotion
- Resilience Promotion: Community
- Self-Care Assistance
- Social Justice Facilitation
- Socialization Enhancement
- Spiritual Growth Facilitation
- Spiritual Support
- Surveillance
- Sustenance Support
- Teaching: Group
- Teaching: Individual
- Telecommunication Consultation
- Touch
- Values Clarification

Flight Nursing

- Anaphylaxis Management
- Artificial Airway Management
- Bleeding Reduction
- Blood Products Administration
- Cardiac Care: Acute
- Caregiver Support
- Code Management
- Defibrillator Management: External
- Defibrillator Management: Internal
- Emergency Care
- Family Presence Facilitation
- Hypovolemia Management
- Infant Care: Preterm
- Intravenous (IV) Insertion
- Intravenous (IV) Therapy
- Invasive Hemodynamic Monitoring

- Laboratory Data Interpretation
- Mechanical Ventilation Management: Invasive
- Mechanical Ventilation Management: Noninvasive
- Medication Administration
- Oxygen Therapy
- Pain Management: Acute
- Patient Identification
- Rapid Sequence Intubation
- Respiratory Monitoring
- Resuscitation
- Sedation Management
- Shock Management
- Shock Management: Cardiac
- Shock Management: Sepsis
- Shock Management: Vasogenic
- Shock Management: Volume

- Shock Prevention
- Technology Management
- Telecommunication Consultation
- Thrombolytic Therapy Management
- Transport: Interfacility

- Triage: Disaster
- Ventilation Assistance
- Vital Signs Monitoring
- Wound Care

Forensic Nursing

- Abuse Protection Support
- Anxiety Reduction
- Calming Technique
- Communicable Disease Management
- Consultation
- Counseling
- Crisis Intervention
- Deposition
- Documentation
- Documentation: Meetings
- Emergency Care
- Emotional Support
- Environmental Management: Violence Prevention
- Examination Assistance
- Family Integrity Promotion
- Forensic Data Collection

- Grief Work Facilitation
- Health Care Information Exchange
- Health Screening
- Health System Guidance
- Human Trafficking Detection
- Incident Reporting
- Laboratory Data Interpretation
- Patient Identification
- Patient Rights Protection
- Postmortem Care
- Sexual Assault Trauma Care
- Referral
- Risk Identification
- Specimen Management
- Substance Use Prevention

Gastroenterological Nursing

- Abdominal Massage
- Airway Management
- Airway Suctioning
- Anesthesia Administration
- Aspiration Precautions
- Bowel Incontinence Care: Encopresis
- Bowel Management
- Calming Technique
- Constipation Management
- Diarrhea Management
- Diet Staging
- Diet Staging: Weight Loss Surgery
- Distraction
- Emotional Support
- Enema Administration
- Enteral Tube Feeding
- Flatulence Reduction
- Infection Control
- Intravenous (IV) Insertion
- IV Therapy
- Medication Administration: Intramuscular (IM)

- Medication Administration: Intravenous (IV)
- Medication Administration: Oral
- Medication Administration: Rectal
- Nasogastric Intubation
- Nausea Management
- Nutritional Counseling
- Ostomy Care
- Pain Management: Acute
- Pain Management: Chronic
- Sedation Management
- Self-Efficacy Enhancement
- Specimen Management
- Surveillance
- Swallowing Therapy
- Technology Management
- Total Parenteral Nutrition (TPN) Administration
- Tube Care: Gastrointestinal
- Vital Signs Monitoring
- Vomiting Management
- Wound Care

Genetics Nursing

- Active Listening
- Anticipatory Guidance
- Anxiety Reduction

- Coping Enhancement
- Counseling
- Crisis Intervention

- Documentation
- Emotional Support
- Environmental Management: Community
- Environmental Risk Protection
- Family Integrity Promotion
- Family Mobilization
- Family Support
- Genetic Counseling
- Grief Work Facilitation
- Health Care Information Exchange
- Health Coaching
- Health Literacy Enhancement
- Health Policy Monitoring
- Health Screening
- Laboratory Data Interpretation
- Multidisciplinary Care Conference
- Normalization Promotion
- Parent Education: Childrearing Family
- Parent Education: Infant
- Patient Rights Protection
- Preconception Counseling
- Pregnancy Termination Care
- Referral
- Risk Identification: Genetic
- Self-Efficacy Enhancement
- Support Group
- Teaching: Disease Process
- Values Clarification

Gerontological Nursing

- Abuse Protection Support: Elder
- Active Listening
- Activity Therapy
- Behavior Management
- Bibliotherapy
- Bowel Incontinence Care
- Bowel Management
- Caregiver Support
- Case Management
- Communication Enhancement: Hearing Deficit
- Communication Enhancement: Visual Deficit
- Constipation Management
- Coping Enhancement
- Delirium Management
- Dementia Management
- Dementia Management: Bathing
- Dementia Management: Wandering
- Discharge Follow-Up
- Dressing
- Dying Care
- Ear Irrigation
- Emotional Support
- Enema Administration
- Comfort Management
- Discharge Planning: Home Preparation
- Exercise Promotion
- Exercise Therapy: Ambulation
- Family Involvement Promotion
- Financial Resource Assistance
- Fluid/Electrolyte Management
- Foot Care
- Functional Ability Enhancement
- Grief Work Facilitation
- Hair and Scalp Care
- Health Literacy Enhancement
- Insurance Authorization
- Lower Extremity Monitoring
- Medication Administration
- Medication Deprescribing
- Medication Prescribing
- Medication Reconciliation
- Nutrition Management
- Pain Management: Chronic
- Patient Rights Protection
- Positioning
- Prescribing: Diagnostic Testing
- Prescribing: Nonpharmacologic Treatment
- Pressure Injury Prevention
- Prompted Voiding
- Rectal Prolapse Management
- Relocation Stress Reduction
- Reminiscence Therapy
- Respite Care
- Self-Care Assistance
- Self-Efficacy Enhancement
- Skin Care: Absorbent Products
- Social Justice Facilitation
- Urinary Habit Training
- Urinary Incontinence Care
- Validation Therapy
- Wound Care: Nonhealing

HIV/AIDS Care Nursing

- Acid-Base Management
- Anxiety Reduction
- Bed Rest Care
- Caregiver Support
- Case Management
- Cognitive Restructuring
- Communicable Disease Management
- Coping Enhancement

- Counseling
- Decision-Making Support
- Diarrhea Management
- Dying Care
- Electrolyte Management
- Electrolyte Monitoring
- Emotional Support
- Energy Management
- Exercise Promotion
- Family Integrity Promotion
- Family Involvement Promotion
- Family Support
- Financial Resource Assistance
- Fluid Management
- Fluid Monitoring
- Functional Ability Enhancement
- Health Education
- Health Screening
- Health System Guidance
- Hyperthermia Management
- Infection Control
- Infection Protection
- Insurance Authorization
- Medication Administration
- Medication Management
- Medication Management: Medical Cannabis
- Medication Reconciliation
- Memory Training
- Mood Management
- Multidisciplinary Care Conference
- Nausea Management
- Neutropenic Precautions
- Pain Management: Chronic
- Patient Rights Protection
- Resilience Promotion
- Resilience Promotion: Community
- Risk Identification: Infectious Disease
- Self-Care Assistance
- Social Justice Facilitation
- Teaching: Disease Process
- Teaching: Individual
- Teaching: Prescribed Medication
- Teaching: Procedure or Treatment
- Values Clarification
- Vital Signs Monitoring
- Wound Care

Holistic Nursing

- Abdominal Massage
- Active Listening
- Acupressure
- Animal-Assisted Therapy
- Anticipatory Guidance
- Anxiety Reduction
- Aromatherapy
- Art Therapy
- Autogenic Training
- Bibliotherapy
- Biofeedback
- Body Image Enhancement
- Calming Technique
- Caregiver Support
- Cognitive Restructuring
- Coping Enhancement
- Counseling
- Dance Therapy
- Decision-Making Support
- Emotional Support
- Energy Management
- Environmental Management
- Exercise Promotion
- Family Involvement Promotion
- Gardening Therapy
- Guided Imagery
- Healing Touch
- Health Coaching
- Health Education
- Health Screening
- Hope Inspiration
- Humor
- Journaling
- Laughter Yoga
- Massage
- Meditation Facilitation
- Medication Management: Medical Cannabis
- Music Therapy
- Mutual Goal Setting
- Nutritional Counseling
- Phytotherapy
- Presence
- Progressive Muscle Relaxation
- Reiki
- Relaxation Therapy
- Self-Awareness Enhancement
- Self-Efficacy Enhancement
- Self-Esteem Enhancement
- Self-Modification Assistance
- Self-Responsibility Facilitation
- Spiritual Growth Facilitation
- Spiritual Support
- Teaching: Group
- Teaching: Individual
- Therapeutic Touch
- Touch
- Truth Telling
- Values Clarification
- Yoga

Home Health Nursing

- Advanced Care Planning
- Bathing
- Bed Rest Care
- Bowel Management
- Bereavement Care
- Caregiver Support
- Dementia Management: Wandering
- Developmental Enhancement: Infant
- Dressing
- Dying Care
- Electronic Health Record Access Assistance
- Emotional Support
- Comfort Management
- Discharge Planning: Home Preparation
- Fall Prevention
- Family Involvement Promotion
- Functional Ability Enhancement
- Hair and Scalp Care
- Health Coaching
- Health Education
- Home Maintenance Assistance
- IV Therapy
- Lactation Counseling
- Medication Management
- Medication Administration: Continuous Subcutaneous Infusion
- Medication Deprescribing
- Medication Management: Wearable Infusion Device
- Ostomy Care
- Pain Management: Chronic
- Parent Education: Childrearing Family
- Parent Education: Infant
- Parenting Promotion
- Physical Distancing Facilitation
- Prescribing: Nonpharmacologic Treatment
- Quarantine Facilitation
- Referral
- Risk Identification
- Self-Care Assistance
- Self-Care Assistance: Toileting
- Sibling Support
- Skin Care: Absorbent Products
- Smoking Cessation Assistance
- Surveillance: Remote Monitoring
- Teaching: Adolescent Development
- Teaching: Adolescent Nutrition
- Teaching: Adolescent Safety
- Teaching: Early Childhood Development
- Teaching: Early Childhood Nutrition
- Teaching: Early Childhood Safety
- Teaching: Group
- Teaching: Individual
- Teaching: Infant Development 0–3 Months
- Teaching: Infant Development 4–6 Months
- Teaching: Infant Development 7–9 Months
- Teaching: Infant Development 10–12 Months
- Teaching: Infant Nutrition 0–3 Months
- Teaching: Infant Nutrition 4–6 Months
- Teaching: Infant Nutrition 7–9 Months
- Teaching: Infant Nutrition 10–12 Months
- Teaching: Infant Safety 0–3 Months
- Teaching: Infant Safety 4–6 Months
- Teaching: Infant Safety 7–9 Months
- Teaching: Infant Safety 10–12 Months
- Teaching: Middle Childhood Development
- Teaching: Middle Childhood Nutrition
- Teaching: Middle Childhood Safety
- Teaching: Prescribed Diet
- Teaching: Prescribed Medication
- Teaching: Procedure or Treatment
- Teaching: Safe Sex
- Teaching: Toddler Nutrition 13–18 Months
- Teaching: Toddler Nutrition 19–24 Months
- Teaching: Toddler Nutrition 25–36 Months
- Teaching: Toddler Safety 13–18 Months
- Teaching: Toddler Safety 19–24 Months
- Teaching: Toddler Safety 25–36 Months
- Telecommunication Consultation
- Vaccination Management
- Vehicle Safety Promotion
- Urinary Catheterization
- Urinary Catheterization: External
- Vital Signs Monitoring
- Wound Care

Hospice and Palliative Care Nursing

- Active Listening
- Advanced Care Planning
- Analgesic Administration
- Anticipatory Guidance
- Anxiety Reduction
- Aromatherapy
- Bed Rest Care
- Bereavement Care
- Bowel Management
- Caregiver Support
- Case Management
- Constipation Management
- Coping Enhancement
- Decision-Making Support
- Delirium Management
- Dying Care
- Emotional Support
- Endotracheal Extubation: Palliative
- Energy Management
- Environmental Management
- Family Integrity Promotion
- Family Involvement Promotion

- Financial Resource Assistance
- Fluid/Electrolyte Management
- Forgiveness Facilitation
- Grief Work Facilitation
- Healing Touch
- Health Care Information Exchange
- Health System Guidance
- Medication Administration: Continuous Subcutaneous Infusion
- Medication Deprescribing
- Medication Management
- Medication Management: Medical Cannabis
- Multidisciplinary Care Conference
- Neurologic Monitoring
- Nutrition Management
- Pain Management: Acute
- Pain Management: Chronic
- Patient Rights Protection
- Phytotherapy
- Positioning
- Presence
- Pressure Injury Prevention
- Religious Ritual Enhancement
- Reminiscence Therapy
- Respiratory Monitoring
- Respite Care
- Self-Care Assistance
- Skin Surveillance
- Sleep Enhancement
- Spiritual Support
- Support System Enhancement
- Telecommunication Consultation
- Touch
- Urinary Elimination Management
- Values Clarification
- Visitation Facilitation

Infection Control and Epidemiology Nursing

- Bioterrorism Preparedness
- Communicable Disease Management
- Community Health Advocacy
- Documentation: Meetings
- Environmental Management: Safety
- Environmental Risk Protection
- Health Education
- Health Policy Monitoring
- Infection Control
- Infection Control: Intraoperative
- Infection Control Teaching
- Infection Protection
- Latex Precautions
- Learning Facilitation
- Multidisciplinary Care Conference
- Neutropenic Precautions
- Pandemic Precautions
- Physical Distancing Facilitation
- Product Evaluation
- Program Development
- Quality Monitoring
- Quarantine Facilitation
- Research Protocol Management
- Risk Identification
- Risk Identification: Infectious Disease
- Surveillance
- Teaching: Safe Sex
- Vaccination Management

Informatics Nursing

- Collaboration Enhancement
- Competency Management
- Cost Containment
- Critical Path Development
- Decision-Making Support
- Documentation
- Documentation: Meetings
- Electronic Health Record Access Assistance
- Environmental Management: Safety
- Environmental Management: Worker Safety
- Environmental Risk Protection
- Fiscal Resources Management
- Forensic Data Collection
- Health Care Information Exchange
- Health Care Provider Collaboration
- Health Literacy Enhancement
- Health Policy Monitoring
- Health Screening
- Health System Guidance
- Incident Reporting
- Multidisciplinary Care Conference
- Order Transcription
- Product Evaluation
- Program Development
- Quality Monitoring
- Research Protocol Management
- Risk Identification
- Social Marketing
- Supply Chain Management
- Surveillance
- Surveillance: Remote Monitoring
- Surveillance: Video Monitoring
- Technology Management
- Telecommunication Consultation

Infusion Nursing

- Acid-Base Management
- Acid-Base Management: Metabolic Acidosis
- Acid-Base Management: Metabolic Alkalosis
- Acid-Base Management: Respiratory Acidosis
- Acid-Base Management: Respiratory Alkalosis
- Acid-Base Monitoring
- Allergy Management
- Analgesic Administration: Intraspinal
- Blood Products Administration
- Capillary Blood Sample
- Caregiver Support
- Central Venous Access Management: Central Insertion
- Central Venous Access Management: Peripheral Insertion
- Chemotherapy Management
- Dialysis Access Maintenance
- Electrolyte Management
- Electrolyte Management: Hypercalcemia
- Electrolyte Management: Hyperkalemia
- Electrolyte Management: Hypermagnesemia
- Electrolyte Management: Hypernatremia
- Electrolyte Management: Hyperphosphatemia
- Electrolyte Management: Hypocalcemia
- Electrolyte Management: Hypokalemia
- Electrolyte Management: Hypomagnesemia
- Electrolyte Management: Hyponatremia
- Electrolyte Management: Hypophosphatemia
- Electrolyte Monitoring
- Environmental Management: Safety
- Fluid Management
- Fluid Monitoring
- Fluid/Electrolyte Management
- Health Care Information Exchange
- Health Education
- Hyperglycemia Management
- Hypertension Management
- Hypervolemia Management
- Hypotension Management
- Hypothermia Treatment
- Hypovolemia Management
- Incident Reporting
- Infection Control
- Infection Protection
- Intravenous (IV) Insertion
- Intravenous (IV) Therapy
- Invasive Hemodynamic Monitoring
- Laboratory Data Interpretation
- Medication Administration: Continuous Subcutaneous Infusion
- Medication Administration: Intraosseous
- Medication Administration: Intraspinal
- Medication Administration: Intravenous (IV)
- Medication Administration: Ventricular Reservoir
- Medication Management: Wearable Infusion Device
- Nutrition Management
- Nutrition Therapy
- Nutritional Monitoring
- Pain Management: Acute
- Pain Management: Chronic
- Patient-Controlled Analgesia (PCA) Assistance
- Peritoneal Dialysis Therapy
- Phlebotomy: Arterial Blood Sample
- Phlebotomy: Blood Acquisition
- Phlebotomy: Venous Blood Sample
- Product Evaluation
- Quality Monitoring
- Risk Identification
- Supply Chain Management
- Teaching: Prescribed Medication
- Teaching: Procedure or Treatment
- Technology Management
- Thrombolytic Therapy Management
- Total Parenteral Nutrition (TPN) Administration
- Tube Care: Umbilical Line
- Tube Care: Ventriculostomy/Lumbar Drain

Legal Nursing

- Collaboration Enhancement
- Community Health Advocacy
- Consultation
- Decision-Making Support
- Deposition
- Documentation
- Documentation: Meetings
- Electronic Health Record Access Assistance
- Environmental Risk Protection
- Forensic Data Collection
- Health Care Information Exchange
- Health Literacy Enhancement
- Health Policy Monitoring
- Health Screening
- Human Trafficking Detection
- Incident Reporting
- Multidisciplinary Care Conference
- Patient Rights Protection
- Product Evaluation
- Quality Monitoring
- Risk Identification
- Surveillance
- Technology Management
- Telecommunication Consultation

Medical-Surgical Nursing

- Acid-Base Management
- Airway Suctioning
- Artificial Airway Management
- Aspiration Precautions
- Asthma Management
- Bathing
- Bed Rest Care
- Bleeding Reduction: Gastrointestinal
- Blood Products Administration
- Bowel Incontinence Care
- Bowel Management
- Capillary Blood Sample
- Central Venous Access Management: Central Insertion
- Central Venous Access Management: Peripheral Insertion
- Chemical Restraint
- Chemotherapy Management
- Circulatory Care: Arterial Insufficiency
- Circulatory Care: Venous Insufficiency
- Code Management
- Critical Path Development
- Diet Staging
- Discharge Planning
- Documentation
- Dressing
- Electrolyte Management
- Emotional Support
- Enema Administration
- Enteral Tube Feeding
- Fall Prevention
- Family Involvement Promotion
- Family Presence Facilitation
- Feeding
- Fluid/Electrolyte Management
- Functional Ability Enhancement
- Health Literacy Enhancement
- Hyperglycemia Management
- Hyperlipidemia Management
- Hypertension Management
- Hypoglycemia Management
- Hypotension Management
- Incision Site Care
- Infection Control
- Intravenous (IV) Insertion
- Intravenous (IV) Therapy
- Laboratory Data Interpretation
- Mechanical Ventilation Management: Noninvasive
- Medication Administration
- Medication Administration: Continuous Subcutaneous Infusion
- Medication Deprescribing
- Medication Management
- Medication Management: Wearable Infusion Device
- Medication Reconciliation
- Multidisciplinary Care Conference
- Nasogastric Intubation
- Nausea Management
- Neurological Monitoring
- Nutrition Management
- Ostomy Care
- Oxygen Therapy
- Pacemaker Management: Permanent
- Pain Management: Acute
- Pain Management: Chronic
- Patient Identification
- Patient Rights Protection
- Patient-Controlled Analgesia (PCA) Assistance
- Physical Restraint
- Postmortem Care
- Pressure Injury Care
- Pressure Injury Prevention
- Quality Monitoring
- Readmission Prevention
- Respiratory Monitoring
- Seizure Management
- Seizure Precautions
- Self-Care Assistance
- Shock Management
- Shock Prevention
- Skin Care: Absorbent Products
- Skin Surveillance
- Staff Supervision
- Surveillance
- Surveillance: Video Monitoring
- Teaching: Disease Process
- Teaching: Individual
- Teaching: Prescribed Medication
- Teaching: Procedure or Treatment
- Total Parenteral Nutrition (TPN) Administration
- Traction/Immobilization Care
- Tube Care: Chest
- Tube Care: Gastrointestinal
- Tube Care: Urinary
- Ultrasonography: Bladder
- Urinary Catheterization: External
- Urinary Elimination Management
- Urinary Incontinence Care
- Vital Signs Monitoring
- Vomiting Management
- Wound Care
- Wound Care: Nonhealing
- Wound Care: Protection

Midwifery Nursing

- Abuse Protection Support
- Active Listening
- Admission Care
- Amnioinfusion
- Anticipatory Guidance
- Attachment Promotion
- Birthing
- Breast Examination
- Childbirth Preparation
- Decision-Making Support

- Delegation
- Discharge Planning
- Documentation
- Emotional Support
- Environmental Management
- Family Integrity Promotion: Childbearing Family
- Family Planning: Contraception
- Family Planning: Unplanned Pregnancy
- Fertility Preservation
- Health Care Provider Collaboration
- Health Coaching
- Health Education
- Health Screening
- High-Risk Pregnancy Care
- Hormone Replacement Therapy
- Infant Care: Newborn
- Infant Care: Preterm
- Intrapartal Care
- Labor Pain Management
- Lactation Counseling
- Lactation Suppression
- Medication Administration: Intraspinal
- Medication Management

- Medication Prescribing
- Nutritional Counseling
- Pain Management: Acute
- Parent Education: Infant
- Phototherapy: Neonate
- Postpartal Care
- Preconception Counseling
- Premenstrual Syndrome (PMS) Management
- Prescribing: Diagnostic Testing
- Procedural Support: Infant
- Referral
- Risk Identification: Childbearing Family
- Self-Efficacy Enhancement
- Sexual Counseling
- Surveillance: Late Pregnancy
- Suturing
- Teaching: Individual
- Teaching: Infant Development 0–3 Months
- Teaching: Infant Nutrition 0–3 Months
- Teaching: Infant Safety 0–3 Months
- Telecommunication Consultation
- Temperature Regulation: Newborn

Neonatal Nursing

- Acid-Base Management
- Airway Insertion and Stabilization
- Airway Management
- Airway Suctioning
- Analgesic Administration
- Artificial Airway Management
- Attachment Promotion
- Blood Products Administration
- Bottle Feeding
- Caregiver Support
- Central Venous Access Management: Central Insertion
- Circumcision Care
- Critical Path Development
- Discharge Planning
- Documentation
- Electrolyte Management
- Electrolyte Management: Hypercalcemia
- Electrolyte Management: Hyperkalemia
- Electrolyte Management: Hypermagnesemia
- Electrolyte Management: Hypernatremia
- Electrolyte Management: Hyperphosphatemia
- Electrolyte Management: Hypocalcemia
- Electrolyte Management: Hypokalemia
- Electrolyte Management: Hypomagnesemia
- Electrolyte Management: Hyponatremia
- Electrolyte Management: Hypophosphatemia
- Endotracheal Extubation
- Enteral Tube Feeding
- Environmental Management
- Extracorporeal Membrane Oxygenation (ECMO) Therapy
- Comfort Management
- Eye Care
- Family Involvement Promotion
- Family Support
- Feeding

- Fluid Management
- Fluid Monitoring
- Health Care Information Exchange
- Hypovolemia Management
- Infant Care
- Infant Care: Eye Examination Support
- Infant Care: Newborn
- Infant Care: Preterm
- Infection Protection
- Intravenous (IV) Insertion
- Intravenous (IV) Therapy
- Kangaroo Care
- Laboratory Data Interpretation
- Lactation Counseling
- Mechanical Ventilation Management: Invasive
- Mechanical Ventilation Management: Noninvasive
- Mechanical Ventilatory Weaning
- Medication Administration
- Medication Administration: Enteral
- Medication Administration: Eye
- Medication Administration: Intramuscular (IM)
- Medication Administration: Intravenous (IV)
- Medication Administration: Oral
- Medication Management
- Multidisciplinary Care Conference
- Nonnutritive Sucking
- Nutrition Management
- Nutrition Therapy
- Nutritional Monitoring
- Ostomy Care
- Oxygen Therapy
- Pain Management: Acute
- Parent Education: Infant
- Patient Identification
- Phototherapy: Neonate

- Positioning
- Procedural Support: Infant
- Respiratory Monitoring
- Resuscitation
- Resuscitation: Neonate
- Shock Management: Volume
- Sibling Support
- Skin Care: Topical Treatment
- Skin Surveillance
- Sleep Enhancement
- Surveillance
- Technology Management
- Temperature Regulation
- Temperature Regulation: Newborn
- Total Parenteral Nutrition (TPN) Administration

- Teaching: Infant Development 0–3 Months
- Teaching: Infant Nutrition 0–3 Months
- Teaching: Infant Safety 0–3 Months
- Transport: Interfacility
- Transport: Intrafacility
- Tube Care: Chest
- Tube Care: Gastrointestinal
- Tube Care: Umbilical Line
- Tube Care: Urinary
- Urinary Catheterization
- Urinary Catheterization: Intermittent
- Ventilation Assistance
- Visitation Facilitation
- Vital Signs Monitoring
- Wound Care

Nephrology Nursing

- Acid-Base Management
- Bleeding Reduction: Wound
- Capillary Blood Sample
- Case Management
- Comfort Management
- Constipation Management
- Cultural Care Negotiation
- Decision-Making Support
- Delegation
- Dialysis Access Maintenance
- Electrolyte Management
- Electrolyte Monitoring
- Emotional Support
- Environmental Management: Safety
- Family Involvement Promotion
- Financial Resource Assistance
- Fluid Management
- Fluid Monitoring
- Fluid/Electrolyte Management
- Health Care Provider Collaboration
- Health Literacy Enhancement
- Hemodialysis Therapy
- Hyperglycemia Management
- Hypertension Management
- Hypervolemia Management
- Hypoglycemia Management
- Hypotension Management
- Hypovolemia Management

- Infection Control
- Infection Protection
- IV Therapy
- Laboratory Data Interpretation
- Medication Administration
- Medication Management
- Multidisciplinary Care Conference
- Nausea Management
- Nutritional Monitoring
- Organ Procurement
- Peritoneal Dialysis Therapy
- Point of Care Testing
- Pruritus Management
- Self-Efficacy Enhancement
- Specimen Management
- Teaching: Disease Process
- Teaching: Individual
- Teaching: Prescribed Diet
- Teaching: Prescribed Medication
- Teaching: Procedure or Treatment
- Teaching: Psychomotor Skill
- Technology Management
- Telecommunication Consultation
- Ultrasonography: Bladder
- Values Clarification
- Vital Signs Monitoring
- Vomiting Management

Neuroscience Nursing

- Airway Management
- Anxiety Reduction
- Behavior Management
- Body Image Enhancement
- Bowel Management
- Cerebral Edema Management
- Cerebral Perfusion Promotion
- Chemical Restraint

- Cognitive Stimulation
- Communication Enhancement: Speech Deficit
- Communication Enhancement: Visual Deficit
- Delirium Management
- Delusion Management
- Dementia Management
- Dementia Management: Wandering
- Dysreflexia Management

- Energy Management
- Environmental Management: Safety
- Fall Prevention
- Functional Ability Enhancement
- Hypothermia Induction Therapy
- Intracranial Pressure (ICP) Monitoring
- Medication Administration
- Medication Management
- Neurologic Monitoring
- Pain Management: Acute
- Pain Management: Chronic
- Positioning: Neurologic
- Seizure Management
- Seizure Precautions
- Self-Efficacy Enhancement
- Sleep Enhancement

- Subarachnoid Hemorrhage Precautions
- Surveillance
- Surveillance: Skin
- Surveillance: Video Monitoring
- Swallowing Therapy
- Temperature Regulation
- Thermoregulation Management
- Thrombolytic Therapy Management
- Tube Care: Ventriculostomy/Lumbar Drain
- Ultrasonography: Bladder
- Unilateral Neglect Management
- Urinary Catheterization: External
- Urinary Catheterization: Intermittent
- Urinary Elimination Management
- Vehicle Safety Promotion

Nurse Anesthesiology and Post Anesthesia Care Nursing

- Acid-Base Management
- Acid-Base Monitoring
- Airway Insertion and Stabilization
- Airway Management
- Airway Suctioning
- Analgesic Administration
- Analgesic Administration: Intraspinal
- Anaphylaxis Management
- Anesthesia Administration
- Artificial Airway Management
- Autotransfusion
- Blood Products Administration
- Central Venous Access Management: Central Insertion
- Central Venous Access Management: Peripheral Insertion
- Circulatory Care: Mechanical Assist Device
- Code Management
- Controlled Substance Checking
- Defibrillator Management: External
- Defibrillator Management: Internal
- Documentation
- Dysrhythmia Management
- Electrolyte Management
- Electrolyte Monitoring
- Emergency Care
- Endotracheal Extubation
- Eye Care
- Fluid Management
- Fluid Monitoring
- Fluid Resuscitation
- Health Care Provider Collaboration
- Hyperglycemia Management
- Hypervolemia Management
- Hypoglycemia Management
- Hypothermia Induction Therapy
- Hypothermia Treatment
- Hypovolemia Management
- Incident Reporting
- Infection Control: Intraoperative
- Intracranial Pressure (ICP) Monitoring
- Intravenous (IV) Insertion

- IV Therapy
- Laboratory Data Interpretation
- Laser Precautions
- Latex Precautions
- Malignant Hyperthermia Precautions
- Mechanical Ventilation Management: Invasive
- Medication Administration
- Medication Administration: Intravenous (IV)
- Medication Management
- Medication Prescribing
- Nausea Management
- Oxygen Therapy
- Pacemaker Management: Permanent
- Pacemaker Management: Temporary
- Pain Management: Acute
- Patient-Controlled Analgesia (PCA) Assistance
- Patient Identification
- Phlebotomy: Arterial Blood Sample
- Phlebotomy: Blood Acquisition
- Phlebotomy: Venous Blood Sample
- Pneumatic Tourniquet Management
- Positioning: Intraoperative
- Postanesthesia Care
- Preoperative Coordination
- Prescribing: Diagnostic Testing
- Quality Monitoring
- Rapid Sequence Intubation
- Referral
- Respiratory Monitoring
- Resuscitation
- Sedation Management
- Shock Management
- Surgical Precautions
- Surgical Preparation
- Teaching: Preoperative
- Technology Management
- Transcutaneous Electrical Nerve Stimulation (TENS)
- Triage: Emergency Center
- Ventilation Assistance
- Vital Signs Monitoring

Obstetric Nursing

- Attachment Promotion
- Birthing
- Bleeding Reduction: Antepartum Uterus
- Bleeding Reduction: Postpartum Uterus
- Bottle Feeding
- Cesarean Birth Care
- Childbirth Preparation
- Circumcision Care
- Electronic Fetal Monitoring: Antepartum
- Electronic Fetal Monitoring: Intrapartum
- Family Integrity Promotion: Childbearing Family
- Family Planning: Contraception
- Grief Work Facilitation: Perinatal Death
- Health Literacy Enhancement
- High-Risk Pregnancy Care
- Hypertension Management
- Infant Care
- Infant Care: Newborn
- Intrapartal Care
- Intrapartal Care: High-Risk Delivery
- IV Therapy
- Invasive Hemodynamic Monitoring
- Labor Induction
- Labor Pain Management
- Labor Suppression
- Lactation Counseling
- Medication Administration
- Medication Administration: Intraspinal
- Pain Management: Acute
- Parent Education: Infant
- Parenting Promotion
- Phototherapy: Neonate
- Postpartal Care
- Pregnancy Termination Care
- Prenatal Care
- Procedural Support: Infant
- Resuscitation: Fetus
- Resuscitation: Neonate
- Risk Identification: Childbearing Family
- Substance Use Treatment
- Surveillance: Late Pregnancy
- Teaching: Individual
- Teaching: Infant Development 0–3 Months
- Teaching: Infant Nutrition 0–3 Months
- Teaching: Infant Safety 0–3 Months
- Temperature Regulation: Newborn

Occupational Health Nursing

- Active Listening
- Allergy Management
- Anticipatory Guidance
- Anxiety Reduction
- Asthma Management
- Bioterrorism Preparedness
- Cardiac Care: Rehabilitative
- Case Management
- Communicable Disease Management
- Counseling
- Crisis Intervention
- Decision-Making Support
- Defibrillator Management: External
- Discharge Follow-Up
- Ear Care
- Emergency Care
- Emotional Support
- Environmental Management: Community
- Environmental Management: Safety
- Environmental Management: Violence Prevention
- Environmental Management: Worker Safety
- Environmental Risk Protection
- Exercise Promotion
- Fall Prevention
- Family Support
- Health Coaching
- Health Education
- Health Literacy Enhancement
- Health Screening
- Health System Guidance
- Infection Control Teaching
- Infection Protection
- Insurance Authorization
- Nutritional Counseling
- Pandemic Precautions
- Parent Education: Adolescent
- Parent Education: Childrearing Family
- Prenatal Care
- Quarantine Facilitation
- Referral
- Respiratory Monitoring
- Risk Identification
- Smoking Cessation Assistance
- Social Marketing
- Substance Use Prevention
- Substance Use Treatment
- Teaching: Group
- Teaching: Individual
- Technology Management
- Telecommunication Consultation
- Triage: Disaster
- Vaccination Management
- Vehicle Safety Promotion
- Vision Screening
- Weight Management
- Weight Reduction Assistance
- Wound Care

Oncology Nursing

- Advanced Care Planning
- Analgesic Administration
- Anxiety Reduction
- Bereavement Care
- Bleeding Precautions
- Bowel Management
- Caregiver Support
- Central Venous Access Management: Central Insertion
- Central Venous Access Management: Peripheral Insertion
- Chemotherapy Management
- Comfort Management
- Coping Enhancement
- Dance Therapy
- Discharge Follow-Up
- Dying Care
- Energy Management
- Family Involvement Promotion
- Financial Resource Assistance
- Fluid Management
- Healing Touch
- Hope Inspiration
- Hyperthermia Management
- Infection Control
- Infection Protection
- Intravenous (IV) Insertion
- Laboratory Data Interpretation
- Massage
- Medication Administration
- Medication Management
- Medication Management: Medical Cannabis
- Medication Management: Wearable Infusion Device
- Music Therapy
- Nausea Management
- Neutropenic Precautions
- Nutrition Management
- Nutritional Monitoring
- Pain Management: Acute
- Pain Management: Chronic
- Peripheral Sensation Management
- Phytotherapy
- Preparatory Sensory Information
- Radiation Therapy Management
- Reiki
- Relaxation Therapy
- Self-Efficacy Enhancement
- Spiritual Support
- Stem Cell Infusion
- Support Group
- Teaching: Disease Process
- Teaching: Procedure or Treatment
- Therapeutic Touch
- Urinary Elimination Management
- Vomiting Management
- Wound Care: Nonhealing

Ophthalmic Nursing

- Active Listening
- Communication Enhancement: Visual Deficit
- Consultation
- Contact Lens Care
- Discharge Follow-Up
- Discharge Planning
- Dry Eye Prevention
- Emotional Support
- Eye Care
- Eye Irrigation
- Fall Prevention
- Family Involvement Promotion
- Hypoglycemia Management
- Incision Site Care
- Infection Control
- Infection Control: Intraoperative
- Intravenous (IV) Insertion
- Intravenous (IV) Therapy
- Laser Precautions
- Medication Administration
- Medication Administration: Intraocular Disk
- Medication Administration: Eye
- Medication Administration: Intramuscular (IM)
- Medication Administration: Oral
- Pain Management: Acute
- Preoperative Coordination
- Sedation Management
- Self-Care Assistance
- Surgical Assistance
- Surgical Preparation
- Surveillance
- Teaching: Disease Process
- Teaching: Individual
- Teaching: Preoperative
- Teaching: Prescribed Medication
- Teaching: Procedure or Treatment
- Teaching: Psychomotor Skill
- Telecommunication Consultation
- Vision Screening
- Vital Signs Monitoring

Orthopedic Nursing

- Amputation Care
- Analgesic Administration
- Autotransfusion
- Bathing
- Bed Rest Care
- Blood Products Administration
- Cast Care: Maintenance
- Cast Care: Wet
- Constipation Management
- Controlled Substance Checking
- Cough Enhancement
- Critical Path Development
- Delirium Management
- Discharge Planning
- Embolus Care: Peripheral
- Exercise Promotion
- Exercise Therapy: Ambulation
- Exercise Therapy: Joint Mobility
- Fall Prevention
- Functional Ability Enhancement
- Heat/Cold Application
- Incision Site Care
- Infection Control
- Intravenous (IV) Insertion
- Intravenous (IV) Therapy
- Lower Extremity Monitoring
- Medication Administration
- Medication Administration: Intramuscular (IM)
- Medication Administration: Intravenous (IV)
- Medication Administration: Oral
- Pain Management: Acute
- Pain Management: Chronic
- Patient-Controlled Analgesia (PCA) Assistance
- Physical Restraint
- Positioning
- Positioning: Wheelchair
- Preparatory Sensory Information
- Pressure Injury Prevention
- Self-Care Assistance
- Self-Care Assistance: Transfer
- Skin Care: Topical Treatment
- Skin Surveillance
- Splinting
- Teaching: Individual
- Teaching: Preoperative
- Teaching: Prescribed Exercise
- Teaching: Prescribed Medication
- Teaching: Procedure or Treatment
- Traction/Immobilization Care
- Tube Care: Urinary
- Urinary Retention Care
- Wound Care
- Wound Care: Closed Drainage
- Wound Care: Protection

Otorhinolaryngology and Head/Neck Nursing

- Airway Insertion and Stabilization
- Airway Management
- Airway Suctioning
- Allergy Management
- Analgesic Administration
- Anxiety Reduction
- Artificial Airway Management
- Aspiration Precautions
- Asthma Management
- Bleeding Reduction: Nasal
- Body Image Enhancement
- Chemotherapy Management
- Communication Enhancement: Hearing Deficit
- Communication Enhancement: Speech Deficit
- Critical Path Development
- Discharge Planning
- Ear Care
- Ear Irrigation
- Exercise Therapy: Balance
- Infection Control: Intraoperative
- Intracranial Pressure (ICP) Monitoring
- IV Therapy
- Mechanical Ventilation Management: Noninvasive
- Medication Administration
- Medication Administration: Inhalation
- Medication Administration: Nasal
- Nasal Irrigation
- Oral Health Maintenance
- Oral Health Promotion
- Oral Health Restoration
- Pain Management: Acute
- Pain Management: Chronic
- Positioning: Intraoperative
- Postanesthesia Care
- Preoperative Coordination
- Radiation Therapy Management
- Self-Efficacy Enhancement
- Smoking Cessation Assistance
- Surgical Assistance
- Surgical Precautions
- Surgical Preparation
- Swallowing Therapy
- Teaching: Preoperative
- Teaching: Prescribed Diet
- Teaching: Prescribed Exercise
- Teaching: Prescribed Medication
- Teaching: Procedure or Treatment
- Telecommunication Consultation
- Tube Care
- Wound Care

Pain Management Nursing

- Abdominal Massage
- Analgesic Administration
- Analgesic Administration: Intraspinal
- Behavior Contracting
- Biofeedback
- Case Management
- Central Venous Access Management: Central Insertion
- Central Venous Access Management: Peripheral Insertion
- Comfort Management
- Controlled Substance Checking
- Coping Enhancement
- Decision-Making Support
- Discharge Planning
- Distraction
- Dying Care
- Energy Management
- Exercise Promotion
- Guided Imagery
- Healing Touch
- Health Care Information Exchange
- Health Care Provider Collaboration
- Health Coaching
- Health Education
- Health Policy Monitoring
- Heat/Cold Application
- Humor
- Infection Control
- Insurance Authorization
- IV Therapy
- Laughter Yoga
- Massage
- Medication Administration
- Medication Administration: Continuous Subcutaneous Infusion
- Medication Management
- Medication Management: Medical Cannabis
- Medication Management: Wearable Infusion Device
- Medication Reconciliation
- Meditation Facilitation
- Multidisciplinary Care Conference
- Music Therapy
- Mutual Goal Setting
- Pain Management: Acute
- Pain Management: Chronic
- Patient-Controlled Analgesia (PCA) Assistance
- Phytotherapy
- Product Evaluation
- Progressive Muscle Relaxation
- Quality Monitoring
- Referral
- Reiki
- Relaxation Therapy
- Sedation Management
- Self-Efficacy Enhancement
- Self-Esteem Enhancement
- Spiritual Support
- Support Group
- Surgical Assistance
- Surgical Preparation
- Surveillance
- Teaching: Prescribed Medication
- Teaching: Procedure or Treatment
- Therapeutic Touch
- Touch
- Transcutaneous Electrical Nerve Stimulation (TENS)
- Yoga

Pediatric Nursing

- Abuse Protection Support: Child
- Adolescent Care
- Asthma Management
- Caregiver Support
- Child Care
- Developmental Enhancement: Infant
- Discharge Planning
- Documentation
- Ear Irrigation
- Emotional Support
- Environmental Management: Safety
- Eye Irrigation
- Family Involvement Promotion
- Family Presence Facilitation
- Feeding
- Fluid/Electrolyte Management
- Genetic Counseling
- Health Education
- Human Trafficking Detection
- Hyperthermia Management
- Infant Care
- Infant Care: Newborn
- Infant Care: Preterm
- Intravenous (IV) Therapy
- Medication Administration
- Medication Management: Wearable Infusion Device
- Multidisciplinary Care Conference
- Normalization Promotion
- Nutrition Management
- Oxygen Therapy
- Pain Management: Acute
- Pain Management: Chronic
- Parent Education: Adolescent
- Parent Education: Childrearing Family
- Parent Education: Infant
- Parenting Promotion
- Procedural Support: Infant
- Respiratory Monitoring
- Risk Identification
- Risk Identification: Genetic

- Surveillance
- Teaching: Adolescent Development
- Teaching: Adolescent Nutrition
- Teaching: Adolescent Safety
- Teaching: Early Childhood Development
- Teaching: Early Childhood Nutrition
- Teaching: Early Childhood Safety
- Teaching: Infant Development 0–3 Months
- Teaching: Infant Development 4–6 Months
- Teaching: Infant Development 7–9 Months
- Teaching: Infant Development 10–12 Months
- Teaching: Infant Nutrition 0–3 Months
- Teaching: Infant Nutrition 4–6 Months
- Teaching: Infant Nutrition 7–9 Months
- Teaching: Infant Nutrition 10–12 Months
- Teaching: Infant Safety 0–3 Months
- Teaching: Infant Safety 4–6 Months
- Teaching: Infant Safety 7–9 Months
- Teaching: Infant Safety 10–12 Months
- Teaching: Middle Childhood Development
- Teaching: Middle Childhood Nutrition
- Teaching: Middle Childhood Safety
- Teaching: Sports-Injury Prevention
- Teaching: Toddler Nutrition 13–18 Months
- Teaching: Toddler Nutrition 19–24 Months
- Teaching: Toddler Nutrition 25–36 Months
- Teaching: Toddler Safety 13–18 Months
- Teaching: Toddler Safety 19–24 Months
- Teaching: Toddler Safety 25–36 Months
- Teaching: Toilet Training
- Technology Management
- Temperature Regulation: Newborn
- Therapeutic Play
- Total Parenteral Nutrition (TPN) Administration
- Trauma Therapy: Child
- Vaccination Management
- Vehicle Safety Promotion
- Vital Signs Monitoring

Pediatric Hematology/Oncology Nursing

- Active Listening
- Adolescent Care
- Advanced Care Planning
- Analgesic Administration
- Anxiety Reduction
- Bleeding Precautions
- Blood Products Administration
- Bereavement Care
- Calming Technique
- Caregiver Support
- Case Management
- Central Venous Access Management: Central Insertion
- Central Venous Access Management: Peripheral Insertion
- Chemotherapy Management
- Coping Enhancement
- Decision-Making Support
- Child Care
- Dying Care
- Family Integrity Promotion
- Family Involvement Promotion
- Family Mobilization
- Family Presence Facilitation
- Family Process Maintenance
- Fluid/Electrolyte Management
- Genetic Counseling
- Grief Work Facilitation
- Hope Inspiration
- Hyperthermia Management
- Infection Protection
- IV Initiation
- IV Therapy
- Medication Administration: Continuous Subcutaneous Infusion
- Medication Administration: Intramuscular (IM)
- Medication Administration: Intravenous (IV)
- Medication Administration: Oral
- Multidisciplinary Care Conference
- Nausea Management
- Neutropenic Precautions
- Normalization Promotion
- Pain Management: Acute
- Pain Management: Chronic
- Parent Education: Childrearing Family
- Procedural Support: Infant
- Radiation Therapy Management
- Sedation Management
- Sibling Support
- Stem Cell Infusion
- Teaching: Adolescent Development
- Teaching: Adolescent Nutrition
- Teaching: Adolescent Safety
- Teaching: Disease Process
- Teaching: Early Childhood Development
- Teaching: Early Childhood Nutrition
- Teaching: Early Childhood Safety
- Teaching: Infant Development 0–3 Months
- Teaching: Infant Development 4–6 Months
- Teaching: Infant Development 7–9 Months
- Teaching: Infant Development 10–12 Months
- Teaching: Infant Nutrition 0–3 Months
- Teaching: Infant Nutrition 4–6 Months
- Teaching: Infant Nutrition 7–9 Months
- Teaching: Infant Nutrition 10–12 Months
- Teaching: Infant Safety 0–3 Months
- Teaching: Infant Safety 4–6 Months
- Teaching: Infant Safety 7–9 Months
- Teaching: Infant Safety 10–12 Months
- Teaching: Middle Childhood Development
- Teaching: Middle Childhood Nutrition
- Teaching: Middle Childhood Safety
- Teaching: Prescribed Medication
- Therapeutic Play
- Total Parenteral Nutrition (TPN) Administration
- Trauma Therapy: Child
- Vomiting Management

Perioperative Nursing

- Active Listening
- Anaphylaxis Management
- Anxiety Reduction
- Autotransfusion
- Blood Products Administration
- Critical Path Development
- Delegation
- Discharge Planning
- Documentation
- Electrolyte Management
- Emotional Support
- Comfort Management
- Environmental Management: Safety
- Environmental Management: Worker Safety
- Fluid Monitoring
- Health Care Provider Collaboration
- Hypothermia Induction Therapy
- Infection Control: Intraoperative
- IV Initiation
- IV Therapy
- Laser Precautions
- Latex Precautions
- Malignant Hyperthermia Precautions
- Oxygen Therapy
- Pain Management: Acute
- Patient Identification
- Patient Rights Protection
- Pneumatic Tourniquet Management
- Positioning: Intraoperative
- Postanesthesia Care
- Preceptor: Employee
- Preoperative Coordination
- Presence
- Pressure Injury Prevention
- Product Evaluation
- Quality Monitoring
- Rapid Sequence Intubation
- Sedation Management
- Self-Care Assistance: Transfer
- Shock Management
- Skin Care: Donor Site
- Skin Care: Graft Site
- Skin Surveillance
- Specimen Management
- Supply Chain Management
- Surgical Assistance
- Surgical Instrumentation Management
- Surgical Precautions
- Surgical Preparation
- Suturing
- Teaching: Preoperative
- Technology Management
- Temperature Regulation: Perioperative
- Touch
- Transport: Intrafacility
- Vital Signs Monitoring
- Wound Care

Plastic Surgery Nursing

- Analgesic Administration
- Bleeding Precautions
- Body Image Enhancement
- Counseling
- Decision-Making Support
- Emotional Support
- Guided Imagery
- Heat/Cold Application
- Incision Site Care
- Infection Control
- Infection Protection
- Insurance Authorization
- Intravenous (IV) Therapy
- Journaling
- Laser Precautions
- Medication Administration
- Medication Administration: Intraocular Disc
- Pain Management: Acute
- Patient-Controlled Analgesia (PCA) Assistance
- Patient Identification
- Preoperative Coordination
- Preparatory Sensory Information
- Pruritus Management
- Sedation Management
- Self-Care Assistance
- Skin Care: Donor Site
- Skin Care: Graft Site
- Skin Care: Topical Treatment
- Skin Surveillance
- Sleep Enhancement
- Surgical Instrumentation Management
- Teaching: Individual
- Teaching: Preoperative
- Values Clarification
- Vital Signs Monitoring
- Wound Care
- Wound Care: Protection

Psychiatric/Mental Health Nursing

- Abdominal Massage
- Abuse Protection Support
- Active Listening
- Anger Control Assistance
- Anxiety Reduction
- Area Restriction
- Assertiveness Training
- Behavior Management: Inattention and Hyperactivity
- Behavior Management: Self-Harm
- Behavior Management: Sexual
- Behavior Modification
- Behavior Modification: Social Skills
- Bibliotherapy
- Body Image Enhancement
- Body Search
- Calming Technique
- Caring Interaction Development
- Case Management
- Chemical Restraint
- Cognitive Restructuring
- Consultation
- Coping Enhancement
- Counseling
- Crisis Intervention
- Dance Therapy
- De-Escalation Management
- Delusion Management
- Dementia Management
- Dementia Management: Bathing
- Dementia Management: Wandering
- Eating Disorders Management
- Electroconvulsive Therapy (ECT) Management
- Elopement Precautions
- Environmental Management: Violence Prevention
- Family Involvement Promotion
- Family Therapy
- Fire-Setting Precautions
- Gardening Therapy
- Grief Work Facilitation
- Guided Reflection
- Guilt Work Facilitation
- Hallucination Management
- Health Coaching
- Health Literacy Enhancement
- Human Trafficking Detection
- Impulse Control Training
- Journaling
- Life Skills Enhancement
- Limit Setting
- Listening Visits
- Medication Administration
- Medication Management
- Medication Prescribing
- Milieu Therapy
- Mood Management
- Motivational Interviewing
- Pass Facilitation
- Phototherapy: Mood Regulation
- Physical Accompaniment
- Physical Restraint
- Prescribing: Diagnostic Testing
- Reality Orientation
- Readmission Prevention
- Relapse Prevention
- Reminiscence Therapy
- Resilience Promotion
- Resilience Promotion: Community
- Seclusion
- Self-Awareness Enhancement
- Self-Care Assistance
- Self-Esteem Enhancement
- Social Justice Facilitation
- Substance Use Prevention
- Substance Use Treatment: Alcohol Withdrawal
- Substance Use Treatment: Drug Withdrawal
- Suicide Prevention
- Support Group
- Surveillance: Video Monitoring
- Therapeutic Play
- Therapy Group
- Transgender Hormone Therapy

Radiology Nursing

- Airway Management
- Airway Suctioning
- Allergy Management
- Analgesic Administration
- Anxiety Reduction
- Aspiration Precautions
- Bleeding Precautions
- Bleeding Reduction
- Blood Products Administration
- Calming Technique
- Cardiac Risk Management
- Cerebral Perfusion Promotion
- Circulatory Precautions
- Code Management
- Discharge Planning
- Dysrhythmia Management
- Embolus Care: Peripheral
- Embolus Care: Pulmonary
- Embolus Precautions
- Emergency Care
- Emotional Support
- Environmental Management: Safety
- Examination Assistance
- Fluid Management
- Fluid Monitoring
- Fluid/Electrolyte Management

- Fluid Resuscitation
- Health Care Information Exchange
- Health Screening
- Incident Reporting
- Infection Control
- Infection Protection
- Intravenous (IV) Insertion
- Intravenous (IV) Therapy
- Laser Precautions
- Latex Precautions
- Medication Administration
- Medication Administration: Intravenous (IV)
- Neurologic Monitoring
- Oxygen Therapy
- Pacemaker Management: Permanent
- Pain Management: Acute
- Pain Management: Chronic
- Preparatory Sensory Information
- Quality Monitoring
- Radiation Therapy Management
- Referral
- Relaxation Therapy
- Research Protocol Management
- Respiratory Monitoring
- Resuscitation
- Sedation Management
- Shock Prevention
- Smoking Cessation Assistance
- Staff Supervision
- Teaching: Individual
- Teaching: Procedure or Treatment
- Technology Management
- Telecommunication Consultation
- Touch
- Tube Care
- Tube Care: Chest
- Tube Care: Gastrointestinal
- Tube Care: Urinary
- Ultrasonography: Bladder
- Urinary Catheterization
- Ventilation Assistance
- Vital Signs Monitoring

Rehabilitation Nursing

- Amputation Care
- Behavior Management
- Body Image Enhancement
- Body Mechanics Promotion
- Bowel Management
- Case Management
- Communication Enhancement: Speech Deficit
- Coping Enhancement
- Decision-Making Support
- Discharge Planning
- Dressing
- Embolus Precautions
- Emotional Support
- Energy Management
- Discharge Planning: Home Preparation
- Environmental Management: Safety
- Exercise Promotion: Strength Training
- Family Involvement Promotion
- Family Support
- Financial Resource Assistance
- Functional Ability Enhancement
- Health Coaching
- Health Education
- Hope Inspiration
- Learning Facilitation
- Life Skills Enhancement
- Medication Management
- Memory Training
- Multidisciplinary Care Conference
- Mutual Goal Setting
- Normalization Promotion
- Nutrition Management
- Pain Management: Chronic
- Positioning
- Positioning: Wheelchair
- Pressure Injury Care
- Pressure Injury Prevention
- Relapse Prevention
- Relocation Stress Reduction
- Self-Care Assistance
- Self-Efficacy Enhancement
- Self-Responsibility Facilitation
- Socialization Enhancement
- Swallowing Therapy
- Teaching: Individual
- Ultrasonography: Bladder
- Unilateral Neglect Management
- Urinary Catheterization: External
- Urinary Elimination Management
- Wound Care: Nonhealing

School Nursing

- Abuse Protection Support: Child
- Adolescent Care
- Active Listening
- Allergy Management
- Analgesic Administration
- Anger Control Assistance
- Anticipatory Guidance
- Anxiety Reduction
- Asthma Management
- Bleeding Reduction

- Bleeding Reduction: Wound
- Calming Technique
- Caregiver Support
- Child Care
- Commendation
- Contact Lens Care
- Coping Enhancement
- Counseling
- Crisis Intervention
- Decision-Making Support
- Delegation
- Documentation
- Emergency Care
- Emotional Support
- Eye Care
- Family Integrity Promotion
- Family Involvement Promotion
- Family Support
- First Aid
- Grief Work Facilitation
- Health Care Information Exchange
- Health Coaching
- Health Education
- Health Literacy Enhancement
- Health Screening
- Health System Guidance
- Heat/Cold Application
- Humor
- Hyperthermia Management
- Infection Control
- Learning Facilitation
- Learning Facilitation
- Medication Administration: Oral
- Medication Management
- Medication Management: Wearable Infusion Device
- Multidisciplinary Care Conference
- Nutritional Counseling

- Pain Management: Acute
- Pain Management: Chronic
- Parent Education: Adolescent
- Parent Education: Childrearing Family
- Patient Rights Protection
- Referral
- Resilience Promotion
- Resilience Promotion: Community
- Self-Efficacy Enhancement
- Self-Esteem Enhancement
- Skin Surveillance
- Social Marketing
- Socialization Enhancement
- Spiritual Support
- Substance Use Prevention
- Suicide Prevention
- Support Group
- Teaching: Adolescent Development
- Teaching: Adolescent Nutrition
- Teaching: Adolescent Safety
- Teaching: Early Childhood Development
- Teaching: Early Childhood Nutrition
- Teaching: Early Childhood Safety
- Teaching: Individual
- Teaching: Middle Childhood Development
- Teaching: Middle Childhood Nutrition
- Teaching: Middle Childhood Safety
- Teaching: Sports-Injury Prevention
- Telecommunication Consultation
- Touch
- Vaccination Management
- Values Clarification
- Vehicle Safety Promotion
- Vision Screening
- Vital Signs Monitoring
- Wound Care

Spinal Cord Injury Nursing

- Active Listening
- Airway Suctioning
- Artificial Airway Management
- Bathing
- Behavior Management
- Body Image Enhancement
- Bowel Management
- Caregiver Support
- Case Management
- Chest Physiotherapy
- Circulatory Precautions
- Coping Enhancement
- Discharge Planning
- Dressing
- Dysreflexia Management
- Emotional Support
- Family Involvement Promotion
- Feeding
- Financial Resource Assistance
- Fluid Management
- Functional Ability Enhancement

- Health Care Information Exchange
- Hope Inspiration
- Infection Protection
- Lower Extremity Monitoring
- Mechanical Ventilation Management: Invasive
- Mechanical Ventilation Management: Noninvasive
- Mechanical Ventilation Management: Pneumonia Prevention
- Medication Management
- Multidisciplinary Care Conference
- Mutual Goal Setting
- Nutrition Management
- Pain Management: Acute
- Pain Management: Chronic
- Pass Facilitation
- Peripheral Sensation Management
- Positioning
- Positioning: Wheelchair
- Pressure Injury Care
- Pressure Injury Prevention
- Relocation Stress Reduction
- Self-Care Assistance

- Self-Care Assistance: Toileting
- Self-Care Assistance: Transfer
- Teaching: Disease Process
- Teaching: Group
- Teaching: Individual
- Teaching: Prescribed Medication
- Teaching: Psychomotor Skill
- Thermoregulation Management
- Traction/Immobilization Care

- Transfer
- Tube Care: Urinary
- Ultrasonography: Bladder
- Urinary Bladder Training
- Urinary Catheterization
- Urinary Catheterization: External
- Urinary Catheterization: Intermittent
- Wound Care: Nonhealing

Transplant Nursing

- Acid-Base Management
- Case Management
- Coping Enhancement
- Counseling
- Decision-Making Support
- Electrolyte Management
- Electrolyte Monitoring
- Emotional Support
- Family Integrity Promotion
- Family Involvement Promotion
- Family Support
- Financial Resource Assistance
- Fluid Management
- Fluid Monitoring
- Hyperglycemia Management
- Hypertension Management
- Hypoglycemia Management
- Hypotension Management
- Infection Control
- Infection Protection
- Insurance Authorization

- IV Therapy
- Laboratory Data Interpretation
- Medication Administration
- Medication Management
- Medication Reconciliation
- Multidisciplinary Care Conference
- Neutropenic Precautions
- Organ Procurement
- Pain Management: Chronic
- Patient Identification
- Patient Rights Protection
- Stem Cell Infusion
- Support Group
- Surveillance
- Teaching: Disease Process
- Teaching: Individual
- Teaching: Prescribed Medication
- Teaching: Procedure or Treatment
- Values Clarification
- Vital Signs Monitoring
- Wound Care

Travel Health Nursing

- Anxiety Reduction
- Behavior Modification
- Capillary Blood Sample
- Communicable Disease Management
- Coping Enhancement
- Decision-Making Support
- Delegation
- Discharge Follow-Up
- Documentation
- Documentation: Meetings
- Electronic Health Record Access Assistance
- Emotional Support
- Examination Assistance
- First Aid
- Health Care Provider Collaboration
- Health Coaching
- Health Education
- Health Literacy Enhancement
- Health Screening
- Health System Guidance
- Human Trafficking Detection

- Medication Administration: Intradermal
- Medication Administration: Intramuscular (IM)
- Medication Administration: Oral
- Medication Administration: SQ
- Medication Management
- Medication Prescribing
- Nutritional Counseling
- Pandemic Precautions
- Physical Distancing Facilitation
- Point of Care Testing
- Prescribing: Diagnostic Testing
- Prescribing: Nonpharmacologic Treatment
- Quarantine Facilitation
- Referral
- Risk Identification
- Risk Identification: Infectious Disease
- Sleep Enhancement
- Surveillance
- Teaching: Disease Process
- Teaching: Individual
- Teaching: Prescribed Diet

- Teaching: Prescribed Medication
- Teaching: Procedure or Treatment
- Transport: Interfacility
- Triage: Emergency Center
- Triage: Telecommunication
- Vaccination Management
- Vision Screening
- Vital Signs Monitoring

Urologic Nursing

- Active Listening
- Analgesic Administration
- Behavior Modification
- Biofeedback
- Bladder Irrigation
- Body Image Enhancement
- Caregiver Support
- Case Management
- Chemotherapy Management
- Dialysis Access Maintenance
- Fluid/Electrolyte Management
- Infection Control: Intraoperative
- Intravenous (IV) Therapy
- Latex Precautions
- Medication Administration
- Medication Management
- Ostomy Care
- Pelvic Muscle Exercise
- Pessary Management
- Positioning: Intraoperative
- Preoperative Coordination
- Preparatory Sensory Information
- Prompted Voiding
- Radiation Therapy Management
- Skin Care: Absorbent Products
- Specimen Management
- Surgical Assistance
- Surgical Precautions
- Surgical Preparation
- Teaching: Disease Process
- Teaching: Individual
- Teaching: Preoperative
- Teaching: Prescribed Medication
- Teaching: Procedure or Treatment
- Temperature Regulation: Perioperative
- Tube Care
- Tube Care: Urinary
- Ultrasonography: Bladder
- Urinary Bladder Training
- Urinary Catheterization
- Urinary Catheterization: External
- Urinary Catheterization: Intermittent
- Urinary Elimination Management
- Urinary Habit Training
- Urinary Incontinence Care
- Urinary Retention Care
- Wound Care

Vascular Nursing

- Amputation Care
- Circulatory Care: Arterial Insufficiency
- Circulatory Care: Venous Insufficiency
- Circulatory Precautions
- Discharge Planning
- Embolus Care: Peripheral
- Embolus Care: Pulmonary
- Embolus Precautions
- Exercise Promotion: Strength Training
- Exercise Therapy: Ambulation
- Exercise Therapy: Joint Mobility
- Exercise Therapy: Muscle Control
- Foot Care
- Grief Work Facilitation
- Health Screening
- Hypertension Management
- Hypotension Management
- Incision Site Care
- Infection Protection
- Leech Therapy
- Lower Extremity Monitoring
- Medication Management
- Nail Care
- Nutrition Management
- Pain Management: Acute
- Pain Management: Chronic
- Peripheral Sensation Management
- Pressure Injury Care
- Pressure Injury Prevention
- Risk Identification
- Self-Care Assistance
- Skin Care: Donor Site
- Skin Care: Graft Site
- Skin Care: Topical Treatment
- Smoking Cessation Assistance
- Teaching: Individual
- Teaching: Prescribed Exercise
- Unilateral Neglect Management
- Wound Care
- Wound Care: Nonhealing

Women's Health Obstetric and Neonatal Nursing

- Abuse Protection Support
- Abuse Protection Support: Domestic Partner
- Anticipatory Guidance
- Behavior Modification
- Body Image Enhancement
- Breast Examination
- Coping Enhancement
- Counseling
- Decision-Making Support
- Emotional Support
- Exercise Promotion
- Family Planning: Contraception
- Family Planning: Infertility
- Family Planning: Unplanned Pregnancy
- Fertility Preservation
- Health Coaching
- Health Education
- Health Literacy Enhancement
- Health Screening
- Health System Guidance
- Hormone Replacement Therapy
- Labor Pain Management
- Listening Visits
- Medication Management
- Nutritional Counseling
- Pelvic Muscle Exercise
- Pessary Management
- Preconception Counseling
- Pregnancy Termination Care
- Premenstrual Syndrome (PMS) Management
- Risk Identification
- Self-Efficacy Enhancement
- Social Justice Facilitation
- Teaching: Disease Process
- Teaching: Individual
- Teaching: Safe Sex
- Telecommunication Consultation
- Urinary Bladder Training
- Weight Management
- Weight Reduction Assistance

Wound, Ostomy, and Continence Nursing

- Abdominal Massage
- Acid-Base Management
- Bowel Incontinence Care
- Circulatory Care: Arterial Insufficiency
- Circulatory Care: Venous Insufficiency
- Electrolyte Management
- Emotional Support
- Family Involvement Promotion
- Fluid/Electrolyte Management
- Incision Site Care
- Infection Control
- Lower Extremity Monitoring
- Medication Administration: Skin
- Medication Management
- Multidisciplinary Care Conference
- Nutrition Management
- Ostomy Care
- Pain Management: Chronic
- Pressure Injury Care
- Pressure Injury Prevention
- Self-Care Assistance
- Skin Care: Absorbent Products
- Skin Care: Topical Treatment
- Skin Surveillance
- Teaching: Disease Process
- Teaching: Procedure or Treatment
- Urinary Catheterization: External
- Urinary Elimination Management
- Urinary Incontinence Care
- Wound Care
- Wound Care: Nonhealing
- Wound Care: Protection

## PART FIVE

Estimated Time and Education Level Necessary to Perform NIC Interventions

Estimated Time and Education Level Necessary to Perform NIC Interventions

In this section, we list the estimated time to perform and type of personnel to deliver each of the 614 interventions in this edition of the Classification (see Table 1). The estimates were derived in the following manner:

Step One: The 433 interventions included in the second edition of NIC were rated in 1999 in response to a request from a user who was incorporating NIC into a coding/reimbursement manual.[1] Small groups of research team members rated selected interventions in their area of expertise on (1) education needed for each intervention and (2) time needed for each intervention. Rating group members referred to the NIC second edition[4] for intervention definitions and activities. Each group of raters returned their work to the principal investigators, who, with two other members of the research team, reviewed all the ratings for all interventions for overall consistency.

Step Two: In Fall 2000, ratings were done using the same methodology for the 53 interventions new to the third edition of NIC published in 2000.[5] Changes in interventions from the second to third edition were also examined for their impact on the ratings. Following this, all 486 intervention ratings were reviewed together, and a few of these were modified to be consistent with others in the same class. This information was published in a monograph titled "Estimated Time and Educational Requirements to Perform 486 Nursing Interventions,"[2] produced by the Center for Nursing Classification and Clinical Effectiveness at the College of Nursing, University of Iowa. Portions of the monograph were published in *Nursing Economic$* ("Determining Cost of Nursing Interventions: A Beginning").[3]

Step Three and Ongoing: Since 2002, for each of the new editions of the classification, we estimated the time and education for each of the new interventions using the same criteria.

Education needed is defined as the minimal educational level necessary to perform the intervention in most cases in most states and rated as: (1) assistive (e.g., nursing assistant, certified nursing assistant [CNA], scrub technician), LPN, LVN; (2) RN (basic education, whether baccalaureate,

associate degree, or diploma); or (3) advanced (i.e. advanced practice nurse [APN] is defined as specialized education or training beyond the RN basic education, including a master's degree with or without certification, certificate, or certification in a specialty area, or a doctoral degree (Doctor of Nursing Practice [DNP] or Doctor of Philosophy [PhD]). These categories were selected after thorough discussion. They were chosen over other possibilities because it was felt that the categories allow raters to differentiate among them but are not so fine that raters could not be consistent. The basic types of RN preparation were grouped in one category because this reflects the reality of the practice situation that does not usually differentiate job responsibilities by RN educational preparation.

Time needed is defined as the average time needed to initiate and complete the intervention. This is an average time that can be used to determine reimbursement rates, and assist with development of acuity levels. Time estimates are grouped into five categories: (1) 15 minutes or less, (2) 16 to 30 minutes, (3) 31 to 45 minutes, (4) 46 to 60 minutes, and (5) more than 1 hour.

It is emphasized that the estimates are based on the judgments of those who are familiar with the intervention and the specialty practice area. The ratings included here may differ by practice facility and provider. The estimates provide a starting point for estimating time required, level of provider needed, and cost of nursing care.

References

1. Alternative Link, Inc. (2001). *CAM and nursing coding manual.*
2. Center for Nursing Classification. (2001). *Estimated time and educational requirements to perform 486 nursing interventions.* Iowa City, IA
3. Iowa Intervention Project. (2001). Determining cost of nursing interventions: A beginning. *Nursing Economic$, 19*(4), 146–160.
4. McCloskey, J. C., & Bulechek, G. M. (Eds.). (1996). *Nursing interventions classification (NIC)* (2nd ed.). Mosby.
5. McCloskey, J. C., & Bulechek, G. M. (Eds.). (2000). *Nursing interventions classification (NIC)* (3rd ed.). Mosby.

Table 1	TIME & EDUCATION FOR 614 NIC INTERVENTIONS LISTED ALPHABETICALLY		
Intervention	Code No.	Educational Level	Time Required
Abdominal Massage	1310	RN	16–30 min
Abuse Protection Support	6400	RN	More than 1 hour
Abuse Protection Support: Child	6402	RN	More than 1 hour
Abuse Protection Support: Domestic Partner	6403	RN	More than 1 hour
Abuse Protection Support: Elder	6404	RN	More than 1 hour
Abuse Protection Support: Religious	6408	RN	More than 1 hour
Acid-Base Management	1910	RN	More than 1 hour
Acid-Base Management: Metabolic Acidosis	1911	RN	31–45 min
Acid-Base Management: Metabolic Alkalosis	1912	RN	31–45 min
Acid-Base Management: Respiratory Acidosis	1913	RN	31–45 min
Acid-Base Management: Respiratory Alkalosis	1914	RN	31–45 min
Acid-Base Monitoring	1920	RN	15 min or less
Active Listening	4920	RN	16–30 min
Activity Therapy	4310	RN	46–60 min
Acupressure	1320	Advanced	16–30 min
Admission Care	7310	RN	16–30 min
Adolescent Care	8272	RN	46–60 min
Advanced Care Planning	7300	RN	16–30 min
Airway Insertion and Stabilization	3120	RN	16–30 min
Airway Management	3140	RN	16–30 min
Airway Suctioning	3160	RN	15 min or less
Allergy Management	6410	RN	31–45 min
Amnioinfusion	6700	Advanced	31–45 min
Amputation Care	3420	RN	31–45 min
Analgesic Administration	2210	RN	16–30 min
Analgesic Administration: Intraspinal	2214	Advanced	16–30 min
Anaphylaxis Management	6412	RN	46–60 min
Anesthesia Administration	2840	Advanced	More than 1 hour
Anger Control Assistance	4640	Advanced	16–30 min
Animal-Assisted Therapy	4320	Assistive	16–30 min
Anticipatory Guidance	5210	RN	31–45 min
Anxiety Reduction	5820	Assistive	31–45 min
Area Restriction	6420	Assistive	More than 1 hour
Aromatherapy	1330	RN	15 min or less
Art Therapy	4330	Advanced	46–60 min
Artificial Airway Management	3180	RN	15 min or less
Aspiration Precautions	3200	Assistive	15 min or less
Assertiveness Training	4340	RN	46–60 min
Asthma Management	3210	RN	16–30 min
Attachment Promotion	6710	RN	More than 1 hour
Autogenic Training	5840	Advanced	46–60 min
Autotransfusion	2860	RN	46–60 min
Bathing	1610	Assistive	16–30 min
Bed Rest Care	0740	Assistive	16–30 min
Behavior Contracting	4420	RN	46–60 min
Behavior Management	4350	RN	46–60 min
Behavior Management: Inattention and Hyperactivity	4352	RN	31–45 min
Behavior Management: Self-Harm	4354	RN	31–45 min
Behavior Management: Sexual	4356	RN	31–45 min
Behavior Modification	4360	RN	More than 1 hour
Behavior Modification: Social Skills	4362	RN	More than 1 hour
Bereavement Care	5215	RN	More than 1 hour
Bibliotherapy	4680	Advanced	46–60 min

continued

Table 1	TIME & EDUCATION FOR 614 NIC INTERVENTIONS LISTED ALPHABETICALLY—cont'd		

Intervention	Code No.	Educational Level	Time Required
Biofeedback	5860	Advanced	46–60 min
Bioterrorism Preparedness	8810	Advanced	More than 1 hour
Birthing	6720	Advanced	More than 1 hour
Bladder Irrigation	0550	RN	16–30 min
Bleeding Precautions	4010	RN	31–45 min
Bleeding Reduction	4020	RN	46–60 min
Bleeding Reduction: Antepartum Uterus	4021	RN	46–60 min
Bleeding Reduction: Gastrointestinal	4022	RN	46–60 min
Bleeding Reduction: Nasal	4024	RN	16–30 min
Bleeding Reduction: Postpartum Uterus	4026	RN	46–60 min
Bleeding Reduction: Wound	4028	RN	46–60 min
Blood Products Administration	4030	RN	More than 1 hour
Body Image Enhancement	5220	RN	31–45 min
Body Mechanics Promotion	0140	RN	16–30 min
Body Search	6425	Assistive	15 min or less
Bottle Feeding	1052	Assistive	31–45 min
Bowel Incontinence Care	0410	RN	16–30 min
Bowel Incontinence Care: Encopresis	0412	RN	16–30 min
Bowel Management	0430	RN	31–45 min
Breast Examination	6522	RN	15 min or less
Calming Technique	5880	Assistive	31–45 min
Capillary Blood Sample	4035	RN	15 min or less
Cardiac Care	4040	RN	31–45 min
Cardiac Care: Acute	4044	RN	31–45 min
Cardiac Care: Rehabilitative	4046	RN	More than 1 hour
Cardiac Risk Management	4050	RN	31–45 min
Caregiver Support	7040	RN	More than 1 hour
Caring Interaction Development	5000	RN	More than 1 hour
Case Management	7320	Advanced	More than 1 hour
Cast Care: Maintenance	0762	Assistive	15 min or less
Cast Care: Wet	0764	RN	16–30 min
Central Venous Access Management: Central Insertion	4054	Advanced	31–45 min
Central Venous Access Management: Peripheral Insertion	4220	Advanced	31–45 min
Cerebral Edema Management	2540	RN	More than 1 hour
Cerebral Perfusion Promotion	2550	RN	31–45 min
Cesarean Birth Care	6750	RN	31–45 min
Chemical Restraint	6430	RN	15 min or less
Chemotherapy Management	2240	Advanced	46–60 min
Chest Physiotherapy	3230	RN	16–30 min
Childbirth Preparation	6760	RN	More than 1 hour
Child Care	8274	RN	46–60 min
Circulatory Care: Arterial Insufficiency	4062	RN	15 min or less
Circulatory Care: Mechanical Assist Device	4064	RN	31–45 min
Circulatory Care: Venous Insufficiency	4066	RN	15 min or less
Circulatory Precautions	4070	RN	16–30 min
Circumcision Care	3000	RN	46–60 min
Code Management	6140	RN	31–45 min
Cognitive Restructuring	4700	Advanced	16–30 min
Cognitive Stimulation	4720	Advanced	16–30 min
Collaboration Enhancement	7615	RN	More than 1 hour
Comfort Management	6482	Assistive	15 min or less
Commendation	4364	Assistive	15 min or less
Communicable Disease Management	8820	RN	46–60 min

Table 1	TIME & EDUCATION FOR 614 NIC INTERVENTIONS LISTED ALPHABETICALLY—cont'd		
Intervention	**Code No.**	**Educational Level**	**Time Required**
Communication Enhancement: Hearing Deficit	4974	Assistive	16–30 min
Communication Enhancement: Speech Deficit	4976	RN	31–45 min
Communication Enhancement: Visual Deficit	4978	Assistive	16–30 min
Community Disaster Preparedness	8840	RN	More than 1 hour
Community Health Advocacy	8510	RN	More than 1 hour
Community Health Development	8500	RN	More than 1 hour
Competency Management	7850	RN	More than 1 hour
Conflict Mediation	5020	Advanced	46–60 min
Constipation Management	0450	RN	16–30 min
Consultation	7910	RN	46–60 min
Contact Lens Care	1620	Assistive	15 min or less
Controlled Substance Checking	7620	RN	15 min or less
Coping Enhancement	5230	RN	31–45 min
Cost Containment	7630	RN	31–45 min
Cough Enhancement	3250	Assistive	15 min or less
Counseling	5240	Advanced	46–60 min
Crisis Intervention	6160	Advanced	46–60 min
Critical Path Development	7640	RN	More than 1 hour
Culture Care Negotiation	7330	RN	16–30 min
Cup Feeding: Newborn	8240	Assistive	31–45 min
Cutaneous Stimulation	1340	RN	16–30 min
Dance Therapy	4367	RN	46–60 min
Decision-Making Support	5250	RN	16–30 min
De-Escalation Management	6170	RN	16–30 min
Defibrillator Management: External	4095	RN	31–45 min
Defibrillator Management: Internal	4096	RN	31–45 min
Delegation	7650	RN	15 min or less
Delirium Management	6440	RN	More than 1 hour
Delusion Management	6450	RN	More than 1 hour
Dementia Management	6460	RN	More than 1 hour
Dementia Management: Bathing	6462	Assistive	31–45 min
Dementia Management: Wandering	6466	Assistive	More than 1 hour
Deposition	7930	RN	More than 1 hour
Developmental Enhancement: Infant	8278	RN	46–60 min
Dialysis Access Maintenance	4240	RN	15 min or less
Diarrhea Management	0460	RN	15 min or less
Diet Staging	1020	RN	15 min or less
Diet Staging: Weight Loss Surgery	1024	Advanced	31–45 min
Discharge Follow-Up	8190	RN	15 min or less
Discharge Planning	7370	RN	46–60 min
Discharge Planning: Home Preparation	6485	RN	More than 1 hour
Distraction	5900	Assistive	31–45 min
Documentation	7920	RN	15 min or less
Documentation: Meetings	7926	RN	More than 1 hour
Dressing	1630	Assistive	15 min or less
Dry Eye Prevention	1350	RN	16–30 min
Dying Care	5260	RN	16–30 min
Dysreflexia Management	2560	RN	16–30 min
Dysrhythmia Management	4090	RN	16–30 min
Ear Care	1640	RN	16–30 min
Ear Irrigation	1645	Assistive	15 min or less
Eating Disorders Management	1030	Advanced	31–45 min
Electroconvulsive Therapy (ECT) Management	2570	RN	More than 1 hour

continued

Table 1	TIME & EDUCATION FOR 614 NIC INTERVENTIONS LISTED ALPHABETICALLY—cont'd		
Intervention	**Code No.**	**Educational Level**	**Time Required**
Electrolyte Management	2000	RN	31–45 min
Electrolyte Management: Hypercalcemia	2001	RN	16–30 min
Electrolyte Management: Hyperkalemia	2002	RN	16–30 min
Electrolyte Management: Hypermagnesemia	2003	RN	16–30 min
Electrolyte Management: Hypernatremia	2004	RN	16–30 min
Electrolyte Management: Hyperphosphatemia	2005	RN	16–30 min
Electrolyte Management: Hypocalcemia	2006	RN	16–30 min
Electrolyte Management: Hypokalemia	2007	RN	16–30 min
Electrolyte Management: Hypomagnesemia	2008	RN	16–30 min
Electrolyte Management: Hyponatremia	2009	RN	16–30 min
Electrolyte Management: Hypophosphatemia	2010	RN	16–30 min
Electrolyte Monitoring	2020	RN	15 min or less
Electronic Fetal Monitoring: Antepartum	6771	Advanced	More than 1 hour
Electronic Fetal Monitoring: Intrapartum	6772	Advanced	More than 1 hour
Electronic Health Record Access Assistance	8070	Assistive	16–30 min
Elopement Precautions	6470	Assistive	More than 1 hour
Embolus Care: Peripheral	4104	RN	16–30 min
Embolus Care: Pulmonary	4106	RN	16–30 min
Embolus Precautions	4110	RN	16–30 min
Emergency Care	6200	Assistive	16–30 min
Emergency Cart Checking	7660	Assistive	15 min or less
Emotional Support	5270	RN	16–30 min
Endotracheal Extubation	3270	RN	15 min or less
Endotracheal Extubation: Palliative	1360	RN	15 min or less
Enema Administration	0466	Assistive	16–30 min
Energy Management	0180	RN	16–30 min
Enteral Tube Feeding	1056	RN	16–30 min
Environmental Management	6480	Assistive	31–45 min
Environmental Management: Community	6484	RN	More than 1 hour
Environmental Management: Safety	6486	RN	31–45 min
Environmental Management: Violence Prevention	6487	Assistive	More than 1 hour
Environmental Management: Worker Safety	6489	RN	More than 1 hour
Environmental Risk Protection	8880	RN	46–60 min
Examination Assistance	7680	Assistive	16–30 min
Exercise Promotion	0200	RN	31–45 min
Exercise Promotion: Strength Training	0201	RN	31–45 min
Exercise Promotion: Stretching	0202	RN	31–45 min
Exercise Therapy: Ambulation	0221	Assistive	15 min or less
Exercise Therapy: Balance	0222	RN	16–30 min
Exercise Therapy: Joint Mobility	0224	RN	16–30 min
Exercise Therapy: Muscle Control	0226	Advanced	16–30 min
Extracorporeal Membrane Oxygenation (ECMO) Therapy	4115	Advanced	More than 1 hour
Eye Care	1650	RN	15 min or less
Eye Irrigation	1655	Assistive	15 min or less
Fall Prevention	6490	RN	More than 1 hour
Family Integrity Promotion	7100	RN	More than 1 hour
Family Integrity Promotion: Childbearing Family	7104	RN	More than 1 hour
Family Involvement Promotion	7110	RN	More than 1 hour
Family Mobilization	7120	RN	More than 1 hour
Family Planning: Contraception	6784	RN	31–45 min
Family Planning: Infertility	6786	Advanced	46–60 min
Family Planning: Unplanned Pregnancy	6788	RN	46–60 min
Family Presence Facilitation	7170	RN	More than 1 hour

Table 1	TIME & EDUCATION FOR 614 NIC INTERVENTIONS LISTED ALPHABETICALLY—cont'd		
Intervention	**Code No.**	**Educational Level**	**Time Required**
Family Process Maintenance	7130	RN	More than 1 hour
Family Support	7140	RN	More than 1 hour
Family Therapy	7150	Advanced	More than 1 hour
Feeding	1050	Assistive	16–30 min
Fertility Preservation	7160	Advanced	31–45 min
Financial Resource Assistance	7380	RN	46–60 min
Fire-Setting Precautions	6500	Assistive	More than 1 hour
First Aid	6240	Assistive	16–30 min
Fiscal Resource Management	8550	Advanced	More than 1 hour
Flatulence Reduction	0470	RN	15 min or less
Fluid Management	4120	RN	31–45 min
Fluid Monitoring	4130	RN	16–30 min
Fluid Resuscitation	4140	RN	15 min or less
Fluid/Electrolyte Management	2080	RN	15 min or less
Foot Care	1660	RN	16–30 min
Forensic Data Collection	7940	Advanced	More than 1 hour
Forgiveness Facilitation	5280	RN	16–30 min
Functional Ability Enhancement	1665	RN	31–45 min
Gardening Therapy	4368	RN	More than 1 hour
Genetic Counseling	5242	Advanced	46–60 min
Grief Work Facilitation	5290	RN	31–45 min
Grief Work Facilitation: Perinatal Death	5294	RN	31–45 min
Guided Imagery	6000	RN	31–45 min
Guided Reflection	4730	RN	46–60 min
Guilt Work Facilitation	5300	RN	31–45 min
Hair and Scalp Care	1670	Assistive	16–30 min
Hallucination Management	6510	RN	More than 1 hour
Handoff Report	8140	RN	31–45 min
Healing Touch	1390	Advanced	46–60 min
Health Care Information Exchange	7960	RN	15 min or less
Health Care Provider Collaboration	7685	RN	16–30 min
Health Coaching	5305	RN	31–45 min
Health Education	5510	RN	16–30 min
Health Literacy Enhancement	5515	RN	16–30 min
Health Policy Monitoring	7970	RN	More than 1 hour
Health Screening	6520	RN	46–60 min
Health System Guidance	7400	RN	16–30 min
Heat/Cold Application	1380	RN	15 min or less
Hemodialysis Therapy	2100	Advanced	More than 1 hour
Hemodynamic Regulation	4150	RN	16–30 min
Hemofiltration Therapy	2110	RN	More than 1 hour
High-Risk Pregnancy Care	6800	Advanced	More than 1 hour
Home Maintenance Assistance	7180	RN	31–45 min
Hope Inspiration	5310	RN	16–30 min
Hormone Replacement Therapy	2280	Advanced	16–30 min
Human Trafficking Detection	6525	Assistive	16–30 min
Humor	5320	Assistive	15 min or less
Hyperglycemia Management	2120	RN	More than 1 hour
Hyperlipidemia Management	2125	Advanced	31–45 min
Hypertension Management	4162	RN	31–45 min
Hyperthermia Management	3786	RN	16–30 min
Hypervolemia Management	4170	RN	16–30 min
Hypnosis	5920	Advanced	46–60 min

continued

| Table 1 | TIME & EDUCATION FOR 614 NIC INTERVENTIONS LISTED ALPHABETICALLY—cont'd | | |

Intervention	Code No.	Educational Level	Time Required
Hypoglycemia Management	2130	RN	More than 1 hour
Hypotension Management	4175	RN	31–45 min
Hypothermia Induction Therapy	3790	RN	More that 1 hour
Hypothermia Treatment	3800	RN	More than 1 hour
Hypovolemia Management	4180	RN	16–30 min
Impulse Control Training	4370	Advanced	More than 1 hour
Incident Reporting	7980	RN	16–30 min
Incision Site Care	3440	RN	31–45 min
Infant Care	6820	RN	More than 1 hour
Infant Care: Eye Examination Support	6810	RN	16–30 min
Infant Care: Newborn	6824	RN	More than 1 hour
Infant Care: Preterm	6826	Advanced	More than 1 hour
Infection Control	6540	RN	31–45 min
Infection Control: Intraoperative	6545	RN	More than 1 hour
Infection Protection	6550	RN	31–45 min
Insurance Authorization	7410	RN	16–30 min
Intracranial Pressure (ICP) Monitoring	2590	RN	More than 1 hour
Intrapartal Care	6830	RN	More than 1 hour
Intrapartal Care: High-Risk Delivery	6834	Advanced	More than 1 hour
Intravenous (IV) Insertion	4190	RN	15 min or less
Intravenous (IV) Therapy	4200	RN	15 min or less
Invasive Hemodynamic Monitoring	4210	RN	46–60 min
Journaling	4740	RN	46–60 min
Kangaroo Care	6840	RN	46–60 min
Labor Induction	6850	Advanced	More than 1 hour
Labor Pain Management	6855	RN	46–60 min
Labor Suppression	6860	Advanced	More than 1 hour
Laboratory Data Interpretation	7690	RN	15 min or less
Lactation Counseling	5244	RN	31–45 min
Lactation Suppression	6870	RN	16–30 min
Laser Precautions	6560	Advanced	31–45 min
Latex Precautions	6570	RN	31–45 min
Laughter Yoga	5930	RN	46–60 min
Learning Facilitation	5520	RN	16–30 min
Leech Therapy	3460	RN	46–60 min
Life Skills Enhancement	5326	Advanced	46–60 min
Limit Setting	4380	RN	16–30 min
Listening Visits	5328	RN	46–60 min
Lower Extremity Monitoring	3480	RN	15 min or less
Malignant Hyperthermia Precautions	3840	RN	More than 1 hour
Massage	1480	RN	15 min or less
Mechanical Ventilation Management: Invasive	3300	RN	More than 1 hour
Mechanical Ventilation Management: Noninvasive	3302	RN	More than 1 hour
Mechanical Ventilation Management: Pneumonia Prevention	3304	RN	More than 1 hour
Mechanical Ventilatory Weaning	3310	RN	More than 1 hour
Medication Administration	2300	RN	15 min or less
Medication Administration: Continuous Subcutaneous Infusion	2321	RN	16–30 min
Medication Administration: Ear	2308	Assistive	15 min or less
Medication Administration: Enteral	2301	Assistive	15 min or less
Medication Administration: Eye	2310	Assistive	15 min or less
Medication Administration: Inhalation	2311	Assistive	15 min or less
Medication Administration: Interpleural	2302	Advanced	15 min or less

Table 1	TIME & EDUCATION FOR 614 NIC INTERVENTIONS LISTED ALPHABETICALLY—cont'd

Intervention	Code No.	Educational Level	Time Required
Medication Administration: Intradermal	2312	RN	15 min or less
Medication Administration: Intramuscular (IM)	2313	RN	15 min or less
Medication Administration: Intraocular Disk	2322	Assistive	15 min or less
Medication Administration: Intraosseous	2303	Advanced	15 min or less
Medication Administration: Intraspinal	2319	RN	15 min or less
Medication Administration: Intravenous (IV)	2314	RN	15 min or less
Medication Administration: Nasal	2320	Assistive	15 min or less
Medication Administration: Oral	2304	Assistive	15 min or less
Medication Administration: Rectal	2315	Assistive	15 min or less
Medication Administration: Skin	2316	Assistive	15 min or less
Medication Administration: Subcutaneous	2317	RN	15 min or less
Medication Administration: Vaginal	2318	Assistive	15 min or less
Medication Administration: Ventricular Reservoir	2307	Advanced	15 min or less
Medication Deprescribing	2370	Advanced	16–30 min
Medication Management	2380	RN	16–30 min
Medication Management: Medical Cannabis	2385	Advanced	16–30 min
Medication Management: Wearable Infusion Device	2398	RN	15 min or less
Medication Prescribing	2390	Advanced	15 min or less
Medication Reconciliation	2395	RN	16–30 min
Meditation Facilitation	5960	RN	16–30 min
Memory Training	4760	Advanced	31–45 min
Milieu Therapy	4390	RN	More than 1 hour
Mood Management	5330	RN	31–45 min
Motivational Interviewing	4395	RN	46–60 min
Multidisciplinary Care Conference	8020	RN	More than 1 hour
Music Therapy	4400	RN	15 min or less
Mutual Goal Setting	4410	RN	46–60 min
Nail Care	1680	Assistive	16–30 min
Nasal Irrigation	3316	RN	15 min or less
Nasogastric Intubation	1080	RN	15 min or less
Nausea Management	1450	RN	16–30 min
Neurologic Monitoring	2620	RN	16–30 min
Neutropenic Precautions	6580	RN	16–30 min
Nonnutritive Sucking	6900	Assistive	16–30 min
Normalization Promotion	7200	RN	More than 1 hour
Nutrition Management	1100	Advanced	31–45 min
Nutrition Therapy	1120	RN	16–30 min
Nutritional Counseling	5246	RN	16–30 min
Nutritional Monitoring	1160	RN	15 min or less
Oral Health Maintenance	1710	RN	15 min or less
Oral Health Promotion	1720	RN	15 min or less
Oral Health Restoration	1730	RN	15 min or less
Order Transcription	8060	RN	15 min or less
Organ Procurement	6260	RN	46–60 min
Ostomy Care	0480	Advanced	16–30 min
Oxygen Therapy	3320	RN	15 min or less
Pacemaker Management: Permanent	4091	RN	31–45 min
Pacemaker Management: Temporary	4092	RN	31–45 min
Pain Management: Acute	1410	RN	31–45 min
Pain Management: Chronic	1415	RN	More than 1 hour
Pandemic Precautions	6592	RN	16–30 min
Parent Education: Adolescent	5562	RN	16–30 min
Parent Education: Childrearing Family	5566	RN	16–30 min

continued

Table 1	TIME & EDUCATION FOR 614 NIC INTERVENTIONS LISTED ALPHABETICALLY—cont'd		
Intervention	**Code No.**	**Educational Level**	**Time Required**
Parent Education: Infant	5568	RN	31–45 min
Parenting Promotion	8300	RN	31–45 min
Pass Facilitation	7440	RN	15 min or less
Patient-Controlled Analgesia (PCA) Assistance	2400	RN	16–30 min
Patient Identification	6574	RN	15 min or less
Patient Rights Protection	7460	Assistive	15 min or less
Peer Review	7700	RN	More than 1 hour
Pelvic Muscle Exercise	0560	Advanced	16–30 min
Perineal Care	1750	Assistive	15 min or less
Peripheral Sensation Management	2660	RN	15 min or less
Peritoneal Dialysis Therapy	2150	RN	More than 1 hour
Pessary Management	0630	RN	16–30 min
Phlebotomy: Arterial Blood Sample	4232	RN	15 min or less
Phlebotomy: Blood Acquisition	4234	RN	More than 1 hour
Phlebotomy: Venous Blood Sample	4238	RN	15 min or less
Phototherapy: Mood Regulation	6926	RN	31–45 min
Phototherapy: Neonate	6924	RN	More than 1 hour
Phototherapy: Skin	3510	RN	16–30 min
Physical Accompaniment	6576	Assistive	16–30 min
Physical Distancing Facilitation	6594	RN	15 min or less
Physical Restraint	6580	RN	15 min or less
Phytotherapy	2420	RN	31–45 min
Pneumatic Tourniquet Management	2865	RN	46–60 min
Point of Care Testing	7610	Assistive	15 min or less
Positioning	0840	Assistive	16–30 min
Positioning: Intraoperative	0842	RN	16–30 min
Positioning: Neurologic	0844	Assistive	16–30 min
Positioning: Prone	3330	RN	16–30 min
Positioning: Wheelchair	0846	RN	15 min or less
Postanesthesia Care	2870	RN	46–60 min
Postmortem Care	1770	Assistive	16–30 min
Postpartal Care	6930	RN	More than 1 hour
Preceptor: Employee	7722	RN	More than 1 hour
Preceptor: Student	7726	RN	More than 1 hour
Preconception Counseling	5247	Advanced	More than 1 hour
Pregnancy Termination Care	6950	Advanced	More than 1 hour
Premenstrual Syndrome (PMS) Management	1440	Advanced	16–30 min
Prenatal Care	6960	RN	More than 1 hour
Preoperative Coordination	2880	RN	31–45 min
Preparatory Sensory Information	5580	RN	31–45 min
Prescribing: Diagnostic Testing	8080	Advanced	16–30 min
Prescribing: Nonpharmacologic Treatment	8086	Advanced	16–30 min
Presence	5340	Assistive	16–30 min
Pressure Injury Care	3520	Assistive	16–30 min
Pressure Injury Prevention	3540	RN	16–30 min
Procedural Support: Infant	6965	RN	16–30 min
Product Evaluation	7760	RN	More than 1 hour
Professional Development	7770	RN	More than 1 hour
Program Development	8700	Advanced	More than 1 hour
Progressive Muscle Relaxation	1460	Advanced	16–30 min
Prompted Voiding	0640	Assistive	15 min or less
Pruritus Management	3550	RN	16–30 min
Quality Monitoring	7800	RN	More than 1 hour

Table 1	TIME & EDUCATION FOR 614 NIC INTERVENTIONS LISTED ALPHABETICALLY—cont'd		
Intervention	**Code No.**	**Educational Level**	**Time Required**
Quarantine Facilitation	6596	RN	15 min or less
Radiation Therapy Management	6600	RN	46–60 min
Rapid Sequence Intubation	3340	Advanced	16–30 min
Readmission Prevention	7470	RN	16–30 min
Reality Orientation	4820	Assistive	15 min or less
Recreation Therapy	5360	Assistive	16–30 min
Rectal Prolapse Management	0490	Advanced	16–30 min
Referral	8100	RN	16–30 min
Reiki	1520	Advanced	46–60 min
Relapse Prevention	5235	RN	31–45 min
Relaxation Therapy	6040	RN	31–45 min
Religious Addiction Therapy	5422	RN	46–60 min
Religious Ritual Enhancement	5424	RN	31–45 min
Relocation Stress Reduction	5350	RN	16–30 min
Reminiscence Therapy	4860	Advanced	46–60 min
Reproductive Technology Management	7886	Advanced	More than 1 hour
Research Protocol Management	8130	RN	31–45 min
Resilience Promotion	8340	RN	More than 1 hour
Resilience Promotion: Community	8720	RN	More than 1 hour
Respiratory Monitoring	3350	RN	15 min or less
Respite Care	7260	RN	More than 1 hour
Resuscitation	6320	RN	16–30 min
Resuscitation: Fetus	6972	Advanced	More than 1 hour
Resuscitation: Neonate	6974	Advanced	46–60 min
Risk Identification	6610	RN	46–60 min
Risk Identification: Childbearing Family	6612	RN	More than 1 hour
Risk Identification: Genetic	6614	Advanced	More than 1 hour
Risk Identification: Infectious Disease	6620	RN	16–30 min
Role Enhancement	5370	RN	16–30 min
Safety Huddle	7810	RN	15 min or less
Seclusion	6630	RN	More than 1 hour
Sedation Management	2260	Advanced	More than 1 hour
Seizure Management	2680	RN	16–30 min
Seizure Precautions	2690	RN	15 min or less
Self-Awareness Enhancement	5390	RN	16–30 min
Self-Care Assistance	1800	Assistive	16–30 min
Self-Care Assistance: Toileting	1804	Assistive	15 min or less
Self-Care Assistance: Transfer	1806	Assistive	15 min or less
Self-Efficacy Enhancement	5395	RN	31–45 min
Self-Esteem Enhancement	5400	RN	16–30 min
Self-Hypnosis Facilitation	5922	Advanced	46–60 min
Self-Modification Assistance	4470	RN	46–60 min
Self-Responsibility Facilitation	4480	RN	46–60 min
Sexual Assault Trauma Care	6300	RN	More than 1 hour
Sexual Counseling	5248	Advanced	46–60 min
Shock Management	4250	RN	16–30 min
Shock Management: Cardiac	4254	RN	16–30 min
Shock Management: Sepsis	4255	RN	31–45 min
Shock Management: Vasogenic	4256	RN	31–45 min
Shock Management: Volume	4258	RN	31–45 min
Shock Prevention	4260	RN	16–30 min
Sibling Support	7280	RN	16–30 min
Skin Care: Absorbent Products	3570	Assistive	15 min or less

continued

Table 1	TIME & EDUCATION FOR 614 NIC INTERVENTIONS LISTED ALPHABETICALLY—cont'd		
Intervention	**Code No.**	**Educational Level**	**Time Required**
Skin Care: Donor Site	3582	RN	16–30 min
Skin Care: Graft Site	3583	RN	16–30 min
Skin Care: Topical Treatment	3584	RN	16–30 min
Skin Surveillance	3590	RN	16–30 min
Sleep Enhancement	1850	RN	16–30 min
Smoking Cessation Assistance	4490	RN	46–60 min
Social Justice Facilitation	8740	RN	More than 1 hour
Social Marketing	8750	Advanced	More than 1 hour
Socialization Enhancement	5100	RN	31–45 min
Specimen Management	7820	Assistive	15 min or less
Spiritual Growth Facilitation	5426	RN	31–45 min
Spiritual Support	5420	RN	16–30 min
Splinting	0910	RN	15 min or less
Staff Supervision	7830	RN	More than 1 hour
Stem Cell Infusion	4266	Advanced	More than 1 hour
Subarachnoid Hemorrhage Precautions	2720	RN	15 min or less
Substance Use Prevention	4500	RN	46–60 min
Substance Use Treatment	4510	RN	46–60 min
Substance Use Treatment: Alcohol Withdrawal	4512	Advanced	More than 1 hour
Substance Use Treatment: Drug Withdrawal	4514	Advanced	More than 1 hour
Substance Use Treatment: Overdose	4516	Advanced	More than 1 hour
Suicide Prevention	6340	RN	More than 1 hour
Supply Chain Management	7840	Assistive	16–30 min
Support Group	5430	Advanced	46–60 min
Support System Enhancement	5440	RN	31–45 min
Surgical Assistance	2900	RN	More than 1 hour
Surgical Instrumentation Management	2910	RN	More than 1 hour
Surgical Precautions	2920	RN	More than 1 hour
Surgical Preparation	2930	RN	46–60 min
Surveillance	6650	RN	More than 1 hour
Surveillance: Community	6652	RN	More than 1 hour
Surveillance: Late Pregnancy	6656	Advanced	More than 1 hour
Surveillance: Remote Monitoring	6658	RN	31–45 min
Surveillance: Video Monitoring	6660	Assistive	More than 1 hour
Sustenance Support	7500	RN	31–45 min
Suturing	3620	RN	16–30 min
Swallowing Therapy	1860	RN	31–45 min
Teaching: Adolescent Development 12–21 Years	5670	RN	16–30 min
Teaching: Adolescent Nutrition 12–21 Years	5672	RN	16–30 min
Teaching: Adolescent Safety 12–21 Years	5674	RN	16–30 min
Teaching: Disease Process	5602	RN	16–30 min
Teaching: Early Childhood Development 1–5 Years	5680	RN	16–30 min
Teaching: Early Childhood Nutrition 1–5 Years	5682	RN	16–30 min
Teaching: Early Childhood Safety 1–5 Years	5684	RN	16–30 min
Teaching: Group	5604	RN	More than 1 hour
Teaching: Individual	5606	RN	31–45 min
Teaching: Infant Development 0–3 Months	5655	RN	16–30 min
Teaching: Infant Development 4–6 Months	5658	RN	16–30 min
Teaching: Infant Development 7–9 Months	5656	RN	16–30 min
Teaching: Infant Development 10–12 Months	5657	RN	16–30 min
Teaching: Infant Nutrition 0–3 Months	5640	RN	16–30 min
Teaching: Infant Nutrition 4–6 Months	5641	RN	16–30 min
Teaching: Infant Nutrition 7–9 Months	5642	RN	16–30 min
Teaching: Infant Nutrition 10–12 Months	5643	RN	16–30 min

Table 1	TIME & EDUCATION FOR 614 NIC INTERVENTIONS LISTED ALPHABETICALLY—cont'd		
Intervention	**Code No.**	**Educational Level**	**Time Required**
Teaching: Infant Safety 0–3 Months	5645	RN	16–30 min
Teaching: Infant Safety 4–6 Months	5646	RN	16–30 min
Teaching: Infant Safety 7–9 Months	5647	RN	16–30 min
Teaching: Infant Safety 10–12 Months	5648	RN	16–30 min
Teaching: Infection Control	5649	RN	16–30 min
Teaching: Middle Childhood Development 6–12 Years	5650	RN	16–30 min
Teaching: Middle Childhood Nutrition 6–12 Years	5652	RN	16–30 min
Teaching: Middle Childhood Safety 6–12 Years	5654	RN	16–30 min
Teaching: Preoperative	5610	RN	16–30 min
Teaching: Prescribed Diet	5614	RN	16–30 min
Teaching: Prescribed Exercise	5612	RN	16–30 min
Teaching: Prescribed Medication	5616	RN	16–30 min
Teaching: Procedure or Treatment	5618	RN	16–30 min
Teaching: Psychomotor Skill	5620	RN	16–30 min
Teaching: Safe Sex	5622	RN	16–30 min
Teaching: Sexuality	5624	RN	16–30 min
Teaching: Sports-Injury Prevention	6648	RN	46–60 min
Teaching: Toddler Nutrition 13–18 Months	5660	RN	16–30 min
Teaching: Toddler Nutrition 19–24 Months	5661	RN	16–30 min
Teaching: Toddler Nutrition 25–36 Months	5662	RN	16–30 min
Teaching: Toddler Safety 13–18 Months	5665	RN	16–30 min
Teaching: Toddler Safety 19–24 Months	5666	RN	16–30 min
Teaching: Toddler Safety 25–36 Months	5667	RN	16–30 min
Teaching: Toilet Training	5634	RN	16–30 min
Technology Management	7880	RN	15 min or less
Telecommunication Consultation	8180	RN	16–30 min
Temperature Regulation	3900	RN	31–45 min
Temperature Regulation: Newborn	3910	RN	31–45 min
Temperature Regulation: Perioperative	3902	RN	More than 1 hour
Therapeutic Play	4430	RN	46–60 min
Therapeutic Touch	5465	Advanced	46–60 min
Therapy Group	5450	Advanced	46–60 min
Thermoregulation Management	3920	RN	31–45 min
Thrombolytic Therapy Management	4270	RN	More than 1 hour
Total Parenteral Nutrition (TPN) Administration	1200	RN	16–30 min
Touch	5460	Assistive	15 min or less
Traction/Immobilization Care	0940	RN	15 min or less
Transcutaneous Electrical Nerve Stimulation (TENS)	1540	Advanced	16–30 min
Transfer	0970	Assistive	15 min or less
Transgender Hormone Therapy	2430	RN	31–45 min
Transport: Interfacility	7890	RN	16–30 min
Transport: Intrafacility	7892	RN	31–45 min
Trauma Therapy: Child	5410	Advanced	46–60 min
Triage: Community Disaster	6362	RN	15 min or less
Triage: Emergency Center	6364	RN	15 min or less
Triage: Telecommunication	6366	RN	15 min or less
Truth Telling	5470	RN	16–30 min
Tube Care	1870	Assistive	15 min or less
Tube Care: Chest	1872	RN	15 min or less
Tube Care: Gastrointestinal	1874	RN	15 min or less
Tube Care: Umbilical Line	1875	Advanced	46–60 min
Tube Care: Urinary	1876	Assistive	15 min or less
Tube Care: Ventriculostomy/Lumbar Drain	1878	RN	15 min or less

continued

| Table 1 | TIME & EDUCATION FOR 614 NIC INTERVENTIONS LISTED ALPHABETICALLY—cont'd | | |

Intervention	Code No.	Educational Level	Time Required
Ultrasonography: Bladder	0565	Assistive	16–30 min
Ultrasonography: Obstetric and Gynecologic	6982	Advanced	31–45 min
Unilateral Neglect Management	2760	RN	31–45 min
Urinary Bladder Training	0570	Advanced	16–30 min
Urinary Catheterization	0580	Assistive	15 min or less
Urinary Catheterization: External	0581	Assistive	16–30 min
Urinary Catheterization: Intermittent	0582	Assistive	15 min or less
Urinary Elimination Management	0590	Advanced	31–45 min
Urinary Habit Training	0600	Advanced	31–45 min
Urinary Incontinence Care	0610	RN	31–45 min
Urinary Incontinence Care: Enuresis	0612	RN	16–30 min
Urinary Retention Care	0620	RN	15 min or less
Vaccination Management	6530	RN	16–30 min
Validation Therapy	6670	Advanced	46–60 min
Values Clarification	5480	RN	16–30 min
Vehicle Safety Promotion	9050	RN	More than 1 hour
Ventilation Assistance	3390	RN	15 min or less
Vision Screening	6675	RN	31–45 min
Visitation Facilitation	7560	Assistive	15 min or less
Vital Signs Monitoring	6680	RN	15 min or less
Vomiting Management	1570	RN	16–30 min
Weight Gain Assistance	1240	RN	16–30 min
Weight Management	1260	RN	31–45 min
Weight Reduction Assistance	1280	RN	16–30 min
Wound Care	3660	RN	31–45 min
Wound Care: Burns	3661	RN	More than 1 hour
Wound Care: Closed Drainage	3662	RN	31–45 min
Wound Care: Nonhealing	3664	RN	31–45 min
Wound Care: Protection	3670	Assistive	16–30 min
Wound Irrigation	3680	RN	31–45 min
Yoga	6050	RN	46–60 min

## PART SIX

Nursing Interventions and Nursing Outcomes Linked to Clinical Conditions

Nursing Interventions and Nursing Outcomes Linked to Clinical Conditions

This section provides linkages between six clinical conditions, the Nursing Outcomes Classification (NOC) outcomes and the Nursing Interventions Classification (NIC) interventions (see Tables 1 through 6). This section illustrates how NOC outcomes and NIC interventions can be linked to clinical conditions and used to form a plan of care for an individual with one of these conditions. As noted by Bulechek et al.:

> "A *linkage* is defined as a relationship or association between a clinical condition, a nursing outcome, and a nursing intervention that causes them to occur together in order to obtain a desired outcome or resolution of a person's problem. Linkages facilitate the diagnostic reasoning and clinical decision-making of the nurse by identifying nursing interventions and outcomes that are treatment options for the resolution of the clinical condition. They can also assist those who are designing clinical nursing information systems to structure their databases."[4] (p. 462)

The clinical conditions presented in this section are Coronary Artery Disease, Coronavirus Disease 2019, Hyperlipidemia, Lung Cancer, Substance Use Disorder, and Ulcerative Colitis/Crohn's Disease. Each condition contains a description of the condition including prevalence and mortality, and noting evidence-based recommendations for treatment. All of the conditions in this section are listed in the top 10 health conditions affecting persons in the United States,[29] and most are noted in the top costly health concerns on the Centers for Disease Control and Prevention (CDC) website for the National Center for Chronic Disease Prevention and Health Promotion (NCCDPHP).[6]

The conditions are presented alphabetically using the names identified in the preceding sections. A generic care plan is presented, with varying depth and number of outcomes and interventions provided. In general, the plans do not address consideration of age, gender, socioeconomic status, or culture because these may differ from organization to organization. They do demonstrate the various ways in which NOC outcomes and NIC interventions can be used in the development of generic and individual care plans for persons with any of these six clinical conditions.

NOC outcomes are presented in alphabetical order and not in order of importance or a particular sequence in which they might be used. The NIC are comprehensive and include multiple interventions, again in alphabetical order

but also indicating priorities. The following two levels of interventions are provided for each clinical condition in separate columns:

1. Major Interventions: "these are the most likely or most obvious intervention(s) to impact the outcome listed."[4] (p. 462)
2. Suggested Interventions: "These are interventions that are likely to address the outcome but not as likely as the priority intervention, for the majority of the persons with the condition. These are also interventions that may apply only to some persons with the condition, allowing the nurse to further tailor the plan of care to the individual."[4] (p. 462)

The following steps are suggested when using the linkage list:

1. Factors to consider when selecting outcomes include: "the type of health problem, the nursing or medical diagnoses, patient characteristics, available resources, patient preferences and treatment potential."[28] (pp. 9–10) Moorhead et al. also note when outcome selection is based on the medical diagnoses (or clinical conditions), "nurses should consider the signs and symptoms of the medical diagnosis as well as the causative and other related factors."[28] (pp. 9–10)
2. Review the major nursing interventions for that outcome, for first consideration as the treatment of choice for resolution of a condition.[4]
3. Review the suggested interventions for those that may also be used for resolution of the condition.[4]

Coronary Artery Disease

Coronary artery disease (CAD) occurs when the arteries that supply blood to the heart become damaged, causing the formation of atherosclerotic plaque in the arteries. This in turn leads to obstructed blood flow through these hardened and narrowed arteries. It is the most common type of heart disease and the leading cause of death in the United States for both men and women.[25] Globally, CAD is a primary cause of death, affecting individuals negatively as it reduces their functional skills and self-care abilities and disrupts quality of life.[46] Treatments include helping affected persons to adopt lifestyle adjustments,[46] and develop self-efficacy and increased self-care capacity through continuity of nursing care.[7,36]

Table 1	NIC AND NOC LINKAGES FOR CORONARY ARTERY DISEASE		
Outcome	**Major Interventions**	**Suggested Interventions**	
Activity Tolerance	Activity Therapy Energy Management	Body Mechanics Promotion Exercise Promotion Functional Ability Enhancement Medication Management	Oxygen Therapy Teaching: Prescribed Exercise Weight Management
Health Promoting Behavior	Health Education	Culture Care Negotiation Health Coaching Risk Identification Self-Modification Assistance Support System Enhancement	Teaching: Disease Process Teaching: Prescribed Exercise Teaching: Prescribed Diet Teaching: Prescribed Medication Teaching: Procedure or Treatment
Hypertension Severity	Hypertension Management	Exercise Promotion Fluid Monitoring Hyperlipidemia Management Medication Management Sleep Enhancement	Smoking Cessation Assistance Teaching: Prescribed Diet Teaching: Prescribed Exercise Teaching: Prescribed Medication Weight Reduction Assistance
Participation in Health Care Decisions	Coping Enhancement Decision-Making Support Self-Responsibility Facilitation	Assertiveness Training Health Coaching Health Literacy Enhancement	Health System Guidance Self-Efficacy Enhancement
Respiratory Status	Respiratory Monitoring	Airway Management Chest Physiotherapy Cough Enhancement Energy Management	Oxygen Therapy Ventilation Assistance Vital Signs Monitoring
Self-Management: Coronary Artery Disease	Teaching: Disease Process	Cardiac Risk Management Culture Care Negotiation Energy Management Exercise Promotion Family Involvement Promotion Health Coaching Hyperlipidemia Management Hypertension Management Medication Management Nutritional Counseling	Relaxation Therapy Self-Efficacy Enhancement Self-Modification Assistance Smoking Cessation Assistance Sleep Enhancement Teaching: Prescribed Exercise Teaching: Prescribed Diet Teaching: Prescribed Medication Teaching: Procedure or Treatment Weight Reduction Assistance
Smoking Cessation Behavior	Smoking Cessation Assistance	Coping Enhancement Health Coaching Health Education	Self-Modification Assistance Self-Responsibility Facilitation Teaching: Disease Process
Stress Level	Relaxation Therapy	Anxiety Reduction Gardening Therapy Guided Reflection Laughter Yoga Massage	Meditation Facilitation Reiki Self-Hypnosis Facilitation Yoga
Symptom Control	Teaching: Disease Process	Cardiac Risk Management Culture Care Negotiation Energy Management Health Coaching Hyperlipidemia Management Hypertension Management Nutritional Counseling Relaxation Therapy	Smoking Cessation Assistance Support Group Teaching: Prescribed Exercise Teaching: Prescribed Diet Teaching: Prescribed Medication Teaching: Procedure or Treatment Weight Management
Weight Maintenance Behavior	Weight Management	Behavior Modification Exercise Promotion Health Coaching Medication Management	Nutritional Counseling Teaching: Prescribed Diet Teaching: Prescribed Exercise Weight Reduction Assistance

Coronavirus Disease 2019

Coronavirus disease 2019 (COVID-19) is an infectious respiratory disease caused by the SARS-CoV-2 virus, with symptoms that vary from mild to moderate respiratory illness to serious illness and even death. Older people and those with underlying health conditions like cardiovascular disease, diabetes, chronic respiratory disease, or cancer are most likely to develop serious illness. As of 2021, there were 179 million confirmed cases worldwide[11] and 6.9 million deaths.[45] Initial data indicate a higher proportion of infection in non-White, lower income populations.[33] Treatments include focusing on psychological needs as well as physiological needs,[13,20] attending to respiratory needs and unexpected sequelae,[3,38,41] addressing age-related concerns particularly in vulnerable populations,[15] and encouraging vaccination and infection control practices.[42]

Table 2		NIC and NOC Linkages for Coronavirus Disease 2019	
Outcome	**Major Interventions**	**Suggested Interventions**	
Acute Respiratory Acidosis Severity	Acid-Base Management: Respiratory Acidosis	Acid-Base Management: Respiratory Alkalosis: Acid-Base Monitoring Mechanical Ventilation Management: Noninvasive	Mechanical Ventilation Management: Pneumonia Prevention Positioning: Prone Oxygen Therapy Respiratory Monitoring Ventilation Assistance
Comfort Status	Comfort Management	Anxiety Reduction Calming Technique Medication Management	Pain Management: Acute Progressive Muscle Relaxation Relaxation Therapy
Energy Conservation	Energy Management	Body Mechanics Promotion Pain Management: Acute Functional Ability Enhancement	Self-Modification Assistance Sleep Enhancement Teaching: Prescribed Exercise
Fatigue Level	Sleep Enhancement	Energy Management Medication Management	Massage Positioning
Fear Level	Coping Enhancement	Anxiety Reduction Emotional Support Healing Touch Hope Inspiration	Meditation Facilitation Presence Relaxation Therapy Spiritual Support
Fluid Balance	Fluid Management	Fluid/Electrolyte Management Fluid Monitoring	Vital Signs Monitoring Weight Management
Infection Severity	Risk Identification: Infectious Disease	Health Screening Infection Protection Risk Identification	Social Marketing Teaching: Disease Process Vaccination Management
Immunization Behavior	Vaccination Management	Risk Identification Teaching: Disease Process	Teaching: Procedure or Treatment
Knowledge: Disease Process	Teaching: Disease Process	Health Coaching Health System Guidance Medication Management Risk Identification Teaching: Individual	Teaching: Prescribed Exercise Teaching: Prescribed Diet Teaching: Prescribed Medication Teaching: Procedure or Treatment Vaccination Management
Loneliness Severity	Coping Enhancement	Activity Therapy Emotional Support Family Support Grief Work Facilitation Healing Touch Mood Management	Presence Recreation Therapy Socialization Enhancement Support System Enhancement Telephone Consultation
Medication Response	Teaching: Individual Teaching: Prescribed Medication	Health Education Learning Facilitation	Medication Management Surveillance

Table 2	NIC and NOC Linkages for Coronavirus Disease 2019—cont'd	

Outcome	Major Interventions	Suggested Interventions	
Mechanical Ventilation Response: Adult	Mechanical Ventilation Management: Invasive Mechanical Ventilation Management: Noninvasive	Acid-Base Monitoring Airway Management Artificial Airway Management Mechanical Ventilatory Weaning	Oxygen Therapy Respiratory Monitoring Ventilation Assistance Vital Signs Monitoring
Neurological Status: Consciousness	Neurological Monitoring	Cerebral Perfusion Promotion Medication Management Respiratory Monitoring	Surveillance Vital Signs Monitoring
Nutritional Status	Nutritional Counseling Nutritional Monitoring	Nutrition Management Nutrition Therapy	Teaching: Prescribed Diet
Psychosocial Adjustment: Life Change	Coping Enhancement	Culture Care Negotiation Decision-Making Support Emotional Support Health Coaching Hope Inspiration Life Skills Enhancement	Resilience Promotion Role Enhancement Spiritual Support Support Group Values Clarification
Respiratory Status* Respiratory Status: Airway Patency* Respiratory Status: Gas Exchange* Respiratory Status: Ventilation*	Respiratory Monitoring Airway Management Oxygen Therapy	Acid-Base Monitoring Acid-Base Management: Respiratory Acidosis Airway Management Airway Suctioning Artificial Airway Management Aspiration Precautions Chest Physiotherapy Comfort Management Cough Enhancement Electrolyte Management Energy Management Extracorporeal Membrane Oxygenation Therapy	Fluid Monitoring Mechanical Ventilation Management: Noninvasive Mechanical Ventilation Management: Pneumonia Prevention Medication Management Neurological Monitoring Positioning Positioning: Prone Smoking Cessation Assistance Surveillance Teaching: Procedure or Treatment Ventilation Assistance Vital Signs Monitoring
Risk Control: Infectious Process	Risk Identification: Infectious Disease	Infection Protection Risk Identification	Self-Responsibility Facilitation
Self-Care: Activities of Daily Living (ADL)	Self-Care Assistance	Bathing Dressing Feeding	Self-Care Assistance: Toileting Self-Care Assistance: Transfer
Spiritual Health	Spiritual Support	Dying Care Emotional Support Forgiveness Facilitation Grief Work Facilitation Guilt Work Facilitation	Hope Inspiration Religious Ritual Enhancement Reminiscence Therapy Spiritual Growth Facilitation Values Clarification
Symptom Control	Cough Enhancement Hyperthermia Management	Chest Physiotherapy Comfort Management Energy Management Fluid Management Medication Administration	Nutritional Monitoring Positioning: Prone Respiratory Monitoring Sleep Enhancement Surveillance
Thermoregulation	Hyperthermia Management	Temperature Regulation Fluid Management Fluid Monitoring	Infection Protection Medication Administration

*More than one outcome may apply to a clinical condition.

Hyperlipidemia

Hyperlipidemia is defined as elevated lipid levels within the body, such as cholesterol or triglycerides. Elevated lipid levels may predispose a person to serious illnesses that may lead to death, such as CAD.[19] There are over 3 million adults throughout the United States and Europe that currently have hyperlipidemia, and that number continues to rise.[18] The degree of hyperlipidemia is highest in persons with premature CAD, defined as CAD arising in males before age 55 to 60 years and females before age 65 years.[18] Prevalence is significantly greater among White people than Black people and among men than women.[18] In countries with lower overall rates of obesity and saturated fat consumption, the prevalence of hyperlipidemia and subsequent CAD is lower, when contrasted to rates in Europe and throughout the United States.[21] Treatment is most effective when nursing care includes nonpharmacological and pharmacological measures, with a focus on lifestyle changes.[17,26,35]

Table 3   NIC AND NOC LINKAGES FOR HYPERLIPIDEMIA

Outcome	Major Intervention	Suggested Interventions	
Health Promoting Behavior	Health Education Self-Modification Assistance Teaching: Disease Process	Behavior Modification Commendation Culture Care Negotiation Health Coaching Health Screening Health System Guidance Medication Management	Nutritional Management Risk Identification Self-Responsibility Facilitation Teaching: Prescribed Diet Teaching: Prescribed Exercise Teaching: Prescribed Medication
Knowledge: Lipid Disorder Management	Teaching: Disease Process	Culture Care Negotiation Exercise Promotion Health Education Health Coaching Learning Facilitation Nutritional Counseling	Sleep Enhancement Smoking Cessation Assistance Teaching: Prescribed Exercise Teaching: Prescribed Diet Teaching: Prescribed Medication Weight Management
Medication Response	Teaching: Individual Teaching: Prescribed Medication	Hyperlipidemia Management	Medication Management Surveillance
Nutritional Status	Nutritional Counseling Nutritional Monitoring	Nutrition Management Nutrition Therapy	Teaching: Prescribed Diet Weight Management
Participation in Health Care Decisions	Decision-Making Support Self-Responsibility Facilitation	Health Literacy Enhancement	Mutual Goal Setting Self-Efficacy Enhancement
Risk Control: Lipid Disorder	Hyperlipidemia Management	Laboratory Data Interpretation Teaching: Prescribed Diet	Teaching: Prescribed Exercise Teaching: Prescribed Medication
Self-Management: Lipid Disorder	Self-Efficacy Enhancement Self-Responsibility Facilitation	Exercise Promotion Health Coaching Hyperlipidemia Management Medication Management Nutritional Management	Sleep Enhancement Teaching: Prescribed Exercise Teaching: Prescribed Diet Teaching: Prescribed Medication Weight Management
Stress Level	Anxiety Reduction Meditation Facilitation Relaxation Therapy	Comfort Management Exercise Promotion Gardening Therapy Guided Reflection Reiki	Self-Hypnosis Facilitation Sleep Enhancement Support Group Yoga
Symptom Control	Teaching: Disease Process	Culture Care Negotiation Exercise Promotion Nutritional Counseling Relaxation Therapy Risk Identification Smoking Cessation Assistance	Support Group Teaching: Prescribed Exercise Teaching: Prescribed Diet Teaching: Prescribed Medication Teaching: Procedure or Treatment Weight Management
Weight Maintenance Behavior	Weight Management Nutritional Counseling	Behavior Modification Exercise Promotion Medication Management	Teaching: Prescribed Diet Teaching: Prescribed Exercise Weight Reduction Assistance

Lung Cancer

Lung cancer is defined as any cancer that originates in the lung tissue. It is the leading cause of cancer death and the second most diagnosed cancer in both men and women in the United States, with 1.8 million deaths and 2.21 million cases in 2020.[2] African American males have the highest incidence; Hispanic women have the lowest incidence.[2] Worldwide, the number of smokers increased between 1980 and 2012, as lung cancer rates climbed in developing countries with increased tobacco smoking.[2] Treatment options are improving, but survival remains low. Thus, nursing care is focused on disruptive effects of treatment, adaptation to chronic illness, and preventative measures.[8,12,22,24,44]

Table 4	NIC AND NOC LINKAGES FOR LUNG CANCER		
Outcome	**Major Intervention**	**Suggested Interventions**	
Activity Tolerance	Activity Therapy Energy Management Respiratory Monitoring	Body Mechanics Promotion Comfort Management Environmental Management Exercise Promotion Functional Ability Enhancement Medication Management Meditation Facilitation	Nutrition Management Oxygen Therapy Progressive Muscle Relaxation Self-Care Assistance Sleep Enhancement Teaching: Prescribed Exercise Weight Management
Adaptation to Physical Disability	Mutual Goal Setting Self-Modification Assistance Teaching: Disease Process	Coping Enhancement Counseling Culture Care Negotiation Decision-Making Support Guided Reflection Health Coaching Teaching: Disease Process	Teaching: Infection Control Teaching: Prescribed Exercise Teaching: Prescribed Diet Teaching: Prescribed Medication Teaching: Procedure or Treatment Teaching: Psychomotor Skill
Chemotherapy: Disruptive Physical Effects	Comfort Management	Chemotherapy Management Diarrhea Management Medication Management Nausea Management Neutropenic Precautions	Pain Management: Acute Pain Management: Chronic Progressive Muscle Relaxation Teaching: Infection Control Vomiting Management
Comfort Status	Comfort Management	Calming Technique Coping Enhancement Medication Management Meditation Facilitation	Pain Management: Acute Progressive Muscle Relaxation Relaxation Therapy Respiratory Monitoring
Coping	Coping Enhancement	Commendation Decision-Making Support Emotional Support	Resilience Promotion Support System Enhancement Therapy Group
Depression Level	Mood Management Coping Enhancement Self-Esteem Enhancement	Active Listening Counseling Emotional Support Forgiveness Facilitation	Guilt Work Facilitation Medication Administration Therapy Group
Electrolyte Balance	Electrolyte Management	Acid-Base Management Electrolyte Monitoring	Fluid/Electrolyte Management
Fatigue Level	Energy Management Fall Prevention	Environmental Management Medication Management Mood Management	Self-Care Assistance Sleep Enhancement Surveillance
Fluid Balance	Fluid Management	Fluid/Electrolyte Management Fluid Monitoring	Vital Signs Monitoring Weight Management
Health Beliefs: Perceived Control	Decision-Making Support Self-Efficacy Enhancement	Advanced Care Planning Coping Enhancement Counseling	Health Coaching Journaling Self-Responsibility Facilitation

continued

Table 4	NIC and NOC Linkages for Lung Cancer—cont'd		

Outcome	Major Intervention	Suggested Interventions	
Health Promoting Behavior	Health Education Self-Modification Assistance	Health Coaching Health Screening Risk Identification Self-Awareness Enhancement	Support Group Support System Enhancement Teaching: Infection Control
Hope	Hope Inspiration Spiritual Support	Anxiety Reduction Coping Enhancement Decision-Making Support Dying Care	Emotional Support Grief Work Facilitation Presence Touch
Knowledge: Cancer Management	Teaching: Disease Process Teaching: Procedure or Treatment	Anticipatory Guidance Chest Physiotherapy Cough Enhancement Coping Enhancement Culture Care Negotiation Energy Management Fluid Management Health System Guidance Medication Management Oxygen Therapy Positioning Positioning: Prone	Relaxation Therapy Risk Identification Sleep Enhancement Smoking Cessation Assistance Support Group Teaching: Individual Teaching: Infection Control Teaching: Prescribed Exercise Teaching: Prescribed Diet Teaching: Prescribed Medication Vaccination Management
Medication Response	Teaching: Individual Teaching: Prescribed Medication	Chemotherapy Management Diarrhea Management Learning Facilitation Medication Management Nausea Management	Nutrition Therapy Surveillance Teaching: Disease Process Vomiting Management
Nausea & Vomiting Severity	Nausea Management Vomiting Management	Comfort Management Nutrition Management	Surveillance Weight Management
Nutritional Status	Nutritional Counseling Nutritional Monitoring	Nutrition Management Nutrition Therapy	Teaching: Prescribed Diet Weight Management
Personal Resiliency	Resilience Promotion	Assertiveness Training Coping Enhancement Decision-Making Support Emotional Support Functional Ability Enhancement Health Coaching Health Literacy Enhancement Health System Guidance	Mood Management Mutual Goal Setting Risk Identification Role Enhancement Self-Efficacy Enhancement Self-Esteem Enhancement Self-Responsibility Facilitation Support Group
Post-Procedure Recovery	Energy Management Pain Management: Acute	Analgesic Administration Bed Rest Care Bowel Management Cough Enhancement Fluid Management Incision Site Care Infection Protection Nausea Management Nutritional Monitoring Oral Health Maintenance	Positioning Respiratory Monitoring Self-Care Assistance Self-Efficacy Enhancement Sleep Enhancement Temperature Regulation Urinary Elimination Management Vital Signs Monitoring Wound Care: Closed Drainage
Quality of Life	Hope Inspiration Values Clarification	Coping Enhancement Emotional Support Family Support Mood Management Resilience Promotion	Role Enhancement Socialization Enhancement Spiritual Support Support System Enhancement Sustenance Support

Table 4	NIC and NOC Linkages for Lung Cancer—cont'd		
Outcome	**Major Intervention**		**Suggested Interventions**
Respiratory Status	Respiratory Monitoring Ventilation Assistance	Airway Management Anxiety Reduction Aspiration Precautions Chest Physiotherapy Cough Enhancement	Energy Management Mechanical Ventilation Management: Noninvasive Oxygen Therapy Vital Signs Monitoring
Risk Control: Cancer	Risk Identification	Health Education Health Screening Smoking Cessation Assistance	Teaching: Prescribed Exercise Teaching: Prescribed Diet Teaching: Prescribed Medication

Self-Management:
  Cancer
	Teaching: Disease Process
	Teaching: Procedure or
	  Treatment
		Anxiety Reduction
		Cough Enhancement
		Coping Enhancement
		Culture Care Negotiation
		Energy Management
		Fluid Management
		Health System Guidance
		Medication Management
		Meditation Facilitation
		Oxygen Therapy
		Positioning
			Relaxation Therapy
			Risk Identification
			Sleep Enhancement
			Smoking Cessation Assistance
			Support Group
			Teaching: Individual
			Teaching: Infection Control
			Teaching: Prescribed Exercise
			Teaching: Prescribed Diet
			Teaching: Prescribed Medication
			Vaccination Management

Spiritual Health	Spiritual Support	Active Listening Calming Technique Coping Enhancement Dying Care Emotional Support Forgiveness Facilitation Grief Work Facilitation Guilt Work Facilitation	Hope Inspiration Music Therapy Religious Ritual Enhancement Reminiscence Therapy Self-Esteem Enhancement Spiritual Growth Facilitation Support System Enhancement Values Clarification
Symptom Control	Teaching: Disease Process	Culture Care Negotiation Energy Management Family Involvement Promotion Health System Guidance Nutritional Counseling Relaxation Therapy Resilience Promotion Risk Identification Sexual Counseling	Smoking Cessation Assistance Support Group Teaching: Infection Control Teaching: Prescribed Exercise Teaching: Prescribed Diet Teaching: Prescribed Medication Teaching: Procedure or Treatment Weight Management Yoga
Weight Maintenance Behavior	Weight Management Nutritional Counseling	Behavior Modification Exercise Promotion Health Coaching	Teaching: Prescribed Diet Teaching: Prescribed Exercise Weight Gain Assistance

Substance Use Disorder

Substance use disorder is defined as excessive use of psychoactive drugs, such as alcohol, pain medications, or illegal drugs. Substances or classes of substances for which addictive disorders are recognized include alcohol, caffeine, cannabis, hallucinogens, inhalants, opioids, (e.g., sedatives, hypnotics, anxiolytics), stimulants, and tobacco.[14] Statistics are alarming for this disorder. For example, in 2018 more than 139 million Americans 12 years or older reported alcohol use and 31 million reported illicit drug use.[40] Opioids were involved in nearly 68% of all drug overdose deaths, with substance use costing the United States more than $600 billion annually.[32] Males are more likely to have drug use disorder than females, and White and Hispanic races are more likely.[40] Native Americans have the highest prevalence of substance-related disorder, followed by adolescents of multiple race/ethnicities, adolescents of White race/ethnicity, Hispanics, African Americans, and Asians or Pacific Islanders.[40] Treatment includes detoxification measures[39] with a focus on fostering improved self-care habits to avoid relapse,[16,43] building personal resiliency,[1,27,37] and preventative measures.[9,30,34]

Table 5	NIC AND NOC LINKAGES FOR SUBSTANCE USE DISORDER		
Outcome	**Major Intervention**	**Suggested Interventions**	
Adherence Behavior	Mutual Goal Setting Patient Contracting	Behavior Modification Commendation Counseling Relapse Prevention Self-Modification Assistance Self-Responsibility Facilitation	Support Group Teaching: Disease Process Teaching: Procedure or Treatment Teaching: Psychomotor Skill Values Clarification
Alcohol Abuse Cessation Behavior	Substance Use Treatment	Impulse Control Training Motivational Interviewing Self-Modification Assistance Self-Responsibility Facilitation	Substance Use Treatment: Alcohol Withdrawal Teaching: Disease Process
Depression Level	Mood Management Coping Enhancement Self-Esteem Enhancement	Active Listening Counseling Emotional Support Forgiveness Facilitation	Guilt Work Facilitation Hope Medication Administration Therapy Group
Drug Abuse Cessation Behavior	Substance Use Treatment	Impulse Control Training Medication Management Self-Awareness Enhancement Self-Efficacy Enhancement Self-Responsibility Facilitation	Self-Modification Assistance Substance Use Treatment: Drug Withdrawal Substance Use Treatment: Overdose Support Group
Impulse Self Control	Impulse Control Training Values Clarification	Behavior Management De-escalation Management Health Coaching Hope Mutual Goal Setting Motivational Interviewing	Self-Modification Assistance Self-Responsibility Facilitation Support Group Teaching: Disease Process Teaching: Procedure or Treatment Truth Telling
Medication Response	Teaching: Individual Teaching: Prescribed Medication	Health Education Learning Facilitation	Medication Management Surveillance
Knowledge: Healthy Lifestyle	Health Education Self-Modification Assistance	Coping Enhancement Exercise Promotion Health Screening Nutritional Counseling Risk Identification Self-Awareness Enhancement	Smoking Cessation Assistance Substance Use Prevention Support Group Support System Enhancement Weight Management
Knowledge: Stress Management	Anxiety Reduction Teaching: Disease Process	Comfort Management Exercise Promotion Sleep Enhancement	Smoking Cessation Assistance Support Group Yoga
Personal Resiliency	Resilience Promotion	Coping Enhancement Decision-Making Support Emotional Support Mood Management Role Enhancement	Self-Esteem Enhancement Self-Responsibility Facilitation Social Justice Facilitation Support Group

Table 5	NIC AND NOC LINKAGES FOR SUBSTANCE USE DISORDER—cont'd		
Outcome	**Major Intervention**	**Suggested Interventions**	
Risk Control: Alcohol Use	Coping Enhancement Substance Use Prevention	Behavior Management: Self Harm Impulse Control Training Risk Identification Self-Esteem Enhancement	Self-Modification Assistance Self-Responsibility Facilitation Spiritual Support Support Group
Risk Control: Drug Use	Coping Enhancement Substance Use Prevention	Behavior Management: Self Harm Impulse Control Training Risk Identification Self-Esteem Enhancement	Self-Modification Assistance Self-Responsibility Facilitation Spiritual Support Support Group
Risk Control: Tobacco Use	Coping Enhancement Substance Use Prevention	Behavior Management: Self Harm Impulse Control Training Risk Identification Self-Esteem Enhancement	Self-Modification Assistance Self-Responsibility Facilitation Smoking Cessation Assistance Spiritual Support
Self-Care Status	Self-Care Assistance	Bathing	Dressing
Social Support	Family Involvement Promotion Support System Enhancement	Caregiver Support Family Support Referral Respite Care Relapse Prevention	Socialization Enhancement Social Justice Facilitation Spiritual Support Support Group
Substance Addiction Consequences	Substance Use Treatment	Body Search Caring Interaction Development Coping Enhancement Counseling Decision-Making Support De-Escalation Management Exercise Promotion Family Involvement Promotion Impulse Control Training Infection Protection Patient Contracting Role Enhancement	Self-Awareness Enhancement Self-Esteem Enhancement Self-Modification Assistance Self-Responsibility Facilitation Socialization Enhancement Spiritual Support Substance Use Prevention Support Group Teaching: Disease Process Therapy Group Truth Telling

Ulcerative Colitis/Crohn's Disease

Crohn's disease (CD) and ulcerative colitis (UC) are two major inflammatory bowel diseases (IBDs). CD can affect any part of the gastrointestinal tract, while UC occurs in the large intestine or rectum.[31] UC affects the lining of the colon, whereas CD can affect the layers of the colon wall of the alimentary tract anywhere from the mouth to the anus and may even skip segments.[31] (p.11) At times, it is difficult to distinguish between UC or CD. About 3 million United States adults have CD or UC, with approximately 80,000 that are children.[10] CD is found in all racial groups worldwide, but the highest prevalence rates have been reported in White populations, particularly those of North America and Europe, with significantly lower rates seen in Black and Asian populations.[10] UC is more common in people of eastern and central European (Ashkenazi) Jewish descent, and less common in African Americans, Asians, Hispanics, and Native Americans. Treatment goals focus on complete remission, although this is not as easily accomplished in CD as in UC, leading to nursing care that is focused on symptom management,[5] adaptation to chronic illness,[23] and preventative measures.[10]

| Table 6 | NIC and NOC Linkages for Ulcerative Colitis/Crohn's Disease | | |

Outcome	Major Intervention	Suggested Interventions	
Activity Tolerance	Energy Management	Activity Therapy Environmental Management: Safety Functional Ability Enhancement	Self-Care Assistance Teaching: Prescribed Exercise Vital Signs Monitoring
Adaptation to Physical Disability	Mutual Goal Setting Self-Modification Assistance Teaching: Disease Process	Coping Enhancement Counseling Culture Care Negotiation Health Coaching Teaching: Disease Process	Teaching: Individual Teaching: Prescribed Exercise Teaching: Prescribed Diet Teaching: Prescribed Medication
Bowel Elimination	Bowel Management	Abdominal Massage Constipation Management Diarrhea Management Enema Administration Medication Management	Nausea Management Nutrition Management Pain Management: Acute Vomiting Management
Comfort Status	Comfort Management	Calming Technique Emotional Support Medication Management Meditation Facilitation	Pain Management: Acute Progressive Muscle Relaxation Relaxation Therapy Vital Signs Monitoring
Depression Level	Mood Management Coping Enhancement Self-Esteem Enhancement	Counseling Emotional Support Forgiveness Facilitation	Guilt Work Facilitation Medication Management Therapy Group
Fluid Balance	Fluid Management	Fluid/Electrolyte Management Fluid Monitoring	Vital Signs Monitoring Weight Management
Health Beliefs: Perceived Control	Decision-Making Support Self-Efficacy Enhancement	Assertiveness Training Coping Enhancement Counseling	Health Coaching Journaling Self-Responsibility Facilitation
Knowledge: Inflammatory Bowel Disease Management	Teaching: Disease Process Teaching: Prescribed Exercise Teaching: Prescribed Medication	Comfort Management Culture Care Negotiation Energy Management Exercise Promotion Medication Management Nutrition Management	Self-Modification Assistance Sexual Counseling Sleep Enhancement Smoking Cessation Assistance Support Group Weight Management
Medication Response	Teaching: Individual Teaching: Prescribed Medication Medication Management	Constipation Management Diarrhea Management Nausea Management	Nutritional Counseling Surveillance Vomiting Management
Nutritional Status	Nutritional Counseling Nutritional Monitoring	Nutrition Management Nutrition Therapy Teaching: Prescribed Diet	Weight Gain Assistance Weight Management Weight Reduction Assistance
Psychosocial Adjustment: Life Change	Coping Enhancement	Anticipatory Guidance Behavior Management Culture Care Negotiation Decision-Making Support Emotional Support Hope Inspiration Life Skills Enhancement	Mood Management Relaxation Therapy Resilience Promotion Role Enhancement Self-Esteem Enhancement Spiritual Support Support Group
Self-Management: Inflammatory Bowel Disease	Teaching: Disease Process Teaching: Prescribed Exercise Teaching: Prescribed Medication	Comfort Management Energy Management Exercise Promotion Medication Management Meditation Facilitation Nutrition Management	Self-Modification Assistance Sexual Counseling Sleep Enhancement Smoking Cessation Assistance Vital Signs Monitoring Weight Management

Table 6	NIC AND NOC LINKAGES FOR ULCERATIVE COLITIS/CROHN'S DISEASE —cont'd		
Outcome	Major Intervention	Suggested Interventions	
Social Involvement	Behavior Modification: Social Skills Socialization Enhancement	Family Involvement Promotion Family Support Motivational Interviewing Recreation Therapy Referral	Role Enhancement Spiritual Support Support Group Support System Enhancement Visitation Facilitation
Symptom Control	Teaching: Disease Process	Culture Care Negotiation Energy Management Health Coaching Nutritional Counseling Relaxation Therapy Resilience Promotion Risk Identification	Sexual Counseling Smoking Cessation Assistance Support Group Teaching: Prescribed Exercise Teaching: Prescribed Diet Teaching: Prescribed Medication Weight Management
Weight Maintenance Behavior	Weight Management Nutritional Counseling	Behavior Modification Exercise Promotion Teaching: Prescribed Diet	Teaching: Prescribed Exercise Weight Gain Assistance Weight Reduction Assistance

References

1. Ariss, T., & Fairbairn, C. E. (2020). The effect of significant other involvement in treatment for substance use disorders: A meta-analysis. *Journal of Consulting and Clinical Psychology*, 88(6), 526–540. https://doi.org/10.1037/ccp0000495
2. Bade, B. C., & Cruz, C. S. D. (2020). Lung cancer 2020: Epidemiology, etiology, and prevention. *Clinics in Chest Medicine*, 41(1), 1–24.
3. Behesht Aeen, F., Pakzad, R., Goudarzi Rad, M., Abdi, F., Zaheri, F., & Mirzadeh, N. (2021). Effect of prone position on respiratory parameters, intubation and death rate in COVID-19 patients: Systematic review and meta-analysis. *Scientific Reports*, 11(1), 14407. https://doi.org/10.1038/s41598-021-93739-y
4. Bulechek, G., Butcher, H., Dochterman, J., & Wagner, C. (2013). *Nursing Interventions Classification* (6th ed.). Elsevier.
5. Casey, G. (2017). Inflammatory bowel disease. *Kai Tiaki Nursing New Zealand*, 23(2), 20–26.
6. Centers for Disease Control and Prevention. (2022). *Health and economic costs for chronic diseases. National Center for Chronic Disease Prevention and Health Promotion (NCCDPHP).* https://www.cdc.gov/chronicdisease/about/costs/index.htm
7. Chiang, C.-Y., Choi, K.-C., Ho, K.-M., & Yu, S.-F. (2018). Effectiveness of nurse-led patient-centered care behavioral risk modification on secondary prevention of coronary heart disease: A systematic review. *International Journal of Nursing Studies*, 84, 28–39. https://doi.org/10.1016/j.ijnurstu.2018.04.012
8. Chorattas, A., Papastavrou, E., Charalambous, A., & Kouta, C. (2020). Home-based educational programs for management of dyspnea: A systematic literature review. *Home Health Care Management & Practice*, 32(4), 211–217. https://doi.org/10.1177/1084822320907908
9. Compton, W. M., Jones, C. M., Baldwin, G. T., Harding, F. M., Blanco, C., & Wargo, E. M. (2019). Targeting youth to prevent later substance use disorder: an underutilized response to the US opioid crisis. *American Journal of Public Health*, 109(S3), S185–S189.
10. Davis, S. C., Robinson, B. L., Vess, J., & Lebel, J. S. (2018). Primary care management of ulcerative colitis. *Nurse Practitioner*, 43(1), 11–20. https://doi.org/10.1097/01.NPR.0000527565.05934.14
11. Dessie, Z. G., & Zewotir, T. (2021). Mortality-related risk factors of COVID-19: A systematic review and meta-analysis of 42 studies and 423,117 patients. *BMC Infectious Diseases*, 21(1), 1–28. https://doi.org/10.1186/s12879-021-06536-3
12. dos Santos Cordeiro, V., Migueis Berardinelli, L. M., & da Silva Santos, R. (2018). Chemotherapy in patients with lung cancer: A look on nursing care. *Journal of Nursing UFPE / Revista de Enfermagem UFPE*, 12(10), 2854–2863. https://doi.org/10.5205/1981-8963-v12i10a234745p2854-2863-2018
13. Fan, W.-J., & Liu, X.-L. (2020). Effect of advanced nursing care on psychological disorder in patients with COVID-19: A protocol of systematic review. *Medicine*, 99(27), 1–3. https://doi.org/10.1097/MD.0000000000021026
14. Finnell, D. S., Tierney, M., & Mitchell, A. M. (2019). Nursing: Addressing substance use in the 21st century. *Substance Abuse*, 40(4), 412–420. https://doi.org/10.1080/08897077.2019.1674240
15. Frazer, K., Mitchell, L., Stokes, D., Lacey, E., Crowley, E., & Kelleher, C. C. (2021). A rapid systematic review of measures to protect older people in long-term care facilities from COVID-19. *BMJ Open*, 11(10), e047012. https://doi.org/10.1136/bmjopen-2020-047012
16. Gonzalez, Y., Kozachik, S., & Finnell, D. (2020). Educating ambulatory care nurses to address substance use. *Journal of Nursing Care Quality*, 35(4), 353–358. https://doi.org/10.1097/NCQ.0000000000000466
17. Gorina, M., Limonero, J. T., & Álvarez, M. (2018). Effectiveness of primary healthcare educational interventions undertaken by nurses to improve chronic disease management in patients with diabetes mellitus, hypertension and hypercholesterolemia: A systematic review. *International Journal of Nursing Studies*, 86, 139–150. https://doi.org/10.1016/j.ijnurstu.2018.06.016
18. Grundy, S. M., Stone, N. J., Bailey, A. L., Beam, C., Birtcher, K. K., Blumenthal, R. S., Braun, L. T., DeFerranti, S., Faiella-Tommasino, J., Forman, D. E., Goldberg, R., & Yeboah, J. (2019). 2018 AHA/ACC/AACVPR/AAPA/ABC/ACPM/ADA/AGS/APhA/ASPC/NLA/PCNA Guideline on the management of blood cholesterol: Executive summary: A report of the American College of Cardiology/American Heart Association Task Force on Clinical Practice Guidelines. *Journal of the American College of Cardiology*, 73(24), 3168–3209.

19. Jellinger, P. S., Smith, D. A., Mehta, A. E., Ganda, O., Handelsman, Y., Rodbard, H. W., Shepherd, M. D., Seibel, J. A., & AACE Task Force for Management of Dyslipidemia and Prevention of Atherosclerosis, (2012). American Association of Clinical Endocrinologists' Guidelines for management of dyslipidemia and prevention of atherosclerosis. *Endocrine Practice: Official Journal of the American College of Endocrinology and the American Association of Clinical Endocrinologists, 18*(Suppl 1), 1–78. https://doi.org/10.4158/ep.18.s1.1

20. Johnstone, J., & Duncan, D. (2021). Coronavirus: the 7th C affecting the 6Cs. A focus on compassion, care and touch. *British Journal of Nursing, 30*(15), 928–933. https://doi.org/10.12968/bjon.2021.30.15.928

21. Karr, S. (2017). Epidemiology and management of hyperlipidemia. *The American Journal of Managed Care, 23*(9 Suppl), S139–S148.

22. Liu, X., Wang, Y.-Q., & Xie, J. (2019). Effects of breathing exercises on patients with lung cancer. *Oncology Nursing Forum, 46*(3), 303–317. https://doi.org/10.1188/19.ONF.303-317

23. Lo, C.-H., Khalili, H., Song, M., Lochhead, P., Burke, K. E., Richter, J. M., Giovannucci, E. L., Chan, A. T., & Ananthakrishnan, A. N. (2021). Healthy lifestyle is associated with reduced mortality in patients with inflammatory bowel diseases. *Clinical Gastroenterology and Hepatology: The Official Clinical Practice Journal of the American Gastroenterological Association, 19*(1), 87. https://doi.org/10.1016/j.cgh.2020.02.047

24. Luckett, T., Phillips, J., Currow, D. C., Agar, M., & Molassiotis, A. (2019). Cough in lung cancer: A survey of current practice among Australian health professionals. *Collegian, 26*(6), 629–633. https://doi.org/10.1016/j.colegn.2019.09.002

25. Malakar, A. K., Choudhury, D., Halder, B., Paul, P., Uddin, A., & Chakraborty, S. (2019). A review on coronary artery disease, its risk factors, and therapeutics. *Journal of Cellular Physiology, 234*(10), 16812–16823. https://doi.org/10.1002/jcp.28350

26. Mbue, N. D., Mbue, J. E., & Anderson, J. A. (2017). Management of lipids in patients with diabetes. *Nursing Clinics of North America, 52*(4), 605–619. https://doi.org/10.1016/j.cnur.2017.07.009

27. McPherson, S. M., Burduli, E., Smith, C. L., Herron, J., Oluwoye, O., Hirchak, K., Orr, M. F., McDonell, M. G., & Roll, J. M. (2018). A review of contingency management for the treatment of substance-use disorders: adaptation for underserved populations, use of experimental technologies, and personalized optimization strategies. *Substance Abuse and Rehabilitation, 9*, 43–57. https://doi.org/10.2147/SAR.S138439

28. Moorhead, S., Swanson, E., Johnson, M., & Maas, M. (2018). *Nursing outcomes classification (NOC): Measurement of health outcomes* (6th ed.). Elsevier.

29. Morgan, K. (2018, October 24). *These are the top 10 health conditions affecting Americans.* USA Today. https://www.usatoday.com/story/sponsor-story/blue-cross-blue-shield-association/2018/10/24/these-top-10-health-conditions-affecting-americans/1674894002/

30. Moulahoum, H., Zihnioglu, F., Timur, S., & Coskunol, H. (2019). Novel technologies in detection, treatment and prevention of substance use disorders. *Journal of Food and Drug Analysis, 27*(1), 22–31.

31. Naeck-Boolauky, P., Adio, J., & Burch, J. (2020). Review of normal gastrointestinal tract, ulcerative colitis, proctitis and rectal medication adherence. *British Journal of Nursing, 29*(14), 805–811. https://doi.org/10.12968/bjon.2020.29.14.805

32. National Institute on Drug Abuse, (2018). *Principles of drug addiction treatment: A research-based guide* (3rd ed.). CreateSpace Independent Publishing Platform.

33. Obinna, D. N. (2021). Confronting disparities: Race, ethnicity, and immigrant status as intersectional determinants in the COVID-19 Era. *Health Education & Behavior, 48*(4), 397–403. https://doi.org/10.1177/10901981211011581

34. Phelps, C. L., Paniagua, S. M., Willcockson, I. U., & Potter, J. S. (2018). The relationship between self-compassion and the risk for substance use disorder. *Drug and Alcohol Dependence, 183*, 78–81.

35. Podvorica, E., Bytyci, I., & Oruqi, M. (2020). Ambulatory nurse education improves metabolic profile and physical activity in patients with cardiovascular disease. *International Journal of Nursing Education, 12*(4), 55–61.

36. Posadas-Collado, G., Membrive-Jiménez, M. J., Romero-Béjar, J. L., Gómez-Urquiza, J. L., Albendín-García, L., Suleiman-Martos, N., & Cañadas-De La Fuente, G. A. (2022). Continuity of nursing care in patients with coronary artery disease: A systematic review. *International Journal of Environmental Research and Public Health, 19*(5). https://doi.org/10.3390/ijerph19053000

37. Priddy, S. E., Howard, M. O., Hanley, A. W., Riquino, M. R., Friberg-Felsted, K., & Garland, E. L. (2018). Mindfulness meditation in the treatment of substance use disorders and preventing future relapse: neurocognitive mechanisms and clinical implications. *Substance Abuse and Rehabilitation, 9*, 103–114. https://doi.org/10.2147/SAR.S145201

38. Puslecki, M., Dabrowski, M., Baumgart, K., Ligowski, M., Dabrowska, A., Ziemak, P., Stefaniak, S., Szarpak, L., Friedrich, T., Szlanga, L., Skorupa, P., Steliga, A., Hebel, K., Andrejanczyk, B., Ladzinska, M., Wieczorek, M., Puslecki, L., Smereka, J., Tukacs, M., & Swol, J. (2021). Managing patients on extracorporeal membrane oxygenation support during the COVID-19 pandemic – a proposal for a nursing standard operating procedure. *BMC Nursing, 20*(1), 1–12. https://doi.org/10.1186/s12912-021-00736-7

39. Salmond, S., Allread, V., & Marsh, R. (2019). Management of opioid use disorder treatment: An overview. *Orthopaedic Nursing, 38*(2), 118–128. https://doi.org/10.1097/NOR.0000000000000522

40. Substance Abuse and Mental Health Services Administration, (2019). *Key substance use and mental health indicators in the United States: Results from the 2018 National Survey on drug use and health.* Rockville, MD: Center for Behavioral Health Statistics and Quality, Substance Abuse and Mental Health Services Administration.

41. Swanson, E., Mantovani, V. M., Wagner, C., Moorhead, S., Lopez, K. D., Macieira, T. G. R., & Abe, N. (2021). NANDA-I, NOC, and NIC linkages to SARS-CoV-2 (COVID-19): Part 2. Individual response. *International Journal of Nursing Knowledge, 32*(1), 68–83. https://doi.org/10.1111/2047-3095.12307

42. Thomas, R. E. (2021). Reducing morbidity and mortality rates from COVID-19, Influenza and Pneumococcal Illness in nursing homes and long-term care facilities by vaccination and comprehensive infection control interventions. *Geriatrics (Basel, Switzerland), 6*(2). https://doi.org/10.3390/geriatrics6020048

43. Volkow, N. D. (2020). Personalizing the treatment of substance use disorders. *American Journal of Psychiatry, 177*(2), 113–116.

44. Wang, Y.-Q., Liu, X., Yin, Y.-Y., Ma, R.-C., Yang, Z., Cao, H.-P., & Xie, J.(2019). Effects of home-based exercise training for patients with lung cancer. *Oncology Nursing Forum, 46*(4), E119–E134. https://doi.org/10.1188/19.ONF.E119-E134

45. World Health Organization. (Febrary 23, 2023). WHO Coronavirus (COVID-19) Dashboard. https://covid19.who.int/

46. Yildiz, F. T., & Kaşikçi, M. (2020). Impact of training based on Orem's Theory on Self-Care Agency and quality of life in patients with coronary artery disease. *Journal of Nursing Research (Lippincott Williams & Wilkins), 28*(6), 1–10. https://doi.org/10.1097/jnr.0000000000000406

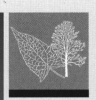

## PART SEVEN

Appendices

Interventions: New, Revised, and Retired Since the Seventh Edition

INTERVENTIONS NEW TO THE EIGHTH EDITION (n=60)

Abdominal Massage
Advanced Care Planning
Bereavement Care
Body Search
De-Escalation Management
Ear Irrigation
Electronic Health Record Access Assistance
Endotracheal Extubation: Palliative
Extracorporeal Membrane Oxygenation Therapy
Eye Irrigation
Gardening Therapy
Guided Reflection
Health Care Provider Collaboration
Human Trafficking Detection
Infant Care: Eye Examination Support
Labor Pain Management
Laughter Yoga
Medication Administration: Continuous Subcutaneous Infusion
Medication Administration: Intraocular Disk
Medication Deprescribing
Medication Management: Medical Cannabis
Medication Management: Wearable Infusion Device
Motivational Interviewing
Neutropenic Precautions
Pandemic Precautions
Phototherapy: Skin
Physical Accompaniment
Physical Distancing Facilitation
Positioning: Prone
Professional Development Facilitation
Quarantine Facilitation
Rapid Sequence Induction and Intubation
Readmission Prevention
Relapse Prevention
Research Protocol Management
Resilience Promotion: Community
Risk Identification: Infectious Disease
Safety Huddle
Shock Management: Sepsis
Skin Care: Absorbent Products
Social Justice Facilitation
Surveillance: Video Monitoring
Teaching: Adolescent Development 12–21 Years
Teaching: Adolescent Nutrition 12–21 Years
Teaching: Adolescent Safety 12–21 Years
Teaching: Early Childhood Development 1–5 Years
Teaching: Early Childhood Nutrition 1–5 Years
Teaching: Early Childhood Safety 1–5 Years
Teaching: Infant Development 4–6 Months
Teaching: Infection Control
Teaching: Middle Childhood Development 6–12 Years
Teaching: Middle Childhood Nutrition 6–12 Years
Teaching: Middle Childhood Safety 6–12 Years
Temperature Regulation: Newborn
Thermoregulation Management
Transgender Hormone Therapy
Ultrasonography: Bladder
Urinary Catheterization: External
Wound Care: Protection
Yoga

INTERVENTIONS REVISED FOR THE EIGHTH EDITION
Label Name Changes (n=32)

Adolescent Care (formerly Developmental Enhancement: Adolescent 8272)
Behavior Contracting (formerly Patient Contracting 4420)
Behavior Management: Inattention and Hyperactivity (formerly Behavior Management: Overactivity/Inattention 4352)
Caring Interaction Development (formerly Complex Relationship Building 5000)

Central Venous Access Management: Central Insertion (formerly Central Venous Access Device Management 4054)
Central Venous Access Management: Peripheral Insertion (formerly Peripherally Inserted Central Catheter [PICC] Care 4220)
Child Care (formerly Developmental Enhancement: Child 8274)

Comfort Management (formerly Environmental Management: Comfort 6482)

Competency Management (formerly Staff Development 7850)

Constipation Management (formerly Constipation/Impaction Management 0450)

Cultural Care Negotiation (formerly Culture Brokerage 7330)

Deposition (formerly Deposition/Testimony 7930)

Discharge Follow-Up (formerly Telephone Follow-Up 8190)

Discharge Planning: Home Preparation (formerly Environmental Management: Home Preparation 6485)

Hyperthermia Management (formerly Hyperthermia Treatment 3786)

Phlebotomy: Blood Acquisition (formerly Phlebotomy: Blood Unit Acquisition 4234)

Phototherapy: Mood Regulation (formerly Phototherapy: Mood/Sleep Regulation 6926)

Pressure Injury Care (formerly Pressure Ulcer Care 3520)

Pressure Injury Prevention (formerly Pressure Ulcer Prevention 3540)

Religious Addiction Therapy (formerly Religious Addiction Prevention 5422)

Resilience Promotion (formerly Resiliency Promotion 8340)

Sexual Assault Trauma Care (formerly Rape-Trauma Treatment 6300)

Surveillance: Remote Monitoring (formerly Surveillance: Remote Electronic 6658)

Teaching: Infant Development 0–3 Months (formerly Teaching: Infant Stimulation 0–4 Months 5655)

Teaching: Infant Development 7–9 Months (formerly Teaching: Infant Stimulation 5–8 Months 5656)

Teaching: Infant Development 10–12 Months (formerly Teaching: Infant Stimulation 9–12 Months 5657)

Teaching: Procedures or Treatments (formerly Teaching: Procedure/Treatment 5618)

Teaching: Sports Injury Prevention (formerly Sports Injury Prevention: Youth 6648)

Telecommunication Consultation (formerly Telephone Consultation 8180)

Triage: Community Disaster (formerly Triage: Disaster 6362)

Triage: Telecommunication (formerly Triage: Telephone 6366)

Vaccination Management (formerly Immunization/Vaccination Management 6530)

Intervention Changes: Major (n=159)

Interventions in this category have substantive changes in definition or addition/revision of multiple activities that further explicate the nursing actions associated with the intervention.

Active Listening 4920
Admission Care 7310
Adolescent Care 8272
Allergy Management 6410
Anaphylaxis Management 6412
Animal Assisted Therapy 4320
Bathing 1610
Behavior Contracting 4420
Behavior Management 4350
Behavior Management: Inattention and Hyperactivity 4352
Behavior Management: Self Harm 4354
Behavior Modification: Social Skills 4362
Blood Products Administration 4030
Body Image Enhancement 5220
Bowel Incontinence Care 0410
Bowel Management 0430
Capillary Blood Sample 4035
Caregiver Support 7040
Caring Interaction Development 5000
Case Management 7360
Central Venous Access Management: Central Insertion 4054
Central Venous Access Management: Peripheral Insertion 4220
Chemical Restraint 6430
Child Care 8274
Circulatory Care: Arterial Insufficiency 4062

Circulatory Care: Mechanical Assist Device 4064
Circulatory Care: Venous Insufficiency 4066
Circumcision Care 3000
Cognitive Restructuring 4700
Comfort Management 6482
Communicable Disease Management 8820
Community Health Development 8500
Competency Management 7830
Conflict Mediation 5020
Constipation Management 0450
Consultation 7910
Cough Enhancement 3250
Counseling 5240
Crisis Intervention 6160
Cultural Care Negotiation 7330
Dementia Management 6460
Dementia Management: Bathing 6462
Dementia Management: Wandering 6466
Deposition 7930
Diarrhea Management 0460
Discharge Follow-Up 8190
Discharge Planning 7370
Discharge Planning: Home Preparation 6485
Documentation 7920
Dressing 1630

Electroconvulsive Therapy Management 2570
Enteral Tube Feeding 1056
Environmental Management 6480
Environmental Management: Community 6484
Environmental Management: Safety 6486
Exercise Promotion: Stretching 0202
Exercise Therapy: Muscle Control 0226
Eye Care 1650
Fall Prevention 6490
Feeding 1050
Financial Resource Assistance 7380
Fiscal Resource Management 8550
Fluid Management 4120
Foot Care 1660
Genetic Counseling 5242
Health Education 5510
Health System Guidance 7400
Home Maintenance Assistance 7180
Hyperglycemia Management 2120
Hyperthermia Management 3786
Infant Care: Newborn 6824
Infection Control 6540
Infection Protection 6550
Intrapartal Care 6830
Intravenous (IV) Therapy 4200
Invasive Hemodynamic Monitoring 4210
Learning Facilitation 5520
Leech Therapy 6430
Lower Extremity Monitoring 3480
Medication Administration 2300
Medication Administration: Ear 2308
Medication Administration: Enteral 2301
Medication Administration: Eye 2310
Medication Administration: Intramuscular 2313
Medication Administration: Intraosseous 2303
Medication Administration: Intraspinal 2319
Medication Administration: Intravenous 2314
Medication Administration: Nasal 2320
Medication Administration: Oral 2304
Medication Administration: Rectal 2315
Medication Administration: Skin 2316
Medication Administration: Subcutaneous 2317
Medication Administration: Vaginal 2318
Medication Administration: Ventricular Reservoir 2307
Medication Management 2380
Medication Prescribing 2390
Medication Reconciliation 2395
Mood Management 5330
Nail Care 1680
Nausea Management 1450
Nutrition Therapy 1120
Oral Health Maintenance 1710

Oral Health Promotion 1720
Oral Health Restoration 1730
Ostomy Care 0480
Oxygen Therapy 3320
Patient Rights Protection 7460
Phlebotomy: Arterial Blood Sample 4232
Phlebotomy: Blood Acquisition 4234
Phototherapy: Mood Regulation 6926
Phototherapy: Neonate 6924
Positioning 0840
Preconception Counseling 5247
Presence 5340
Pressure Injury Care 3520
Pressure Injury Prevention 3540
Program Development 8700
Prompted Voiding 0640
Pruritis Management 3550
Religious Addiction Therapy 5422
Religious Ritual Enhancement 5424
Relocation Stress Reduction 5350
Resilience Promotion 8340
Sedation Management 2260
Self-Care Assistance 1800
Sexual Assault Trauma Care 6300
Skin Care: Topical Treatment 3584
Smoking Cessation Assistance 4490
Spiritual Growth Facilitation 5426
Spiritual Support 5420
Substance Use Prevention 4500
Substance Use Treatment: Alcohol Withdrawal 4512
Surveillance 6650
Surveillance: Community 6652
Surveillance: Remote Monitoring 6658
Teaching: Disease Process 5602
Teaching: Group 5604
Teaching: Infant Development 0–3 Months 5655
Teaching: Infant Development 7–9 Months 5656
Teaching: Infant Development 10–12 Months 5657
Teaching: Prescribed Medication 5616
Teaching: Procedures or Treatments 5618
Teaching: Sports Injury Prevention 6648
Technology Management 7880
Telecommunication Consultation 8180
Temperature Regulation 3900
Triage: Community Disaster 6362
Triage: Emergency Center 6364
Triage: Telecommunication 6366
Tube Care: Gastrointestinal 1874
Urinary Bladder Training 0570
Urinary Catheterization: Intermittent 0582
Urinary Elimination Management 0590
Vaccination Management 6530

Vehicle Safety Promotion 9050
Vital Signs Monitoring 6680
Vomiting Management 1570

Weight Gain Assistance 1240
Wound Care 3660

Intervention Changes: Minor (n=61)

Interventions in this category have additions or revisions of a few activities that enhance the clinical application of the intervention.

Abuse Protection Support 6400
Abuse Protection Support: Religious 6408
Airway Management 3140
Amnioinfusion 6700
Anxiety Reduction 5820
Aromatherapy 1330
Asthma Management 3210
Behavior Management: Sexual 4356
Behavior Modification 4360
Bioterrorism Preparedness 8810
Bottle Feeding 1052
Breast Examination 6522
Community Disaster Preparedness 8840
Cost Containment 7630
Eating Disorders Management 1030
Emotional Support 5270
Environmental Risk Protection 8880
Exercise Promotion 0200
Exercise Promotion: Strength Training 0201
Exercise Therapy: Ambulation 0221
Exercise Therapy: Balance 0222
Exercise Therapy: Joint Mobility 0224
Family Presence Facilitation 7170
Grief Work Facilitation 5290
Hormone Replacement Therapy 2280
Hypoglycemia Management 2130
Incision Site Care 3440
Infection Control: Intraoperative 6545
Intravenous Insertion 4190
Latex Precautions 6570
Medication Administration: Inhalation 2311

Medication Administration: Interpleural 2302
Medication Administration: Intradermal 2312
Memory Training 4760
Music Therapy 4400
Nonnutritive Sucking 6900
Parent Education: Infant 5568
Parenting Promotion 8300
Pelvic Muscle Exercise 0560
Pessary Management 0630
Phlebotomy: Venous Blood Sample 4238
Premenstrual Syndrome 1440
Preparatory Sensory Information 5580
Risk Identification: Genetic 6614
Sibling Support 7280
Skin Care: Donor Site 3582
Skin Care: Graft Site 3583
Sleep Enhancement 1850
Suicide Prevention 6340
Swallowing Therapy 1860
Teaching: Infant Nutrition 0–3 Months 5640
Teaching: Infant Nutrition 4–6 Months 5641
Teaching: Infant Nutrition 7–9 Months 5642
Teaching: Infant Nutrition 10–12 Months 5643
Teaching: Infant Safety 0–3 Months 5645
Teaching: Infant Safety 4–6 Months 5646
Teaching: Infant Safety 7–9 Months 5647
Teaching: Infant Safety 10–12 Months 5648
Urinary Catheterization 0580
Ventilation Assistance 3390
Weight Management 1260

INTERVENTIONS IN THE SEVENTH EDITION THAT WERE RETIRED IN THIS EDITION (n=11)

Bowel Training 0440 (redundant with Bowel Management)
Fever Treatment 3740 (redundant with Hyperthermia Treatment)
Learning Readiness Enhancement 5540 (redundant with Learning Facilitation)
Phlebotomy: Cannulated Vessel 4235 (no longer appropriate nursing care, content assumed into Central Venous Access NICs and IV Insertion NIC)
Physician Support 7710 (new NIC created Health Care Provider Collaboration more in context with current practice)

Research Data Collection 8120 (retired and new NIC created with new focus Research Protocol Management)
Self-Care Assistance: Bathing/Hygiene 1801 (redundant with Bathing)
Self-Care Assistance: Dressing/Grooming 1802 (redundant with Dressing)
Self-Care Assistance: Feeding 1803 (redundant with Feeding)
Self-Care Assistance: IADL 1805 (redundant with Self Care Assistance)
Teaching: Foot Care 5603 (content added to Foot Care)

Guidelines for Submission of a New or Revised NIC Intervention

This appendix contains materials to assist in preparing an intervention to submit for review or to suggest a change to an existing intervention. It is important that a submitter be familiar with NIC and with the guidelines for intervention development and refinement as described below, before developing or revising an intervention.

The new interventions or those you have modified are to be sent by email to: classification-center@uiowa.edu. Submissions will be reviewed, and the final decision for inclusion will be made by the editors. The submitter will receive a letter stating the outcome of the review process. If the decision is for inclusion in NIC, the submitter will be notified and acknowledged in the next edition.

NEW INTERVENTION

Each submission of a **proposed new intervention** should include a label, a definition, activities listed in logical order, four to six references for background evidence that support the intervention, and a rationale for inclusion. All submissions should be in English (United States) and formatted in the same style as currently appears in the NIC. Materials that are too difficult to read or incomplete will be returned to the submitter.

STEP 1 Search relevant literature and select Background Evidence. Core curricula, published practice standards, and evidence-based guideline statements from authoritative groups are preferable sources to use in developing a new intervention. Recognized textbooks (current edition), journal articles, published research, and published narrative, systematic, or integrative reviews; meta-syntheses or meta-analyses (as recent as possible) can be submitted as evidence supporting the intervention and activities. Relevant classic works can be included. List Background Evidence references in APA format. If a website source is used, please follow the most current reference format given by APA.

STEP 2 Create the **intervention label** using the following **general principles for intervention labels**. Intervention labels are concepts.

Use the principles below when selecting names for concepts:

- Names should be noun statements; no verbs.
- Names should preferably be three words or less; no more than five words.
- When a two-part label is required, use a colon to separate the words (e.g., Bleeding Reduction: Nasal).

Avoid colon use unless it is indicated and desired by clinical practice; use a colon to indicate a more specialized area of practice only when there are different activities that require a new intervention.

- Capitalize each word.
- Labels will include modifiers to represent the nurse's actions. Choose modifiers to represent the nurse's actions (e.g., Administration, Assistance, Management, Promotion). The modifier should be selected based on its meaning, how it sounds in relationship to the other words in the label, and its acceptability in general practice. Some of the possible modifiers are listed here:

   Administration: directing the movement or behavior of, having charge of; see also Management

   Assistance: helping

   Care: paying close attention, giving protection, being concerned about

   Enhancement: making greater, augmenting, increasing; see also Promotion

   Maintenance: continuing or carrying on, supporting

   Management: directing the movement or behavior of, having charge of; see also Administration

   Monitoring: watching and checking

   Precaution: taking care beforehand against a possible danger; see also Protection

   Promotion: advancing; see also Enhancement

   Protection: shielding from injury; see also Precaution

   Reduction: lessening, diminishing

   Restoration: reinstating, bringing back to normal or unimpaired state

   Therapy: having a therapeutic nature, healing

NOTE: Some of these terms mean the same thing; a choice of which one to use will depend upon which sounds better in context and whether one is already more familiar and more accepted in practice.

Step 3 Create a **definition**. A definition for an intervention label is a phrase that defines the concept. It is a summary of the most distinguishing characteristics. The definition, together with the defining activities, delineates the boundaries of nurse behavior circumscribed by the label. The following **general principles for definitions of interventions** assist in developing definitions of interventions:

1. Use phrases (not complete sentences) that describe the behavior of the nurse and can stand alone without examples.
2. Avoid using terms for the patient and nurse, but when a term must be used, *person* is preferred rather than *client* or *patient*.
3. For those phrases that begin with a verb form, consider the situation and choose either the -ion form (e.g., limitation) or the -ing form (e.g., limiting).
4. Avoid the use of any of the terms in the intervention label in the definition.

Step 4 Create **activities** and list them in logical order. Activities are actions that a nurse does to implement the intervention. Use the following **general principles for activities**:

- Begin each activity with a verb. Possible verbs include assist, administer, explain, avoid, inspect, facilitate, monitor, and use. Use the most active verb that is appropriate for the situation. Use the term *monitor* rather than *assess*. Monitoring is a type of assessment but is done post-diagnosis as part of an intervention rather than as preparation for making a diagnosis. Avoid the terms *observe* and *evaluate*.
- Use the term *instruct* instead of *teach*.
- Keep the activities as generic as possible (e.g., instead of saying, "place on Kinair bed", say "place on therapeutic bed"). Eliminate brand names.
- Avoid combining two different ideas in one activity unless they illustrate the same point.
- Avoid repeating an idea; when two activities are saying the same thing, even in different words, eliminate one.
- Focus on the critical activities; do not worry about including all supporting activities. The number of activities depends on the intervention, but, on average, use a one-page list.
- Word similar activities the same across interventions.
- Word activities so they are clear without referring to the person or the nurse. If the person must be referred to, use the term *person* in preference to *client*, *patient*, or other terms. Use the terms *family members* or *significant others* rather than *spouse*. Use the word *health care provider* rather than *physician*.
- Add the phrase "as appropriate," "as necessary," "as prescribed" or "as needed" to the end of those activities that are important but used only on some occasions.
- Check for consistency between the activities and the label's definition.
- Arrange the activities in the order in which they are usually carried out, when appropriate.
- Instructional activities are listed last.

Step 5 Describe a **rationale for inclusion** of a new intervention and include it in the submission. The submitter should *note how the proposed new intervention differs from existing interventions*. If a new intervention would call for changes in existing interventions, these changes should also be submitted.

REVISED INTERVENTION

Each submission of a **revised intervention** should include a label, a definition, activities, background evidence, and a rationale for revision. All submissions should be in English (United States) and formatted in the same style as appears in the NIC. Each submission of a revised intervention should indicate how the proposed changes related to the existing intervention. To do so, use a **track changes** feature of a word processing software. If a major revision is made, retype with changes clearly identified and make sure your submission is easy to understand. Materials that are too difficult to read or incomplete will be returned to the submitter.

Step 1 Update the **Background Evidence** with four to six references. Core curricula, published practice standards, and evidence-based guideline statements from authoritative groups are preferable. Recognized textbooks (current edition), journal articles, published research, and published narrative, systematic, and integrative reviews; meta-syntheses or meta-analyses (as recent as possible) can be submitted as evidence supporting the intervention and activities. Relevant classic works can be included. List Background Evidence references in APA format. If a website source is used, please follow the most current reference format given by APA.

Step 2 Consider the **label and definition**. The aim is to make as *few* changes to the definition or label as possible. Should, however, accepted practice or official statements of standards change, those changes need to be reflected in the terminology. When revising the labels and/or definitions, use the **general principles for intervention labels** and **general principles for definitions of interventions** described earlier.

Step 3 Update the **activities**. Most changes in practice will be reflected in this section. Updating the activities includes deleting an activity if it is no longer relevant, editing an activity to bring it up to date or add clarity, and writing a new activity. To update activities, use the following **general principles for activities**:

- Begin each activity with a verb. Possible verbs include assist, administer, explain, avoid, inspect, facilitate, monitor, and use. Use the most active verb that is appropriate for the situation. Use the term *monitor* rather than *assess*. Monitoring is a type of assessment but is done post-diagnosis as part of an intervention rather than as preparation for making a diagnosis. Avoid the terms *observe* and *evaluate*.

- Keep the activities as generic as possible (e.g., instead of saying "Place on Kinair bed" say "Place on therapeutic bed"). Eliminate brand names.
- Avoid combining two different ideas in one activity unless they illustrate the same point.
- Avoid repeating an idea; when two activities are saying the same thing, even in different words, eliminate one.
- Focus on the critical activities; do not worry about including all supporting activities. The number of activities depends on the interventions, but on average, use a one-page list.
- Word similar activities the same across interventions.
- Use the word *instruct* instead of *teach*.
- Word activities so they are clear without referring to the patient or the nurse. If the patient must be referred to, use the term *person* in preference to *client, patient* or other terms. Use the terms *family members* or *significant others* rather than *spouse*. Use the word *health care provider* rather than *physician*.
- Add the phrase "as appropriate," "as necessary," "as prescribed" or "as needed" to the end of those activities that are important but used only on some occasions.
- Check for consistency between the activities and the label's definition.
- Arrange the activities in the order in which they are usually carried out, when appropriate. In general, instructional activities occur at the end of the intervention.

Step 4 Provide a **rationale** for the revisions you are submitting. Each submission for a **revised intervention** should indicate how the proposed changes relate to the existing intervention. Provide a **compelling rationale** if any changes to the definition or label are proposed.

Please supply the following information as you want it to appear in the book.

Print your name and credentials: _____

Employment title: _____

Place of employment: _____

Address: _____

City, State, Zip Code, Country: _____

Email Address: _____

Please send this form along with your proposed new or revised intervention(s) to:

Center for Nursing Classification & Clinical Effectiveness
NIC Review
The University of Iowa
College of Nursing 407 CNB
Iowa City, IA 52242-1121
(319) 335-7051
classification-center@uiowa.edu

Timeline and Highlights for NIC

1985

Nursing Interventions: Treatments for Nursing Diagnoses, edited by Bulechek and McCloskey and published by W. B. Saunders, is one of the first two books to define independent nursing interventions.

1987

Intervention research team formed by Joanne McCloskey and Gloria Bulechek at the University of Iowa.

1990

The Iowa Research Team led by Joanne McCloskey and Gloria Bulechek, and including Mary F. Clarke, is funded by a research grant from the National Institute of Nursing Research (1990–1993).

First publication about Nursing Interventions Classification (NIC) appears in print in the *Journal of Professional Nursing*.

1991

American Nurses Association (ANA) recognizes NIC.

1992

The first edition of *Nursing Interventions Classification (NIC)* is published by Mosby.

The *Nursing Clinics of North America* publishes an entire volume (Nursing Interventions, 27[2]. Philadelphia: W.B. Saunders) on the initial survey research on the interventions in the first edition of NIC.

Nursing Interventions: Essential Nursing Treatments, edited by Bulechek and McCloskey, is published by W. B. Saunders.

1993

NIC is added to National Library of Medicine's Unified Medical Language System Meta thesaurus.

The second NIC intervention grant is funded by NINR (June 1993–1997; extended to 1998) with Joanne McCloskey and Gloria Bulechek as the co-principal investigators.

NIC is included in the International Council of Nurses (ICN) *International Classification for Nursing Practice* (Alpha version).

Publication of *The NIC Letter* begins at the University of Iowa.

1994

Cumulative Index to Nursing and Health Care Literature (CINAHL) and Silver Platter add NIC to their indexes.

The Joint Commission on Accreditation of Health Care Organizations (JCAHO) includes NIC as a means to meet standard on uniform data collection.

The National League for Nursing (NLN) makes a video describing the development and testing of NIC.

An institutional effectiveness grant for preparing PhD candidates and postdoctoral students is funded at The University of Iowa, with Joanne McCloskey and Meridean Maas as directors.

The Nursing Classifications Fund is established at The University of Iowa to provide ongoing financial support for the continued development and use of NIC and NOC.

1995

The Center for Nursing Classification (the Center) at the University of Iowa is approved (December 13) by the Iowa Board of Regents (without funding) to facilitate the ongoing research and implementation of NIC and NOC. A fundraising advisory board for the Center is established and members are appointed.

1996

Mosby publishes the second edition of *Nursing Interventions Classification (NIC)*.

The first meeting of the Center's fundraising advisory board is held.

The ANA's *Social Policy Statement* includes the NIC definition of an intervention.

The first vendor signs licensing agreement for NIC and NOC.

NIC is linked to the Omaha classification and distributed in a monograph published by the Center.

1997

The NIC Letter becomes *The NIC/NOC Letter*.

The first joint international North American Nursing Diagnosis Association (NANDA), NIC, NOC Conference is held in St. Charles, Illinois.

1998

NIC submits information to American National Standards Institute Health Informatics Standards Board (ANSI HISB) for Inventory of Clinical Information Standards.

The NIC/ NOC Letter is sponsored by Mosby-Yearbook.

Multiple translations of NIC are processed (Dutch, Korean, Chinese, French, Japanese, German, and Spanish).

The Center for Nursing Classification receives 3 years of support from the College of Nursing at The University of Iowa (1998–2001), is given space on the fourth floor of the College of Nursing, and Joanne McCloskey is appointed director.

NIC interventions are linked to NOC outcomes in monograph published by the Center.

1999

The First Institute on Informatics and Classification is held at the University of Iowa.

Nursing Interventions: Effective Nursing Treatments, edited by Bulechek and McCloskey, is published by W.B. Saunders.

2000

Mosby publishes the third edition of *Nursing Interventions Classification (NIC)*.

The NNN Alliance is created, with Dorothy Jones and Joanne Dochterman* as co-chairs.

NIC and NOC linked with Resident Assessment Protocols (RAP) and Outcome and Assessment Information Set (OASIS).

The Second Institute on Informatics and Classification is held.

2001

The book that links the three languages—*Nursing Diagnoses, Outcomes, Interventions: NANDA, NOC, and NIC Linkages*—is authored by the NIC and NOC principal investigators and published by Mosby.

A NNN Invitational Common Structure Conference is funded by the National Library of Medicine (Joanne Dochterman and Dorothy Jones, principal investigators) and held in Utica, Illinois in August.

An effectiveness grant is funded (NINR & Agency for Healthcare Research and Quality [AHRQ]) for large database research with the use of NIC (Marita Titler and Joanne Dochterman). This is the first such grant to fund nursing effectiveness research in which a clinical database with nursing standardized language is used. Mary F. Clarke is appointed to the research team.

* Joanne McCloskey changed her name to Joanne Dochterman in 1999

NIC is registered in Health Level Seven (HL7).

The Third Institute on Informatics and Classification is held

2002

The NNN Alliance holds an international conference on nursing language, classification, and informatics in Chicago, Illinois. This is a replacement for NANDA's biennial conference. A White Paper on the development of a common structure for NANDA, NIC, and NOC is presented to conference participants.

Systematized Nomenclature of Medicine (SNOMED) licenses NIC for inclusion in its database.

The Center for Nursing Classification expands name to Center for Nursing Classification and Clinical Effectiveness; endowment reaches $600,000.

The Fourth Institute on Informatics and Classification is held.

A 4-hour long web course on standardized languages, NANDA, NIC, and NOC, is offered by the Center for Nursing Classification and Clinical Effectiveness at the University of Iowa.

A second institutional training grant for PhD candidates and postdoctoral students in effectiveness research is funded at The University Iowa by NINR, with Joanne Dochterman and Martha Craft-Rosenberg as directors.

The position of Center Fellow is established (to assist in the ongoing development of NIC and NOC), and about 30 people are appointed for a 3-year terms, including Mary F. Clarke.

NIC celebrates its 10th anniversary.

2003

ANA publishes the Common Taxonomy of Nursing Practice in a monograph, *Unifying Nursing Languages: The Harmonization of NANDA, NIC and NOC* (edited by Joanne Dochterman and Dorothy Jones).

The first meeting of the CNC Fellows held on April 11th at the University of Iowa College of Nursing.

NANDA, NIC, NOC software program based on linkage book *Nursing Diagnoses, Outcomes, and Interventions: NANDA, NOC and NIC Linkages* - CD-ROM is produced by Mosby.

The Center for Nursing Classification and Clinical Effectiveness receives the Sigma Theta Tau International Award for Clinical Scholarship.

The Fifth Institute on Nursing Informatics & Classification is held.

Elizabeth Swanson and Howard Butcher join the CNC Executive Board.

Howard Butcher accepts appointment as NIC editor.

A Spanish version of the web course, *NIC and NOC 101: The Basics*, translated by Patricia Levi is offered by the Center.

2004

The fourth edition *Nursing Interventions Classification* and the third edition *Nursing Outcomes Classification* are published by Mosby.

The NNN Alliance holds the second international conference on nursing language, classification, and informatics in Chicago Illinois.

Joanne Dochterman retires as Director of the Center and Sue Moorhead is appointed Director effective July 1st.

Cheryl Wagner joins the NIC team as a doctoral student.

A monograph, *Guideline for Conducting Effectiveness Research in Nursing and Other Health Care Services*, authored by Marita Titler, Joanne Dochterman, and David Reed is published by the Center.

The Center for Nursing Classification and Clinical Effectiveness endowment reaches $700,000.

2005

NIC and NOC are incorporated into the University of Iowa Gerontological Nursing Interventions Research Center (GNIRC) evidence-based practice guidelines.

The Sixth Institute on Nursing Informatics and Classification is held.

Center Fellows are re-appointed for 3-year term beginning July 1st. Additional fellows nominated and appointed, including Cheryl Wagner.

The Center for Nursing Classification & Clinical Effectiveness celebrated its 10th anniversary in December.

The second Annette Scheffel Fundraising event held December 2nd with a reception and a live and silent auction.

2006

The second edition *NANDA, NOC, and NIC Linkages: Nursing Diagnoses, Outcomes, and Interventions* is published by Mosby.

The NNN Alliance holds the third international conference on nursing language, classification, and informatics in Philadelphia, Pennsylvania.

Five new Center Fellows were appointed at the annual meeting in April.

American Nurses Association (ANA) recognition of NIC and NOC is renewed.

2007

The Seventh Institute on Nursing Informatics and Classification is held June 11–13.

The Center offers first research grant for $10,000.

2008

The fifth edition *Nursing Interventions Classification* and the fourth edition *Nursing Outcomes Classification* are published by Mosby Elsevier.

Joanne Dochterman retires from the CNC Executive Board.

The Eighth Institute on Nursing Informatics & Classification is held June 9–11.

The Center becomes an affiliate member of The Alliance for Nursing Informatics (ANI).

2009

CNC submits materials to ANA for Biennial Recognition process.

CNC offers first postdoctoral fellowship for $10,000.

2010

Center offers the first teleconference to Ile Ife, Nigeria, March 14–19.

The Ninth Institute on Nursing Informatics and Classification is held June 9–11.

Major renovation to the Center is completed with update of electronic equipment to facilitate the upkeep of the classifications.

2011

Cheryl Wagner accepts appointment as NIC editor.

Elsevier creates NIC/NOC Facebook site and a quarterly newsletter.

2012

The third edition *NOC and NIC Linkages to NANDA-I and Clinical Conditions: Supporting Critical Reasoning and Quality Care* is published by Elsevier Mosby.

The 20th anniversary of *Nursing Interventions Classification* and the 15th anniversary of *Nursing Outcomes Classification* are celebrated along with the *NANDA International* 40th anniversary at the NANDA-I conference in Houston, Texas.

2013

The sixth edition *Nursing Interventions Classification* and the fifth edition *Nursing Outcomes Classification* are published by Mosby Elsevier.

The 10th Institute on Nursing Informatics and Classification is held June 13–14.

Sharon Sweeney, Administrative Coordinator, completes 10 years of service to the Center for Nursing Classification and Clinical Effectiveness.

2014

A webinar, *Transforming Nursing Education, Research, and Practice using the Nursing Interventions Classification*, was sponsored and produced by Elsevier.

2015

The Center for Nursing Classification and Clinical Effectiveness celebrates 20 years as an Iowa Board of

Regents Center to facilitate the ongoing research and implementation of NIC and NOC.

2016

Multiple translations of NIC are available (Chinese, Dutch, German, Italian, French, Japanese, Korean, Norwegian, Portuguese, Spanish). Elsevier Japan begins to process licenses for Japanese language.

Howard Butcher becomes Series Editor of the Gerontological Evidence-Based Practice Guidelines at the University of Iowa Csomay Center (previously Gerontological Nursing Interventions Research Center) and integrates NIC interventions and NOC outcomes into each revised evidence-based guideline.

2017

Elsevier expands licensing process to other international offices.

2018

The seventh edition of *Nursing Interventions Classification* and the sixth edition of *Nursing Outcomes Classification* are published by Elsevier.

Noriko Abe is hired as CNC Coordinator (100%).

Celebration of 120th anniversary of Nursing occurs at Iowa.

2019

Joanne Dochterman retires as editor of the NIC but continues as consultant.

Howard Butcher accepts a position as Professor at the Christine E. Lynn College of Nursing at Florida Atlantic University in Boca Raton, Florida.

Karen Dunn Lopez is hired as Director of Research for the Center as part of her appointment as a tenured Associate Professor on August 1st.

NIC and NOC terms are updated in SNOMED Clinical Terms.

Cheryl Wagner is appointed as Adjunct Assistant Professor at the College of Nursing.

2020

Gloria Bulechek retires as editor of the NIC but continues as consultant.

Howard Butcher accepts a position as Director of the PhD program at the Christine E. Lynn College of Nursing at Florida Atlantic University in Boca Raton, Florida.

A Strategic Planning Conference is held in February at the College of Nursing to establish a Strategic Plan for the next 5 years with external consultation support.

Sue Moorhead steps down as Director of the Center and Karen Dunn Lopez becomes the Director on July 1st.

The Center celebrates 25 years as a Board of Regents approved Center in the College of Nursing.

2021

Sue Moorhead retires from the College of Nursing, January 1st.

Three papers linking NANDA-I, NOC, and NIC to care of COVID-19 patients, families, and communities are published in the *International Journal of Nursing Knowledge*.

Elspeth Adriana McMullan is hired in the CNC as a Center Administrator/Research Specialist in September.

Karen Dunn Lopez is inducted as a Fellow of the American Academy of Nursing.

Karen Dunn Lopez becomes the Center representative to the Alliance for Nursing Informatics.

Mary F. Clarke accepts appointment as an editor of NIC.

2022

The 30th anniversary of *Nursing Interventions Classification* and the 25th anniversary of *Nursing Outcomes Classification* are celebrated.

Howard K. Butcher is inducted as a Fellow of the American Academy of Nursing.

2024

The eighth edition of the *Nursing Interventions Classification* and the seventh edition of the *Nursing Outcomes Classification* are published by Elsevier.

In addition to the aforementioned events, NIC and NOC have been presented over the years at numerous national and international conferences in the following countries: Andorra, Australia, Austria, Brazil, Canada, Colombia, Czech Republic, Denmark, England, Estonia, France, Germany, Iceland, Ireland, Italy, Japan, Mexico, Netherlands, Nigeria, Peru, Portugal, Slovakia, Slovenia, Spain, South Korea, Sweden, Switzerland, Taiwan, Turkey, and Wales.

Abbreviations

A-aDO$_2$	Alveolar arterial Oxygen Pressure Difference		EMG	ElectroMyoGram
ABG	Arterial Blood Gas		EOA	Esophageal Obturator Airway
ABO	Blood types **A, B, O**		EOM	ExtraOcular Movement
ACLS	Advanced Cardiac Life Support		EPA	Environmental Protection Agency
ACT	Activated Clotting Time		ET	Endotracheal Tube
ADH	Anti-Diuretic Hormone		FDA	Food and Drug Administration
ADL	Activities of Daily Living		FEV$_1$	Forced Expiratory Volume in 1 second
AED	Automated External Defibrillator		FTE	Full Time Equivalent
AICD	Automatic Implantable Cardioverter Defibrillator		FiO$_2$	Fraction of inspired Oxygen
AIDS	Acquired Immune Deficiency Syndrome		FVC	Forced Vital Capacity
app	Application		GI	GastroIntestinal
ARDS	Adult Respiratory Distress Syndrome		g, gm	gram
AST	ASpartate aminoTransferase		GFR	Glomerular Filtration Rate
AV	AtrioVentricular		HAI	Healthcare Associated Infection
avDO$_2$	arteriovenous Oxygen Difference		HAPI	Hospital Associated Pressure Injury
BE	Base Excess		HCl	HydroChloric Acid
BMI	Body Mass Index		HCO$_3$	Bicarbonate
BP	Blood Pressure		Hct	Hematocrit
BUN	Blood Urea Nitrogen		HEPA	High Efficiency Particulate Air
C	Celsius		Hg	Mercury
Ca	Calcium		Hgb	Hemoglobin
CAUTI	Catheter Associated Urinary Tract Infection		HIV	Human Immunodeficiency Virus
CBC	Complete Blood Count		HOB	Head of Bed
cc	cubic centimeter		HPV	Human Papilloma Virus
CDC	Centers for Disease Control and Prevention		HR	Heart Rate
CI	Cardiac Index		IADL	Instrumental Activities of Daily Living
CK	Creatinine Kinase		ICP	IntraCranial Pressure
CLABSI	Central Line Associated Blood Stream Infection		ICU	Intensive Care Unit
cm	centimeter		IM	IntraMuscular
CNS	Central Nervous System		I&O	Intake and Output
CO	Cardiac Output		IRB	Institutional Review Board
CO$_2$	Carbon dioxide		IV	IntraVenous
COPD	Chronic Obstructive Pulmonary Disease		JVD	Jugular Venous Distention
CPAP	Continuous Positive Airway Pressure		K	Potassium
CPP	Cerebral Perfusion Pressure		L	Liter
CPR	Cardio-Pulmonary Resuscitation		LDH	Lactate DeHydrogenase
Cr	Creatinine		LDL	Low-Density Lipoprotein
CSF	CerebroSpinal Fluid		LOC	Level Of Consciousness
CT	Computed Tomography		mA	milliAmpere
CVAD	Central Venous Access Device		MAP	Mean Arterial Pressure
CVP	Central Venous Pressure		MAR	Medication Administration Record
D$_5$W	Dextrose 5% in Water		MAST	Military AntiShock Trousers
DNA	DeoxyriboNucleic Acid		mEq	milliEquivalant
DVT	Deep Vein Thrombosis		mEq/hr	milliEquivalant per hour
ECG	Electrocardiogram		mEq/L	milliEquivalant per liter
ECMO	ExtraCorporeal Membrane Oxygenation		mg	milligram
ECT	ElectroConvulsive Therapy		mg/dL	milligram per deciliter
EEG	ElectroEncephaloGram		min	minute
EKG	Electrocardiogram		mL	milliliter

mL/kg/hr	milliliter per kilogram per hour
mm	millimeters
mm Hg	millimeters of mercury
mmol/L	millimoles per Liter
mOsm/L	milliosmoles per Liter
MMR	Measles Mumps Rubella
MVV	Maximal Voluntary Volume
Na	Sodium
NG	NasoGastric
NPO	Non Per Os (nothing by mouth)
NSAID	Non-Steroidal Anti-Inflammatory Drug
OSHA	Occupational Safety and Health Administration
OTC	Over the Counter (non-prescription medication)
oz	ounce
PAP	Pulmonary Artery Pressure
PAWP	Pulmonary Artery Wedge Pressure
$PaCO_2$	Partial arterial Carbon dioxide pressure
PaO_2	Partial arterial Oxygen pressure
PCA	Patient-Controlled Analgesia
pCO_2	partial Carbon dioxide pressure
PCWP	Pulmonary Capillary Wedge Pressure
PE	Pulmonary Embolus
PEEP	Positive End Expiratory Pressure
PEG	Percutaneous Endoscopic Gastrostomy
PERF	Peak Expiratory Flow Rate
PERRLA	Pupils Equal Round and Reactive to Light and Accommodation
PFT	Pulmonary Function Tests
pH	Hydrogen ion concentration
PHI	Personal Health Information
PICC	Peripherally Inserted Central Catheter
PMS	Pre-Menstrual Syndrome
PO	Per Os (orally)
PO_4	Phosphate

PPE	Personal Protective Equipment
PRN	Pro Re Nata (as often as necessary)
PT	Prothrombin Time
PTT	Partial Thromboplastin Time
PVC	Premature Ventricular Contraction
Q_{sp}/Q_t	physiologic blood flow per minute/cardiac output per minute
REM	Rapid Eye Movement
Rh	Rhesus antigen
ROM	Range Of Motion
RN	Registered Nurse
SaO_2	Saturation (arterial) Oxygen
SARS-COV-2	Severe Acute Respiratory Syndrome Coronavirus 2
SIADH	Syndrome of Inappropriate AntiDiuretic Hormone
SpO_2	Saturation (peripheral) Oxygen
SPF	Sun Protection Factor
SQ	Subcutaneous
STD	Sexually Transmitted Disease
STI	Sexually Transmitted Infection
SvO_2	Saturation (venous) Oxygen
SVR	Systemic Vascular Resistance
S_3	3rd heart sound
S_4	4th heart sound
TDaP	Tetanus Diphtheria and Pertussis
TENS	Transcutaneous Electrical Nerve Stimulation
THC	Tetrahydrocannabinol
TPN	Total Parenteral Nutrition
V_d/V_t	Physiological dead space/Tidal volume
V/Q scan	Ventilation-Perfusion scan
WBC	White Blood Cell/White Blood Count
WOCN	Wound Ostomy Continence Nurse

Previous Editions and Translations

McCloskey, J. C., & Bulechek, G. M. (Eds.). (1992). *Nursing Interventions Classification* (NIC). Mosby. [336 Interventions]
- Translated into French, 1996, Décarie Éditeur

McCloskey, J. C., & Bulechek, G. M. (Eds.). (1996). *Nursing Interventions Classification* (NIC) (2nd ed.). Mosby. [433 Interventions]
- Translated into Traditional Chinese, 1999, Farseeing
- Translated into Dutch, 1997, Tijdstroom
- Translated into French 2000, Masson
- Translated into Japanese 2001, Nankodo
- Translated into Korean, 1998, Hyun Moon Sa
- Translated into Spanish 2000, Editorial Sintesis

McCloskey, J. C., & Bulechek, G. M. (Eds.). (2000). *Nursing Interventions Classification* (NIC) (3rd ed.). Mosby. [486 Interventions]
- Translated into Dutch, 2002, Elsevier
- Translated into Japanese, 2002, Nankodo
- Translated into Portuguese, 2004, Artmed Editora S.A.
- Translated into Spanish, 2001, Harcourt

Dochterman, J. M., & Bulechek, G. M. (Eds.). (2004). *Nursing Interventions Classification* (NIC) (4th ed.). Mosby [514 Interventions]
- Translated into Italian, 2007, Casa Editrice Ambrosiana
- Translated into Japanese, 2006, Nankodo
- Translated into Norwegian, 2006, Akribe
- Translated into Portuguese, 2008, Artmed Editora S.A.

Bulechek, G., Butcher, H., & Dochterman, J. (Eds.). (2008). *Nursing Interventions Classification (NIC)* (5th ed.). Mosby/Elsevier. [542 interventions]
- Translated into Simplified Chinese, 2009, Peking University Medical Press
- Translated into Traditional Chinese, 2011, Elsevier Taiwan
- Translated into Dutch, 2010, Elsevier Gezondheidszorg
- Translated into Japanese, 2009, Nankodo
- Translated into Portuguese, 2010, Elsevier Editora
- Translated into Spanish, 2009, Elsevier España

Bulechek, G., Butcher, H., Dochterman, J., & Wagner, C. (Eds.). (2013). *Nursing Interventions Classification (NIC)* (6th ed.). Elsevier Mosby. [554 interventions]
- Translated into Dutch, 2016, Bohn Stafleu van Loghum
- Translated into German, 2016, Hogrefe Verlag
- Translated into Indonesian, 2016, CV. Mocomedia/Elsevier
- Translated into Italian, 2020, CV. Casa Editrice Ambrosiana
- Translated into Japanese, 2015, Elsevier Japan
- Translated into Portuguese, 2016, Elsevier Editora
- Translated into Spanish, 2014, Elsevier España
- Translated into Turkish, 2017, Nobel Tip Kitabevler/Elsevier

Butcher, H., Bulechek, G., Dochterman, J., & Wagner, C. (Eds.). (2018). *Nursing Interventions Classification (NIC)* (7th ed.). Elsevier. [565 interventions]
- Translated into Dutch, 2020, Bohn Stafleu van Loghum
- Translated into Indonesian, 2019, CV. Mocomedia/Elsevier
- Translated into Italian, 2020, CV. Casa Editrice Ambrosiana
- Translated into Japanese, 2018, Elsevier Japan
- Translated into Portuguese, 2020, GEN Guanabara Koogan
- Translated into Spanish, 2018, Elsevier España

Index